D1032418

Becoming a Supple Leopard

The Ultimate Guide to Resolving Pain, Preventing Injury, and Optimizing Athletic Performance

Dr. Kelly Starrett
with Glen Cordoza

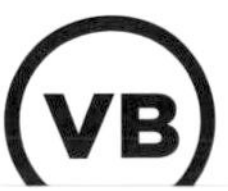

Victory Belt Publishing Inc.
 First edition published 2013
Second edition published 2015

ISBN-13: 978-1628600-83-4

This book is for educational purposes. The publisher and authors of this instructional book are not responsible in any manner whatsoever for any adverse effects arising directly or indirectly as a result of the information provided in this book. If not practiced safely and with caution, working out can be dangerous to you and to others. It is important to consult with a professional fitness instructor before beginning training. It is also very important to consult with a physician prior to training due to the intense and strenuous nature of the techniques in this book.

Interior design by Yordan Terziev and Boryana Yordanova

Printed in Canada.
TC 0818

For Juliet

CONTENTS

Preface to the Expanded and Updated Edition—7

Introduction: A New Human Performance Epoch—14

PART 1
PRINCIPLES AND THEORY

Chapter 1: Midline Stabilization and Organization (Spinal Mechanics)—33
Prioritizing spinal mechanics is the first and most important step in rebuilding and ingraining functional motor patterns, optimizing movement efficiency, maximizing force production, and avoiding injury. In order to safely and effectively transmit force through your core and into your extremities, you need to organize your spine in a neutral position and then create stability throughout that organized system by engaging the musculature of your trunk, which is known as bracing. This is the basis of midline stabilization and organization. This chapter explains why it's important to prioritize spinal mechanics over everything else—and how to organize and brace your spine in an optimal position.

Chapter 2: One-Joint Rule—56
The premise of the one-joint rule is simple: When you are working from a braced neutral position, flexion and extension should occur only in your hips and shoulders, not in your spine. Your hips and shoulders are designed to support and accommodate large loads and dynamic movements, and movement should always be initiated from those primary engines. In fact, it's easier to think of your hips and shoulders as a single joint because they are governed by the same principles—hence the name "one-joint rule."

Chapter 3: Laws of Torque—63
In order to create safe and stable positions for your joints as well as preserve a braced neutral spinal position, you have to create tension in your hips and shoulders and, by extension, your elbows, knees, wrists, and ankles. You do so by generating torque, which is expressed through external rotation (rotating your limb away from your body) and internal rotation (rotating your limb toward the center of your body).

Chapter 4: Body Archetypes and the Tunnel—91
The functional positions for the hips and shoulders can be categorized into seven basic configurations: four for the shoulders and three for the hips. These seven body archetypes, which represent the start and finish positions for most exercise movements, encompass all the range of motion and motor control that you need to be a fully functional human being. Consider the body archetypes and the tunnel concept as a blueprint for assessing movement and positional competency and range of motion restrictions.

Chapter 5: Movement Hierarchy—117
The movement hierarchy categorizes exercise movements based on stabilization demands and complexity. It provides a framework for building efficient, transferable movement patterns and skill progressions—from simple to more advanced exercises—and for modifying strength and conditioning movements based on skill, fitness level, and mobility.

Chapter 6: Mobility: A Systematic Approach—130
There is no one-size-fits-all approach when it comes to correcting range of motion restrictions, addressing tight muscles, and treating achy joints. To account for all positional and movement-related problems, soft tissue stiffness, and joint restriction, you need to combine techniques and take a systematic approach. What's more, you need to perform basic, routine maintenance on your body—that is, spend 10 to 15 minutes a day working on your mobility. In this chapter, you'll find a template for improving range of motion, resolving pain, and treating sore muscles. Equally important, you'll learn how and when to mobilize.

PART 2

CATEGORIES OF MOVEMENT

PART 3

MOBILIZATION TECHNIQUES

AREA MAP

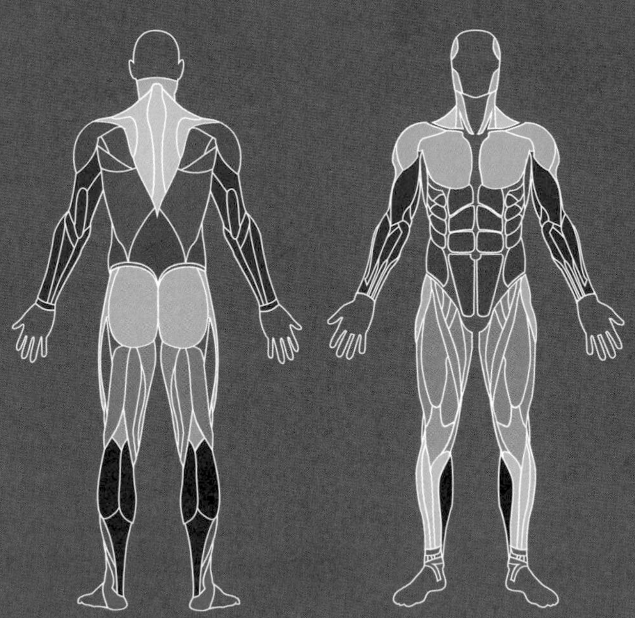

PART 4
MOBILITY PRESCRIPTIONS

PREFACE TO THE EXPANDED AND UPDATED EDITION

When I began writing *Becoming a Supple Leopard* back in 2011, I had two goals:

1. Create an all-encompassing, open-ended system for human movement that teaches people how to predict and resolve dysfunctional movement patterns that can impede performance and lead to injury or pain.

2. Give people the tools they need to perform basic, routine maintenance on their bodies so that they have a model for preventing, treating, and resolving injury and pain, as well as improving mobility (joint and tissue restrictions).

Becoming a Supple Leopard (BASL) hit stores in April 2013 and was an immediate success, selling more than 100,000 copies in the first few months and making the *Wall Street Journal* and *New York Times* bestseller lists. From *The View* to *60-Minute Sports,* the ideas and methods from the book have reached audiences I never could have imagined. From elite military forces to professional sports teams, the concepts, movements, and mobility techniques have been tested at the highest levels. The system has worked equally well for children and weekend warriors. From universities and elementary schools to corporate giants like Google, the original principles and techniques have been broken down into their simplest forms, making the practices available to everyone, regardless of age, body type, or fitness level.

Although I accomplished my goals with the original book, working and testing the ideas in these environments has enriched my system in unexpected ways. The system has evolved. It's better and stronger than ever before—which is one of the main reasons for publishing this expanded and updated edition. These changes have dramatically improved the system, making the concepts and techniques much easier to learn, digest, and implement.

The truth is, I wrote *BASL* with athletes and coaches in mind. And I was focused on performance. Pain resolution and injury prevention have always been part of the conversation, and I do believe that the original book provided the tools to treat and resolve chronic pain and prevent injury, but, admittedly, the book was not organized in a way that catered to novices or laypersons. This time around, it is. Whether you're a deskbound weekend warrior or an athlete competing at the highest levels, the original practices have been refined and improved, making them accessible to everyone.

The second reason for publishing this expanded and updated edition is you, the reader. The reviews posted on Amazon and other bookseller websites provided me with invaluable feedback. The comments and questions posted on my blog and social media pages also played a key role in the evolution of the system. This confluence of feedback and constructive criticism helped me turn *BASL* into a more comprehensive, detailed manual, for which I am very grateful.

So What's Changed?

To improve the overall quality, readability, and navigability of the book, I've made a lot of changes. Let's start with what's been added to the book.

This edition contains more than 80 pages of new content, including nearly 50 new mobility techniques. Chapter 4, "Body Archetypes and the Tunnel" (which begins on page 91) is a new chapter on assessing range of motion and movement quality. I've also added a whole new part devoted to mobility prescriptions that you can use to treat positional restrictions, pain, and tweaks (see part 4, beginning on page 442).

Another small yet significant addition is the "Chapter Highlights" section located at the end of each chapter, which summarizes the key takeaways. I've also added illustrations and graphics to support and clarify some of the more complex and salient concepts and techniques. And, as many readers have requested, anatomy images have been infused into the mobility sections as a way of highlighting important muscles, joints, and body parts.

In addition to adding new content, I've made changes to enrich the original text and images. I've reworked each chapter and clarified some language that might have confused or misled readers—specifically the "Laws of Torque" chapter and the ever-controversial "straight foot stance" description and "shove your knees out" cue in reference to the squat.

Finally, dramatic improvements have been made to make navigating the book easier, starting with a detailed index. Colored tabs have been added along the sides of the pages so that you can quickly flip to a specific part. I've even expanded the "A Guide to Using This Book" section, which serves as a road map for reading the book. Even if you've read the first edition, I highly recommend that you review this section first before you delve into the other chapters—see pages 10–12.

The most important change with regard to navigability is the organization of the parts and chapters. In the first edition, I presented the chapters sequentially, which admittedly made browsing difficult. To remedy this issue, I have lumped all the principles and theory into one part and divided the movements and mobilization techniques into two separate parts. This consolidates all the core principles that comprise the system into one section and enables you to browse the techniques based on what you want to work on or which techniques you're interested in learning.

Here's a brief summary of what you can expect to learn in each section:

- **Part 1, Principles and Theory:** This is the most important part of the book because it encompasses the core of my system and lays the groundwork for the movements and mobilization techniques covered in parts 2 and 3, as well as the mobility prescriptions featured in part 4. Here you will learn about the principles for optimal human movement: spinal mechanics, the one-joint rule, and the laws of torque. Think of these chapters as a blueprint for moving safely and effectively through life and sport. In addition, you will learn how to assess and restore range of motion to restricted joints and tissues—and how to identify and resolve common movement errors that can compromise performance and lead to injury. Lastly, you will learn how to progress exercise movements in a way that builds functional and transferable movement patterns, as well as mobility methods for improving range of motion and treating injuries and pain. In short, part 1 contains all the information you will need to understand, implement, and teach my system.

- **Part 2, Categories of Movement:** This part contains all the exercise movements—squats, pushup, clean, and so on—that are used to help test, instill, and progress the principles covered in part 1.

- **Part 3, Mobilization Techniques:** All the mobilization or mobility techniques (also known as "mobs") that comprise my system are contained in this part of the book. Consider the mobilization techniques tools to resolve pain and improve position. These techniques will help you address short and tight muscles, soft tissue and joint capsule restriction, motor control problems, joint range of motion limitations, and neural dynamic issues. To help you navigate, this part is divided into 14 sections based on body areas. For example, area 1 contains all the jaw, head, and neck mobs, and area 2 includes all the upper back mobs. For a full breakdown, flip to page 283.

- **Part 4, Mobility Prescriptions:** To help you piece together the mobilization techniques and devise your own customized mobility program, I've included prescriptions for a variety of movements and common issues. In this part, you will find prescriptions that will help you improve your range of motion for specific positions and movements. There are also prescriptions for treating minor tweaks (injuries), painful joints, and sore muscles. In addition, I've included an all-encompassing mobility template that ensures all body parts are treated and maintained, along with a sample beginner and intermediate 14-day program.

Start Here: A Guide to Using This Book

To maximize your time and get the most out of this book, there are some things you need to know.

First and foremost, understand that there are a couple of ways to approach this book. One way is simply to read it straight through. If you're a serious athlete or a coach, reading the book in its entirety will give you a complete understanding of my system, as well as help you apply the information to your own practice. Although not all the techniques and information will be immediately applicable, reading the entire book will illuminate the interconnectedness of the principles and how they apply to the actions of life, sport, combat, and play. And because all the concepts, movements, and mobility techniques are interrelated, chances are you will find useful applications long after you've finished reading this book.

This book is also designed for browsing. If you've read the first edition or attended my Movement & Mobility Course, or if you've been following the Mobility Project blog at MobilityWOD.com, using the book as a reference tool will prove easy to manage. As I explained in the preface, changes have been made to make the book easier to navigate. For example, by browsing the descriptions in the table of contents, you can quickly identify chapters that are relevant to you. In fact, I highly recommend that you take the time to read those descriptions before proceeding to part 1. It will give you a better understanding of how the book is laid out and what you can expect to learn from each chapter.

However, even if you're familiar with my Movement & Mobility System, I still recommend that you read part 1 straight through before you start jumping around the book. Why, you might ask? Simple: The chapters in part 1 encompass the core principles, philosophy, and application of my system. Certain knowledge and basic skills are necessary for carrying out the movements and mobility techniques featured in parts 2 and 3. If you skip around without reading part 1 first, you will never fully experience the benefits that the system has to offer.

I know that some readers will want to skip right to the mobilization techniques and prescriptions later in the book. And if you have a tight muscle or a painful joint that needs to be dealt with, by all means go there. For example, say you're suffering from low back pain. You can flip to the back of the book, implement the low back pain mobility prescription on page 468, and then get to work on mobilizing using the techniques in part 3. But hear this: You will never get to the bottom of your pain and dysfunction if you don't correct the movement or position that is causing the problem. It's like treating a symptom without addressing the disease. Again, this is why it's imperative that you read all of part 1, especially the first three chapters that describe the movement principles: midline stabilization and organization, the one-joint rule, and the laws of torque.

Consider the movement principles your master blueprint for creating safe and stable positions for all movement. If you practice them in the order presented, you will know how to stabilize your spine in a braced, well-organized position; how to maintain a neutral spine during loaded, dynamic movements; and how to create stability (tension) in your joints to generate maximum force, power, and speed.

Realize that you can immediately apply the movement principles to the actions involved in sport and life. Once you understand the movement principles, you can start to bring consciousness to your position and movement in all situations. Whether you're trapped behind a desk at work, picking up your child, carrying a bag of groceries, or playing a sport, you need to follow the guidelines contained within these chapters.

It's important to note, however, that in order to master the movement principles, you need to practice them in a safe and controlled environment using transferable, full-range strength and conditioning movements. As I will discuss, doing so not only ensures competency across all movement planes, but also makes it easier to detect and correct dysfunctional movement patterns and limitations in mobility.

For example, in chapter 4, "Body Archetypes and the Tunnel," you will learn the basic archetypal shapes (positions within movements) for the hips and shoulders. Although the human body can conform to a wide range of positions and shapes, the functional positions for the hips and shoulders and, by extension, the knees, ankles, elbows, and wrists can be categorized into a few basic configurations. For instance, a squat is an archetypal shape for your hips, knees, and ankles. Arms raised overhead is an archetypal shape for your shoulders. So you take the movement principles, which tell you how to organize your body in safe, stable working positions, and then apply them to the body archetypes. This gives you a template for organizing your hips and shoulders and assessing your range of motion and provides a framework for understanding which position and which body part you need to mobilize. In chapter 5, "Movement Hierarchy," you will learn how to group movements into three categories based on difficulty and complexity, providing a framework for learning the movement principles, progressing as a beginner, and rebuilding when coming off an injury.

In short, the "Body Archetypes" and "Movement Hierarchy" chapters give you the building blocks you need to accurately pinpoint limitations in mobility, as well as isolate archetypal positions of restriction. The mobility systems approach outlined in chapter 6 lays the groundwork for correcting these range of motion issues by providing mobilization methods for resolving and treating pain and improving range of motion.

After you've read part 1, you will have the necessary foundation to implement the strength and conditioning movements in part 2, the mobilization techniques in part 3, and the mobility prescriptions in part 4. Stated differently, once you have a general understanding of my system, you can start navigating the book based on a movement or archetypal shape or mobility technique, or by program. It's important to note that you can navigate the movements by category (difficultly level) or by archetype (shape/position). The mobility techniques are presented by body part or area. To enhance your browsing experience, I recommend that you read the description at the beginning of each of these sections.

Now, I know that the sheer volume of information and techniques in this book can be a bit overwhelming. There's a lot to digest, it's true. But if you exercise the concepts and commit to performing the techniques correctly, you will experience immediate, positive change. You will look, feel, and perform better with fewer occurrences of pain and injury. However, to ensure long-term success, you have to be consistent. Don't get discouraged if you can't squat butt to ankles after 15 minutes of mobilizing, or keep your spine braced in a neutral position as you begin applying the movement principles to actual movements. You didn't start moving poorly and turn into a tight, knotted-up mess overnight; it's going to take time, practice, and a lot of effort to undo the damage and rewire those motor pathways. But it will be worth it, I promise. Eventually, you won't have to think about moving correctly; you just will. You won't even have to think about what or how to mobilize; you'll just do it.

However, to help keep you on track and alleviate potential frustrations, I'll leave you with two important points.

First, remember that your tissues are like obedient dogs. With consistency and time, they will come around. When you reach a block or you're struggling to make positive change, just remember that it's not your muscles' fault; it's you, the inconsistent, disobedient owner, who is to blame. I've never met anyone who hasn't been able to make a ton of change with 15 minutes of daily self-maintenance. Even if you suffer from a congenital deformity like hip dysplasia (this falls into the 1 percent category), there are still areas that can be optimized. The bottom line is that you can always improve and be working toward positive change. You just have to remain consistent and implement the right practices. I recommend that you spend 10 to 15 minutes a day working on your mobility. And never take a day off. Whether you're sore from a workout, stiff from a long car ride, or simply trying to improve your mobility, there is always something to work on or a position that can be improved.

Second, in order to correct the biomechanical errors that compromise your movement efficiency and cause pain, you have to learn how to move correctly. This often means starting from ground zero. You can't just tune out and do work. It's going to take a lot of time and practice before you start unconsciously and automatically moving in good positions. It's also important to realize that performing a movement correctly is more difficult than doing it poorly, because you have to engage more musculature to support good positioning. Just because something is harder doesn't mean it's not better. Resolve now to measure movement on the quality of form, not on the task. If you want to master the basics, you're going to have to rewire the hardware upstairs. And to do that, you're probably going to have to take a few steps backward. But now is as good a time as any to get started, so take a crack at it. Your body will thank you.

The Mobility Project

In 2010, my wife, Juliet, and I started the Mobility Project—an instruction-based movement and mobility video blog (MobilityWOD.com)—with the ambitious goal of filming one video a day for 365 days on subjects ranging from squatting technique to treating low back pain. If you haven't visited MobilityWOD.com, we invite you to start watching and encourage you to join the knowledgeable and supportive community. There are more than 500 free videos (and counting) that encompass everything you will learn in this book. To see these videos, go to MobilityWOD.com or to my YouTube channel, www.youtube.com/user/sanfranciscocrossfit.

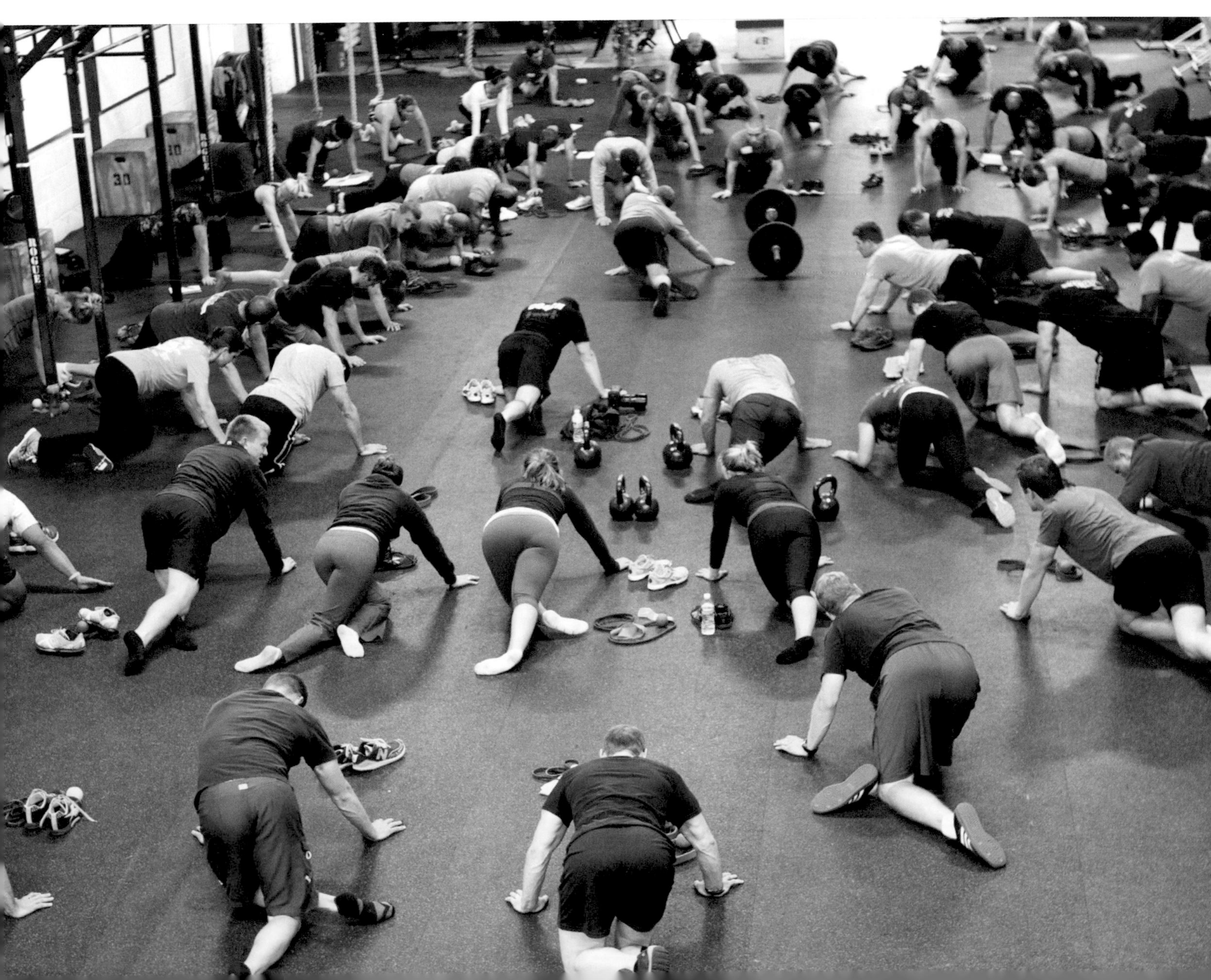

INTRODUCTION:

A NEW HUMAN PERFORMANCE EPOCH

These days, I often find myself crammed into an airplane seat on my way across the country to work with athletes, coaches, professional sports teams, CrossFit gyms, corporations, and elite military forces. Inevitably I end up making small talk with the poor soul imprisoned next to me. Soon enough I get the question: "What do you do?"

Dozens of answers run through my head.

"I make the best athletes in the world better."

"I work with the government to improve our military's force protection and force resiliency."

"I work with athletes and coaches to help them understand and resolve common and preventable losses of torque, force, wattage, and output."

"I'm trying to change the world's movement-based economy from subsistence tension hunting to sustainable, high-yield torque farming."

"I'm fomenting revolution. I'm trying to empower people to live more integrated, pain-free, self-actualized lives."

No, I don't mention anything about torque farming or self-actualization, which I'll spend plenty of time on in the pages to come. I keep it simple. "I'm a teacher," I say.

Typically my seatmate's eyes glaze over, and the conversation sputters to a halt. But once in a while, my seatmate is curious enough to ask the obvious follow-up question—"What do you teach?"—unaware of the depths of my obsession with human movement and performance. But he or she soon finds out.

What I teach—and what you will learn in this book—is an extraordinarily effective Movement & Mobility System. Learn, practice, and apply it and you will understand how to move correctly in all situations. And I mean all. It will serve you at rest and when you are executing a demanding physical feat—say, in an Olympic competition or in a strenuous combat or rescue operation.

This strength and conditioning system is also diagnostic in nature: It can help you predict, identify, and resolve common, transferable movement- and positioning-related errors that can lead to injury and compromise performance.

With enough practice, you can develop yourself to the point where your full physical capabilities are available to you instantaneously. You will develop the motor control and range of motion to do anything at any time. You could ultimately become the human equivalent of a supple leopard—always poised and ready for action. My system gives you the tools to dissolve the physical restrictions that are preventing you from fully actualizing your potential.

Is what I teach new? Yes, and then again, no.

I see myself as one of the latest in a long line of teachers concerned with organizing and optimizing movement to maximize physical performance—consistently and without injury.

Certainly, human beings have explored this subject for eons. There have always been smart, inquisitive people working out the software to the incredible human machine. In fact, I've seen a thousand-year-old image on a coin that shows a man sitting in full lotus—a posture that creates more stability for the spinal system. More recently, some 370 years ago, a famous Japanese swordsman, Miyamoto Musashi, wrote about the importance of keeping your belly firm and your knees and feet in a good position: "Make your combat stance your everyday stance." It is strange yet perfect advice from Musashi's famous text, *The Book of Five Rings*.

The truth is that we already know the safe, stable, and injury-preventing positions for the body. It's no secret. Humans have always been obsessed with figuring out how to optimize movement efficiency, which is why there are so many universally applicable systems that teach us how to move safely and effectively, regardless of the activity. We are the beneficiaries of an incredible convergence of disciplines, theory, science, technology, and expression of how the human body operates.

Although we should be careful not to forget the lessons and systems handed down over time, certain factors have sparked a golden age in human physical performance. People have always been fit and brutally strong, it's true, but extraordinary physical accomplishments are more the norm than the outlier these days. Modern humans are not that much more physically evolved, yet we continue to prove that the impossible is possible. What has changed? What makes modern-day athletes so different from our physically equal predecessors?

Motor control: The conscious and unconscious expression of ideal biomechanics or movement practices. When I say that an athlete doesn't have the motor control to perform a movement, I'm saying that he lacks the technique to perform the movement correctly.

Range of motion: The distance you can move your joint in a given direction. For example, if you are missing overhead range of motion, you're unable to position your arms in the ideal overhead position due to a shoulder joint and/or tissue restriction.

The Golden Age of Physical Performance

What's exciting about being alive today is that we're in the midst of a human performance epoch. Physical mastery is not limited to the few. As I see it, we are experiencing a quantum leap in the quality, reproducibility, and ubiquity of human physical potential. In fact, if we imagine the peak expression of our potential to be some kind of golden ratio, then the current generation of coaches, athletes, and thinkers have achieved the equivalent of a Fibonacci jump at light speed.

It's crazy. I mean, even my mother is gluten-free and casually brags about her latest deadlift personal record.

What's going on? What's so different about the time in which we live?

What's different is that we've seen a convergence of factors create a new golden age in human physical performance. Four key factors are responsible.

What Is a Supple Leopard?

You might ask, "What does it mean to become a supple leopard?" It's a good question that warrants an explanation.

I've long been fascinated with the idea of a leopard: powerful, fast, adaptable, stealthy…badass.

When I was fourteen, I watched the movie *Gallipoli* with my dad. It's about two Australian sprinters who go off to fight in Turkey during World War I. There's a memorable scene at the beginning where Archy, a rising track star, is being trained by his uncle Jack. The pep talk goes like this:

Jack: What are your legs?
Archy: Springs. Steel Springs.

Jack: What are they going to do?
Archy: Hurl me down the track.

Jack: How fast can you run?
Archy: As fast as a leopard.

Jack: How fast are you going to run?
Archy: As fast as a leopard!

Jack: Then let's see you do it!

For whatever reason, the "fast as a leopard" mantra stuck with me. But it wasn't until a Navy SEAL buddy of mine said, "You know, Kelly, a leopard never stretches," that this notion of becoming a supple leopard drifted into my consciousness.

Unlike a human, a leopard doesn't need to prepare for movement. It doesn't need to warm up; it doesn't have to foam-roll; it doesn't have to raise its core temperature—it's just ready. Its full physical capacity is available at all times. A leopard can attack and defend with full power at any moment.

Obviously, we do not share the same physical playing field with leopards. We have to warm up for strenuous activities and learn how to move correctly to avoid injury. But that doesn't mean we can't be working toward the goal of having our full physical capabilities available to us instantaneously, or having the motor control and the range of motion to perform any physical feat at any time. Leopards don't have to work at being supple; they naturally are supple. But many people are brutally tight and missing key ranges of motion that prevent them from moving as pliantly and powerfully as a leopard.

If you want to become a supple leopard, metaphorically speaking, you need to understand how to move correctly in every situation. You also need the tools to deal with stiff and adaptively short tissues that restrict your range of motion. This is exactly what I show you how to do in this book.

First, **the advent of the Internet and modern media** has enabled the global sharing of ideas. Isolated pockets of embodied knowledge are more easily transferred and dispersed. Ten years ago, finding an Olympic-lifting coach required bloodhound-like determination, luck, or both. Today, the clean and the snatch—the two core Olympic-lifting movements—are widespread practices.

Second, for the first time in the modern training era, there is an **unparalleled exchange among different training practices and theories of human movement.** For example, our gym, San Francisco CrossFit, is an interdisciplinary melting pot: physiotherapists hang out with elite powerlifters, Olympic-lifting medalists talk with champion gymnasts, and ballet dancers train with elite endurance coaches. This phenomenon is the strength and conditioning equivalent of the great systems theorist Buckminster Fuller's concept of mutual accommodation: that correctly organized, functionally sound systems are never in opposition. They support one another.

We all share the same basic design and body structure. People's shoulders all work the same way: The principles that govern a stable shoulder position while vaulting in gymnastics are the same in the bench press; how you organize your shoulders to sit in lotus position while meditating is the same way you should organize them when working at your computer. It's just that the same problems have been solved from radically different angles and approaches. Until now.

Third, there is **growing interest in the human body.** While this topic probably merits its own book, there is no doubt that the accessibility of online and mobile tools that make it possible to measure our lifestyle, nutrition, and exercise habits has shifted the responsibility for keeping our bodies in the best shape possible back to where it belongs: on us as individuals. Elite and recreational athletes alike can track and measure nearly every aspect of their performance and biology with little effort and cost. Want to know how that afternoon coffee affects your sleep quality? No problem. Want to fractionate your cholesterol and find out whether you are eating too much bacon? No problem (although I'm pretty sure that it's impossible to eat too much bacon). Whether people are tracking their blood chemistry or their daily step totals or are trying to get to the root of their knee pain, there has been an enormous shift in consciousness leading to a greater sense of self-control. Eating, sleeping, and moving correctly are not gimmicks or fads. The dam has burst, and the personal biological revolution is here.

It's a brave new world. We don't have to wait decades or endure multiple knee surgeries and heart attacks to find out that we're running poorly, eating poorly, sleeping poorly, and training poorly. Peter Drucker—world-renowned management consultant, educator, and author—was right: "What gets measured gets managed."

The fourth and most significant contributing factor to this golden age is the **evolution of strength and conditioning.** People have been lifting heavy weights, moving quickly, and working very hard to real effect for some time. The difference today is that a good strength and conditioning program covers all the elements of human movement. That is, an intelligently structured strength and conditioning program gives you full range of motion in your joints, limbs, and tissues; the motor control to express those ranges; and the ability to do so under actual physical load, metabolic demand, cardiorespiratory demand, speed, and stress. In addition, coaches are combining functional movement disciplines like powerlifting, Olympic weightlifting, and gymnastics (bodyweight) training into one training arena, which pretty much covers the entire spectrum of positions and movements that the body can adopt. This means that every movement performed in the gym has a transferable application to sport and life. Couple this complete physical paradigm and the cross-disciplinary exchange with the number of people now using a common language of movement, and you have the largest scale model experiment in human movement in the history of the world.

Let's put this in perspective. In the 11 years that our gym, San Francisco CrossFit, has been open, we've facilitated nearly 100,000 athlete training sessions encompassing all forms of functional movement training, both as isolated modalities (such as powerlifting, Olympic lifting, gymnastics, and running mechanics) and in combination (for example, CrossFit). The sheer volume of pattern recognition that this is capable of generating is staggering—it could take a single clinician or coach a lifetime to accumulate. Now multiply this by thousands of locations and suddenly a well-balanced strength and conditioning program becomes the world's most potent diagnostic tool with unmatched test and retest capabilities. This accumulated wisdom is what has given rise to my system. The gym is a laboratory.

We are able to eliminate correlates for human movement and performance and replace them with actual human movement. Take the active straight-leg raise test, for example. It's a common tool that physical therapists use to assess hamstring range of motion. Here's how it works: You lie on your back and raise your leg by flexing your hip. Although the active straight-leg raise test highlights hamstring range of motion (among other things), it doesn't look like a movement that you would perform in life or sport. This is what makes it a correlate for human movement.

The deadlift, on the other hand, not only tests hamstring range of motion, but also highlights motor control competency within the context of actual human movements that we perform daily. Stated differently, you don't have to demonstrate an active straight-leg raise; you just need to demonstrate that you can pick something up off the ground while keeping your spine organized and flat (in other words, a deadlift). This is how you bring it down to the bare essentials.

Realize what a huge shift in thinking this is.

In the past, it has been difficult to understand the nuances of poor technique and biomechanics as expressed by athletes. Why do middle-aged guys so readily tear their Achilles while playing pickup basketball? Because it's hard for them to detect the underlying poor movement patterns while they're playing. They're changing shapes, transitioning from one position to another at high speeds. (Anecdotally, basketball is the most dangerous sport that a middle-aged man can play.)

To prevent these injuries, you need a tool to make the invisible visible. You need to go into the lab (the gym) and assess their movement patterns using functional strength and conditioning movements before a catastrophe occurs—an ACL tear, herniated disc, or torn rotator cuff. In addition, you need a model that allows you to identify the problem, be it motor control or mobility.

By consistently and systematically exposing yourself to the rigors of full-range functional movements with optimal motor control (this is exactly what I will show you how to do in part 2), you can quickly identify faulty technique; motor inefficiency; poorly integrated movement patterns; holes in strength, speed, and metabolic conditioning; and restrictions in mobility.

Best of all, the tool you use to detect and prevent injury is the same tool needed to improve performance. The middle-aged "tore my heel cord" syndrome is a lot less likely to happen if you understand how to stabilize your joints in a good position and if your ankle is regularly exposed to full-range-of-motion movements like pistols or overhead squats.

But there's even more to it. The modern strength and conditioning environment has not only become the most complete way to systematically test and retest athletic performance and to diagnose movement inefficiencies and dysfunction; it has also created a formal, universal language of human movement. In short, if you understand the principles that govern full-range strength and conditioning exercises and can apply them in a low-risk environment (like a gym), you can apply them to the activities and positions of life, sports, dance, combat, and play.

For example, if you understand how to organize your spine and stabilize your hips and shoulders while performing a deadlift or clean, you have a ubiquitous model for picking something up off the ground. If you understand how to create a braced neutral spine (see chapter 3) and generate torque off a bar when performing a pull-up (see chapter 5), you will have no problem applying the same principles when climbing a tree. You can start to connect the dots between the safe, stable positions you practice in the gym to the movements you perform outside the gym.

And here's the rub: If you only climb trees, it may be impossible to know whether you are working in the safest and most efficient positions—with stable shoulders and a stable trunk—unless you also do formal pull-ups. In other words, it's a lot harder to identify whether you are moving in a safe, stable position when climbing a tree than when performing a pull-up in the gym, even though both activities abide by the same fundamental movement principles (more on that in part 1). So, in addition to being a lab in which to identify, diagnose, and treat poor movement practices, the gym is a safe and controlled environment in which we can layer these ubiquitous, transferable concepts to accelerate learning and reduce the potential for injury.

Moreover, the creation of a common movement language based on formal strength and conditioning principles is why there can suddenly be so much interdisciplinary, movement-based discussion and collaboration. We are able to move beyond "people should train in gymnastics" to "people should train in gymnastics because the handstand position easily teaches shoulder stability and organization and has the same finish position and shoulder demands as the jerk." The universality of "formal" human movement is easily understood by coaches and athletes alike, and it is easy to track and test changes in positional quality by measuring the very thing we are chasing in the gym anyway—performance. This is precisely why we keep track of work output, wattage, poundage, reps, and time.

Brilliant people have spent their entire lives developing systems that help us understand how and why humans move the way we move and have the ailments we do. Do these systems work? Of course—to varying degrees and with varying applications.

Should we discard them? No, of course not. But there is a significant disconnect between older models of human movement and our current understanding about how best to maximize our physical potential. To bridge the gap, we need a model that covers all the bases—that is, a blueprint for moving correctly in all situations, detecting and correcting common position and movement errors, and understanding how to perform routine maintenance on your body in order to improve range of motion and resolve pain. This is the premise of my movement and mobility system.

Lagging Indicators: Signs That You Have Been Moving Incorrectly

As I've said, we can learn a lot from traditional systems like yoga. They are certainly effective in some regards, but they don't target every aspect of a person's athletic profile. There's transferable application, sure, but it's not universally applicable across the entire spectrum of human movement. What we need is a model that not only teaches us how to move correctly in all situations, but also tells us when we are doing something wrong...before the onset of pain or injury.

But how do you know that you have some sort of musculoskeletal problem? More specifically, how do you know when your body is not operating at its full potential? The average athlete typically uses cues like pain, swelling, loss of range of motion, decreased force, or numbness and tingling. The conversation with yourself begins something like this: "When I run lately, my knee hurts. I wonder what's wrong with my knee?" Though typical, there are many errors in this line of thought.

The first is that pain and other symptoms of injury are lagging indicators. For example, swelling might indicate tissue overuse or strain from poor mechanics. But swelling is an after-the-fact sign. The tissue damage has already occurred. It's helpful to have a diagnostic tool that can highlight dysfunction and let you know that something is wrong, but only if it is applicable before the fact.

Imagine if you had to wait for your car's engine to blow up to know when you should add oil, or if a soldier had to wait for his weapon to jam in the middle of a firefight to know when to perform some preventative maintenance. That would be ridiculous, right? But in general terms, this is how modern sports medicine operates. We wait until something is broken, sometimes horribly so, before we expect a physician or physiotherapist to fix it. This paradigm keeps orthopedic surgeons very busy.

You can imagine what the doctor thinks when you come into his or her office with a hole in your kneecap from years of poor movement practices and overly tight tissues. Seriously? That bone in your knee was designed to last 110 years, and you managed to wear a hole in it in 20 (true story). Imagine waiting until you are suffering from unrelenting back pain and having your leg go numb to find out that you used poor spinal mechanics to carry a 100-pound pack as a young Marine (also a true story).

Like a light switch that's designed to last for tens of thousands of on-and-off cycles, our bodies are set up for millions of movement cycles. Millions! But every time you squat, bend over, or walk in a compromised position, you burn through those cycles at an accelerated rate. So by the time you've worn a hole in your kneecap, herniated a disc, or torn your labrum, chances are good that you've gone through millions of poor movement cycles. In other words, your tissues and joints didn't just wear out; your body put up with your bad positions and movements for millions of cycles. Everyone is different—genetics, training volume, and other lifestyle factors have a profound impact—but if you learn to move in the way the body is designed to move, you will put less stress on your system, reducing the number of cycles you burn through.

The second issue is that the human animal is set up for survival. Your central nervous system controls the flow of sensory and mechanical information for your entire body. It's not an accident that the pain and movement pathways in the brain stem are one and the same. If you bang your finger, the first thing you do is start moving it around. Why? You can't hear the pain signal along with the movement signal. This elegant system keeps people moving and surviving because it literally relegates those pesky pain signals to background noise, which you can't hear until you stop moving. Put another way, movement (sensory input) overrides the pain signal so that you can continue exercising and training. No wonder your shoulder starts to throb when you lie down to go to sleep. Your brain is no longer receiving any movement signal input; all it is getting now is full-blown pain.

Now imagine training like an athlete your whole life, spending countless hours ignoring the pain signals that your body is sending while you train and compete. There is little chance that you can actually hear the pain of tissue injury and failure amid all that movement and other pain noise. Pain doesn't work during periods of high movement load and peak output. Add stress to the equation, and it's a recipe for disaster. If you've ever been in a fight, you know that one of the great secrets of fighting is that you probably won't feel any immediate pain. Professional fighters will tell you that they feel violent impacts and concussions but don't immediately feel pain. Humans are designed to be able to take the hit, keep fighting, and deal with the consequences later.

Exercise presents a similar scenario. When you start to lose position and compromise your tissues—like rounding your back during a deadlift—you may not feel it at the time, especially if you're under competition stress. However, just as a fighter feels the abuse from combat after the adrenaline has worn off, your back will scream in pain when you cool down from a workout in which you did 20 improperly executed deadlifts. Just as you could say that the more skilled fighter usually suffers less damage and as a result doesn't feel as much—if any—pain after the battle, the better you are at deadlifting, the less likely you are to tweak your back.

The third and most notable problem with our current thinking is that it continues to be based on a model that prioritizes task completion above everything else. It's a sort of one-or-zero, task-done-or-not, weight-lifted-or-not, distance-swum-or-not mentality. This is like saying, "I deadlifted 500 pounds, but I herniated a disc," or, "I finished a marathon, but I wore a hole in my knee." Imagine this sort of ethic spilling over into the other aspects of your life: "Hey, I made you some toast! But I burned down the house."

Hang out at the end of any local marathon and you'll notice a significant number of finishers who are obviously suffering. They look as if they'd been hit by cars and stricken by disease. Yes, you say, but they finished. And this is true. Being obsessed with task completion certainly has its place, like in the Olympic finals, a world championship, or a military mission. But even then, there may be a heavy price to pay. Couple this task-priority blindness with an overly simplified system of pain indicators, and it's easy to understand how athletes can dig themselves into some pretty deep holes.

Many athletes go about their business this way for decades, spending their genetic inheritance, getting their daily workout done without pain, until one day it's game over. You can lift with a rounded back and sit in a chair in a slouched position—until one day you can't. So how do you keep from harming yourself? You need a set of leading indicators—observable, measurable, and repeatable diagnostic tools that enable you to predict potential problems before they manifest as recognizable disorders. The good news is that we already possess this information. It's called training.

Training as a Diagnostic Tool

Human movement, and by extension the body's positions within those movements, is really just a combination of biomechanics and movement technique. By exposing people to a broad palette of movements and making them express body control through full, normal ranges of motion, we are able to expose holes and inefficiencies in their motor control and mobility (more on that in chapter 5).

This means that while you are training for a stronger set of legs or a bigger set of lungs, you are simultaneously thinking in terms of diagnostics. The deadlift is no longer just a matter of picking up something heavy from the floor. Rather, it becomes a dynamic question: Do you have the capacity to keep your spine efficiently braced and stable and express full posterior-chain range of motion while picking up something and breathing hard in a stressful environment? We don't need to develop an entirely new set of correlate or diagnostic movements to understand what is happening when you lift something off the ground. We simply need to see and understand what's happening during the movement you are performing—that is, you have to understand why you are performing the movement and how to do it correctly.

Repurposing your training so that it also serves as a diagnostic tool is useful on many other fronts as well. First, it's efficient. Systematically and effectively assessing and screening for movement problems can be an enormous moving target at best and a colossal exercise in misplaced precision at worst. Any system or set of tools that helps us better understand what's going on under the hood is a good thing. Here's the key: Any good assessment tool, even one that's built on movement correlates rather than actual movement, needs to be easily scalable, meaning that the movement or exercise can be adjusted and applied to all athletes, regardless of age, body type, or skill level. It needs to be topical, addressing the issues that the coach is seeing that day, with that set of athletes, with those movements. Ultimately, it has to be able to render changes that both the coach and the athlete can observe, measure, and repeat. Over time, this daily combination of training and assessment frees the coach and the athlete to work through and discover problems systematically.

What you have to remember is that human movement is complex and nuanced. Marrying the diagnostic process to the training process ensures that no stone will go unturned. However, you can't train every movement or energy system that you may use in a single training session. Nor do you need to assess and address every deficiency in a single day. It's a lifelong process of identifying problems, fixing them, and then exposing more holes in your athletic profile with more challenging stimuli. This is how we become better athletes.

This model, based on the movements and training of the day, has the added benefit of being psychologically manageable in scope and practice. Anyone can fix one problem at a time. But the typical list of dysfunctions for the average athlete is just that: a list. The most important thing you can do is to train and address problems along the way. Small, consistent positional interventions don't create extreme, additional time demands on the athlete or the coach. The priority remains training, not resolving what is probably a laundry list of dysfunction in one training session.

I have yet to meet an athlete with perfect motor control, mobility, and biomechanical efficiency. Hell, most of the really successful athletes I know are dumping huge amounts of torque, bleeding horrendous amounts of force, and missing key corners in their range of motion. Yet they are still the best in the world. A 10- or 15-minute intervention performed on the spot, within the context of the athlete's current training, is manageable and sustainable. The modern training session is a little miracle. It's a frantic, compressed session of teaching, nutritional and lifestyle counseling, strength work, skill work, metabolic conditioning, and mobility work. Layering complex, time-demanding, full-body diagnostic movements and interventions on top of a cramped training session, especially if you're training several athletes at once, will only make you throw your hands up and revert to a wait-until-they-break model. But if a coach is able to program a few specific fixes (mobilization techniques—see part 3) for the demands of the day's movements, then the coach wins, and the athlete is able to embody the connection between mobilization and improved positioning. Athletes are both greedy and smart—greedy in that they will do whatever it takes to get better in the shortest amount of time possible, and smart in that they will repeat specific practices and interventions that improve their performance or take away their pain.

The second benefit of using training exercises as a diagnostic tool is that it shifts the issue of lost or poor positioning from the realm of injury prevention to the realm of performance. This shift has a twofold implication. The first is that it diverts your focus from task completion. "Well, I didn't get hurt, my knees aren't in pain, and I have an Olympic gold medal, so why should I care about injury prevention?" But, if you focus on output, you are in a constant state of chasing performance, of eking out small changes in position, efficiency, work output, poundage, and wattage. Our goal isn't just to make the best athletes in the world. Our goal is to make the best athletes in the world better.

These are the metrics that matter, because functioning well is never a force production or work output compromise. You don't have to choose between safety and a world record, sacrificing one for the other. If you chase performance first, you get injury prevention in the bargain. If you obsess over the reasons behind poor positioning, you get better mechanical advantage, improved leverage, and more efficient force production. For example, improved hip mechanics may mean a change in the total range of motion of the hip, but when it translates into a world-record squat, it actually means a little more. When a rower is able to improve her thoracic extension, she will sit taller on the seat and have better shoulder control. But when she notices greater wattage output and decreased times, she is a believer and will reproduce the phenomenon herself.

Using the training movements of the day as an instantaneous and ongoing diagnostic screening tool serves athletic development in other ways as well. For example, assessing an athlete for mechanical dysfunction with common screening processes is primarily a snapshot of that athlete on that day. It's not uncommon to run into athletes who have recently acquired tissue stiffness after a brutal training micro-cycle, tournament, or prolonged mission. Programming diagnostic/mobility work based on a well-rounded strength and conditioning program's daily movement is a roving, built-in, periodized system. Nothing is missed as long as you are performing movements that express full range of motion and motor control within those ranges. This leads to another useful change in the conceptual framework of what the gym can and should be.

The Gym Is Your Lab

The modern gym should be considered a human performance laboratory. Your goal in the gym should be to exceed any strength, speed, or metabolic demand that you might need in life, sport, or a shift on the SWAT team. It should also be the place where you hunt out every positional inefficiency, poor mechanical tendency, and default or compensatory movement pattern. Where else can you safely expose your movement and tissue dysfunctions? The gym/lab is a controlled environment in which you can safely and systematically layer skill progressions while simultaneously addressing mechanical and range-of-motion issues.

The hallmark of any good strength and conditioning program is twofold:

1. To consistently and routinely challenge both the strength and the fitness components of your constitution

2. To express motor control under a wide variety of demands and situations, which have transferable application to both sport and life

If the strength and conditioning program continuously challenges your position with the additional stresses of actual load, metabolic demand, speed, and competition, there is little doubt that your conditioned tendency, default motor patterns, and true physical self will be revealed.

I'll use a simple example to help illustrate my point. In our gym, we regularly see athletes who can correctly perform an overhead squat with a PVC pipe. This is the most challenging iteration of a squat because it has high hip and ankle demands: The athlete must keep his torso upright and his shoulders stable while his arms (the load) are locked out overhead. But what if we have that same person run 400 meters, then overhead squat with anything heavier than a barbell for more than a few repetitions, all while competing against someone else? We end up with a totally different athlete. And all we did was add a little volume, intensity, stress, and metabolic demand to the overhead squat. Very quickly and very safely, we make the invisible visible.

I'll discuss more on how to safely test the quality of movement using such methods (see chapter 5, "Movement Hierarchy"), but for now it's important to understand why these tests help you optimize performance and resiliency. The point is that the person who aces the quick test sometimes falls apart under real-life working conditions. You just have to adjust load, volume, and intensity to match the person's abilities and capacities—not only to expose holes in the their movement profile, but also to make her stronger, faster, more explosive, and generally more capable. In other words, if you have perfect form and fast times, you need to up the weight, volume, and metabolic demands, as well as introduce movements that require a higher degree of motor control and mobility. You should be seeking thresholds where you begin to break down, and use that not only as a tool for gauging movement quality and technique, but also as a way to get stronger, faster, and more efficient.

There are great athletes who can buffer their movement dysfunctions—meaning that they can hide their mobility restrictions and poor technique—for short periods, but regularly lose effective positioning when they begin to fatigue even a little. But if an athlete has the mobility and motor control to maintain a stable spine, hips, and knees during a high intensity workout of heavy front squats and running, then that athlete is more likely to be able to reproduce that efficient positioning when it matters most (say, in the last 500 meters of the Olympic rowing final).

As I said, the gym is the lab. It's practically impossible for a coach to follow around hundreds of athletes while they're engaged in their actual sport in order to spot movement errors. That coach would not only have to be a world-class expert in hundreds of sports and have perfect timing—catching the athlete just when he or she happens to break down—but also need the skill set to correct those faults within the context of that particular sport. Fortunately, you don't have to be an expert in every training modality to identify and fix problems that are specific to your chosen sport. All you need to do is repurpose the training movements so that they also serve as diagnostic tools. You are then able to observe and highlight every aspect of your movement quality and fix the suboptimal pieces, all while operating within a safe and controlled environment.

This moves strength and conditioning to the heart of athletic development and the heart of any human performance model. A program that is organized around challenging movement capacities with load, speed, cardiorespiratory/metabolic demand, and stress leaves very few body and capacity dysfunction stones unturned. For example, I regularly work with world-class athletes who cannot perform the most basic light deadlifting, squatting, or pushups without defaulting into a horribly dysfunctional position. It's not surprising that these same athletes have trouble maintaining decent spinal or shoulder positioning at the end of a workout or competition. If you understand the principles of midline stabilization and shoulder torque development—both of which are covered in this book—you will be able to apply those principles to another set of movement demands. Running is just maintaining a braced neutral spine (see page 36) while falling forward and extending the hip. And rowing looks an awful lot like performing a light deadlift (page 196) while breathing really, really hard. This insight is invaluable.

To reach your full athletic potential and reduce the risk of injury and pain, you need to prepare yourself physically for the demands of your sport (even if this sport is life or combat) and be your own chief movement and mobility diagnostician. This is the reason for training and practicing functional movements in the gym/lab: it prepares you for the acquisition of new skills and tasks. If you have full range of motion in your joints and tissues and you understand the movement principles, you're literally a blank canvas. It doesn't matter if you've never wrestled or played football before: If you understand how to get organized—how to stabilize your trunk (chapter 2) and create torque in your extremities (chapter 3)—then you enter the playing field with a distinct advantage.

Remember, classical strength and conditioning movements (gymnastics, Olympic lifting, powerlifting, sprinting, etc.) are the vocabulary of human movement. Sport doesn't look exactly like squatting and bench pressing. But if we connect the dots, drawing attention to the principles inherent in these movements, you can go out and apply those principles to the new set of variables that is sport and life. For example, if a football player understands how to set his feet and create hip torque while performing a squat, he'll be able to find the stable and effective hip, knee, and ankle position when he sets up in a three-point stance. Conversely, if the coach observes that the athlete loses effective knee stability at the bottom of a squat, that pattern will probably present itself as a more vulnerable and less effective knee position during play.

Here's another way to think about it: Learning how to move correctly in the gym is like learning how to read and write in school, in that you get a formal education and become fluent. The bad news is that you're going to have to invest some time and learn the basics. The good news is that it's never too late.

You Are an Incredible Healing Machine

The human body has an immense capacity to heal itself. At any age, and in nearly any state, the human animal is capable of an incredible amount of tissue repair and remodeling. Clearly torn ACLs don't magically reattach, and herniated lumbar discs are slow to heal, but the human body will take a ton of abuse for a really long time before it finally gives up the fight.

The fact is our bodies will put up with our silly movement and lifestyle choices because they have a freakish amount of functional tolerance built in. We shouldn't, however, make the classic error of confusing this miraculous genetic inheritance with a tacit rationalization for eating, sleeping, or moving however we please. And here is the larger point: Most of the typical musculoskeletal dysfunction that people deal with is really just preventable disease.

When thinking about movement dysfunction, it's useful to classify pain and injury into four categories, which I've organized here according to frequency of occurrence.

Those factors that account for 2 percent of the dysfunction in a typical gym:

- Pathology (something serious is going on with your system)
- Catastrophic injury (you got hit by a car)

Those factors that account for 98 percent of the dysfunction in a typical gym:

- Overtension (missing range of motion)
- Open-circuit faults (moving in a bad position)

Pathology

Pathology is dealt with through traditional medicine, and it accounts for a whopping 1 percent or less of the typical problems we see in the gym. But any good coach or practitioner is thinking on this level during any conversation with an athlete: "I don't think it's just back pain you're experiencing. It sounds like you have the makings of a kidney infection." Or: "I don't think you're overtrained. Based on that bright red ring around that suspicious bite on your arm, you may need to get checked out for Lyme disease." These are both real-life examples, and why a good clinician always asks about changes in bladder or bowel function, unaccounted-for weight loss or gain, night sweats, dizziness, fever, nausea, or vomiting—just to make sure that "knee pain" isn't "knee cancer." We tell our coaches that if something doesn't fit about the way athletes are talking about their musculoskeletal issues, they should always refer them to their physicians.

Catastrophic Injury

This category includes getting hit by a car, jumping downwind out of an airplane at night and landing on a stump, or having a 300-pound lineman roll into your knee. Catastrophic injury is where modern sports medicine excels; reconstruction and injury management capabilities are at an all-time high. Bad things are going to happen to people working to their limits in their respective fields. Fortunately, catastrophic injury also falls into the 1 percent bucket.

So if we have accounted for only about 2 percent of the typical movement dysfunction we see in the gym, where does the other 98 percent reside? Simple: It resides within the preventable disease categories of overtension and open-circuit faulting.

Overtension

I regularly observe athletes who lack significant ranges of motion. For example, it's not uncommon to see an Olympic medalist missing 50 percent or more range of motion in the anterior-chain system of the hips and quadriceps.

Imagine having dinner with a good friend and noticing that he can't bend his elbow past 90 degrees.

"What's wrong with your elbow?" you'd ask.

"Oh, nothing," he'd say. "I just set the bench press world record. But my neck and wrist kill me every time I eat."

This example would be silly except that it is not unusual. In general, though, the problem occurs in less socially crippling joint/tissue systems like the ankle, shoulder, and hip. And don't just think of flexion (bending) and extension (straightening). Full range of motion has to include the body's rotational capacities as well. Move your hand to your face as if you are going to eat. Is there resistance in this range of motion? There shouldn't be. Your limbs and joints should get stiff near end range and then suddenly stop. They should not be limited in range or be excessively stiff through the full range of motion. Either of these symptoms indicates that your joints or muscles are overtensioned. Put simply, you're missing normal ranges of motion as a result of your tight tissues.

In nearly every athlete I evaluate for position and movement compensations or for injured and painful tissues, I find an obvious and significant restriction in the joints or tissues immediately above or below the site of dysfunction. If you have ankle pain, chances are good that your calves are tight and are pulling on your ankles, limiting your range of motion. If you have knee pain, chances are good that your quads, hips, hamstrings, and calves (all the musculature that connects to your knee) are brutally tight. It's no mystery why you have pain: You can't get into the correct positions or move with good form because you're missing key ranges of motion. Mitigating an overtensioned system by using mobilization techniques feeds "slack" to the site, reducing localized joint pain by improving the efficiency of the system. I call this the "upstream/downstream approach," and you will learn more about it in chapter 6.

It's important to note that the traditional thinking of overtensioned tissues pairing, like "tight hamstrings causing low back pain," typically lays the lion's share of blame on the "short muscle" aspect of the system. But it's not that simple. Muscle "length" is a far more complex phenomenon comprising, among other things, intramuscular stiffness, neurodynamics, motor control, hip and joint mechanics, and even hydration. What ultimately matters, however, is that an overtensioned system needs to be remedied—by addressing position and range-of-motion restrictions. This is exactly what I will teach you how to do in the pages to come.

Open-Circuit Faults

This category encompasses most of the serious athletic trauma in the world of strength and conditioning. Injuries like torn ACLs, flexion-related herniated discs, torn biceps tendons, labral tears of the hip and shoulder, and torn Achilles tendons belong in this category.

Your body is a simple mechanical system composed of "wet" biological tissues. It operates best when it is able to create ideal, stable positions before it generates freakish outputs of power. Most people are familiar with the maxim that functional movement begins in a wave of contraction from core to sleeve, from trunk to periphery, from axial skeleton to peripheral skeleton. This principle is a good example of the body operating best when all its circuits are closed—spine stable and braced, hips stable, shoulders stable, feet straight, etc.—before movement is initiated. The problem is that the body is always able to generate force, even in poor positions. This is not unlike being able to get away with driving your car with no oil in the engine or with a flat tire. Sure, you can do it temporarily; it just gets expensive. Your body will always default to a "secondary" or "second order" system of stabilization, with a rounded back, internally rotated shoulders, collapsed knees and ankles, etc. This is what I mean by "open-circuit" and "movement compensation": When you compensate into a poor position because you're missing range of motion or lacking motor control, stability and as an extension force and power, leak from the system at the open circuit site. So if you round your back when picking something up off the ground, the bend of your back is the open circuit.

Here's an example: Children with cerebral palsy have damaged motor-control systems. They are cognitively intact; they just have aspects of movement that aren't well controlled within the brain. Yet these children are able to ambulate despite this damage. Their bodies are clever enough to default to a collapsed arch and ankle, internally rotated and valgus knee, internally rotated and impinged hip, and overextended lumbar spine (this is a movement compensation because they are unable to get into the ideal position). They are able to leverage their tissues into secondary positions of stability that turn out to be quite functional—until those tissues wear out.

CLOSED CIRCUIT

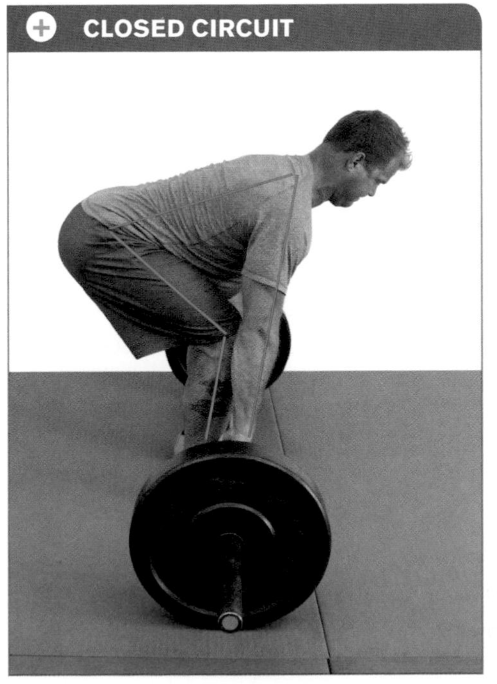

OPEN CIRCUIT

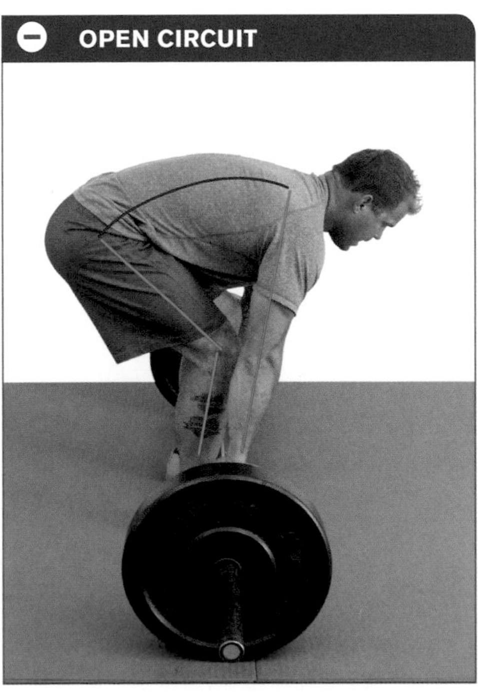

Examples of Open/Closed Circuits

In the closed circuit photo, I've established a stable position, giving me optimal power and reducing the chance of injury. In the open circuit photo, I am in an unstable position, which not only leaks power, but also can lead to a number of injuries, such as a herniated disk.

These positions should look familiar to anyone watching a heavy front squat gone wrong. If you don't or can't create a stable position from which to generate force, your body will provide one for you. You don't need to address your ankle or hip range of motion; your body will address it by turning your feet out. You don't need to work on restoring anterior hip range of motion; your body will overextend at the lumbar spine.

Open-circuit faults include:

- Rounded back
- Shoulders rolled forward
- Overextended lumbar spine
- Feet turned out or collapsed arches
- Head tilted up or down
- Elbows flared out

Herein lies the problem: We have confused functionality with physiology. Positions that have served us functionally—like jumping and landing with feet like a duck's—quickly become a liability when speed, load, or fatigue is introduced. Sure, you can lift heavy loads with a rounded back (the default spinal-stability position) for a long, long time, but at some point your tissues will fail, resulting in injury. Eventually those "off-label" tissue uses with which you exercised and moved so freely will expire.

The implications of this concept are incredible. Most ACL injuries are preventable, especially in children. Most shoulder dislocations are preventable. Most herniated discs are preventable. Remember, your tissues are designed to last 110 years. You just have to know what the stable, tissue-saving, catastrophe-avoiding positions are. And you have to practice them. A lot. Not only that, but you also have to align the other aspects of your lifestyle. I'm talking about hydration, food quality, sleep, and other factors that wreak havoc on tissue health and compromise athletic performance.

You Cannot Make Basic Adaptation Errors

As I said earlier, I will teach you the safest and most effective body positions so that you can optimize performance and resolve pain and dysfunction. But before moving on to the actual movement principles, diagnostics, categories of movement, and mobilizations, it's important for you to understand that lifestyle errors have a direct impact on how well or how poorly you move. Let's address these now and set the foundation for your success.

You cannot make basic lifestyle errors and expect your body to be able to absorb the consequences when you are working in a performance-biased paradigm. For example, it is possible to make fundamental errors in hydration, nutrition, sleep, and stress and not suffer any direct impact on your elliptical biceps training. However, every athlete at the top of his or her game can make direct correlations between these errors and the potential for creating significant decreases in performance outputs. Being dehydrated by even 2 percent can cause a 5 to 10 percent decrease in VO2 output (think aerobic capacity). Less than six hours of sleep? Say hello to elevated blood glucose levels (think prediabetes). Stressed out? Forget about getting a healthy adaptation response to that crushingly difficult workout—you will simply get crushed.

The less obvious implication of lifestyle maladaptation is on tissues. Connective tissue, menisci, spinal discs, fascia, articular cartilages, tendons, and ligaments all suffer from the immediate and downstream effects of unhealthy lifestyle choices. Managing and optimizing the lifestyle aspects of sports performance are certainly beyond the scope of this book, but I would be remiss if I did not mention that I regularly observe significant changes in athletes' mobility (and ultimately position) when they begin to address and correct these vital aspects.

Adaptation errors include:

- No warm-up or cool-down
- Sleep deprivation
- Dehydration
- Poor nutrition
- Prolonged sitting
- Stress

It's easy to feel overwhelmed when you consider how complicated human movement can be and how many different aspects of your life directly affect movement mechanics and tissue health. But underlying all this beautifully complex technology is a simple truth: Your body has an amazing capacity to deal with poor mechanics. Again, your body can generate huge amounts of force and endure a ton of punishment in spite of your bad technique and tissue restrictions. You can move fast, lift heavy, and sit all day with poor technique and still perform well. But eventually your body will tell you that you're doing something wrong. And it doesn't just whisper in your ear; it rams the message down your throat by zapping your ability to generate force and opening the floodgates to pain. If you're currently facing injury and pain, don't wait for tomorrow to start moving correctly. The damage is reversible. If you're healthy, don't wait until you're injured or in pain to start taking care of your body. The time is now.

PART 1 PRINCIPLES AND THEORY

My goal in this book is to provide a blueprint for moving safely and effectively in all situations—and to teach you how to perform basic, routine maintenance on your body. This section serves as that blueprint. It sets the stage for the techniques covered in parts 2 and 3, as well as the mobility prescriptions outlined in part 4.

In chapter 1, you'll learn about spinal mechanics, the reasons why you should prioritize midline stabilization over everything else, and how to properly brace your spine in a neutral position. Then you'll learn what it means to get "organized" into a good position, why that is important, and how to do it correctly. You'll learn how much range of motion you need to optimize athletic performance and how to resolve common positional and movement faults that can impede performance and lead to injury. Finally, you will learn how to progress exercise movements in a way that builds functional and transferable movement patterns, as well as mobility methods for improving range of motion and resolving pain. It's all here, so let's get started.

MIDLINE STABILIZATION AND ORGANIZATION (SPINAL MECHANICS)

Prioritizing spinal mechanics is the first and most important step in rebuilding and ingraining functional motor patterns, optimizing movement efficiency, maximizing force production, and avoiding injury. In order to safely and effectively transmit force through your core and into your extremities, you need to organize your spine in a neutral position and then create stability throughout that organized system by engaging the musculature of your trunk, which is known as bracing. This is the basis of midline stabilization and organization. This chapter explains why it's important to prioritize spinal mechanics over everything else—and how to organize and brace your spine in an optimal position.

Throughout history, advanced thinkers have harped on the importance of organizing the spine in a good position, tightening the body, bracing the abdomen, and stabilizing the trunk. The "core to extremity" concept is not new. It's a well-known fact that if you don't organize and brace your spine optimally—in a neutral position with your head aligned over your shoulders and your ribcage balanced over your pelvis—you can't effectively transmit energy to the primary engines of your hips and shoulders (more on that in chapter 3). This results in staggering losses of stability, force, and power and opens the floodgates to pain and injury.

Yet the spine remains the weak link. In my physical therapy practice, I see trunk-related errors and weaknesses even among the world's best athletes. And these athletes know that a braced, well-organized spine is the key to moving safely and effectively.

So the question is, why do we regularly see so many fundamental spinal sins that impede performance and invite injury? There are a few reasons.

For starters, people tend to focus on completing a movement or lift with little or no regard for spinal mechanics. As I discussed in the introduction to this book, it's possible to generate huge amounts of force from a bad position without immediate, overtly negative consequences. I've seen athletes lift enormous loads from rounded and overextended spinal positions and walk away uninjured, grinning from ear to ear. This isn't always bad, and by that I mean that it may be a conscious choice made by a professional athlete who has measured what he stands to gain against the cost. Consider a powerlifter who chooses to round his upper back to break the deadlift world record. Although he loses shoulder stability and leaks power through his spinal system, rounding his upper back reduces the distance that he has to lift the weight. He knows damn well that he's flirting with potential injury, but he's willing to take the risk. The key is that he must practice lifting in a good position so that when he chooses to round his upper back, it is a conscious choice and not a default motor pattern.

This is a very important distinction to understand, because patterns repeated in practice will reveal themselves at game time and during daily life activities. Rounding your back for a deadlift will ensure that you pick things up off the ground with a flexed spine. Your overextended pushup position will transfer to overextension in your running. Sure, athletes in competition, warriors under extreme stress, and even desk jockeys will fatigue and eventually default to less efficient working positions. But—and this message is critical—prioritizing good spinal mechanics in training not only ingrains functional and efficient movement patterns, but also helps you buffer those lapses into overextension and flexion that inevitably occur. The problem is that people who aren't aware of these fundamental truths will default to compromised form when training, which in turn develops and reinforces faulty body mechanics that exact payment during the physical actions of sport and life.

The fact is that we do a great job of celebrating the completion of 50 pushups, but we haven't done a good job of identifying the loss of proper spinal positioning during those pushups. You will make a few movement errors under cardiorespiratory and metabolic load (fatigue), but you still have to be safe and be able to correct those errors. If it's for the world championship, by all means win. But recognize training as training. Again, we need to move away from the practice-makes-perfect paradigm and realize that practice makes *permanent*. If you lift with a back that looks like a snake that's been hit by a car, you've taught yourself to generate force from

Neutral Spinal Position and Spinal Faults

neutral spinal position

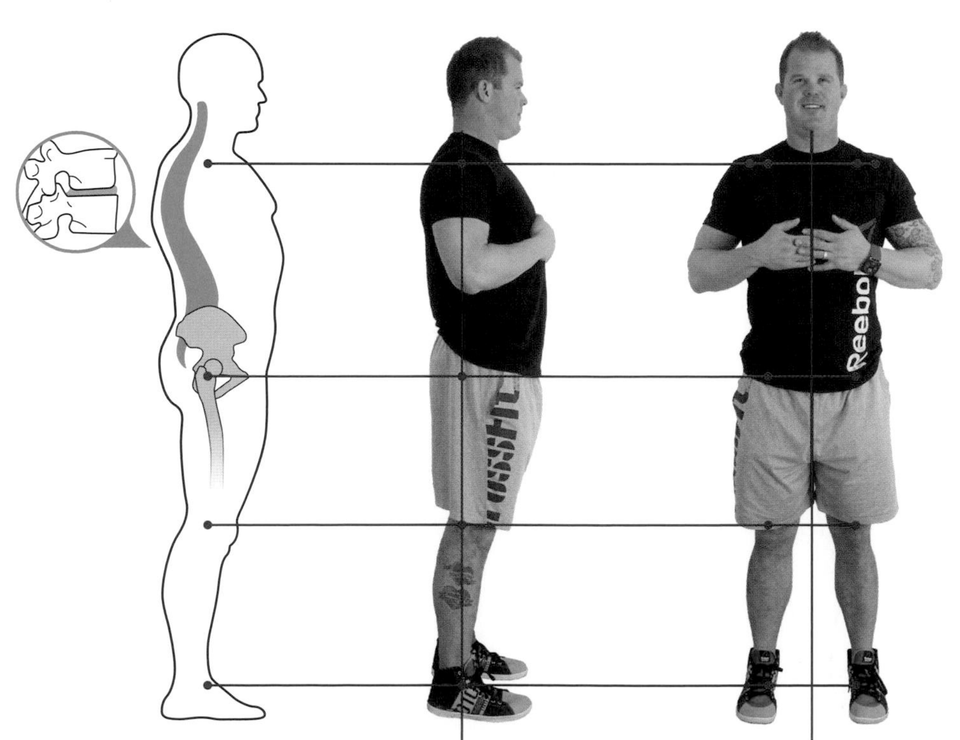

that broken spinal position. And exercise is only half of it. If you sit, stand, or walk with an overextended or rounded back, chances are you will have trouble organizing your spine in a good position during loaded or dynamic athletic movements. The best defense is not to make those errors in the first place.

Another problem that keeps athletes from prioritizing spinal mechanics is that they simply lack a model for organizing and bracing the spine in a good position. While trainers talk obsessively about core strength, posture, and bracing, they seldom teach athletes how to organize and brace the spine as an independent sequence. Instead, they attempt to ingrain midline stabilization as athletes practice complex movements. Now, you can certainly develop midline stability by practicing complex movements, but unless you organize and brace your spine in a neutral position prior to moving, you're much more likely to break into a less than optimal spinal position. You see this with kids who practice gymnastics or martial arts at a young age. They intuitively brace the spine to match the dynamic demands of the sport, but they aren't taught how to set up in the best position possible. So they brace their spine by engaging the musculature of the trunk, but they don't always organize the spine in a neutral position—that is, with the pelvis, ribcage, shoulders, and head in alignment.

Coaches who understand the importance of spinal position often cue athletes to get tight or flatten their back, but those cues don't really work. Although the belly should be tight and the back should look flat, those cues don't teach athletes anything about organizing the spine in a good position. When midline stabilization isn't taught by itself, poor bracing strategies are often the result. And poor bracing strategies ultimately lead to a host of biomechanical compromises, such as an overextended or flexed spine or rounded shoulders.

flexion spinal fault

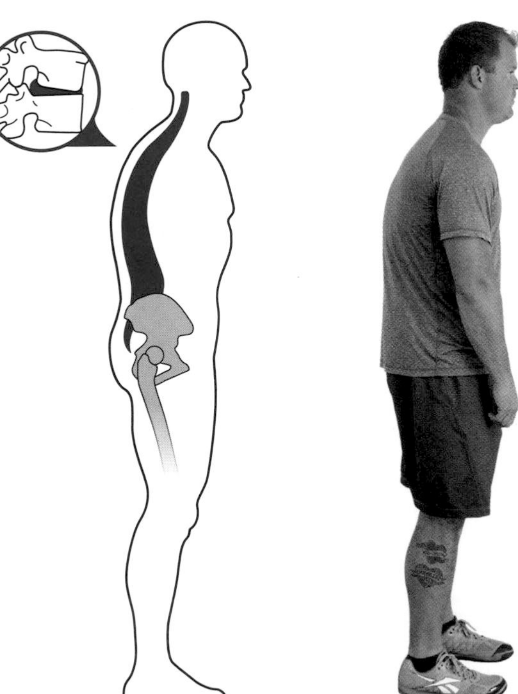

overextension spinal fault

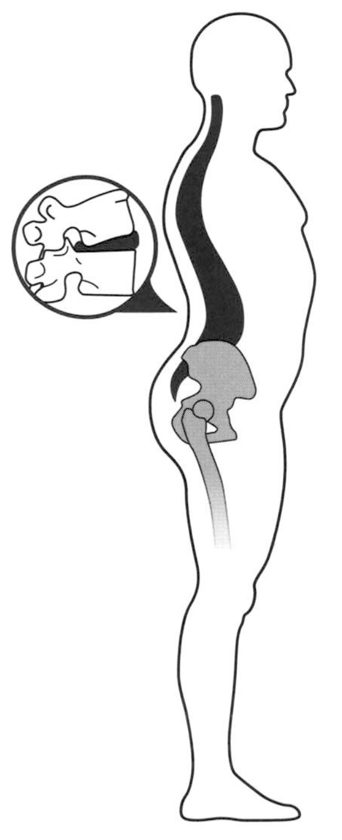

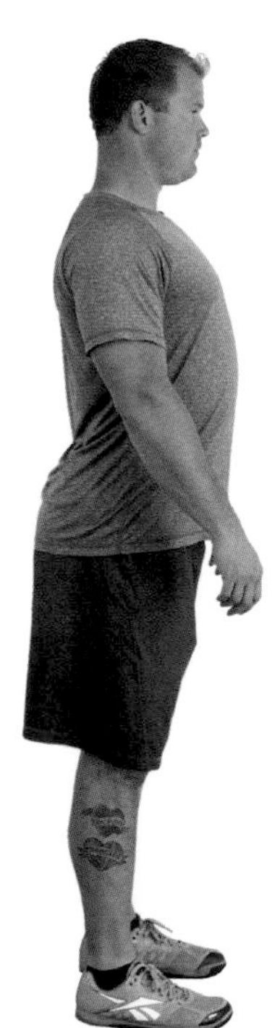

A Braced Neutral Spine: The Key to Moving Safely and Effectively

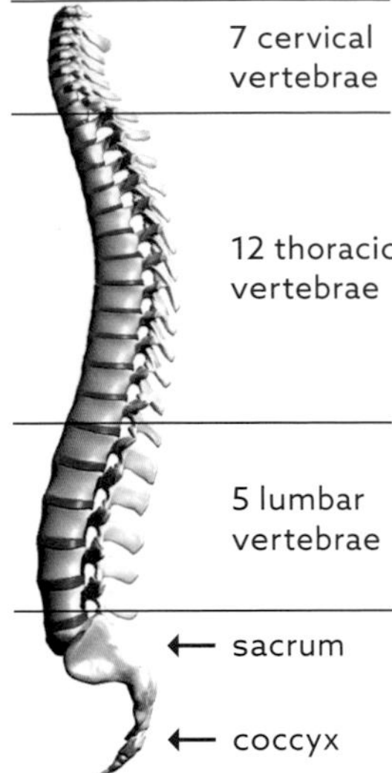

There is a blueprint for organizing and stabilizing your spine in a neutral position: It's called the bracing sequence. But before I delve into that, you should understand the reasons for organizing your spine in a neutral position—and why you need to prioritize spinal mechanics over everything else.

The functional positions of the spine (as well as the shoulders and hips) can be categorized into a few basic configurations:

- braced neutral
- global flexion
- global extension
- braced flexion
- braced extension

The braced neutral position is the optimal base position for most human movements. By braced neutral, I mean that your ribcage is balanced over your pelvis, your ears are aligned with your shoulders, and you're engaging the musculature of your trunk to stabilize the position. It is the most utilitarian position for the spine because it allows you to handle load safely and transmit force efficiently. For the majority of movements, you do not want your spine to deviate from this neutral position.

To understand why, it's important to realize that the spine is divided into three regions: cervical, thoracic, and lumbar. Each region consists of individual bones called vertebrae, which function a lot like hinges. But these hinges are not meant to bend individually. Rather, they are meant to bend as part of a global arch through the entire spinal system (more on that later). In fact, anytime one or two vertebral segments hinge or express a greater degree of motion in relation to the rest of the spine—whether it's the head (cervical spine), the base of the ribcage (thoracic spine), or the pelvis (lumbar spine)—force production is limited and your ability to stabilize your hips and shoulders is compromised. This is what I refer to as a local extension or local flexion spinal fault.

To clarify this concept, think of your trunk and spine as a chassis for the primary engines of your hips and shoulders. If your spine is in a bad position, it is impossible to create a safe, functionally stable hip, knee, ankle, or shoulder position. This is why you want to fix spinal positioning before you go after the poor mechanics or tissue restrictions in your shoulders or hips: You'll never fix those big engines if the chassis is broken. Put another way, it doesn't matter what's going on at your shoulder, elbow, knee, or ankle, whether it is a motor control or a

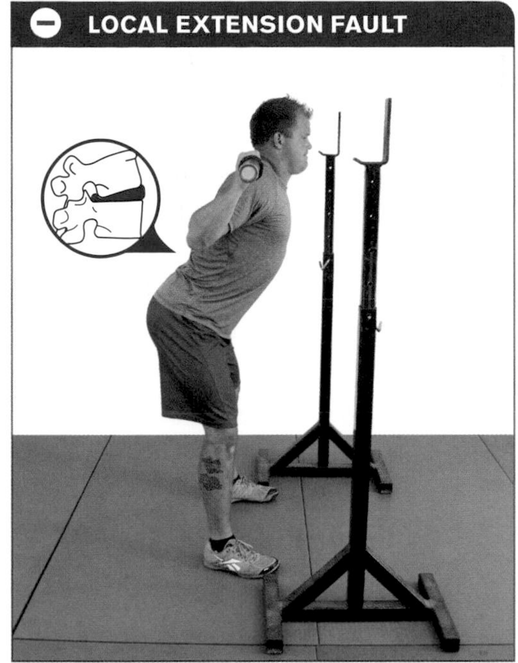

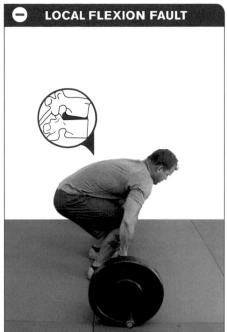

mobility issue: If your spine is out of whack, you're never going to be able to fix the problem.

When you organize your spine in a neutral position, with each spinal segment in perfect alignment, force can travel efficiently and uninterrupted through the kinetic chain. You're also in an optimal position to handle the compression forces acting on your spine. When you're standing, sitting, or moving, your spine is carrying and supporting the weight of your upper body. To manage the load effectively, the structures of your trunk need to be balanced and stable. If you hinge from one or two vertebral segments, the weight of your upper body compresses that hinge, creating a shear force across that spinal segment. Stated differently, there is off-axis pressure that causes structural strain, or shear. So if you assume a position in which one or two vertebral segments are out of alignment, you create a shear force across the bend of that spinal segment.

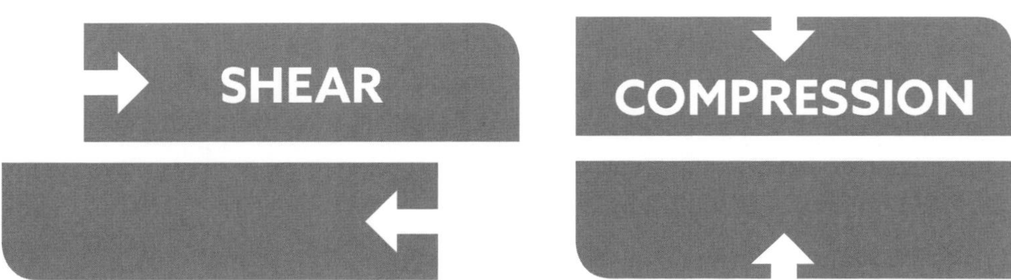

In short, the moment you deviate from a neutral spinal position, you lose stability and with it the flow of potential force. This is why you have to think of the spine as a continuum. If you try to generate force while one section of your spine is unstable, you're doomed. Add an axial load (a force compressing your spine), and it's a recipe for disaster. In the short run, it can shut down force production and open the door to a minor spinal tweak (injury), and in the long run, it may result in spondylolisthesis, herniated discs, pars fractures, and stenosis.

It's important to realize that injury to the central nervous system (spinal cord) is one of the greatest threats to the human body. If you injure the meniscus in your knee, you can still soldier on—it might not be all that pleasurable, but you can go on with your life. If you herniate a disk or injure a facet joint, on the other hand, it's game over: Your whole mechanical system shuts down. You are unable to run, lift, move quickly, or reproduce. And it's not a minor interruption, either; injuries to the spine are a hard bell to unring. The healing process is long and brutally slow. In my practice, if an athlete has a spinal tweak, it takes a minimum of two days to get that athlete back into training. And that's for a minor positional fault. I regularly get calls from athletes who have missed a week or two after a minor spinal tweak. This is two weeks of missed preparation (not to mention two weeks of less-than-optimal living) because of a simple and preventable trunk-related error. Still think that extra back squat with an overextended lumbar spine was worth it? (To learn a how to self-treat a spinal tweak, flip to the low back tweak pain prescription on page 468.)

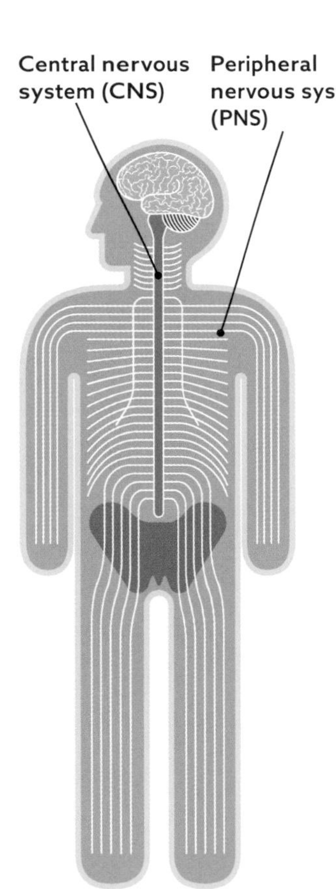

Another common consequence resulting from poor bracing is reduced range of motion. That's right: A disorganized spine can limit your mobility. I regularly run into athletes who look as if they have horribly restricted posterior chain tissues—specifically hamstrings—when in reality it's a disorganized spine that is holding them back. Old-school thinking would have us fix the problem by mobilizing those stiff cables running down the backs of the legs. While doing so may in fact improve hamstring range of motion, it might not alleviate back pain or improve lifting mechanics.

What you need to understand is that your nerves are a fixed length; they do not stretch. So when you put a kink in your spinal cord (CNS) and then load the nerve root—the initial segment of a nerve leaving the CNS—your body recognizes the position as a liability and tightens the surrounding musculature to limit your range of motion. For example, say you commit a lumbar overextension spinal fault. The moment you overextend, you load some of the lower nerve roots in your lumbar spine and by extension the peripheral nerves—those that connect the CNS to your limbs and organs—that exit into your legs. When that happens, your quadriceps, your hamstrings, and even your calves tighten to protect your nervous system, a phenomenon I refer to as neural tension. I've found that if I simply organize an athlete's spine into a braced neutral position, range of motion improves by 30 to 40 percent. This is why I prioritize midline stabilization and good movement mechanics over mobilization techniques, because what often looks like tight musculature is really just the body protecting the nervous system.

Finally, an organized, braced neutral spine allows you to transition from one functional position to another. Remember, you rarely perform only one movement. Whether you're playing sports or just going about your day, you are constantly transitioning from one position to another. And you're constantly rotating. Consider a basketball player who needs to jump, land, cut, and then jump again, or an athlete playing a rotational sport like baseball or golf. If that player starts out in an overextended or flexed position, every position and movement that follows is compromised. Understand that rotation and speed magnify small positional errors around the spine. To ensure safe, optimal, and transferable movement patterns, you need to start in a braced neutral position and maintain that position as you rotate or transition into your next position. This is why you need a model for organizing your spine in the best possible position at the start.

The Bracing Sequence

The bracing sequence is the bedrock from which all safe, dynamic, and high-volume athletic movement is generated. Consider it a new weapon to practice with and master as you apply it to all the positions and movements of sport and life. You need to have a conscious plan for bracing your spine in a neutral position, and the bracing sequence is a step-by-step template that will give you the same results every time.

The idea is to make the bracing sequence instinctual so that you can reproduce the same neutral, stable position in any situation. Go through this sequence anytime you're setting up for a dynamic movement, picking something up, or squatting, or simply to fix your posture. Ingraining it will take time, however. In the beginning, it might take 20 to 30 percent of your mental RAM just to keep your shoulders in a stable, externally rotated position, your abs tensed, and your spine neutral. But you have to cultivate the mindset that anything other than a braced neutral spinal position is feasting on your athletic potential and opening the door to pain or injury.

Stabilizing Your Head and Jaw

People do some crazy things with their jaws in an attempt to stabilize their head and neck system. What you have to remember is that your jaw is a large open circuit right in the middle of a complex and very important kinetic chain. To avoid defaulting into a compensated head or neck position (i.e., Olympic-lifter yawn), you need a strategy for setting your jaw in a good position.

The general recommendation is to relax your face, pin your tongue to the roof of your mouth, jamming it behind your teeth, and close your jaw. This will allow you to create tension in your jaw without clenching, opening your mouth, shortening your neck flexors, or compromising breathing mechanics. It's that simple. There are even companies that build specific mouthguards to help facilitate this!

The Bracing Sequence, Step by Step

START
COMPROMISED POSITION

STEP 1
Screw your feet into the ground.

STEP 2
Squeeze your butt.

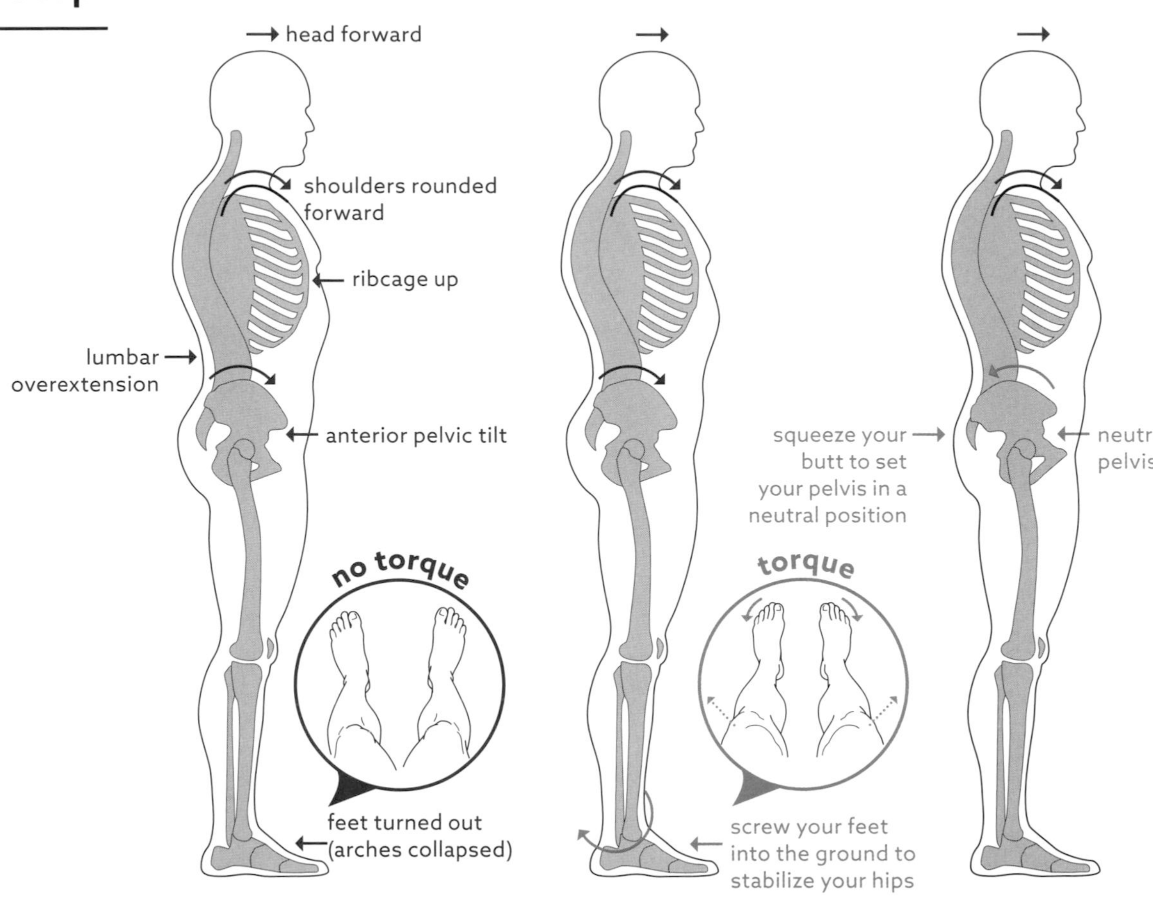

START: To highlight each step, let's start the bracing sequence from a poor yet common posture: the overextended spinal fault with forward head on neck, rounded shoulders, and turned-out feet. *Note:* It doesn't matter what position you start the bracing sequence in—whether you're rounded forward or overextended—the end result should be the same.

STEP 1: Position your feet directly under your hips and parallel to each other. Externally rotate from your hips by screwing your feet into the ground—more specifically, keeping your feet straight, screw your left foot into the ground in a counterclockwise direction and your right foot into the ground in a clockwise direction. *Note:* You're not turning your feet outward; you're just exerting force in an outward direction.

STEP 2: Set your pelvis in a neutral position by squeezing your butt (which you can do concurrently with step 1). You will always end up in the right position because those glutes were engineered to support your pelvis and spine. You don't need to keep your butt at full tension; just activate your glutes and then reduce the tension to maintain a neutral pelvic position.

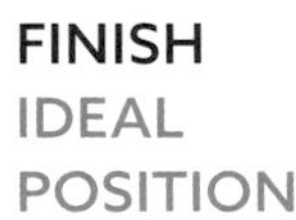

STEP 3
Take a deep breath in.

STEP 4
Balance your ribcage over your pelvis and get your belly tight as you exhale.

STEP 5
Set your head and shoulders in a neutral position.

FINISH
IDEAL POSITION

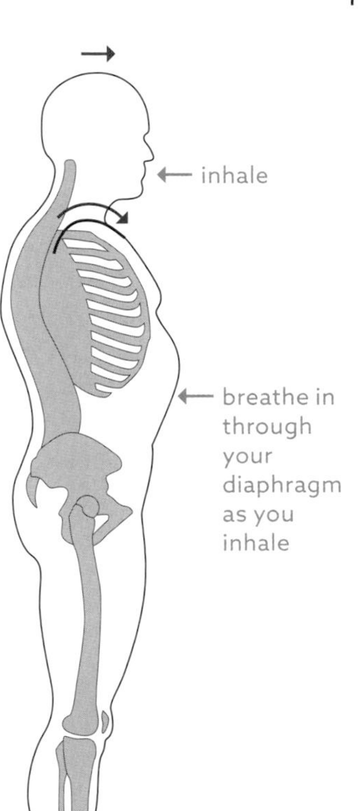
inhale
breathe in through your diaphragm as you inhale

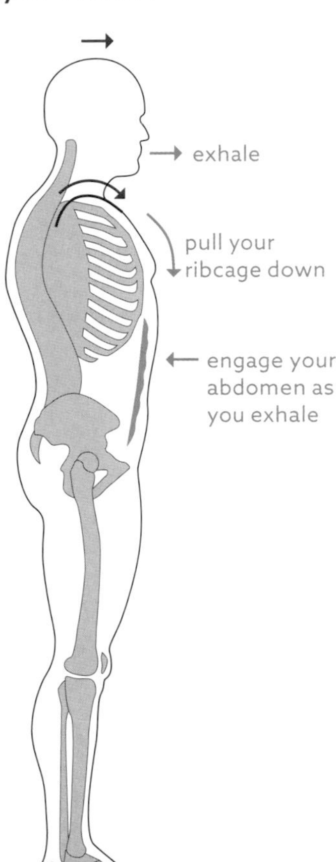
exhale
pull your ribcage down
engage your abdomen as you exhale

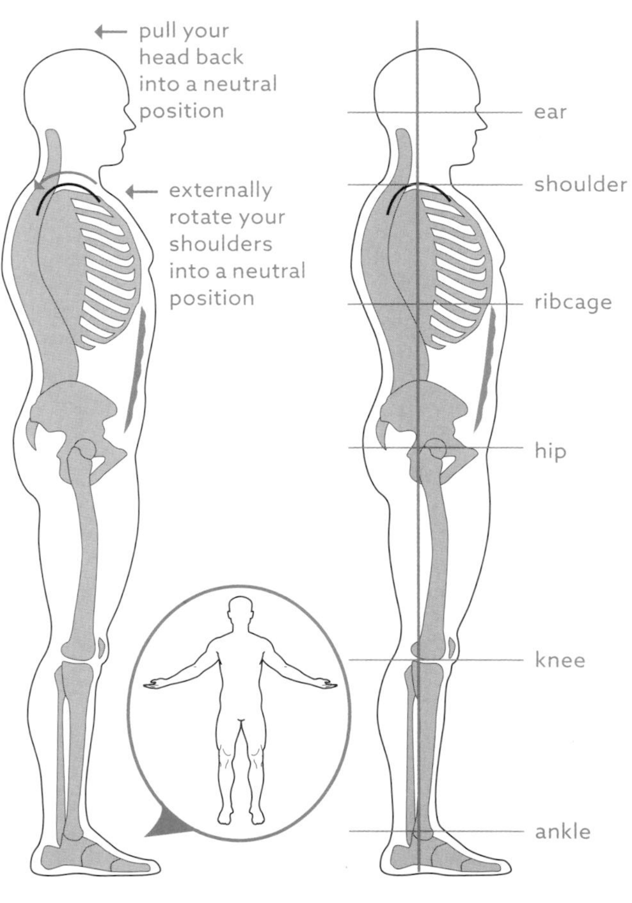
pull your head back into a neutral position
externally rotate your shoulders into a neutral position
ear
shoulder
ribcage
hip
knee
ankle

STEP 3: Lock your pelvis and ribcage in place by using your abdominals. You can't move with your butt squeezed, so you need to lock in the position by engaging your abs. Think about it like this: Glutes set position, and abs brace position. You need at least 20 percent tension in your abs to set and maintain a braced neutral spine for basic positions like sitting, standing, and walking. To execute this step, continue squeezing your glutes and take a big breath in through your diaphragm (belly).

STEP 4: As you let the air out, balance your ribcage over your pelvis and tighten your belly, stiffening as you exhale. It's not sucking in or hollowing. It's not even drawing in; it's stiffening in place as you exhale. As the musculature of your trunk compresses toward your midline, you create intra-abdominal pressure around your spine, resulting in a more rigid lever. The idea is to breathe into that tight space as if you were putting compressed air into a steel tank. You don't make the tank tight around the air; you put the air into the rigid tank.

STEP 5: Draw the heads of your arm bones back, spreading your collarbones wide as you externally rotate your shoulders and turn your palms toward the sky. As you do so, center your head over your shoulders, focusing your gaze straight ahead. Think about aligning your ears over your shoulders, hips, and ankles.

FINISH: To complete the sequence, let your arms fall to your sides, keeping your thumbs pointed forward and your shoulders externally rotated. The goal is to align your ears over your shoulders, your ribcage over your pelvis, and your hips over your knees and ankles.

The Two-Hand Rule

To bring awareness to the bracing sequence, I developed a simple and effective method to highlight spinal positioning. I call it the two-hand rule. This technique not only helps you get into a neutral position, but also helps you identify where you are losing form. Note that you can apply the two-hand rule to everyday life positions like standing, sitting, and lying down. It can also be used with basic bodyweight movements like squatting, walking, and running.

Here's how it works: Take one thumb and put it on your xiphoid process (sternum)—keeping your fingers splayed and your palm facing down. Pin your other thumb on your pubic bone, creating two parallel planes. The key is to keep your hands on the same horizontal plane as your ribcage and pelvis so that any deviation from neutral will be reflected in a change in hand position. If your hands move farther apart, you're overextended. If your hands move closer together, you're rounded forward.

You can apply the two-hand rule to daily life positions like standing, sitting, and lying down, as well as to basic bodyweight movements like squatting, walking, and running.

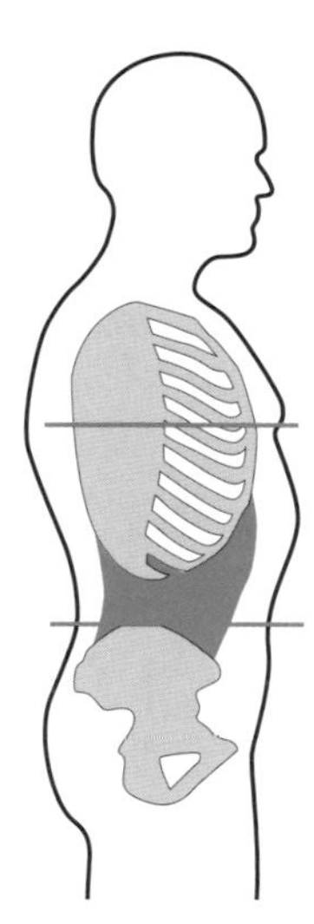

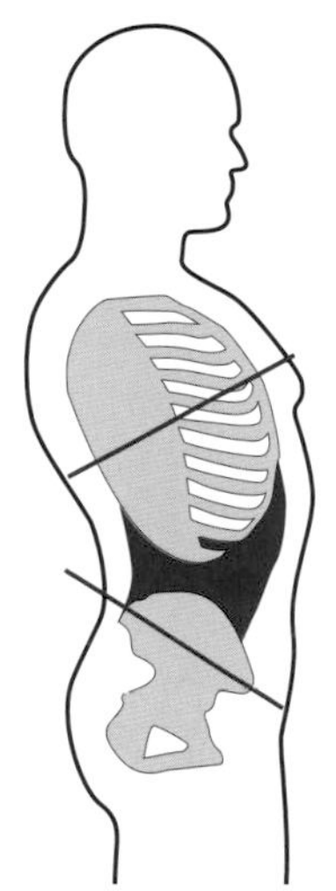

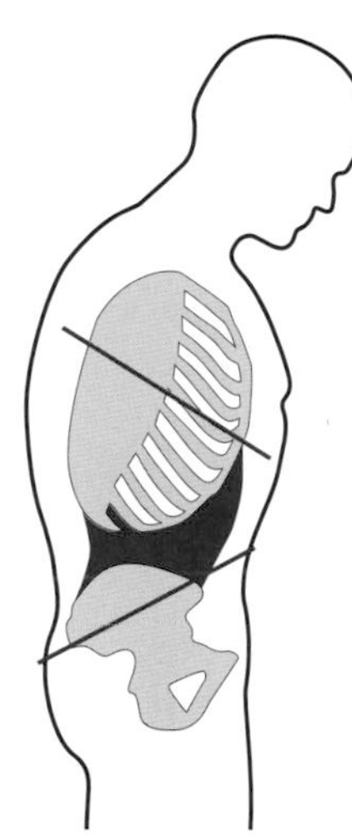

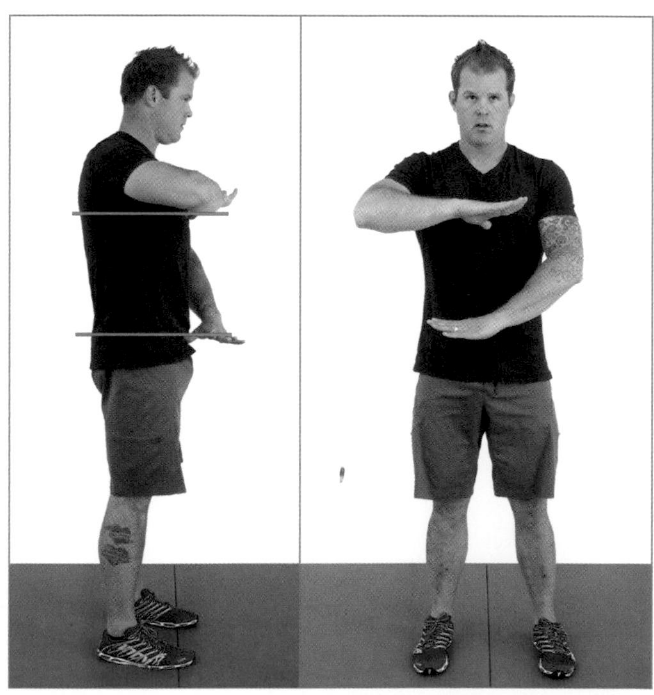

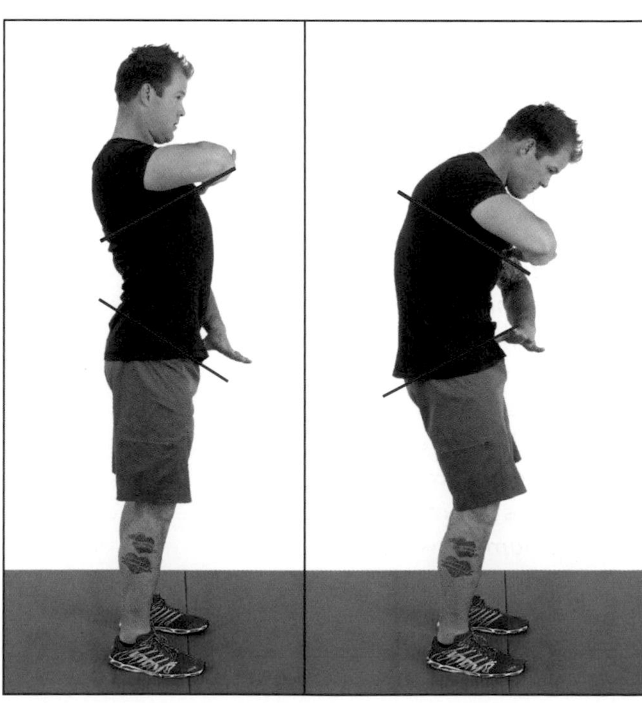

Although you should think of the spine as one contiguous, stable structure with the same nervous system running through it, dividing it into parts is a convenient way to spot and feel spinal faults. This is why the two-hand rule is so effective: It brings a heightened sense of awareness to the reference points of the pelvis and ribcage.

There is one problem with this model, however. It misses a key reference point that is every bit as important as the pelvis and ribcage: the head. When using the two-hand rule to bring awareness to the bracing sequence and to spot spinal faults, don't forget that the head is an essential factor. If your head is out of position—meaning that it's tilted forward or backward—you compromise your spinal position and lose the ability to stabilize your hips and shoulders.

The Tony Blauer test is a perfect example of this. As you can see below, the moment you deviate from a neutral head position, you lose the ability to maintain a braced neutral spine. And this is not limited to the head. Anytime one or two vertebral segments hinge or express a greater degree of motion in relation to the rest of the spine—whether it's the head, ribcage, or pelvis—creating a stable carriage is impossible.

TONY BLAUER TEST

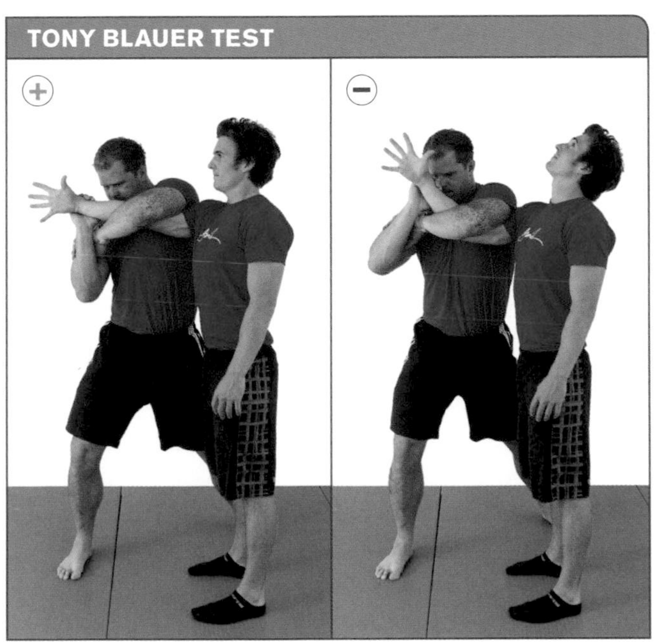

NEUTRAL HEAD

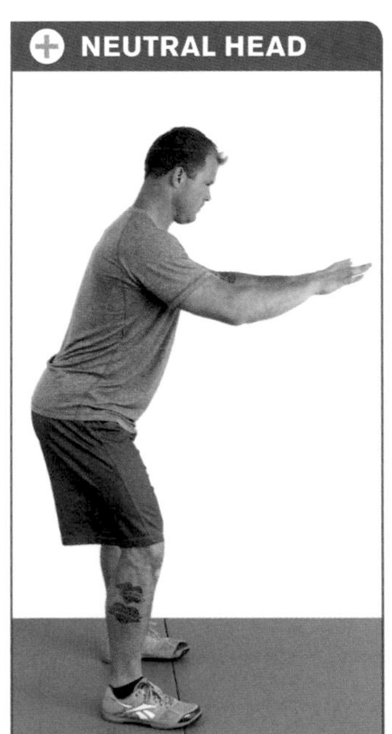

HEAD FAULT

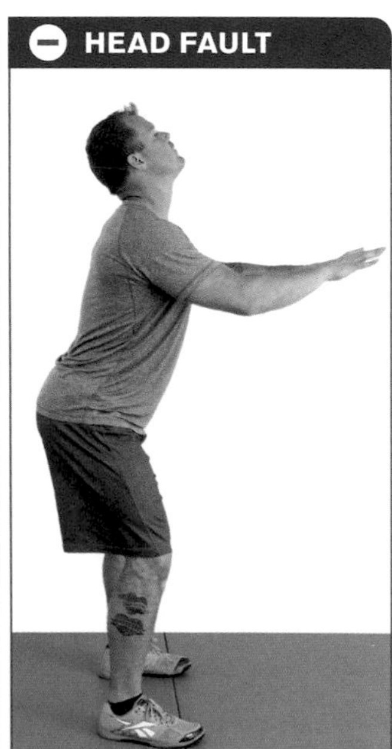

I've established a figure-four lock on Carl's right arm. With his arm straight, spine neutral, fingers splayed, and shoulder externally rotated, I can't bend his arm. But the instant he looks up or down or deviates from a neutral head position, his arm bends. This drill really helps illuminate the fact that breaking a neutral head position throws a kink in the entire system and destabilizes the structures downstream, making it impossible to maintain an integrated position. The same thing occurs during a squat. The moment you throw your head back, you default into an overextended position.

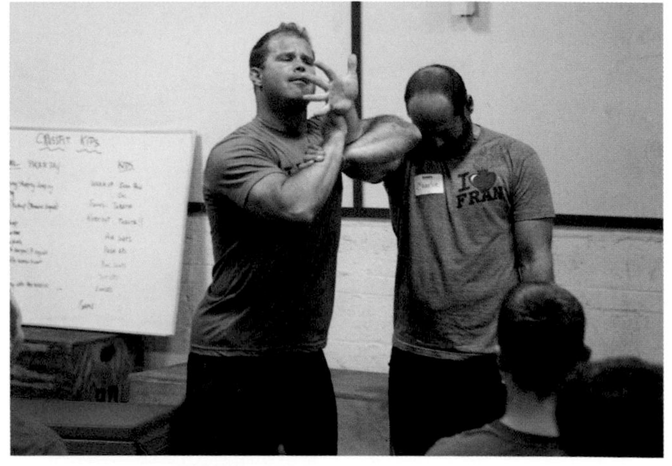

IDEAL STANDING POSITION

Braced Neutral Standing Position

Now that you have a model for organizing your spine in a neutral position and you can spot common spinal faults, you can start to apply the bracing sequence to fundamental positions like standing and sitting. Whether you're at work, chatting with a friend at the gym, or standing at attention, the basic setup is always the same: feet straight, back flat, belly tight, head neutral, and shoulders externally rotated in a stable position. Don't be that guy who stands with his arms crossed, shoulders rolled forward, back slouched, feet turned out, etc. If you care about how you look, feel, and perform, start paying attention to the quality of your standing position.

What is an ideal position for your arms, you might ask? Simple: You can position your arms any way you want as long as your shoulders are in an externally rotated, stable position. Internally rotating your shoulders (rolling them forward) puts strain on your spinal system, pulling you into a flexed position. If you're just standing around, you can adopt what I call an active standing position. In the photo below left, I've placed my hands on my chest, which puts my shoulders in a comfortable yet stable position. This is just a personal preference. With my hands up and in front of my body, I can do pretty much anything: defend, attack, text, whatever. But I'm not advocating that you stand around with your hands on your chest all the time. It's just one example of an effective standing position that gives you movement options. Again, the key is to remain in a braced neutral position with your shoulders stable and then move from there.

The other issue here is that it's impossible to stand for long periods with your butt squeezed and your abs tight. At some point, your muscles will fatigue, causing you to default to a weakened position. (No wonder your leg goes numb, your knees ache, and your back is cooked after you stand all day!) The easiest way to take a load off your lumbar spine and reduce trunk tension is to prop your foot up on something. You still want to maintain a moderate amount of tension, with the glute of your grounded leg activated, but placing your foot on a short stool reduces the amount of tension required to keep your pelvis in a neutral position. You can also lean your butt against a stool to give your legs a rest.

CAPTAIN MORGAN POSE

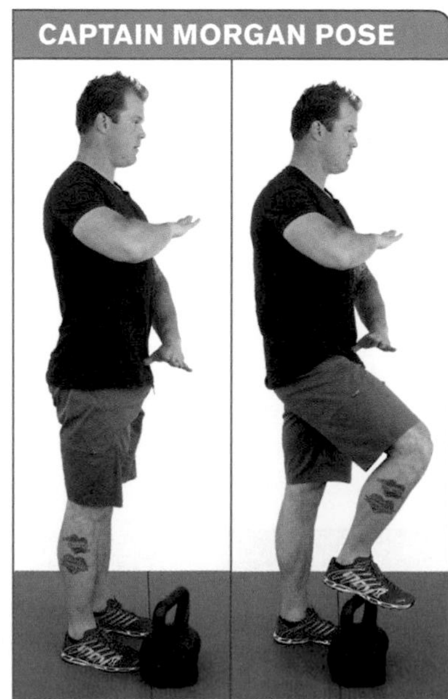

The idea is to vary your position as often as possible to avoid fatigue, focusing on staying in a neutral position while you transition from one position to another. Think about it like this: Your best working position is your next one, which is a hint to move often.

Remember that standing is a technique in and of itself. Just because you have a workstation that enables you to stand doesn't mean that you are immune to muscle stiffness and back pain. Certainly, standing is loads better than sitting, and it opens up your hips and turns on the musculature of your legs, but it's not a cure-all. You need to practice the bracing sequence and remain conscious of your position at all times.

Pelvic Floor Dysfunction in Women

Whenever you're in an overextended position, your pelvic floor turns off, which can unleash problems galore, especially in women. For example, when women jump and land, especially when doing double-unders (passing a jump rope under the feet twice per jump), they sometimes have trouble controlling their bladder. Fixing this problem is simple: Squeeze your butt to set your pelvis in a neutral position, and then get your belly tight to brace the position. You'll find that a lot of the issues related to pelvic floor dysfunction spontaneously resolve themselves once you lock your pelvis in a neutral position.

JUMPING WITH A NEUTRAL SPINE

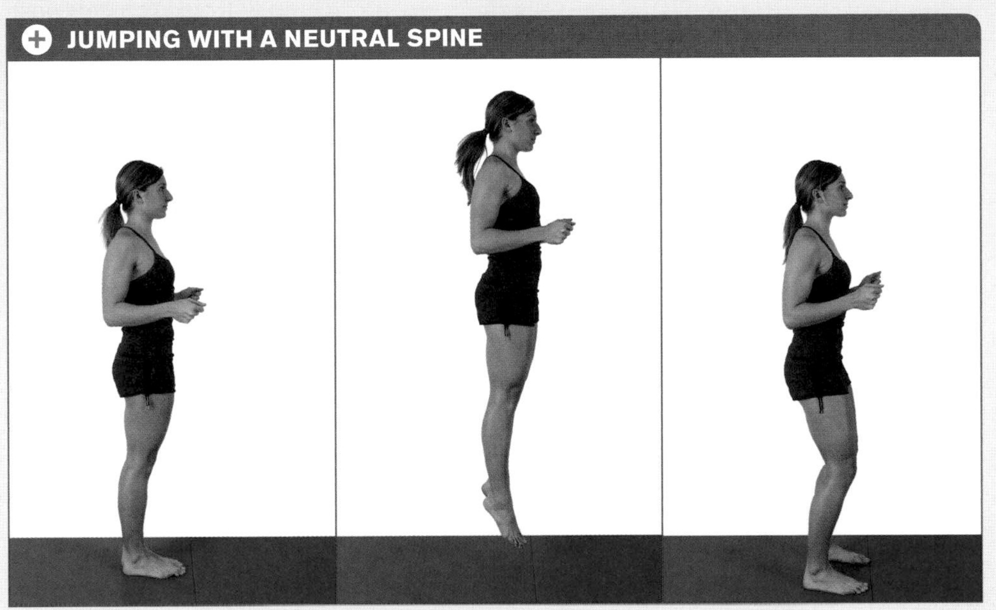

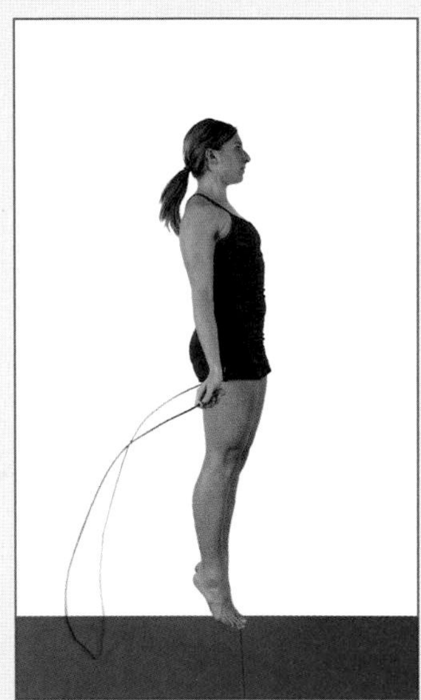

Whether you're performing double-unders or jumping up and down, you want to go through the bracing sequence, keep your shoulders back, and maintain abdominal tension to keep your pelvis locked in a neutral position.

LUMBAR OVEREXTENSION SPINAL FAULT

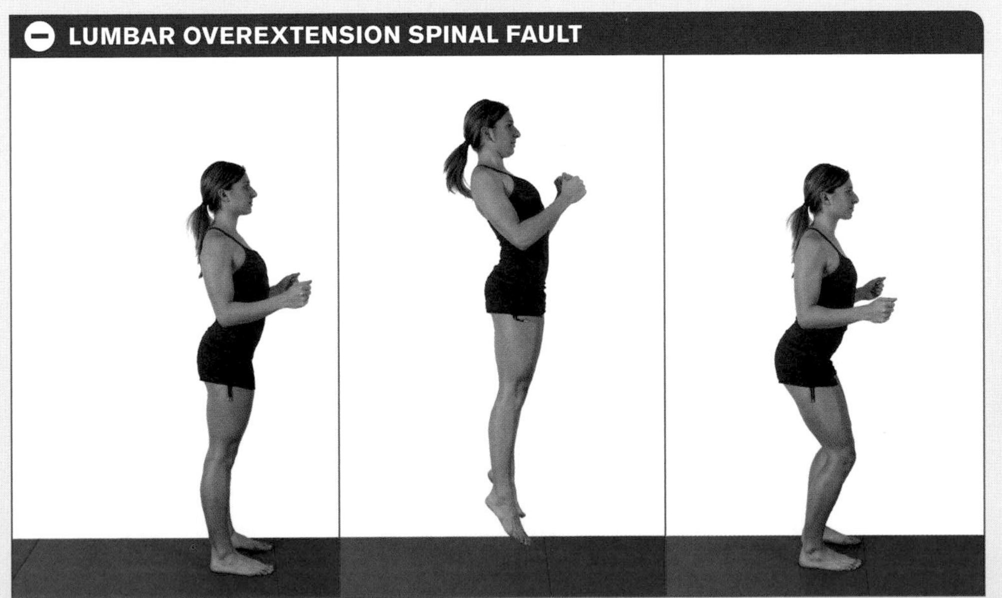

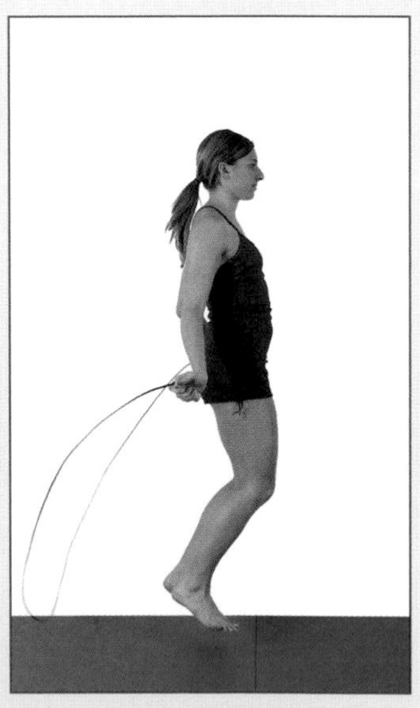

If your abs are not tensed, maintaining a neutral spinal position is nearly impossible. You will automatically default to an overextended position—a mechanism for low back pain and a host of other problems.

Braced Neutral Sitting Position

I have a saying: Sitting is death. It causes muscle tightness, but that's not all. Long periods of sitting devour your athletic performance potential. This is even more true for those who spend seven to nine hours a day sitting in compromised positions. It should come as no surprise when you feel like a broken-down mess after sitting on a plane, in a car, or at a desk. You've forced yourself into a toxic position that feasts on your athletic potential and wreaks havoc on your health.

It's not hard to see why experts are now referring to sitting as a disease. In fact, recent research suggests that long periods of sitting can be as harmful to your health as smoking. The trouble is, you can't avoid sitting. So how do you prevent or at least reduce the damage caused by extended periods of sitting?

BRACED NEUTRAL

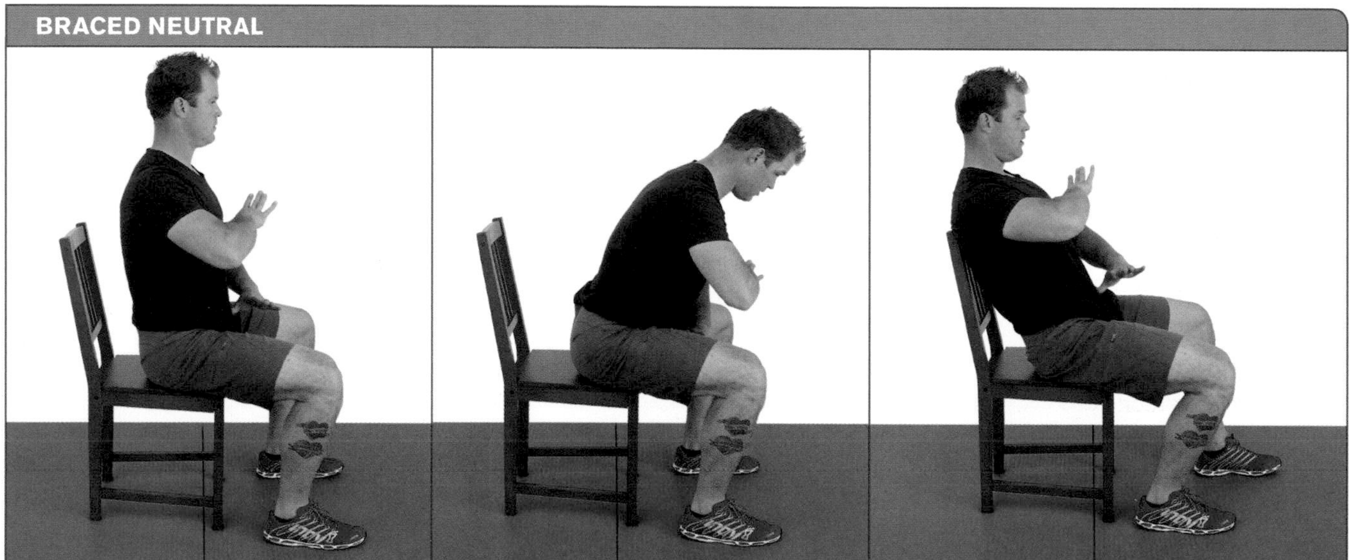

You're not limited to sitting perfectly upright: You can also lean forward or backward while maintaining a braced neutral spine.

TEXTING FAULT

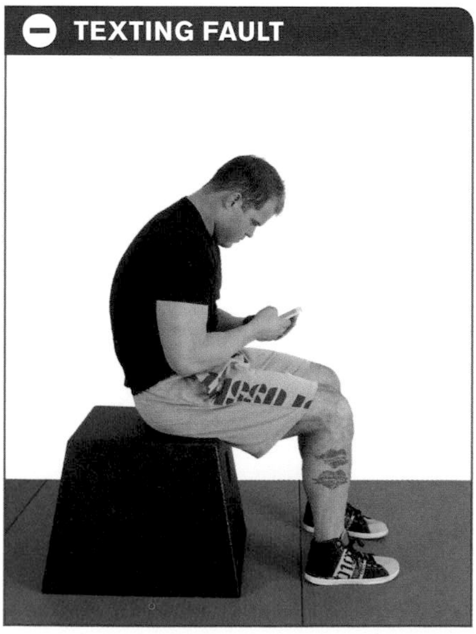

CORRECT TEXTING POSITIONS

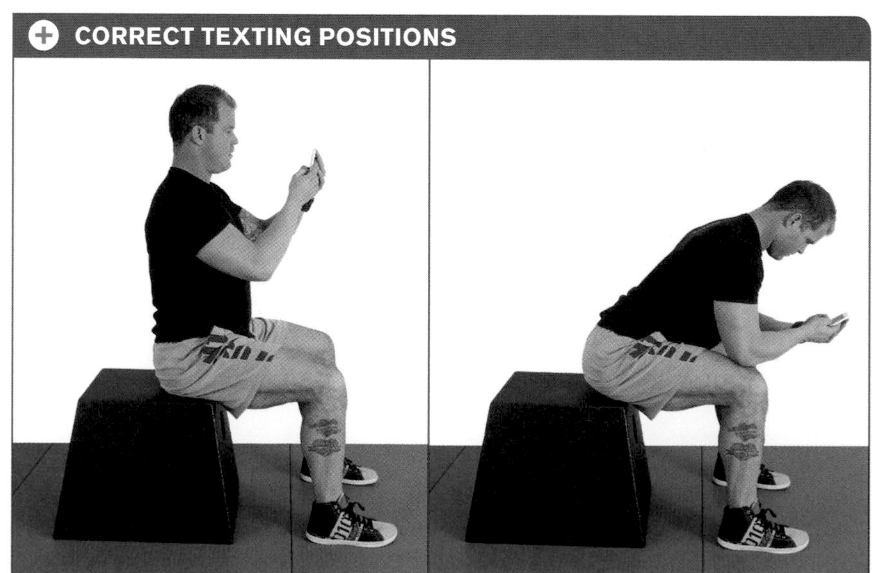

For starters, you need to learn how to sit. Sitting—like standing—is one of the most technically challenging things we do. Yet most of us are clueless when it comes to how to sit well.

In order to stabilize your spine in a neutral position, you have to get organized while standing by following the bracing sequence. (*Note:* A basic understanding of how to box squat—see page 176—also plays a key role in organizing your body to sit.) Once seated, you need to keep at least 20 percent tension in your abs to maintain a rigid spine. And herein lies the problem: Keeping your abs engaged at 20 percent is extremely taxing. All the research indicates that it's not muscular strength, but muscular endurance, that dictates loss of spinal position. This is why so many people tweak their back at the end of a run or workout. It also helps explain why most people collapse into a horribly rounded or overextended position after only a couple minutes of sitting. It's more comfortable because it doesn't require any work. Maintaining a stable position, on the other hand, takes focus and abdominal endurance.

The best way to keep from defaulting into a bad position and avoid the negative health effects that stem from prolonged sitting is to stand and reorganize yourself every 10 to 15 minutes. It's almost impossible to remain in a good static position for longer than 20 minutes. I know—this is not always a realistic option. But if you're trapped behind a desk and you want to heal your body and reach the performance goals you're entitled to, you have to do the work. You have to make sacrifices. Think about it like this: Every time you stand up and sit down is an opportunity not only to move, which is the main goal, but also to practice the bracing sequence, work on your squatting technique, and develop muscular endurance. While you're answering emails, you can also ingrain good movement mechanics and improve your athletic performance.

People often make the mistake of trying to correct their spinal position while seated. The moment you sit down, the large muscles of your butt go to sleep. This not only places additional stress on your spine, but also makes it difficult to stabilize your pelvis in a neutral position. So if you fail to address the bracing sequence before you sit down, you don't keep your belly tight, or you round or overextend your spine once seated, fixing your position from your chair is difficult. For example, say you're sitting in front of your computer working and after a few minutes you start to slouch. After answering a few emails, you become aware of how bad your posture is (or you just become uncomfortable), so you try to fix it by flattening your back. Although it may seem as if you're rectifying the problem, all you're doing is going from a flexed position to an overextended one—see the illustration on the following page. Again, in order to correct your position, it's best to stand up, go through the bracing sequence, and then sit down with your spine locked in a neutral position.

Pelvic Rotation

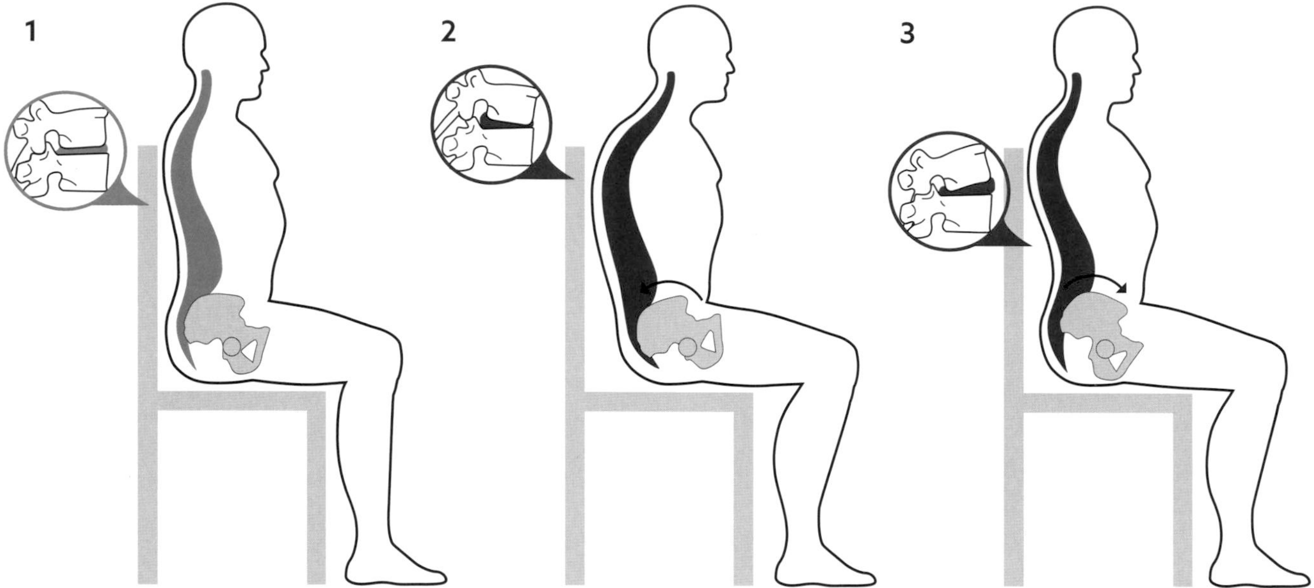

If you find that you've rounded forward and try to correct that by straightening your back, you'll probably end up in an overextended position. Instead, stand up, run through the bracing sequence, and then sit back down, keeping your back flat and your belly tight.

Another helpful strategy is to change your position as often as possible. You don't need to stay locked in an upright seated position all the time. You can lean backward and forward while remaining in a good position. What's more, you should always be looking for opportunities to move. Try creating games that force you to move every time you perform a certain activity. Kneel in front of the computer to open up your hips while browsing the Internet, walk around while talking on the phone, or even mobilize at your desk (the chair and desk are excellent props for mobility work). When you're watching TV, make it a habit to mobilize during commercials or, even better, during the entire show or movie. The point is that you usually have options at your disposal that don't involve sitting. And you should explore those options whenever possible.

In addition to getting up and changing your position, you need to work on restoring function to the tissues that become adaptively short and tight after long periods of sitting. As a rule, for every 30 minutes of continuous sitting you do, you should mobilize for 4 minutes. For example, you could do the Couch Stretch—a brutal hip opener that you can find on page 391—for 2 minutes on each side every half hour. The idea is to tackle the areas that become restricted, specifically your glutes, psoas and other hip flexors, thoracic spine, hamstrings, and quads (to mention a few). Think of it as a mobilization penalty based on sitting time.

These are just ideas to get your creative juices flowing. It doesn't matter how much you mobilize, stand, or change your position or what kind of chair, keyboard, or mouse you have: If you're hanging out in a bad position, you will continue to experience the same consequences. That said, using some kind of lumbar support (which is particularly useful during long car rides) will definitely give your low back a break and put you in a better position. But nothing replaces or is as important as treating sitting as a skill.

Abdominal Tension

In order to maintain a braced neutral spine, you need to keep your abdominals tensed. The minimum tension required for basic standing and sitting positions is about 20 percent of your peak (it varies from person to person). However, the moment you add dynamic movement or axial load (a force compressing your spine), you need to increase your abdominal tension to avoid rounding or flexing your spine. For example, if you're running around the block or doing pushups, you might need about 40 percent tension to maintain a good spinal position. But if you're going for a max deadlift, you will need 100 percent abdominal tension.

Perhaps you have trouble relating to numbers like 20 percent or 40 percent. You might find it helpful to rate abdominal tension on a scale from 1 to 10, with 1 being little to no tension and 10 being maximum tension. On this scale:

- Sitting in a chair requires a 2 (20 percent).
- Doing pushups or running around the block requires a 4 (40 percent).
- Doing a max back squat, deadlift, or a 50-meter sprint requires a 10 (100 percent).

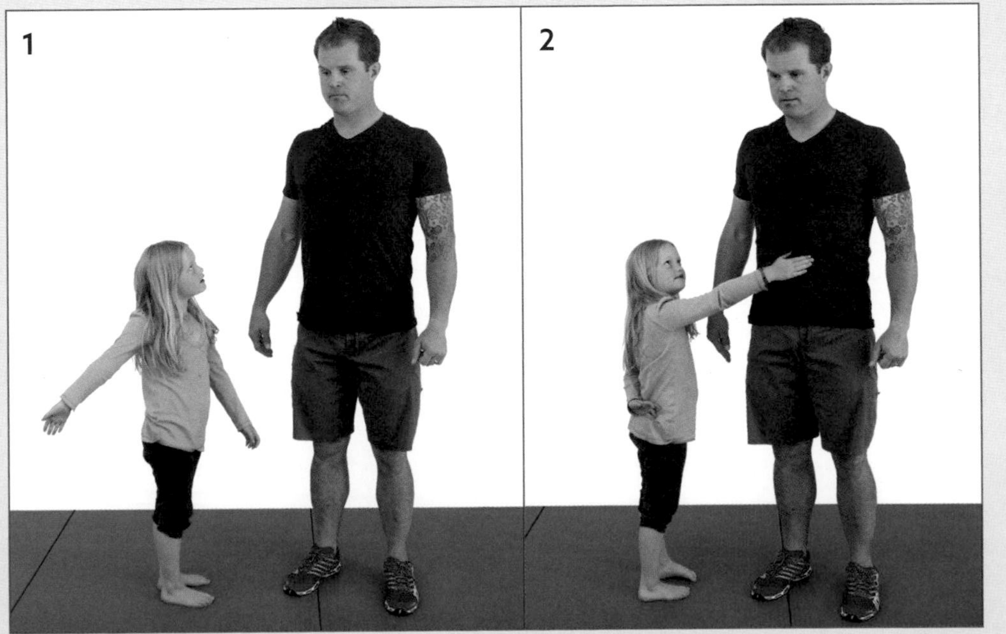

Belly-Whack Test

Like the two-hand rule, the belly-whack test is a way to bring consciousness to the braced neutral position and the 20 percent constant tension concept. It's simple: You should always have enough abdominal tone to take a whack to the belly. We do this at our gym and around the house. If you've got a spongy middle, you'll get caught right away.

In short, the tension necessary to maintain a braced, well-organized spine largely depends on the action and the load on your spine. And it's different for everyone. The percentages I offer are merely examples. If you're not used to maintaining a braced neutral spine, it may feel like you're engaging your trunk at about 50 percent of your full capacity just to support and maintain a balanced, upright position. But with time and practice, it will seem effortless. In fact, when you practice putting your bones in a good position, you'll notice that your musculature turns on automatically, making it feel very natural and efficient.

Active Straight-Leg Test

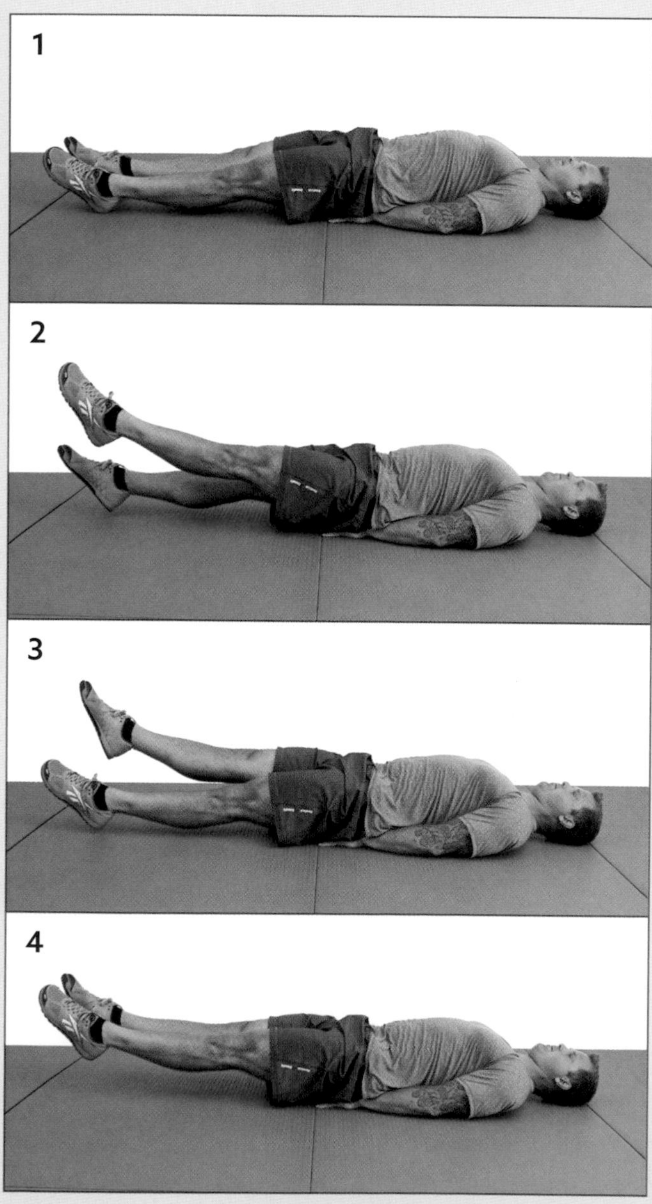

The active straight-leg test helps illuminate the role your glutes play in maintaining a neutral spinal position. If you lie on your back and raise your legs off the ground with your butt offline, you will immediately default to an overextended position. This test is also a safe and easy way to test your bracing strategy. Without adding weight or using any equipment, you can effectively challenge your ability to breathe and maintain abdominal tension with a braced neutral spine.

To execute this test, lie on the ground and go through the bracing sequence (pages 40–41). Next, lift one leg at a time off the ground (you can use the two-hand rule), and then both legs. With each step, you will have to increase the level of tension in your abs in order to maintain a neutral spinal position.

1. Lie on your back. Squeeze your butt, pull your legs together, and point your toes. Then take a big breath and get your belly tight as you exhale. Think about stiffening your belly around your spine as you let out air. An important distinction worth noting here is that I'm not telling you to push your low back into the ground. The key is to squeeze your butt and then engage your abs to lock in a neutral spinal position.

2. Keeping your toes pointed, your legs straight, and your low back flush with the ground, raise your left leg. Pointing your toes makes it easier to activate your glutes.

3. Lower your left leg and raise your right leg off the ground. Again, there should be no change in spinal position.

4. To increase the stabilization demand, raise both legs off the ground.

Just so we're clear, I'm talking about abdominal tension as it relates to actions of sport and life, not meditating in the full lotus. Again, we humans are rarely in one position for very long, and if we are, the lack of movement is probably causing damage or putting strain on the body. Having a baseline level of tension in your abs not only helps you maintain a neutral spinal position, but also preps you for your next movement. Think of it like driving a car: It's much more efficient to go from 20 mph to 60 mph than it is to hit 60 mph from a dead stop. Keeping 20 percent abdominal tension gives you inertia so that you can ramp up to meet the demands of your next movement.

The key is to understand how and when to cycle up to peak tension based on your activity. A cobra doesn't cruise around with its head up and hood flared all the time: It hits peak tension when it's getting ready to strike. Similarly, you don't want to walk around with 100 percent abdominal tension or attempt a high-rep, heavy back squat with your ab tension at 20 percent. Knowing how much tension you need to maintain a braced neutral position is a skill that requires a ton of practice and consciousness. The better you are at it, the less energy and thought you have to put into managing abdominal tension. Like learning how to breathe correctly, it becomes instinctual over time.

Breathing Mechanics

As discussed in the bracing sequence section, to create a braced neutral spinal position you breathe in through your diaphragm (belly) and then engage your abs as you exhale, as illustrated on the following page. But maintaining this diaphragmatic breathing pattern is extremely difficult in positions that require high tension or involve an enormous load. What usually happens when people don't have a model for getting into a braced neutral position is that they inhale and then hold their breath, which is not only ineffective, but also costly.

Imagine taking in a huge breath and then engaging your abdominals with all that air trapped inside. Do you think you could perform a high-rep back squat while keeping your spine rigid? Better yet, could you take a punch to the gut? Not a chance. You can use your diaphragm to stabilize your trunk, but the moment you have to breathe, you surrender your spinal position. So it might work for a max-effort deadlift, but you're doomed after the first rep, or the moment you have to breathe. You can imagine how this bracing strategy plays out when you do anything highly aerobic. With your diaphragm jammed down to stabilize your spine, you have only one breathing option: to breathe using only your neck and chest. Taking these very shallow breaths restricts respiration and makes it difficult to create and maintain stability.

This is why it's so important to do high-rep back squats and lift heavy objects while under cardiorespiratory stress. In addition to challenging your capacity to maintain a braced neutral position while breathing hard, it mimics the real-life scenarios we face as athletes, soldiers, firefighters, and so on.

Now, it's important to understand that if you're bracing correctly—with your belly tight and your spine neutral—you won't need to put conscious effort into breathing

Diaphragmatic Breathing

1

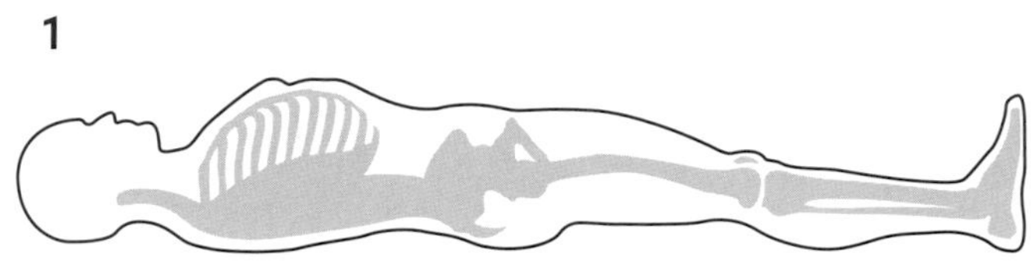

2

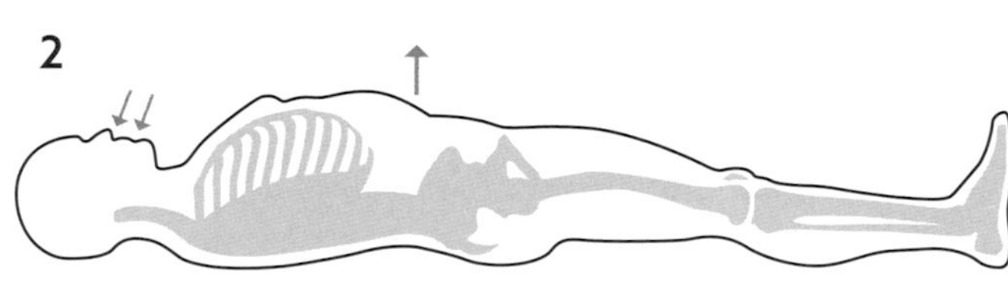

3

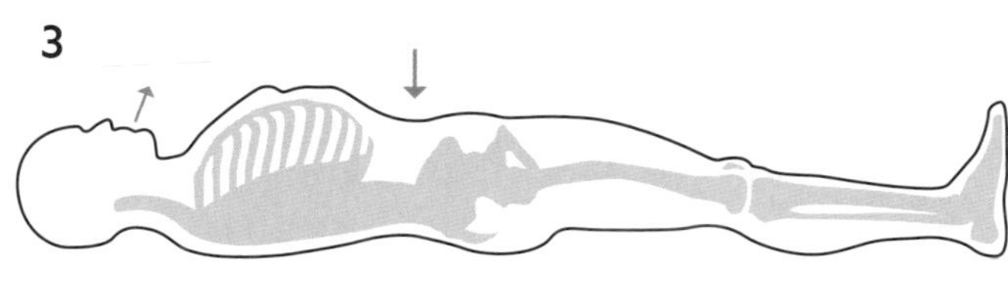

If you lie on your back and put your hand on your stomach, you should feel your belly rise and descend as you inhale and exhale. This is diaphragmatic breathing. When you're braced correctly, you will automatically default to this breathing pattern.

through your diaphragm. It's a self-regulating system. Breathing through your diaphragm is the most effective way to preserve a stable position, plain and simple.

For example, elite gymnasts in moments of peak tension and strongmen under enormous loads take short, concise breaths through the diaphragm—diaphragmatic gasps—and reconstitute trunk stiffness every time they exhale. They never lose spinal stiffness, disengage the abdomen, or stop breathing through the diaphragm. Rather, they keep their trunk stiff while continuing to breathe into that compressed system: take a short breath in, exhale into tension, take a short breath in, and exhale into tension, all while keeping the belly tight. When you're in kickass mode, you will inevitably use your sternum and chest to help facilitate breathing, but as long as you prioritize bracing and diaphragmatic breathing, your body will take care of the rest.

However, diaphragmatic breathing is difficult if you're in an overextended or flexed position. You end up breathing through your chest, laboring for each breath. Now imagine hanging out all day in a disorganized position with your diaphragm turned off. That's roughly 20,000 compromised breaths in a single day. You should take this stressed breathing pattern very seriously because it can compromise sleep, recovery, performance, and more. Fortunately, it's pretty easy to fix. By simply addressing your spinal position (and maybe doing some gut smashing to free up your diaphragm—see pages 363–364), you can easily and effectively restore optimal breathing function.

The same pattern applies to all sports: When you restore position, you restore function. When you improve position, you improve function.

CHEST AND NECK BREATHING FAULT

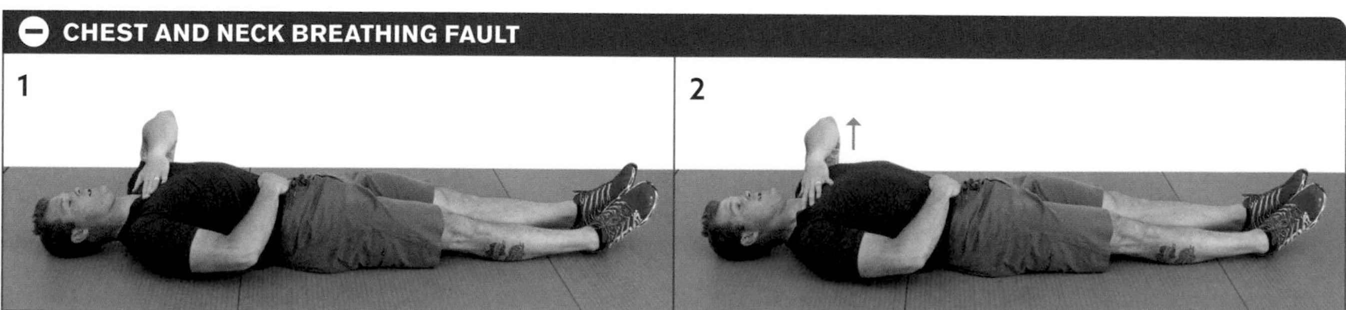

If you're keeping your belly tight but not breathing diaphragmatically, your breath will be confined to your chest and neck, compromising performance, recovery, and more.

Braced Extension and Flexion

A braced neutral spine is ideal for the majority of human movements—squatting, pulling, running, jumping, and so forth. However, there are situations where assuming a flat-back position is impossible. For example, if you have to lift a keg or some other super-heavy, awkward object, good luck trying to get into anything but a braced flexed or braced extended position. Is it ideal? No way. It is technically a compromised position, but it's the only position that works in these circumstances. And you need to be able to pick up heavy, awkward objects and not mess up your back. It's part of being a fully functional human being.

To avoid injury and optimize your position, it is critical that you pay attention to the details. When you lift something from a flexed or extended position, you have to brace in that arched position and maintain that bracing through the full range of the movement. And this is where people get confused. Braced flexion or extension is characterized by a greater global arch, usually in the thoracic spine. All the same rules apply. You're not changing your spinal position under load or during the movement, and you're not committing a local extension fault. Rather, you brace and stabilize your thoracic spine in a slightly flexed or extended position at the start (the thoracic spine is better able to handle braced flexion loads than the lumbar spine), and you maintain that fixed shape throughout the movement.

BRACED FLEXION

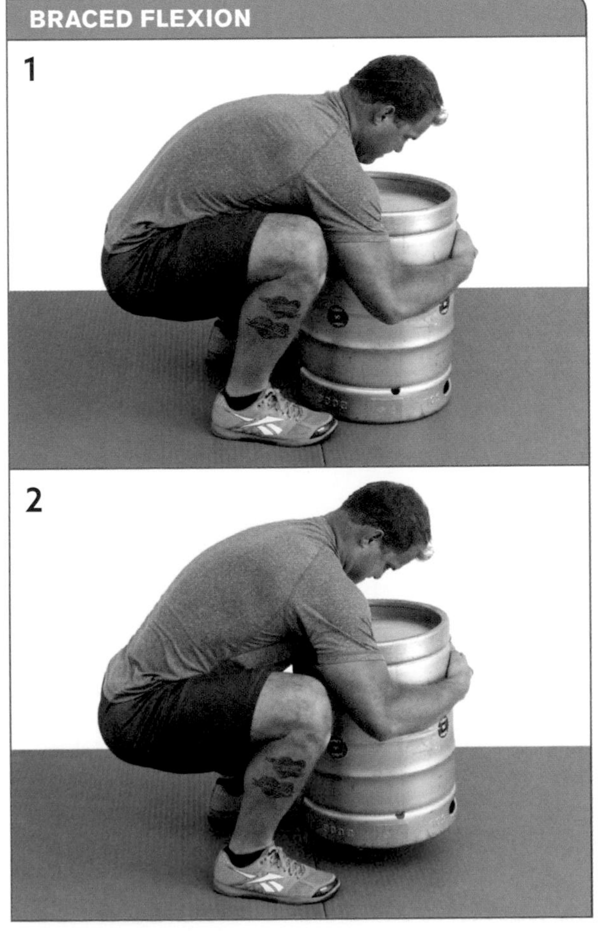

BRACED EXTENSION

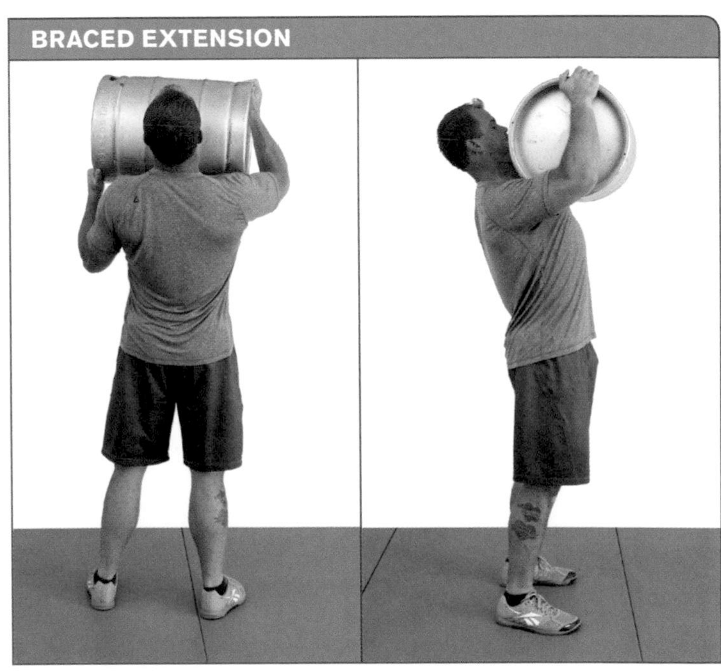

In the photos at left, notice that there is a global arch in my upper back. I get braced against the keg and maintain that position as I lift the keg off the ground. The same rules apply to extension. If you have to load something onto your chest and then lift it overhead, focus on keeping your butt squeezed to stabilize your low back.

Global Extension and Flexion

Other situations require you to flex and extend into globally arched positions. After all, you can't move around with your spine stiff and straight all the time. In order to perform the dynamic actions of sport, you need to be able to create flexion and extension throughout your entire system—see below. Imagine a volleyball player's spike, a tennis player's serve, or a pitcher throwing a 100 mph fastball. In all these movements, the athlete is essentially using the spine as a whip, creating a global opening and closing, or flexing and extending, throughout the entire spinal system.

As with braced extension and flexion, these positions are expressed as a continuum of flexion and extension throughout the entire spine. There is rarely an axial load on the spine, and you're not flexing or extending at a single joint (thereby committing a local extension fault). When you tumble, somersault, or do a backflip, you're creating a global arch, which is very challenging. This is why the cobra pose in yoga is so difficult—you must extend to create a global arch. It's no wonder that most people extend at only one or two segments of the lumbar or cervical spine. It's easier.

Although it's hard to learn these globally extended and flexed, dynamic, high-speed positions, there are things you can do in the gym to develop motor control and highlight the mobility dysfunction that may be preventing you from getting into ideal positions when it matters most. This is why it's useful to implement movements like the kipping pull-up (page 252): They not only teach you how to create dynamic, globally arched positions, but also ensure full range of motion in your spine. Even swinging from a bar can be used as a diagnostic. If you can't get into these large global shapes, you should ask yourself a very important question: What's going on? You might need to work on your motor control, mobility, or both.

GLOBAL FLEXION

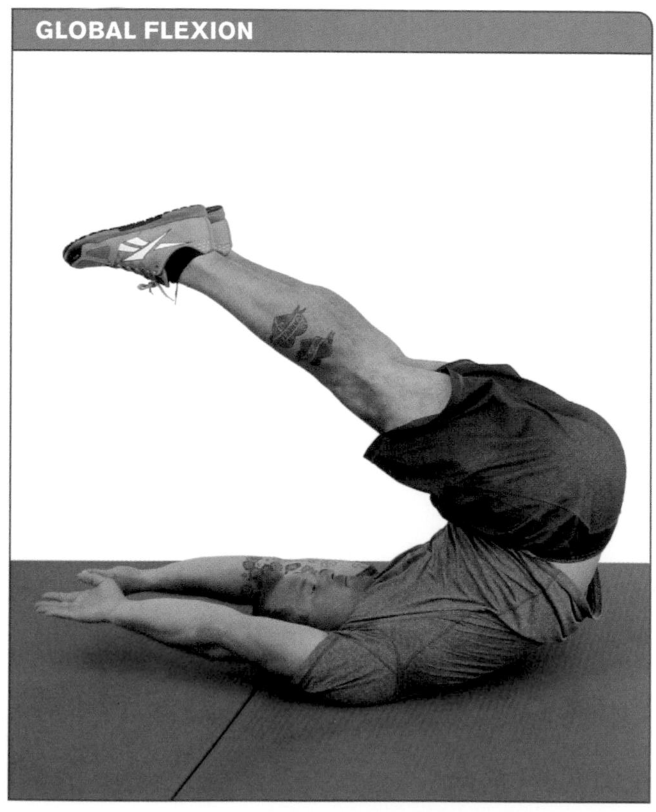

GLOBAL EXTENSION AND GLOBAL FLEXION

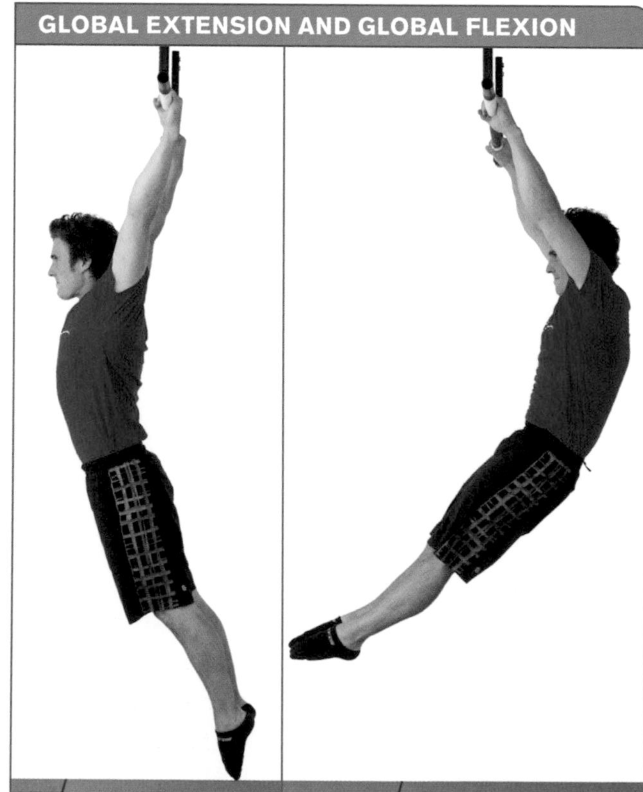

Chapter Highlights

- Poor spinal mechanics lead to a host of biomechanical compromises and increase the potential for injury.
- Organizing your spine in a braced neutral position means that your ears are aligned over your shoulders, your ribcage is balanced over your pelvis, and you're engaging the musculature of your trunk to stabilize (brace) the position.
- A braced neutral spine is the base position for most movements. It is the most utilitarian position for the spine because it allows you to handle load safely and transmit force efficiently.
- People typically default into mechanically unstable spinal positions for three reasons:
    1. *They have a task-completion, get-the-job-done mindset.*
    2. *They've ingrained poor positions and movement patterns in their training and daily life.*
    3. *They don't have a reproducible, all-encompassing bracing strategy that transfers to the majority of movements.*
- Anytime you see flexion or extension occur at a single spinal segment (an isolated part of your spine), it's an error. This is what I call a local extension or local flexion spinal fault. When you commit a local extension spinal fault, you overextend from your lumbar spine (think tilting your pelvis forward). When you commit a local flexion spinal fault, you flex from your thoracic spine, round your shoulders forward, and position your head out in front of your body.
- The bracing sequence is the blueprint for organizing your spine in a braced neutral position. You should run through the bracing sequence every time you set up to perform a movement, get ready to sit down, or need to reset your posture. Here's the step-by-step setup in a nutshell:
    1. *Stand with your feet straight and your posture upright. Squeeze your butt and externally rotate from your hips to set your pelvis in a neutral position.*
    2. *Align your ribcage over your pelvis.*
    3. *Engage your abdomen to lock in the position.*
    4. *Pull your shoulders back into a stable position and align your ears over your shoulders, hips, and ankles.*
- Sitting and standing are skills that take practice. Use the bracing sequence to set your posture and maintain a neutral position while sitting and standing.
- The two-hand rule is a model that brings awareness to your ribcage and pelvic relationship.
- In order to maintain a braced neutral spine, you need to keep your abdominals tensed. The tension necessary to maintain a braced, well-organized spine depends on the action and the load on your spine. You need at least 20 percent tension in your abs to set and maintain a braced neutral spine for basic positions and movements. Increase abdominal tension to match the demands of the movement.
- The functional positions of the spine can be categorized into a few basic configurations: braced neutral, global flexion, global extension, braced flexion, and braced extension.
- When you're in a braced neutral position, you want to breathe diaphragmatically by pulling air in through your belly while keeping your abs engaged. Don't hold your breath. Think about keeping your belly tight and breathing into that tight space as if you were putting compressed air into a steel tank.

2

ONE-JOINT RULE

The premise of the one-joint rule is simple: When you are working from a braced neutral position, flexion and extension should occur only in your hips and shoulders, not in your spine. Your hips and shoulders are designed to support and accommodate large loads and dynamic movements, and movement should always be initiated from those primary engines. In fact, it's easier to think of your hips and shoulders as a single joint because they are governed by the same principles—hence the name "one-joint rule."

All the movements featured in this book are what are commonly referred to as "functional movements." I define a functional movement as one that requires you to prioritize spinal mechanics and initiate movement from your hips and shoulders. When you squat, for example, you brace your spine first, and then initiate the movement by sitting your hips back slightly and flexing your knees and ankles.

For an exercise movement that you perform in the gym to be considered functional, it should be transferable, meaning that it is applicable to real-world activities and caters to your individual goals as an athlete. Take the squat as an example. Learning how to squat teaches you how to stabilize your hips in a good position and provides a blueprint for sitting down and getting up out of a chair. It also builds strength and power, critical attributes that all athletes must acquire. And because there are several iterations of the squat—air squat, back squat, front squat, overhead squat, and so on—you can adapt the technique to suit your sport or individual goals. This is why I recommend that everyone learn and practice category 1 functional movements. The squat, deadlift, pushup, strict press, and pull-up (to mention a few) enable you to assess motor control and mobility in a safe, controlled environment, as well as instill positions and movements that resemble the positions and movements that you employ in sport and in life. Most important, a functional movement should not increase the potential for injury. After 1 rep or 100, you should come out unharmed. While the goal is to use functional movements to detect and correct poor movement patterns and mobility restrictions, it should not come at the cost of lost performance or injury.

I offer this definition of functional movement for two reasons:

1. It helps explain the selection of movements featured in part 2—and why you should take the time to learn and practice them.
2. It crystallizes midline stabilization as the first and most important aspect of movement.

Midline Stability Basic Movement Test

When I teach a seminar to a new group of athletes, coach someone for the first time, or rehab an athlete coming off an injury, I always take a spine-first approach. The problem, however, is not necessarily getting athletes to prioritize midline stabilization. Rather, it is getting them to maintain a stable, well-organized trunk during complex, loaded athletic movements. In fact, most athletes grasp the midline stabilization concept and have no trouble maintaining a braced neutral spine in static positions. It's not until I ask them to change shapes—bend from the hips, move from the shoulders, or set up in an unfamiliar position—that the flaws in their bracing strategy become apparent.

This is why I teach the bracing sequence first and then challenge an athlete's ability to support a neutral spine with two basic hip and shoulder movements:

- **Hip Hinge Test:** Bend over and touch your toes, which requires you to hinge from your hips.
- **Overhead Test:** Raise your arms overhead—either when standing or while lying down—which expresses movement through your shoulders.

Although these are simple tests, a lot of people struggle. They simply can't keep their head, ribcage, and pelvis in alignment as they move their hips and shoulders. What is it that makes moving with a neutral spine so challenging for some people?

HIP HINGE TEST

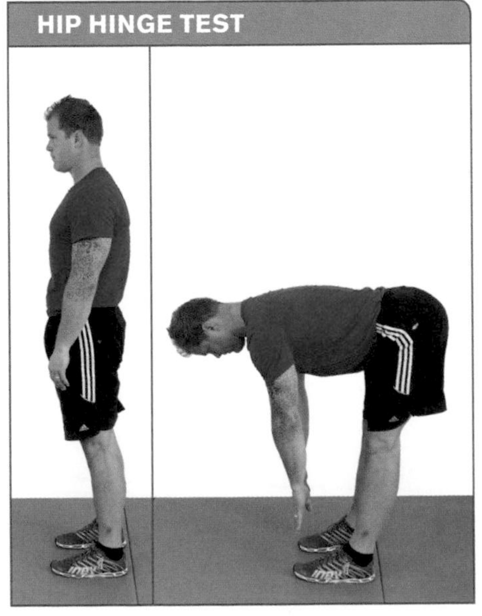

OVERHEAD TEST

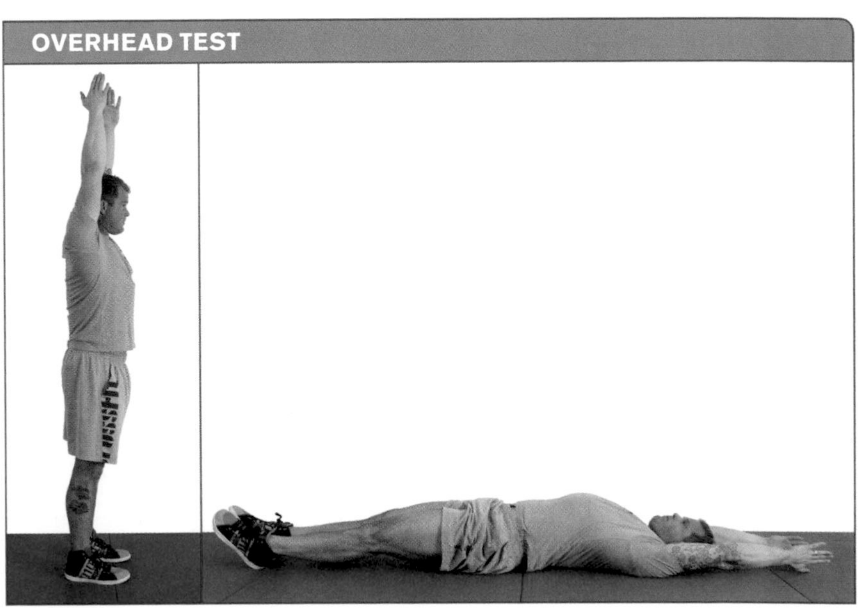

The reality is that most people have never practiced moving with a braced neutral spine. Heck, most people don't even know that flexing and extending the spine is potentially harmful. People spend their entire life using their spine as a hinge, rounding their back every time they need to bend over or tilting their ribcage back anytime they raise their arms above chest level. While these spinal faults may seem relatively harmless, they add up over time and become movement patterns. This is why so many people struggle to keep their back flat when simple movements are introduced: Initiating movement from their back has been hardwired into their motor program.

This problem becomes even bigger when formal training exercises are added, because those exercises require you to maintain spinal stiffness through a full range of motion. In other words, you need to be able to lower into the bottom of a squat, press a barbell overhead, and set up for a deadlift without defaulting into a flexed or overextended spinal position.

When you think about it, the test is really just an extension of the two-hand rule (see pages 42–43): Flexion or extension anywhere in the spine is an error. This gives you an easy template for spotting spinal faults. Anytime your spine changes shape during a loaded movement, you know that you didn't set up correctly or you don't have the motor control or mobility to get into or maintain the correct position.

Remember, your spine is not designed to handle loaded flexed or extended positions. The musculature surrounding your spine is designed to create stiffness—again, so that you can effectively transmit energy from your hips and shoulders.

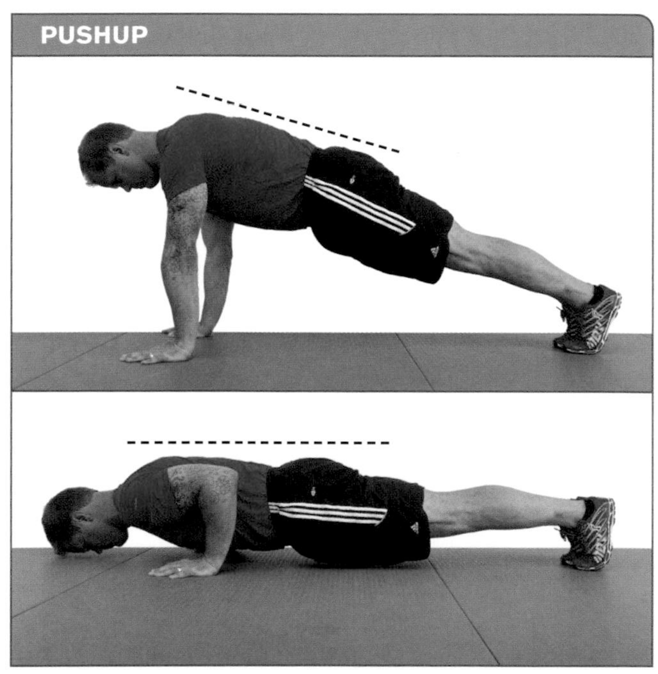

The majority of movements require you to keep your spine in a neutral position through the entire range of motion. If you are performing a pushup, for example, movement should occur in your shoulders and elbows, not in your spine.

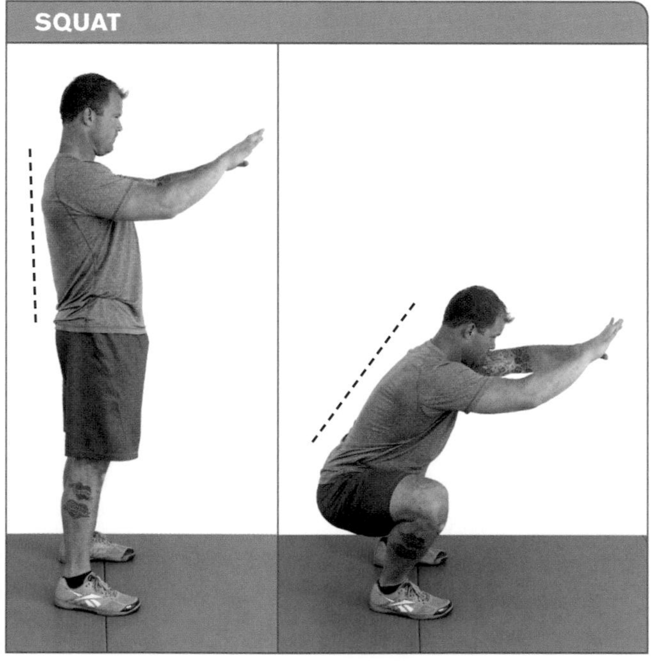

If you are performing a squat, movement should occur in your hips and knees. Again, there should be no movement in your spinal system.

Load Order Sequencing: Initiating Movement from Your Primary Engines

As you will learn in chapter 3, the process for creating a stable shoulder position is the same as the process for creating a stable hip position—that is, the hips and shoulders abide by the same laws of torque. This is because they function in much the same way. Both are ball-in-socket joints, have a ton of rotational capacity, and are designed to handle freakish amounts of flexion and extension load. In fact, as you start applying the principles of midline stabilization and torque to your hips and shoulders, it becomes easier to think of them as a single joint because they are governed by the same principles—hence the name "one-joint rule."

In chapter 3, you will learn how to create tension and organize your hips and shoulders in a good position to avoid movement errors. But first it's important to understand that for the majority of movements—specifically formal training movements—you want to load the primary engines of your hips and shoulders first, because the tissues and joints that get loaded first during movement get loaded maximally during movement. In other words, the joint you move first will carry the lion's share of the load (your weight plus any weight you're lifting) as you execute the movement. For example, if you initiate a squat by flexing your knees first, your knees will be loaded maximally as you lower into the squat, which is not ideal. If you drive your hips back as you initiate the squat, on the other hand, your hips will be loaded maximally, which is the correct technique. Similarly, if you initiate a pushup by driving your elbows back, your elbows will be loaded maximally. But if you initiate the movement by keeping your forearms vertical, your shoulders and chest will be loaded maximally, which is ideal.

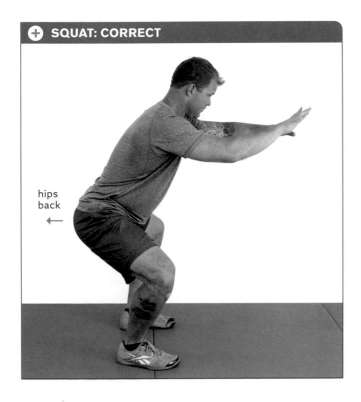

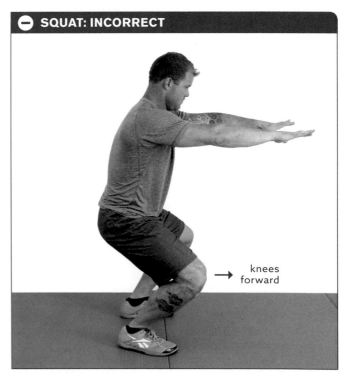

PUSHUP: CORRECT

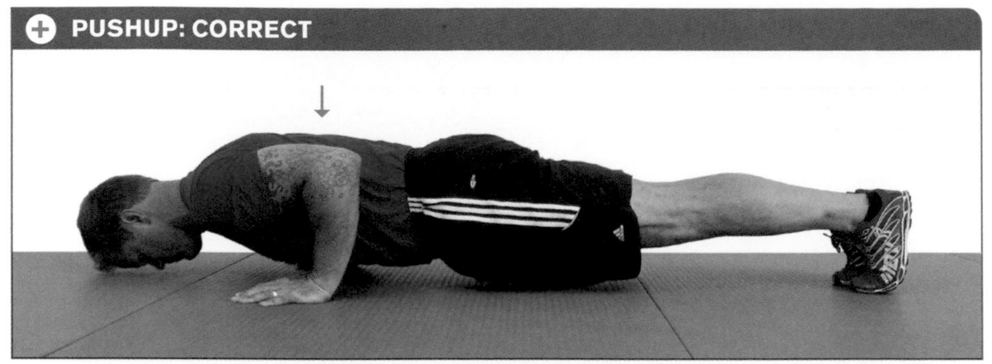

PUSHUP: INCORRECT

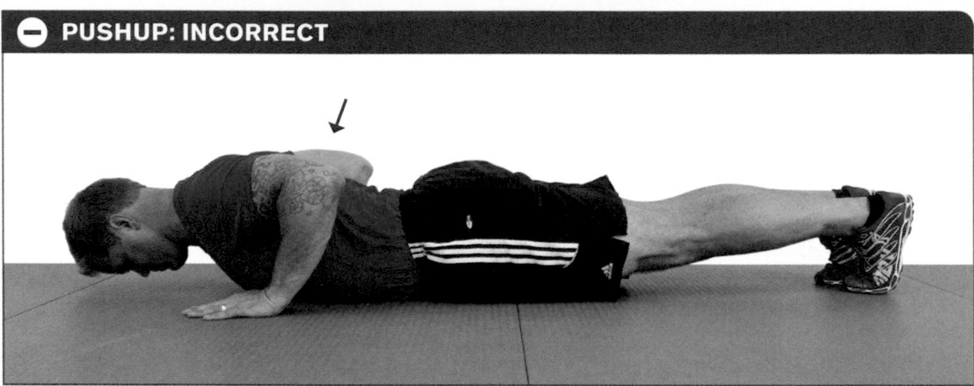

This concept as it relates to formal training exercises will become clearer once you start reading and implementing the movements in part 2, especially the squat, deadlift, and pushup.

To improve your understanding of the load order sequencing idea, let's apply it to daily movements like getting up out of a chair and standing up from a deep squat. In both of these situations, you're essentially starting in a squat position, loading your hips to initiate the movement, and then extending your knees to stand up. Keeping your shins vertical and allowing your chest to drop forward slightly creates tension and transfers your weight to your hips. This is what I mean by "loading" your hips. If you drive your knees forward, you will increase the shear forces across the soft tissue within the knee joint, specifically the patellar tendon and ACL.

GET UP FROM A CHAIR: CORRECT

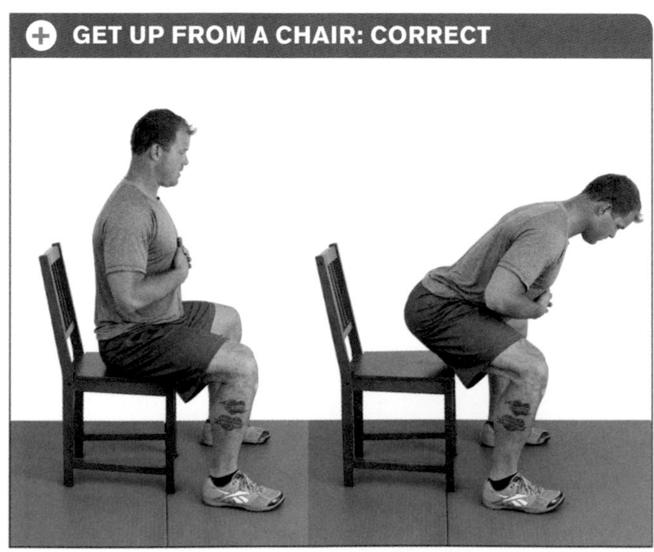

GET UP FROM A CHAIR: INCORRECT

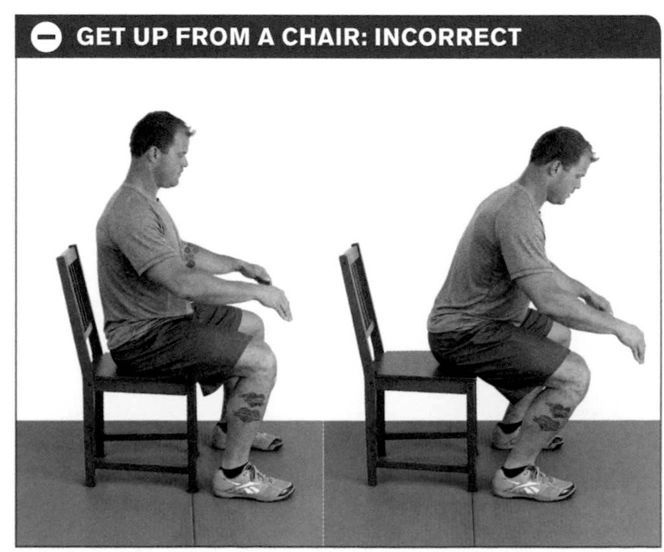

STAND UP FROM A DEEP SQUAT: SCENARIO 1

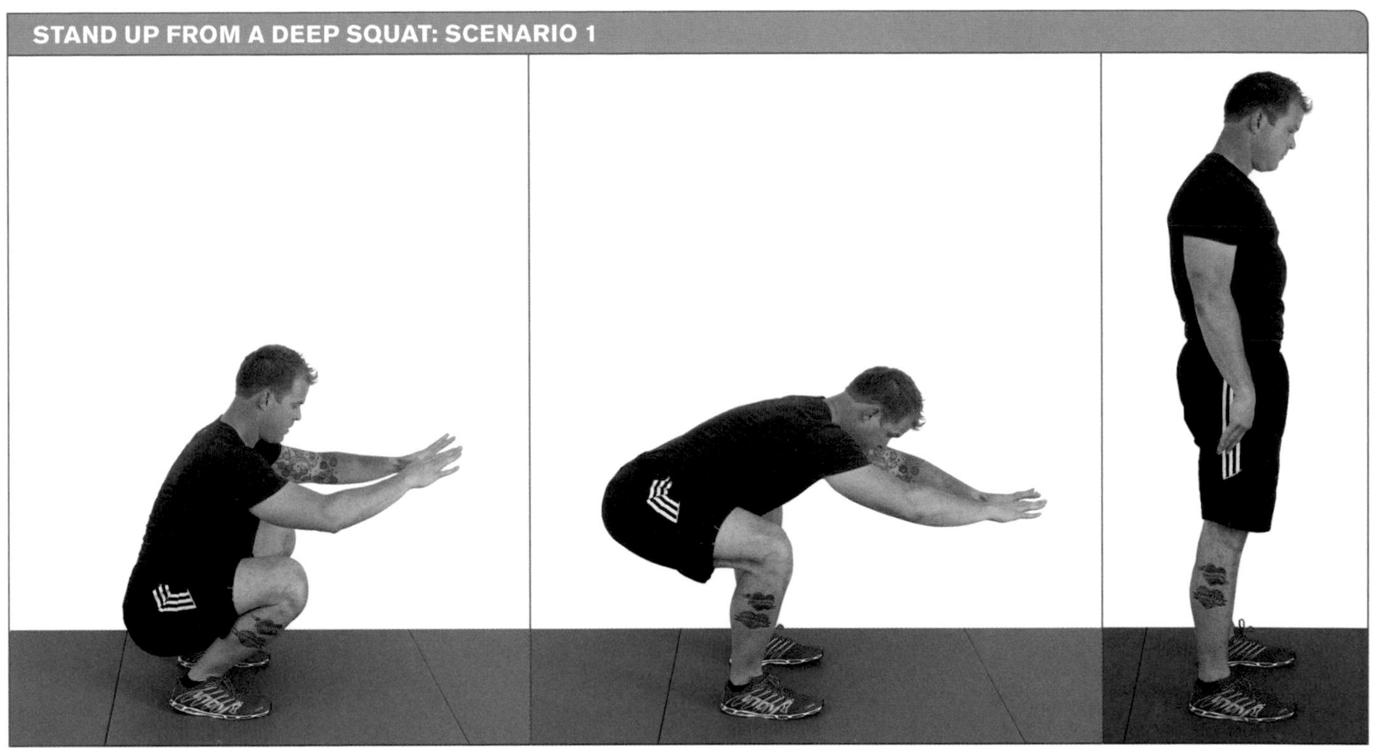

In this scenario, I start in a full squat. If I were to stand straight up, I would transfer a ton of weight to my knees instead of my hips. So before I stand, I get my shins vertical and drive my hips backward. With my primary engine loaded, I can stand up and avoid any unneeded strain on my knees.

STAND UP FROM A DEEP SQUAT: SCENARIO 2

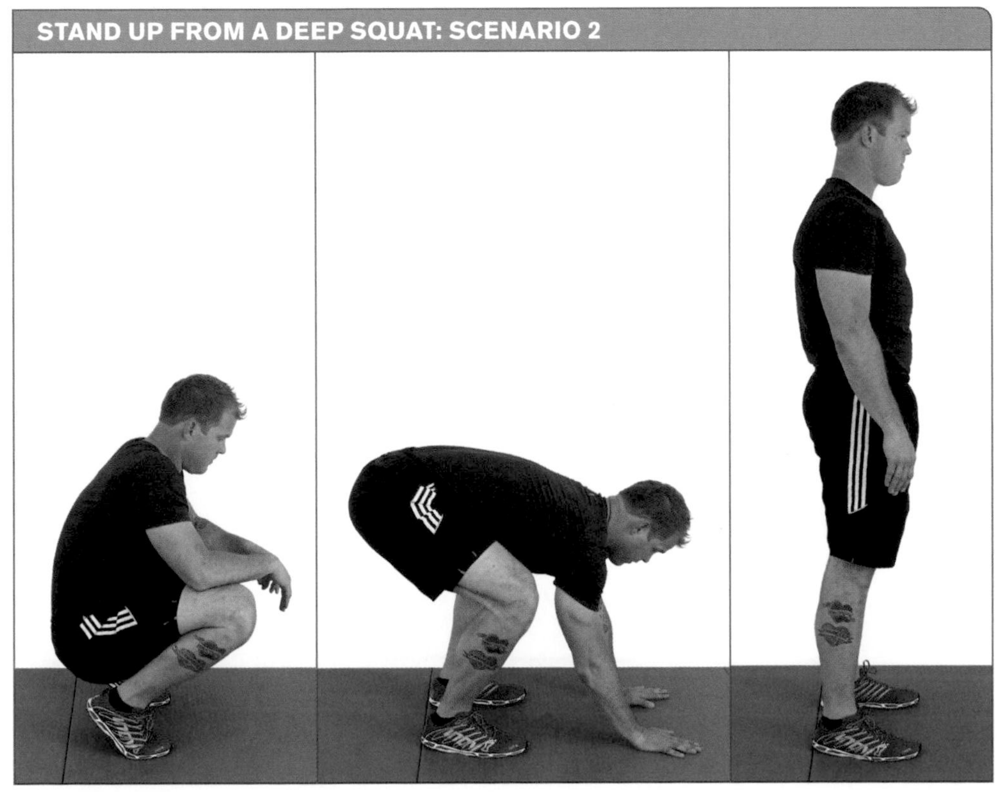

If you're missing range of motion, then you will probably have to come up onto the balls of your feet when you squat to the ground. In this scenario, you need to create tension in your hips by shifting your weight back and getting your shins as vertical as possible before you stand up. To do so, place your hands on the ground to support the weight of your upper body, elevate your hips, and get your feet flush with the floor. As with the previous scenario, this transfers your weight into your hips instead of your knees.

Another simple yet relevant example is standing up from a kneeling position. Rather than transfer your weight forward, which would load your weight onto your front knee, you load your hips by shifting your weight back. Elevating your hips spreads out the load and allows you to stand up using the power of your legs and hips. If you were to stand up by driving your front knee forward (which is the most common technique), you would load the majority of your weight over your front knee.

STAND UP FROM A KNEELING POSITION

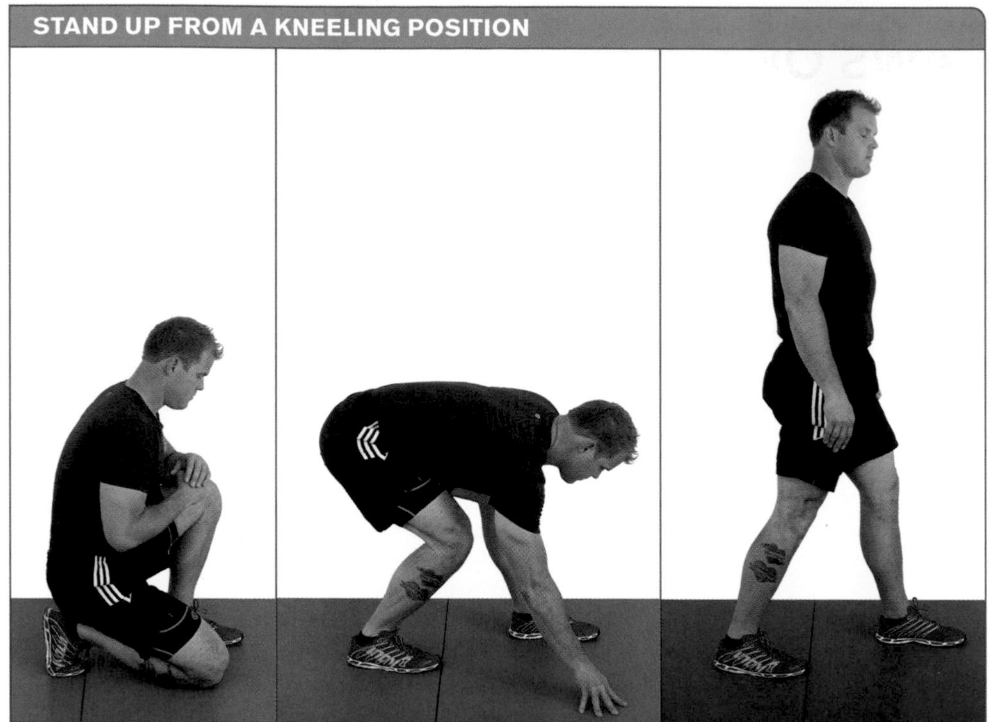

To summarize, your hips and shoulders function in much the same way, and they (not your spine) are designed to handle flexion and extension loads. For this reason, you should always try to load as much weight as possible into your primary engines while using your accessory joints (knees, elbows, etc.) to adjust for position. No doubt, maintaining an organized spine during loaded athletic movements is very difficult. Keeping your back flat during a heavy deadlift, overhead press, or squat is no joke; it takes skill and a keen understanding of how these systems work. The fact is, you can't just brace your spine and then move from your hips and shoulders and expect everything to be okay. Hip and shoulder stability doesn't happen automatically. To stabilize your limbs in a good position and preserve spinal stability, you need to create tension in your hip and shoulder systems. You do so by generating torque, which is the subject of the next chapter.

Chapter Highlights

- For an exercise to be considered a functional movement, it must prioritize spinal mechanics, have transferable application to real-life activities, and express full ranges of motion.
- The hips and shoulders are ball-in-socket joints designed to handle flexion and extension load. They are governed by the same principles and abide by the same laws of torque, hence the "one-joint rule."
- Flexion and extension should occur only in the hips and shoulders, not in the spine.
- Initiate movement from your hips and shoulders first, because the tissues and joints that get loaded first get loaded maximally during movement. This is the basis of the load order sequence.

LAWS OF TORQUE

In order to create safe and stable positions for your joints as well as preserve a braced neutral spinal position, you have to create tension in your hips and shoulders and, by extension, your elbows, knees, wrists, and ankles. You do so by generating torque, which is expressed through external rotation (rotating your limb away from your body) and internal rotation (rotating your limb toward the center of your body).

Consider a powerlifter setting up underneath a bar loaded with 800 pounds to perform a back squat. To move such a staggering amount of weight and avoid collapsing under the load, he has to brace his spine and generate torque by externally rotating his hips and shoulders. To create tension in his upper back and set his shoulders in a stable, tight position, he grips the bar just outside his shoulders' width and then twists his hands into the bar as if he were trying to bend it in half. To stabilize the structures of his lower body, he creates an external rotation force from his hips by screwing both feet into the ground—keeping his feet straight and parallel to each other—as if he were trying to spread a crack in the floor. Bracing his spine and generating torque in this manner is the only way the powerlifter can complete the lift without injury. If his knees collapsed inward or his back bent with 800 pounds perched on his shoulders, not completing the lift would be the least of his worries.

In short, torque enables the powerlifter to stabilize his position and minimize variability in movement—meaning that he can keep his back flat and maintain tension in his hips and shoulders, preventing potentially disastrous movement faults. If he does not generate torque, his body will find stability for him by defaulting into a bad position. I call this "tension hunting." When you fail to generate torque, you create an open circuit that your body closes down immediately by committing a local extension spinal fault, flaring out at the elbows, or collapsing your ankles and knees inward. (In part 2, you'll learn more about these common faults and how to correct them.)

What is torque, you might ask? Torque is turning force. It's the amount of energy that you need to turn a wrench or open a jar. When it comes to the human body, I use the word *torque* to describe the turning force generated by the hips and shoulders, which causes the limbs to rotate.

Another way to think of torque is as a rotational force being applied to an object. For example, when you internally or externally rotate from your hip or shoulder while keeping your hand or foot anchored to a surface such as the floor or an object such as a barbell, you're generating torque. This rotational force turns on the musculature that stabilizes your joints in good positions.

To help you understand how torque works and familiarize you with some common strength and conditioning cues for generating torque, let's look at four basic examples.

Create torque in your hips by screwing your feet into the ground.

If you've experimented with the bracing sequence on pages 40–41, you already know what it feels like to generate torque. When you externally rotate from your hips while keeping your feet straight and rooted to the floor, you can feel the tension in your lower body: Your glutes fire, your hips lock into place, and your feet come into an arch. This is how you generate torque from your hips while standing. It is also the most stable position for your ankles, knees, and hips. As a reminder, "screw your feet into the ground" means that you exert an outward force with your feet while keeping them in the same position. You're not turning them outward; you're just exerting force in an outward direction.

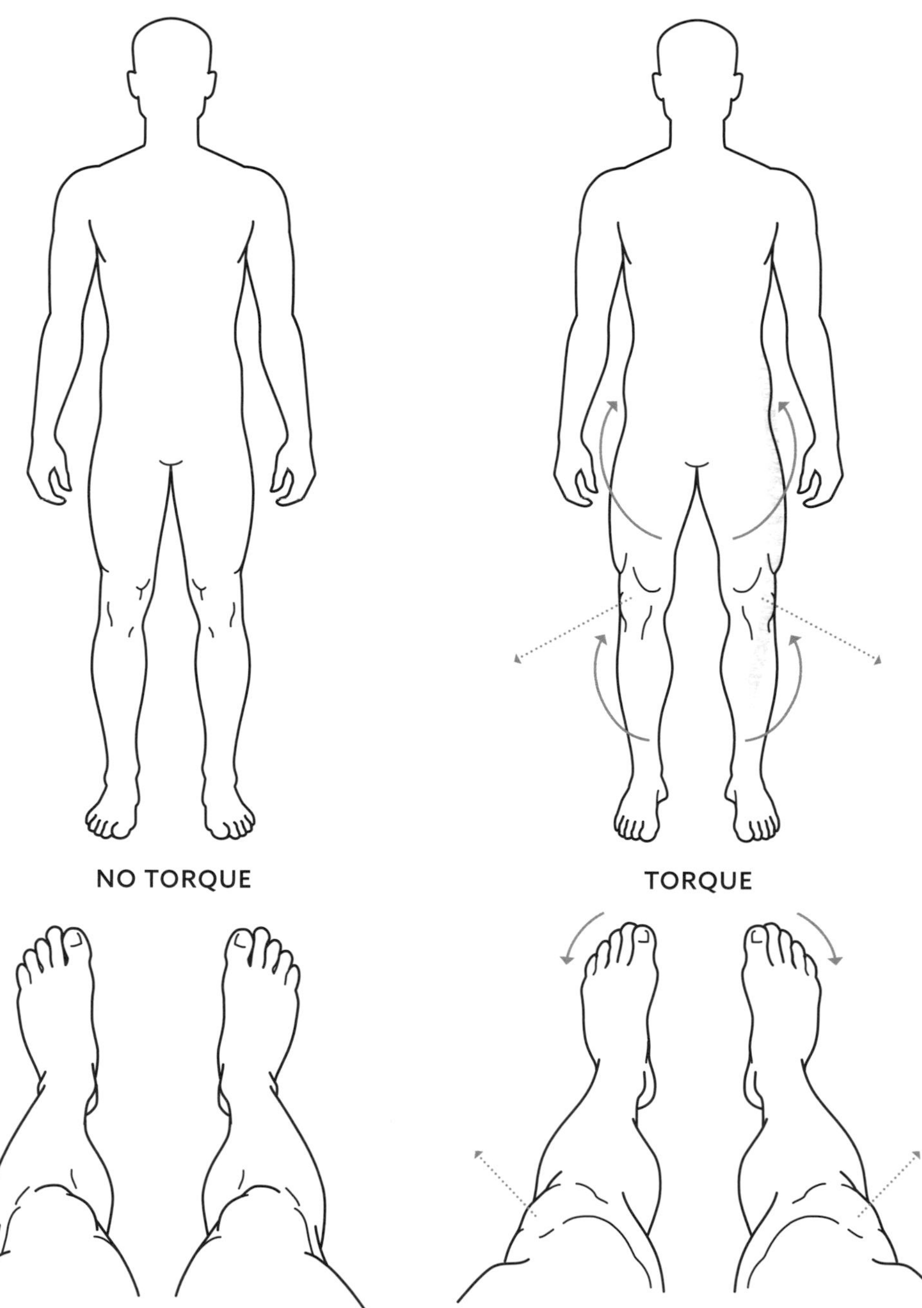

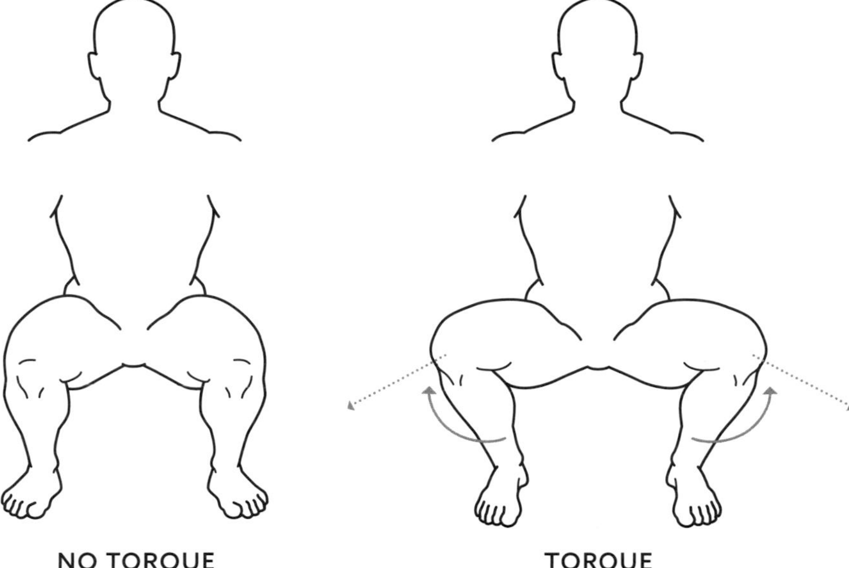

In the gym, coaches often tell athletes to drive their knees out as they descend into the bottom position of the squat. This is to cue hip external rotation or torque. So when a coach tells you to shove your knees out as you squat, what he's really telling you to do is to externally rotate your hips to create a stable position for your hips, knees, and ankles. I'll talk more about the "knees out" cue as it relates to squatting in part 2—see page 168. For now, I want you to see and understand that driving your knees out is how you create torque and stability when squatting.

Create torque in your hips by driving your knees out.

Strength and Conditioning Torque Cues

Universal cues for creating a stable hip position:

- Screw your feet into the ground.
- Spin your feet as if they were on dinner plates.
- Spread the floor.
- Shove your knees out.

Universal cues for creating a stable shoulder position:

- Break (bend) the bar.
- Keep your elbows in.
- Armpits forward (when pressing overhead).
- Elbow pits forward (when doing a pushup).

These common strength and conditioning cues remind us of two things:

1. Our bodies are set up for rotation.
2. We need to generate a rotational force in order to create stable positions from which to move.

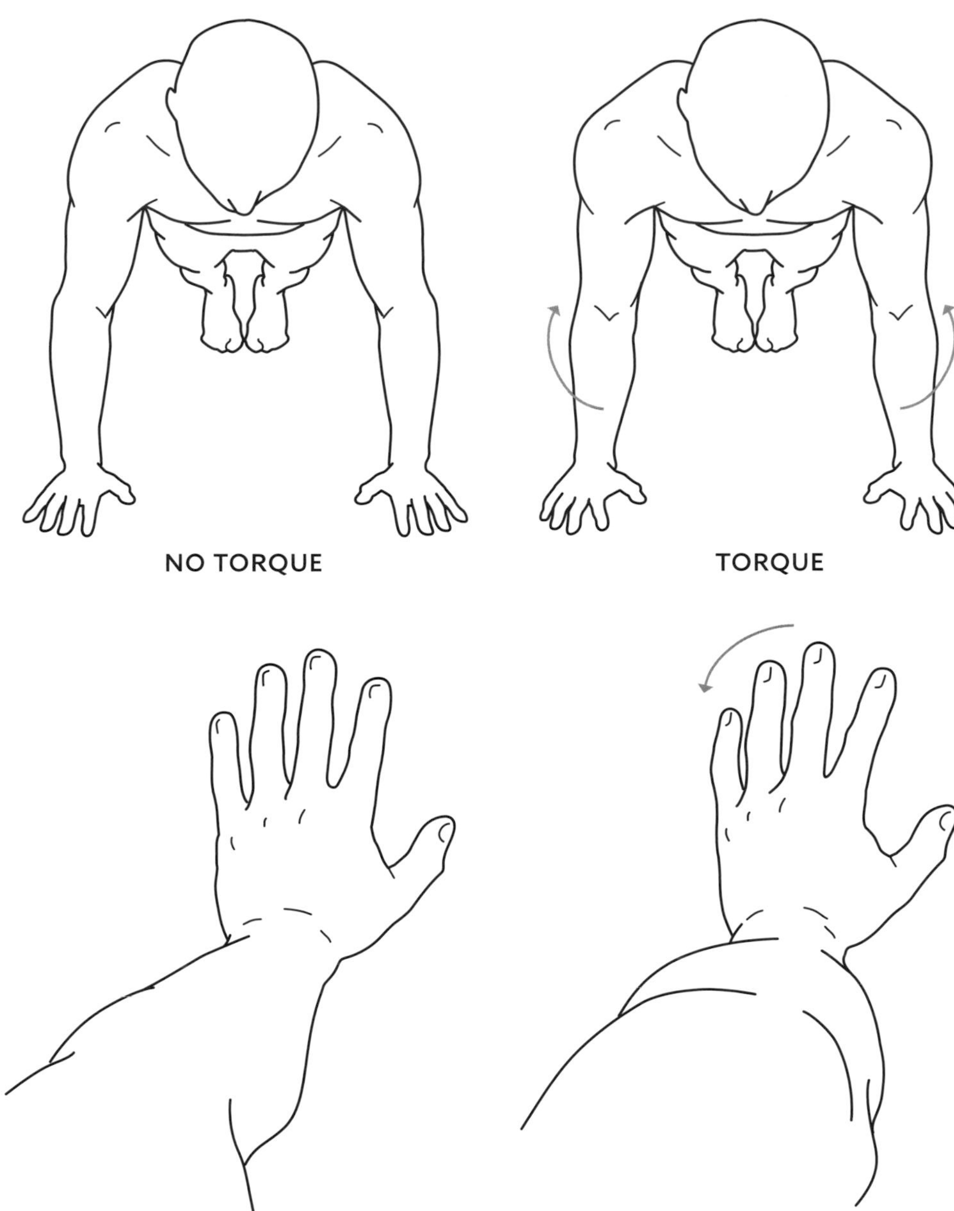

Create torque in your shoulders by screwing your hands into the ground.

Just as screwing your feet into the ground stabilizes your hips, screwing your hands into the ground stabilizes your shoulders. For example, if you're setting up for a pushup, you screw your left hand into the ground in a counterclockwise direction and screw your right hand into the ground in a clockwise direction. Again, you're not turning them outward; you're just exerting an outward rotational force. This is how you create torque to stabilize your wrists, elbows, and shoulders in a good position when you're pressing against a solid surface like the floor.

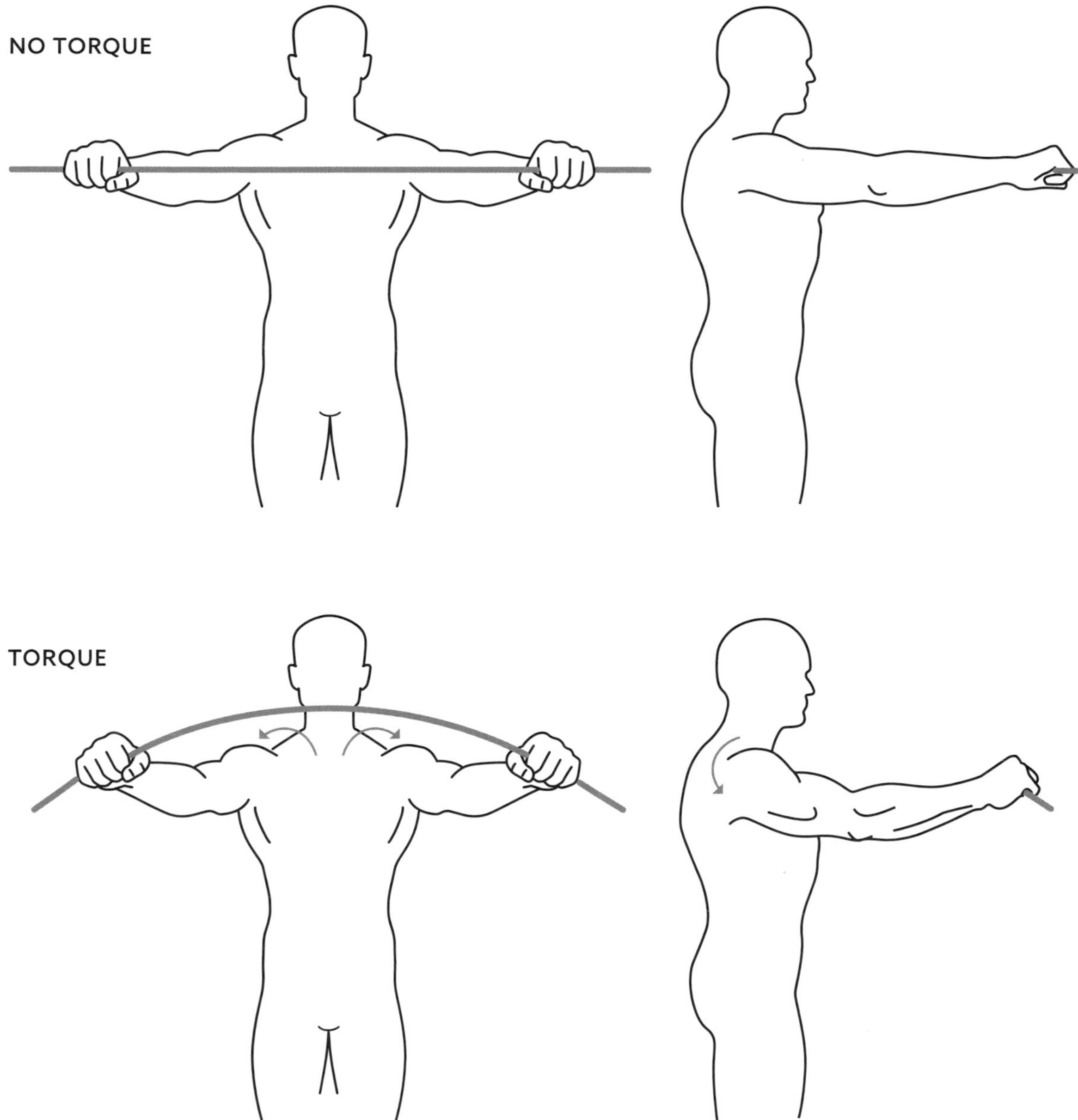

Imagine trying to bend or, better yet, break a pliable stick in half while holding it out in front of your body. To accomplish this task, you need to twist both hands into the stick—rotating your left hand in a counterclockwise direction and your right hand in a clockwise direction—while externally rotating your shoulders. This is exactly how you stabilize your shoulders when you grasp an object such as a barbell. In fact, coaches have been cueing athletes to "break the bar" as a way of stabilizing the shoulders for ages. If you're setting up for a bench press or shoulder press, actively trying to bend the bar creates torque, which stabilizes your wrists, elbows, and shoulders in a good position.

Create torque in your shoulders by breaking the bar.

Torque = Tension/Stability

As I mentioned in chapter 2, your hips and shoulders are ball-in-socket joints that are very similar in function. This is why the cues for creating stable shoulders are essentially the same as those for creating stable hips. Screwing your feet into the ground stabilizes your hips, while screwing your hands into the ground stabilizes your shoulders. Exactly why do you need to generate a rotational force to create stability in the primary engines of your hips and shoulders? Simple: There is slack within these ball-in-socket joints that allows for the full movement of your limbs. To make the joint stable and maintain a braced neutral spine, you need to wind up, twist, and spiral your limb into your hip or shoulder socket. In other words, when you create torque, you activate the musculature to support the joint. When you fail to create torque, you essentially hang on your tissues and rely on your tendons and ligaments to support the position.

ONE-JOINT BODY

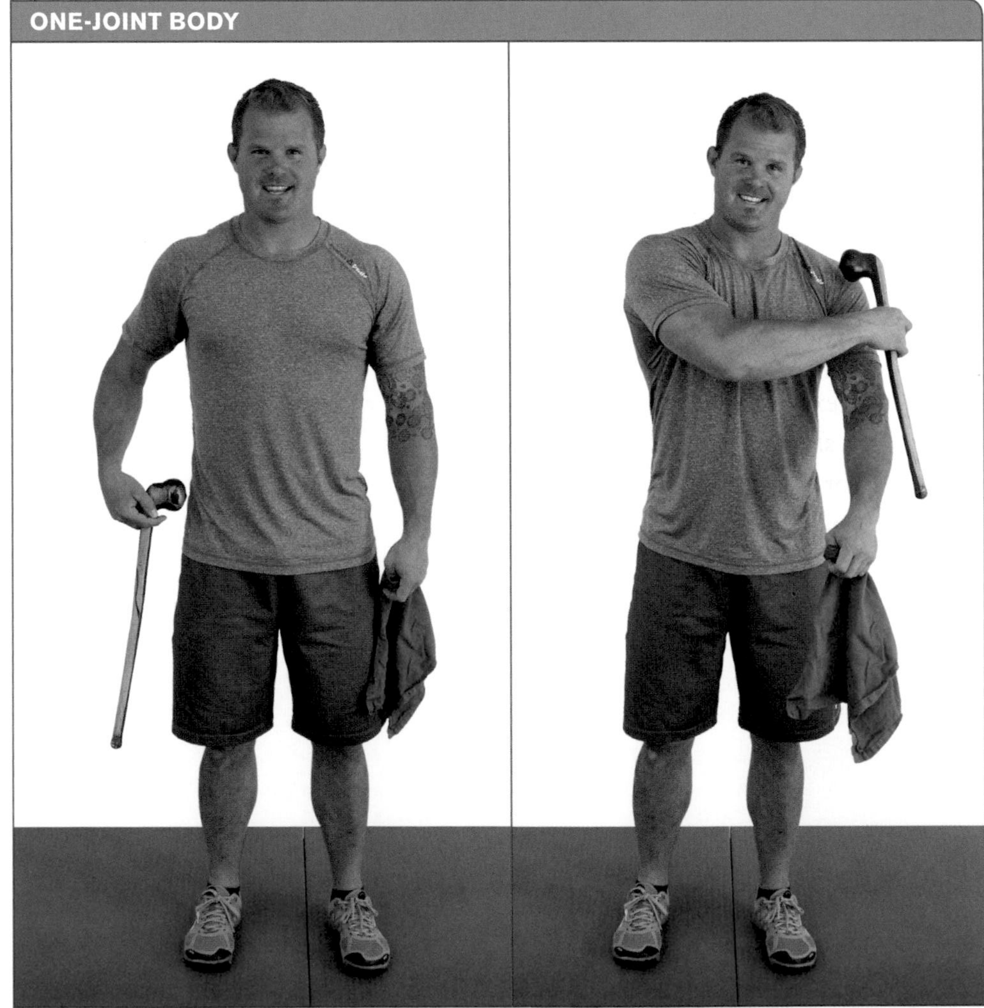

I'm using a club as a model for both the femur (upper leg bone) and the humerus (upper arm bone).

Here's a simple example to help you understand how this works. In the photos below, I've wrapped a rag around the head of a club and bundled up the loose cloth in my opposite hand. When the rag is wrapped snugly around the head of the club, there is still space around the head, which means that it can be pulled and manipulated in different directions—and also means that there can be no torque (rotation). Now imagine that the club is the head of your femur (upper leg bone) or humerus (upper arm bone), and the rag is the joint capsule. As long as there is slack in that rag or joint capsule, your shoulders, hips, and downstream joints will never get into tight, stable positions. The results are—you guessed it—huge losses of power and an increased risk of injury.

When there is no torque, there is slack within the joint capsule, making it impossible to get the joint into a functionally stable position.

CAPSULAR SLACK

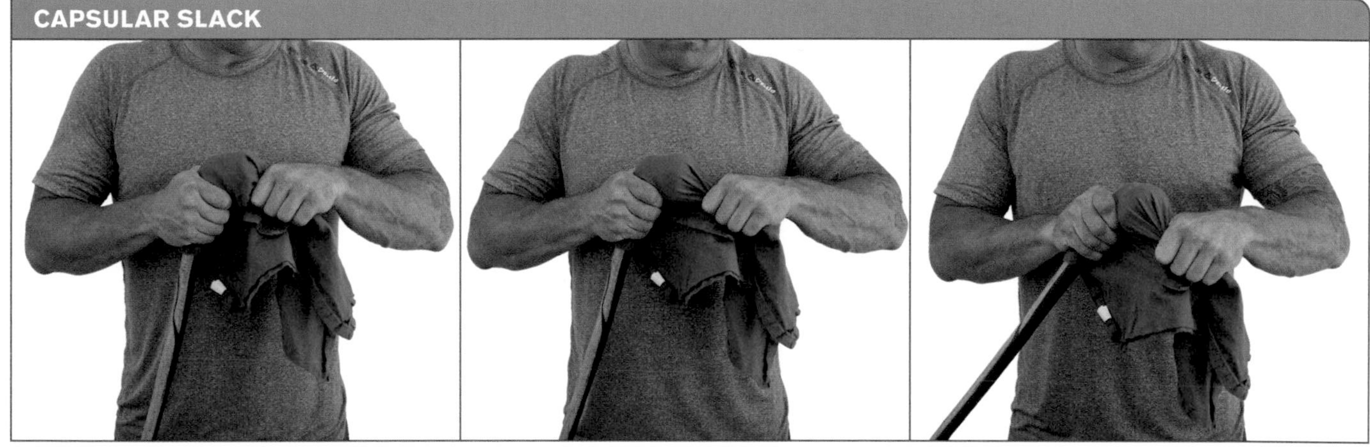

Adding rotation takes up all the capsular slack within the socket, making the joint very tight and stable. The point is that these attachments are set up to create torsional stability. This is why it's so important to have full rotation range of motion in your primary engines. In fact, you can probably get away with missing a little bit of flexion and extension range of motion, but if you're missing rotation at the hips and shoulders, your body will default into structurally stable yet inefficient positions. For example, when your shoulders roll forward, your shoulder joints are stable, but you're in a compromised position.

The act of creating a rotational force to stabilize the joint is not limited to your hips and shoulders; it applies to your ankles, knees, elbows, and wrists as well.

Adding rotation takes up all the capsular slack within the socket, making the joint very tight and stable.

CAPSULAR STABILITY

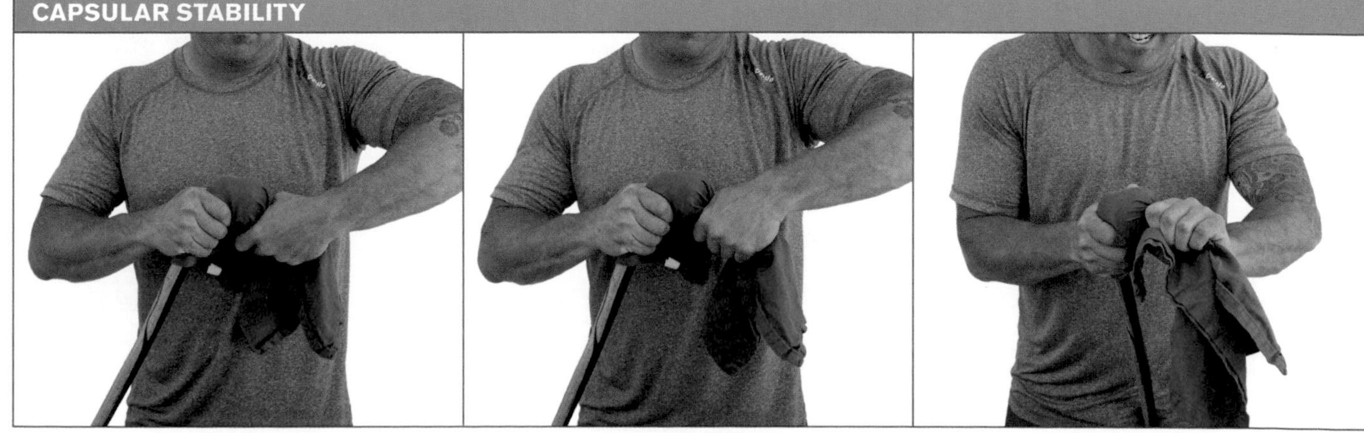

Let's examine the structure of your anterior cruciate ligament (ACL). Your ACL attaches to your femur and tibia (lower leg bone) and is one of the major ligaments that cross your knee. Its role is to prevent your tibia from rotating independently of your femur. It's important to note that although your hips and shoulders function in much the same way, your arms have independent rotational capacities at the elbows. (Fundamental movements like feeding and grabbing would be difficult without those capacities.) Your knees do not: You can't internally and externally rotate at the knee as you can at the elbow.

ACL HAND MODEL

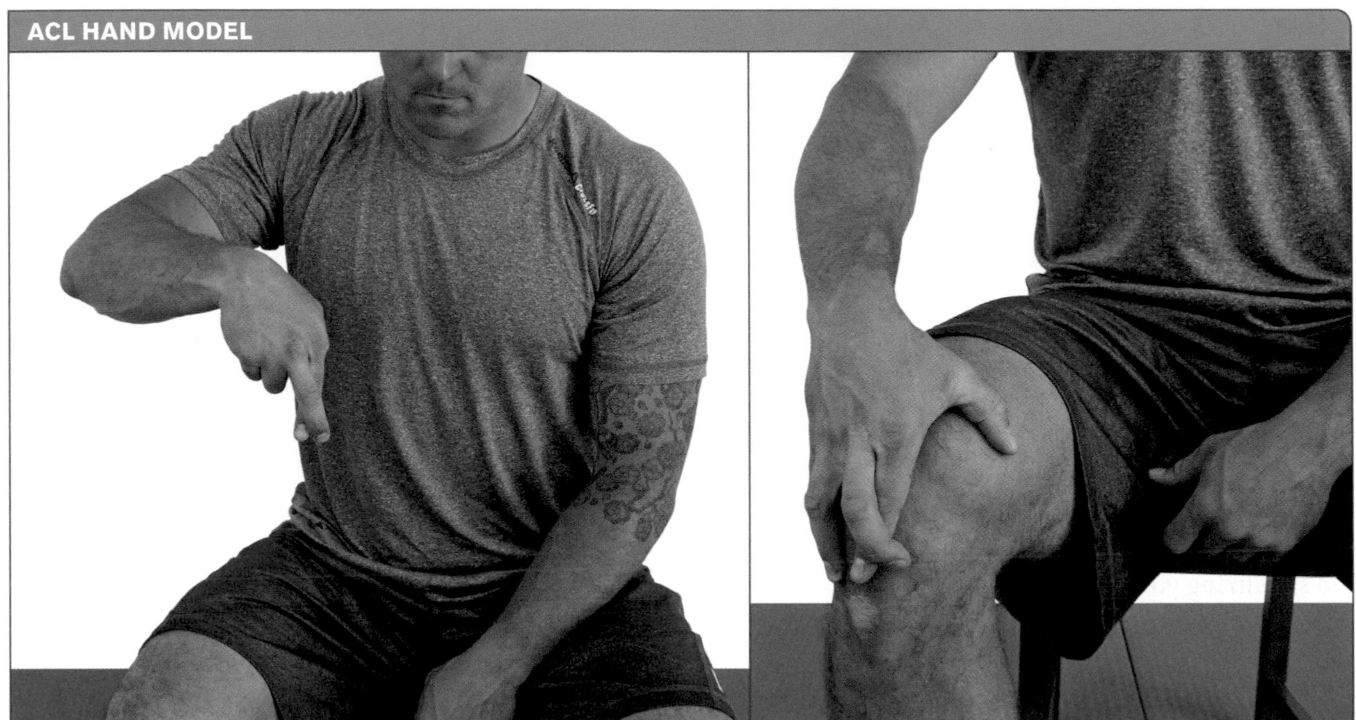

To illustrate how this works, cross your right middle finger over your index finger. This is a crude model of how your ACL crosses through your knee joint.

ACL STABILITY TEST

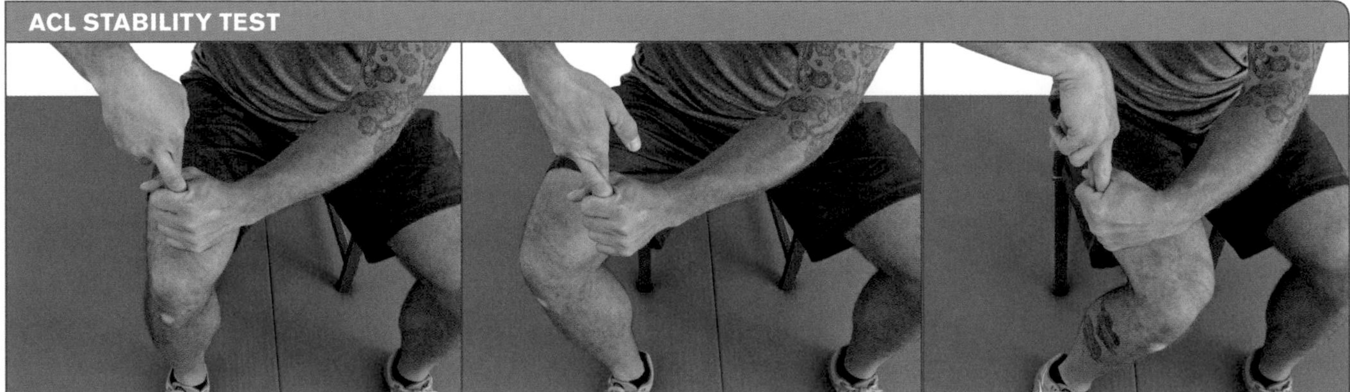

Next, wrap your left hand around your crossed fingers and externally rotate your right hand, creating a force that tightens your fingers. If you internally rotate your right hand, your fingers loosen and come apart. The former is the stable position for your knee, the latter the unstable one. This unstable position can cause the ACL to tear.

The point is that the *right* kind of rotation will set your knee in a more stable position, dramatically reducing your potential for injury. But the *wrong* kind of rotation will put your knee in a disastrous position, increasing the odds of injury sooner or later. The key takeaway is this: Your body will not leave you unstable; it recognizes instability as a liability and would rather close down that open circuit in the wrong way than leave you all loosey-goosey. This is why generating torque is so important: You take up the capsular slack within the ball-in-socket joints and create tension in the muscular system, which helps stabilize the joint in a strong position.

So if generating rotational force is so important, then why aren't more coaches teaching this principle of movement?

As with midline stabilization, torque has long been a part of the athletic conversation, but no one has given it a name. Instead, coaches have relied heavily on torque-generating movement cues like "screw your feet into the ground" and "break the bar" as a way of prompting athletes to create tension in their joints. While these cues serve an important purpose and remain useful, they don't tell the athlete why or how to implement the technique correctly. It's like telling athletes to "get tight" as a way of teaching them how to brace the spine in a neutral position. It doesn't work.

To instill safe, stable positions from which to move, you need more than just movement cues. You need a model that explains why and how these systems work. This is the premise behind both the midline stabilization principle and the laws of torque: The former tells you why spinal mechanics is important and provides a blueprint for organizing and stabilizing your spine in a good position, and the latter explains the importance of creating torque and provides a blueprint for organizing and stabilizing your hips, shoulders, and other joints in good positions. Put simply, these principles are models for creating global stability and tension throughout the body, which is key to moving safely and effectively.

Understand that midline stabilization and the laws of torque work together. If you don't have an organized spine, it is difficult to generate torque or transmit force to your primary engines. Conversely, if you don't generate enough torque, you can't stabilize your trunk in a good position. When both of these factors are in proper alignment, meaning that your trunk is organized and you're applying the right amount of torque through your joints, your ability to generate maximum force—safely and without risk of injury—improves dramatically.

However, it's important to understand that there are two ways to generate torque: You can internally rotate or externally rotate. The right kind of rotation sets your joint in a mechanically stable position, and the wrong kind puts your joint in a bad position. So how do you know when you should generate external rotation torque and when you should generate internal rotation torque? The answer can be summarized by the two laws of torque.

The Two Laws of Torque

The two laws of torque are as follows. Consider them your guide for organizing and stabilizing your extremities in good positions:

Law #1: If your hips or shoulders are in flexion (which decreases the angle of the joint), you create an external rotation force (away from your body).

Examples: squat/pulling positions, front rack, overhead press

Flexion and external rotation cover the broad spectrum of human movements. Squatting, pressing, and pulling movements that occur in front of the body, overhead, and in squatting positions (hips back, knees and ankles bent) involve flexion and require external rotation to create stability. Turning the key in the ignition, screwing in a light bulb, and drawing a bow are all examples of external rotation. This is why being a lefty sucks when you have to screw or unscrew something. (Internally rotating with your left hand to tighten a screw is a weak movement.)

Most torque-related strength and conditioning cues involve creating an external rotation force, like screwing your feet or hands into the ground or breaking the bar.

LAW 1: EXAMPLES OF FLEXION AND EXTERNAL ROTATION

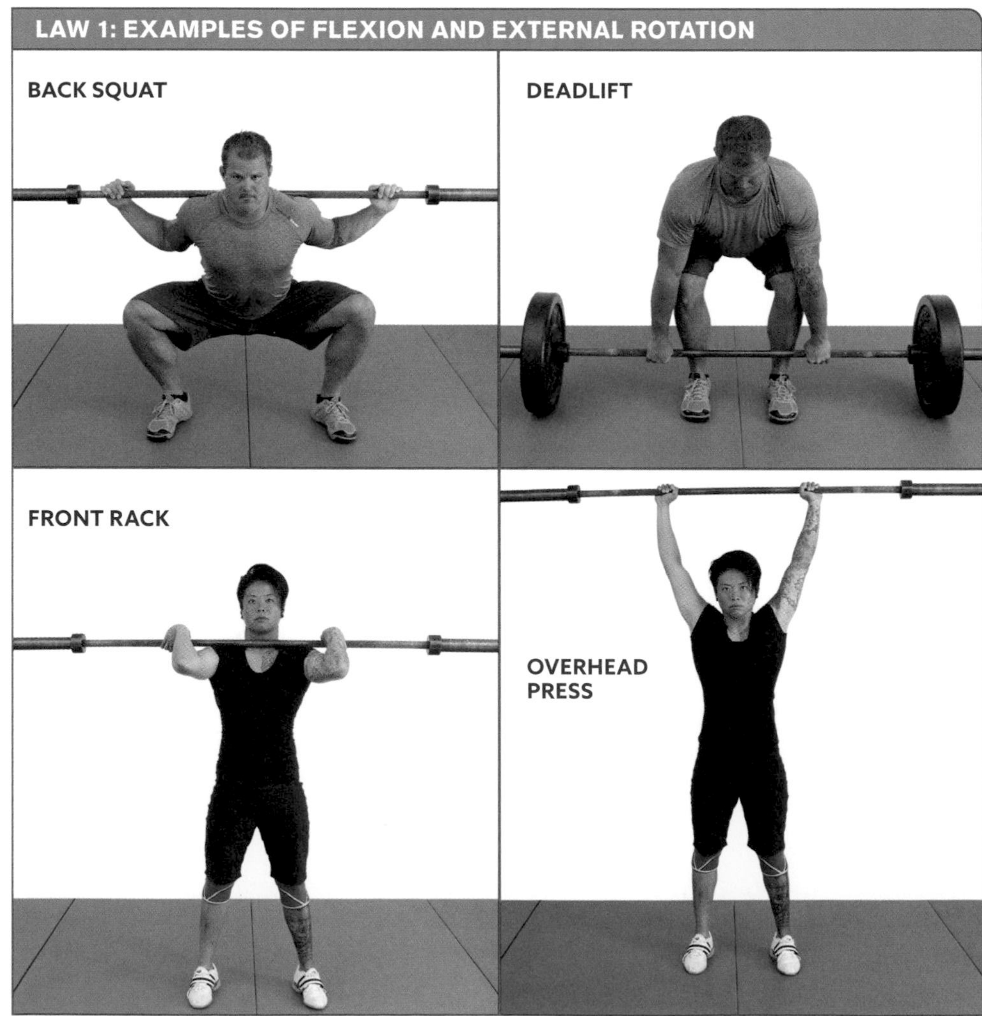

Law #2: If your hips or shoulders are in extension (which increases the angle of the joint), you create an internal rotation force (toward the center of your body).

Examples: split-jerk, arms swinging behind you while jumping

In most situations, you enforce the second law of torque when your foot or hand is positioned behind your body. The most obvious examples are when you swing your arms back while jumping and when your leg tracks behind your body while walking, running, or lunging. This law also comes into play in sports that involve a lot of rotation, like boxing, golf, and baseball, and in any type of throwing movement (in a split or staggered stance, you want to internally rotate your rear leg).

For example, when a technically proficient boxer throws a cross—a straight punch with the rear hand—he will screw (internally rotate) his rear foot into the ground as he rotates his hips and upper body. With his ankle, knee, and hips in the most stable position possible, he can effectively harness the energy traveling through the kinetic chain, maximizing the power of his strike.

This law sometimes confuses people because there are movements in which the shoulders are in extension but the arms are in flexion (bent at the elbows), such as the bench press, dip, and pushup, as well as the arm swing in running. To stabilize your shoulders during these movements, you need to generate an *external* rotation force. Think of it like this: If your shoulders are in extension but your elbows are bent (in flexion), you generate an external rotation force.

LAW 2: EXAMPLES OF EXTENSION AND INTERNAL ROTATION

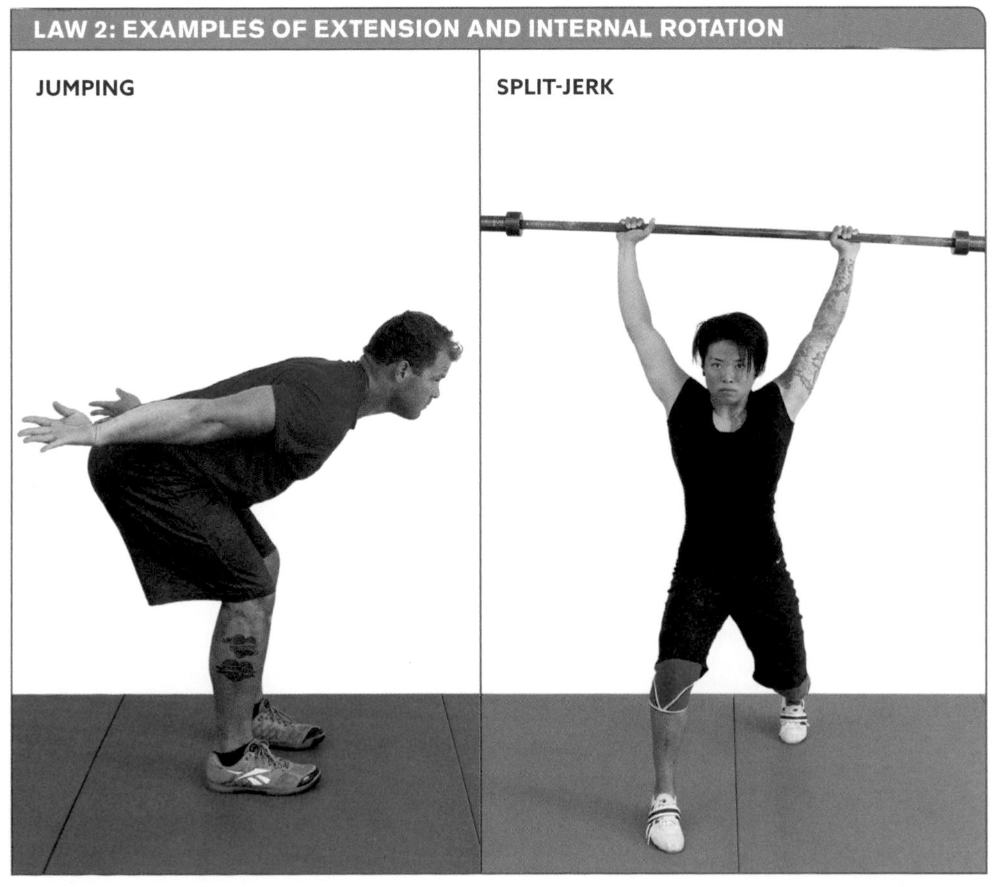

LAW 2: SHOULDER EXTENSION AND ARM FLEXION

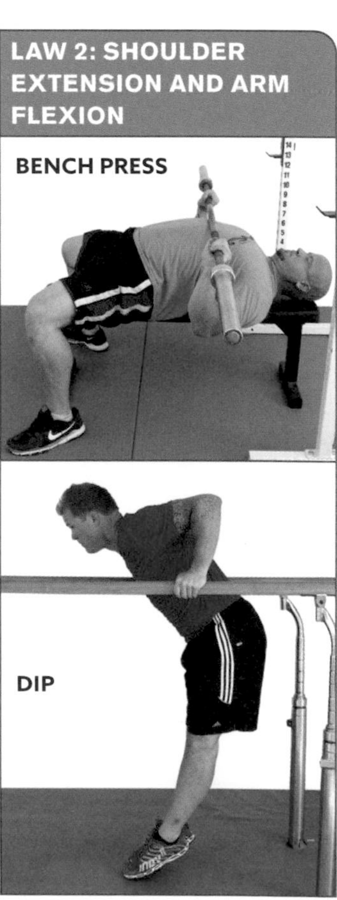

Torque Tension

Now that you understand the concept of generating torque, let's discuss the amount of torque that you need to generate in order to maintain tension in your system. As with bracing your midline (see page 36), you want to create just enough tension to support the demand of your position or movement so that you can maintain a mechanically stable position. So if you're just standing around or performing basic bodyweight movements, you might need to apply only 10 to 20 percent of your total torque capacity. In other words, you generate just enough torque to avoid force bleeds and injury-inviting movement faults.

A common mistake is to exaggerate the action of torque and generate way more than needed, which can compromise form in the same way as not generating torque at all. This is perhaps most common when people are first starting to experiment with this concept—especially when it comes to the squat.

Like most strength and conditioning coaches, I typically use a bodyweight (air) squat (page 162) as a diagnostic tool for assessing movement competency and range of motion. When I teach the laws of torque as they relate to this common bodyweight movement, I typically use cues like "drive your knees out" and "screw your feet into the ground" so that the athletes externally rotate from the hips. As with a lot of coaching cues, this set of cues is often misinterpreted as "drive your knees out and screw your feet into the ground as hard as you can." People tell me all the time how generating torque destroys their ability to squat or causes knee and ankle pain.

Here's what is probably happening: These athletes are creating too much torque. If you try to generate an external rotation force from your hips with 100 percent of your capacity, you're creating more tension than is necessary for carrying out the movement. When that happens, the movement becomes labored and visibly awkward. (The same thing happens when you exaggerate midline stabilization. If you're bracing your spine to 100 percent tension while performing a bodyweight movement like a squat or pushup, chances are the movement will feel slow and tight, as if you're lacking range of motion.) Again, you need only enough rotation to combat the forces that are pulling you into a bad position. Remember the stability maxim: If you don't create stability in the right way, your body will find stability for you by defaulting to a bad position. So you want to apply enough tension to support a good position, but not so much that you compromise the movement. It's a delicate balance that takes time and practice to master.

Another way to think about torque tension is to match it with your midline stabilization strategy: If your torque and midline tension levels aren't in sync or your midline stabilization strategy is weak, your spine will sag the moment you start applying an external rotation force. Let's say, for example, that you set up for a pushup with trunk tension at a 2 out of 10 and try to apply torque through your hands at a 5. Your spine will respond by overextending. You need to apply just enough torque to maintain a flat back. For bodyweight movements, you don't need that much torque to keep your belly tight to maintain good form, but as you increase the load or add speed, you have to increase both torque and trunk tension to match the demands of the movement.

The laws of torque can be confusing, so I've put together some tests that help illustrate the function and application of torque. If you're questioning the role of torque, especially as it relates to hand and foot position, I highly recommend that you review this section and try some of the tests. If you already grasp the concepts of torque and midline stabilization, feel free to skip to the next chapter.

Torque Tests

The two laws of torque give you a general blueprint for creating tension and stabilizing your joints in a good position. In part 2, I apply these laws to a broad spectrum of transferable strength and conditioning movements. But first, let's test this movement principle by using two simple, universally transferable movements: the pushup and the squat.

In this section, I use the pushup to illustrate how to create stability in your shoulders (see "Shoulder Stability Torque Tests") and the squat to demonstrate how to create stability in your hips (see "Hip Stability Torque Tests"). It's important to realize that these two bodyweight movements are more than just training exercises: If you understand how to set up for a pushup, you have a model for stabilizing your shoulders for any movement that requires pressing or pulling. In the same way, if you understand how to squat correctly, you have a universal model for creating stability and torque in your hips, knees, and ankles anytime your hips and legs are in flexion.

In the following pages, I provide a series of tests to help you develop the connection between midline stabilization and torque and understand how your setup or start position dictates your capacity to move optimally. As you perform these tests, I want you to pay close attention to the orientation of your hands and feet as it relates to generating torque.

As I will make clear, the more you turn your hands or feet away from your body, the less torque you can generate. And the less torque you generate, the less stability you have. Coaches sometimes tell athletes to adopt a more open foot or hand stance because it gives them a greater degree of hip and shoulder range of motion. Turning your feet out to perform a squat allows you to circumvent some range of motion limitations you have in your hips and ankles, and turning your hands out to perform a pushup allows you to circumvent some range of motion limitations in your shoulders and wrists. But it also compromises your ability to generate torque and ingrains a dysfunctional pattern that will bleed into other movements and positions.

This is the crux of the problem that many people fail to recognize. You can get away with squatting and pressing with your feet and hands turned out when the weight and speed demand is relatively low because the midline stabilization and torque demands are low. But when you add weight and speed and the midline stabilization and torque demands increase, things start to fall apart. With your feet or hands turned out, you simply can't generate enough torque to meet the demands of the movement. So you can imagine how this limitation starts to pose problems when you transition from a bodyweight squat to more complex and load-bearing movements, like jumping and landing, the back squat, and the Olympic lifts.

Shoulder Stability Torque Tests

When I teach the laws of torque in my seminars, I typically start at the shoulders and use the pushup as my diagnostic movement. By putting people in the top of a pushup, I can safely and effectively illuminate the two central tenets of stability. People immediately realize that if they're disorganized at the trunk (not braced in a neutral position), they can't get organized at the shoulders. Conversely, if their shoulders are rolling forward or they can't lock out their elbows, they struggle to achieve a flat back.

Pushup Butt Acuity Test

The pushup butt acuity test is the first application of midline stabilization and torque that I introduce. To perform this test, simply get into the pushup start position by making your hands as parallel as possible—positioning them underneath your shoulders—and pinning your feet together.

Next, go through the bracing sequence: Squeeze your butt, align your ribcage over your pelvis, and get your belly tight. The key is to make sure that your wrists, elbows, and shoulders are aligned and your feet are together. A lot of people mistakenly spread their feet apart, not realizing that they're just cheating range of motion. This makes it difficult to engage the glutes and stabilize the trunk.

After you establish a well-organized pushup start position, the next step is to disengage your glutes and then try to maintain a flat back. If you can sequence multiple full-range pushups, you'll probably need to do 5 to 10 pushups—one set with your butt online and another with it offline—to get the desired effect. What you will find is that the latter setup (with your glutes offline) is not nearly as stable because there's a domino effect: If your glutes are disengaged, it's difficult to organize your spine in a good position. This gives you two important pieces of information:

1. When your butt is offline, you're susceptible to spinal faults.
2. A broken midline makes it difficult to generate sufficient torque, placing additional strain on your shoulders. The difference is shocking.

+ ENGAGED

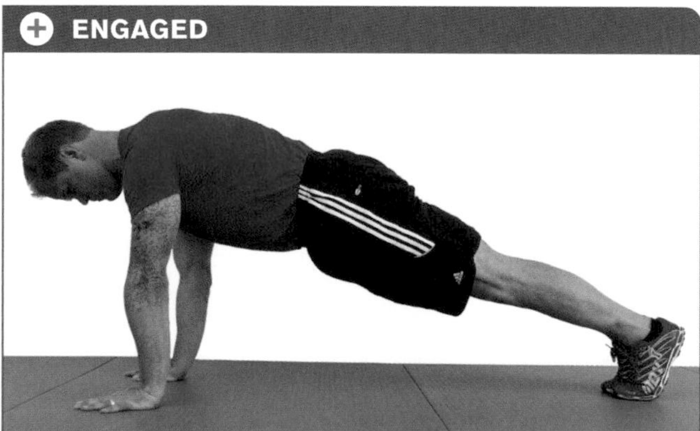

When your butt is squeezed, it's easier to keep your back flat.

− DISENGAGED

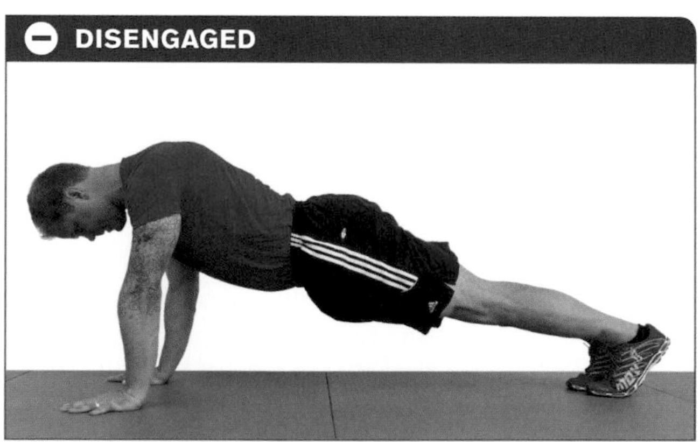

When you disengage your glutes, it's harder to preserve a neutral spinal position, especially as you start sequencing multiple pushups.

Open-Hand Torque Test

The second test uses one of the most common strength and conditioning cues as it relates specifically to the pushup: screwing your hands into the ground. This is how people really start to understand how important torque is in stabilizing the trunk. With the pits of your elbows forward and the heads of your shoulders externally rotated, it's much easier to keep your back flat. Moreover, this test teaches you about the connection between hand position and the amount of torque you can generate.

Here's how it works: You start with your hands parallel (or as straight as you can get them), and then create torque by screwing your hands into the ground. You should feel your shoulders stabilize and your upper back tense. Once you have a sense of what if feels like to create torque with your hands straight, turn your hands out slightly, while trying to create torque and keeping your back flat. You will realize that the more you turn out your hands, the harder it is to create torque and stabilize your trunk. Once you get to 45 degrees, cultivating torque is simply untenable. At this point, your shoulders start to sag and your spine bends because you're in such a low-torque environment. If you turn your hands out as if you were doing a planche (a difficult gymnastics move in which the entire body is held parallel to the ground, like a high pushup without using the feet), keeping your trunk stiff and stable becomes even harder. Maintaining this position with zero torque is very difficult and explains why doing a planche pushup, even when your feet are on the ground, is so hard. It takes not only extreme mobility, but also extreme strength.

The takeaway is this: To create a stable platform for your shoulders and thoracic spine (the middle segment), you have to create torque through your hands. If you put your hands in a position in which you can't create torque, it's hard to stabilize and generate force. Remember, I'm not just talking about the pushup; I'm talking about the entire gamut of pressing and pulling exercises. Adopting an open-hand position (hands turned out) in the pushup ensures that you will adopt the same hand position when you block, push a car, do a burpee—you name it.

Get into the pushup start position. With your fingers pointed straight ahead and splayed, screw your hands into the ground. Then turn your hands out slightly and try to generate torque. You will find that you can't create nearly as much torque with your hands turned out. As you turn your hands out even farther, you will completely lose the ability to cultivate torque, making it a supreme challenge to stabilize your shoulders and trunk. And if you turn your hands backward, you can't create any torque at all.

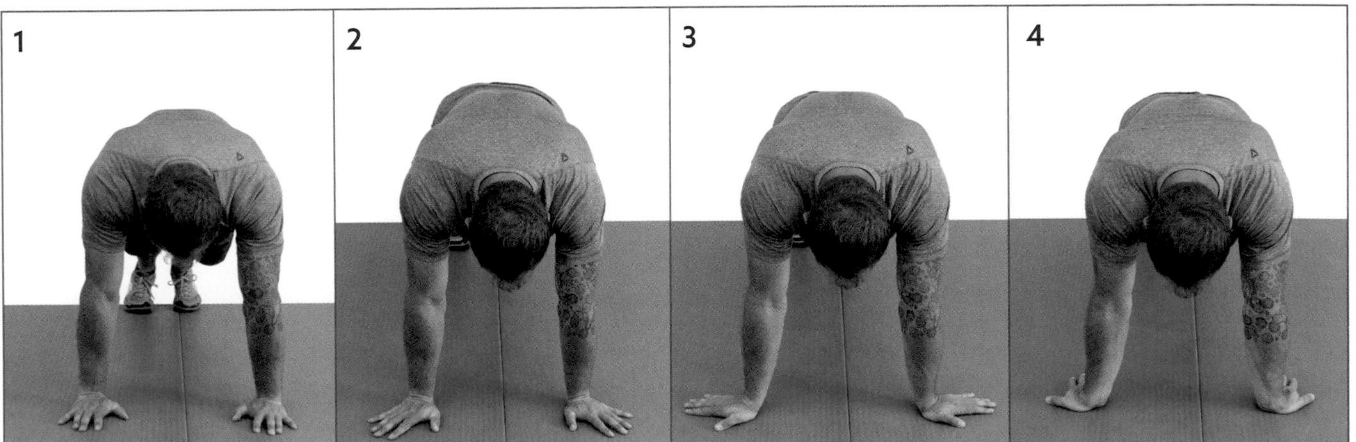

Screwing your hands into the ground creates external rotation in your shoulders, but turning your hands outward robs you of your ability to generate torque.

Ring Pushup Torque Test

If you really want to look under the hood of shoulder stabilization, do pushups on the rings. Your understanding of bracing and torque, or the lack thereof, will instantly become clear: You can see whether you're in a good or bad position because it's so much harder to stabilize your shoulders and trunk on the rings.

The ring pushup start position also teaches you that you need to create torque early and often. It's difficult to reclaim torque at the bottom of a pushup, particularly on the rings—you have to arrive with torque. This is why coaches cue athletes to "break the bar" at the top of the bench press: It optimizes shoulder position when the bar is lowered to the chest.

This test helps you understand that if you set yourself up in a good position with adequate torque and an organized spine, chances are good that you will perform the movement with perfect technique. And if you set up properly, a lot of the mid-range problems and discomfort that people experience—like shoulder pain—will disappear. The fact is, a lot of torque-related movement errors go unnoticed when performing pushups from the ground because the demands are so low. This is what makes the rings such a valuable tool. It takes a high level of torque to stabilize your shoulders and trunk in a good position. If you don't generate enough external rotation, your shoulders will roll forward and your back will sag.

Note: Unlike a regular pushup, where you have a base of support and can screw your hands into the ground to create external rotation, with the ring pushup you have to physically rotate your hands. Your right thumb should be at 1 o'clock and your left thumb at 11 o'clock.

+ ENGAGED/TORQUE

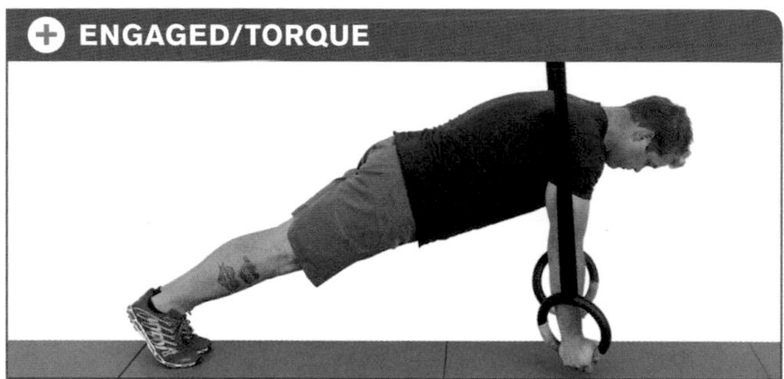

Get into a good pushup position by squeezing your butt, engaging your abdominals, and getting your back flat. To create torque, you still have to generate an external rotation force, but unlike performing pushups from the ground, cultivating torque on the rings is a lot harder. To put your shoulders in a good position, you have to turn your hands out so that your thumbs are pointing away from your body. Your right thumb should be at 1 o'clock and your left thumb at 11 o'clock.

− DISENGAGED/NO TORQUE

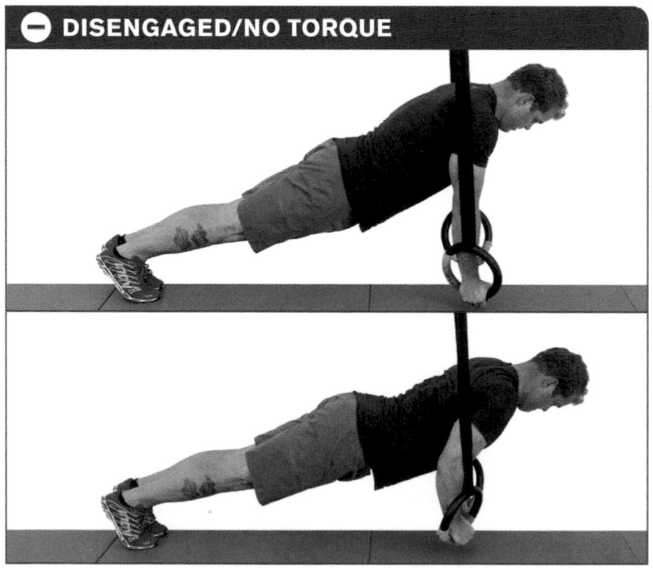

If you don't externally rotate your hands, you can't create torque. And if you can't create torque, you can't organize your spine, your elbows will flare out, and your shoulders will default into a rounded position. The moment you disengage your glutes, you will feel your hips sag, pulling you into an overextended position.

Hip Stability Torque Tests

Like the pushup, the squat has a broad range of applications. If you understand how to create torque while squatting, you have a global model for hip stability that is germane to the vast majority of movements. In addition, the squat illustrates that your setup—specifically your foot position, or stance—dictates your ability to generate torque upstream in your ankles, knees, hips, spine, and shoulders.

Remember, your joints need to be in a position to facilitate rotational force *before* you start moving. As these squat torque tests will prove, a straight or neutral foot position is ideal for generating maximum torque—see the sidebar "Clarifying the Neutral (Straight) Foot Stance" on page 82.

The trouble is that there has been a historical disconnect between foot position and stabilization through torque. For years, coaches have taught athletes to turn their feet out—like a duck's—when they squat, which opens up the hip joint and allows the athletes to drive their knees out farther and lower into the bottom of the squat more easily. What coaches and athletes have failed to realize is that you can create room in the hip joint through external rotation torque: by positioning your feet straight (parallel), screwing your feet into the ground, and driving your knees out. Although this technique requires more mobility, it enables you to maximize torque and still free the head of your femur (open up your hip joint).

However, most people don't have the range of motion required to perform a full-range butt-to-ankles squat. Turning their feet out enables them to get the job done, but that quick fix comes at a cost: It instills a dysfunctional movement pattern that carries over to other activities. Squat with a duck-footed stance, and chances are you will also stand, walk, jump, land, and pull with a duck-footed stance. And what do you think will happen when you go for a one-rep max back squat? Or spontaneously receive weight in the bottom of a squat during an Olympic lift? Or plant to change directions in a basketball game? This is what will happen: You will express the same movement pattern that you've been practicing, dramatically increasing your risk for injury.

Another problem with the open-foot stance is that it makes it difficult to generate torque and stabilize your body. What often happens as a result is that your ankles collapse and your knees spiral inward, creating a valgus (twisting and shearing) force across your joints. This is how athletes lose force through their hips, and it is the primary culprit in ACL tears.

When I teach the neutral foot position as it relates to the squat, I say that you can squat in any position as long as you can create arches in both feet. If your foot sustains an arch, you will be able to generate sufficient torque. It just so happens that straight and neutral is the best foot position for achieving this ideal arch. The more you turn out your feet, the more likely it is that your arches will collapse.

For example, if you lower into a squat but reach the end of your ankle range of motion before you complete the exercise—meaning that you can't flex any deeper as you move into the bottom position—you have to start tension hunting, which is expressed by ankles collapsing inward. Although this collapse makes your ankles structurally stable, it compromises the integrity of your upstream joints. You are, in effect, depending on your ligaments and tissues to support you. To ensure optimal

+ NEUTRAL FOOT

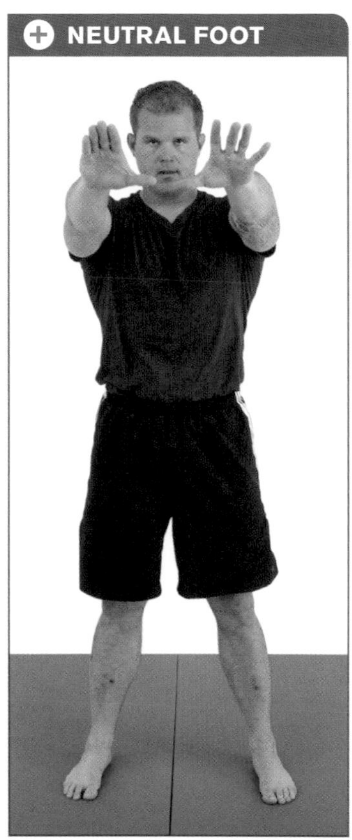

– OPEN FOOT

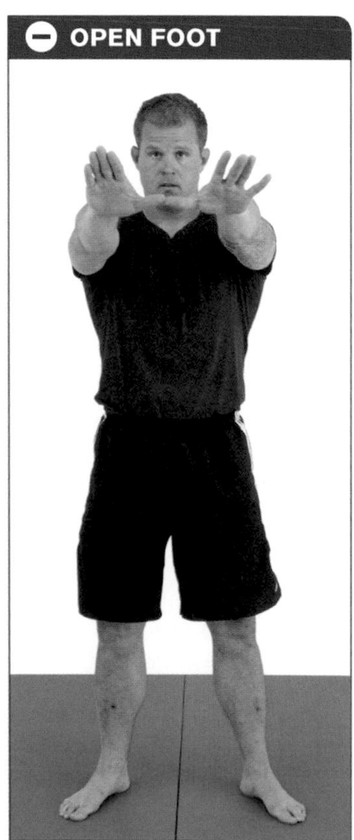

positioning of your ankle joint, you need to create an arch in your foot, which is expressed through external rotation torque.

Here's the deal: While you can get away with squatting with your feet turned out when working with body weight and low volume, the house of cards is going to collapse the moment the weight, speed, or volume increases.

As with the shoulder stability torque tests, the goal of the subsequent demonstrations is to drive home the relationship between torque and midline stability, as well as to illustrate why a neutral foot position is ideal for maximizing torque.

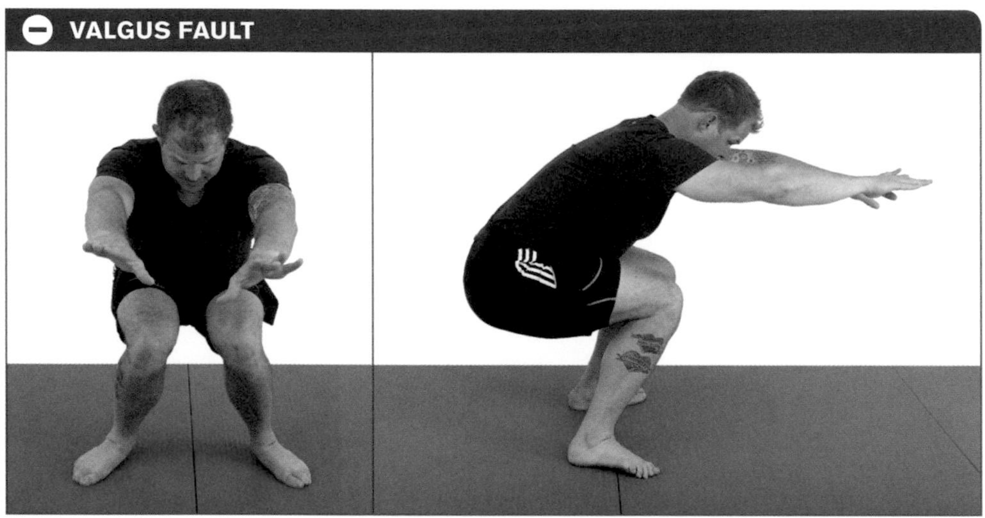

Your arch is largely a phenomenon of this mechanical system—bones, ligaments, tendons, and connective tissues—derived from the external rotation of your hip. Heel aligned with the Achilles (straight), or heel cord matching the calf, is ideal. If your feet are straight and you externally rotate at the hips, your feet will come into a natural arch. You can lift more weight and jump with more force. Oh, and it also happens to be the safest position from which to move.

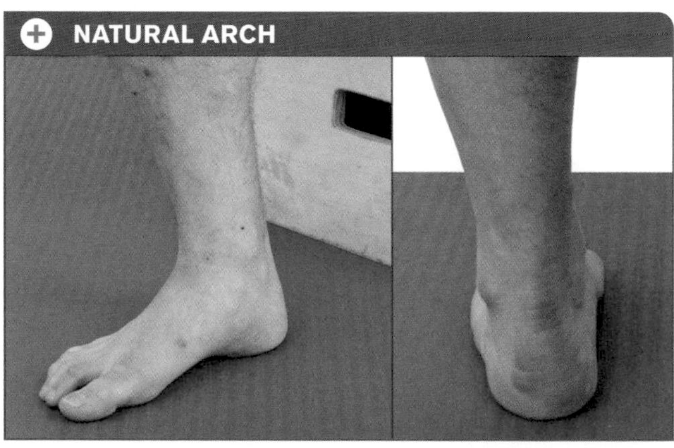

This oblique load on the Achilles is one of the mechanisms for Achilles rupture, Achilles tendinopathy, and ACL tears. One way to mitigate off-axial oblique loads on your Achilles is to get your foot into a straighter position.

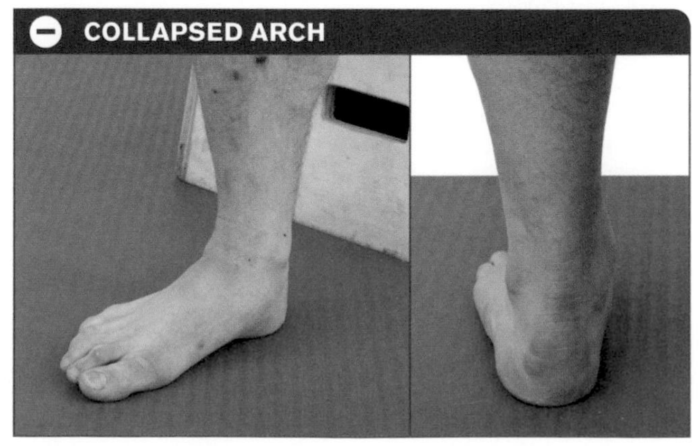

Open-Foot Torque Test

When I teach people about creating a stable hip position, I start with the open-foot torque test because it's easy to make the connection between a neutral foot position and torque.

To execute this test, stand with your feet directly under your hips, or roughly shoulder width apart, go through the bracing sequence, and then screw your feet into the ground as if you were trying to spread the floor apart. Create as much external rotation force as possible, and squeeze your butt as hard as you can without letting your big toes come up off the ground. When you externally rotate at the hips, your feet come into an arch—connective tissue contracts, bones align properly, and muscles are activated—which is the ideal position.

After you carry out the torque test with your feet straight, turn your feet out about 45 degrees and repeat the process. You won't be able to cultivate the same amount of torque, your feet won't come into an arch, and you won't be able to activate your glutes to the same degree.

Now, it's important to mention that you can turn your feet out *slightly*—between 0 and 12 degrees—and still generate a sufficient amount of torque. However, as you venture into the 30-degree range, there is no torque to be had. The drop-off rate is radical.

Let me be clear: The more parallel your feet are, the more stable your position. You can turn your feet out slightly and still create torque, but not as much. It might not matter a great deal during bodyweight squats or low-intensity exercise, but when you add a metabolic demand or load, your inability to generate torque will result in a biomechanical compromise of some kind. And you must know by now that a biomechanical compromise is a green light to injury.

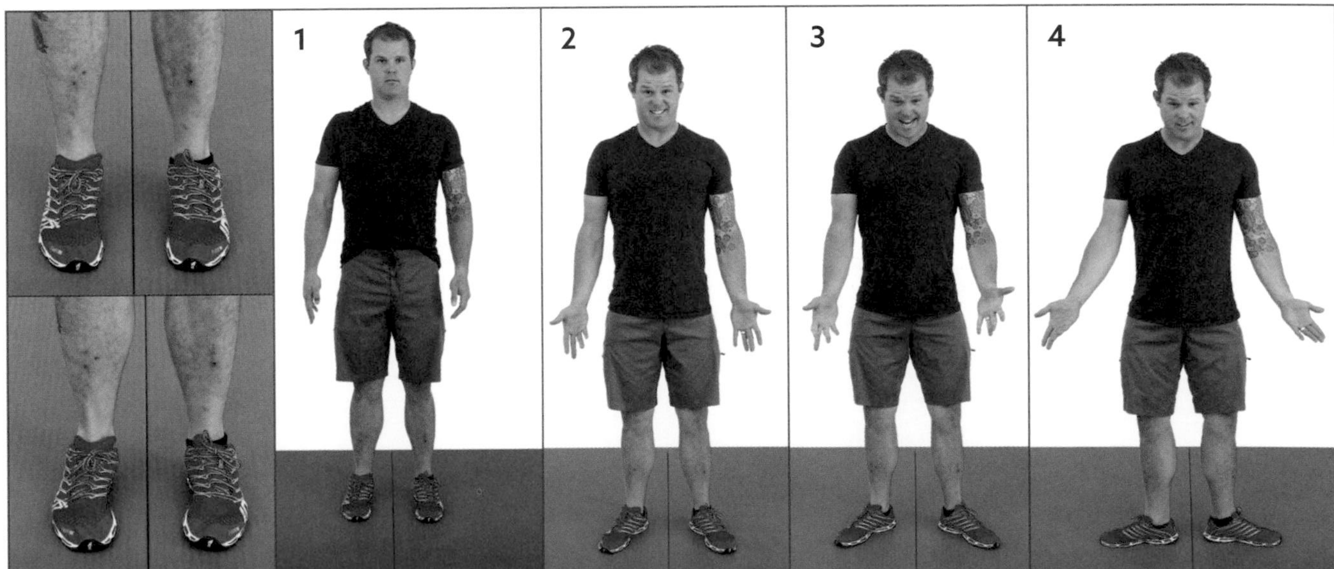

Start with your feet parallel, go through the bracing sequence, and then screw your feet into the ground, creating an external rotation force. You'll notice that your shoes curve. This is your feet coming into an arch. Next, turn your feet out slightly and repeat the process. As your feet venture outward, you'll notice that you can't generate torque, create an arch, or activate your glutes.

Clarifying the Neutral (Straight) Foot Stance

When I say "neutral foot position," I'm advocating for feet straight—toes pointing forward and feet parallel to each other. This is what I consider an ideal stance. However, you can get away with a slightly turned-out stance without compromising your ability to generate torque. But there's a fine line. As you can see in the diagram below, I believe that between 0 and 12 degrees is sufficient for generating maximum torque. If you have limited ankle and hip mobility, turning your feet out slightly—no more than 12 degrees—will probably feel more comfortable and enable you to squat to deeper ranges. However, you should still be working toward a straighter foot stance as your mobility improves.

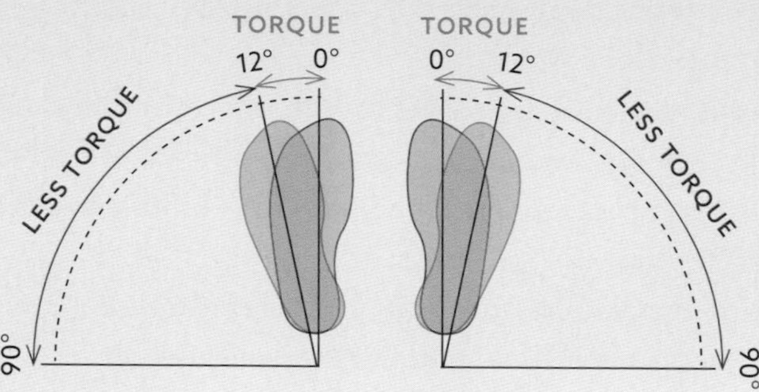

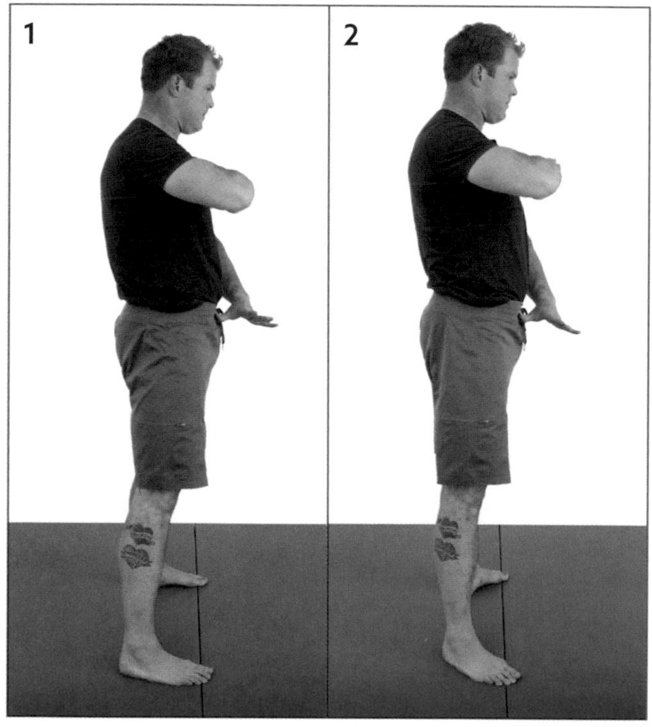

Go through the bracing sequence with your feet as straight as possible, squeezing your butt as hard as you can. Then turn your feet out and do the same thing. You'll notice that you can't activate your glutes to stabilize your pelvis, which creates an unstable spine.

Butt Acuity Test

The butt acuity test helps elucidate the relationship between a straight-foot stance and your ability to activate your glutes. With your feet parallel, you can maximize torque and squeeze your butt to stabilize your pelvis in a neutral position. However, if you turn your feet out, not only do you lose the ability to generate torque, but you also can't engage your glutes, which creates an unstable pelvic position.

As you experienced during the pushup, if you fail to create torque through your hands or you're in a position in which you can't generate a rotational force, your ribcage tilts. A similar thing happens during the squat, but instead of your ribcage tilting, your pelvis tilts. If you have zero torque, you have to create stability in some other way. In the squat, it's created by the pelvis moving forward, which is the mirror action of your ribcage tilting back.

This explains why so many people overextend when they squat and why people experience so much low back pain. In a low-torque environment—where the body can't generate stability—they default to bone-on-bone stability, which is the overextension spinal fault (see page 35).

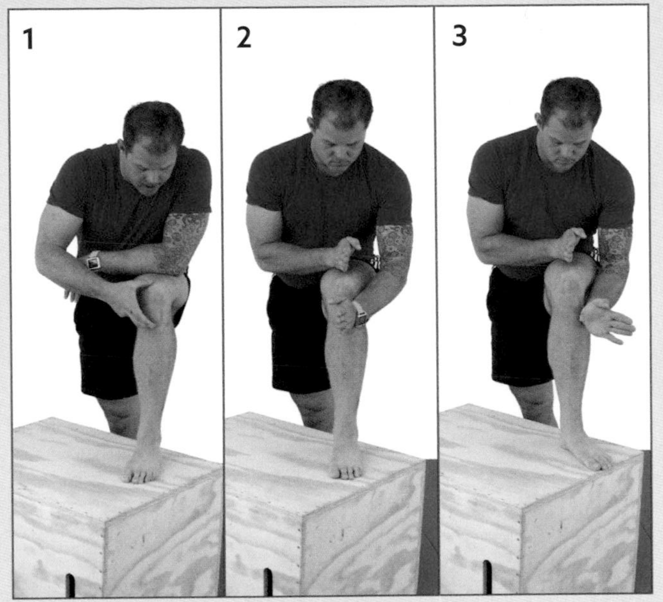

Patellar Alignment

To generate the most force and avoid knee pain, your kneecap and the insertion of the quad ligament on your shin need to be as parallel as possible (photo 2). When you turn your feet out, the quad ligament gets pulled off-axis (photo 3). That's what my hand positions illustrate. With your foot straight, your kneecap tracks straight up and down over your quad, which is optimal.

Base of Support Test

Another problem with turning your feet out is that it limits your base of support. You go from the full length of your foot to about half its length, compromising your forward and backward balance and stability. If you squatted with skis on your feet, you would never fall forward or backward. But if you turn your feet out, you instantly lose that balance and stability.

This is another reason why you see athletes' knees tracking inward. It's not just because they have zero torque; it's because they have zero forward and backward stability. When your feet are straight, your knees don't track as far inward, even when you fail to create torque (see "Torqueless Squat Test" on page 87).

This loss of stability becomes an even bigger issue when you perform Olympic lifts. For example, say you receive a snatch a little bit out in front of or behind your body. With your feet straight, you can adjust your position because you have a large base of support. But if your feet are turned out, regaining your balance is difficult.

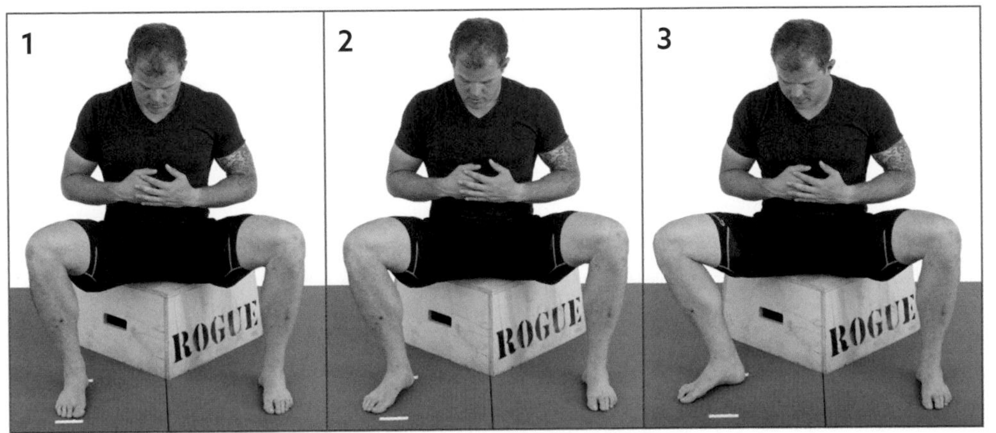

When your foot is straight, you have a large base of support. When you turn your foot out, however, you lose around 30 percent of the length of your foot.

Monster Walk Test

The monster walk is a common warm-up exercise in which you wrap a band above your knees and walk sideways while in a quarter or half squat. What's interesting is that people don't walk with their feet angled out when they do this drill; their feet are always straight. Why? Because it's impossible to keep your knees from collapsing inward as you walk laterally. To remain stable, you have to maintain the position that gives you the most stability, which you accomplish by keeping your feet straight.

Wrap a band just above your knees, parallel your feet, and then reach your hamstrings and hips back, lowering into a quarter squat. Because your feet are straight, you can generate more torque and drive your knees out farther, giving you more balance and stability as you sidestep.

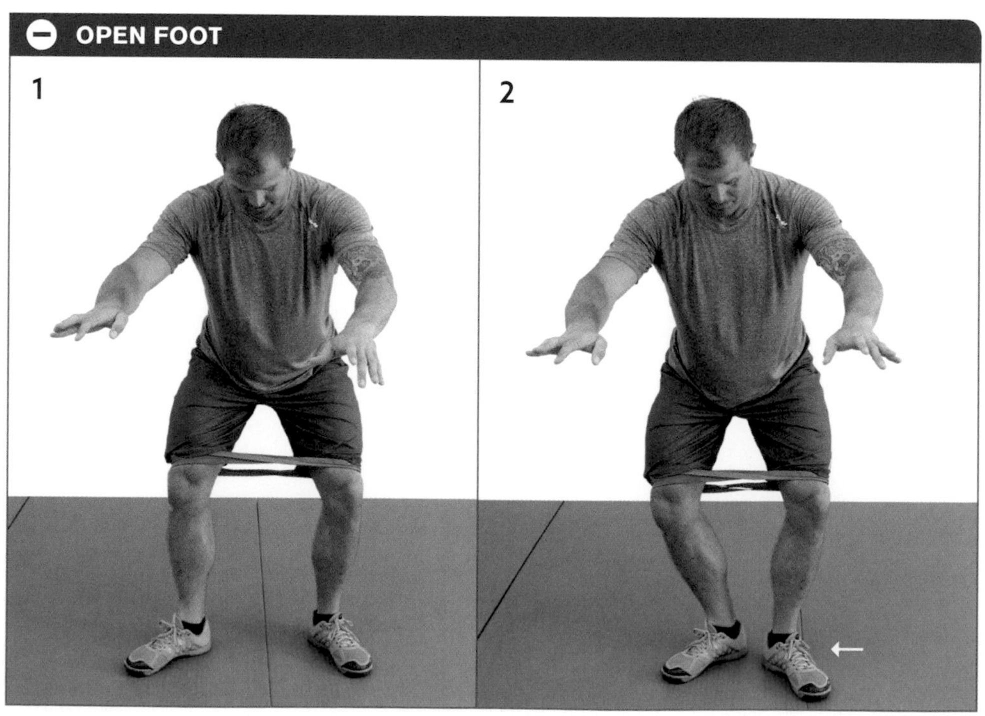

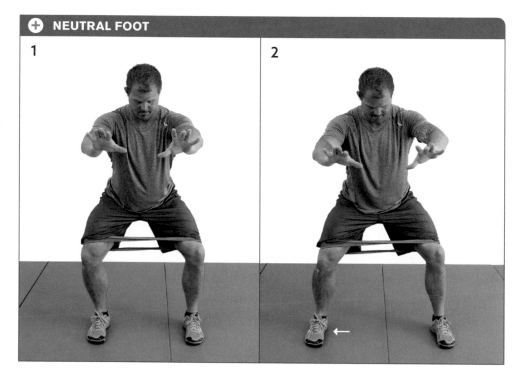

When you attempt this exercise with an open foot stance, you can't generate enough torque to drive your knees out. The band literally pulls your knees together. This makes it difficult to get into a stable position and maintain your balance as you sidestep.

Monster Squat Test

Squatting with a band wrapped around your knees is another illuminating exercise. Again, when your feet are straight, it's easier to generate torque and drive your knees out. The moment you adopt a duck-footed stance and squat, driving your knees out becomes a lot harder. It feels like a less stable, weaker position. And the band does a great job of highlighting that fact.

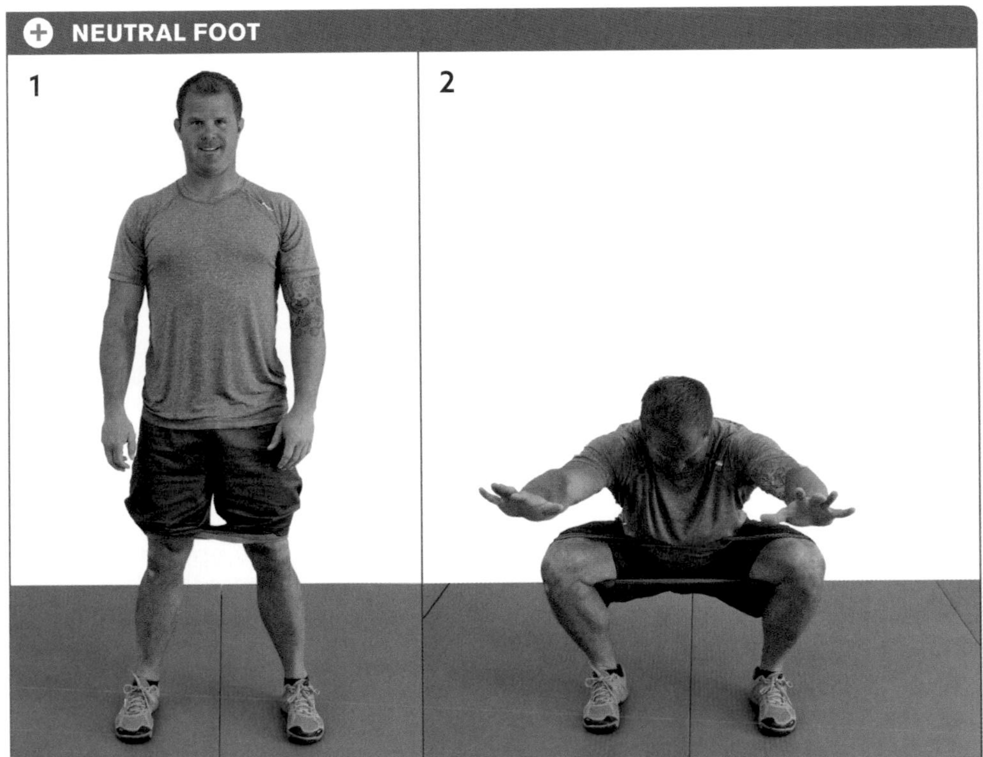

With your feet parallel, it's easier to counter the pressure of the band and squat in a good position.

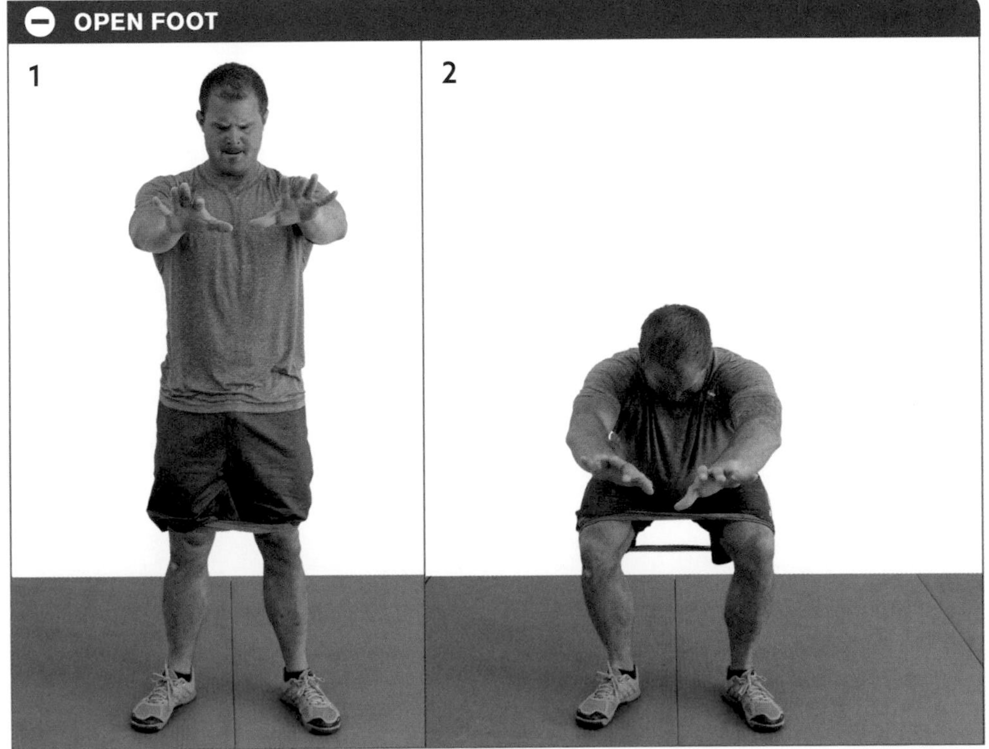

When you squat from an open-foot stance, you can't generate sufficient torque and drive your knees out to counter the band's resistance.

Stable Foot Position Test

This test helps illustrate that with your feet straight, you don't need to drive your knees out that far to achieve ankle stability. However, the more you turn your feet out, the farther out you have to drive your knees to achieve that natural arch and stable ankle position, which at a certain point becomes unattainable.

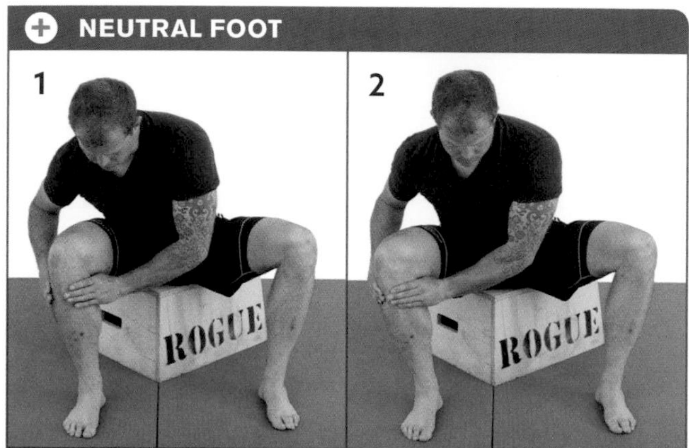

Place your foot in a neutral position and then drive your knee out. You have to push your knee out only slightly to create a natural arch.

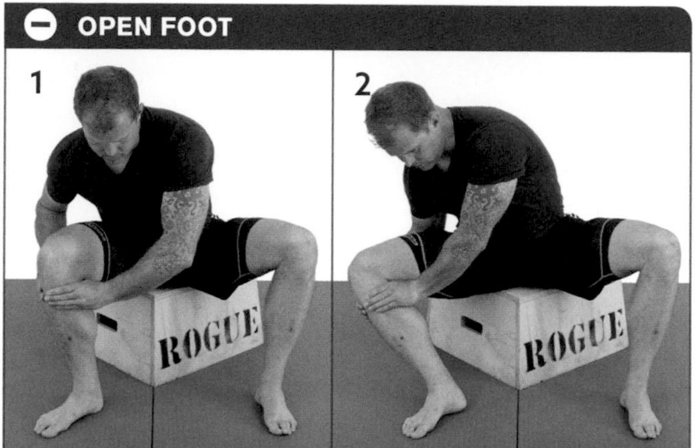

Now turn your foot out and drive your knee out until your foot comes into an arch. You have to drive your knee out a lot farther to achieve that arch.

External Rotation Test

This test illustrates the amount of external rotation that you can create at your hip with your feet parallel, as well as how limited the range of motion in your hip is with your feet turned out.

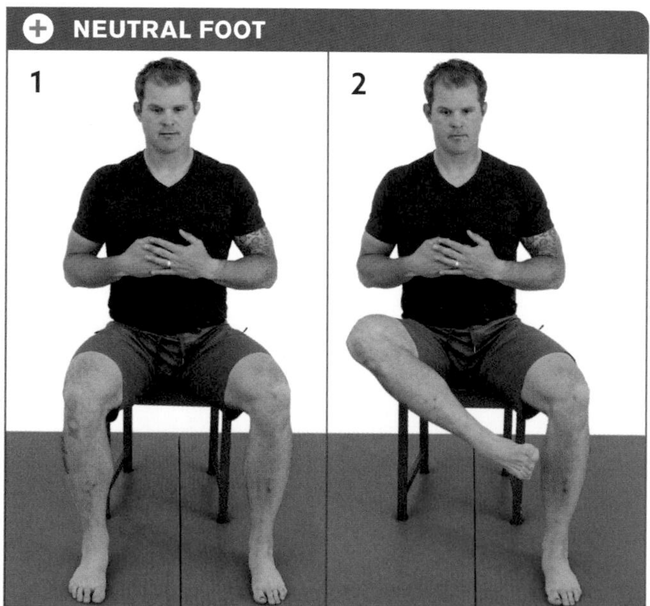

Sit in a chair, position your feet straight, and pull your foot toward your opposite hip. This is an expression of hip external rotation.

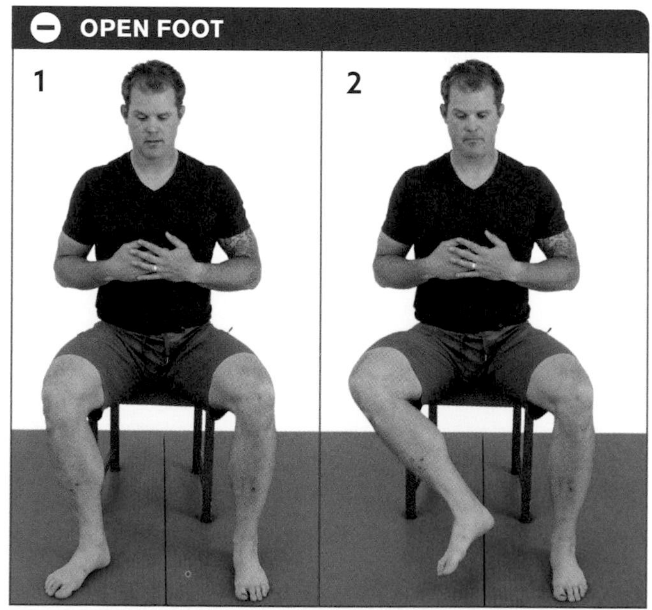

Now turn your foot out and do the same thing. You will find that you can't lift your foot as high or create as much external rotation at your hip.

Torqueless Squat Test (Ankle Collapse Test)

Keeping your feet straight limits end-range valgus collapse, while turning your feet out increases valgus collapse. In other words, when your feet are straight, you can prevent your knees from collapsing inward as you descend into the bottom of a squat much more effectively than when your feet are turned out.

You can test this in one of two ways: Either squat with your feet straight and then with them turned out without creating any torque, or sit on a chair and simply drive your knees inward with your feet straight and then again with your feet turned out. The latter test is much easier, but you should try both to see how they feel, and then imagine being in these positions under a heavy load or while sprinting down a field and then changing directions.

The bottom line is that you need to be able to survive a bad position in case the load is too heavy or you make a mechanical or motor control error. It happens. But if you're in a good position, you can at least mitigate the negative outcome.

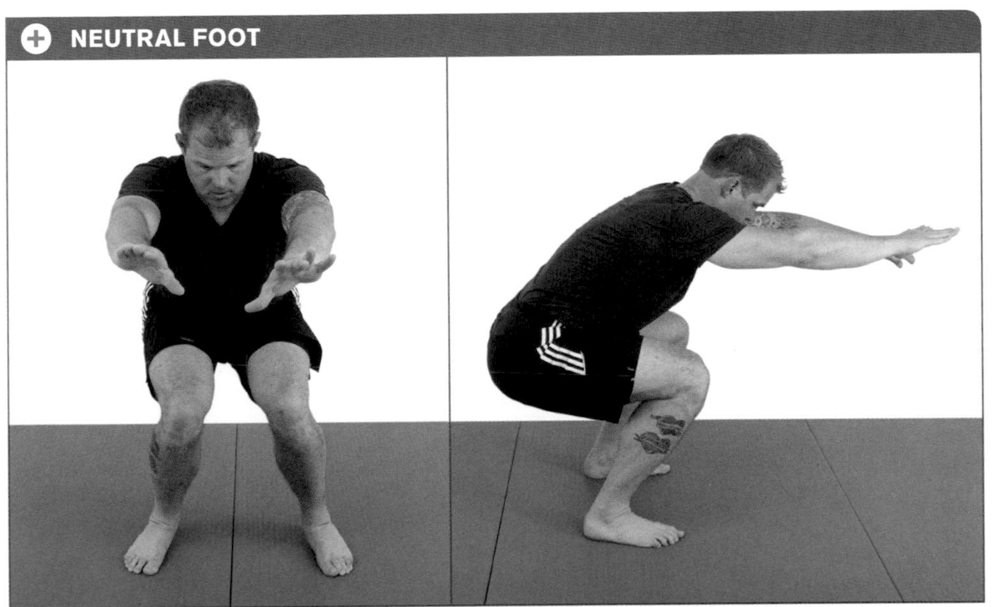

When your feet are straight, you can mitigate the valgus force on your ankles and knees when you fail to create torque during a squat. It's also easier to keep your shins vertical and maintain your balance because you have a larger base of support.

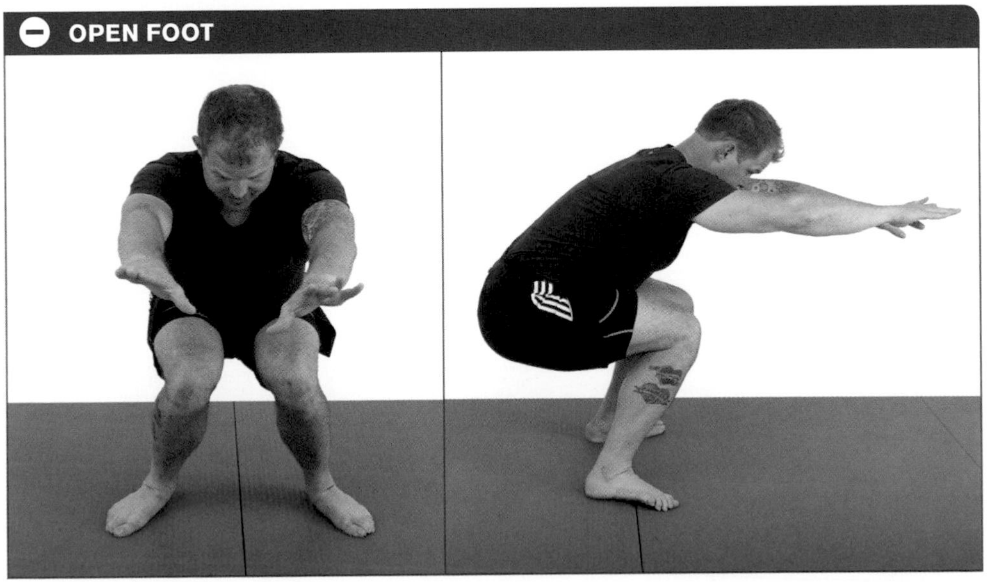

With your feet turned out, your ankles collapse to a much greater degree. Get into this position, and the sketchiness of this valgus force will become immediately apparent.

Ankle-Collapse Test

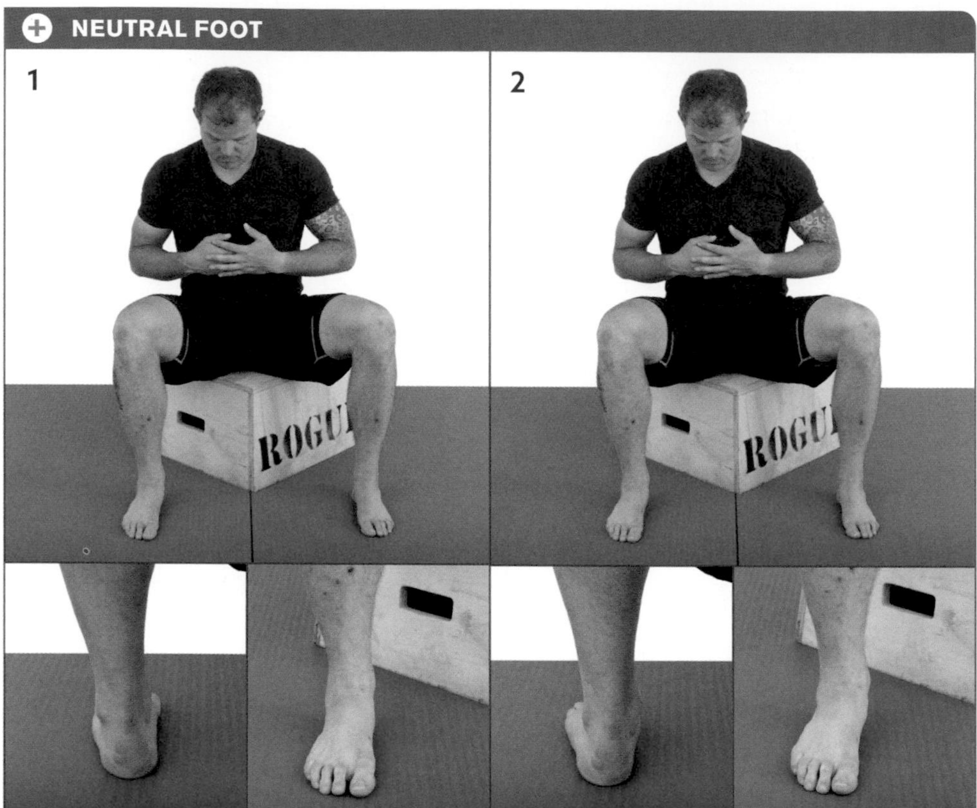

Sit on a box with your toes pointed forward and try to collapse your arches.

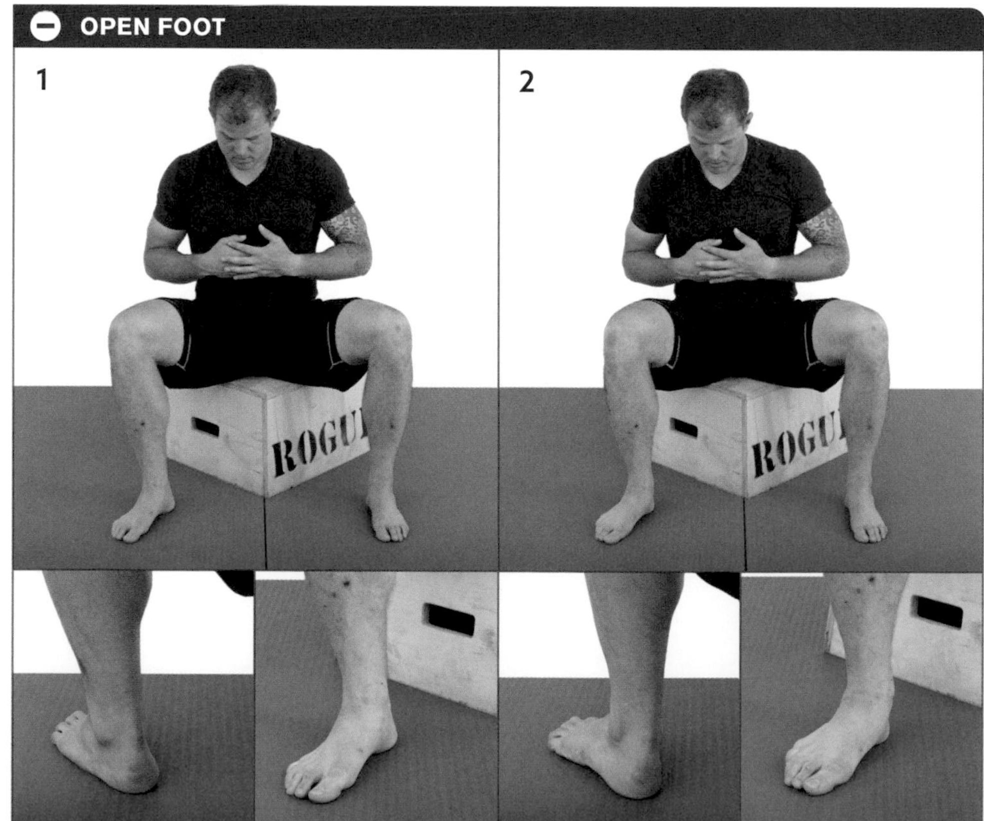

Now turn your foot out and collapse your arch. As you can see, it's a much more dramatic collapse.

Chapter Highlights

- *Torque,* as it's used in this book, describes the action of stabilizing your joints in a good position by creating a rotational force from your hips and shoulders.
- To make your joint stable, you need to rotate your limb into your hip or shoulder socket. This is how you generate torque: You externally or internally rotate from your hips or shoulders while keeping your hands or feet stationary (anchored to a surface or object such as the floor or a barbell).
- In order to stabilize your joints in a good position and preserve a braced neutral position, you need to create global stability. You do so by:
  - *Creating an organized, stable framework for your trunk (movement principle #1)*
  - *Initiating movement from your primary engines (movement principle #2)*
  - *Generating a torsion force through your extremities (movement principle #3)*
- Generating torque not only sets your joints in a good position, but also engages the surrounding musculature, which helps support and maintain optimal joint positioning. When you fail to create torque, you rely on your tendons and ligaments to support the position.
- If you don't create tension and stability in your hips and shoulders by generating torque, your body will find stability for you by defaulting into a bad position. This is called tension hunting.
- The two laws of torque provide a template for organizing and stabilizing your hips, shoulders, and other joints in good positions:

  Law #1: If your hips or shoulders are in flexion (which decreases the angle of the joint), you create an external rotation force (away from your body).

  Law #2: If your hips or shoulders are in extension (which opens the angle of the joint), you create an internal rotation force (toward the center of your body).
- To maintain a mechanically stable position during movement, you create just enough torque to match the demand of your position or movement. You need only enough rotation to combat the forces that are pulling you into a bad position.
- Hand and foot position dictate the amount of torque that you can generate. The more you turn your hands or feet away from your body, the less torque you can generate and the less stability you have.
- Adopting an open-foot stance during a squat not only diminishes your ability to generate torque, but also ingrains a dysfunctional pattern that carries over to other sports. Squat with an open-foot stance and chances are you will stand, walk, jump, land, and pivot with an open-foot stance.
- Positioning your hands and feet straight or turned out slightly—between 0 and 12 degrees—is ideal. Turning your hands or feet past 30 degrees will diminish your ability to generate torque, compromising your mechanics.
- The more parallel your feet and hands are, the more stable your position. You can turn your feet or hands out slightly and still create torque, but not as much.

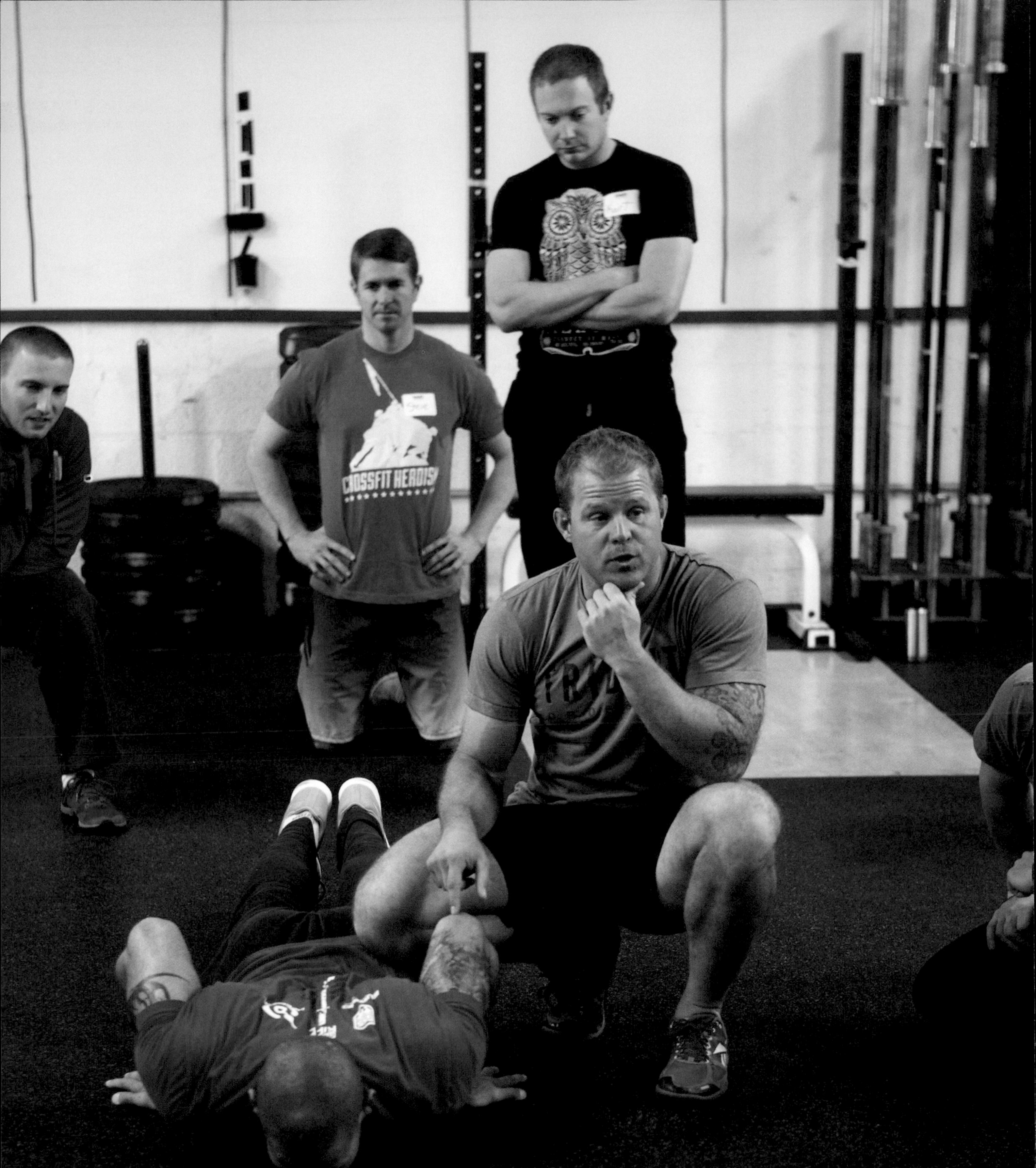

BODY ARCHETYPES AND THE TUNNEL

The functional positions for the hips and shoulders can be categorized into seven basic configurations: four for the shoulders and three for the hips. These seven body archetypes, which represent the start and finish positions for most exercise movements, encompass all the range of motion and motor control that you need to be a fully functional human being. Consider the body archetypes and the tunnel concept as a blueprint for assessing movement and positional competency and range of motion restrictions.

Although strength and conditioning movements function as diagnostic and evaluative tools (more on that in chapter 5, "Movement Hierarchy"), pinpointing mobility restrictions can be tricky, especially when you combine multiple movements into a high-intensity workout. In that situation, it's difficult to know whether you are missing range of motion or are faulting due to factors like speed, load, and fatigue. What's more, strength and conditioning movements are complex and technical. Performing them correctly—which I will show you how to do in part 2—requires a lot of skill and practice.

To make assessing and understanding range of motion easier, I created the body archetypes template, which categorizes components of movements into seven distinct shapes. These archetypes represent the safe, stable positions for the shoulders and hips and encompass the entire range of motion for nearly every movement. In this chapter, you'll learn about these basic body archetypes and how they can help you solve common errors related to motor control, biomechanics, and range of motion.

If you examine the illustrations on the next two pages, you'll notice that the shoulders and hips don't do that many things. Whether you're playing sports, lifting weights, or just going about your day, chances are you're adopting or expressing movement from one or more of these seven archetypal positions. If you can express competency in these positions, you have the building blocks to create safe, stable positions for most movements.

SHOULDER ARCHETYPES

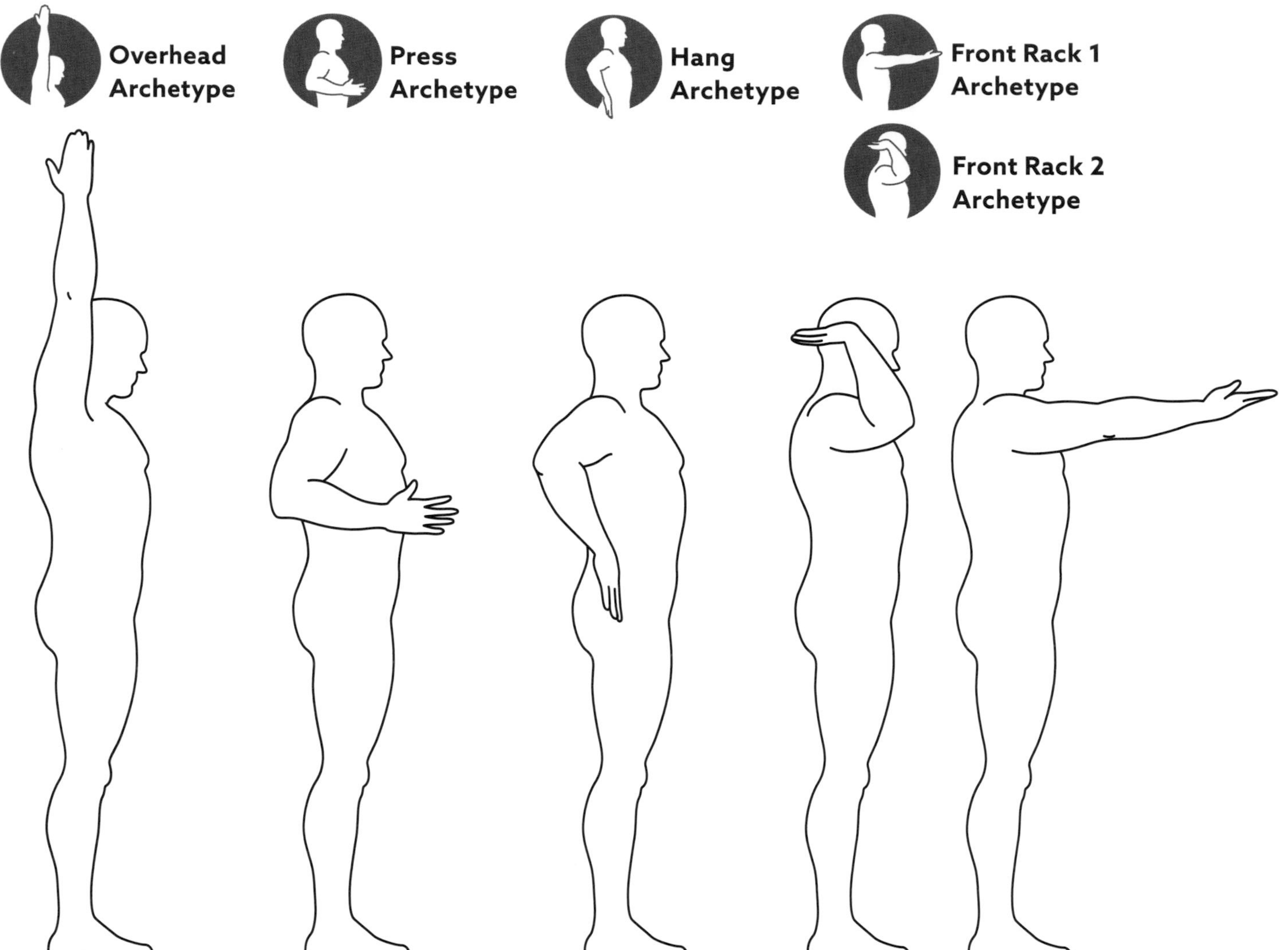

The overhead archetype encompasses all movements that require you to stabilize your arms over your head: strict press, snatch, hanging from a bar, throwing, etc.

Anytime you perform a pushup or bench press or reach your arm behind your body, you're stabilizing your shoulders in the press archetype.

Movements that require you to stabilize your shoulders with your arms at your sides fall into the hang archetype. This includes the setup for the deadlift and clean.

The front rack archetype captures the stable position for your shoulders when you're talking on the phone, carrying a load on your shoulder, or pushing or resisting a force with your arms extended out in front of your body. There are two basic shapes associated with this archetype: arms bent and arms extended straight out in front of you.

HIP ARCHETYPES

Squat 1 Archetype

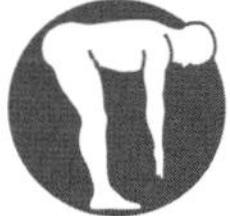

Squat 2 Archetype

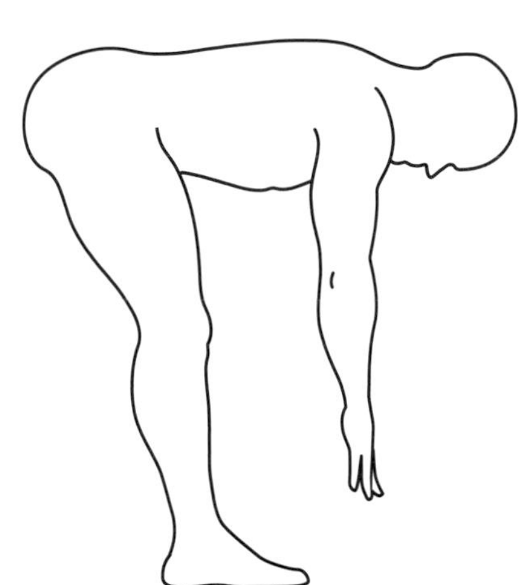

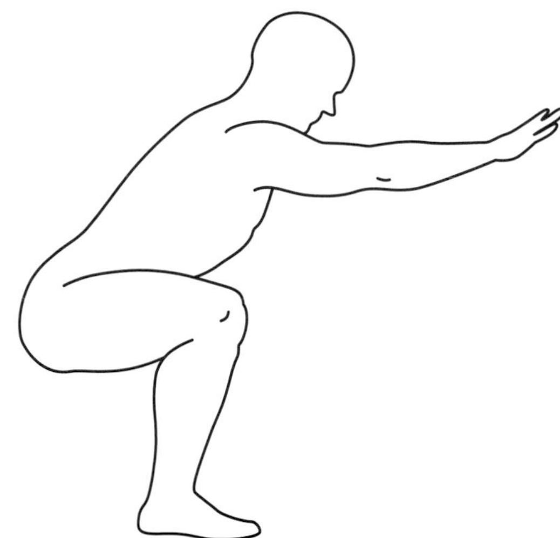

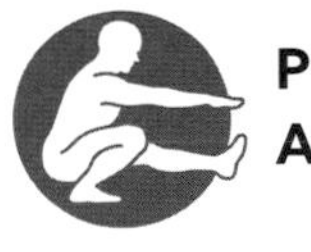

Pistol Archetype

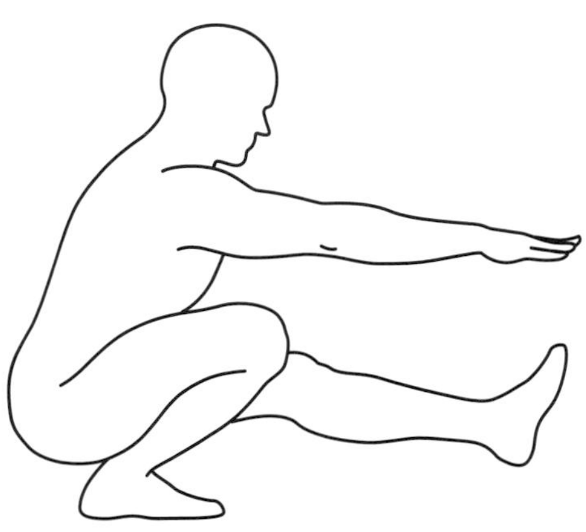

Lunge Archetype

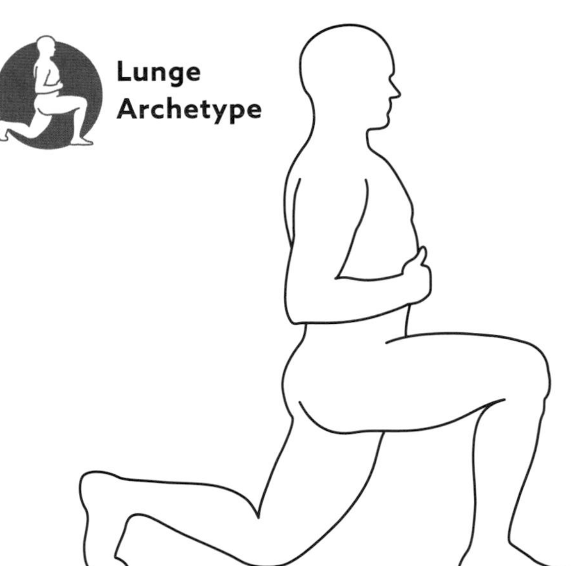

The squat archetype encompasses movements that require you to hinge from the hips, such as bending over to pick something up and squatting down to sit in a chair. There are two basic shapes associated with this archetype: the hips-below-knee-crease squat and the deadlift.

The pistol archetype captures full hip flexion and full ankle dorsiflexion range of motion. Getting up from a seated position and stepping up onto or lowering yourself down from an elevated platform are two common examples of this archetype in action.

The lunge archetype encompasses movements in which one leg is positioned behind your body, such as running, throwing, punching, and swinging.

These archetypal shapes serve another important purpose: They encompass the start and finish positions for the majority of movements performed in the gym. Just to be clear, "start" and "finish" always refer to the top or bottom positions of a movement.

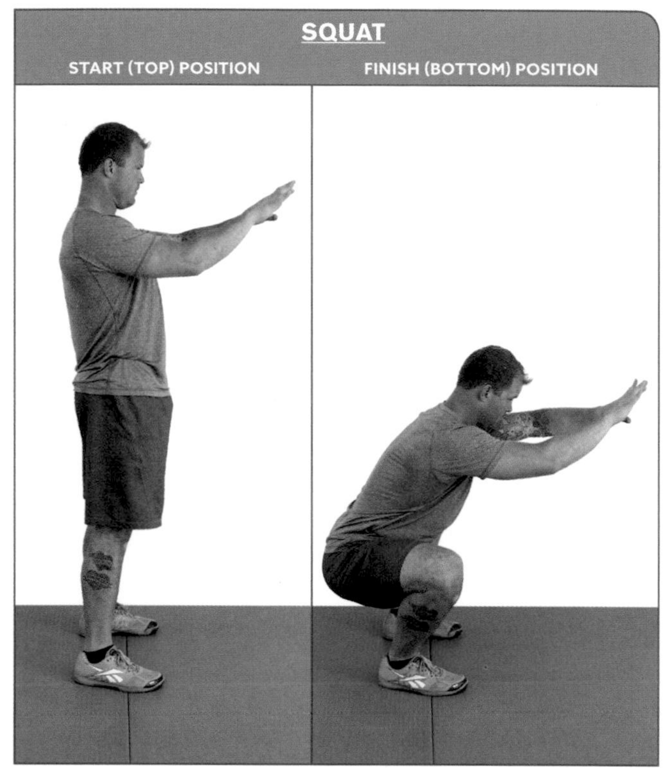

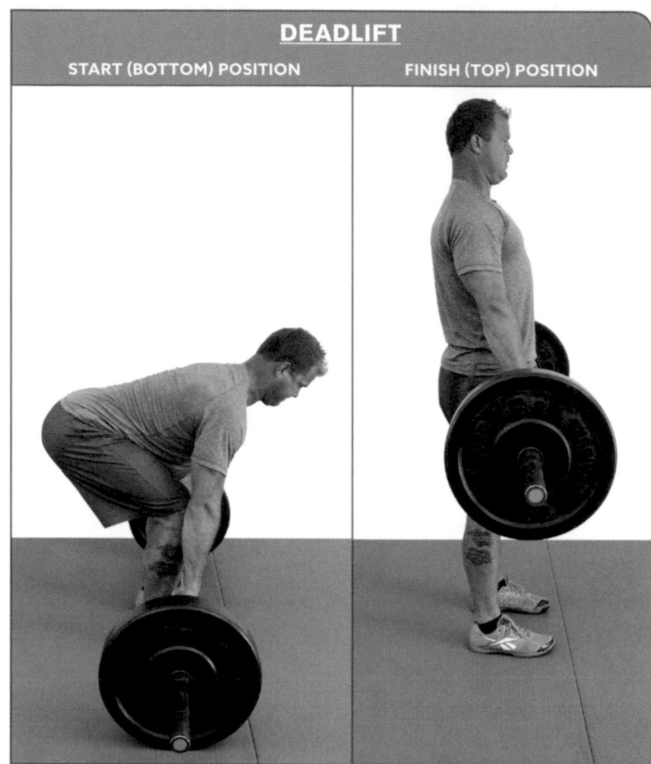

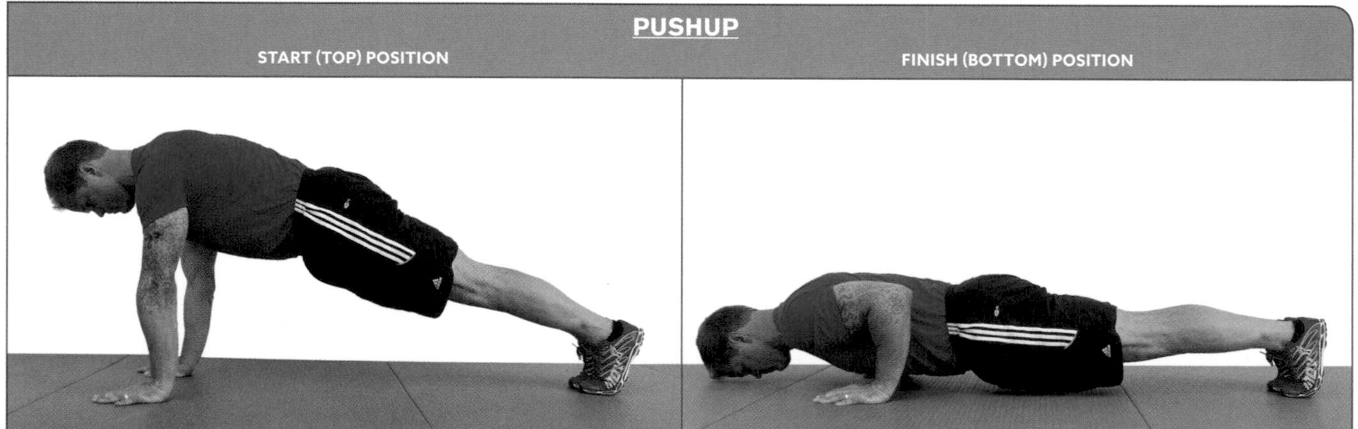

Viewing movement in this light—breaking it down into positional archetypes or start and finish positions—is useful for several reasons.

For starters, it helps shorten the learning curve for those who are new to strength and conditioning movements. Again, every exercise has one or more of the archetypes built into it: an overhead squat includes the overhead and squat archetypes, while a strict overhead press includes a front rack and overhead archetypes. If you understand each archetype, you have a template for starting and finishing every movement in an optimal position. The interconnectivity of human movement also becomes much easier to see, because all you're doing is transitioning from one archetypal shape to another. As stated earlier, performing a movement correctly requires a ton of practice, but simply knowing how and where you need to start and finish will accelerate the learning process because you have only seven positions to learn and memorize.

Think about it like this: Your front rack position for the front squat should look like your receiving position for the clean. Whether you're front squatting or power cleaning, you want to practice the same patterns and skills for the same archetypal shape. Conversely, you want to be very careful not to create wrong patterns for the same archetype. For example, pulling with a rounded back when you deadlift increases the chance that you will pull with a rounded back when you clean or when you pick up a bag of groceries. Doing pushups with your shoulders rounded forward increases the chance that you will bench press or push a car with rounded shoulders. In a nutshell, having flaws with an archetype in one exercise increases your chance of injury while performing not only that particular exercise, but also every other movement that involves that archetype. Performing an archetype correctly every time will help ensure that when you add a new movement with the same archetype, you will perform it correctly. This concept is called the "one-pattern."

The body archetypes template is also a great way to test technique and evaluate range of motion. At the end of this chapter, you'll find quick tests for each archetypal shape. These simple tests allow you to assess range of motion and positional competency from a static position with minimal movement variables and low strength demands, which is much safer and in some cases more accurate than trying to diagnose mobility issues that occur during a workout or when movements are performed with speed. This is particularly helpful when it comes to assessing range of motion, because there are two components that you always have to consider: the rotational element and the flexion/extension element. The static quick tests will help you differentiate between rotational limitations and flexion/extension restrictions.

Finally, breaking movement down into archetypes and performing the quick tests will help you determine which joint(s), muscle(s), or position(s) you need to mobilize. For example, say you attempt the pistol quick test on page 112 and fall on your butt. This is a pretty clear indication that you're missing ankle (dorsiflexion) range of motion. Fortunately, it's easy to perform mobilization techniques that will improve dorsiflexion. All you have to do is choose techniques that focus on the restricted area and/or position, in this case the ankle and the pistol shape.

The body archetypes add another layer of detail to the language of human movement, because now you can talk about movement within the context of start and finish positions. Without a knowledge of archetypes, you might know simply that you experience pain while bench pressing or doing pushups. However, knowing that the start and finish positions of both exercises involve two particular archetypes, you can isolate the pain to either the push archetype (finish) or the front rack archetype (start), and then use parts 3 and 4 of this book to begin piecing together a prescription. To help with this, I have included archetype icons next to many of the mobilization techniques described in part 3. If you see a pressing icon, for example, you will know that the technique helps with the pressing archetype. If you see a front rack icon, you will know that the technique helps improve the front rack archetype.

In summary, categorizing strength and conditioning movements into start and finish position archetypes shortens the learning curve for novices and, more important, provides a template for assessing movement quality and identifying mobility restrictions. At the end of this chapter, I elaborate on each archetype, detailing the correct mechanics and common faults, as well as provide quick tests so that you can assess your range of motion and motor control for each archetypal position. But before I do that, it's important to address a conceptual tool that I call the tunnel. The tunnel concept brings intention and purpose to the movement principles and works in conjunction with the body archetypes template to help you identify, diagnose, and correct movement and mobility problems.

The Tunnel Concept

Having a tunnel mindset means understanding that you have to start a movement (enter the tunnel) in a good position in order to finish the movement (exit the tunnel) in a good position. If you don't start right, you won't finish right. And if you don't finish right, your next position will be compromised.

Here's why: Once you are under load or have to bring speed or tension to the equation, it's difficult to organize yourself into a good position. Let's say, for example, that you load a barbell onto your shoulders to perform a back squat but fail to brace your spine in a neutral position before taking the weight out of the rack. With the weight compressing your spine, it's much harder to organize your trunk in a braced neutral position.

This is why it's so important to prioritize your setup *before* you start moving. Again, the position in which you enter the tunnel (start a movement) dictates how you will exit the tunnel (finish the movement). If you take the time to get yourself organized—brace your spine in a neutral position, hinge from your hips and shoulders, and create torque—chances are good that you will enter and exit the tunnel in a good position. But if you enter the tunnel in a bad position, you have only two options: continue moving in a compromised way or restart the movement in a good position.

Identifying the Problem

The tunnel concept forces you to begin your movement assessment with your start position and make sure that you are setting up correctly. When I evaluate an athlete's movement, I always look at his start position first, because I recognize that a poor setup can contribute to faults in the finish position. In fact, what often looks like a finish position problem is more often than not a start position error.

Here's an example to help illustrate this point. A while back, I worked with a champion Olympic lifter who was having a hard time locking out his arms in the snatch. His coach had implemented a slew of drills to help with his finish position, but nothing seemed to work. It turned out that he was missing shoulder internal rotation, which caused his shoulders to round forward during the pull (the early phase of the lift). This is why he was having such a hard time stabilizing his shoulders and locking out his arms overhead. He was entering the tunnel in a bad position, which predisposed him to a bad finish. As I've said before: Start out in a compromised position, finish in a compromised position. I cleaned up his shoulders and restored normal range to the tissues that were restricting the joints, and the problem with his finish position vanished. He could have done a million drills to improve his lockout without ever getting to the root of the issue.

The point is that a lot of athletes and coaches mistakenly focus on drills aimed at improving the finish position when the real problem is the start. So if you are having trouble completing a movement, immediately assess your setup (start position) and make sure that you're not making a motor control error or missing key ranges of motion. In the same sense, if your setup is good but you are still having problems with the finish, chances are excellent that it is a mobility issue.

As you start putting together mobility prescriptions, use the body archetypes template in conjunction with the tunnel concept to help focus your time on the areas requiring the most attention. Remember, these are merely tools that force you to evaluate your position from both sides of a movement. In fact, the start and finish are the places to begin your diagnosis when you are deconstructing a movement problem using the body archetypes template.

Let's say that you lose your balance and can't maintain a good position when you perform the pistol archetype quick test. Unless you can't fully extend your hips, you can rule out the start position as the limiting factor. The next step is to see if you can get into a good finish position, which is the bottom of the pistol (squat). You don't even have to perform the movement; you just have to squat down and extend your leg out in front of your body. If you fall over or can't get into a stable, well-organized finish position, you know that your ankles are tight (among other things). Now you can focus on mobilizations that target your position(s) of restriction.

The Finish Position Error

The tunnel concept also gives you a template for evaluating circular or repetitive movements like running and swimming. Consider a runner who is having problems with her landing—her foot contacting the ground. Her coach might prescribe any number of running techniques and motor control drills to improve her foot position. And these drills might work for the initial foot contact. But if the athlete is missing range of motion in her anterior hip, or her calf or ankle is super-tight, her leg will externally rotate into an unstable position. (This is an example of the second law of torque, page 73.) She may be able to keep her foot straight at the start, but as her leg swings behind her and externally rotates, she lands with an open foot. She enters a brand-new tunnel from a compromised position. In this scenario, it's not a start position problem; it's a finish position problem. The finish position—leg swinging back—dictates how well the athlete will start her next stride and enter the next tunnel of movement.

Here's what this means for you: Your finish position dictates your ability to transition into the next rep, which is your new start position. And this is true of all transitory movements—whether you're jumping, landing, and then cutting, or transitioning from one position to the next: If you exit a tunnel of movement in a bad position, you will enter the next tunnel in a compromised position.

Another fault worth mentioning is not hitting the finish position of a movement. When performing multiple repetitions at high intensity, people tend to cut the movement short by stopping just shy of the finish position. For example, say you're performing push-presses at high speed. If you're being rewarded based on speed and number of repetitions, you might fail to lock out your arms overhead at the end of a repetition, compromising the start position for your next repetition.

You can't just tune out and do the work. Sport, combat, and life don't work like that. You have to train smart and hard, with consciousness. This is what training is for. Resolve now to change your criteria from quantity to quality and judge your movement based on form, not on how many repetitions you can complete.

Archetype Quick Tests

In this section, I explain the seven body archetypes and demonstrate the common faults associated with each shape. I also include two types of quick tests that you can use to assess your range of motion. The first is done without weight or equipment and can be used to safely and quickly assess range of motion. The problem is, it doesn't tell you anything about your motor control or your ability to get into a stable position. This is why I've included a second, loaded quick test. These tests are performed under load (with weight) or resistance, or in a position that increases the difficulty. The idea is to use the basic quick test to assess range of motion and then use the loaded quick test to more accurately evaluate range of motion and motor control.

Here's an example to help illustrate how this works. Say you're testing the overhead archetype. Start by trying to get into the position as demonstrated in the photos: Lock out your arms overhead while keeping your spine neutral and your shoulders externally rotated. If you pass the basic quick test—meaning that you can get into the position as described and demonstrated—the next step is to challenge the position with one of the loaded quick tests by hanging from a bar or holding a dumbbell or kettlebell overhead.

In short, use the basic quick test to see if you can get into a good position. If you pass that test, challenge the position with load or resistance. If you're unable to get into a good position due to a joint restriction or you exhibit one of the common faults, flip to the body archetypes mobility prescriptions in part 4. There you will find a list of mobilization techniques that you can use to reclaim the range of motion required to get into each of the seven body archetypes.

Although the quick tests serve an important function, they are not definitive. While they will illuminate common movement faults, they function primarily as tools for detecting and correcting range of motion restrictions and teaching basic positioning. You may pass the pistol basic quick test, which suggests that you have full ankle range of motion, but this doesn't tell you anything about your strength or your ability to move into or from that position. The bottom line is this: To build efficient movement patterns, you need to practice moving from archetype to archetype, which is just another way of saying that you need to perform actual movements—which I will show you how to do in the pages to come. Think of the quick tests as clinical guidelines for understanding hip and shoulder positioning and function. If you don't pass the quick tests, ask yourself, "What's the problem—and how do I fix it?"

When I implement these quick tests in the gym, I make sure that the athlete adheres to the movement principles (midline stability and torque) and doesn't experience pain in the position. If he commits one of the common faults, I know that one of two things is likely causing the error: Either he doesn't understand how to perform the technique properly (motor control), or he doesn't have the range of motion to get into a good position. In some cases, it's a combination of both.

In part 2, I highlight common faults associated with specific training movements. As you will see, the faults associated with each archetype are the same faults that occur when you express that archetype during movement. For example, if your elbows fly out and your shoulders roll forward during the press archetype quick test, you can bet that the same unstable shoulder position will rear its ugly head when you perform actual pressing movements, like the bench press or pushup. I recommend that you use the quick tests to highlight these faults so that when you start applying the movement principles to strength and conditioning exercises and developing a well-balanced program, you already know which positions you need to work on and which areas you need to mobilize.

With this information in hand, you can start using the movement hierarchy (explained in chapter 5)—which is a method for categorizing exercise movements based on stabilization demands and movement complexity—to further test motor control competency and build efficient, transferable movement patterns.

It's important to note that in part 2, I offer tips for correcting faults from a motor control perspective. If you can't get into certain body archetypes because you are missing range of motion, turn to the body archetypes mobility prescriptions in part 4.

SHOULDER ARCHETYPES

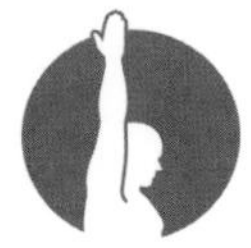

Overhead

Common examples:
Reaching/pressing overhead, hanging, throwing

Start position examples:
Pull-up, muscle-up

Finish position examples:
Strict press, push-press, snatch balance, overhead squat, snatch, jerk

The overhead archetype is an expression of full flexion and external rotation of the shoulders, which encompasses any position or movement that requires you to stabilize your arms over your head. Common examples are pressing or reaching overhead, hanging, and overhead throwing movements.

The truest expression of overhead competency is holding a dumbbell or kettlebell overhead. This not only highlights overhead range of motion, but also tests motor control to a higher degree. Why, you might ask? You're not creating torque off a fixed object, so you have to find the stability through external rotation, which is purely motor control. There's no hiding your dysfunction.

Hanging from a bar is another great way to test overhead range of motion. In fact, hanging from a bar with a chin-up grip (palms facing toward your body) is one of the easiest ways to test overhead range of motion because it automatically winds your shoulders into an externally rotated position. If you see any common faults, you can assume that you're missing shoulder external rotation and flexion.

Basic Quick Test

Keeping your spine neutral, raise your arms overhead. Your ears should be visible from the side, your elbows straight, and your shoulders externally rotated. To cue shoulder external rotation, point your thumbs back and get your armpits forward.

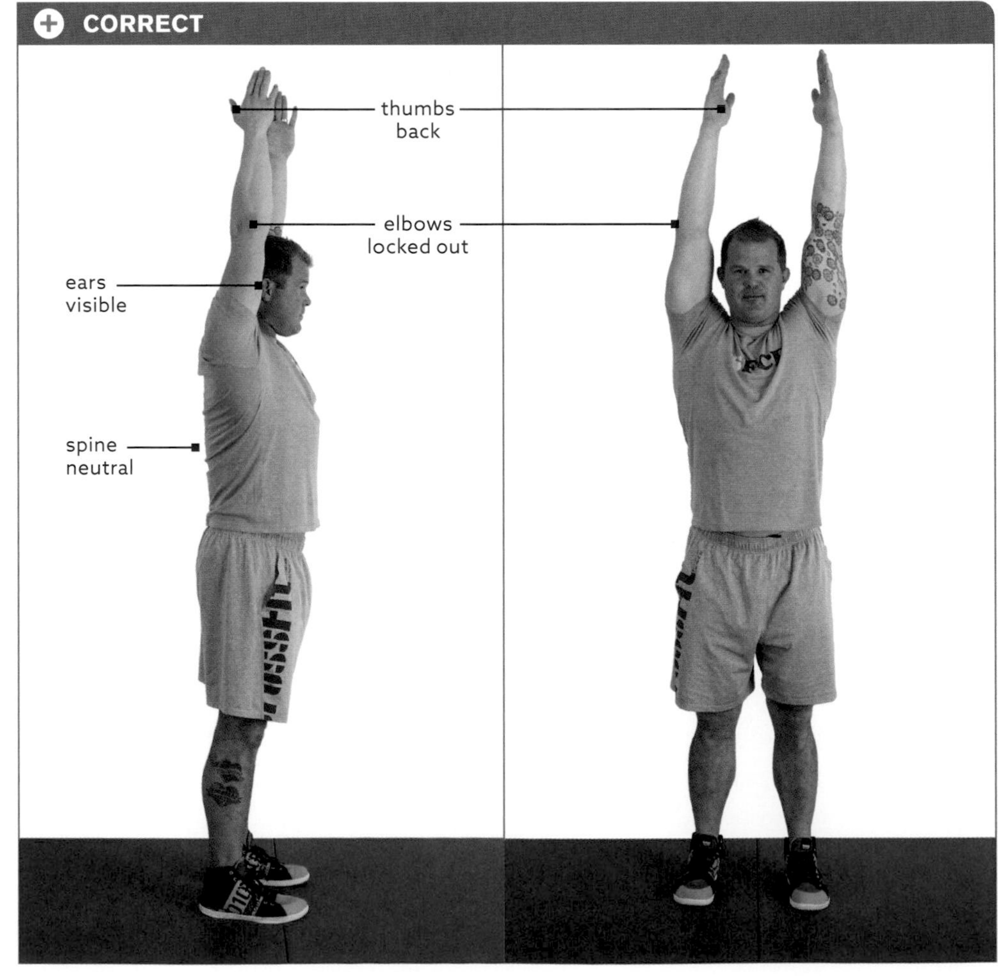

COMMON FAULTS

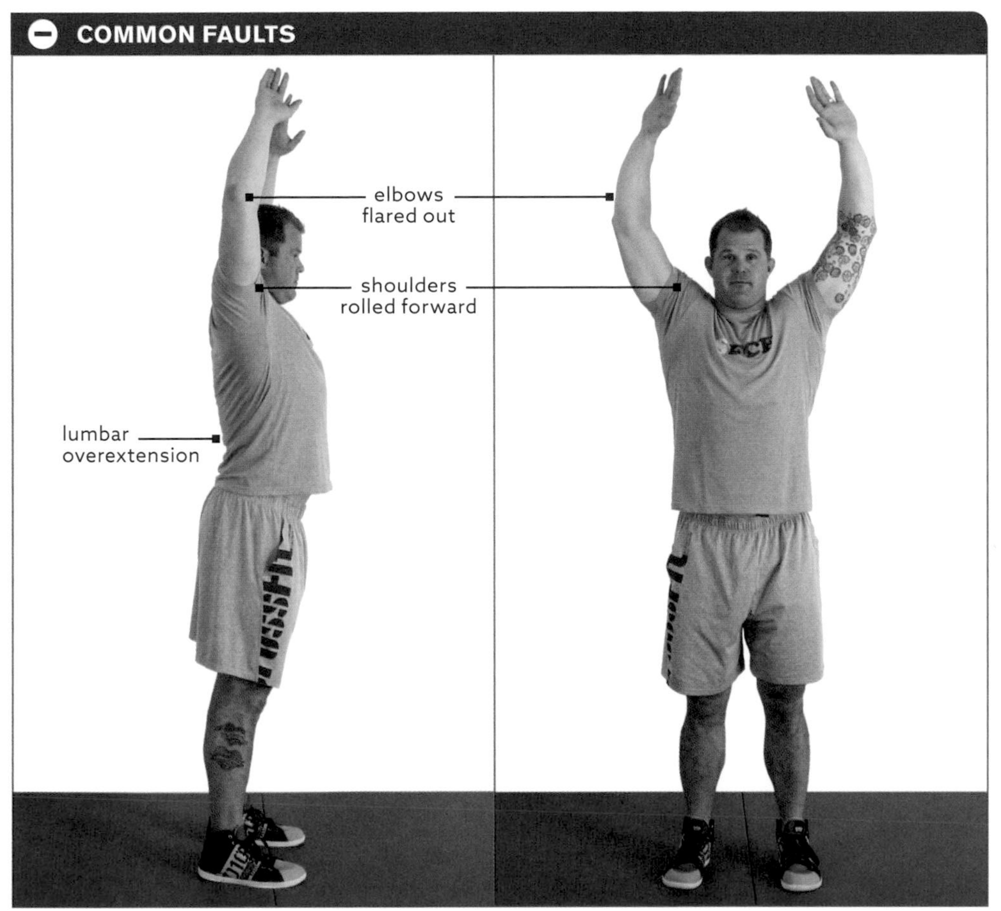

If you're missing shoulder range of motion or you fail to brace your spine, you may overextend by tilting your ribcage back and your pelvis forward. If your triceps are stiff, locking out your elbows is difficult. Missing shoulder rotation range of motion is expressed by rolling the shoulders forward and flaring the elbows out.

Loaded Quick Tests

DUMBBELL OVERHEAD TEST

OVERHEAD TEST

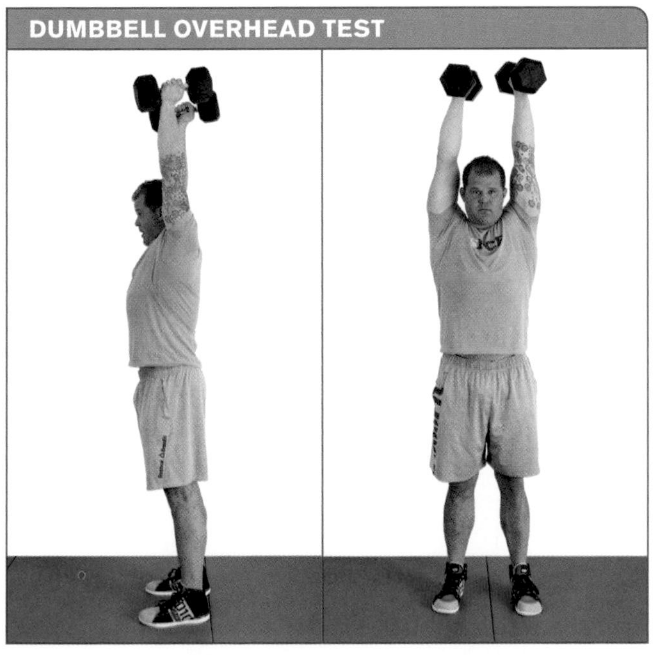

HANG TEST (chin-up grip and pull-up grip)

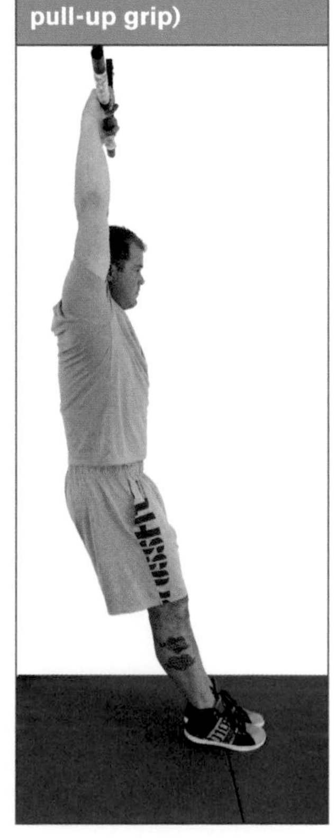

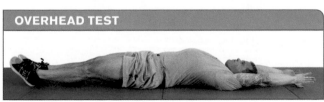

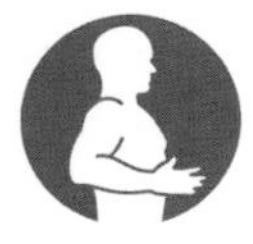

Press

Common examples:
Reaching behind your body, jumping, getting up off the ground from your belly

Start position example:
Burpee

Finish position examples:
Pushup, bench press, dip, row

The press archetype looks like the bottom of a pushup, bench press, dip, or burpee. The idea is to position yourself in the bottom of a pushup or, even better, the bottom of a dip, without letting your shoulders roll forward or your elbows flare out to the sides. This is a great way to test stabilization for the shoulders when your arms move behind your body, which is expressed by internal rotation and extension.

Realize that in all movements that involve shoulder extension (arms behind the back), internal rotation plays a huge role. Having internal rotational capacity is what enables you to keep your shoulders pulled back and externally rotated into a stable position. An example is when people run with their elbows flared out and their hands crossing their body from side to side instead of moving from front to back. That's a dead giveaway that they're missing extension and internal rotation, which is the stable shoulder position.

Remember, you need total capsular range of motion (internal and external rotational capacity) in order to move like a normal human. If you're missing shoulder internal rotation range of motion, you will end up internally rotated—in the dreaded rolled-forward shoulder position that we're always trying to avoid.

When it comes to exercise movements, the press archetype is primarily a finish position (think about the bottom position of a pushup or bench press). The only time it comes into play in the middle of a movement is during a burpee, when you sprawl your hips and chest to the ground. The press archetype is expressed as a start position anytime you get up off the ground from your belly (think surfing). It is also a common start position in close-quarter contact sports, like wrestling, jiu-jitsu, and football.

Basic Quick Test

From a braced neutral stance, draw your elbows behind your body while keeping your forearms parallel to the ground. Keep your shoulders in a stable position and your elbows aligned with your wrists.

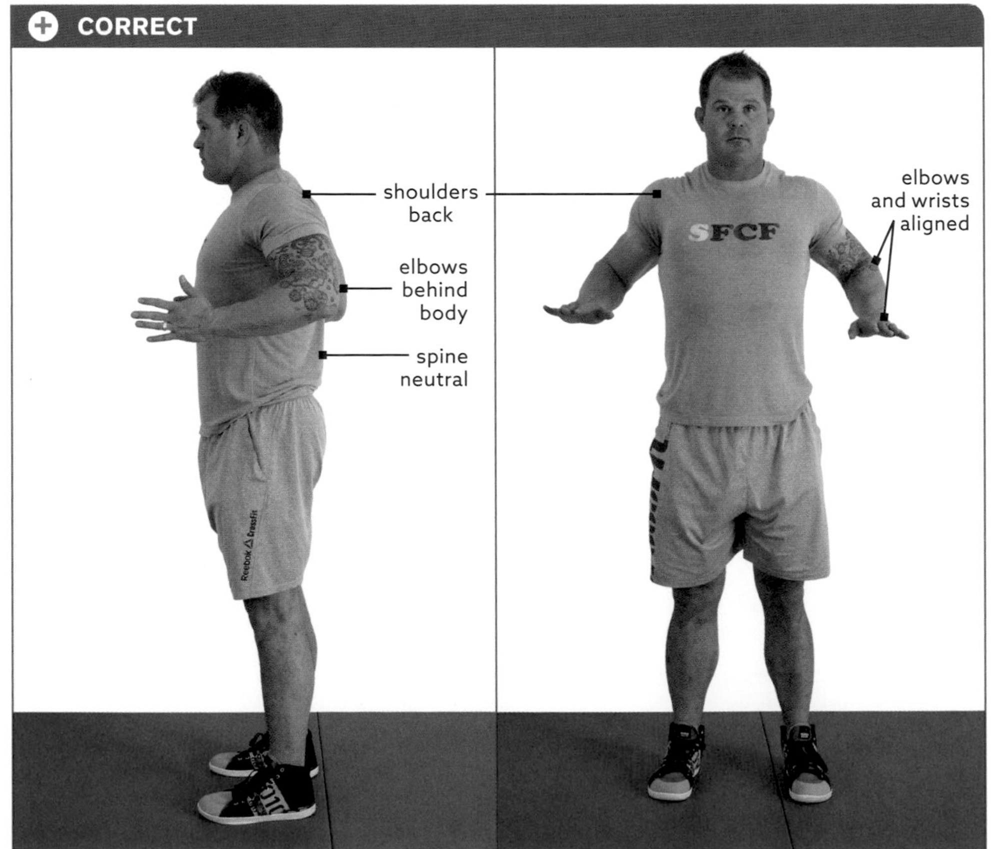

COMMON FAULTS

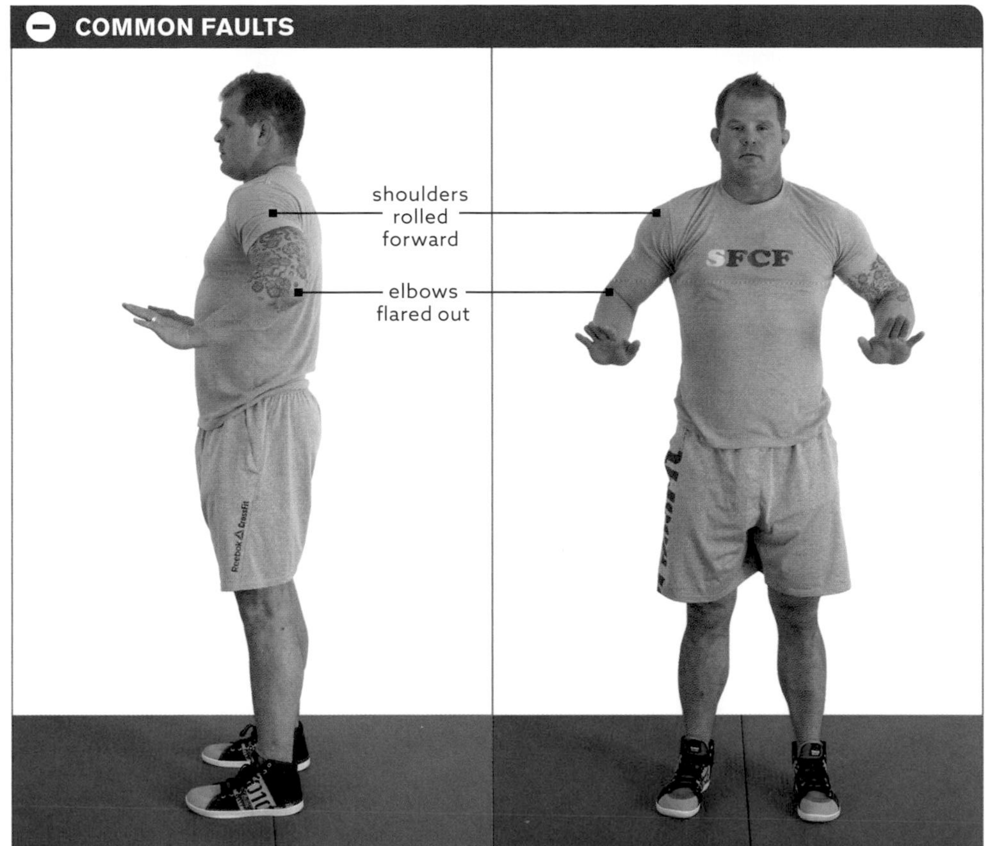

If your shoulders roll forward, your elbows flare out, or you can't get your elbows behind your body, it is an indication that you are missing shoulder extension.

Loaded Quick Tests

PUSHUP TEST

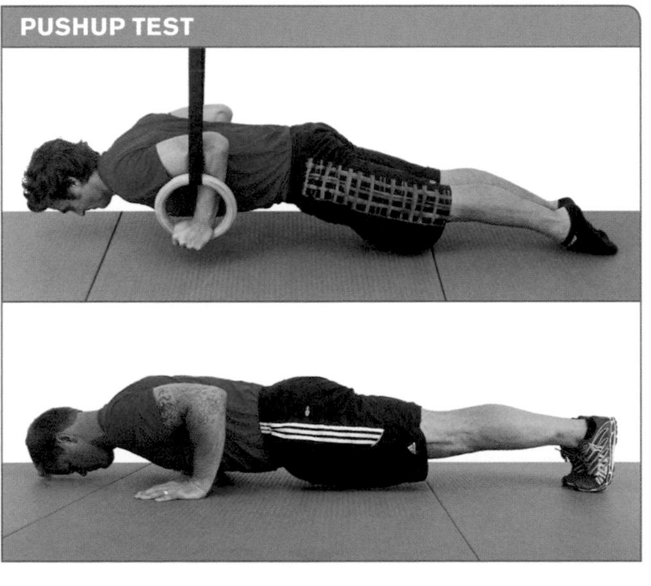

DIP TEST

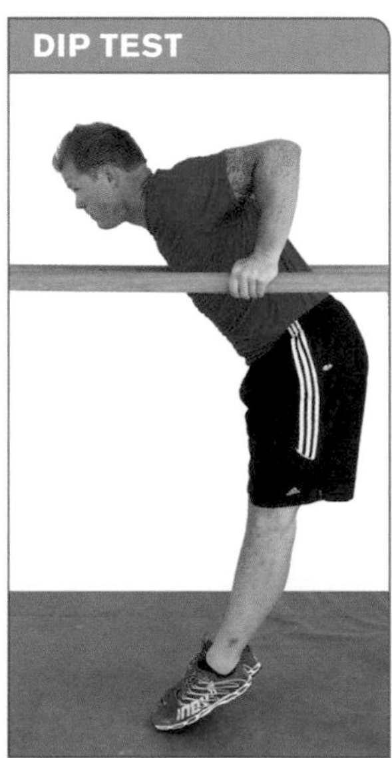

PLANCHE TEST

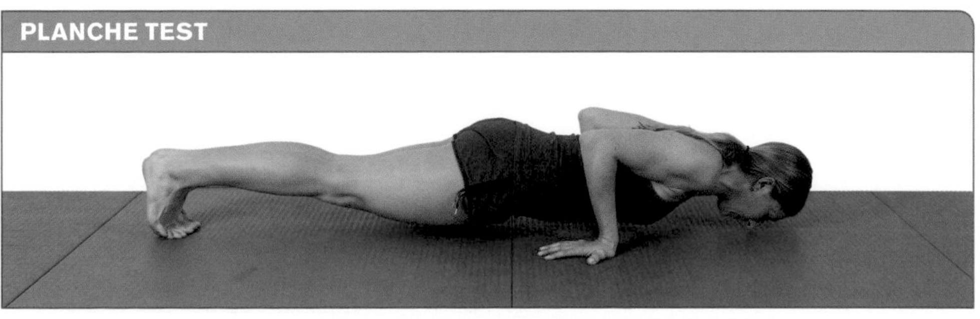

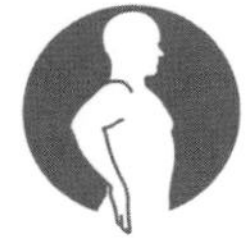

Hang

Common examples:
Standing with your hands at your sides or in your pockets, carrying something at your side or behind your back

Start position examples:
Setup position for the deadlift, clean, and snatch

Finish position example:
Deadlift

Basic Quick Test

With your arms hanging at your sides, externally rotate your shoulders and then elevate your elbows. The goal is to position your wrists behind your torso and lift your elbows up to chest level. Don't cheat by shrugging or tilting your ribcage back. Keep your shoulders and spine neutral.

The hang shoulder archetype encompasses all movements and positions for your shoulders when your arms are down by your sides. This includes the resting position for your shoulders when your arms are hanging at your sides; the setup position for pulling movements like the deadlift, clean, and snatch; and the finish position for most throwing movements (think pitching). You see this archetype during the pull phase in swimming and during the secondary pull phase of Olympic lifts—it is the transitory position that occurs when you go from the pulling phase (pulling the bar upward) to the receiving phase (dropping underneath the bar to receive the weight).

As with the other shoulder archetypes, the goal is to keep your shoulders externally rotated in a stable position: If you're missing internal rotation, your shoulders will compensate forward.

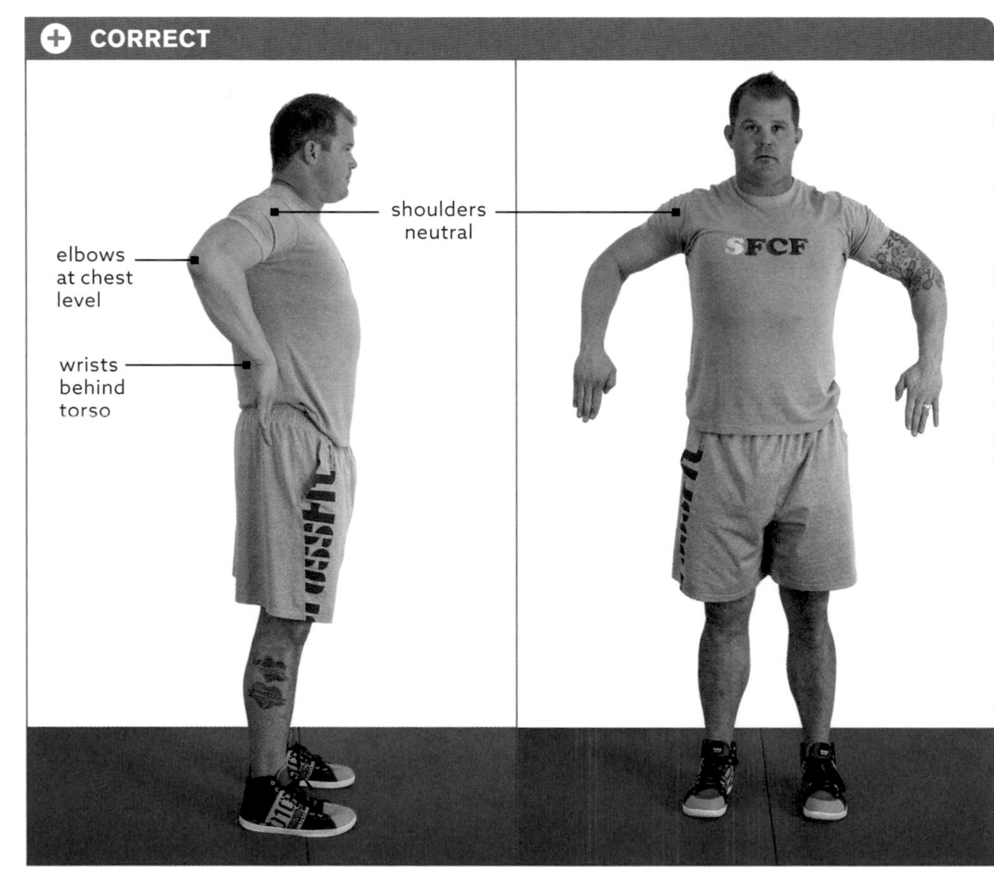

COMMON FAULTS

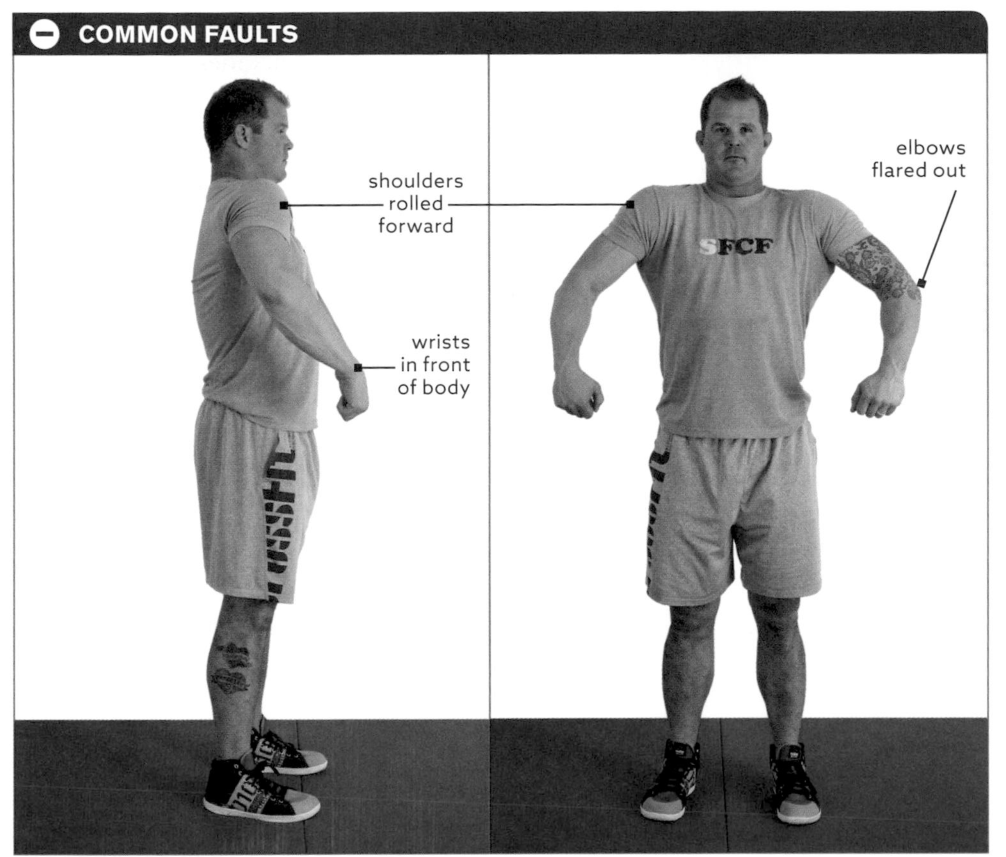

If you're missing range of motion, your shoulders will compensate forward and your elbows will flare out. If you can't elevate your elbows or get your wrists behind your torso, it is an indication that you're missing shoulder internal rotation.

Loaded Quick Tests

HIGH PULL TEST

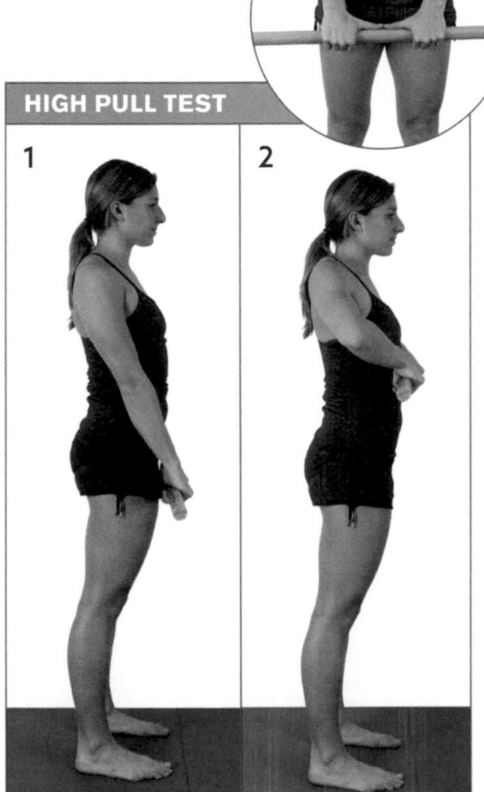

BEHIND THE BACK TEST

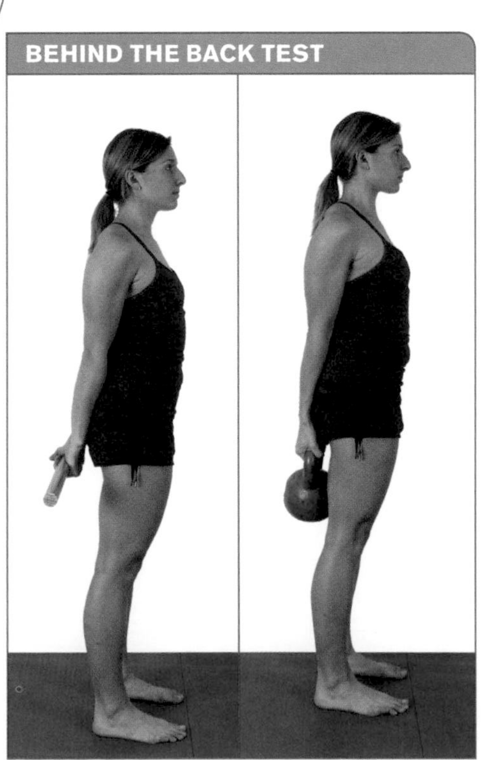

DUMBBELL CARRY TEST

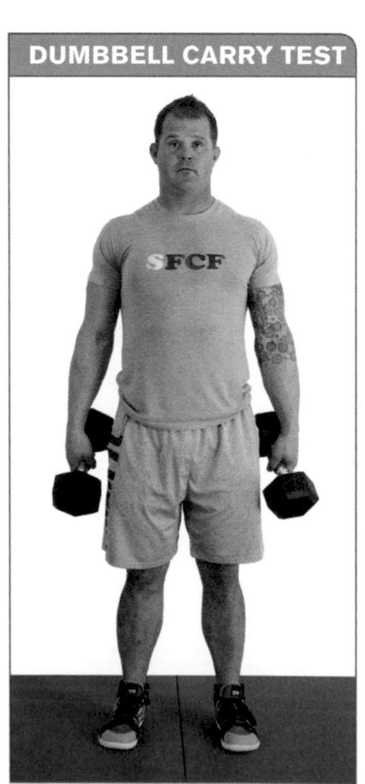

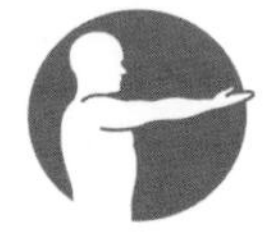

Front Rack

Common examples:
Pushing or resisting a force with your arms extended in front of your body, talking on the phone, holding a large object at chest level, carrying something on your shoulder

Start position examples:
Front squat, strict press, push-press

Finish position examples:
Clean, pull-up

There are two shapes associated with the front rack archetype:

1. Arms extended straight out in front of you (Front Rack 1)
2. Arms bent (Front Rack 2)

Front Rack 1 captures the stable position for your shoulders when you're pushing or pulling with your arms extended out in front of your body. Front Rack 2 captures the stable position for your shoulders when you're carrying a load on your shoulders, holding something at chest level, or talking on the phone. The front rack archetype is also buried in a lot of gym-based movements. You start in Front Rack 1 when you set up for the pushup and bench press. You come into Front Rack 2 as the start position for the front squat and overhead press and the finish position for the pull-up and clean. Remember, your elbow moves independently of your shoulder. So when your arm is extended (straight) or stretched out in front of you—say, in the start position for the pushup—you're expressing the same stable front rack shoulder position.

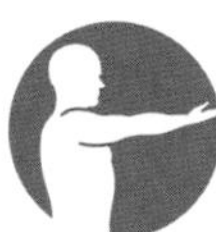

FRONT RACK 1

Basic Quick Test

Keeping your elbows straight, raise your arms to shoulder level. Then externally rotate your shoulders. The goal is to get your palms and the pits of your elbows to face the ceiling. This is position 1.

If you can't lock out your arms or externally rotate your shoulders in position 1—get your elbow pits and palms to face the ceiling—chances are you're missing critical internal and external rotation range of motion in your shoulders.

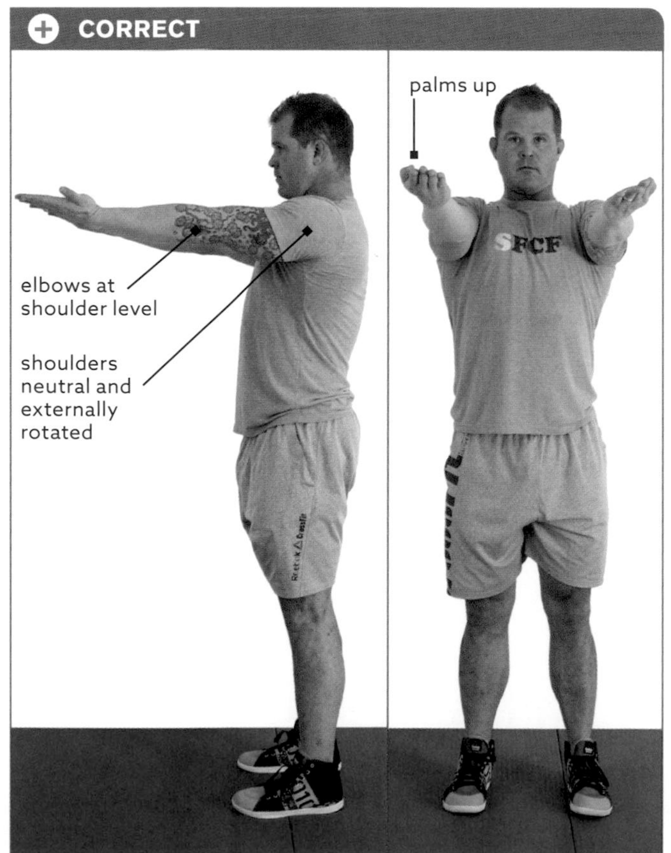
CORRECT
palms up
elbows at shoulder level
shoulders neutral and externally rotated

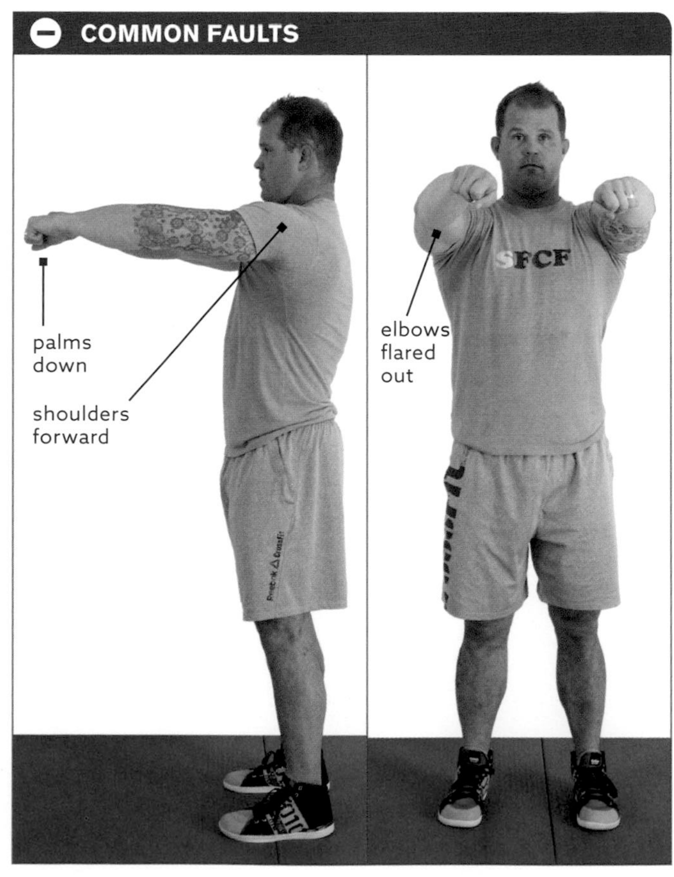
COMMON FAULTS
palms down
shoulders forward
elbows flared out

Loaded Quick Tests

PUSHUP FRONT RACK 1 TEST

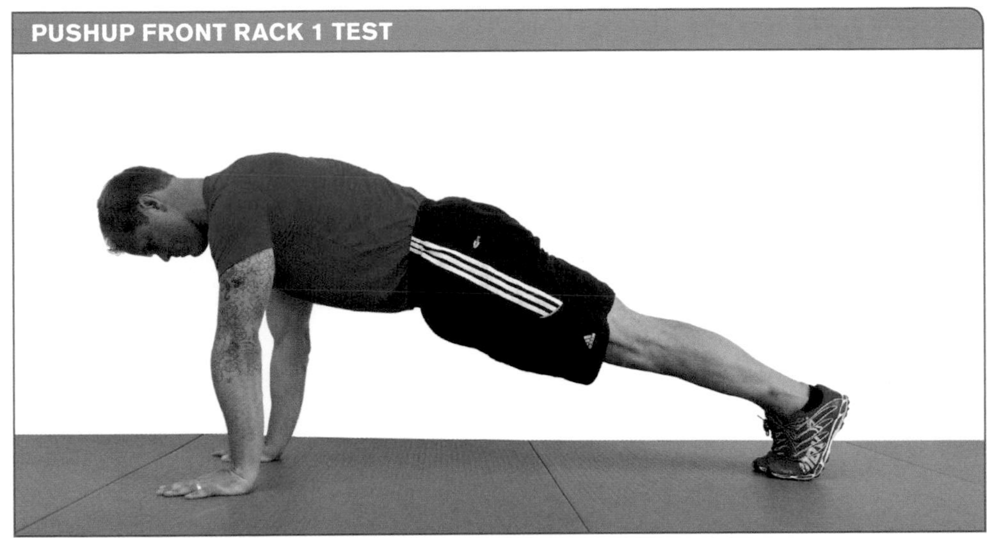

RING PUSHUP FRONT RACK 1 TEST

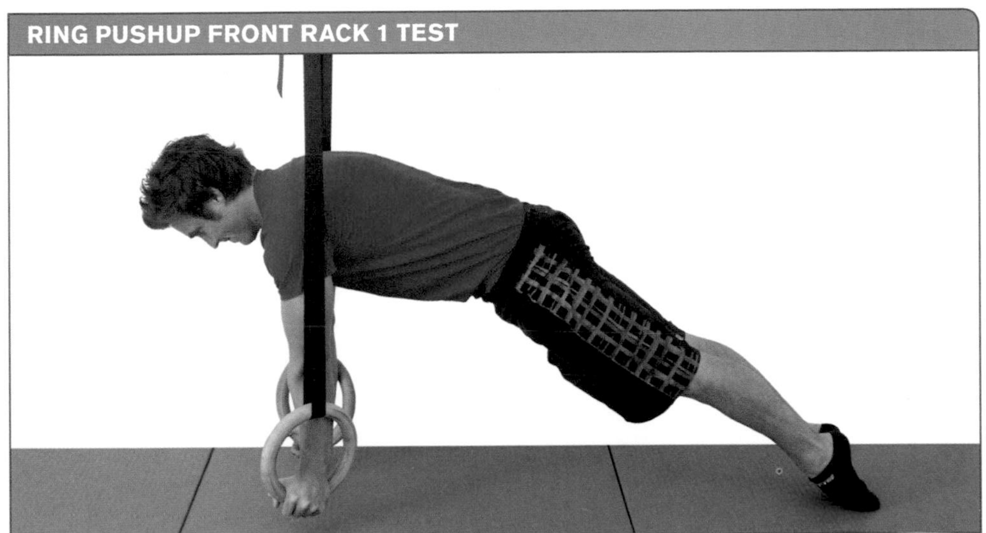

PLANCHE PUSHUP FRONT RACK 1 TEST

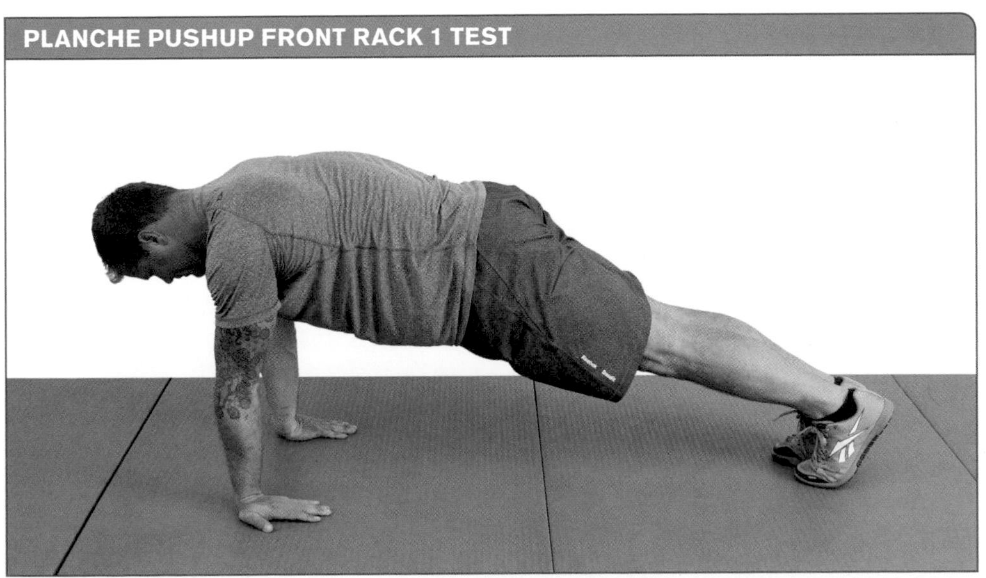

FRONT RACK 2

Basic Quick Test

From position 1, bend your elbows—keeping your shoulders externally rotated—and then turn your hands so that your palms face the sky. You should be able to elevate your elbows to shoulder height while maintaining the same stable shoulder position.

If your wrists collapse inward or your elbows flare out in position 2, you're probably missing shoulder rotation range of motion and/or elbow flexion and wrist extension.

CORRECT

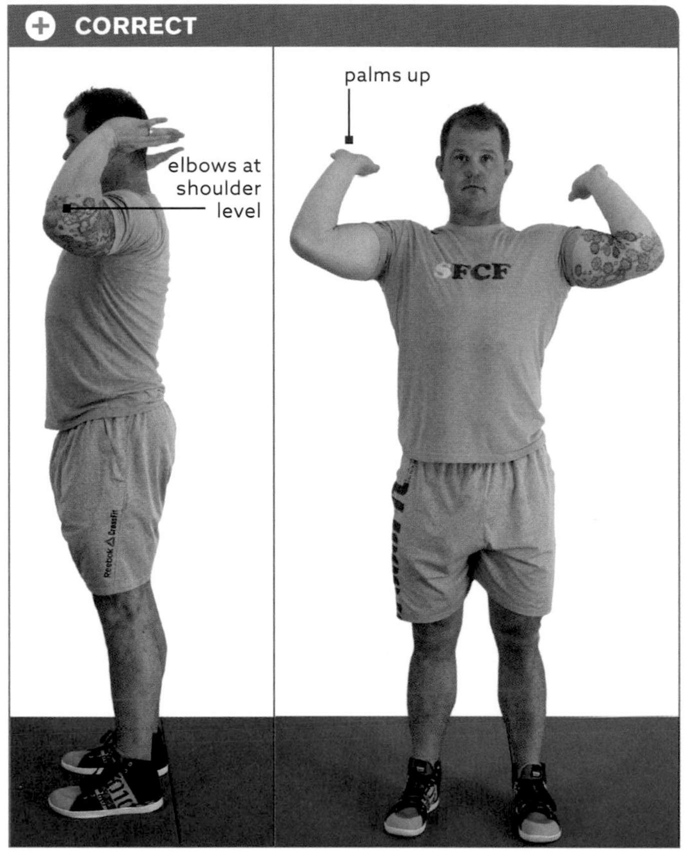

COMMON FAULTS

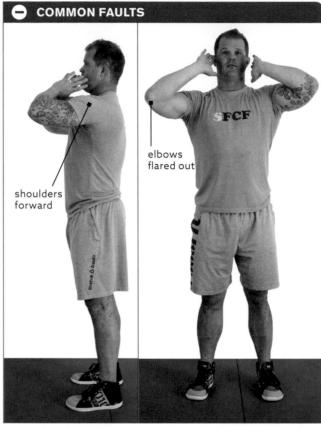

Loaded Quick Tests

KETTLEBELL FRONT RACK 2 TEST

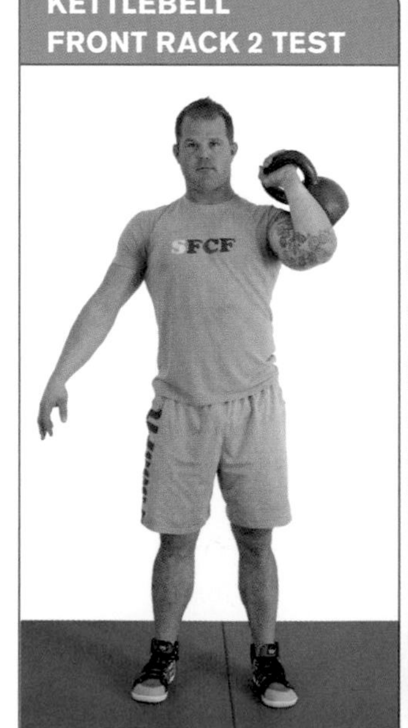

DUMBBELL FRONT RACK 2 TEST

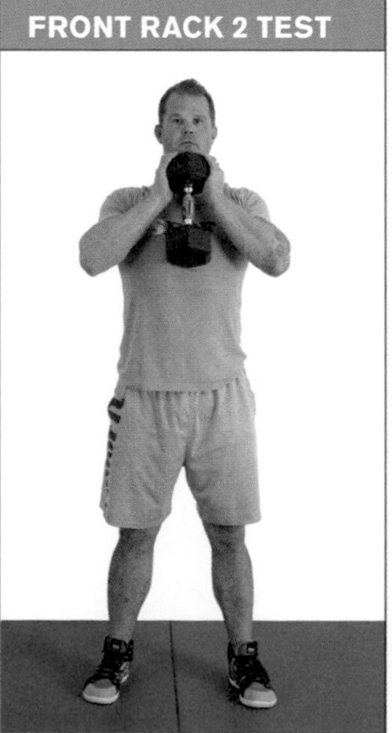

BARBELL FRONT RACK 2 TEST

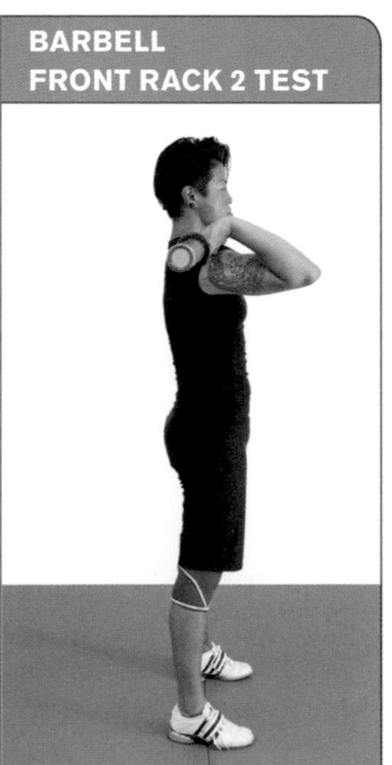

HIP ARCHETYPES

The squat archetype is one of the most fundamental human shapes. Most of the movements performed in the gym and in life involve some iteration of the squat. It doesn't matter how your feet are oriented—wide or narrow stance—or whether your torso is upright or tilted forward, the function and position of your hips are relatively the same; this archetype always captures flexion and external rotation of the hips.

When it comes to gym movements, the squat archetype is part of the deadlift, the squat (front squat, back squat, etc.), and the setup for Olympic lifts. There are two basic tests for this archetype: the hips-just-below-knee-crease squat and the deadlift. The differences are the orientation of your torso and the degree of knee or leg flexion. These distinctions are important because both positions, though similar in shape, test range of motion in different areas: The squat tests hip external rotation and hip, knee, and ankle flexion, while the deadlift tests range of motion for posterior chain straight-legged movements—specifically your hips and hamstrings.

Notice that I've created separate icons for the squat and deadlift positions. This will help you distinguish which position is involved in the movements laid out in this book, as well as identify which mobilizations will help you improve the different ranges of motion. However, it is important to remember that both positions are part of the squat archetype, and when it comes to flexion and external rotation of the hips, they are one and the same.

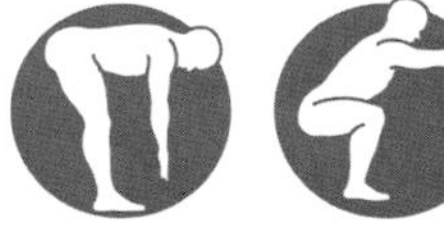

Squat

Common examples:
Getting into and out of a chair, lowering yourself to the ground and standing back up, bending over, lifting something up off the ground

Start position examples:
Clean and snatch setup, deadlift setup, jumping

Finish position examples:
Squat, jumping and landing

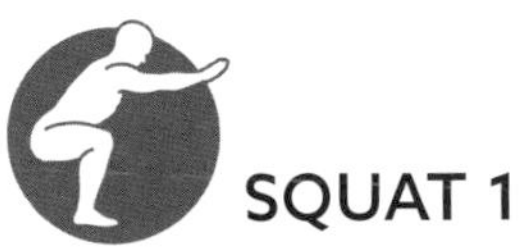

SQUAT 1

CORRECT

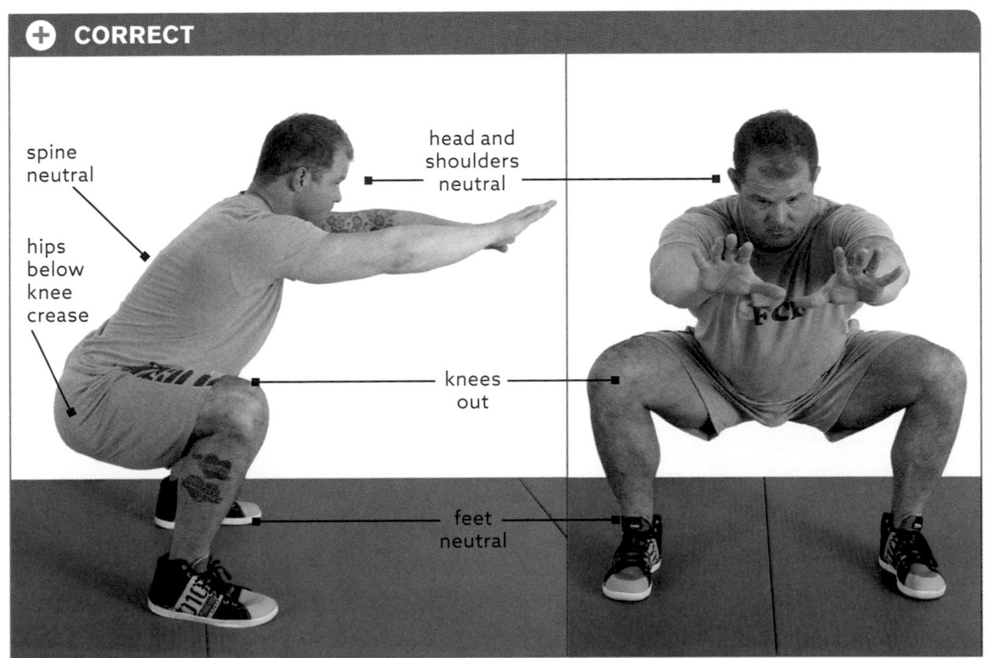

Basic Quick Test

Start by positioning your feet straight—between 0 and 12 degrees—and just outside your shoulders' width. Initiate the movement by driving your hamstrings back and tilting your torso slightly forward. Lower your elevation by bending your knees, trying to keep your shins as vertical as possible. To create torque, drive your knees out while keeping your feet in contact with the ground.

If you fail to brace your spine and create torque through your hips, you will probably see one or more of the following faults: lumbar overextension, knees caving inward, and collapsed arches. Such faults can also be a result of joint restrictions. For example, if you're unable to drive your knees out, drop your hips below your knee crease, keep your back flat, or create a stable arch through your feet, you're probably missing key ranges of hip flexion, hip external rotation, and ankle dorsiflexion (to mention a few possibilities).

COMMON FAULTS

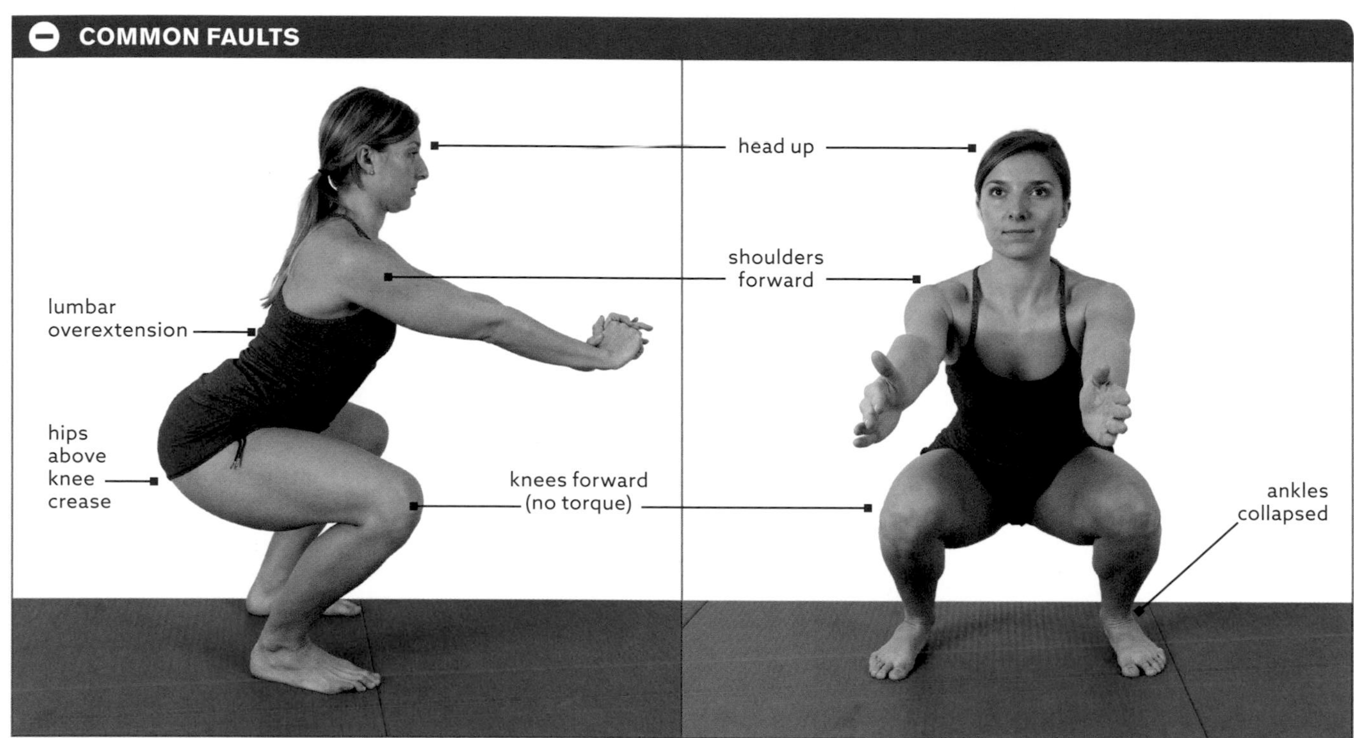

Loaded Quick Tests

BARBELL BACK SQUAT TEST

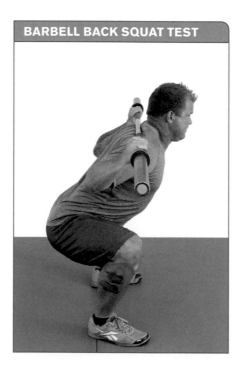

OVERHEAD BOX SQUAT TEST

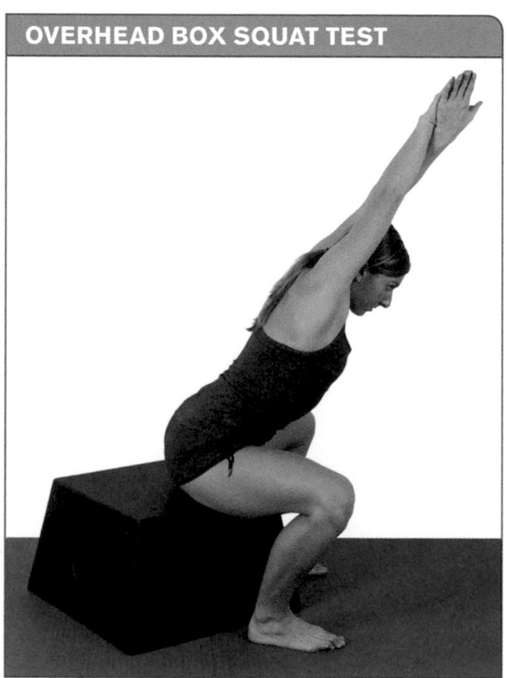

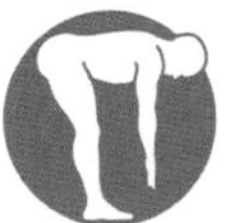

SQUAT 2 (DEADLIFT/PULLING POSITION)

Maintaining a braced neutral spine, drive your hamstrings back and tilt your torso forward, allowing your arms to hang. As you hinge from your hips, bend your knees slightly. Keep your back flat, shoulders neutral, and shins vertical. The goal is to get your torso parallel to the ground, or your hips flexed at a 90-degree angle.

If you are missing posterior chain range of motion—specifically in the hamstrings—you will tend to round your back and allow your shoulders to compensate forward.

Basic Quick Test

CORRECT

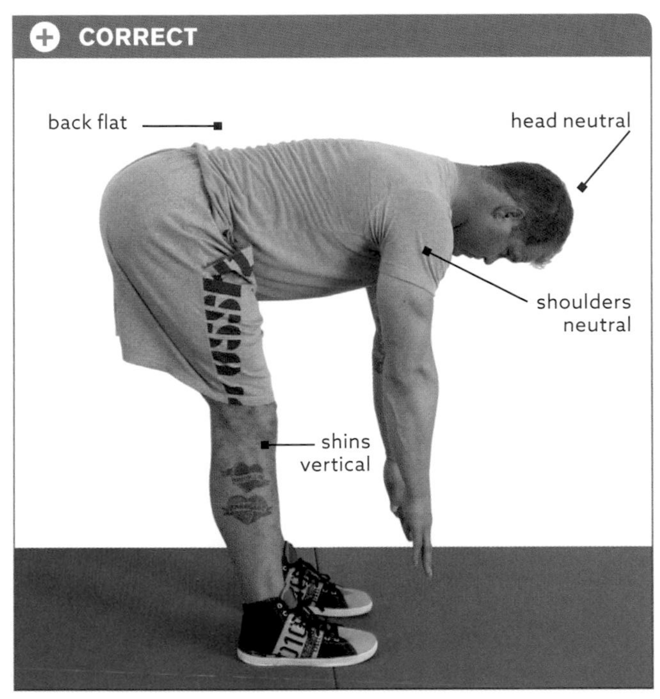

COMMON FAULTS

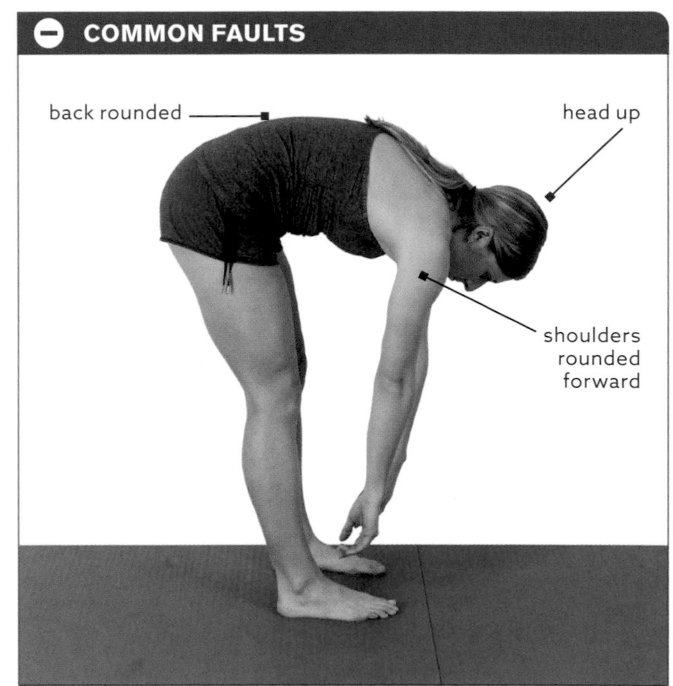

Loaded Quick Tests

KETTLEBELL DEADLIFT TEST

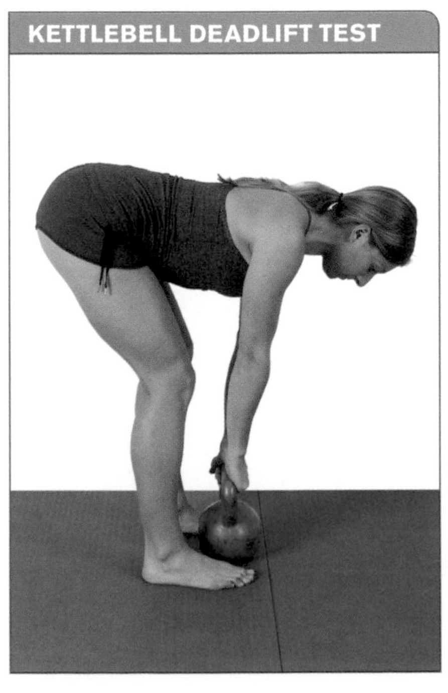

DEADLIFT SETUP TEST

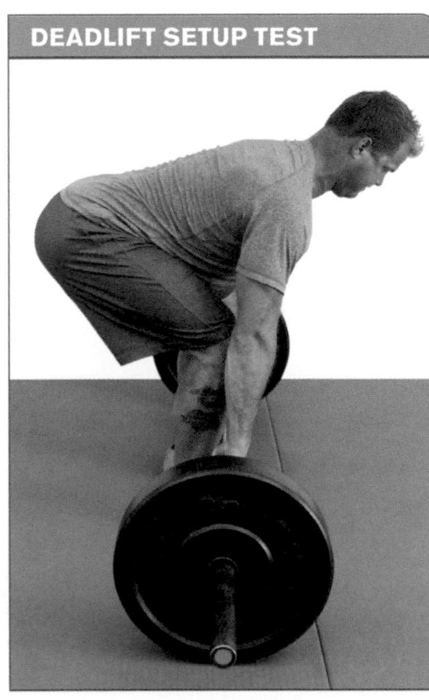

SNATCH SETUP TEST

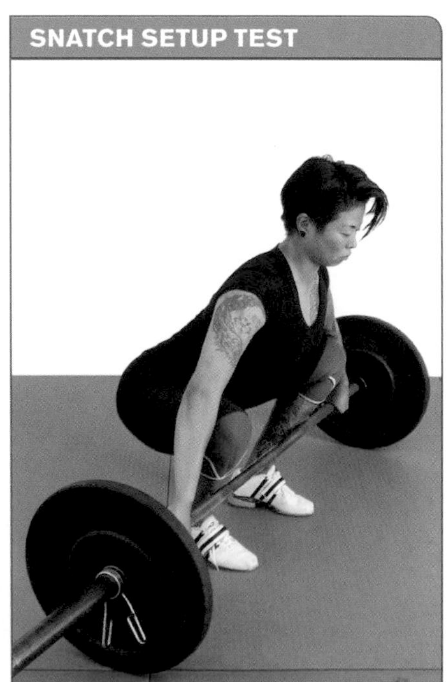

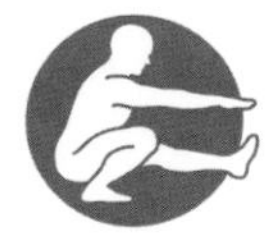

Pistol

Common examples: *Getting up off the ground from a seated position, stepping up onto or lowering yourself down from an elevated platform*

The pistol shape captures all the ankle mobility you need to be a fully functional human being. It requires full hip flexion plus full ankle dorsiflexion. So, if you can get into the pistol shape, chances are you have full ankle dorsiflexion and full hip flexion range of motion. Stated differently, the pistol is the fullest expression of a deep squat. When you squat with your feet apart, for example, you never take your hips or ankles into full flexion. The pistol archetype, on the other hand, expresses full range of motion around the primary engines and the associated joints (knees and ankles).

Anytime you're low to the ground—say, when getting up from the seated position or while gardening or break-dancing—you're expressing a close iteration of this archetype. Like the previous quick tests, realize that the pistol shape is mainly a diagnostic tool for testing deep hip and ankle mobility. It doesn't matter if you can perform an actual pistol (single-leg squat), but you should be able to get into this basic shape without falling on your butt.

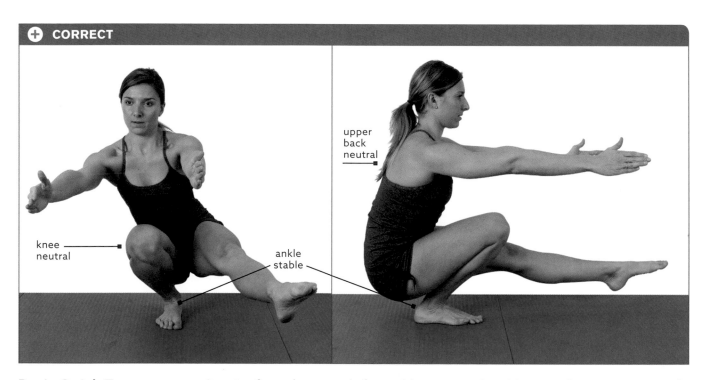

Basic Quick Test

Starting from the ground—from either a seated position or a deep squat—extend one leg out in front of your body, balancing all your weight on your opposite leg. The goal is to keep your foot and knee neutral while keeping your back as flat as possible.

If you're unable to keep your heel flush with the ground or you fall backward on your butt, it's a safe bet that you're missing hip flexion and ankle dorsiflexion. The knee tracking inside the ankle and a collapsed arch are also indicative of missing hip and ankle range of motion.

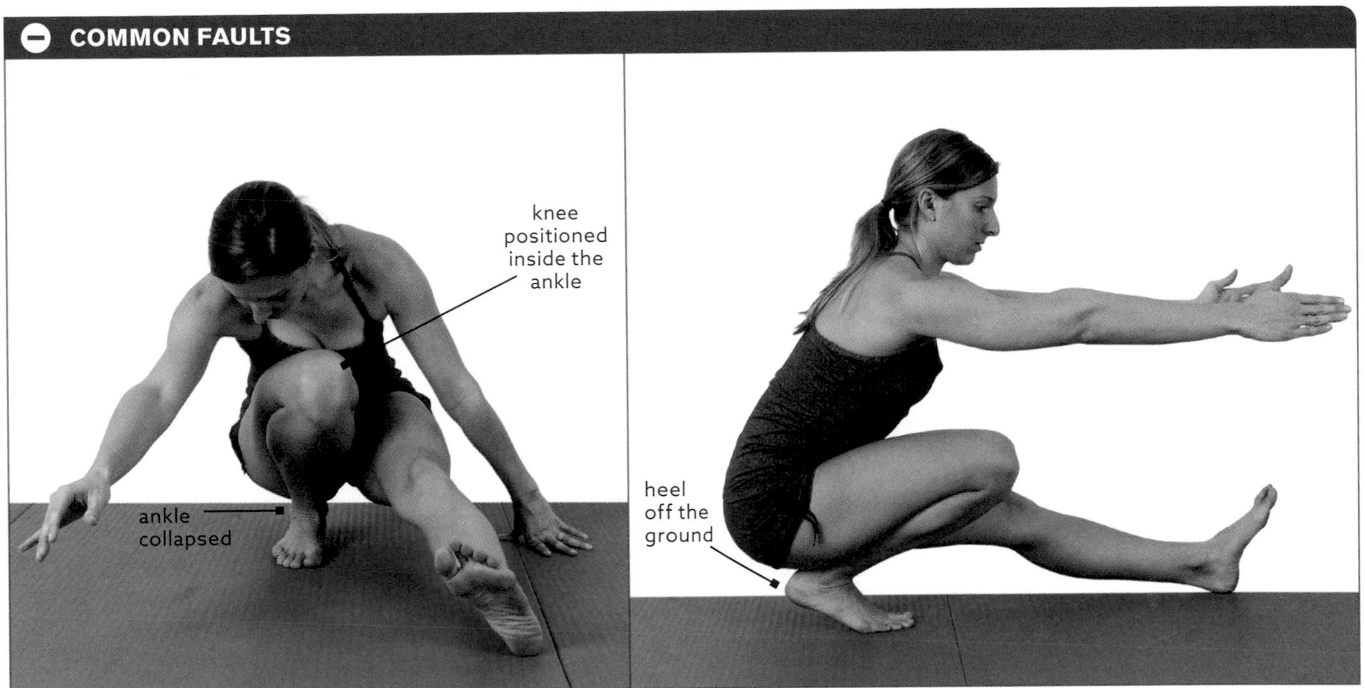

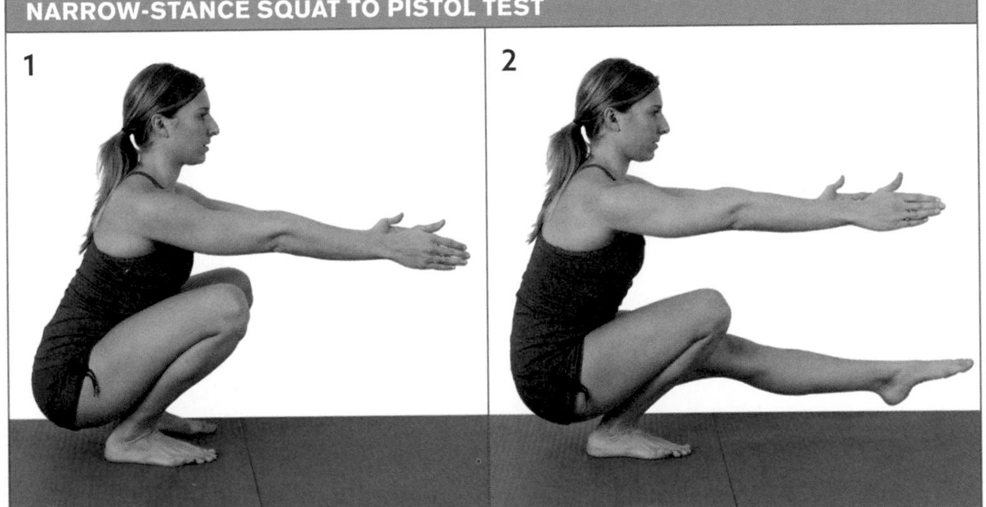

Loaded Quick Test

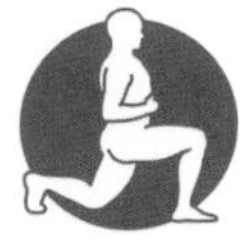

Lunge

Common examples:
Running, walking up stairs, climbing uphill, kneeling

Finish position example:
Split-jerk

Basic Quick Test

Starting from a square stance, take a large step forward and lower your rear knee to the ground. That knee should track behind your hip, and your lead shin should remain vertical.

The lunge archetype captures extension and internal rotation of the hip. Anytime your leg is behind your body—whether you're running, lunging, throwing, fighting, etc.—you're expressing a close iteration of this archetype. The split-jerk and the lunge are the best exercise movement examples of this shape.

The archetype quick test for the lunge primarily highlights hip and ankle mobility. Specifically, it tests hip extension and internal rotation, as well as toe dorsiflexion. If you're missing range of motion in this position, you'll tend to see your rear foot collapse and turn out, which is characteristic of missing hip internal rotation. If you're missing hip extension, you'll tend to see overextension through your lumbar spine. Although this archetype isn't expressed in training as often as the squat archetype, it's important to be able to express competency in the lunge position because it is conducive to so many sport and life movements.

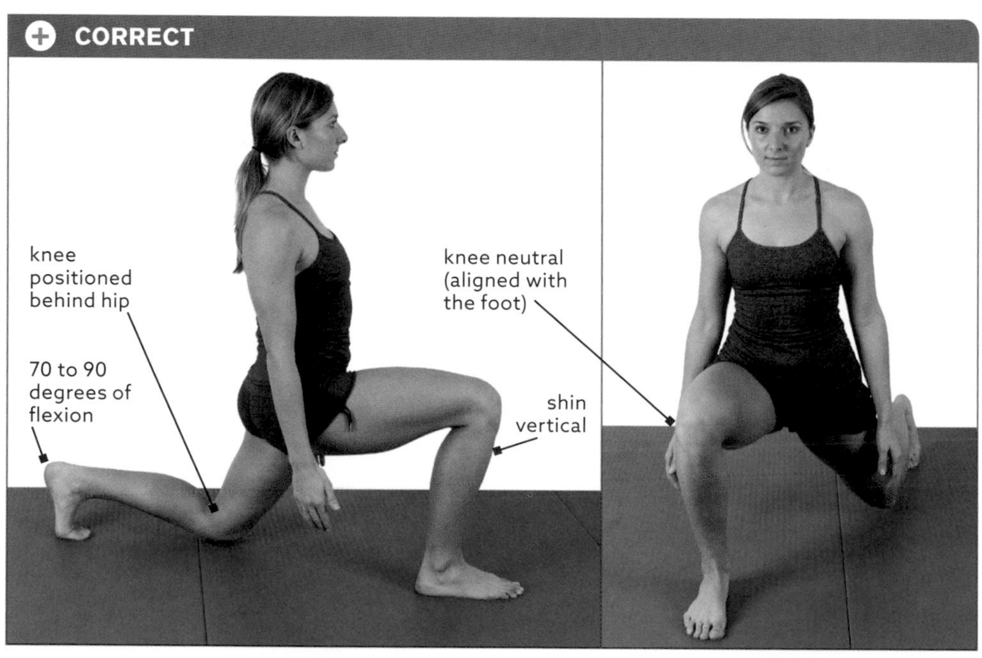

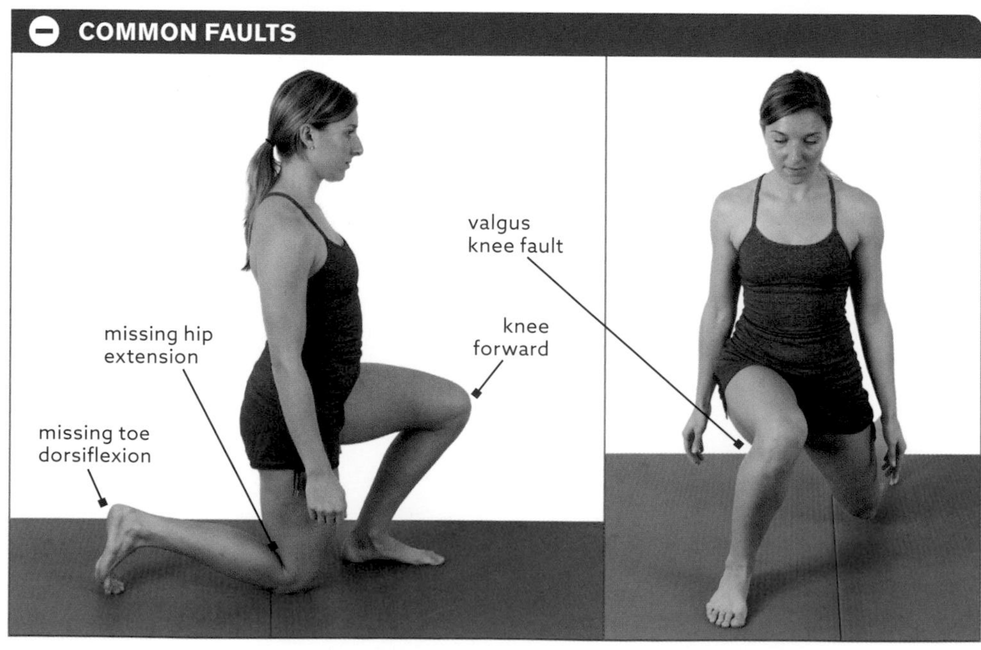

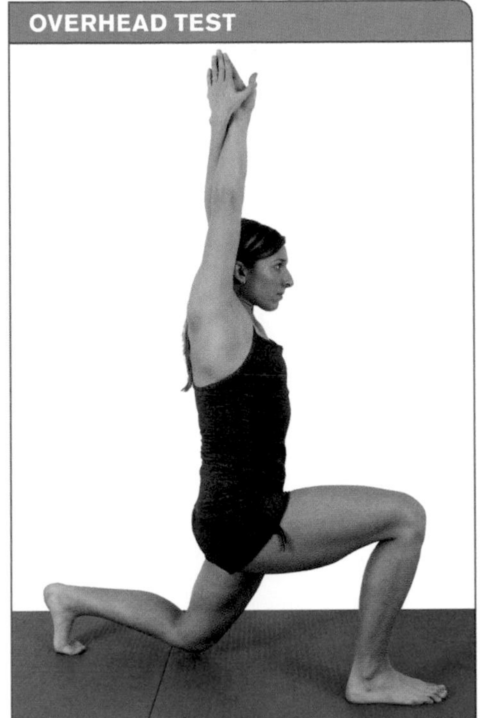
OVERHEAD TEST

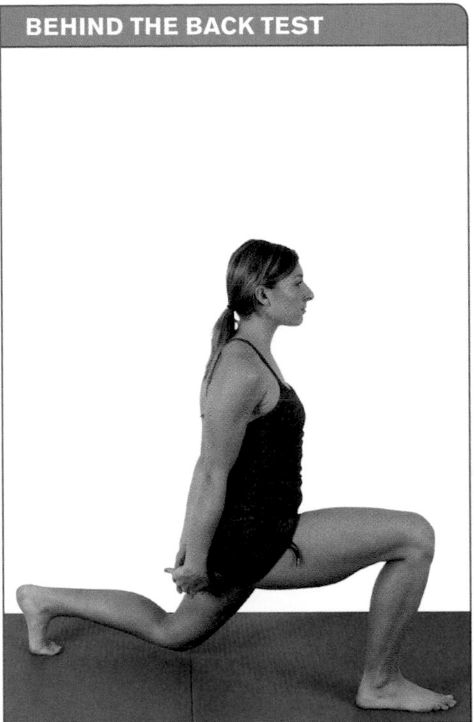
BEHIND THE BACK TEST

Loaded Quick Tests

Chapter Highlights

- The seven body archetypes represent the stable positions for the hips and shoulders and encompass the entire range of motion for most shoulder and hip movements.
- The body archetypes categorize exercise movements into the most common start and finish positions. This provides a template for organizing your hips and shoulders, shortens the learning curve for novices, helps you identify mobility restrictions and weak positions, and helps you determine which joint(s), muscle(s), or position(s) you need to mobilize.
- The premise of the tunnel concept is this: You have to start a movement (enter the tunnel) in a good position in order to finish the movement (exit the tunnel) in a good position. The tunnel concept forces you to begin your movement assessment at your start position and make sure that you are setting up correctly.
- When correcting a movement fault, always prioritize technique (motor control) first by correcting your position. If you are unable to assume a stable position because you're missing range of motion, address your mobility by targeting the areas that are restricting your movement.

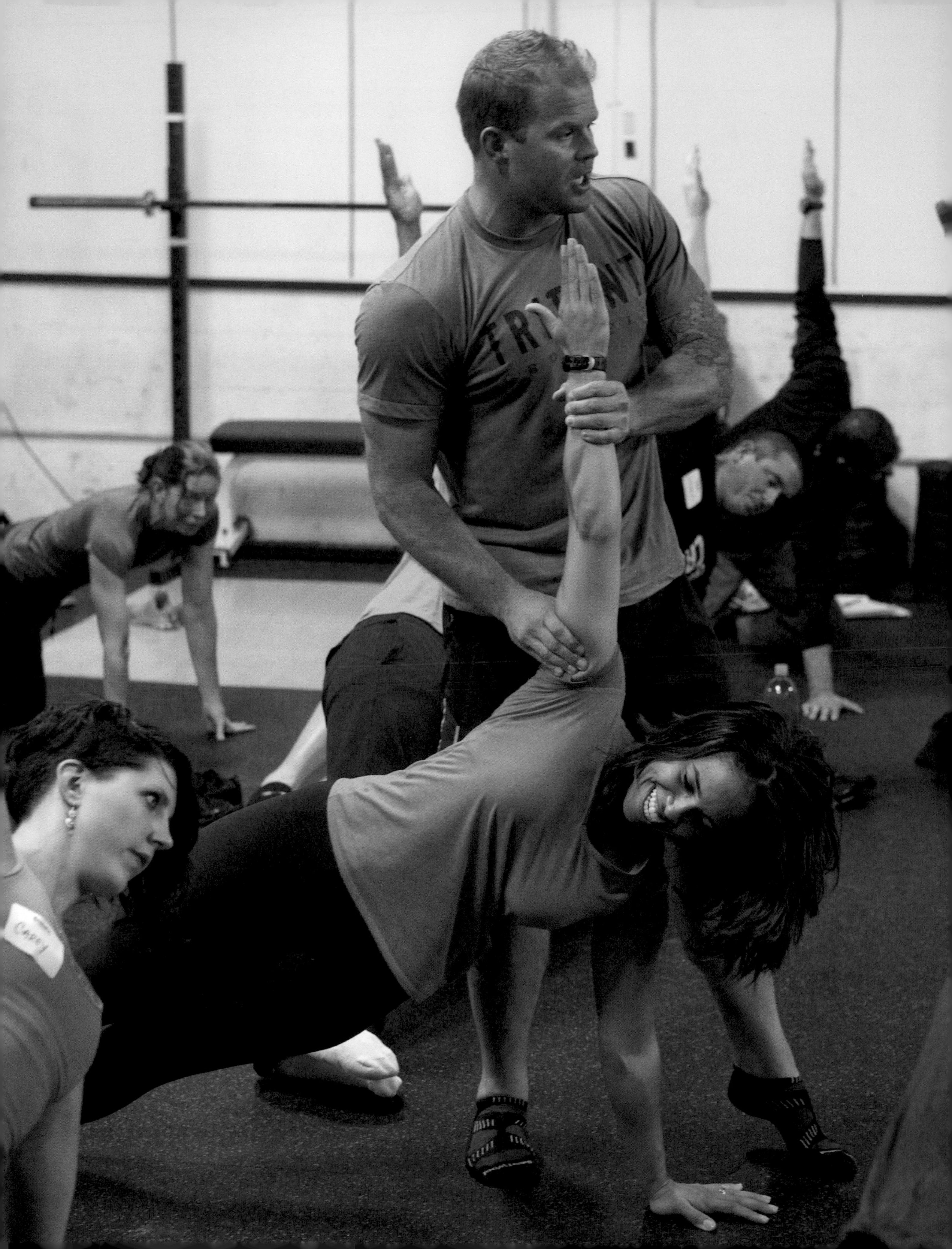

Movement Hierarchy

The movement hierarchy categorizes exercise movements based on stabilization demands and complexity. It provides a framework for building efficient, transferable movement patterns and skill progressions—from simple to more advanced exercises—and for modifying strength and conditioning movements based on skill, fitness level, and mobility.

Once you understand the basic organizing principles that govern spine and joint stability (outlined in chapters 1 through 3) and the body archetypes (outlined in chapter 4), the next step is to put them to work in a safe and controlled environment (the gym) using full-range, transferable strength and conditioning movements. Let's quickly revisit why this is so important.

As I've discussed, learning functional movements gives you a universal language for all human movement. That is, if you're fluent in full-range strength and conditioning movements—squatting, deadlifting, pressing, pulling, etc.—you have universal models for moving safely and effectively regardless of what you're doing. For example, if you understand the principles that govern a deadlift, you have embodied the knowledge to pick up anything off the ground safely and efficiently. If you can perform a push-press and a squat correctly, you understand how to jump and land with your torso upright—like when you rebound a basketball—without destroying your knees. If you can stabilize your shoulders during a pull-up, you will have no trouble creating that same stable shoulder position while climbing a tree or rock wall.

But here's the rub: Just because you can perform functional movements in the gym doesn't necessarily mean that you can apply them elsewhere. You may be able to do a pull-up in the gym, for example, but you may not have the technique to climb a tree. However, if you understand what's going on when you do a pull-up, it's easier to climb a tree safely because you know how to create torque and trunk stability. So as long as you understand how the movement principles work and you develop reproducible motor control patterns, you have a model for reconstituting organized, stable, and efficient positions in any environment. Whether you're windsurfing, shooting, fighting, dancing, or playing football, you have a transferable template for movement that is both safe and effective.

Human movement, however, is complex. To ingrain practical, universal movement patterns, you need to incorporate strength and conditioning exercises that translate to all forms of movement. In addition, you need a model for identifying and resolving dysfunctional movement patterns, unstable positions, and range of motion restrictions that hinder athletic performance and increase the potential for pain and injury. Put simply, you have to treat strength and conditioning movements as tools for improving life and sport performance and turn the gym into a movement assessment laboratory.

The trick is to progress exercise movements in a way that instills good mechanics, accelerates athletic performance, decreases the potential for injury, and highlights movement and mobility dysfunction.

Skill Progressions and Movement Complexity

When I first started thinking about skill progressions and movement complexity, I looked at it through a rehabilitation lens. I asked myself, How do I rebuild functional movement patterns after injury or surgery? More specifically, how do I layer movement progressions within the framework of strength and conditioning in order to instill good, transferable movement patterns?

Here's what I did: First, I introduced the movement principles. Then I applied them to basic, scalable, full-range movements like the squat, deadlift, pushup, and pull-up.

If an athlete demonstrated competency with those basic movements, I would start to challenge the stability of his position by adding load and metabolic demand, and then by introducing more upright positions. For example, if the athlete could back squat with good form, I might introduce the front squat or overhead squat or simply have him run 400 meters—to get him breathing heavily—and then perform multiple air squat repetitions.

The final step was to challenge the athlete's motor control and test his mobility under stress. I did so by adding speed and introducing more complex movements, like Olympic lifts and burpees. I realized that by systematically progressing movements—from basic to more advanced—I could not only rehab an injured athlete, but also build efficient movement patterns in both novices and elites. Putting all this together, I turned a simple template for rehabbing athletes post-injury into a system for understanding movement complexity and skill progressions. I call this system the movement hierarchy. It's a way to categorize and progress movement so that you have a model for:

- Regaining performance after surgery or injury
- Modifying and customizing movement progressions
- Understanding movement complexity
- Illuminating movement errors
- Identifying mobility restrictions

Categorizing Complex Movement

You don't need to be a movement expert to differentiate simple exercises from more advanced ones. Even someone new to strength and conditioning can see that Olympic lifts are more complex than power lifts: Olympic lifts require you to transition from one position to another with speed, while power lifts involve minimal movement and are performed slowly. We tend to categorize movement based on the speed at which the movement is performed, the strength required to perform the movement, and the number of transitions—that is, the number of positions that comprise the movement. But there's another subtle yet key distinction to consider when classifying movement complexity, and that is the difficulty of maintaining a stable position throughout the entire movement.

This is perhaps best explained by way of example. When you perform a power lift—say, a deadlift—you can create and maintain torque throughout the entire range of the movement. In other words, you never lose connection with torque. You go from a grinding start to a grinding finish and maintain tension for the duration of the movement. An Olympic lift, on the other hand, has a transitional element in which you go from one archetype to a completely different archetype. During this transitional phase, you momentarily lose tension and break your connection with torque. It is these two elements—changing shape and having to cultivate stability (torque) in a new position—that make Olympic lifts so much harder than power lifts.

In short, when it comes to categorizing movement, I look at the stabilization component, which is the ability to stay connected to the movement via the action of torque, and the number of archetypal shapes that comprise the movement. Using these criteria, I have created three movement categories.

Let's examine each category and how you can use it to systematically progress movement, highlight motor control weaknesses, and navigate the exercise movements in part 2.

Default Movement

As I've said before, the positions you assume at work or while going about your life will impact the way you move in the gym. If you walk around with your back overextended, chances are good that you will default into that same position while squatting. Your environment also affects movement efficiency. For example, I noticed that in first grade my oldest daughter's classmates had started to heel-strike. (Landing on your heel is less than optimal when running and can lead to a ton of problems.) They didn't seem to do this in kindergarten. What happened?

Well, they had been wearing cushioned shoes and sitting in chairs long enough to create an adaptation, and it turned into their default movement pattern. This is why it's so important and difficult to get to the root of movement issues and take the time to reverse-engineer patterns that have been hardwired over years of conditioning. If you sit in a chair, you have to spend extra time working on your posture. If you wear high heels, you have to focus on your foot position and calf mobility. Remember, biomechanical pathologies are treatable at any time or stage of development. But it takes time, consciousness, and a ton of practice. It starts with understanding the movement principles and then practicing and applying them to every facet of your life.

Category 1 Movements

Category 1 movements represent basic squatting, pressing, and pulling techniques: squat, deadlift, pushup, bench press, strict press, and pull-up. Movements that fall into this category have relatively low speed demands, express normal or full ranges of motion, and closely resemble the actions of daily life. If you are a beginner, are coming off an injury, or simply want to focus on movements that have the most carryover to everyday activities, you should spend most of your time in the gym focusing on category 1 movements.

All these exercises share a common sequence: They start in a position of high stability (PHS)—a braced neutral position from which you can maximize torque in your hips and/or shoulders—and maintain that stable position throughout the entire range of motion. This is how you classify a category 1 movement.

POSITION OF HIGH STABILITY (PHS)

WITH CONNECTION

POSITION OF HIGH STABILITY (PHS)

- **Position of High Stability (PHS):** A braced, well-organized position that allows you to create and maintain maximum stability through your hips and shoulders.
- **Connection:** Maintaining a torsion force through the entire range of motion while moving at a slow speed.

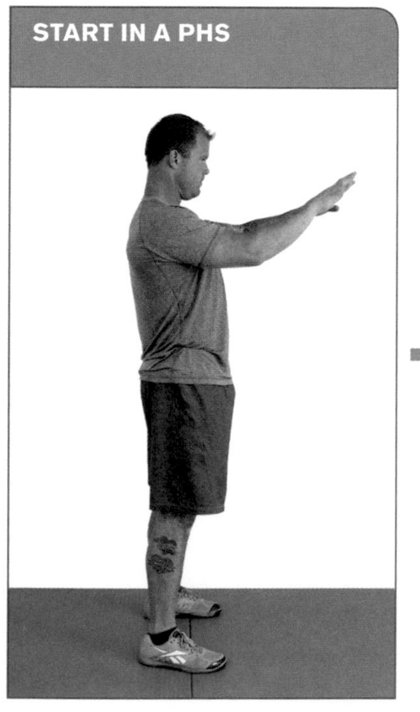

START IN A PHS

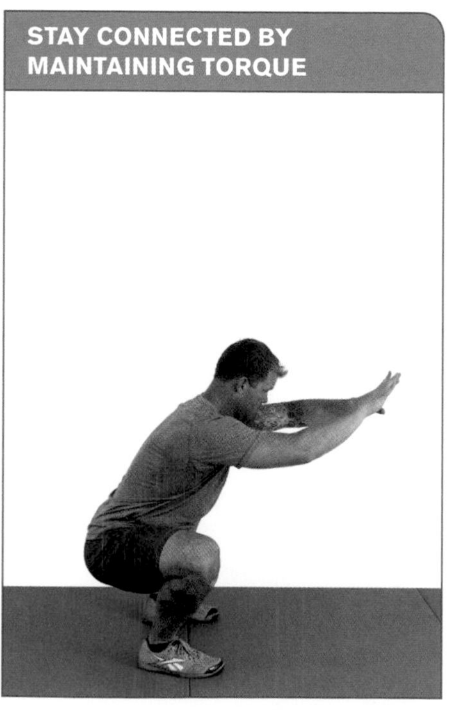

STAY CONNECTED BY MAINTAINING TORQUE

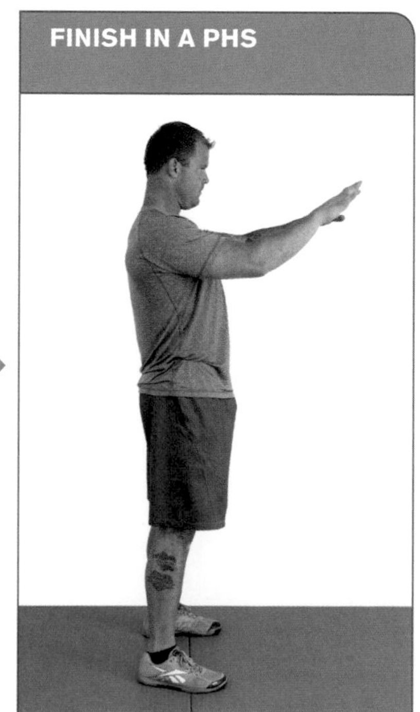

FINISH IN A PHS

Let's use the air squat as an example. You begin in a PHS (top position), lower your body into a squat (bottom position), and complete the movement in the same PHS (top position). You go from one shape to another shape, and then back to the original shape. Because your feet remain in contact with the ground, you can maintain a torsion force through the entire range of the movement. This torsion force keeps you connected to the movement.

Category 2 Movements

Like category 1 movements, category 2 movements take you from a PHS to a PHS, but instead of maintaining connection (torque) throughout the entire movement, there is a speed element between the beginning and the end of the movement.

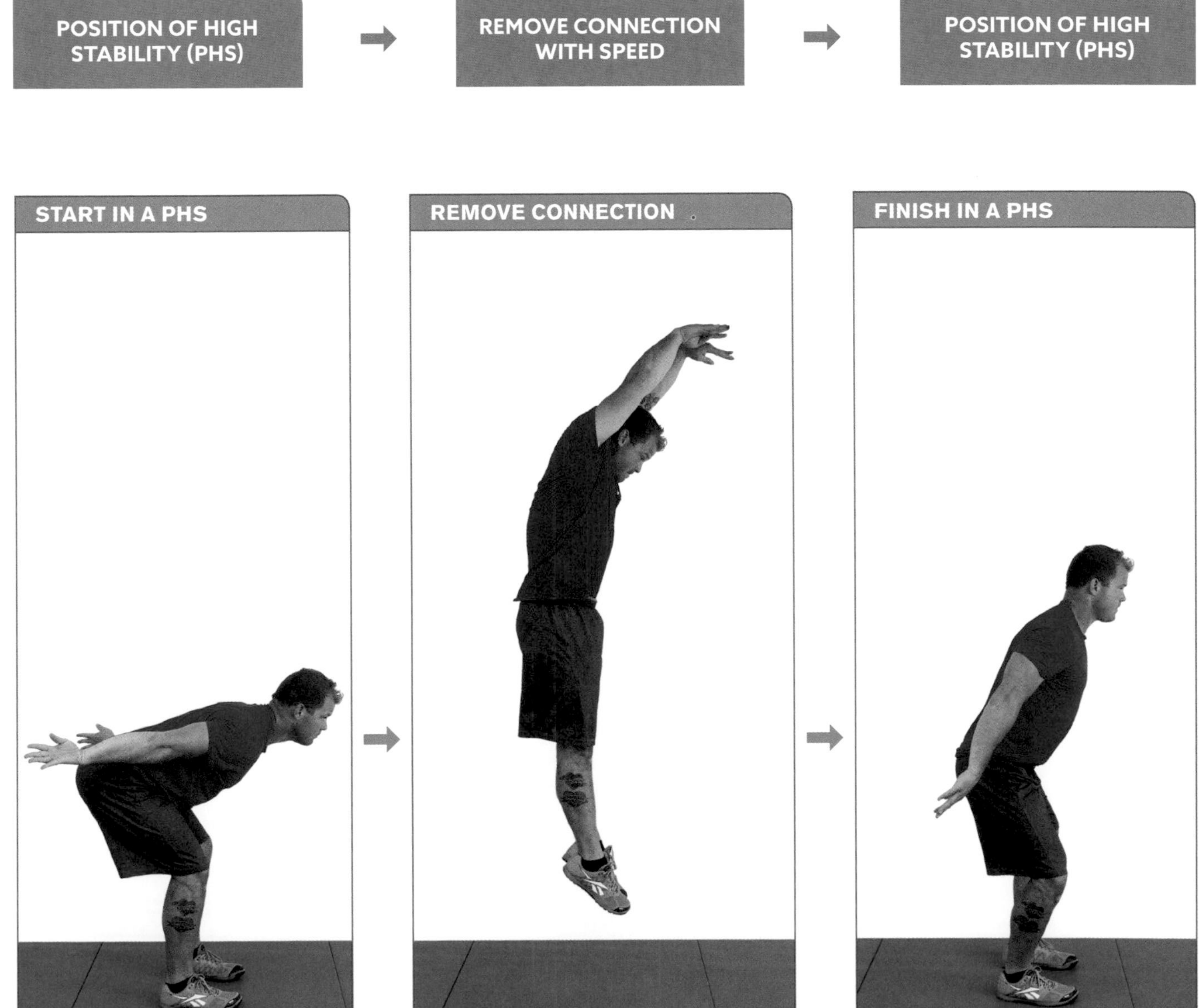
POSITION OF HIGH STABILITY (PHS)
REMOVE CONNECTION WITH SPEED
POSITION OF HIGH STABILITY (PHS)
START IN A PHS
REMOVE CONNECTION
FINISH IN A PHS

Jumping and landing is a perfect example. You start in a PHS, remove connection (torque) as you jump, and then spontaneously stabilize your spine and generate torque to finish in a PHS. You start and finish in the same position, but removing torsion force and adding speed—jumping into the air—increases the motor control and mobility demands of the movement. Other examples of category 2 movements include running, wall ball, rowing, and the snatch balance.

It's a lot harder to hide weaknesses as you progress into category 2 movements. Movement dysfunction and mobility restrictions can be hidden behind the veil of category 1 movements, so you have to constantly challenge motor control and range of motion capacities by adding speed—either in the form of multiple repetitions or by introducing category 2 movements—adding load (weight), or adding a metabolic demand.

As I've discussed, in order to improve as an athlete, you have to work hard to find weaknesses in your movement profile. It's not enough to move fast, lift heavy, or perform a lot of repetitions within category 1. As you move closer to the actions of sports, you need to be able to spontaneously arrive in safe and stable positions so that you can seamlessly transition into your next movement.

Category 3 Movements

Category 3 movements closely resemble the actions of sports: You move fast, combine multiple archetypes into one movement, and change direction rapidly—for example, going from a pull to a press (as in a muscle-up), cutting, jumping, and then landing in a different position. Formally defined, a category 3 movement starts in one position, removes the connection (torque), and arrives in a completely different position. Put another way, you need to be able to spontaneously generate stability while transitioning from one archetype to another.

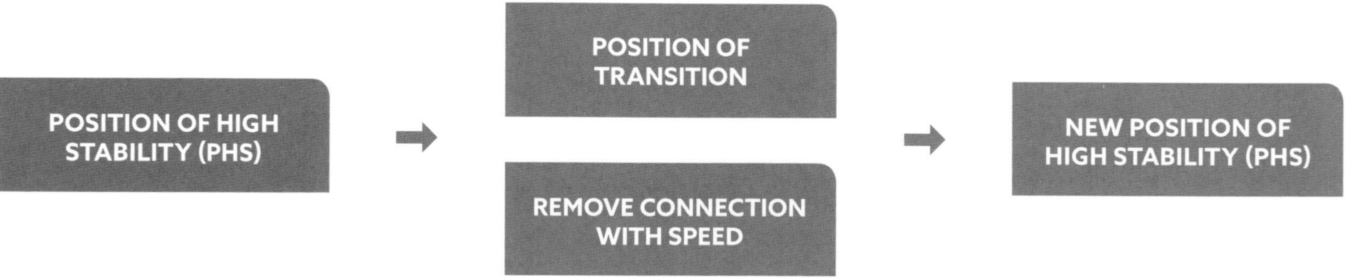

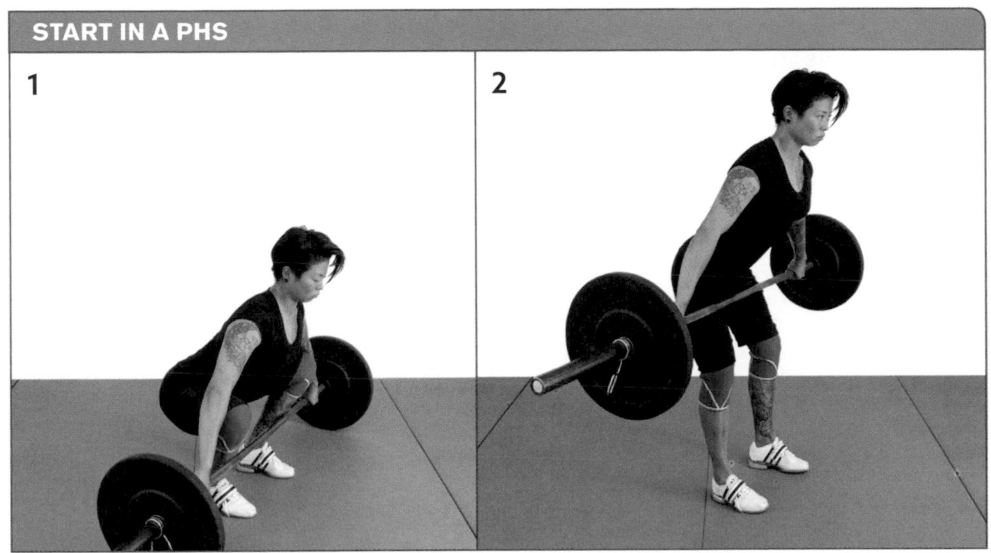
START IN A PHS
1
2

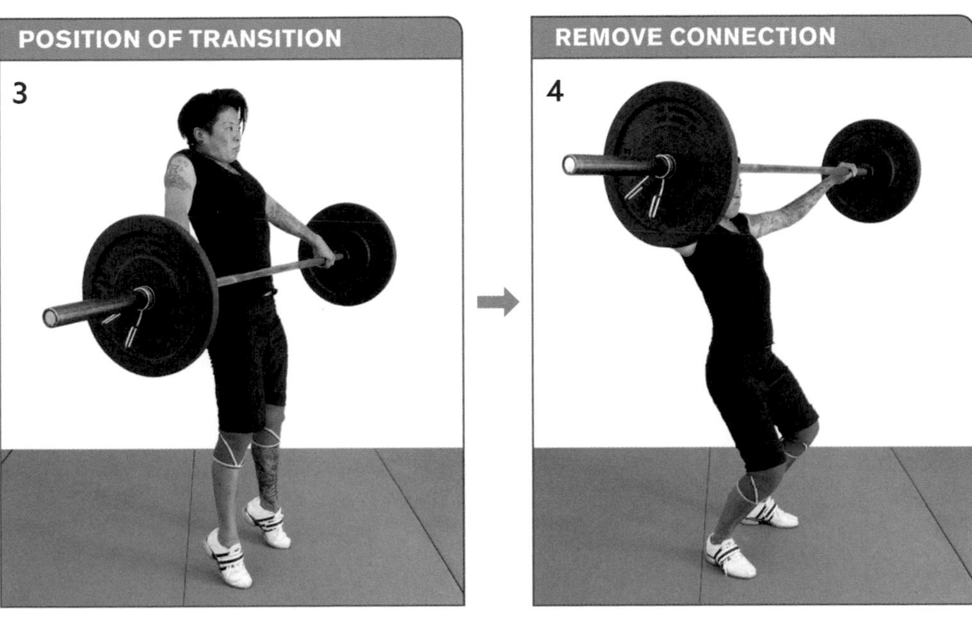
POSITION OF TRANSITION
3
REMOVE CONNECTION
4

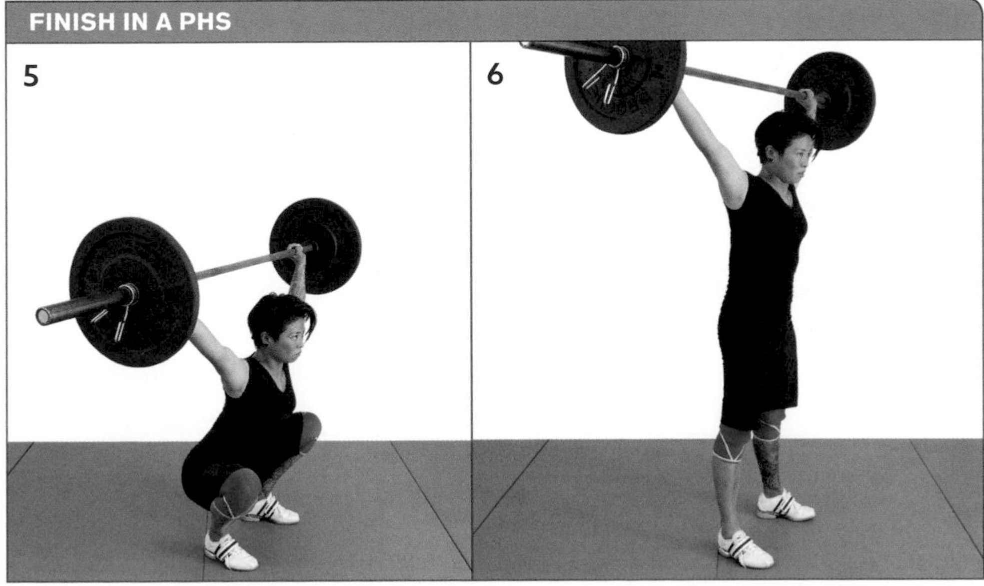
FINISH IN A PHS
5
6

One of the most difficult and easily recognizable category 3 movements performed in the gym is the snatch. As you can see in the photos on the previous page, you start in a pulling position (hang archetype), open your hips into full extension, and then drop into the bottom of a squat with your arms overhead (overhead archetype). As the bar travels upward, there is a moment of weightlessness when you lose torque with the ground and the bar: This is the position of transition. Receiving the weight in the bottom of the overhead squat is your PHS. You go from one shape, which is a position of transition (a pulling position), remove the connection, and then arrive in a completely different shape (the overhead squat), or PHS.

As with category 2 movements, technique tends to fall apart when you start implementing these full-range movements. The simple fact is that these changes of direction are very challenging. You can't disguise poor movement patterns or limited ranges of motion.

The bottom line is that you need to train category 1 movements like the squat, deadlift, and pushup to gain proficiency with the movement principles. But if you want to improve your athleticism and really highlight your understanding of midline stabilization and torque, you should work on category 3 movements like Olympic lifts.

Upright-Torso Demands

The orientation of your torso is another way to categorize complex movements within the framework of the movement hierarchy. It's simple: The more upright your torso, the more motor control, range of motion, and stabilization are required to carry out the movement.

The squat variations shown opposite provide a crude example of how an upright torso increases the difficulty of a movement. The back squat is the simplest because you can tilt your torso slightly forward, giving your hips, hamstrings, and ankles some room to breathe. But if you increase the verticality of your torso in the form of a front squat, right away you will start to see weaknesses in your athletic profile. You will have a much harder time keeping your back flat, your knees out, and your shins vertical. The overhead squat is the toughest of the squat iterations because you have to keep your torso perfectly upright to avoid defaulting into an unfavorable position.

Although each squat variation requires you to stabilize the barbell and organize your shoulders in a different position, the orientation of your torso adds to the difficulty of the lift. Even doing a high-bar back squat (a squat with your torso upright) in place of a low-bar back squat (a squat with your torso tilted forward) creates new challenges in terms of motor control and mobility.

When I teach my Movement & Mobility Course, I highlight this concept by asking the attendees to go through a three-squat series. This series turns into a simple category 1 movement screen for spotting problems and challenging the athletes with higher degrees of motor control and mobility.

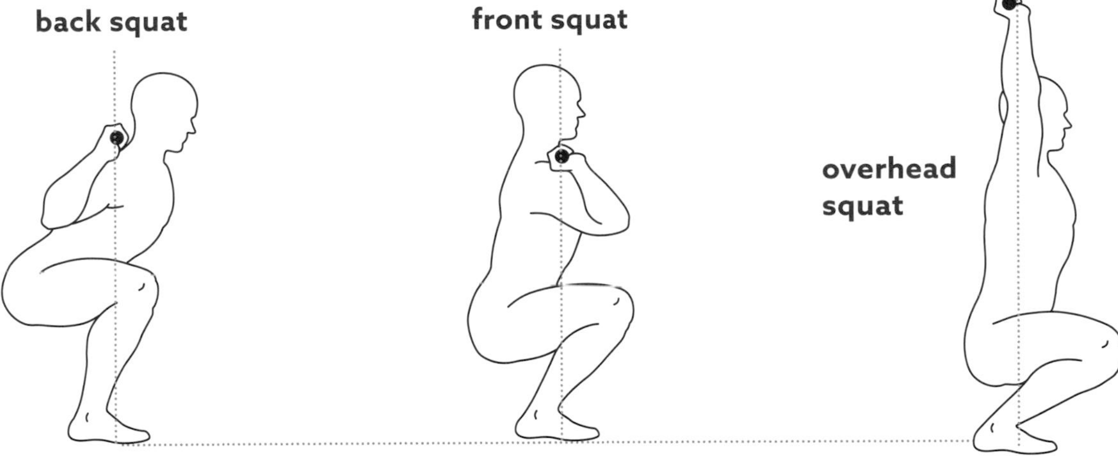

AIR SQUAT

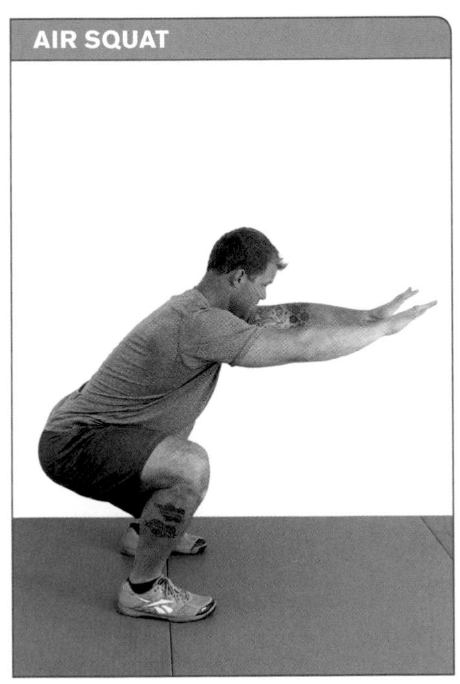

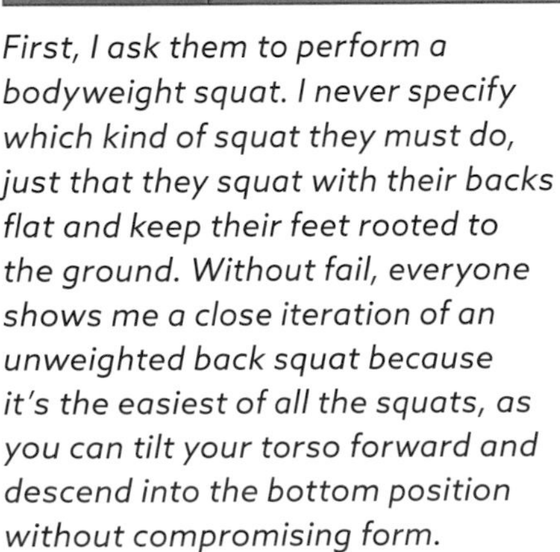

First, I ask them to perform a bodyweight squat. I never specify which kind of squat they must do, just that they squat with their backs flat and keep their feet rooted to the ground. Without fail, everyone shows me a close iteration of an unweighted back squat because it's the easiest of all the squats, as you can tilt your torso forward and descend into the bottom position without compromising form.

HANDS BEHIND HEAD

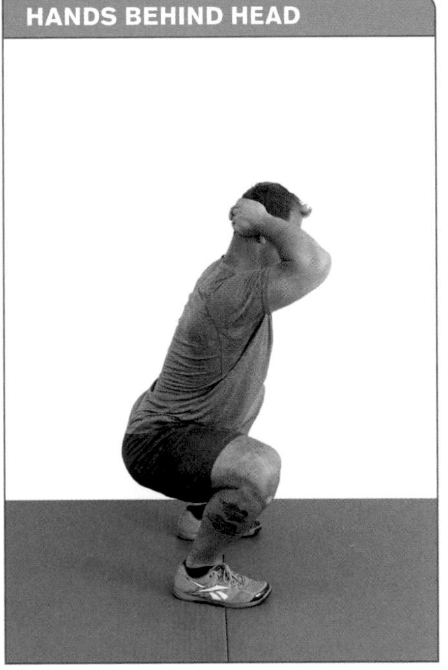

Next, I ask them to put their hands behind their heads, which forces their torsos into a more upright position, and squat again. This is the equivalent of going from a back squat to a front squat. At this point, people start to compensate by rounding forward and going up onto the balls of their feet because more range of motion is required to perform the movement correctly.

ARMS LOCKED OUT OVERHEAD

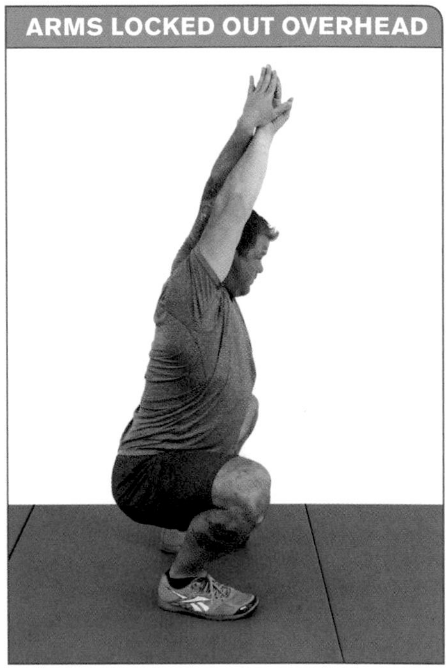

Finally, I ask them to squat with their arms locked out overhead, which is essentially an unweighted overhead squat. And this is where people start defaulting into some pretty wonky positions to keep their torsos upright, hips externally rotated, and arms overhead. Obviously, you can still tilt your torso forward while keeping your hands overhead. However, to get the most out of this exercise, you need to increase the verticality of your torso with each subsequent squat.

Scaling: How to Modify and Customize Movement

When it comes to learning or teaching movement progressions, you need to understand how to alter or customize a movement based on fitness level, mobility, and skill. To do so, you need to understand how to perform the movement correctly, as well as understand why some movements are more complex than others. Imagine having someone perform snatches early in her ACL surgery rehab. That would be silly. Similarly, you wouldn't ask someone to perform a full snatch without first introducing the overhead squat and the snatch balance.

Progressing movement is a systematic process that requires an understanding of movement complexity and the abilities and mobility restrictions of the individual. In other words, you need to be able to scale movement within the context of the movement hierarchy to ensure good technique and continual growth. This is what I mean by "scaling." You can increase the difficulty of a movement by scaling up or decrease the difficulty by scaling down.

Here's an example: Say you can deadlift with good form, meaning that you can keep your back flat and your hips stable (see page 196). To challenge your position, you can scale up by increasing the weight, performing multiple repetitions, or adding a stress stimulus (for example, run 400 meters and then perform multiple deadlift repetitions). Conversely, if you can't set up correctly for a deadlift due to a mobility restriction (such as tight hamstrings), you can scale down by shortening the movement and elevating the bar off the ground. Although this modification shortens the range of motion (ideally, you want to be able to perform the full range of the movement), it allows you to focus on form. As you develop motor control and improve your mobility, you can start to scale up by increasing the range of motion (lifting the weight from the floor) or by adding speed, load, or volume to the modified start position.

Scaling a movement or even a workout is a subtle and complex process that takes knowledge, planning, and experience. A good coach who knows how to scale up or down based on your ability and fitness level should play a vital role in this process. In the absence of a coach (and even in the presence of a coach), you've got to listen to your body and prioritize form over everything else. If you can perform a movement without fault, scale up. If your form starts to break down or you don't have the mobility to get into or maintain a good position, scale down.

Scaling Up (Make a Movement Harder):

- **Speed example:** Perform as many repetitions as possible in 20 seconds.
- **Volume example:** Increase the number of sets or repetitions.
- **Load example:** Increase the weight incrementally.
- **Upright Torso Demands example:** Progress from a back squat to an overhead squat.
- **Intensity/Metabolic Demand example:** Combine multiple movements into a high-intensity workout (for example, run 400 meters and then perform 25 air squats without resting).

Scaling Down (Make a Movement Easier):

- **Shorten the Movement example:** Decrease the range of motion.
- **More Points of Contact example:** Create an additional base of support (such as holding onto a pole as you lower into a squat).
- **Decrease Load example:** Use a band to assist with the movement.

Whether you're layering exercises to rehab after injury or surgery or you're trying to expose restrictions in mobility and technique, creating movement progressions is easy if you understand the movement hierarchy. You should be able to identify the universal shapes of stability (body archetypes). You should be able to incorporate transferable, full-range strength and conditioning movements in a way that instills good movement patterns for athletes at all ability levels (movement hierarchy). Finally, you should be able to spot mobility restrictions, understand what is happening, and know how to fix it. This is exactly what you will learn how to do in the next chapter.

Programming for the Hypermobile Athlete

Hypermobile athletes have excessive range of motion, or too much mobility (aka double-jointedness). Most ballet dancers, contortionists, and yogis fall into this category. These are people who can effortlessly and painlessly move beyond what is considered normal range of motion—like an elbow or knee joint bending in the opposite direction. Now, you may think that being very flexible is a great gift, but ask anyone who has hypermobility in their joints, and they will tell you that they would rather be stiff. Here's why.

People who have hypermobility in their joints—that is, the tissues holding the joints together are overstretched or loose—have a hard time getting into stable positions. Stated differently, it's a lot harder for a hypermobile athlete who has Gumbylike mobility to get into positions of high stability. They don't have the proprioceptive input (the ability to sense how far they are stretching and moving) that tells them where the stable position is.

Most people don't have this problem because their stable position is also their end range position. What's more, most people work at the limits of their mobility every time they exercise. It's a tried-and-true method for improving range of motion and maintaining stability in the joints during movement. Consider an athlete who drives her knees out as far as possible during a max-effort back squat. As you know, this action takes up all the capsular slack in the hips, creating a stable ankle, knee, hip, and spinal position. Not the case for the hypermobile athlete. If someone with hypermobility does this—drives her knees out as far as she can—she'll put excessive strain on the tissues holding her joints together, mainly her ligaments. Put simply, it's a recipe for disaster.

While the movement principles still apply to hypermobile athletes, certain movements and models of training are simply not appropriate for people who fall into this category. In our gym, for example, we modify movements for people who have hypermobility in their joints, especially category 2 and category 3 movements: We might program overhead squats instead of snatches or front squats instead of power cleans. In short, we remove or de-emphasize the speed element and focus on building strength and proficiency with basic squatting, pressing, and pulling movements.

It's important to note that you can still program "speed," but you should do so with movements that don't take the joints to "end range" (like stationary cycling). And when it comes to scaling up or increasing the difficulty of a movement, you can still increase volume and load, but do so using category 1 movements.

To help you better understand how to program for a hypermobile athlete, I've outlined three simple guidelines. If you have hypermobility in your joint(s) or you're a coach who is working with a hypermobile athlete, use these guidelines as a template for training.

1. Prioritize motor control and strengthen muscles around the joint(s) by focusing on category 1 movements and avoiding potentially harmful category 2 and 3 movements.

2. Using the body archetypes as a guide, learn what normal ranges of motion are for basic positions like the squat and the press. Also, consider experimenting with the archetype quick tests on pages 98–115.

3. Focus on sliding surface mobilization techniques and avoid end-range muscle dynamic mobilizations (anything that resembles stretching) and joint capsule mobilizations (banded flossing). The last thing you want to do is stretch an already overstretched tissue or joint. Soft tissue smashing and other sliding surface mobilizations are fair game.

Hypermobility can occur at a single joint (shoulder) or body region (lumbar spine) or at all the joints for a host of reasons: Genetics, bone structure, muscle structure, poor movement patterns, overstretching (think yogis), and injuries (dislocations) can all cause hypermobility in the joints, for example. Bottom line: You need to take all forms of hypermobility seriously.

My goal is to equip you with the knowledge to correct movement faults and address your own range of motion problems. However, that doesn't mean you do it alone; having someone analyze your movement and keep you honest is key. You're way more likely to pay attention to your foot position when you stand and your posture when you sit if someone else is holding you accountable. You need a coach, and you need a training partner—people who understand this material and will call you out when you're hanging out in lousy positions or moving poorly. You need someone who will offer tips on how to correct the problem and help prescribe specific mobility remedies based on your issues. I call this the MWOD Fight Club Drill. The idea is to make an agreement—whether it is with your coach, training partner, significant other, or kid—always to be in a good position. You can't run, and you can't hide.

MWOD Fight Club Drill

Chapter Highlights

- The movement hierarchy provides a template for modifying strength and conditioning movements—from simple to more complex exercises—based on stabilization demands and complexity. In short, it's a way to categorize and progress movement so that you have a model for:
  - *Regaining performance after surgery or injury*
  - *Modifying and customizing movement progressions*
  - *Understanding movement complexity*
  - *Illuminating movement errors*
  - *Identifying mobility restrictions*
- When it comes to categorizing movement, you need to consider the stabilization component, which is the ability to stay connected to the movement via the action of torque, and the number of archetypal shapes that comprise the movement.
- There are three movement categories:
  - ***Category 1 movements*** *are basic movements (squat, deadlift, push-up, etc.) that have low speed demands, express full ranges of motion, and closely resemble the actions of daily life.*
  - ***Category 2 movements*** *are similar to category 1 movements, but instead of maintaining connection (torque) throughout the entire movement, there is a speed element between the beginning and the end of the movement.*
  - ***Category 3 movements*** *closely resemble the actions of sports: You move fast, combine multiple archetypes into one movement, and change direction rapidly.*
- The orientation of your torso is another way to categorize complex movements within the framework of the movement hierarchy. The more upright your torso, the more motor control, range of motion, and stabilization are required to carry out the movement.

6

Mobility: A Systematic Approach

When it comes to correcting range of motion restrictions, addressing tight muscles, and treating achy joints, there is no one-size-fits-all approach. To account for all positional and movement-related problems, soft tissue stiffness, and joint restriction, you need to combine techniques and take a systematic approach. What's more, you need to perform basic, routine maintenance on your body—that is, spend 10 to 15 minutes a day working on your mobility. This is exactly what I've outlined in this chapter. Here you'll find a template for improving range of motion, resolving pain, and treating sore muscles. Equally important, you'll learn how and when to mobilize.

"You need to stretch!"

You've heard it a million times: the perplexing assertion that you're not stretching enough, and that's why you're injured, sore, slow, or clumsy. Think of your first coach admonishing you to stretch after practice, or your gym teacher preaching about the importance of stretching. Your back hurts? No problem! Just stretch your hamstrings and you'll feel better. You can't get into a good squat position because your quads are tight? Just stretch them out!

Conventional wisdom tells us that if we want to optimize athletic performance, improve mobility, prevent muscle soreness, and reduce the potential for injury, we have to stretch. For a long time, stretching has been a catchall modality for dealing with soreness and pain, range of motion restrictions, and joint troubles. But here's the problem: *Stretching doesn't work by itself.* It doesn't improve position, it doesn't improve performance, it doesn't eliminate pain, and it doesn't prevent injury. That's why, when you dutifully complied with your coach's order to stretch after class or practice, you didn't become a better athlete or stop getting injured.

Just to clarify: When I say "stretching," I'm referring specifically to end-range static stretching, or hanging out in an end-range position with zero intention. I'm talking about purposeless stretching. Consider the classic hamstring stretch: You sit on the ground with your legs extended in front of you, reach for your toes, and then hang out and hope that something happens. This type of stretching can theoretically "lengthen" your hamstrings, but it doesn't tell you or your coach anything about your motor control or your ability to get into good positions. In other words, taking your hamstrings to end range and keeping them there is not going to help you run faster or change your capacity to deadlift more weight. Yet when most people have a tissue or joint restriction that prevents them from getting into a good position, they think, "Man, I need to stretch more!"

Here's an analogy: If you pull on both ends of a T-shirt, what happens after a minute or so? It becomes all stretched out, right? What do you think happens when you take your beautiful tissues to end range and keep them there? They get all stretched out, just like your pitiful T-shirt. Imagine lengthening your hamstrings and then sprinting down a field or attempting a max-effort deadlift without developing the strength or motor control to handle that new end-range position. You might as well get down on your knees and beg to be injured. "Lengthening" a muscle is not a bad thing if you have the motor control to support that end-range position and you are expressing that end-range position with load-bearing, full-range exercises. This is why we deadlift, squat, and practice full-range functional movements in the gym. Put simply, performing exercise movements such as those covered in part 2 not only improves your range of motion, but also helps you develop motor control in newly developed ranges of motion gained by performing mobilizations.

The issue is not that static stretching lengthens the muscle. The issue is that it addresses (albeit poorly) only one aspect of your physiological system—your muscle. It doesn't address the positions of your joints or what's going on at those joints. It doesn't address sliding surface function—that critical interplay between your skin, nerves, and muscles. And it doesn't address motor control. Any of these things can look like tight musculature. And that's why "stretching it" is the good old-fashioned Band-Aid that we have always applied. But if stretching muscles works so well, why do we still see so much dysfunction and pain?

Stretching is not the answer. Instead, you need to deal systematically with each of the problems that are preventing you from getting into ideal positions and moving correctly. That's what I'm going to cover in this chapter. I want to show you a system for addressing all the components that limit your ability to get into safe and stable positions. This way, you'll be able to solve your particular problem(s) and see measurable improvement.

Few people think in terms of body systems because the "just stretch it" paradigm remains so prevalent. It's time to move beyond this simplistic, outmoded notion of flexibility and start thinking about the factors that impede position and how position relates to performance. To help people make this transition, I have deleted the word *stretching* from my vocabulary and replaced it with *mobility*—or *mobilization.*

I define mobilization as a movement-based, full-body approach that takes into account all the elements that limit movement and performance. These elements might include short and tight muscles, soft tissue and joint capsule restriction, motor control problems, joint range of motion dysfunction, and neural dynamic issues (tissues that do not slide over the nerves correctly). In short, mobilization is a tool for improving your capacity to move and perform efficiently.

This perspective gives me a clean slate from which to talk about movement restrictions in a more holistic way. The idea is to get you to stop thinking that stretching is important. Are you ready for this? *Stretching is not important.* Position and the application of position through movement are what matter most. If you can't get into a good position because you have a tissue restriction of some kind, stretching alone won't give you the results you want. What *will* give you results is a system that helps you figure out which variables are compromising your ability to move correctly and then identify effective modalities and techniques to resolve them.

A Movement-Based Approach

There is no single one-size-fits-all modality when it comes to correcting range of motion restrictions or tight muscles. In fact, it's best to combine techniques and take a systematic approach so that you can address all positional and movement-related problems, soft tissue stiffness, and joint restrictions at once.

It's like this: A chiropractor, orthopedist, osteopath, or joint-nutty physiotherapist cannot solve all the issues in your tissues and joints. Neither can a massage therapist or other body worker. A strength and conditioning coach might be a genius when it comes to teaching perfect movement, but that is only one variable in the equation. Does this mean that you shouldn't work with a coach, consult a doctor, or get a massage? Absolutely not! You should seek the expertise of professionals in various fields so that you know which modalities work for you.

I find that few people have a model for performing basic maintenance on the human body. When someone comes to me for treatment, I always ask, "What have you done to alleviate the problem?" And nine times out of ten, he will shrug and admit, "Nothing."

You need a go-to safe plan so that you can take responsibility for your own dysfunction. And that safe plan starts with position and movement.

To reiterate, you should always go after positional and movement mechanics first and treat the symptoms afterward. There are several reasons for this:

For starters, if you can get into a good position and move with good form, mechanical inefficiencies disappear, which means that a lot of potential overuse injuries will be nipped in the bud. It's like curing a disease without having to treat the symptoms.

Second, when you have good movement and motor control, your body can deal with tissue restrictions and weather bad mechanics longer. The bottom line is that you can't mobilize (apply a mobilization technique) and resolve all your problems at once. It's an all day, every day endeavor. Change takes time. But if you understand how to move correctly, you can at least mitigate movement errors that have the potential to cause injury and buy yourself some time to work on the compromised tissues.

Third, your body adapts to whatever positions and movements you put it in throughout the day—whether you're driving or doing burpees. If you move with good form and allow your joints and tissues to assume stable positions, you will ingrain functional motor patterns and have fewer tissue and joint restrictions. However, if you slouch or overextend while doing whatever needs doing in your life, your body will adapt to those poor positions, causing your tissues to become adaptively and functionally short, resulting in biomechanical compromise. By "adaptively and functionally short," I mean that when a joint is in a bad position, the surrounding musculature will adapt to that working position. For example, if you sit in a chair every day, your hip flexors will become adaptively short and stiff over time—see "Skin-Pinch Test" below. With that understanding, you can devise an antidote: Implement mobilization techniques that target the fronts of your hips to undo the destructive nature of sitting, and convert to a standing workstation. Standing in a good position rather than sitting eliminates the need to mobilize the same stiff tissues over and over again. Instead, you can spend your time fixing other positions and addressing other issues.

Skin-Pinch Test

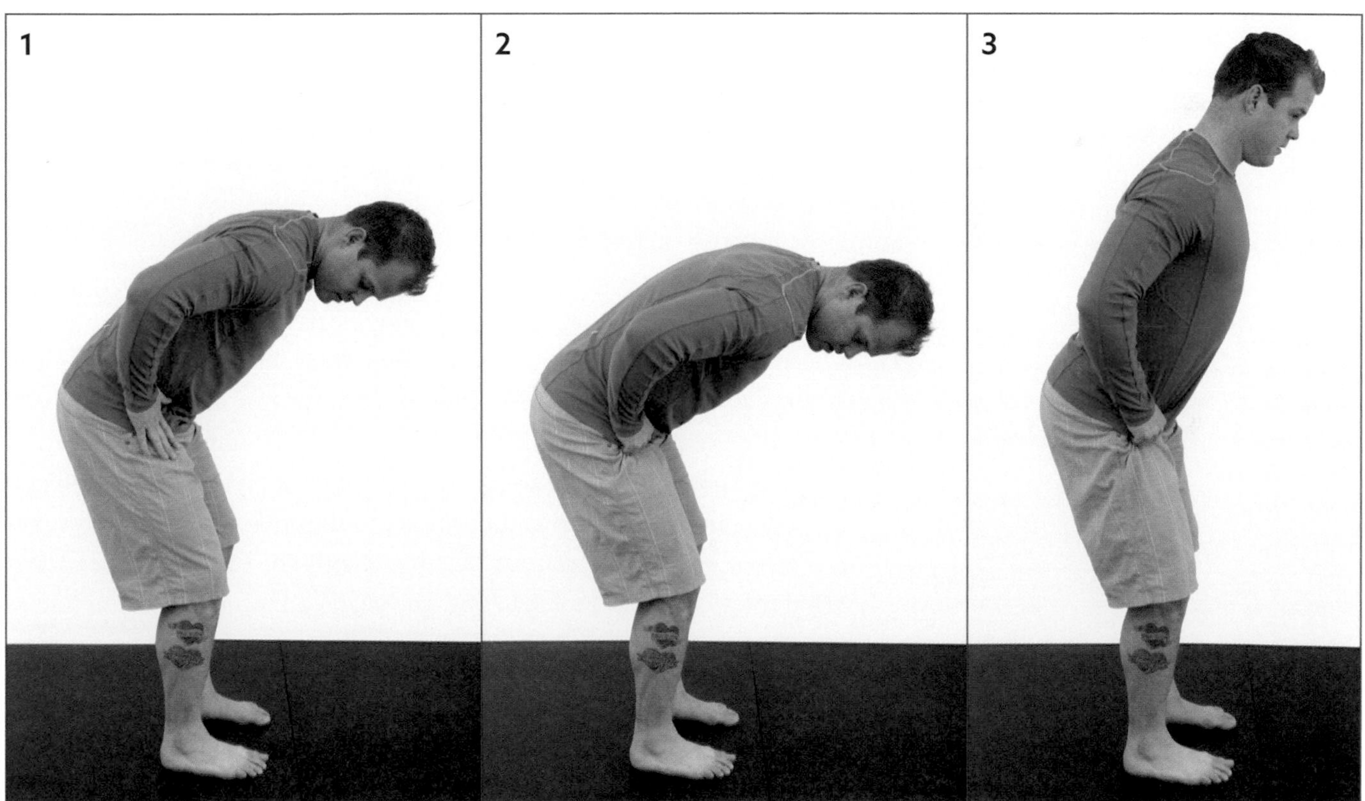

The skin-pinch test is a simple test that you can do to illuminate how your body compensates to adaptively short tissues. Stand up, hinge from your hips, and grab a handful of skin around your hip flexors. Now stand up. What happens? You have to overextend and keep your knees bent to lift your torso upright. This is exactly what happens when you sit for long periods. Your hip flexors start to reflect your working position, becoming adaptively short and stiff.

I'll use a simple example to help clarify my point. Consider an athlete training for a half-marathon who experiences hip pain 6 miles into a run. The fact that she doesn't experience pain until 6 miles, maybe 40 minutes, into her run means either that she is not strong enough to maintain good form for a prolonged period or that her body can mitigate her poor mechanics for only 6 miles. It's not a mobility-related restriction; it's a movement problem. Implementing a mobilization technique to address the pain is important, but only in the short term. It might provide immediate relief, but it won't prevent her hip pain from flaring up the next time she goes out for a long run. Simply mobilizing her hip is like taking a pill that masks the symptom but does not actually cure the disease.

What this athlete really needs to do is address her running mechanics and make sure that she's strong enough to maintain good form throughout the run. Once she learns how to run with correct form and develops the strength to maintain good form, her hip won't get tight and achy. And even if her hip does tighten up (hips inevitably get tight during long runs), she can prolong the onset of pain or maybe even prevent it altogether by moving efficiently.

The fourth reason for prioritizing position and movement is that they guide your mobility program. Put another way, they dictate the position(s) you have to change and the position(s) you need to mobilize. Otherwise you're just guessing. For example, say you can't get your knees out or maintain a rigid spine at the bottom of a squat. This is what I call a "position of restriction." To improve the bottom of the squat, it makes sense to mobilize in a position that looks like the bottom of a squat. Similarly, if you're unable to raise your arms overhead, you should probably mobilize in a position with your arms overhead. (In part 3, I include archetype icons next to many of the mobilization techniques for easy reference.)

You also need to take into account good movement mechanics as you mobilize, which is possible only if you understand what good positions look like. You will never maximize the benefits of mobility if you don't understand how to organize your body in a good position. For example, say you're missing the capacity to stabilize your shoulders in a good overhead position. To improve your shoulder function, you need to not only mobilize your shoulders with your arms overhead, but also cue external rotation. If you mobilize only the overhead component, you'll miss the most important stabilization piece, which is rotation. Similarly, if you understand that your spine should not round or overextend during a squat, you can carry that idea over to mobility (you never want to round or overextend your back while performing mobilization techniques).

Correct human movement is not open to debate. Technique is not some theoretical idea about the best way to move; it provides the means to fully express movement potential in the most stable positions possible. If you understand what those positions are, you will be able to incorporate all the elements—joints, fascia, musculature, and so on—automatically engaging several systems at once, meaning that you will address tissue restriction at the joint and in the muscle.

The question is: How do you go about addressing range of motion once you've taken motor control off the table? To answer this question, you have to take a closer look at the mobility systems at work.

The Mobility Systems

Although most mobilization techniques encompass more than one system, it's helpful to understand how each system works. This is the mobility system checklist:

- Joint mechanics
- Sliding surface dysfunction
- Muscle dynamics

The idea is to use mobilization techniques that address each system and work through the checklist until you've corrected your positions of restriction and resolved your pain.

Joint Mechanics

When I treat someone in my physical therapy practice, I always address technique before I do any kind of mobility work. That is, I highlight the faulty mechanics that caused the problem and then demonstrate the motor control fix. However, if it's clear that the person is missing major ranges of motion—meaning that I've taken motor control off the table as a limiting factor—I tend to go after the joint first, because if I can set the joint in a good position, a lot of the problems (like soft tissue restriction and sliding surface dysfunction) automatically go away.

Say I'm treating an athlete who has anterior shoulder pain because he is missing internal rotation, meaning that his shoulders are consistently rounded forward. This puts the external rotators of his shoulders in a state of constant stretch and causes his pecs to become adaptively and functionally short. I can mobilize the long, stiff musculature that is overstretched and weak and restore normal range of motion to the shortened tissues of his pecs, but until I resolve the dysfunctional mechanics of his shoulders, weakness and tightness in those tissues will always be an issue.

A much more effective approach is to put his shoulders in a good position. And that starts with mobility in the thoracic spine. If I don't fix his spinal position, I will never get to the bottom of his dysfunctional shoulder position. Restoring suppleness to his thoracic spine creates the right conditions for his shoulders to assume a good position. His external rotators will likely turn back on, and his pecs will return to their normal working state. When you put a joint into a good position, all the affiliated muscles turn on the way they're supposed to, and pain tends to disappear.

The question is: How do you mobilize a joint? There are a few tools that you can use to reset a joint into a good position, which I will discuss shortly. But before I delve into the techniques, let's discuss the component that compromises joint mobility and ultimately joint stability—the joint capsule.

When it comes to joint restriction, one of the first things you have to look at is the joint capsule. The joint capsule is a ligamentous sac (thick and leathery fibrous tissue that connects bones and cartilage at a joint) that surrounds the joint. This sac creates an internal environment for freedom of movement. It also helps create stability, keeping the joint from overstretching.

What people tend to forget (or don't fully understand) is that this strong, supportive sac can get tight and adaptively short when the joint is held in bad positions for prolonged periods, which ultimately affects joint range of motion and tissue health. If your shoulders are consistently rounded forward, chances are good that your shoulder joint capsules are extremely tight. Similarly, if you sit for extended periods, the fronts of your hips will become adaptively short and tight. What happens? You can't pull your shoulders back into a stable, externally rotated position, and you can't fully extend your hips. Now, you can mobilize your pecs to feed slack to your shoulders, and you can try to lengthen the fronts of your hips, but that mobility work deals only with the musculature; it does not account for what is happening in the joint capsules.

To help you understand this concept, imagine a rubber band that is fat on one end and skinny on the other. If you pull on that rubber band from both ends, what happens? The skinny part stretches, but you get only a little bit of stretch at the thick end. Similarly, your tissues will stretch at their weakest point. This is why people feel a big stretch in the backs of their knees when they stretch their hamstrings; the weakest end of the hamstring muscle is where it inserts behind the knee. Well, your joint capsule represents the thickest part of the rubber band. In order to effect change within a joint capsule, you need to create space within the joint. You do so by creating a banded distraction (see the photos on the next page)—meaning that you use a band to create space and facilitate movement around the joint. Physical therapists have done this manually for a long time, but the band enables you to do it yourself.

BANDED DISTRACTIONS

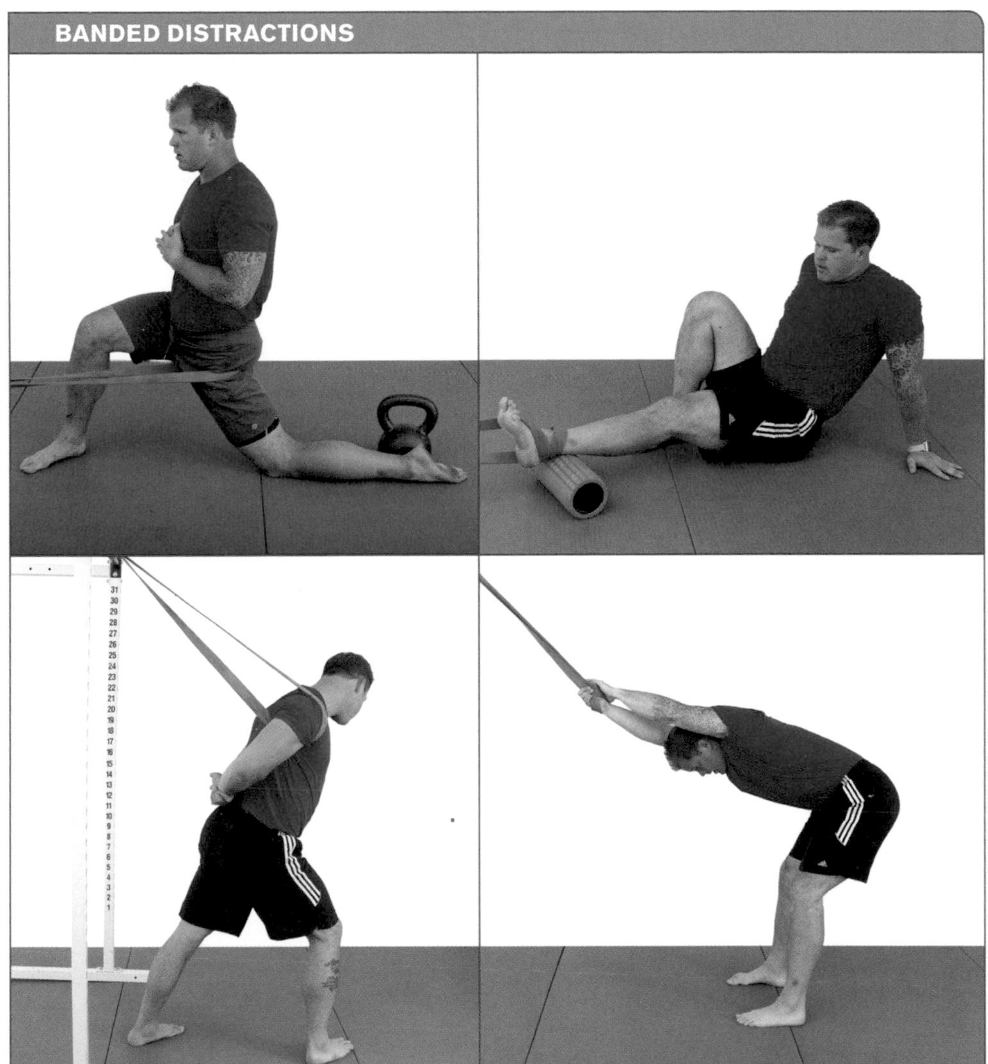

You can create a banded distraction from your hip, ankle, shoulder, or wrist.

As you can see in the photos above, the band can be used in two ways:

1. You can hook it around your hip or shoulder.
2. You can hook it around your ankle or wrist.

The former allows you to pull the joint surfaces apart so that you can reset the joint into a good position; the latter helps encourage motion through the joint capsule so that you can restore intra-joint articulation (how the joint moves inside the joint capsule) and put your joint in a good position.

The third way to address joint capsule restriction is simply to force the joint into a good position and then add rotation. For example, if you're having some funky shoulder pain or restriction, try forcing your humerus into the back of the socket—using a band or kettlebell—and then externally and internally rotate your arm, as shown on the following page. This will reset your shoulder into a good position and help you reclaim rotation range of motion.

Floor-pressing a heavy kettlebell while actively pulling your shoulder to the back of the socket will help reset your shoulder in a good position. Internally and externally rotating your arm will help restore rotation range of motion.

SHOULDER CAPSULE MOBILIZATION

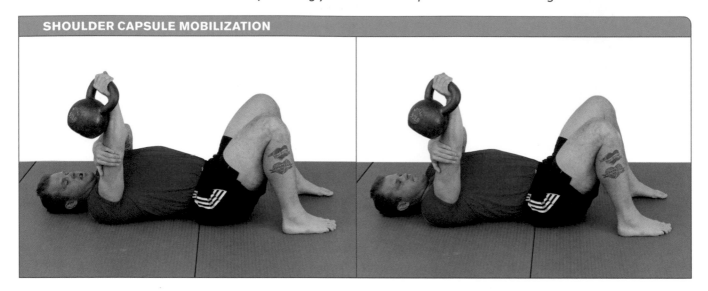

Another way to treat a stiff or painful joint is to create a gapping or compression force around the compromised area. Going back to my hinge analogy, if there's a tight hinge on a door, there will be a little pile of hinge dust. The flexion gapping method, which is used only at the elbow and knee joints, decompresses some of the joint surfaces and restores motion. Pulling the joint apart helps blow away the "hinge dust" and resets the joint in a good position. You can also wrap the dreaded yet magical VooDoo Floss Band around the joint for a similar effect (see page 146 for more on that).

Remember, if you are not actively mobilizing your joint capsules, you're leaving a huge chunk of tissue restriction on the table.

FLEXION GAPPING

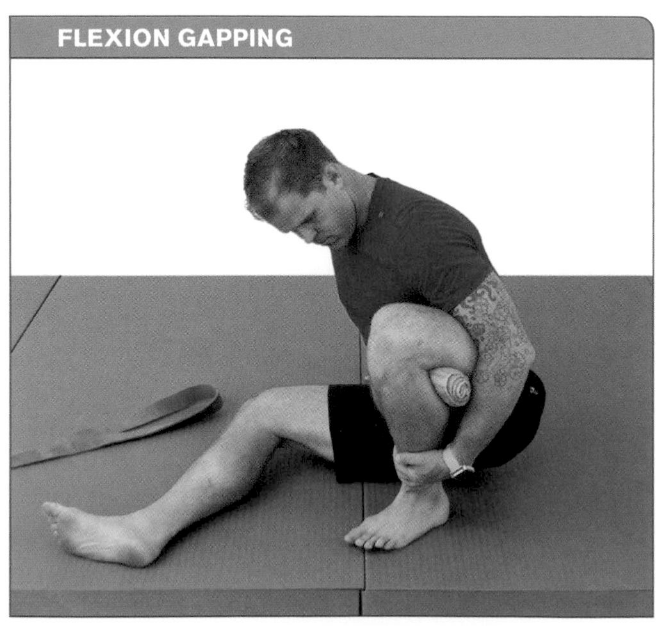

Rolling up a towel and placing it in the crevice of your knee is one way to create a gapping effect to restore motion and decompress some of the joint surfaces that restrict flexion range.

Sliding Surface Dysfunction

After you check joint mechanics off the list, the second mobility system that you should address is sliding surface dysfunction.

Sliding surface is a catchall phrase that I use to describe how the different components, structures, and systems of the body relate to one another. To ensure suppleness, your tissues—skin, nerves, muscles, and tendons—should all slide and glide over each other. Your skin should slide over the underlying surface layers (bones, tendons, muscles), your nerves should slide through your nerve tunnels (muscles), and your tissues should slide around your joints.

To test this idea, take your index and middle fingers, press down on the top of your opposite hand—keeping your hand open—and move your skin around in all directions, as shown below. See how the skin slides over the underlying bones and tissues? To a lesser degree, this is how your skin ought to slide over all the surface layers of your muscles, tendons, and bones.

For example, if you pull your toes toward you in dorsiflexion, you should be able to pinch or slide the skin over the back of your Achilles tendon. You can also test the surfaces around the outside of your knee, thigh, and ankle and around the tip of your elbow. If your skin does not glide freely over what's underneath it, you've basically created an external cast. Imagine wearing a really tight pair of jeans and then trying to squat to full depth. Not going to happen, right? If you have sliding surface dysfunction, your skin and muscle tissue is like those really tight jeans. When you sit for prolonged periods, for example, your glute muscles stick to one another and become unresponsive, which limits their ability to contract. This is why people who sit extensively have trouble fully activating their glutes to stabilize the pelvis and achieve a neutral spinal position.

SLIDING SURFACE HAND TEST

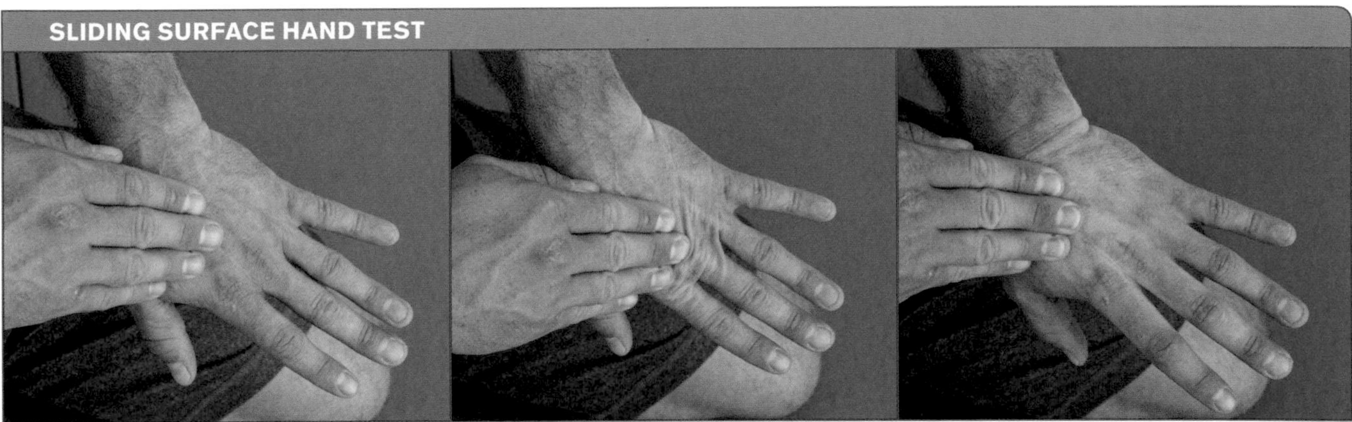

Your skin should slide unrestricted over the back of your hand.

Although you don't have as much skin elasticity around your joints, your skin should still slide unrestricted over your elbow and the outside of your knee, thigh, ankle, and heel cord.

SLIDING SURFACE TEST

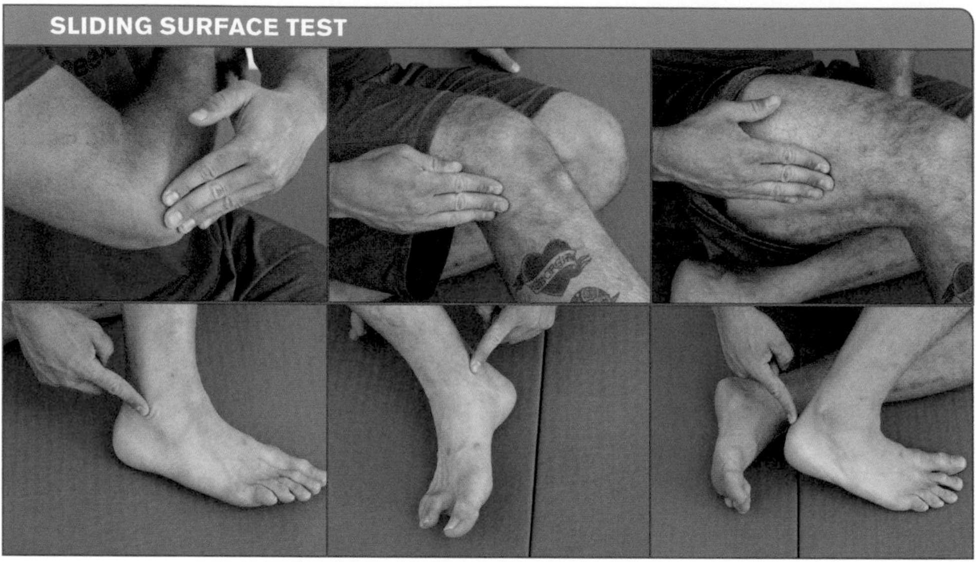

To restore sliding surfaces, you have to release that skin from the underlying tissue or bone using mobilization methods like the pressure wave and smash and floss (see pages 142–151) and techniques like the Ball Whack (see page 432). There are a number of different tools that you can use, the most common being a lacrosse ball, roller, or VooDoo Floss Band. You can also have a Superfriend smash your quads and big muscle groups by creating a shear force—grinding pressures—across the muscle, as demonstrated on page 387. What you have to remember is that sliding surface dysfunction can cause a ton of problems down the road, and no amount of stretching will alleviate it. The only way to unadhere matted-down tissue is to unglue the skin, connective tissue, and superficial and deeper layers of muscle using large shearing forces.

Muscle Dynamics

If I'm running a diagnostic on someone and I'm working sequentially through the mobility checklist, by the time I fix motor control (position or movement errors), clear joint capsule restriction, and restore sliding surface function to overly tight tissues, I've usually restored normal range of motion, and I haven't had to stretch anything. This is why muscle dynamics is the last system on the mobility checklist.

Let me say here that the muscle dynamics component uses mobilization techniques that look a lot like traditional stretches. But let me be clear: Muscle dynamics is not stretching as I've classified it. You're not just pushing the tissue to end range and hanging out for a while, hoping that something changes. Rather, you're using an active model—applying tension at end range—to help facilitate change in the tissue (lengthen the tissue) and restore some muscle contraction. And, more important, you're always biasing or emphasizing positions that look like the positions you're trying to correct. If you're restricted in the bottom of the squat, for example, you want to mobilize in a position that looks like the bottom of the squat.

I use the muscle dynamics system to lengthen muscles or increase range of motion in athletes who need to get into extreme positions, like dancers, gymnasts, and martial artists. Don't confuse this with growing new muscle. I say this because I've seen people fall into the trap of thinking that they can grow new muscle by stretching. The fastest way to grow or lengthen muscle is to perform full-range loaded movements. If your hamstrings are "tight," for example, deadlifting and squatting will not only stimulate hamstring growth, but also build motor control and strength at new end ranges.

When you restore range or function to a joint or tissue, you need to reflect that change in your training. If you improve your overhead shoulder range of motion by 5 percent and use that new range in the gym, you are much more likely to retain that range of motion. It's not a mysterious process.

When muscles are working within limited ranges of motion, they become functionally and adaptively short. Consider an elite cyclist who spends half his day on a bike. His ankles are locked in a neutral position, and his hips are stuck in a closed position. By the time he gets off his bike after a long ride, his muscles have adapted to that working position. This is where muscle dynamics and mobilization methods like contract and relax—forcing tissue to end range, contracting the muscle, and then relaxing to get a little more range—fit into my paradigm of solving problems. If you're stuck in a car for two hours, undo the sitting by spending some time at end-range hip extension (using the contract and relax method) to restore normal length to the tissue. That doesn't mean hanging out in a static position, but actively oscillating in and out of end-range tension and using a band to approximate your hip into a good position.

When possible, always mobilize in a shape that closely resembles the position you're trying to change.

My general rule is to prioritize motor control, joint capsule work, and banded flossing (see page 144) before training, and to save the sliding surface and muscle dynamic end-range mobilization techniques for after training. This way, your tissues are warmed up and prepped for the mobility work. I hear athletes say that they're afraid to stretch before they work out, and that's a reasonable fear. Doing static end-range splits before you squat heavy is probably not a good idea.

Now that you understand the mobility systems and you have a blueprint for solving problems, let's take a closer look at the methods you'll use.

MUSCLE DYNAMICS (SQUAT MOBILIZATION ITERATION)

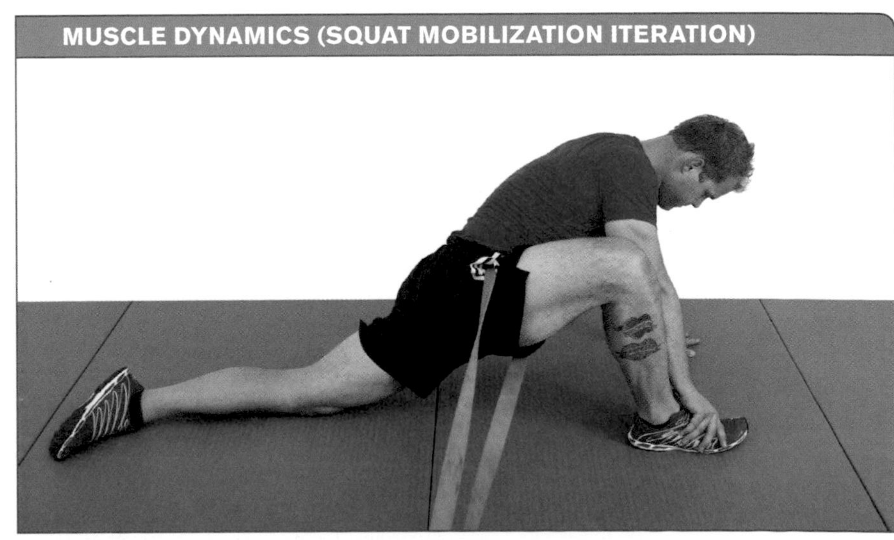

Mobilization Methods

It's important to realize that a dynamic relationship exists between the mobility systems and mobilization methods. If a joint capsule is altered by a joint capsule mobilization, for example, the soft tissue surrounding the joint will probably be affected as well. Similarly, if you restore sliding surfaces to your tissue by using a smashing technique, your joint mechanics and muscle dynamics will probably improve, too. But just as a carpenter has a specific tool for each specific job, there are specific mobilization methods for specific systems. Some techniques focus on improving position, and others are meant to restore length to shortened tissue. In addition, some mobilizations offer a more acute, pinpointed approach, and others address entire muscle groups.

In short, you need to utilize different mobilization methods so that you can cover all the different components of your restriction. So don't limit yourself to just one technique. Most of these methods can be used in combination. Say you're working on restoring sliding surface function to your glutes. You can use the contract and relax method to sink into the deeper layers of tissue, pressure wave across the stiff musculature, and then smash and floss over the knotted-down tissue. Mix and match in the way that effects the greatest amount of change in the shortest time.

Pressure Wave

Best for:
Restoring sliding surfaces, treating sore or tight muscles, releasing trigger points, improving muscle contraction

Do this:
Post workout, at night before bed, anytime you're trying to down-regulate (relax), during sliding surface mobilizations

The pressure wave is a focused approach for working through deeper layers of muscle and connective tissue. It's like using a chisel to pick away knotted-up pockets of tissue, as opposed to using a sledgehammer to break up large muscle masses. It's also a great method for addressing trigger points—tight areas within the muscle tissue that can cause pain in other parts of the body. As I will discuss shortly, your muscles should feel supple and pliable to the touch when relaxed. If you feel a "knot" or tight ropy band in the muscle and it's tender to the touch, that is what's commonly referred to as a trigger point. A trigger point not only causes pain at the site of the knot, but also can refer pain elsewhere in the body and restrict range of motion. Pressure waving into a trigger point is a great way to get the muscle to relax and return to normal function.

To execute this technique, lie on a ball or roller while remaining completely relaxed—the goal is to sink into the deepest levels of your muscle tissue. Next, create a pressure wave by slowly rolling the target area over the ball or roller using the full weight of your body. This is the equivalent of a structural integration therapist or Rolfer pressing an elbow slowly down the length of your hamstrings or quads. Go slowly, and keep the full weight of your body distributed over the ball or roller so that your tissues have a chance to relax into the ball. As a rule, the slower you move, the more pressure you will be able to handle and the more positive effects your tissues will receive. If you move fast and keep your muscles engaged as you roll, your efforts will be futile.

Get all your weight over the ball or roller and slowly roll the tissues you're trying to change over the object, creating a pressure wave across the knotted-up area.

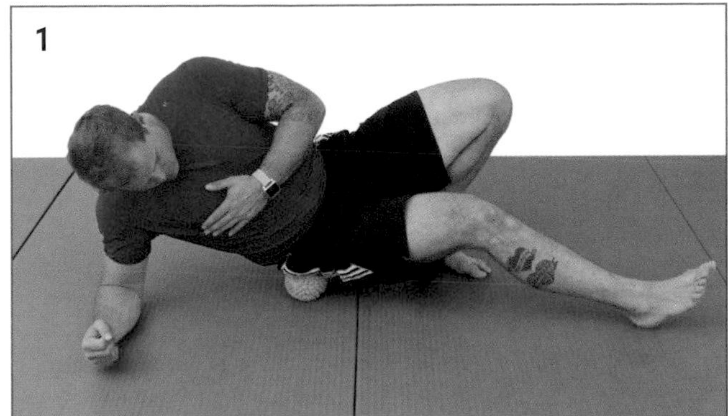

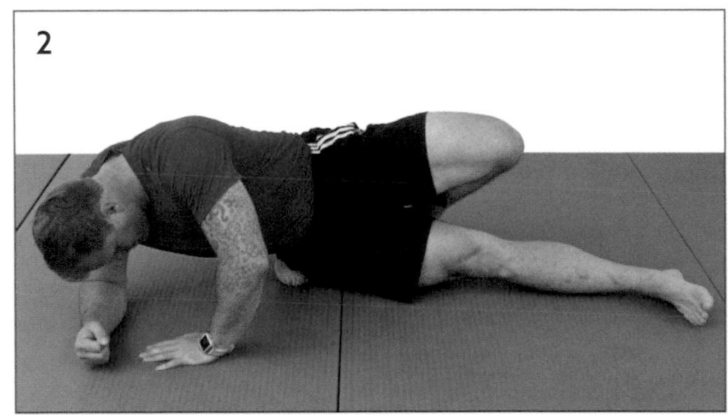

Contract and Relax

Best for:
Improving range of motion to shortened tissues during muscle dynamics mobilizations, getting deeper compression during sliding surface mobilizations, improving muscle contraction

Do this:
Post workout, anytime you're trying to lengthen tissue to end range or get a deeper compression when smashing

The contract and relax method is based on the scientifically established use of proprioceptive neuromuscular facilitation (PNF) stretching. You can use this method to improve mobility or restore normal range of motion to shortened tissue, or to get deeper compression during sliding surface mobilizations. Here's how it works:

- If you are focusing on muscle dynamics, build tension by engaging the muscle and surrounding musculature at end range for 5 seconds, release the tension, and then move into a new range for 10 seconds.
- If you are focusing on sliding surface function, identify a tight area (an area in which you can't surrender your full weight on a ball or roller) and then engage that muscle for no less than 5 seconds. After 5 seconds of tension, relax, allowing the affected tissue to sink deeper into the ball or roller.

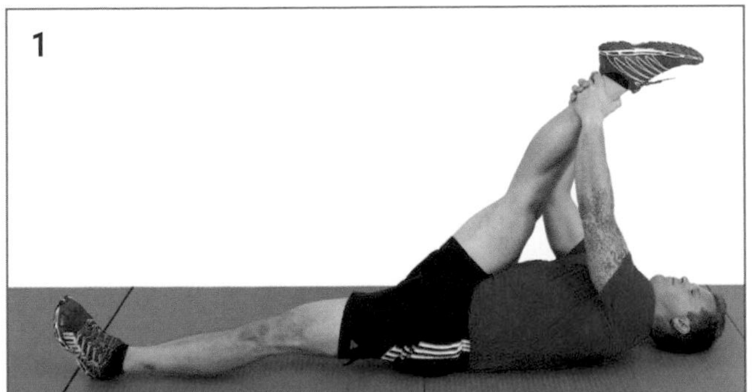

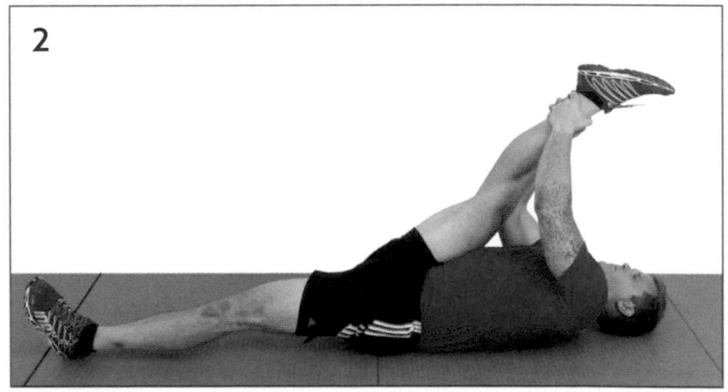

Using your hands to keep your leg in the same place, create tension by driving your leg away from you and hold that tension for 5 seconds. After 5 seconds, release the tension and move into a new range for 10 seconds.

Best for:
Mobilizing the joint capsule (creating movement or space within a joint), clearing an impingement, improving muscle dynamics and joint mechanics, improving range of motion

Do this:
Before training, after training, or between sets (so if you're doing five sets of heavy squats, you might throw in a quick banded mobilization after one or more of those sets)

Banded Flossing

The easiest way to deal with muscle stiffness is to bring the joint into a good position by using a band, and then to create movement through the joint, which I refer to as "flossing." (*Note:* "Flossing" refers to movement.) Remember, your tissues adapt to your working positions. So if you sit all day, not only will your hip flexors become adaptively short, but the head of each femur will also move to the back of the hip capsule instead of remaining in the center of it, where it belongs. And every time you perform deep flexion-based movements, the head of your femur will hit the edge of your acetabulum (hip socket). This is why you may feel an impingement or pain in the front of your hip when you squat or mobilize in positions that close that joint. Using a band to create a distraction—meaning that you create space or movement within the joint—will pull the head of your femur back to the center of the joint capsule and effectively clear that impingement so you can move into newly challenged ranges without discomfort.

Using a band also helps you manage joint capsule restriction. Because the joint capsule is so thick and robust, you need a little extra tension to affect change. Going back to the rubber band analogy, you need to account for the thick end of the rubber band to create an equal stretch throughout the muscle. This is exactly what the band enables you to do.

By creating a lateral or posterior distraction, you can effectively clear hip impingements, allowing you to move into deeper flexion ranges, as well as account for joint capsule restriction.

CLEARING HIP IMPINGEMENT

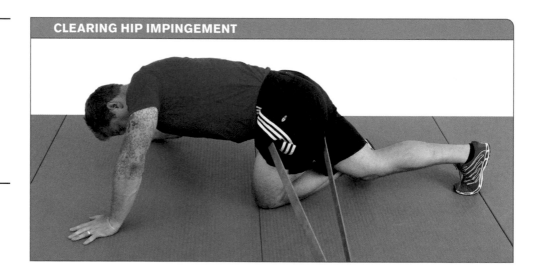

The band also allows you to "floss" around restricted joints and tissues, which happens to be one of the best ways to prepare for dynamic or loaded movements. Say you're trying to mobilize the front of your hip. The first step is to wrap a band around the back of your upper thigh and create an anterior distraction by pulling your hip forward. The next step is to get into the lunge position and perform split squats by lowering and raising your back knee. If you don't feel anything, guess what? You probably have full range of motion. But if you find that you can't get your hip into extension or you feel a big stretch in the front of your hip, chances are that your hip capsule is restricted. Although mobility work doesn't technically count as a warm-up for movement, banded flossing mobilizations like the Banded Hip Extension Lunge squat are great preparation for loaded and dynamic movements.

BANDED FLOSSING

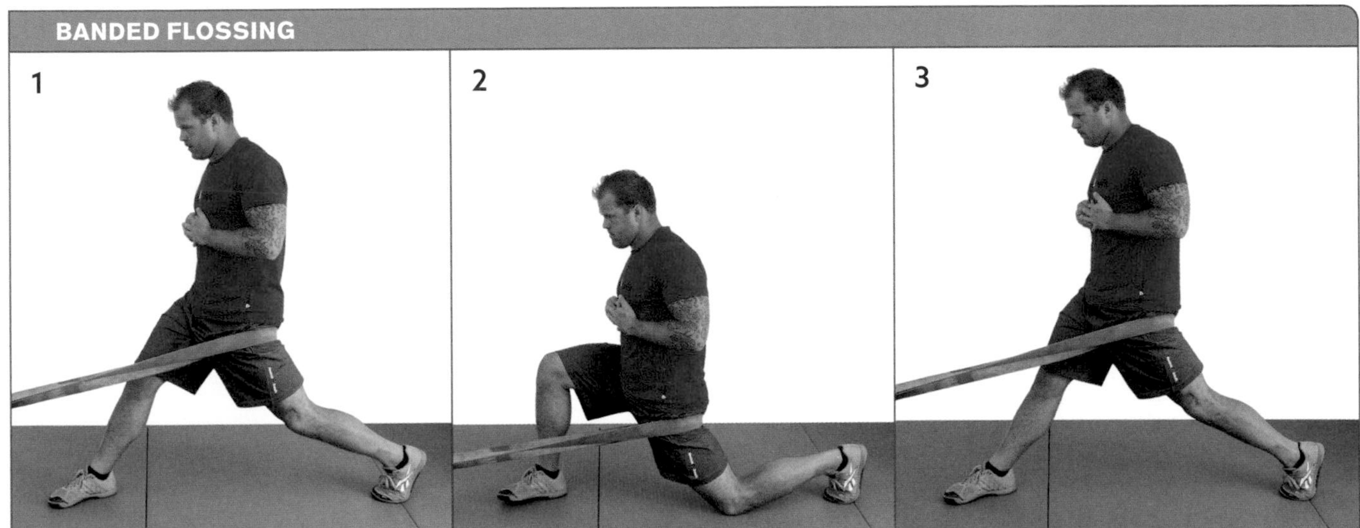

By mobilizing tissues within the context of full-range movement, you can restore normal range of motion to short and stiff tissues and affect multiple tissue systems.

Smash and Floss

The smash and floss method allows you to "tack" down or apply pressure to an area of painfully knotted tissue. Once you have applied a smash to the affected tissue, you "floss," or move, the limb around in every direction through as much range of motion as possible. This method is very similar to active-release treatment (ART), trigger-point therapy, or shiatsu, in that it focuses on restoring sliding surfaces by using movement to unglue the deep mechanical restrictions in the tissue.

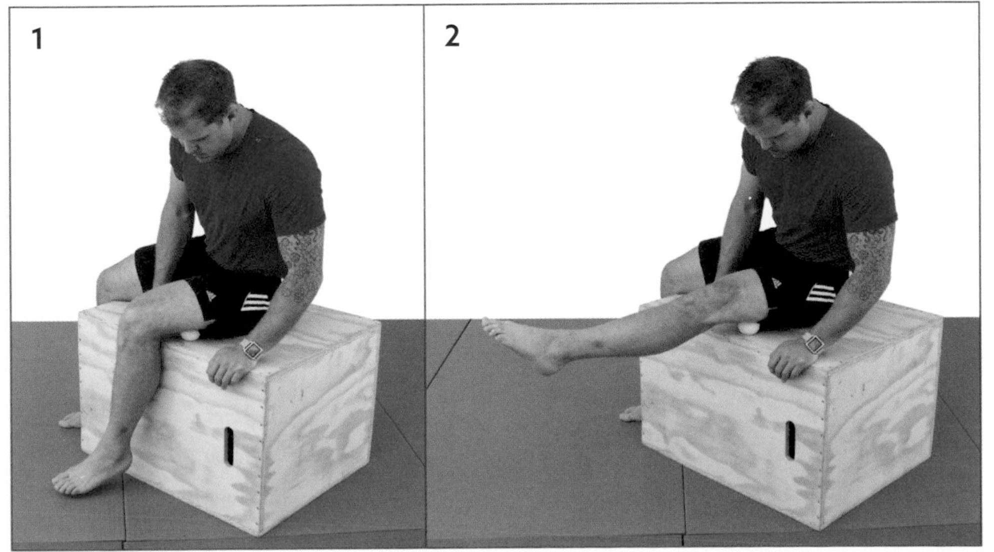

After identifying a tight area, get maximal pressure (weight) over a ball, roller, or barbell, then move your limb through as much range of motion as possible, thereby flossing the compressed tissues.

Tack and Twist

Tack and twist is another great move for restoring sliding surface function. You smash a ball—preferably a softer ball that has some grippiness to it—into the tissue to tack it down and then give the ball a twist. This technique helps you brush through stiff tissue as well as move blood into areas where circulation is relatively weak, like the heel cord or wrist.

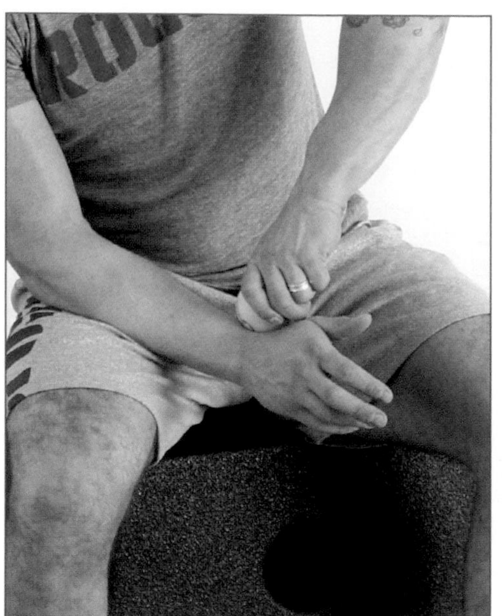

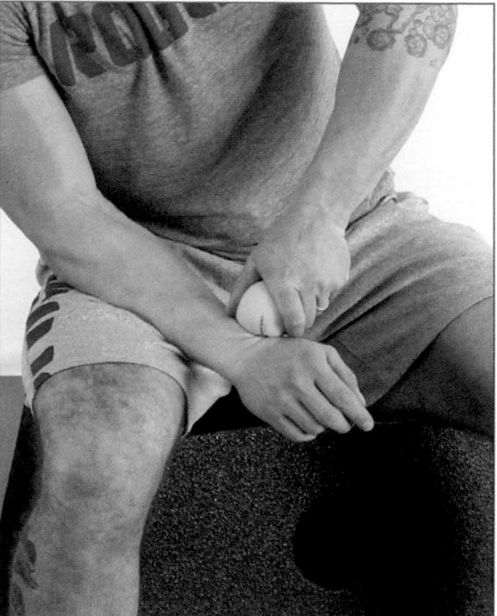

To perform the tack and twist, press a ball into the target area and then take up the skin and soft tissue slack by twisting the ball.

Best for:
Restoring sliding surfaces, releasing trigger points, removing scar tissue, clearing a swollen or inflamed joint, improving range of motion and joint mobility in a position of restriction, improving muscle contraction

Do this:
Before training, when you have a swollen joint, when you want to treat a painful trigger point or joint

VooDoo Floss Band Compression (VooDoo Flossing)

VooDoo Floss Band compression, or VooDoo Flossing, is an intermittent, compression-based joint mobilization method that incorporates all the mobility systems simultaneously. In my opinion, it's the most powerful and effective method for restoring position and range of motion. (*Note:* A VooDoo Floss Band is a stretch band engineered specifically for compression-based mobilization techniques. You can buy one at MobilityWOD.com. Another option is to improvise by cutting a bicycle tire tube in half.)

To do it, you wrap a band around the joint or restricted tissue—creating a large compression force a few inches below and a few inches above the area—move your limb in every direction for two or three minutes, and then remove the band. I typically put a 75 percent stretch across the area I'm working on and 50 percent around the remaining area. For example, if I'm VooDoo Flossing around my suprapatellar pouch (the front of my knee), I put a 75 percent stretch over the front and 50 percent around the back. Wrap with a half-inch overlap (half the width of the band). If

VOODOO FLOSSING IN A POSITION OF RESTRICTION

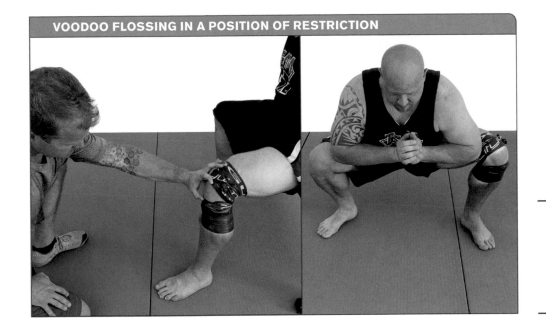

VooDoo Flossing allows you to mobilize in the position you're trying to change (such as the bottom of a squat).

you've got a length of band left over when you're done wrapping, you can make an X over the target area for an additional shearing effect.

What's great about VooDoo Flossing is that you can mobilize in the position you're trying to alter. Rolling out your quad will certainly improve your position, but you're not mobilizing within the context of functional full-range movement. For example, if you wrap your quads and then squat, you're able to change the mechanics in some of the tissues that may be restricting your squat. If you wrap your knee and then squat, you're loading the joint and encouraging improvement in every system while getting into your position of restriction.

Here's the deal: You can only guess what you're changing because VooDoo Floss Band compression works on so many different levels. Wrapping a band around a joint or chunk of scar tissue and introducing movement creates a global shearing effect—restoring sliding surface function to the underlying tissues—and the bulk of the band creates a flexion gapping force at the joint, which can help restore range of motion to the joint. Not only that, but when you release the compression, blood floods into poorly saturated joints and tissues. In short, VooDoo Flossing will help restore sliding surface function to matted-down tissue, resolve joint pain, and radically improve muscle contraction. If you're limited by position or have knee or elbow pain (this method is my first stop for treating tennis elbow), wrap a band around the joint or restricted area and force the tissue through the full range of motion.

VooDoo Flossing is also one of the best methods for dealing with a swollen joint or swollen tissue. Swelling blows out a lot of the proprioceptors (sensory receptors within the body that respond to position and movement), presses on nerve endings, causes acute pain, and degrades joint mechanics. You should take swelling very seriously. Compressing the joint pushes swelling back into the lymphatic system, where it can be drained from the body.

It's important to note that the technique for wrapping a swollen joint is slightly different. To flush out ankle swelling caused by a sprain, for example, start as close to the tip of the foot as you can, wrapping with about a half-inch overlap (half the width of the band) and keeping about a 50 percent stretch in the band all the way around the swollen ankle. The keys are to begin wrapping a few inches below the swollen area, leave no skin exposed, and keep even tension in the band. Once the foot is wrapped (compressed), move it around for a couple of minutes. Take off the band to give the tissue a few minutes to rebound and recover, and then wrap it again. Repeat this process for about 20 minutes (2 or 3 cycles) or until you stop experiencing change. It's insanely effective. By using this method, you can restore an ankle the size of a grapefruit to normal size and completely relieve the pain. In my opinion, VooDoo Floss Band compression is the best remedy for inflammation and pain in an injured joint.

The general rule for VooDoo Flossing a swollen joint is to wrap toward the heart. So if you're wrapping an ankle, you start at the toes and wrap up the leg. However, when you're using VooDoo Floss Band compression to mobilize a joint or matted-down scar tissue, it doesn't really matter whether you wrap from high to low or low to high—just start a few inches below or above the target area.

VOODOO FLOSSING SWOLLEN JOINTS

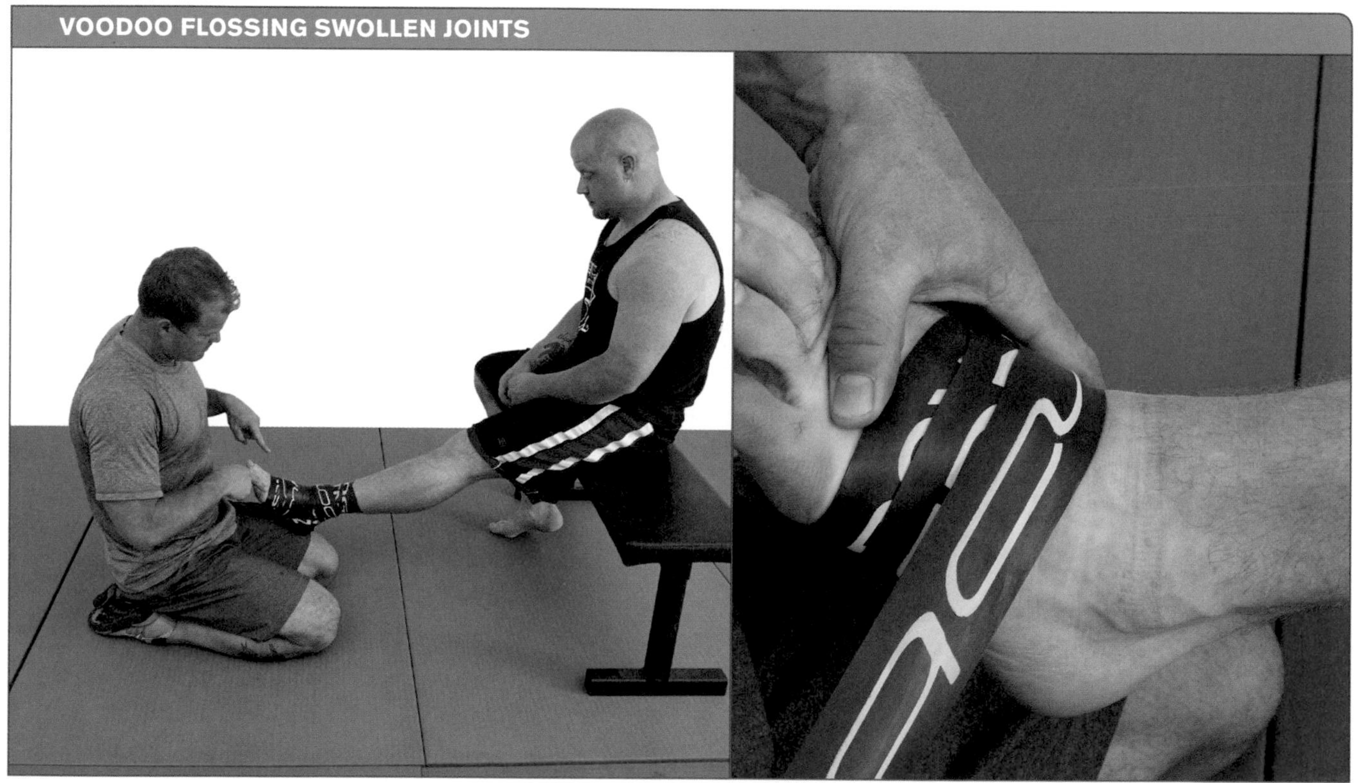

To VooDoo Floss a swollen joint, start as far down on the limb as possible, wrapping toward the heart, and create a 50 percent stretch in the band around the swollen area. The goal is to cover the entire area, keeping a half-inch overlap as you wrap.

VOODOO WRAPPING TECHNIQUE: ELBOW

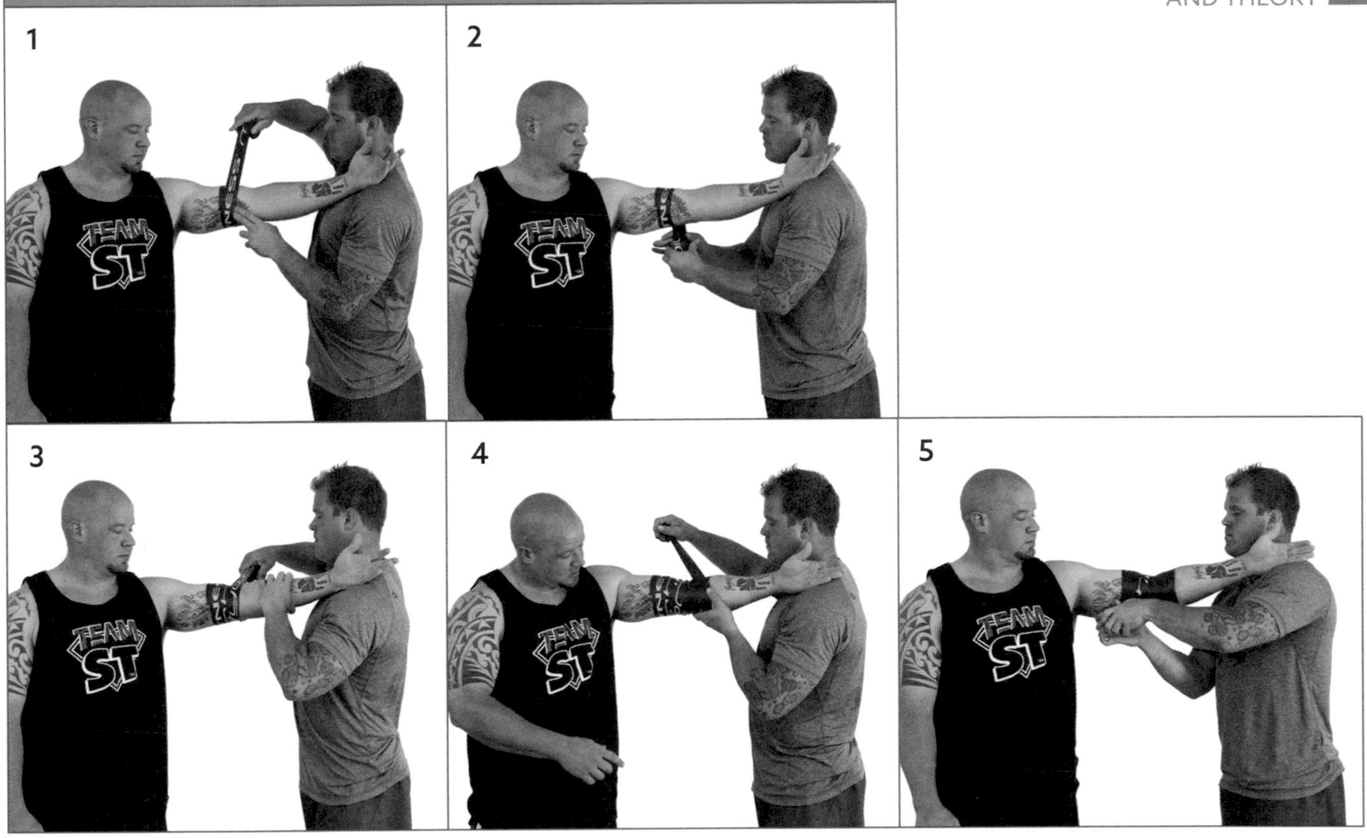

To wrap a joint or section of restricted tissue, start a few inches below or above the target area, keeping a half-inch overlap in the band. Continue wrapping until you cover the area you are trying to change. If you have extra band, form an X by wrapping across the entire area. On your final loop, create extra stretch so that you can tuck the end piece underneath the band. The tension will keep the band in place. Once wrapped, move the limb through as much range of motion as possible.

VOODOO WRAPPING TECHNIQUE: QUADRICEPS

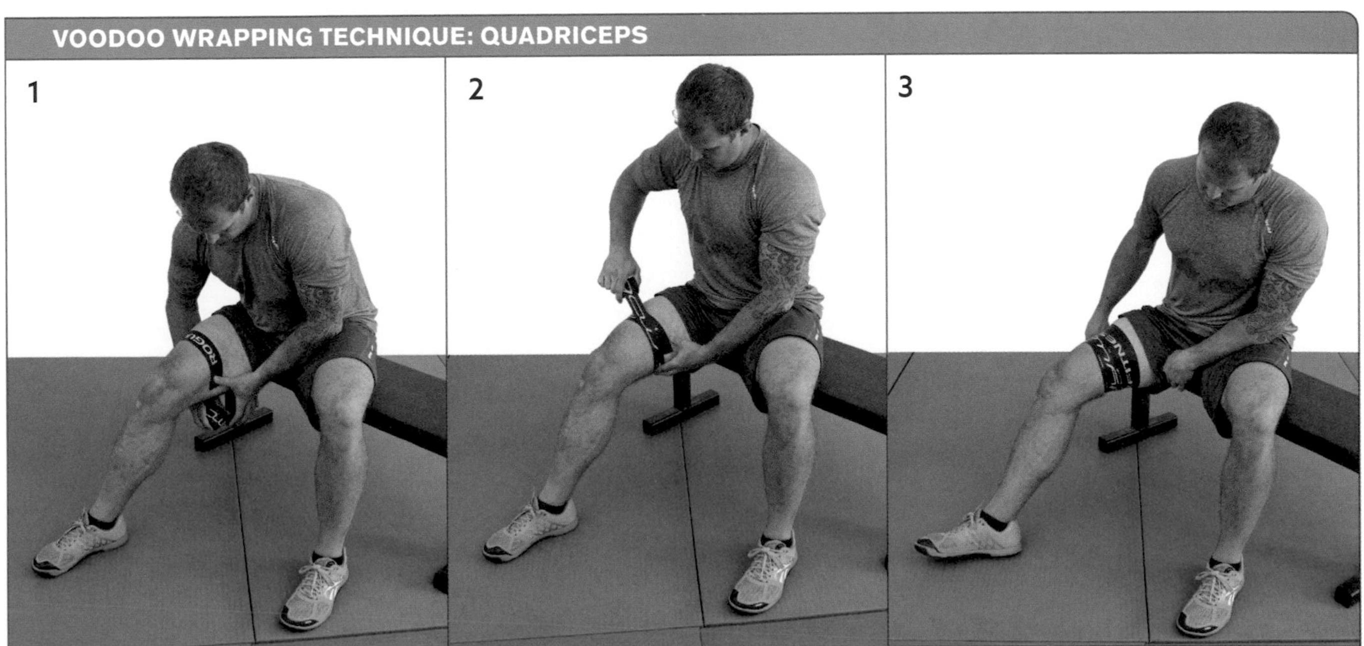

Just so you know, VooDoo Flossing can be a bit uncomfortable. But don't worry; despite the discomfort, it will not harm the joint or tissue in any way. If you end up with some red marks on your skin (I call them leopard stripes), don't panic—that's just the superficial layers of skin being pulled. You'll live.

There are some general guidelines to follow, however. For starters, if you start to go numb or feel a tingly pins-and-needles sensation, or your skin turns a zombie-like color, take the band off. This usually happens at around the two-minute mark. In most cases, you will feel a tingly sensation before your hand or foot turns white, so when you hit this stage, act fast. Another warning sign is suddenly feeling very claustrophobic. You need to respect these sketchy feelings and signs. As with most mobilization methods, VooDoo Flossing is pretty intense, but you should be able to differentiate between discomfort and numbness, tingling, or claustrophobia.

SAFETY CHECK

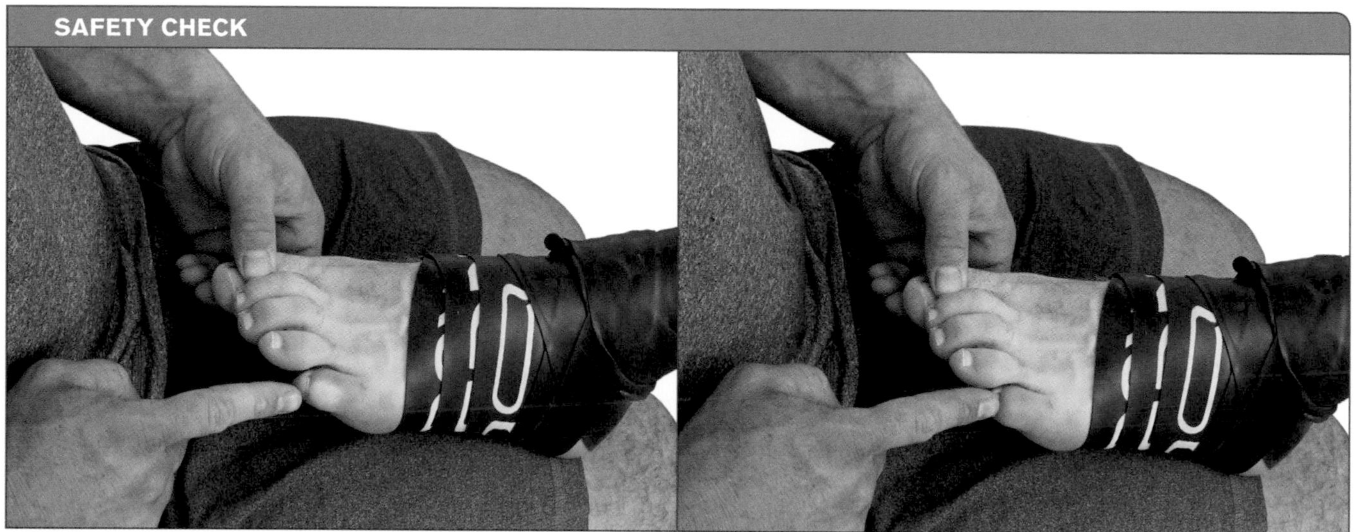

When you touch the skin, it should turn white and then return to normal—like touching sunburned skin. If you touch the skin and color doesn't return, it's time to take the band off.

INCREASED BLOOD FLOW

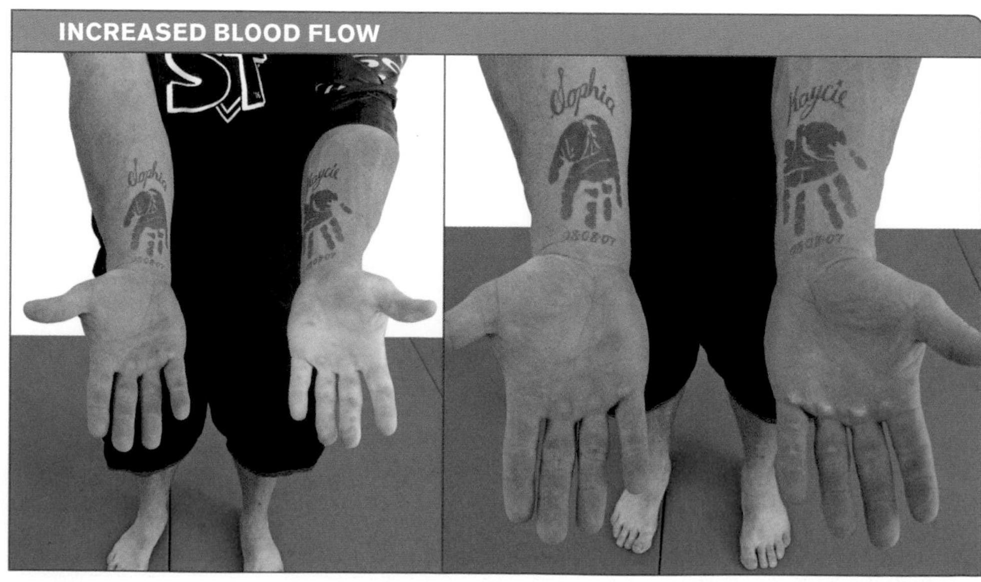

When you take the band off, your skin will turn the color of a dead person. But within a few seconds, you'll notice increased blood flow into the area.

As you reach the two-minute mark, your skin will turn the color of a dead person. While this is normal, it's also warning sign that you should take the band off. Once the band is removed, you'll notice increased blood flow into the area within a few seconds.

LEOPARD STRIPES

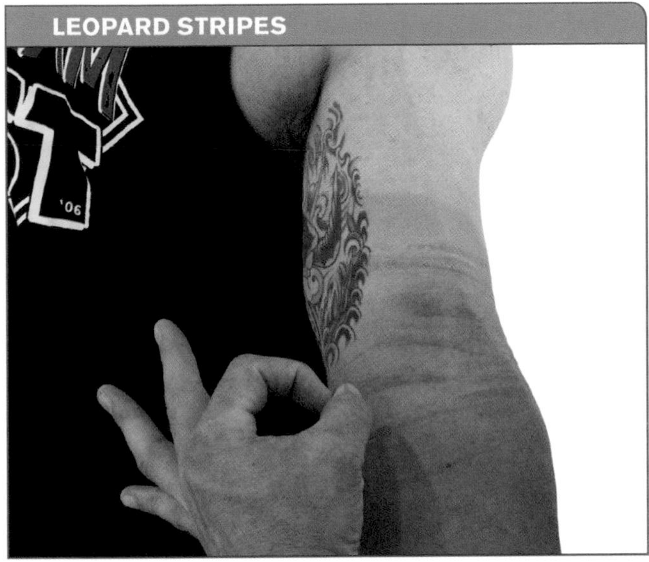

The band will pinch your skin, leaving red lines across your skin. Don't flip out. They will disappear after a few minutes.

Flexion Gapping

Flexion gapping helps eliminate joint capsule restriction and restore flexion range of motion to the knee and elbow. You should be able kiss your forearm to your biceps and get your calf flush with your hamstring without effort. If you have to move your head toward your hand to feed yourself or turn your feet out so that you can drop into a deep squat, you're missing flexion range of motion in your secondary engines (knees and elbows). An easy way to blow away the hinge dust and restore normal range to the joint is to roll up a towel, jam it behind your knee or elbow, and then create a compression or flexion force over the fulcrum. You can also use a band to create that gapping effect, as illustrated in the middle photo below.

Best for:
Creating space within a joint, restoring flexion range of motion to the knee and elbow

Do this:
Before or after a workout, if you're missing flexion range of motion in your knee or elbow

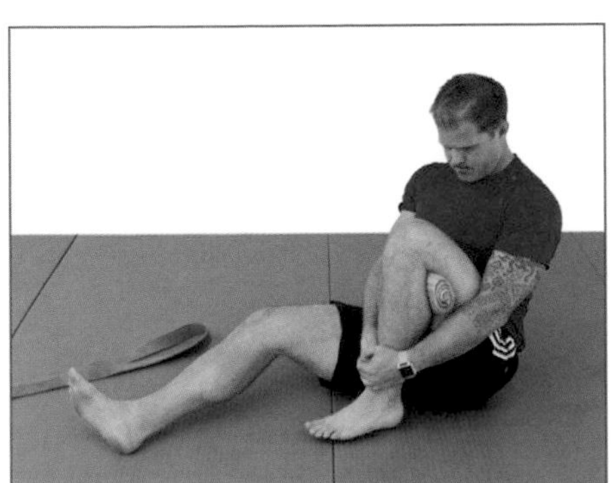

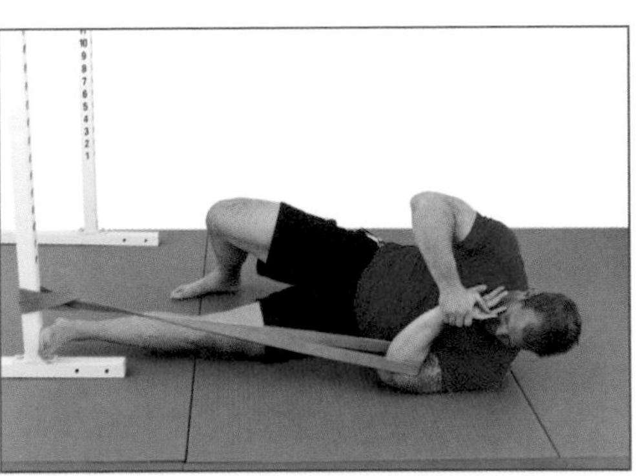

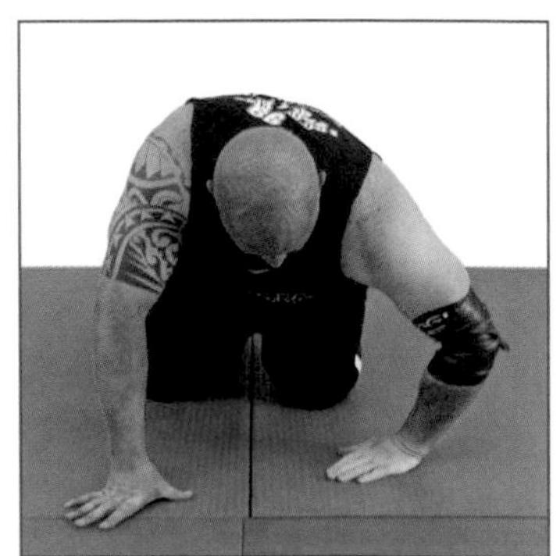

You can create a gapping force by rolling up a towel or by creating a distraction with a band. VooDoo Flossing also creates a gapping effect.

Three Rules for Resolving Pain

Identifying your position(s) of restriction is the best way to address tissue dysfunction and solve mechanical problems as they relate to movement. If you're struggling to drive your knees out in the bottom of a squat, for example, it makes sense to mobilize in that position of restriction. But what if you tweak your knee or back or get hurt playing a sport?

Even if you maintain good form and move with perfect technique, pain and injury are an inherent reality, especially if you play and train at a high level. Joints get tweaked and tissues get stiff—it's the nature of being a physically active human being. This is why it's important to have a template not only for solving mechanical problems, but also for resolving and treating pain.

But I'm getting ahead of myself. Let me take a moment to describe what I mean when I say "tweak."

To be clear, a tweak is not a serious injury. It's a catchall phrase for strains, sprains, and minor movement faults that give way to painful muscle spasms: You're in a bad position or your muscles are tight, you move wrong, you tweak a joint, and that leads to pain symptoms. For example, say you hurt your back picking something up with a rounded back, or you hurt your shoulder pressing something overhead with rounded shoulders. You may think, "Oh shit, I just herniated a disc," or, "I just tore my rotator cuff." But let's be honest: You don't know exactly what you did. All you know is that you're hurt and in pain. Don't get me wrong, if you feel like you're seriously injured, don't mess around. Go see a doctor and get yourself checked out. But if all you did was tweak something—because your muscles are too tight or you are in an unstable position—you can probably address the issue yourself by following these three simple rules:

1. If something is not in the right place, put it in the right place.
2. If something is not moving, get it moving.
3. Work upstream and downstream of the problem.

As a physical therapist, my first order of business when addressing a tweak is to reset the joint into a good position. As I alluded to earlier in the chapter, if I can set the joint in a good position, a lot of the problems (like joint pain and muscle spasms) go away. If you just go after the spasm and never put the joint into a good position, on the other hand, the pain will persist. So if you tweak your shoulder, you need to get your shoulder into a good position (put it in the right place) and move into pain-free ranges (get it moving) by using mobilization techniques that focus on joint mechanics. If you're treating your shoulder, for example, you could employ VooDoo Floss Band compression (page 146) and the Shoulder Capsule Mobilization (page 310). This will clear joint impingements, flush out inflammation, restore sliding surfaces, and get fresh blood into poorly perfused tissue. After you've put the joint into a good position with movement, you can work to break the spasm or tissue restriction that is reinforcing the bad motor pattern using the upstream-downstream approach.

The upstream-downstream approach is simple: Mobilize the tissue upstream (above) and downstream (below) of the problem.

What's great about this approach is that you don't need to know anything about movement or anatomy to take care of yourself. Just target the muscles and tissues above and below the restricted area. It's that simple. And yes, you can certainly mobilize at the site of pain. However, where the rats get in is not necessarily where they chew. If you have tight calves and quads, for example, those tissues will pull on your knees, restricting range of motion and compromising mechanics. Remember that you are encased in a web of fascia—a sheet or band of fibrous connective tissue covering, separating, or binding together the muscles, organs, and soft structures of the body—that transmits movement throughout your body. So if your calf, quad, or hamstring is tight, the fascia surrounding the musculature will also be tight. And if the fascia is tight, it will pull on your knee, compromising your ability to get into stable positions. By mobilizing the tissues above and below your knee—the quad, suprapatellar pouch, hamstring, calf, and shin—you can feed slack to the tensioned joint and restore normal function to the muscles and fascia tugging on your knee.

The only drawback with the upstream-downstream approach is that it's predicated on a lagging indicator, meaning that you spent time moving incorrectly before your body started transmitting the pain signal. Ideally, you want to identify and deal with restrictions *before* they devolve into pain. The problem is that it's easy to circumvent or assimilate bad mechanics until your body starts hurting. So figure out where you are restricted and then work on restoring and improving range of motion there before the area becomes a source of trouble.

To help you treat common tweaks and resolve pain using the mobilization techniques featured in this book, I've included several sample prescriptions for joint tweaks and pain in part 4.

Programming for Mobility

To reiterate, there are two ways to approach mobility work:

1. Identify your position or area of restriction and mobilize within the context of the position you're trying to improve.

2. Mobilize upstream and downstream of a painful area.

Now that you have a basic template, let's discuss how to program (construct an individualized prescription) for mobility.

To begin, it's important to understand that there are no days off (see "The Seven Rules of Mobility," beginning on page 156). You need to commit 10 to 15 minutes every single day to mobilizing. If you can do more, great, but 10 to 15 minutes is the minimum requirement. We modern humans are very busy, yet we still need to carve out time to work on position and improve tissue function. Although 15 minutes of mobility work may not seem like much, it adds up to 105 minutes over a week, which is a significant amount of time.

What should you do within that 10- or 15-minute time frame? Here are four general guidelines to help you devise an individualized mobility program:

1. Resolve issues with painful joints and tissues first, and then focus on positions of restriction. If you imagine a target, your painful joints and tissues should be at the center of that target every time you mobilize, and work on those areas should comprise a good portion of your designated 10- to 15-minute block of time. Spend the rest of the time focusing on a restricted position that you're trying to improve (such as the bottom of a squat) or undoing any damage you might have incurred from your day, like being buckled into an office chair.

2. Make a "problems" list. When it comes to programming for mobility, it helps to know what you need to work on and—equally important—why. Here's what I recommend: Make a detailed list of issues that could potentially be solved or treated using mobilization techniques (such as shoulder pain or missing range of motion in the bottom of the squat). Keep it simple and limit it to things that are actionable and specific to you or your sport. Lastly, make sure that you understand why the problems on your list need to be resolved. This attaches meaning and value to your prescription or the mobility program that you create. Stated differently, understanding *why* you're doing something—whether you're trying to improve a position of restriction or resolve pain—gives your mobility session purpose. This is how you stay motivated to mobilize, which, let's face it, nobody really wants to do.

3. Spend no less than 2 minutes in each position. Research unquestionably asserts that it takes at least 2 minutes to make soft-tissue change, which means that 2 minutes is your minimum therapeutic dose per position. For example, if you're doing the Couch Stretch (page 391), you need to spend no less than 2 minutes mobilizing each hip. However, my rule as a therapist is to work on a restricted area until there's improvement or I realize that there's no more improvement to be had in the session. This could mean 2 minutes or 10 minutes. So don't be in a rush to move on if you haven't experienced positive change in the tissue.

4. Choose 3 or 4 mobilization techniques or areas/positions to mobilize. Don't get overly ambitious and try to mobilize in 10 different positions. Most people can handle only 3 or 4 mobilization techniques per session.

Now that you understand some of the basic rules that guide mobility programming, let's apply them to a hypothetical athlete who is having shoulder pain and has trouble getting into the bottom of a squat. As with the four mobility guidelines, I'm including this template to help you better understand how to construct a personalized mobility program or prescription.

Mobilize the Shoulders:

- Shoulder Capsule Mobilization (page 310): 2 minutes on each arm
- Overhead Banded Distraction (page 301): 2 minutes on each arm

Mobilize the Bottom of the Squat:

- Single-Leg Flexion with External Rotation (page 370): 2 minutes per side

Undo Damage from Sitting:

- Super Couch (page 393): 2 minutes per side

Total time: 16 minutes

Remember, programming for mobility changes from day to day, depending on your current areas of restriction, the movements you're performing, and the positions you're hanging out in. The key is to constantly work on your position and spend the necessary time doing basic body maintenance. It's also helpful to develop a list of problems or issues that you want to improve or change.

In part 4, I provide several prescriptions and more elaborate examples—for specific positions of restriction, dealing with pain, etc.—to give you a better understanding of how to build an individualized mobility program.

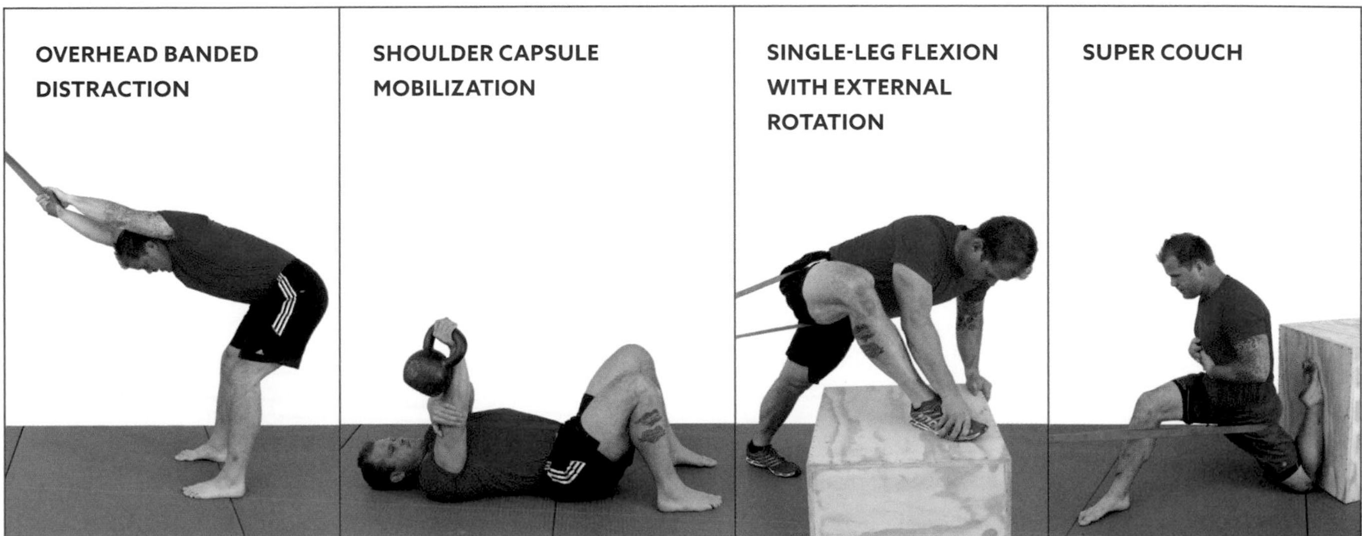

The Seven Rules of Mobility

To optimize your time and keep you safe, I've laid out seven fundamental rules for implementing the mobilization techniques. Consider these seven rules of mobility as general guidelines for performing basic maintenance on your body.

Test and Retest

Everything you do should have observable, measurable, and repeatable results. Otherwise, your time would be better spent watching reality TV. Think of testing and retesting as a diagnostic tool for measuring improvement within the context of movement and/or pain.

Here's how it works: Say you're trying to improve your squat. Before you start smashing your quads or mobilizing your calves, get into the bottom of a squat and assess your areas of restriction. Next, perform some mobility techniques on the tissues that you think might be holding you back from achieving optimal form. For example, if you think your tight calves are the problem, do some calf mobilizations and then retest the bottom of your squat. Can you drive your knees out farther? Can you keep your back flat? If you mobilized the right area and implemented the appropriate techniques, you should experience or observe measurable improvement. If you can't see improvement, then you have irrefutable, the-world-is-round evidence that there wasn't a problem in that area, which means that you need to start targeting another area.

Mobilizing should improve your ability to get into a good position, optimize movement, and reduce or banish pain. Testing and retesting lets you know whether what you are doing is actually working. Also, utilizing your new range of motion right away in an actual movement helps your brain keep track of that new range.

If It Feels Sketchy, It's Sketchy

Mobilizing restricted tissue is uncomfortable—there's no getting around that fact. If you've ever subjected your quads to some smashing on a roller, you know what I'm talking about. But unless your entire quad is as stiff as wood, only certain sections will hurt. When you hit a patch of restricted tissue, it's agony, but as soon as you move past it, the pain is over. That's because supple tissue doesn't elicit a pain response under pressure.

But there's a difference between discomfort—even intense discomfort—and harmful pain. If you think you're injuring yourself, you probably are. If something feels like it's tearing, something probably is tearing. If you experience hot, burning pain, your body is telling you that something is not right. If you're getting a horrible hip impingement, guess what? You have a horrible hip impingement. Don't keep mobilizing into the problem, because it will only make the problem worse.

What I'm trying to say is that ungluing stiff, restricted tissue can be uncomfortable, but it shouldn't feel like you're causing more damage than is already there. It's up to you to know the difference and listen to your body. Having a glass of wine can make mobilizing a little more tolerable, but getting drunk and passing out on a lacrosse ball is never a good idea. And if you roll around on that lacrosse ball for an hour (before you pass out!), you're going to bruise your precious tissues.

I often say, "Don't go into the pain cave." People have an immense capacity to hurt themselves, ignore pain, and travel to places of extreme suffering. And that's how they end up hurting themselves while mobilizing. This is what I must say to you: Stand at the entrance of the pain cave, but do not enter the pain cave. Mobility should be uncomfortable but not unbearable.

No Days Off

It's important to understand that there is no distinction between lifting heavy in the gym and picking up a pillow. Both require conscious awareness of positioning and how best to organize your body. No matter what you are doing throughout the day, you should always be thinking about improving your position and movement mechanics, as well as spend at least 10 to 15 minutes performing basic body maintenance. Likewise, you don't want to take a day off from good nutrition or miss a night of sleep. Of course, there will be times when you can't eat perfectly, exercise, or get eight hours of sleep. But you should cultivate a habit of always being in a good position, regardless of what you're doing.

The fact is, if you want to play and train at a high level, you cannot slack off for even one day. You have to think about your position constantly, whether you are at work, playing a sport, lifting, or lounging around. This is the basis of the No Days Off rule.

Here's a simple example to help illustrate my point. A DEA agent buddy of mine told me about a friend who used to walk past his trunk every time he got out of the car. It didn't matter whether he was on or off duty, or whether he had parked at a grocery store, at home, or at a restaurant—he would walk all the way around the car and past his trunk every single time. He did it because he kept his rifle in his trunk and wanted to ingrain the pattern of approaching his trunk into his motor program. That way, if he ever found himself in a dodgy firefight, he wouldn't hesitate or think—he would automatically find himself by his trunk, ready to grab his rifle.

Remember, your body is an adaptation machine. If you spend a few minutes a day working on improving your position, you will improve your position. But if you take a few days off, you will get stiff, and your movement and position will reflect that adaptation. Even if you're taking a day off from the gym, you should never take a day off from mobilizing. In fact, a lot of muscle soreness and tissue stiffness aggregate the day after training, and those are the days when you really need to work on restoring normalcy to those tissues. For this reason, it's best to break up mobility into short doses. Doing so gives you plenty of time to effect change within the context of movement, and, more important, it is manageable over the long haul.

Make Mobility Realistic

As I've said before, the average person isn't going to know what I'm talking about if I tell him that he needs to improve hip flexion and external rotation. But if I tell him that he needs to mobilize the bottom of the squat, he can immediately make the connection between the position he needs to mobilize and the position he's trying to change. This makes it easy to start thinking about how to approach mobility. If you're missing overhead range of motion, it makes sense to mobilize in a position with your arms overhead and externally rotated.

The key is to prioritize mobilization techniques that approximate real-life situations. Instead of stretching your hamstrings while lying on your back, for example, get a band around your hip and hinge from the hips while standing up, which looks a lot like deadlifting. The more you can replicate what you're trying to change, the more you will improve your position.

Always Mobilize in a Good Position

Committing an overextension spinal fault or mobilizing with your shoulder in an unstable position is not going to get you the results you're looking for. In fact, all you're doing is encouraging bad positions and ingraining poor mechanics. Keep the movement principles in mind as you mobilize. If your ankles collapse, your knees cave inward, your back rounds, or you overextend at your lumbar spine, reset and fix your position.

Don't Get Stuck in One Position; Explore Your Business

Think of the mobilizations as basic guides. Although I demonstrate how to perform each mobilization with proper technique, you are not limited to performing them exactly as indicated in the photos. You know where you're tight and restricted better than anybody else. As long as you maintain good form and avoid defaulting into bad positions, you should feel free to explore your dysfunction and move into newly challenged areas. I call this "informed freestyle." If you're mobilizing your anterior hip, for example, you might rotate your body to the side or put your arm overhead. The key is to target the areas that feel the tightest.

Don't Make a Pain Face

We have a saying around our gym: Don't make a pain face while mobilizing. For one, it shortens your neck flexors, causing restriction along the athletic chain. Second, you don't want to associate pain with a weird face because those things get mapped together in your body. If you grimace every time you roll out your quads, what expression do you think you'll make when your quads start burning during a workout? In a competitive environment, you don't want to give away how much you are suffering. Your opponent will see that and use it to his advantage. This is why athletes practice relaxing their faces when they're uncomfortable. When you mobilize, you're making a conscious choice to improve yourself, so you may as well embrace it.

Lastly, making weird faces while you're lying on a ball can be pretty creepy—you don't want to freak people out.

Chapter Highlights

- End-range static stretching does not work. To maximize physical performance and reduce the potential for injury, you need to take a systematic approach by addressing every aspect of your physiological system. This includes short and tight muscles, soft tissue and joint capsule restriction, motor control dysfunction, and joint range of motion limitations.
- Always prioritize motor control first, and treat systems using mobility techniques afterward.
- Mobilization (mobility) is a movement-based, full-body approach that takes into account all the elements that limit movement and performance. Consider the mobilization techniques as tools for improving motor control and range of motion and maintaining joint and tissue health.
- You need to address three aspects of your physiological system by using mobilization techniques: joint mechanics, sliding surfaces, and muscle dynamics.
- Joint mechanics techniques help restore function to a joint. You can use three different methods to address joint mechanics:

  1. *Pull the joint surfaces apart by using a band or creating a gapping effect.*
  2. *Force the joint into a stable position.*
  3. *Compress the joint.*

- Sliding surface techniques improve the interplay between your skin, nerves, and muscles. These include foam rolling and lacrosse ball smashing.
- Muscle dynamics techniques lengthen tissues to end range. It is an active model in that you're emphasizing movement and applying tension at end range.
- As a general rule, prioritize motor control, joint capsule work, and banded flossing before training, and save sliding surface and muscle dynamic end-range mobilization techniques for after training.
- The mobilization methods include pressure wave, contract and relax, banded flossing, VooDoo Floss Band compression, and flexion gapping. You need to utilize different mobilization methods so that you can cover all the different components of your restriction.
- There are two ways to approach mobility work:

  1. *Identify your position or area of restriction and mobilize within the context of the position you're trying to improve.*
  2. *Mobilize upstream and downstream of (above and below) a painful area.*

- There is no one-size-fits-all mobility program. It is subjective to the individual and changes from day to day, depending on what is tight or restricted, what movements you're performing, and what positions you're hanging out in.
- When it comes to devising an individualized mobility program, there are three general rules:

  1. *Resolve issues with painful joints and tissues first, and then focus on positions of restriction.*
  2. *Spend no less than 2 minutes in each position.*
  3. *Choose 3 or 4 mobilization techniques or areas/positions to mobilize.*

- The seven rules of mobility serve as general guidelines for performing basic maintenance on your body. They include Test and Retest, No Days Off, and Don't Make a Pain Face.

PART 2

CATEGORIES OF MOVEMENT

Now that you understand the movement principles, you know how to brace your spine in a well-organized position, and you've learned how to create torque through the primary engines of your hips and shoulders, it's time to put your knowledge to work. In this section, you will learn how to perform category 1, category 2, and category 3 functional movements.

Remember, category 1 movements have the most carryover to everyday life activities, while category 2 and 3 movements are more conducive to the actions of sport. Whether you're a novice or an elite athlete, you should take the time to master the category 1 movements. If you want to improve your athleticism and highlight movement errors, implementing category 2 and 3 movements is a great idea.

To help you identify and fix common faults, I highlight what *not* to do when performing certain exercises and offer simple tips and cues for correcting and avoiding motor control errors. If you're unable to get into a good position because you're missing range of motion, check the body archetype icon(s) located next to the movement fault, and then refer to the body archetypes mobility prescriptions in part 4.

I want to emphasize one more thing before you dive in: Although the photo sequences illustrate proper form, you may have to modify the techniques based on your mobility, body type, and skill level. In other words, use the photos as a visual reference, but don't freak out if you can't get into the exact positions demonstrated. Your squat may not look like my squat, and that's okay. The key is to take a principle-based approach and prioritize form over everything else.

POSITION OF HIGH STABILITY (PHS) → WITH CONNECTION → POSITION OF HIGH STABILITY (PHS)

CATEGORY 1 MOVEMENTS

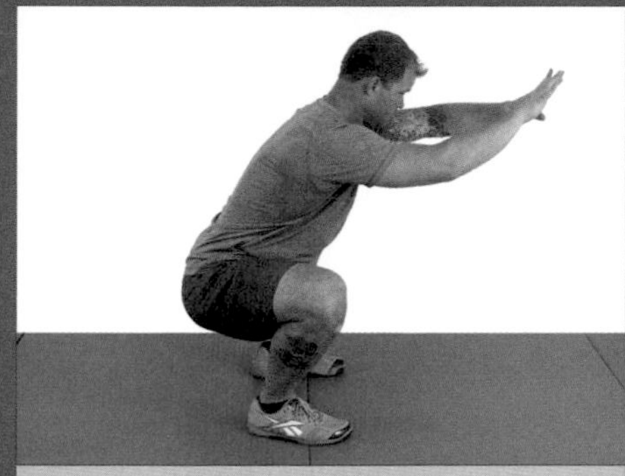
AIR SQUAT (P 162)

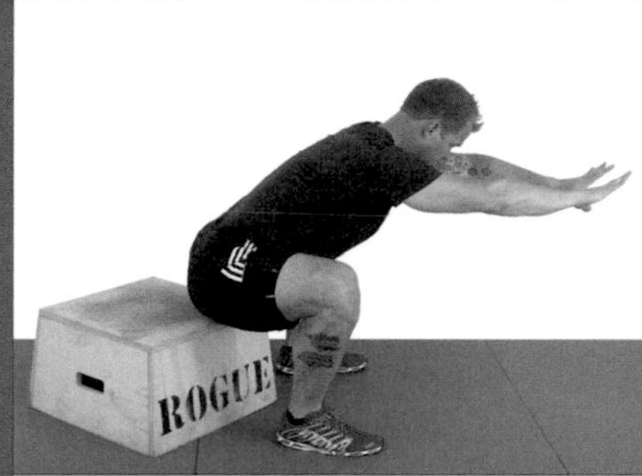

BOX SQUAT (P 176)

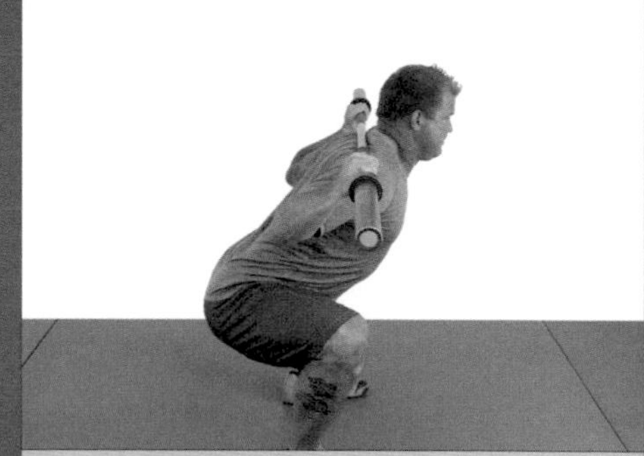
BACK SQUAT (P 178)

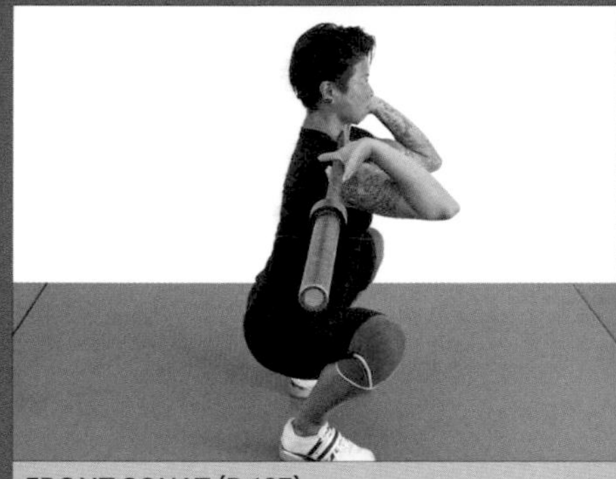
FRONT SQUAT (P 187)

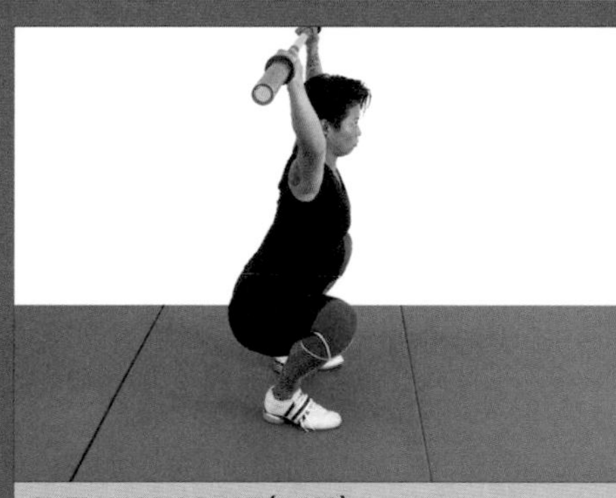
OVERHEAD SQUAT (P 192)

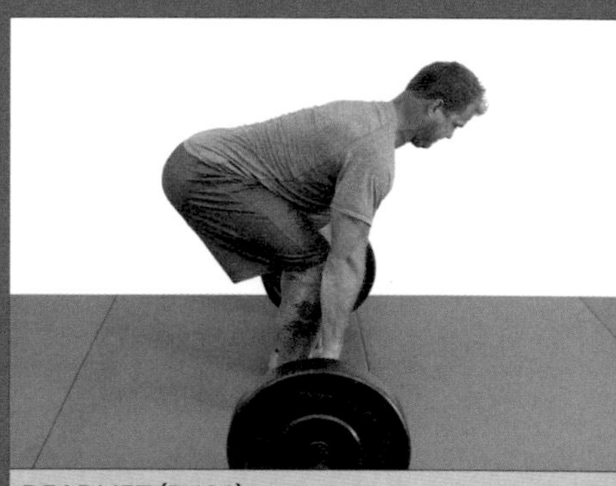
DEADLIFT (P 196)

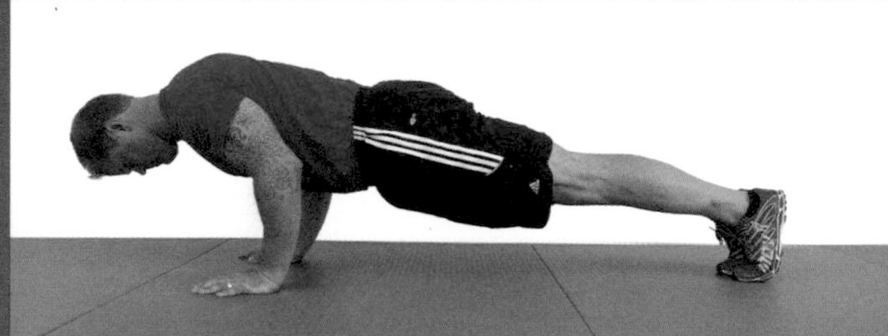
PUSHUP (P 204)

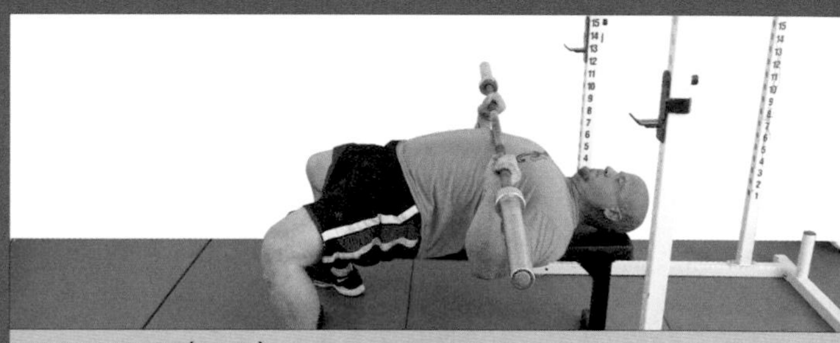
BENCH PRESS (P 209)

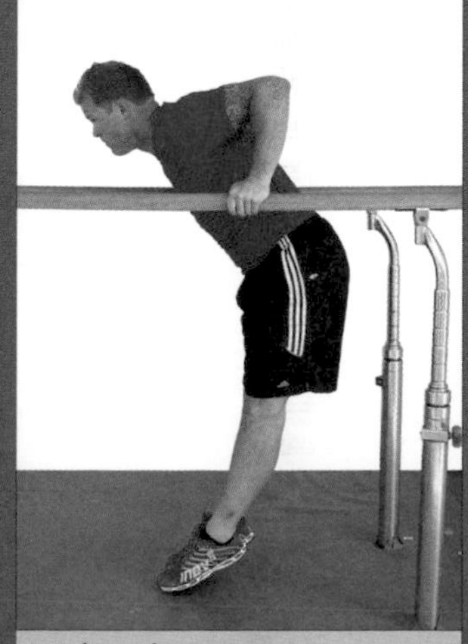
DIP (P 216)

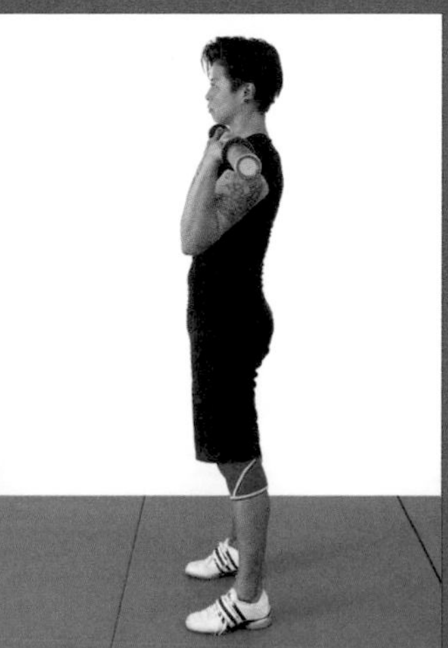
STRICT PRESS (P 220)

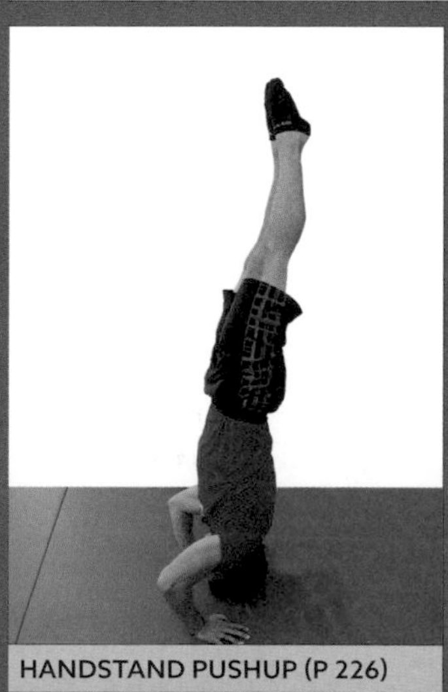
HANDSTAND PUSHUP (P 226)

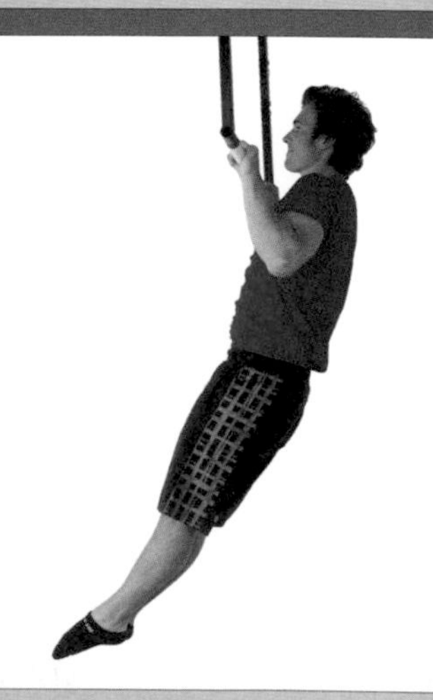
PULL-UP (P 229)

Squat 1
Archetype

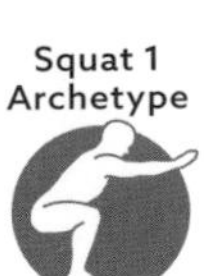

This movement contains the squat archetype. To improve common restrictions associated with this movement, visit the squat archetype prescription in part 4.

AIR SQUAT

Squatting and walking: If there are two movements that you shouldn't take for granted, they are how to squat and how to walk. Think about how many times you sit down and stand up and how much you walk in a typical day. Walk and squat with poor mechanics every day for years on end, and it shouldn't come as much of a surprise when your knees and back glow with chronic pain and a doctor starts describing the modern wonders of joint replacement. Don't even get me started on how walking and squatting poorly will gut your athletic potential.

How a person walks can tell you a lot. The squat, however, is the looking glass. A full-range, hips-below-knee-crease air squat is an omnipotent diagnostic tool for identifying and correcting universal movement and mobility problems. The bottom line is this: If you want to optimize your performance and protect your knees and low back, it's imperative that you learn how to squat and walk (see page 174) correctly.

In this section I break down the squat in detail. I also highlight common squatting faults and provide motor control and mobility fixes so that you can identify and correct these compromising movement errors.

It's important to note that squatting styles—techniques for squatting—differ dramatically from coach to coach and athlete to athlete. The squatting technique that I demonstrate in this section works in conjunction with the movement principles, making it biomechanically safe, efficient, and universally applicable. However, your squat may not look like my squat due to differences in mobility and anthropometry (measurements and proportions of the human body). The keys are that your spine is neutral and your hips, shoulders, knees, and ankles are in a stable position: Your feet have an arch, your knees go up and down along the same path, and you're externally rotating from your hips.

It's also important to note that there are many types of squats: air squat, box squat, back squat, front squat, overhead squat (to mention a few). In the coming pages, I examine the efficacy and technique for each type, as well as the critical principles at work in all types of squatting. But first it's important to touch on the squat stance.

Squat Stance

As with squatting technique, your squat stance—which is the distance between and positioning of your feet—will vary depending on your mobility and what you're trying to achieve. For example, if you are trying to break the world record for the squat, a wide stance is the ticket. It allows you to keep your torso upright—a requirement when handling enormous loads—and squat the equivalent of a Volkswagen. But if you are using the squat as an exercise to improve health and athletic performance, you need a stance that expresses a full range of motion, reveals problems, and transfers to other athletic movements.

For most people, positioning the feet just outside the shoulders will accomplish that goal. This all-purpose squat stance has universality in sports—think of the ready position of a linebacker or tennis player or a fighter's combat stance. From this position you can tackle more advanced exercises—the front squat, overhead squat, and Olympic lifts—without having to adjust your feet. Remember the Miyamoto Musashi quote that I referenced in the introduction to this book: "Make your fight stance your everyday stance; make your everyday stance your fight stance." Another way of thinking about this is to make your squat stance your everyday stance and make your everyday stance your squat stance.

Here's the deal: You want to establish a squat stance that best fits your goals as an athlete and enables you to practice good form. Depending on who you are and what you're trying to accomplish, you might adopt a wide stance with your feet positioned well outside your shoulders' width, an all-purpose stance with your feet positioned just outside your shoulders, or a narrow stance with your feet positioned underneath your hips. I mostly use an all-purpose stance, but on occasion I experiment with a wide stance to change up the stimulus.

The key is to understand why you would use one stance over another. To keep things simple, let's divide the squat stance into two classes: the all-purpose stance and the wide stance. The former—as I said above—is transferable, meaning that it applies to a wide range of movements. In addition, you're moving your hips and ankles through a full range of motion. This makes the all-purpose stance a valuable diagnostic tool and helps you develop motor control and strength in ranges of motion that are conducive to sport and life. However, if you're missing range of motion, squatting with your feet narrow may prove difficult. The closer together your feet are positioned, the more hip and ankle range of motion you need to complete the movement.

The wide-stance squat is used primarily by powerlifters and people with mobility restrictions. With your feet positioned outside shoulder width, your hips and ankles don't have to flex to the same degree to reach a full-depth, hips-below-knee-crease squat. This allows you to handle larger loads because it helps you keep your torso upright. So if you want to squat the most weight possible, you are prone to overextension spinal faults (see page 170), or you're missing critical ankle and hip range of motion, adopting a wide stance is a good option. Understand, however, that a wide stance does not have the same transferability or evaluative benefits of the all-purpose stance. If mobility is the only limiting factor, I recommend starting with a wider stance and working toward an all-purpose stance as your mobility improves.

WIDE STANCE

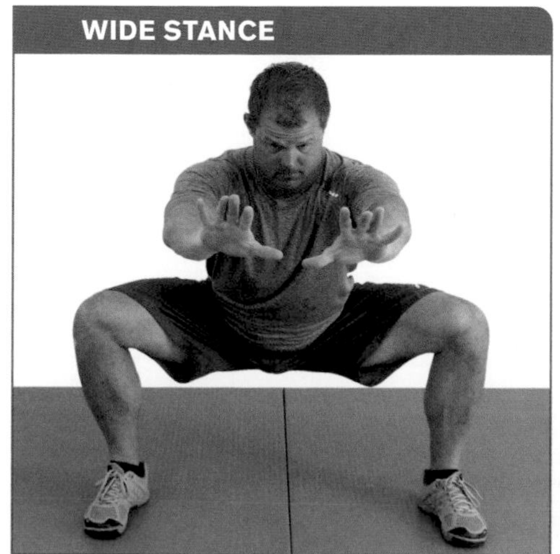

ALL-PURPOSE STANCE

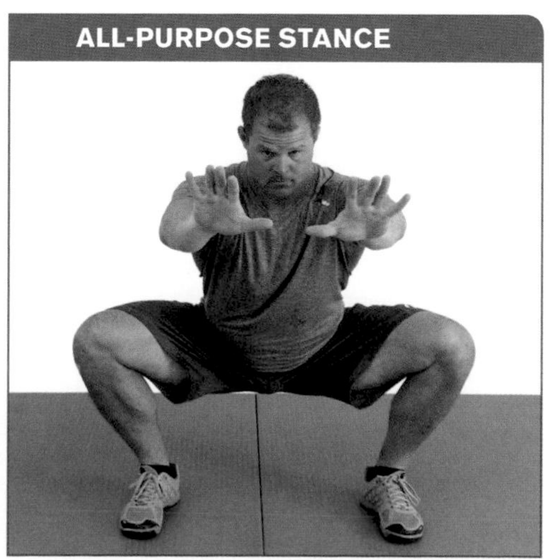

As an interesting side note, a wide stance is also good for people who have too much range of motion. I'm referring specifically to hypermobile athletes (see page 128) who are so flexible that they have a hard time stabilizing and creating tension in their joints. Adopting a wide stance and positioning your feet straight creates tension in the system. This helps people who have too much slack in their joints find stability and avoid potentially harmful movement errors.

In short, the idea is to adopt a squat stance that is conducive to your body type and fitness goals. Both stances have their pros and cons, and both are useful and worth learning. The most important things are to adhere to the principles of squatting.

Principles of Squatting

When it comes to squatting, the idea is to create a stable hip, knee, and ankle position and then maintain that position as you descend and rise. The principles of squatting help you achieve that goal. Consider these principles general guidelines for optimal squatting technique. You can apply these principles to all types of squats—front squat, back squat, overhead squat, etc.

Keep Your Shins as Vertical as Possible

Keep your shins as vertical as possible as you descend and rise out of the squat. Vertical shins allow you to channel the power of your hips and hamstrings and consequently unload weight from your knees. If you fail to keep your shins vertical and your knees lurch forward over your feet, you will lose power from your posterior chain and increase the shear and twisting forces to the soft tissues within the joint, especially the cartilage, patellar tendon, and anterior cruciate ligament (ACL).

Your knees will inevitably track forward as you descend into the bottom of the squat, especially the narrow-stance butt-to-ankles squat. The idea is to delay this motion for as long as you can as you descend and immediately think about getting your shins vertical as you rise out of the bottom position. This will help you keep tension in your hips and hamstrings, thereby maximizing power and minimizing movement faults.

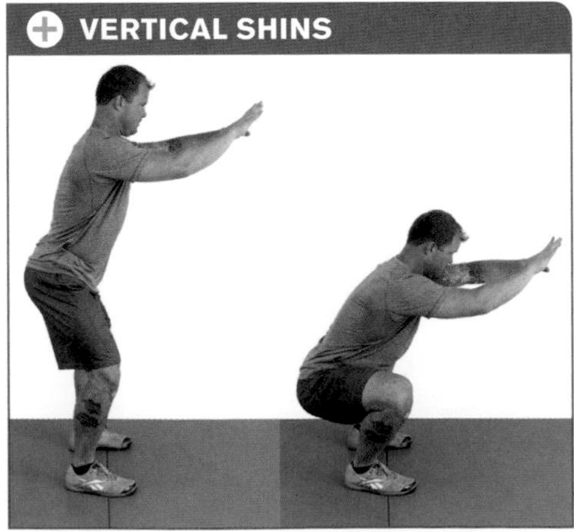

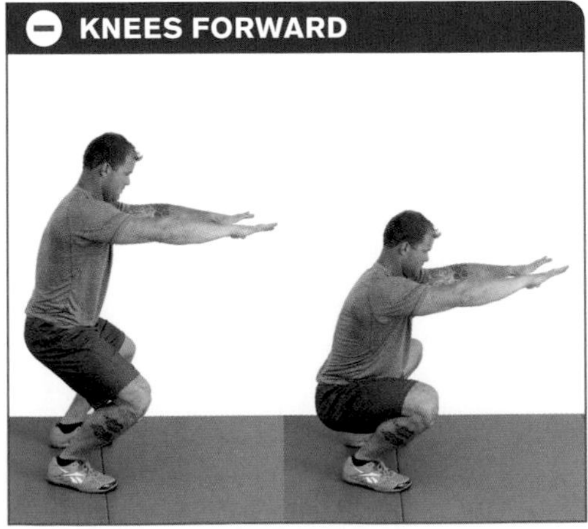

Load Your Hips and Hamstrings

In part 1, I discussed the one-joint rule and load order sequence, which helped elucidate why you want to initiate movement from your hips and shoulders. Loading your hips and hamstrings is an extension of these concepts.

When you initiate the squat, you always want to start by loading your hips and hamstrings. You do so by tilting your torso forward and driving your hamstrings back. This loads the right muscle groups, allows you to hinge from your hips with your spine neutral, and maintains proper torque through your arms and legs. Put simply, it fortifies your posture so that you don't break at the lumbar spine.

A lot of athletes mistakenly keep their chest up and reach their butt back as a way to keep their shins vertical, which causes an overextension fault (aka anterior pelvic tilt). To avoid this fault, think about sitting your hamstrings back as you initiate the movement. If you think about reaching your butt back instead, you're more likely to default into an overextended position.

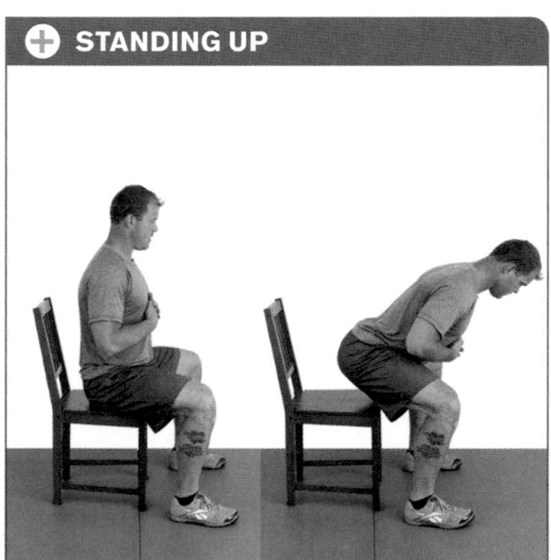
+ STANDING UP

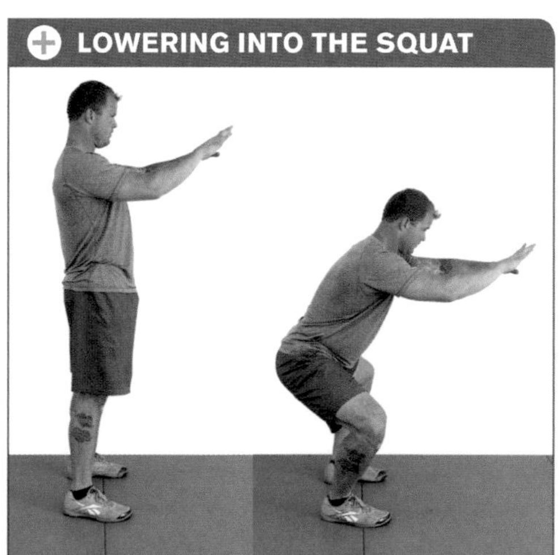
+ LOWERING INTO THE SQUAT

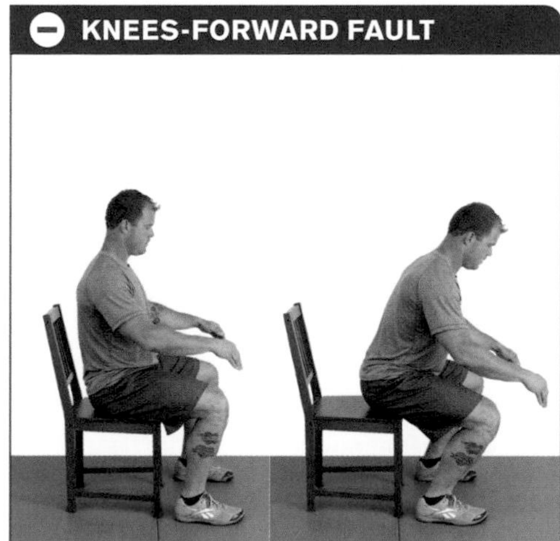
− KNEES-FORWARD FAULT

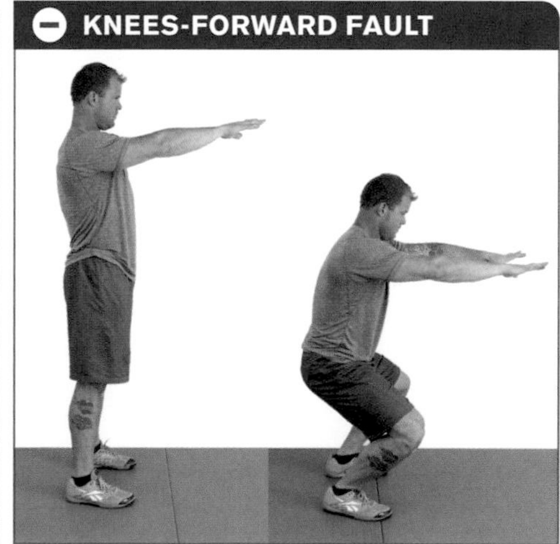
− KNEES-FORWARD FAULT

Distribute Your Weight in the Center of Your Feet

To create and maintain maximum torque, imagine screwing your feet into the ground with your weight distributed over the center of your feet—not the balls of your feet, not your heels, not the outsides of your feet—with your mass right in front of your ankles.

When learning how to squat, people often roll up onto the balls of their feet. This fault stems from a lack of technique, range of motion, or both. Many coaches try to cure the problem by having beginners shift their weight to their heels. The problem with this fix is that it opens the door to other weight-distribution faults as the athletes develop. Centering your weight on your heels makes it difficult to create the torque necessary for full stability. This habit will likely transfer to other movements as well. Imagine trying to make a big Olympic lift or dunk a basketball with your weight on your heels. It's not going to happen.

When you center your weight in front of your ankles—keeping your entire foot in contact with the ground—and create external rotation torque from your hips, you should see a solid arch in your foot. This is what I mean by a stable foot and ankle position.

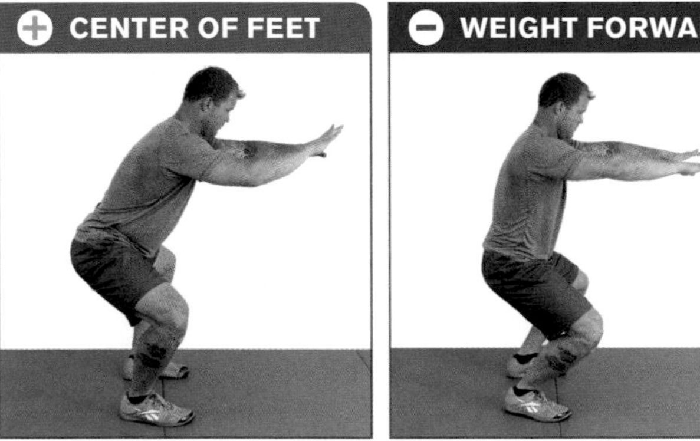

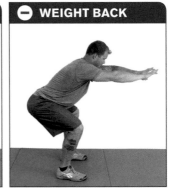

Maintain a Neutral Knee Position

Ideally, your knees should remain neutral, meaning that they stay on the same vertical path as you descend and rise out of the squat. Stated differently, your knees should track up and down along the same plane. It bears repeating that a valgus knee collapse—which occurs when your knee twists inward—is the primary mechanism for knee injuries, specifically ACL tears. Coaches (myself included) typically cue against this common movement error by telling athletes to drive their knees out. Although this cue prompts external rotation, it does not accurately or effectively explain what your knees should be doing when you squat—see "Clarifying the 'Knees Out' Squat Cue" on page 168.

For example, notice in the photos on the following page that my knees move outward as I squat. This is because I'm creating external rotation from my hips. This is a critical point to understand. Shoving your knees out and rolling onto the outsides of your feet is an error that can wreak havoc on your knees and ankles.

Realize that I have full hip range of motion, which is expressed visibly by a knees-out position. If you're in a wide stance or you don't have full hip range of motion, your knees may not track outward. Don't try to shove your knees out past your feet if you don't have the mobility. And don't worry if your knees are not tracking over your feet.

For years, coaches have taught athletes to keep their knees aligned with their feet when they squat. Now, if your feet are turned out and you're creating external rotation from your hips, your knees will track over your feet. But if you have full range of motion and you're squatting in a position that allows you to maximize torque—feet straight or just slightly turned out—your knees may track outside of your feet. The key, therefore, is to limit side-to-side knee movement by creating and maintaining enough external rotation torque to maintain a neutral knee position.

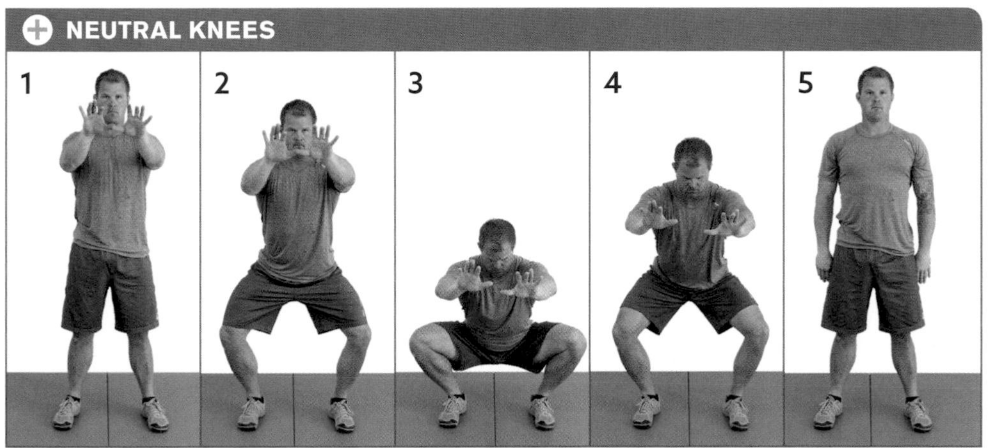

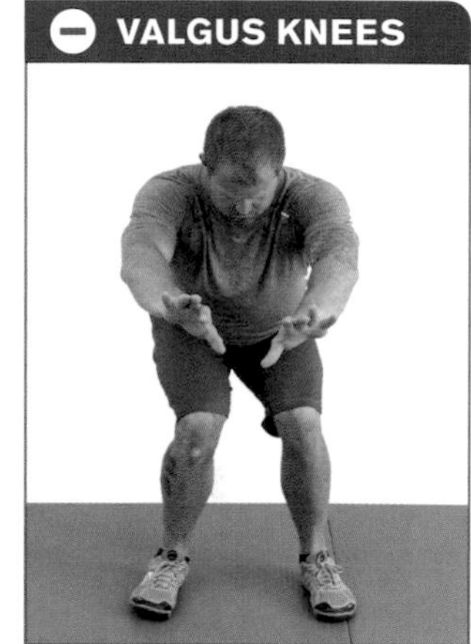

Create Stable Shoulders

The position of your arms will vary depending on the type of squat you're doing. Regardless, always set your shoulders in a stable position by creating force from external rotation.

If you're setting up for an air squat, pull your shoulders back while turning your thumbs toward the inside of your body.

If you're setting up for a barbell lift, screw your hands into the bar—your right hand clockwise and your left hand counterclockwise—as if you were trying to snap the bar in half. The resulting tension will stabilize your shoulders and turn on the muscles across your upper back, resulting in a braced neutral spine. This all-powerful ready position becomes more critical the more weight you're dealing with.

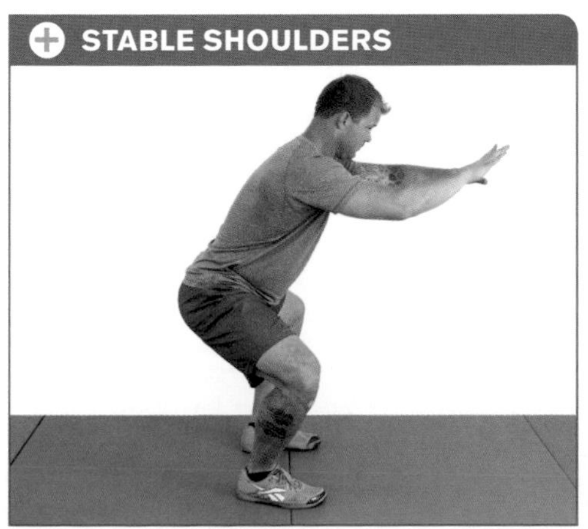

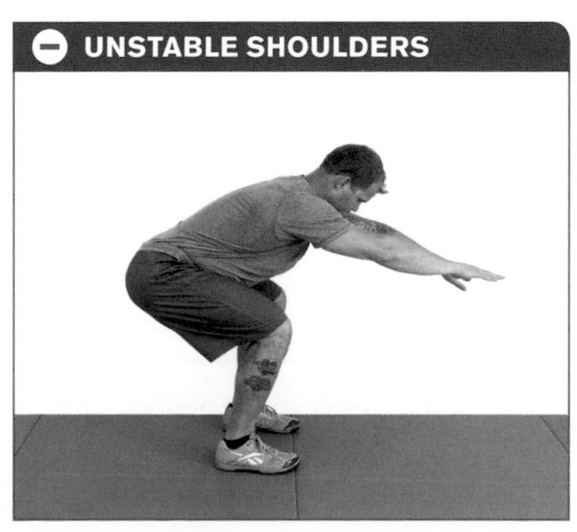

Clarifying the "Knees Out" Squat Cue

When I teach someone how to squat, I often tell the person to drive her knees out to cue external rotation from the hips. But let me be clear: "Knees out" is not a model for squatting; it's not a technique; and it's not a methodology. Like saying, "Screw your feet into the ground," telling someone to shove her knees out is simply a cue to encourage the athlete to stabilize her hips by creating external rotation.

Remember, the idea is to put your ankles, knees, hips, and back in a stable position. I've found that cueing people to screw their feet into the ground and drive their knees out prompts hip external rotation, which stabilizes the structures upstream and downstream of the hips. However, it's important to realize that this cue does not perfectly describe squatting technique. Like all coaching cues, it can be used incorrectly and is often misinterpreted.

For example, coaches often mistakenly use the knees-out cue when someone's knees are starting to track inward during a squat. While this cue prompts hip external rotation and may prevent the knees from tracking farther inward, it violates one of the principles of squatting, which is to keep your knees neutral throughout the entire range of the movement. In such a situation, you want to drive through the center of your feet and stand up, not drive your knees out. In fact, reclaiming a knees-out position as you rise out of the squat will cause your pelvis to wobble—when your knees come in, your pelvis dumps forward, and when your knees move out, your pelvis rotates backward—creating shear across your lumbar spine. The knees-out cue is also sometimes misinterpreted as shoving your knees out as hard as possible. This error can cause all sorts of faults—like rolling onto the outsides of your feet—and can lead to knee and ankle problems.

In the air squat sequence, you'll notice that my knees are in fact out. Again, this is because I have full hip range of motion. My knees translate outward because that's how far I need to position my knees to take up all the rotational slack in my hips and ankles. If you do not share the same mobility, your knees probably won't translate out as far as mine do.

To reiterate a key point from chapter 3, you want to create just enough torque to match the demands of the movement. If you're trying to shove your knees out as hard as you can during a bodyweight squat, it's going to feel awkward and cause problems. But if you shove your knees out (create hip external rotation) just enough to combat the forces trying to pull your knees inward, the movement will feel fluid and you will avoid potentially harmful faults.

In conclusion, the knees-out cue is just something I say to remind people to create hip external rotation and avoid a knees-in fault. So try not to misconstrue this cue to mean something else. I suppose you could say "not knees-in," but that would only cause further confusion.

Remember, a cue is a verbal indicator that is specific to a particular moment or action. In other words, don't worry if your knees don't track out as far as mine do. Rather, focus on organizing your spine in a neutral position, creating torque, and adhering to the principles of squatting.

Air Squat Sequence

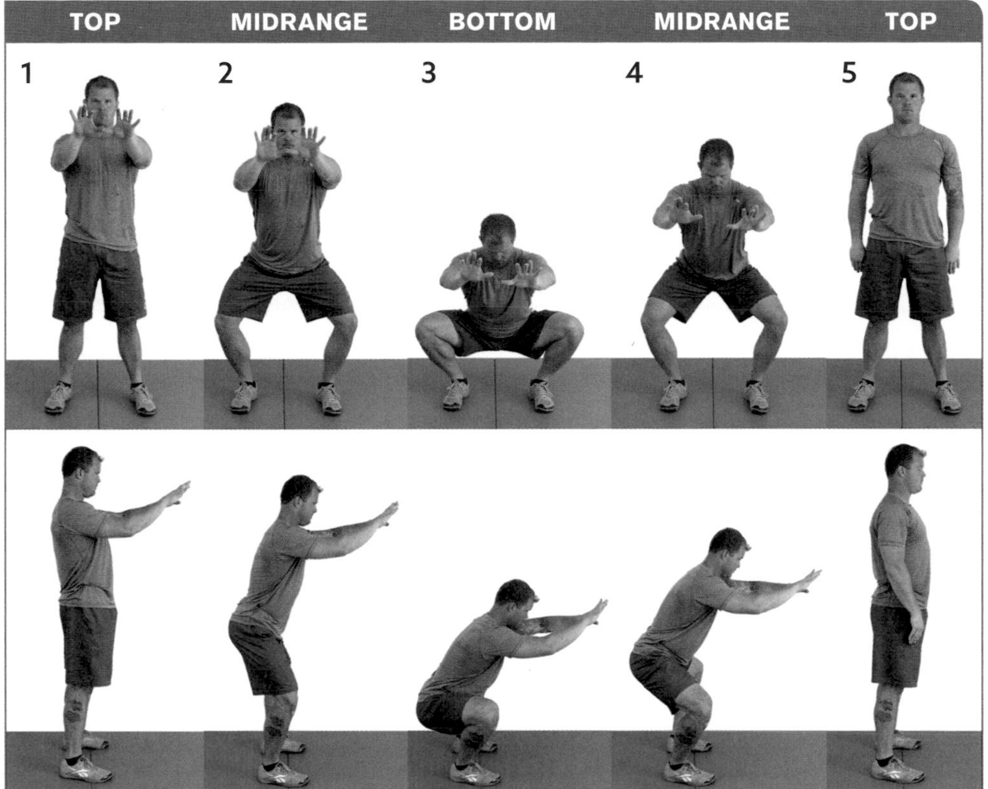

1. To set up for the squat, establish your stance with your feet straight or just slightly turned out, somewhere between 5 and 12 degrees. Then go through the bracing sequence: Squeeze your butt; align your head, ribcage, and pelvis; and get your belly tight. With your spine in a braced neutral position, screw your feet into the ground as if you were trying to spread the floor. To be more specific, screw your left foot into the ground in a counterclockwise direction and your right foot in a clockwise direction, keeping both feet straight and in contact with the ground. Next, set your shoulders in a stable position and tighten your upper back by raising your arms, pulling your shoulders back, and externally rotating your hands slightly. Look forward to maintain a neutral head position and keep your weight centered over the fronts of your ankles.

2. Reach your hamstrings back—keeping your shins as vertical as possible—drive your knees out laterally, and start lowering into the bottom position. To help maintain tension and maximize torque, think about pulling yourself into the bottom position rather than dropping into the bottom position.

3. As your hip crease drops below knee depth, you should feel very stable. In other words, there should be no slack in the system. Your back should be tight, your knees at the limits of their external rotation range, and your hips at peak tension. You may need to adjust your knees slightly forward to reach full depth. The key is to maintain as much external rotation force as necessary to maintain neutral knee and ankle positions.

4. Still making a conscious effort to externally rotate from your hips, pull your shins back to vertical and extend your hips and knees. Rise out of the bottom position in the same way you entered: with your spine neutral and your shoulders and upper back tight. It's the same as descending, but in the reverse order.

5. As you stand up, reclaim a stable top position by squeezing your butt. This sets your pelvis in a neutral position and prepares you for the next movement or repetition.

Knees-Forward Fault

MOTOR CONTROL FIX:

Isolate the first 6 inches of the squat.

Initiate the squat by sitting your hamstrings back (load your hips and hamstrings), keeping your shins as vertical as possible.

Keeping your abs braced and your spine neutral, tilt your torso slightly forward as you descend.

Initiating the squat by driving your knees forward instead of pushing your hips back is a common load order sequencing error. Sometimes people try to keep their torso upright and avoid a lumbar overextension fault, resulting in a knees-forward position. Usually it's a minor technique (motor control) fault that is easily fixed by focusing on the first 6 inches of the squat.

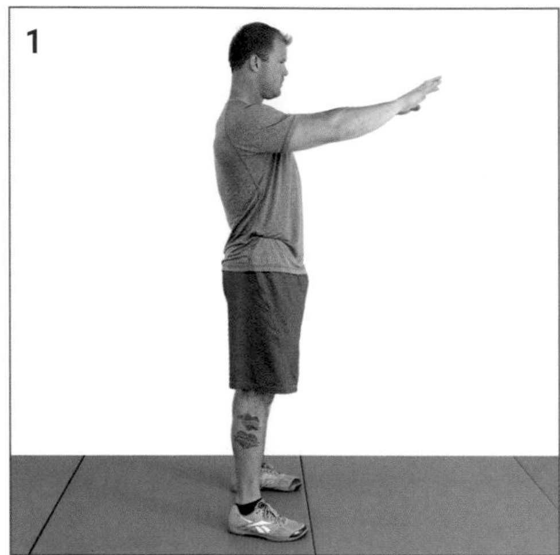

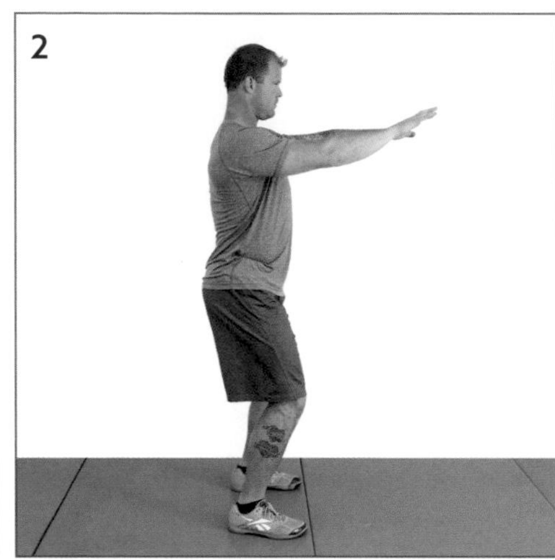

Overextension Spinal Fault: The Dreaded Low-Back Pump-Out

MOTOR CONTROL FIX:

Isolate the first 6 inches of the squat.

Initiate the squat by sitting your hamstrings back and tilting your torso slightly forward.

Keep your belly tight, shoulders back, and shins as vertical as possible while maintaining external rotation torque from your hips.

Failing to organize your spine in a neutral position with your belly muscles tight will cause you to collapse into an overextended position as you initiate the squat. The moment you lose control of your pelvis, you lose stability throughout the chain. Screwing your feet into the ground and driving your knees outward won't matter; power will bleed from your system. This fault is also characterized by a gross reversal of the pelvis in the bottom position (see the butt wink fault on page 173).

Most people have enough mobility to initiate the first 6 inches of the squat, so correcting this fault becomes a learning-related task. However, if your anterior hip structures (hip capsules, hip flexors, and quads) are brutally tight, you are more likely to default into an overextended position to feed slack to your hip system.

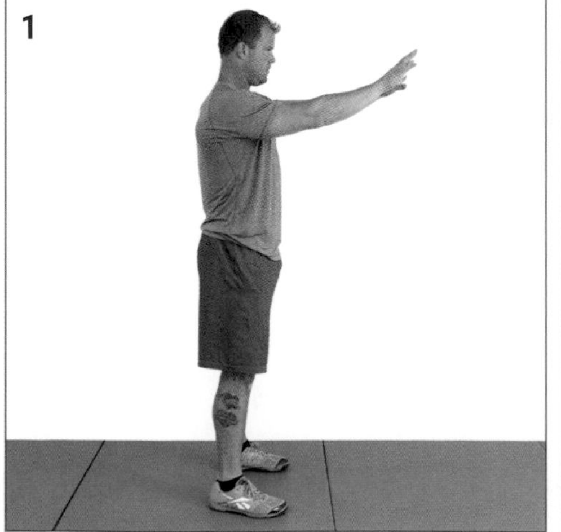

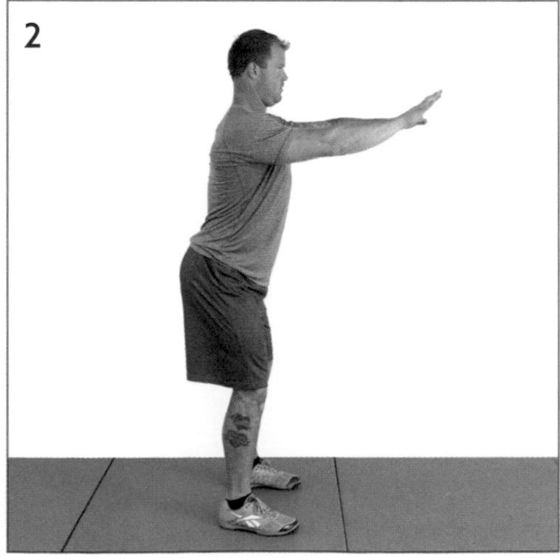

Valgus-Knee Fault

Before you begin a squat, you want to tighten your core, squeeze the muscles of your butt, and create an external rotation force from your hips by screwing your feet into the ground. If you fail to create this stability, your knees will cave in, creating a twisting shear force across those structures. This is called valgus knee collapse. Remember, if you fail to create torque at the start of the squat, your body will have to create stability somewhere else, which is expressed through this fault.

Turning out your feet past the 12- to 15-degree range increases your vulnerability to this problem. Wide-angled feet also make it more difficult to produce torque that will stabilize your knees.

The motor control fix is simple: Screw your feet into the ground in the top position and focus on driving your knees out as you lower into the bottom position. Past the 6-inch point, however, mobility limitations in your ankles, hips, and upper legs will play a part.

It's interesting to note that there are coaches and athletes out there who advocate a knees-in squat. Although you can certainly squat with your knees in and remain pain-free, you're inviting injury and ingraining a movement pattern that does not effectively transfer to other activities. You may get away with it for a while, but as studies have shown, the valgus knee fault is a mechanism for injury—specifically ACL tears. This is why I teach people to squat with their knees tracking up and down along the same vertical path.

Squat 1 Archetype

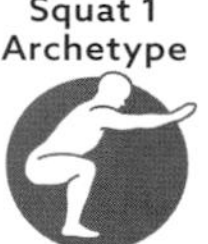

This fault is associated with the squat archetype. For a mobility fix, visit the squat archetype prescription in part 4.

MOTOR CONTROL FIX:

Create external rotation hip torque by screwing your feet into the ground and shoving your knees out.

Focus on keeping your knees neutral so they track up and down along the same vertical path.

MOBILIZATION TARGET AREAS:

Anterior chain (hips and quads)

Posterior high chain (glutes)

Medial chain (adductors)

Calves and heel cords

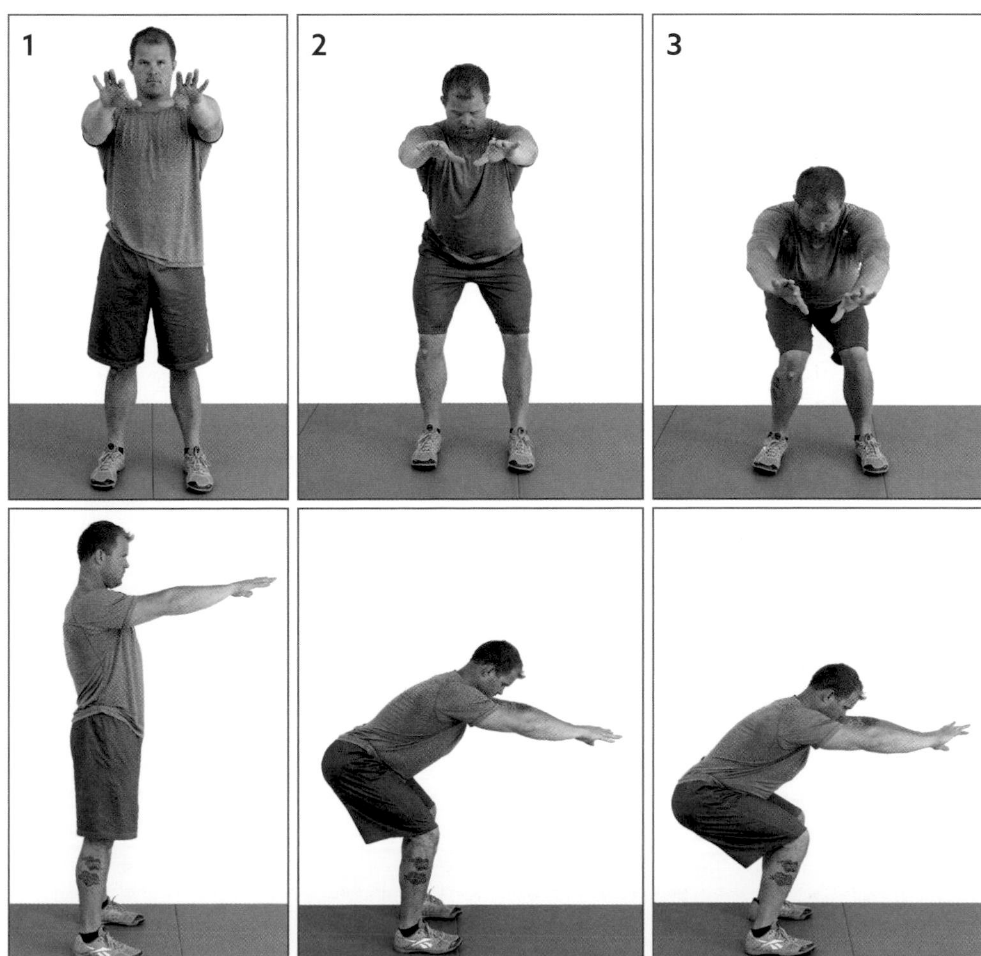

Range of Motion Squat Tests: Ruling Out the Ankles

When you can't get into an ideal position because you're missing key ranges of motion, you have to ask yourself: Where is the problem? Is it my ankles, quads, or anterior hips? Chances are it's a system of systems, meaning that it's a combination of tight tissues. This is why I take a systems approach to dealing with these problems by using simple tests to rule out specific areas of the body.

For example, the ankle wall and pistol test are two ways to see whether you have full ankle range of motion or are missing critical corners. What's great about these tests is that you don't have to memorize the anatomy or joint measurement of a full range of motion; all you have to do is determine whether you can you get into the pistol position. Yes or no?

Ankle Wall

The ankle wall and pistol test both tell you whether you have full ankle range of motion, but the ankle wall lets you know more specifically where you are coming up short. For example, say you lower into the squat with your feet together, keeping your back flat as you descend. If you're missing ankle range of motion, you will literally hit a wall, at which point you will either lose your balance and fall backward or compensate into a rounded position. In either case, the moment you hit the wall is the limit of your ankle range of motion.

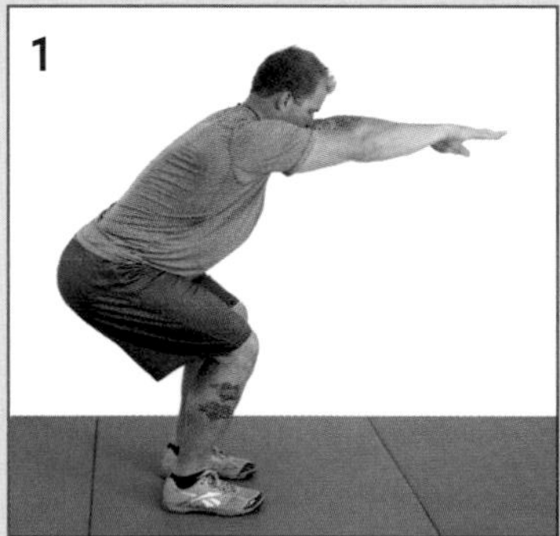
1

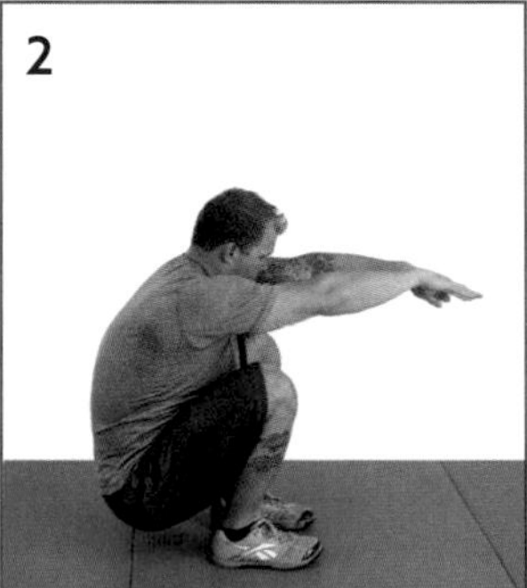
2

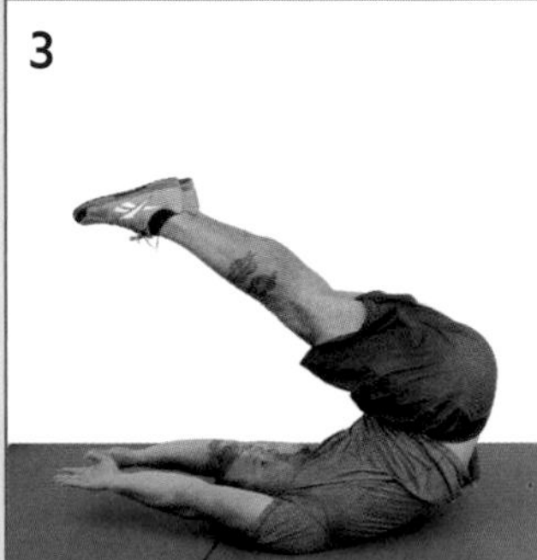
3

Pistol Test

Nothing we do as human beings requires more ankle range of motion than being in the bottom position of the single-leg squat (pistol). If you can lower into a squat with your back flat and extend one of your legs out in front of your body while keeping your grounded foot neutral, you have full dorsiflexion range of motion in your ankle.

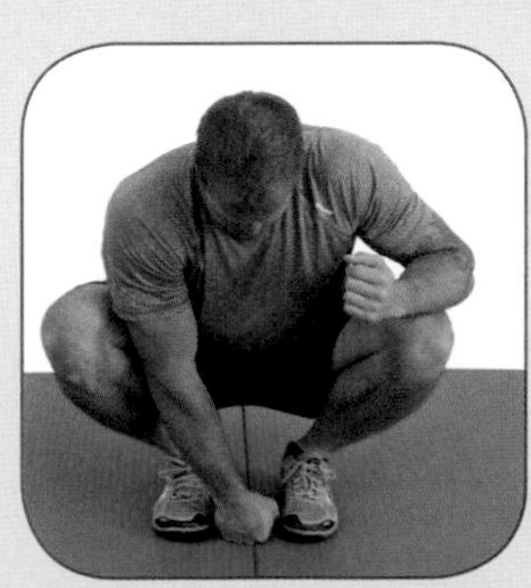

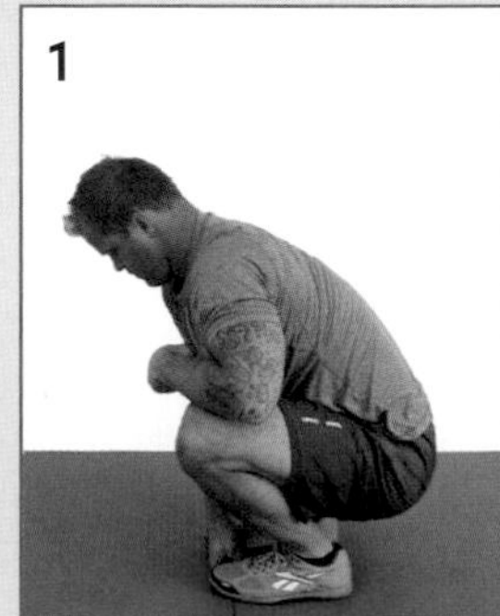
1

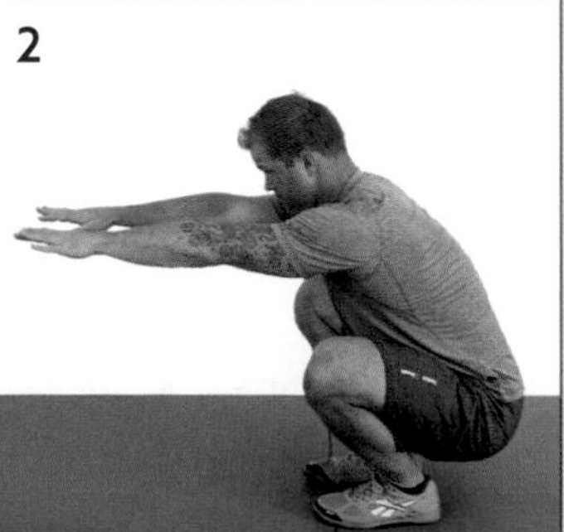
2

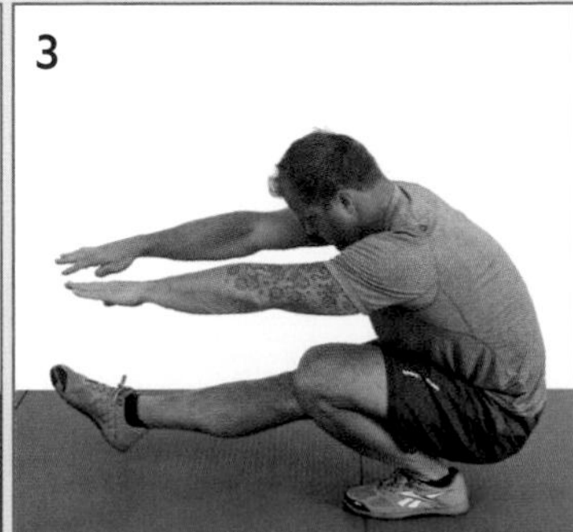
3

Lumbar Reversal Fault (The Butt Wink)

The butt wink fault occurs when your pelvis tucks underneath your body near the bottom of the squat. Here's what typically happens: First, you reach back with your butt, overextending from your lumbar spine and tilting your pelvis forward. Then, as you lower into the bottom of the squat, your pelvis tilts back, tucking underneath your body like a dog with its tail between its legs. When you stand up, your pelvis tilts forward again into the same overextended position.

Whether it's a motor control error or a mobility limitation such as tight hamstrings, the butt wink is something you should take very seriously. It is responsible for more low back pain and spinal tweaks than any other squatting fault described in this section. The reason this fault is so harmful is that you're creating shear across the structures of your lumbar spine three times during the movement: your pelvis tilts forward, then backward, and then forward again. Add a loaded barbell to the mix and it's a recipe for disaster. You can also commit this fault while sitting: If you sit in an overextended position, round forward, and then try to sit up straight again, you're committing the exact same error.

If you're susceptible to this fault, here's the plan: You need to create and maintain midline stability and torque. If you commit a lumbar overextension fault as you initiate the squat, stop the movement, rack the weight (if you're squatting with weight), and reset your position. If you have tissue restrictions that compromise your movement, reduce the depth of your squat and address your adductor and hamstring mobility. Remember, you never want to compromise safe form for depth. To see how this fault translates to sitting, flip to the box squat technique on page 176.

Squat 1
Archetype

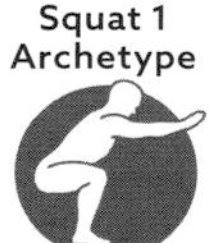

This fault is associated with the squat archetype. For a mobility fix, visit the squat archetype prescription in part 4.

MOTOR CONTROL FIX:

Squeeze your butt and stabilize your spine in the top position, and maintain midline stability as you descend.

Initiate the squat by driving your hamstrings back, not your butt.

Create and maintain hip external rotation torque as you lower into and rise out of the squat, making sure that your knees track up and down along the same path.

Implement a box squat to decrease range of motion (squat depth).

MOBILIZATION TARGET AREAS:

Anterior chain (hips and quads)

Posterior high chain (glutes)

Posterior low chain (hamstrings)

Calves and heel cords

Trunk

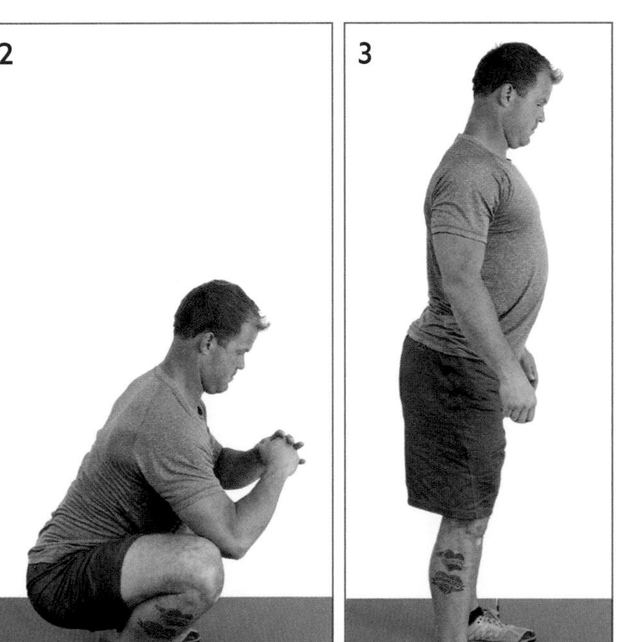

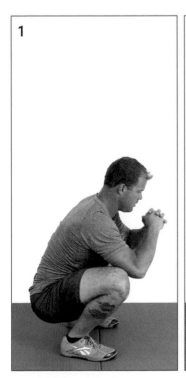

Walking and Stepping Mechanics

Walking

Walking is a complex movement. I could spend a lot of time breaking down the joint positions and phases of walking, but that is beyond the scope of this book. And it isn't necessary. When it comes to walking, just keep your feet straight and your spine neutral. It's that simple.

If you turn out your feet out as you walk, your ankles will collapse into an unstable position with every step. This is a mechanism for bunions and a lot of foot- and knee-related problems. And just think of the number of duty cycles you go through. Again, the key is to get organized before you start moving. Go through the bracing sequence (see pages 40–41) and focus on keeping your feet straight.

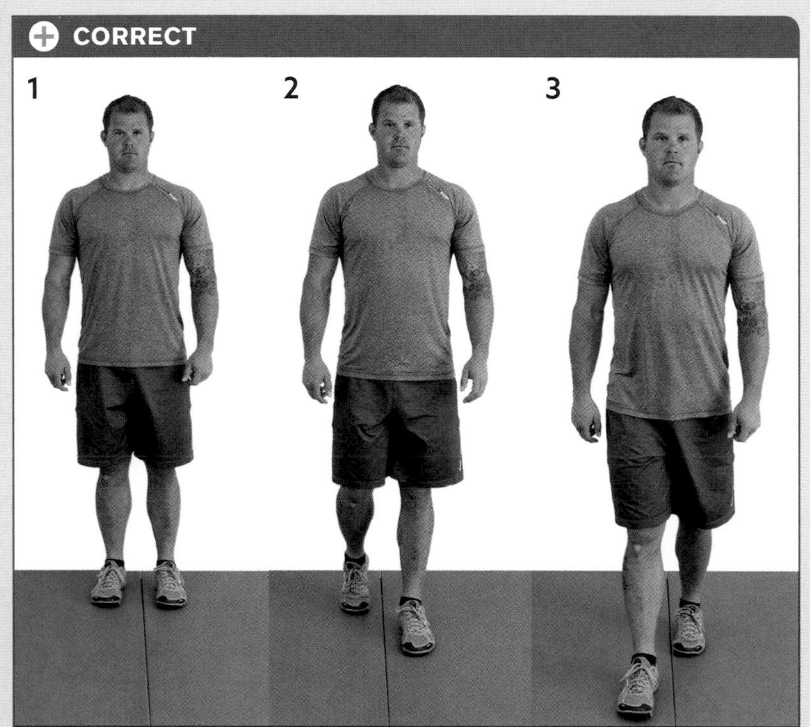

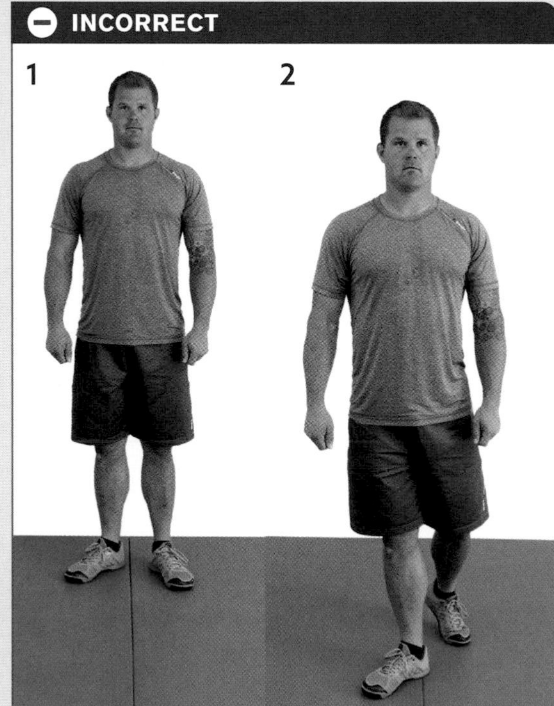

Stepping

Stepping onto an elevated platform and walking up and down stairs share all the same principles as squatting. Think of it as a single-leg upright squat. You want to keep your torso vertical, spine neutral, knees out, and feet arched (neutral). The higher the step, the more you have to hinge from the hip. Regardless of the height, the key to success is to keep your shin as vertical as possible.

When people have problems walking up and down stairs or stepping onto a box, it's because the knee is translating forward and the ankle is collapsing inward. It's the equivalent of initiating a squat with zero stability. There's no torque at the hip, so they overextend, and the downstream structures shift into a wrenched position. The solution is simple: Keep your foot straight, drive your knee out, and maintain a well-organized, stable trunk.

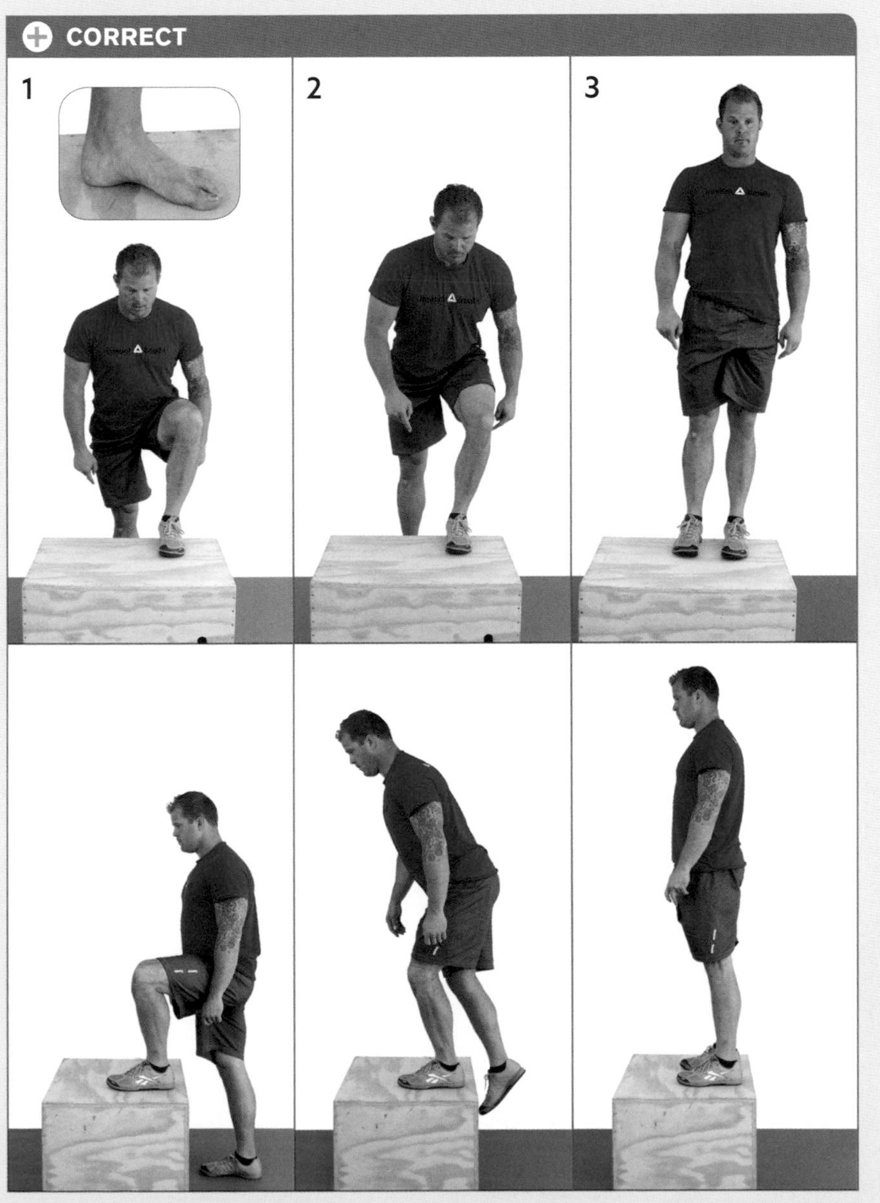

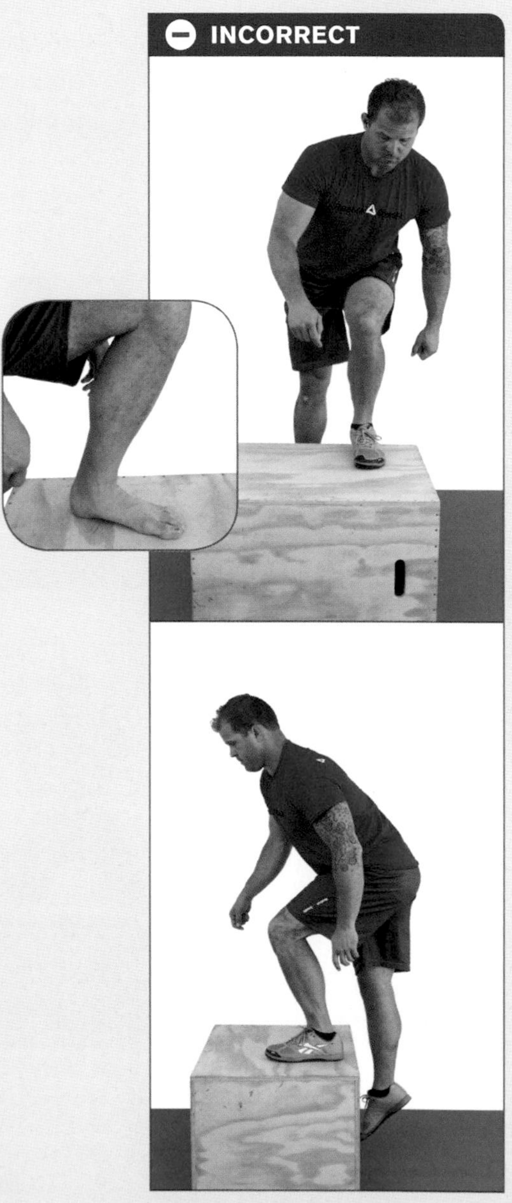

Squat 1
Archetype

This movement contains the squat archetype. To improve common restrictions associated with this movement, visit the squat archetype prescription in part 4.

BOX SQUAT

The box squat is a movement that average people perform thousands of times a week. Every time you sit down or get up from a chair, couch, or toilet, you perform a close iteration of this squat.

Although the air squat is the first movement that I teach to novice athletes—it's my way of teaching fundamental squatting principles—most people don't have the mobility to squat to full depth (even though it's something every human being should be able to do). If squatting butt-below-knee-crease is not a viable option, positioning a box at knee level or slightly higher is a great way to teach squatting mechanics.

Unlike the air squat, the box squat allows you to fix problems that you may not be aware of. For example, say you're struggling to load your hips and hamstrings and pull your knees back to get your shins vertical. Having a stable target like a box or chair to reach for is an easy way to reverse the knees-forward fault and ingrain functional movement patterns. In addition, you can focus on spinal mechanics and weight distribution in the bottom position without worrying about falling over. In short, it's a simple way to scale the depth of the squat without compromising form.

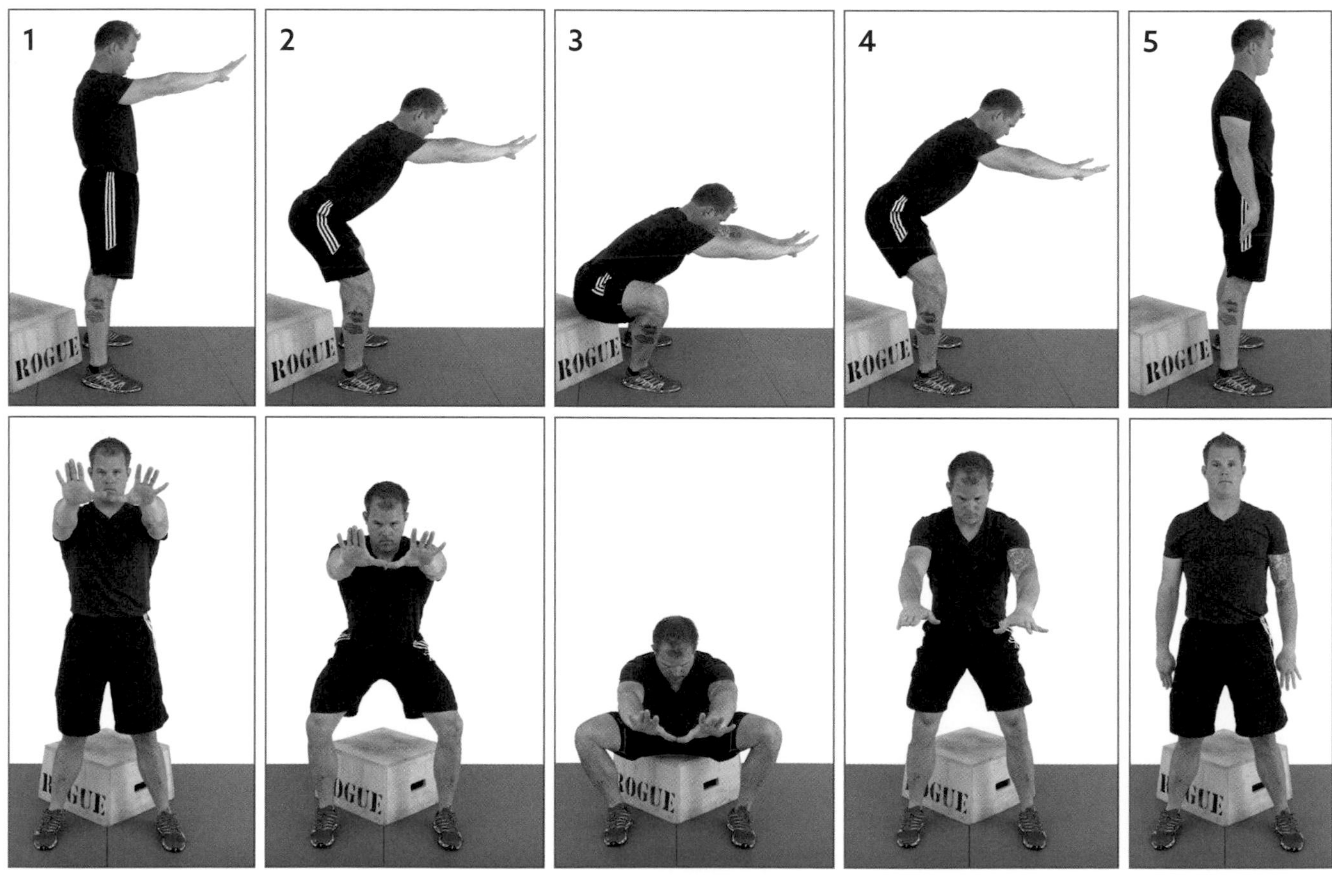

1. Assume your squat stance. Position your heels a few inches from the box, with a corner angled between your legs. Then screw your feet into the ground to create torque, squeeze your butt, stabilize your midline, and set your shoulders in a stable position.

2. Keeping your shins vertical and your back flat, sit your hamstrings back and hinge forward at the hips.

3. Lower your butt to the box, maintaining tension in your hips, hamstrings, and back as you sit your butt down.

4. Drive out of the bottom position the moment your butt touches down.

5. Reestablish the top position.

Standing Up Out of the Bottom Position

When you execute the box squat as an exercise, you never completely release the tension in your hips and hamstrings. The moment your butt touches down, you reverse the sequence by standing back up. However, if you're having trouble in the bottom position, pausing on a box or chair is an excellent way to work on standing up with good mechanics. It gives you a new start position and allows you to focus on getting your shins vertical, shoving your knees out, and keeping your back flat as you rise out of the bottom position.

If you are starting from a seated position, the key is to keep your belly tight and reload your hips and hamstrings by hinging forward at the hips, just as you would when initiating the squat.

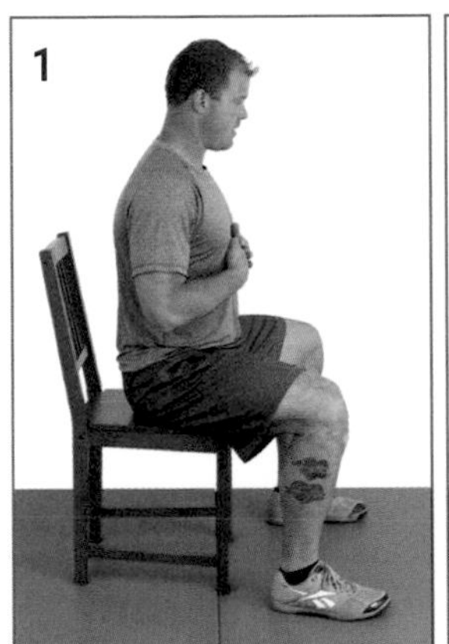

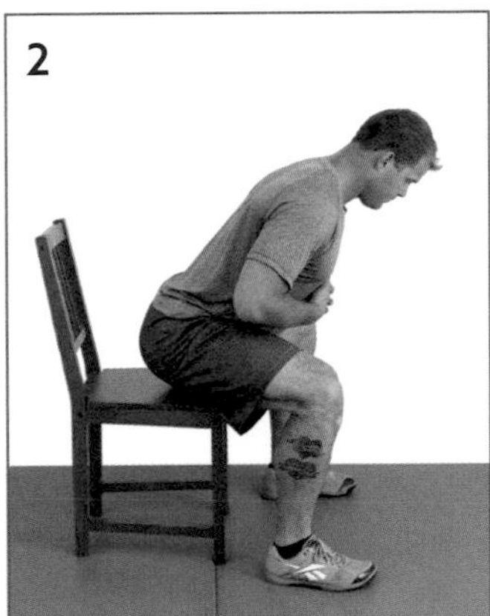

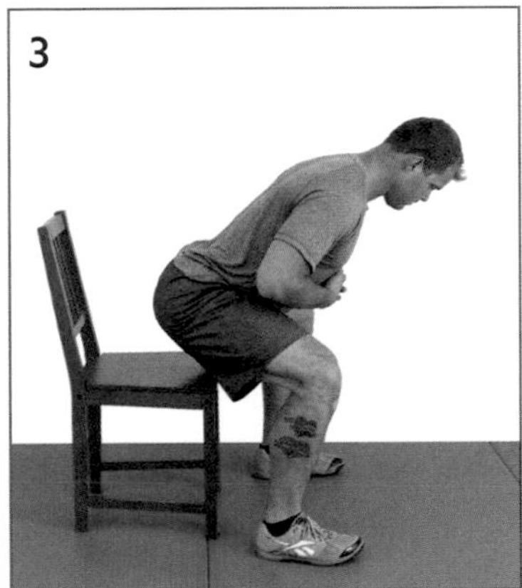

1. Sitting is just a box squat with a long pause in the bottom position. Even if you remain seated for an extended period, your back stays flat, shins vertical, and knees out.
2. When you stand up, reclaim tension by loading your hips and hamstrings by hinging forward at the hips.
3. Keeping your back flat, shove your knees out and stand up, just as you would when performing a squat.

Knees-Forward Chair Fault

If your knees come forward as you get up out of a chair, it's usually one of two things: either you are not comfortable creating tension in your hips and hamstrings as you stand up, or you haven't created sufficient torque. As with the air squat, driving your knees forward out of the bottom position is primarily a motor control error.

If I notice that an athlete's knees come forward every time he squats out of the bottom position, I'll have him sit on a box or chair and put my hand in front of his knee. Every time his knee touches my hand, I'll have him sit back to the box and try again. In addition to illuminating the fault, this simple tactic brings consciousness to the movement, dramatically reducing the probability of committing this error.

MOTOR CONTROL FIX:

Create torque by screwing your feet into the ground and driving your knees out.

Hinge forward with a flat back, load your hips and hamstrings, and get your shins as vertical as possible.

Have someone position her hand just in front of your knee to bring consciousness to the movement.

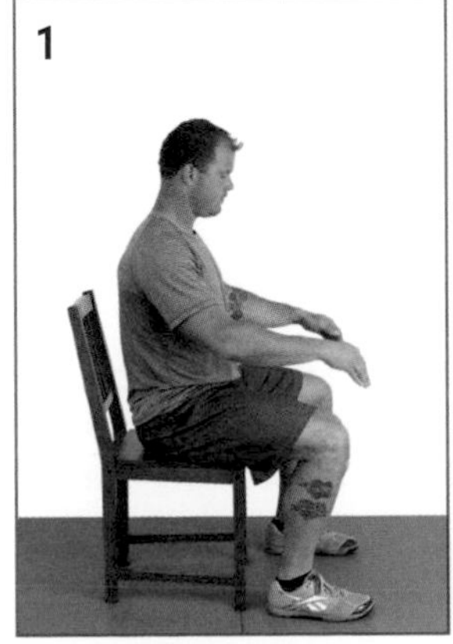

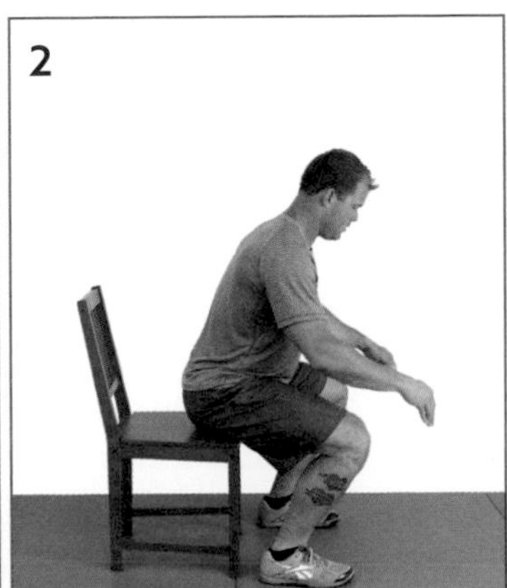

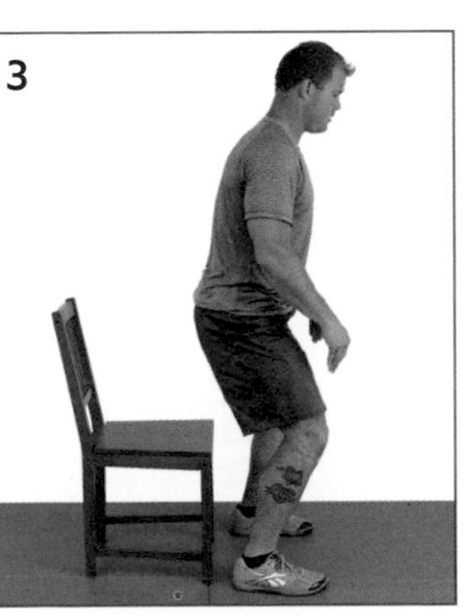

Squat 1 Archetype

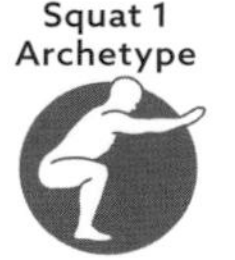

Front Rack 2 Archetype

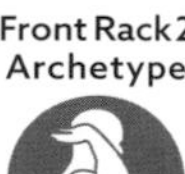

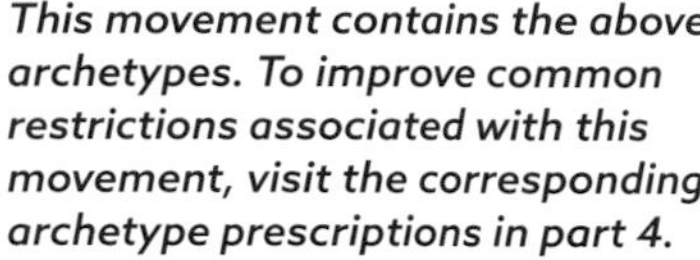

This movement contains the above archetypes. To improve common restrictions associated with this movement, visit the corresponding archetype prescriptions in part 4.

BACK SQUAT

Once you understand the universal laws of squatting and you've practiced the movement with the air squat and box squat, you need to up the ante on your positions and add a load. With additional weight on your torso and hips, small errors that may go unnoticed in the air squat and box squat become obvious, making the back squat another way to diagnose poor movement patterns. Not only that, but adding a barbell to the equation changes the levels of trunk stiffness and torsion force that are applied to the movement, which translates to more complex actions.

This is the idea: If you're air squatting, you might be managing 30 to 40 percent torque and tension levels. While this is great for simple tasks, the stabilization demands don't transfer to more dynamic movements. For example, jumping and landing or squatting with a heavy load requires much higher levels of trunk stiffness and torsion force. If you never challenge your setup and movement with larger loads, it's difficult to generate higher levels of force.

The back squat involves a lot of complex steps: Take the barbell out of the rack, walk back and assume a squat stance, execute the movement, walk forward, and re-rack the weight. It takes skill, practice, and razor-sharp focus to perform each step correctly. To ingrain the correct movement pattern and reduce errors, it's important to go through the same load order sequence. The idea is to minimize the variability of your movement so that you can preserve the quality of your position with each transitory step. If you take the bar out of the rack 17 different ways, you're going to start your squat 17 different ways.

This is not to say that you shouldn't change the position of the bar or change your squat stance from time to time. Those changes are fine—just be sure to practice the same setup every time you lift. If you step back with your left foot first, then do so every single time. That way, when you're tired, under stress, or in competition, you won't make fundamental mistakes because you've ingrained the same motor pattern over and over again. It's instinctual.

To shorten your learning curve, I've broken down the back squat into three phases: the lift-out (taking the barbell out of the rack), the walk back, and then the squat. It's worth mentioning that the lift-out and the walk back are universal steps used in lifts that require you to take a barbell out of a rack—the front squat, overhead squat, strict press, push-press, push-jerk, and split-jerk.

Phase 1: Lift-Out (6-Inch Squat)

Anytime you take a barbell out of a rack, you have to set your shoulders and get your belly tight before adding a load to your spine. It's a perfect example of the tunnel concept (see page 96): If you take the bar out of the rack and your spine is disorganized or your hips are in a bad position, it's impossible to reclaim a good position.

The first phase, which is essentially a 6-inch vertical squat, sets the tone for the rest of the lift. Most injuries and missed lifts relate to errors made in this phase, so it's imperative that you do it right. If you don't perform a good lift-out, reset the bar and start over. And make sure to set the rack to a height that allows for a good lift-out, which is roughly chest level.

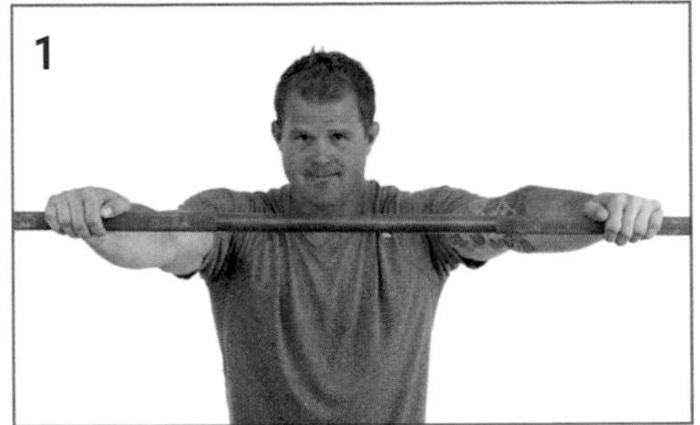

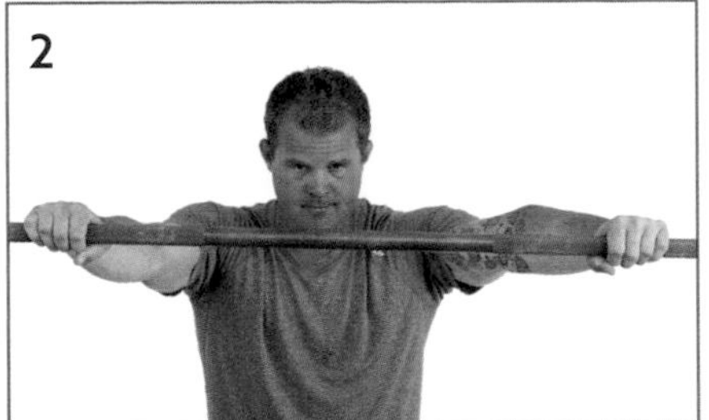

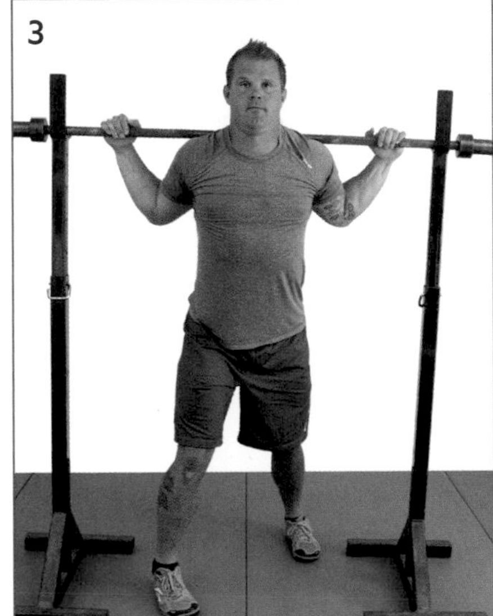

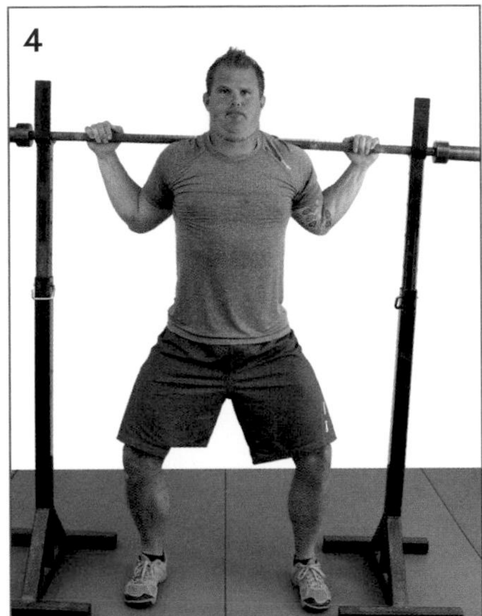

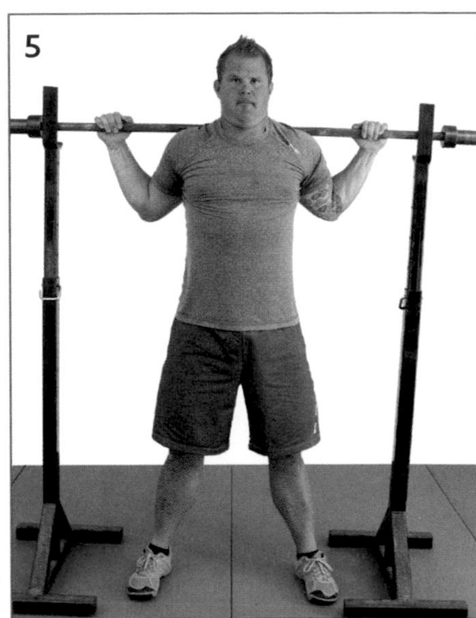

1. Find a comfortable distance for your grip. I like to position my hands just outside shoulder width. As with stance, grip distance is different for everyone and is predicated on mobility and frame size. The key is to form a grip that allows you to create sufficient external rotation force and tension in your upper back and shoulders. Put simply, it allows you to keep your wrists straight and your elbows underneath your shoulders.

2. Once you set your hands, create torque in your shoulders. To do so, pull back on the barbell and create an external rotation force by generating torque off the bar. Imagine trying to break or bend the bar with your hands. You can hook your thumbs under or over the bar. I prefer the thumb-under grip because it allows me to generate a stronger torsion force off the bar.

3. With your shoulders set and your upper back tight, step underneath the bar, positioning it somewhere on the mass of your deltoids, otherwise known as the spine of your scapula. (To learn more about barbell positioning, see "Jesse Burdick's Back Squat Shelf Test" on page 182 and the high-bar back squat on page 183.) Whether the bar is high or low, your goal is the same: create enough torque in your shoulders and tension in your upper back to maintain a good position. As you step under the bar, screw your foot into the ground to create a stable hip position. Take your time. The bar isn't just riding on your back. You want to make it part of your body.

4. Step underneath the bar with your opposite foot and assume your squat stance. The goal is to create tension in your upper back and get your torso as vertical as possible. To do so, press your neck back into the bar, eyes level at the start. Then twist your arms, bringing your elbows down underneath the bar, pulling your shoulders back, and maintaining as much external rotation torque as possible. As you do this, squeeze your butt, get your belly tight, align your ribcage over your pelvis, screw your feet into the ground, and shove your knees out as far as you can.

5. With your spine in a braced neutral position, shoulders and back tight, and torso as vertical as possible, extend your knees and lift the weight out of the rack.

Phase 2: Walk Back

Walking with a significant amount of weight on your back is a tricky endeavor. This is why the lift-out is so important; it sets up the efficacy of the walk back. If you lift out with a disorganized spine, walking back is only going to make your bad position worse.

To prevent this, execute a good lift-out and walk back in the same pattern every time you back squat. For example, after I lift the weight out of the rack, I always step back with my left foot, step back with my right foot, and then establish my squat stance. The steps are short and deliberate. Don't walk 10 feet from the rack, look down at your feet as you establish your stance, or do anything that will compromise the stiffness of your trunk and upper back.

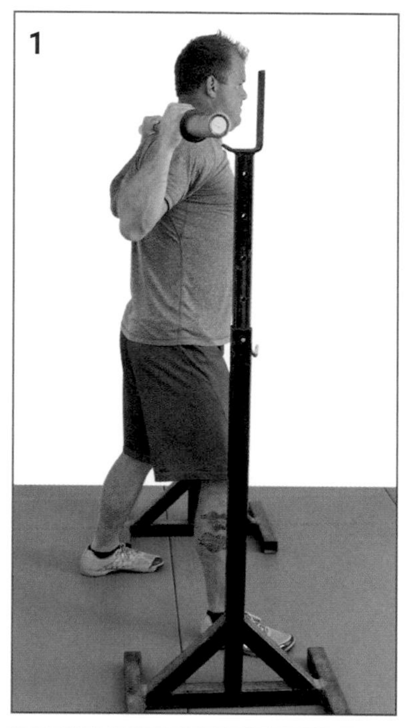

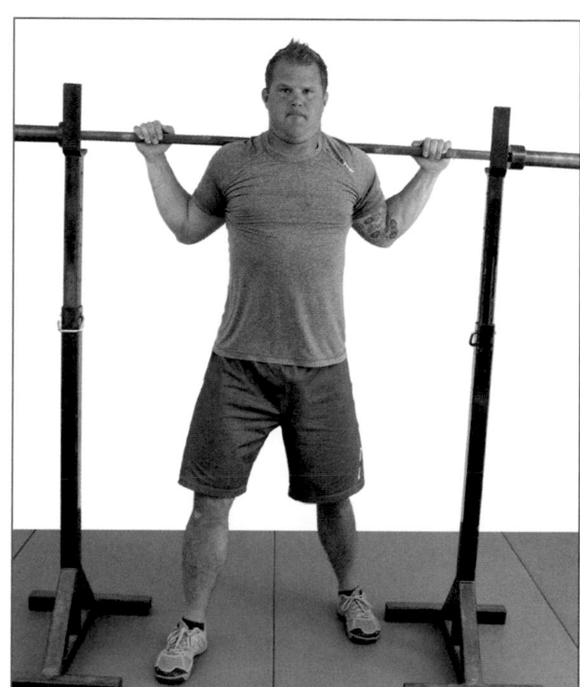

After you've lifted the bar out of the rack, step straight back. The key is to take a short, straight step. Unless you're transitioning into a wider stance, try to keep the same distance as your lift-out stance to reduce the variability of your movement. All the same rules apply: belly tight, spine neutral, and back and shoulders on tension.

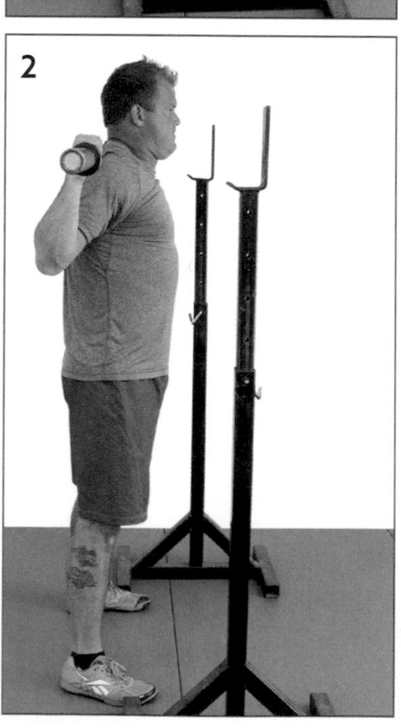

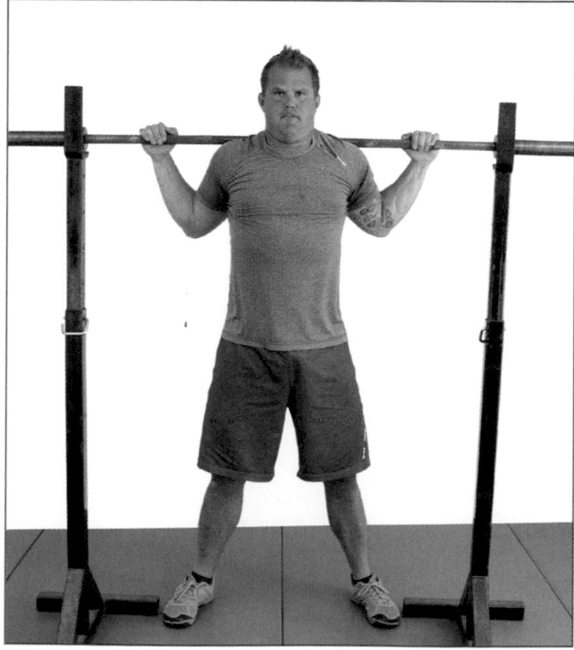

Step back with your opposite foot. Try to position your feet in your squat stance as you step back. The less you have to shift and adjust your stance, the better.

Phase 3: Squat

After you've taken the weight out of the rack, walked back, and established your squat stance, you're ready to perform the third phase of the sequence: the squat. Aside from managing a heavier load and organizing your arms in a different position, you perform the back squat in the same manner as the air squat.

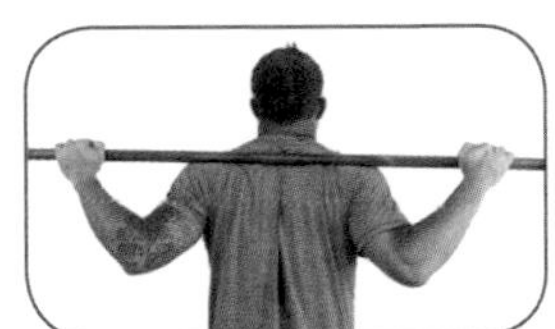

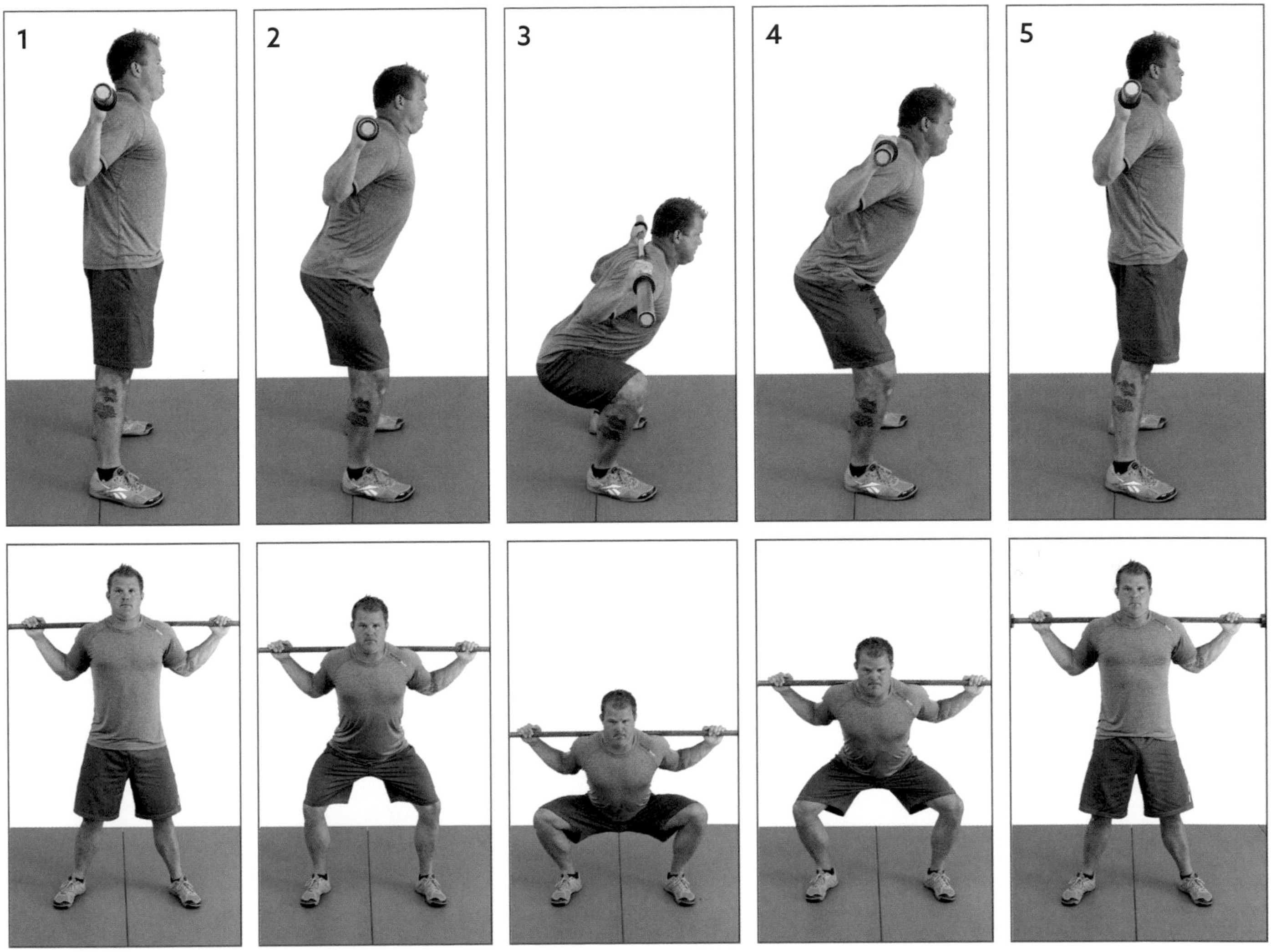

1 2 3 4 5

1. Once you've established your squat stance, squeeze your butt, screw your feet into the ground, and turn your knees out. Your shoulders and upper back should be tight, with wrists straight, head pressed back, and elbows positioned underneath or slightly behind the bar to support the load. Nothing should have changed from the lift-out phase.

2. Keeping your back flat and your shins as vertical as possible, reach your hamstrings back.

3. Still driving your knees out, lower into the bottom position until your hips pass below your knee crease or your thighs are parallel with the floor. To maintain hip stability, think about pulling yourself into the bottom position.

4. The moment you reach end range, stand up, keeping your spine, knees, and feet neutral.

5. As you stand up, squeeze your butt and reestablish the start position.

Jesse Burdick's Back Squat Shelf Test

There are many possible positions for the bar on your back, but all are ultimately categorized as low-bar or high-bar. The low-bar back squat allows you to tilt your torso forward and load tension in your posterior chain (hamstrings and hips). The high-bar back squat requires a more upright torso and shifts more of the demand onto your quadriceps. The former is typical of most powerlifters (although the only way to support 1,000-plus pounds on your back is with an upright torso), while the latter is common with Olympic lifters. While it's good to learn and practice both variations, you're probably going to gravitate toward one or the other, which is fine as long as you can perform both.

The best back squatters in the world adopt a more "low-ish" position for the bar while squatting. The key is to find a comfortable and tight position for the bar on your upper back. To find the sweet spot, perform this simple test:

Position a PVC pipe or bar on your back with your hands spaced far enough apart that you can get your wrists vertical and your elbows underneath the bar. Then slide the bar up and down the meat of your upper back (thoracic spine) and shoulders (deltoids and scapula) to find the tightest position. For some people, that is a high-bar position, while for others it is a low-bar position. (For most people, it's just above the scapula and on the deltoids.) You don't want it too high on your neck above your traps (cervical spine) or below the meat of your external rotators (backs of your shoulders). Remember, you should have enough range of motion to place the bar anywhere. But when it comes time to have a squat-off dance fight, adopt the best and most effective position for you.

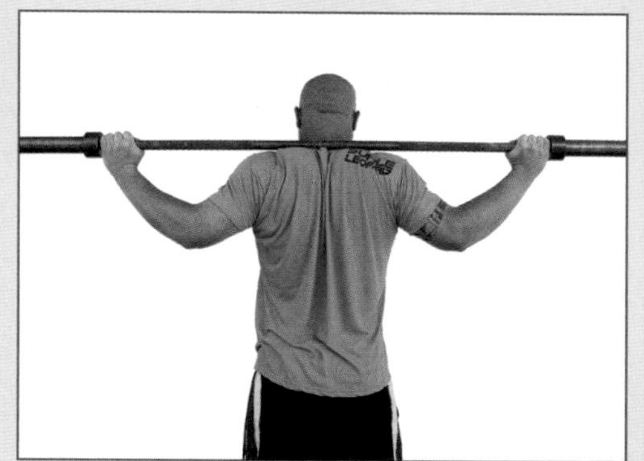

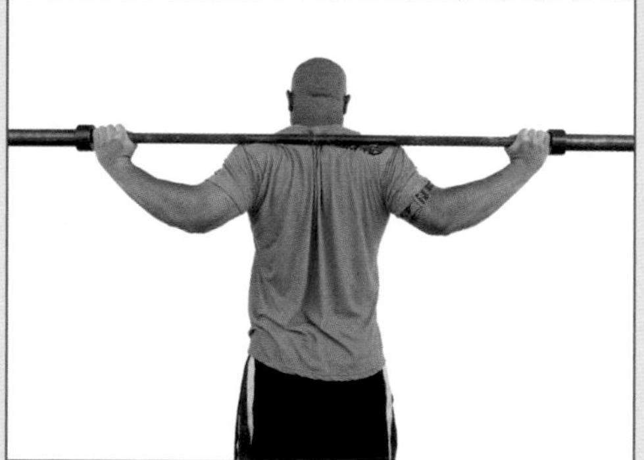

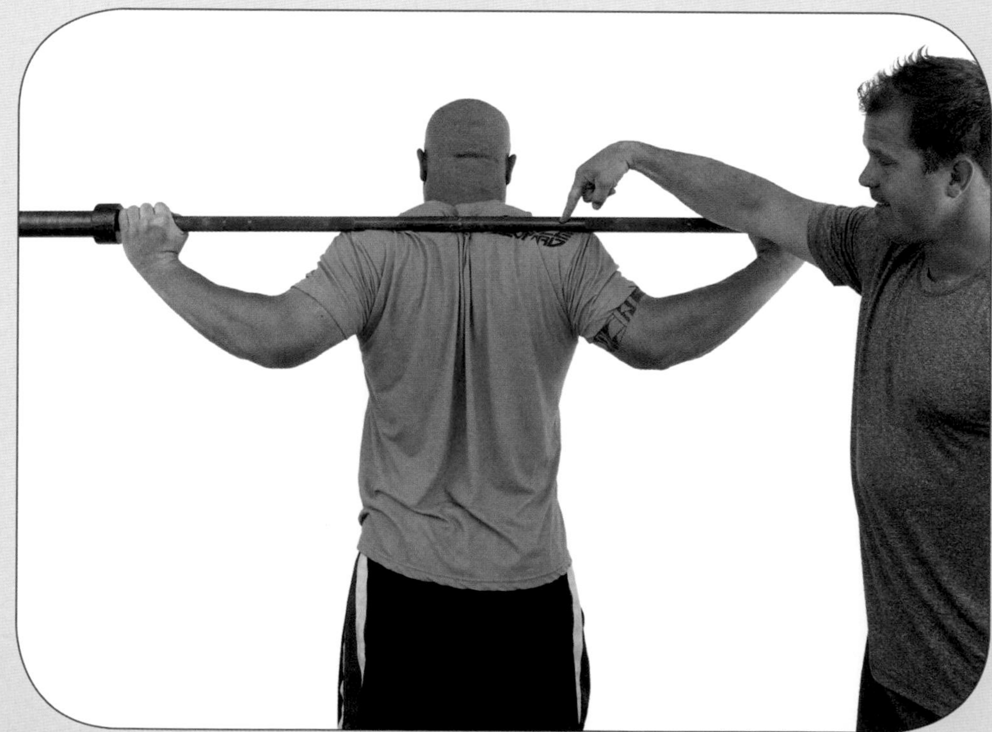

High-Bar Back Squat

If you're just learning how to back squat, I recommend sticking with either the low-bar or the high-bar variation. However, for the intermediate generalist athlete, there's no reason not to learn how to back squat with the bar in different positions. In fact, if you fall into that category, you should switch your stance, change the position of the bar, and change the thickness and weight of the bar often.

Remember, strength and conditioning is a tool for learning and scaling complex movement patterns in a controlled environment. With the bar higher on your back, you have to position your torso in a slightly different manner, providing a slightly different squat stimulus. Put simply, this gives you a brand-new motor pattern to solve.

Unlike the low-bar back squat, which allows you to load your hips and hamstrings and drop your torso slightly forward, the high-bar back squat forces your torso upright, loads more weight onto your quads, and increases the range of motion demands on your hips and ankles. You're abiding by the same principles, but now you're forced to adapt to a new position—see "Mark Bell's Underloading Method" on the next page.

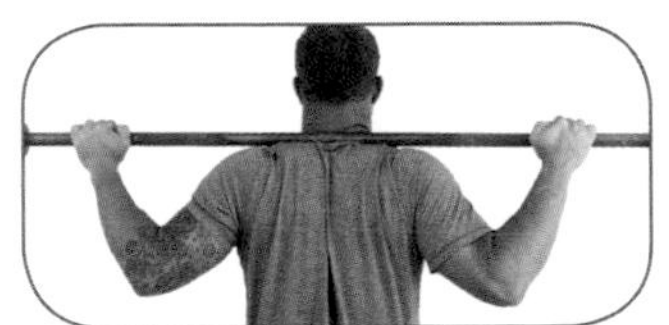

1
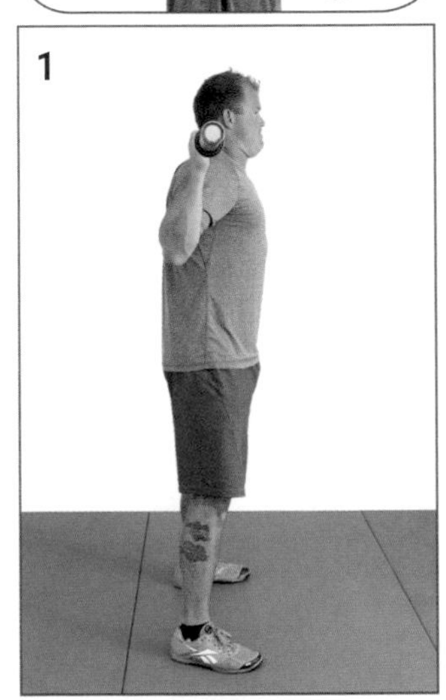

2
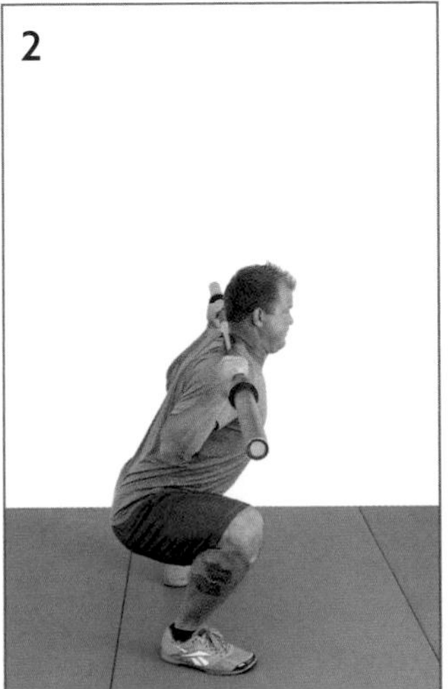

3
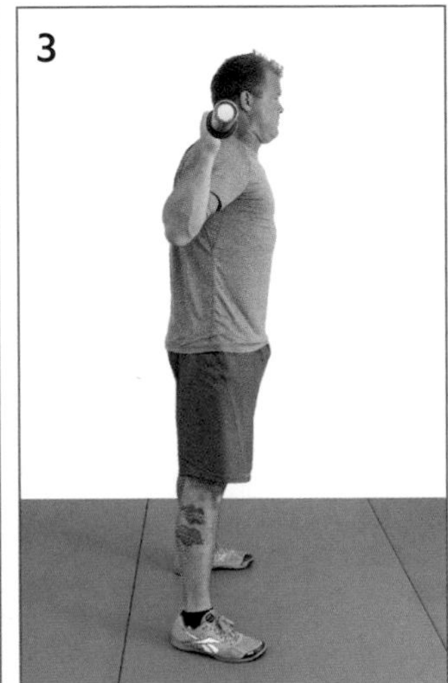

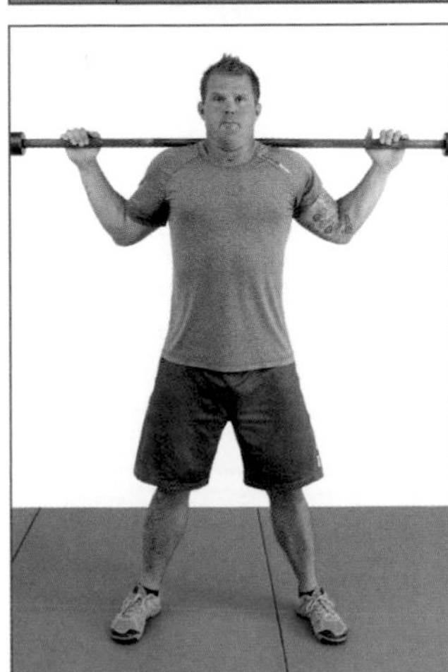

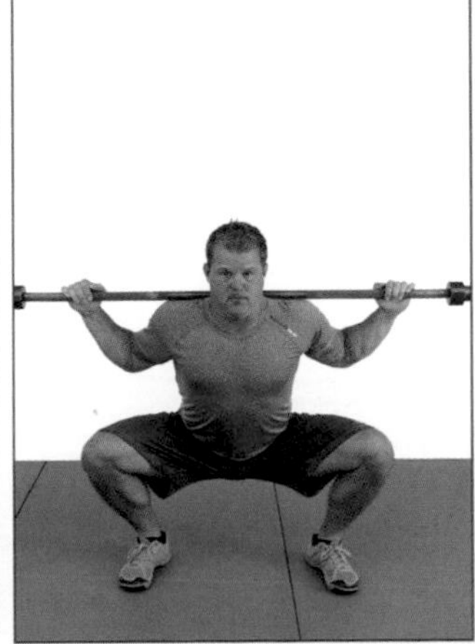

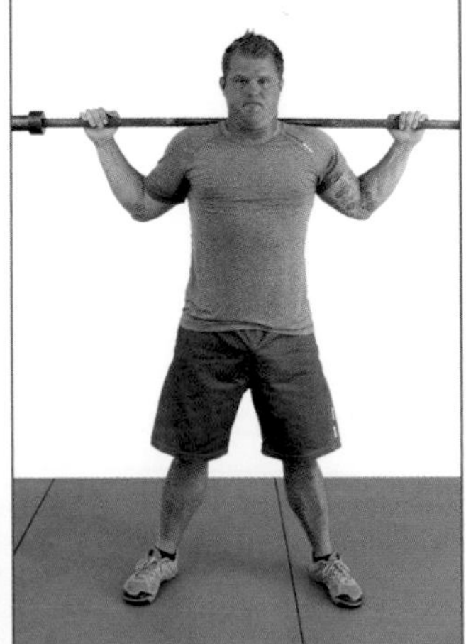

1. Other than the position of the bar, the setup (lift-out and walk back) for the high-bar back squat is exactly the same as the setup for the low-bar back squat. Notice that the bar is positioned just below the base of my neck in the region between my cervical spine and thoracic spine.

2. Keeping your torso upright, shins as vertical as possible, and spine neutral, lower into the bottom position.

3. Reestablish the top position.

Grip Fault (Broken at the Wrists)

Front Rack 2
Archetype

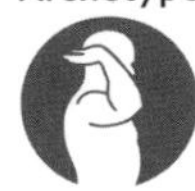

This fault is associated with the front rack archetype. For a mobility fix, visit the front rack archetype prescription in part 4.

MOTOR CONTROL FIX:

Find the shelf of your upper back—see Jesse Burdick's Back Squat Shelf Test on page 182—and make sure that your wrists are straight and your elbows are positioned underneath or just behind the bar.

Press your head back into the bar to create a neutral upper back.

If you're missing range of motion, adjust your grip by sliding your hands out until you can get your wrists in line with your arms.

MOBILIZATION TARGET AREAS:

Thoracic spine

Anterior shoulders and chest

Posterior shoulders and lats

Downstream arms (elbows and wrists)

If you're missing internal rotation in your shoulders or extension in your thoracic spine, you lose the ability to pull your shoulders back and brace your spine in a neutral position. As you can see in the photos below, this fault is characterized by rounding forward into a flexed position and breaking at the wrists. If you're not supporting the weight with your shoulders and wrists in a good position, your elbows end up taking the brunt of the load. Experiencing murderous elbow pain while back squatting? This might be the problem.

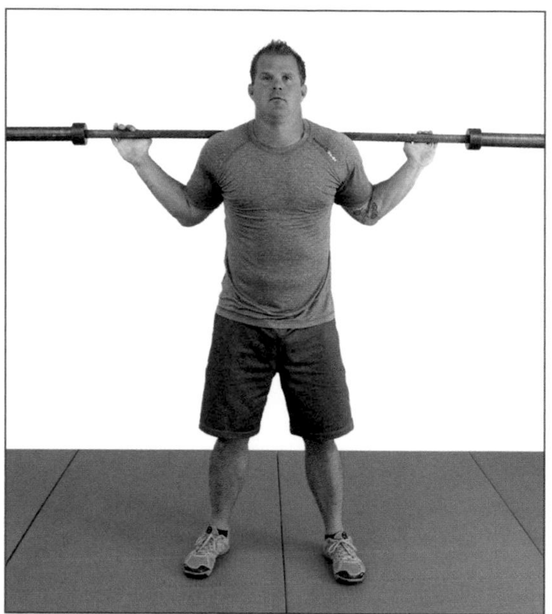

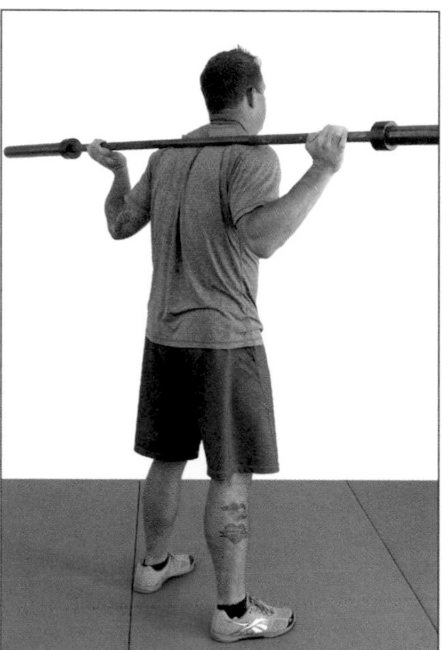

Mark Bell's Underloading Method

Underloading is a concept that Mark Bell—elite American powerlifter and supercoach—uses to train athletes by introducing new positions.

Here's an example: Say you're trying to get stronger with the deadlift. Rather than add weight, increase the speed of the lift, or manipulate the set and rep scheme, Mark will challenge range of motion or position. He does so by making you pull from a deficit, changing the bar position, changing your grip, or changing the bar type. Without adding any additional load, he increases the difficulty of the movement. This is a clever way to help lifters progress without having to make the weight heavier. It's also a great way to teach people how to apply the rules of movement and the load order sequence for a movement in a new position. It builds athletes who can adapt to new positions and quickly understand when they're in a bad position and what they need to do to adjust.

Grip Fault (Elbows High)

Lifting your elbows and pressing the bar into your upper back is another common grip fault that is characterized by poor shoulder and thoracic mobility. As with the previous grip fault, failing to create a stable bar platform forces you into a forward flexed position, places strain on your elbows, and opens the door to other movement errors down the line.

Note: This fault is not limited to athletes with poor mobility. A lot of people mistakenly elevate their elbows in an attempt to create upper back tension. This is simply a motor control error that needs to be addressed in the setup.

Front Rack 2 Archetype

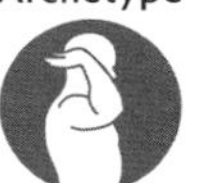

This fault is associated with the front rack archetype. For a mobility fix, visit the front rack archetype prescription in part 4.

MOBILIZATION TARGET AREAS:

Thoracic spine

Anterior shoulders and chest

Posterior shoulders and lats

Downstream arms (elbows and wrists)

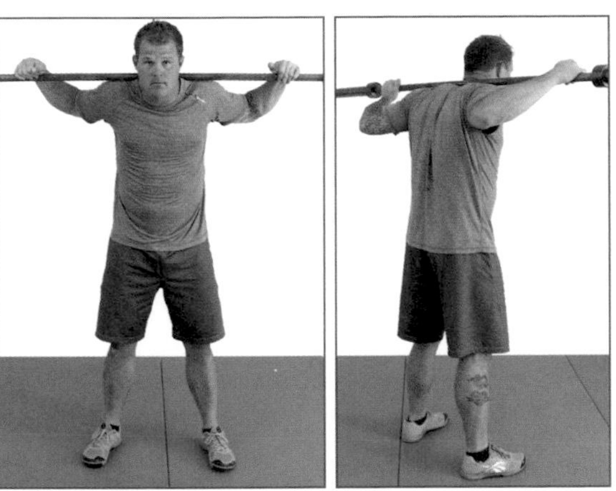

MOTOR CONTROL FIX:

Find the shelf of your upper back—see "Jesse Burdick's Back Squat Shelf Test" on page 182—and make sure that your wrists are straight and your elbows are positioned underneath or just behind the bar.

Press your head back into the bar to create a neutral upper back.

If you're missing range of motion, adjust your grip by sliding your hands out until you can get your wrists in line with your arms.

Head Fault (Checking Stance)

Coaches often tell beginners to look down to check the orientation of their feet while warming up. And with good reason: If the positions of your feet are different—if one foot is turned out more than the other—it wreaks havoc with your ability to generate power and creates an uneven force across your spine. While this isn't a big deal when the weight is light, it ingrains a bad habit that will inevitably cause breaks in spinal position. This is why it's so important to have defined motor patterns—meaning you step back the same way into the same stance every single time—so that you don't have to sacrifice neck position to look down.

MOTOR CONTROL FIX:

When you're first learning how to squat and walk back, try not to exaggerate looking down.

Walk back using the same sequence every time, and practice with a light load until you feel comfortable.

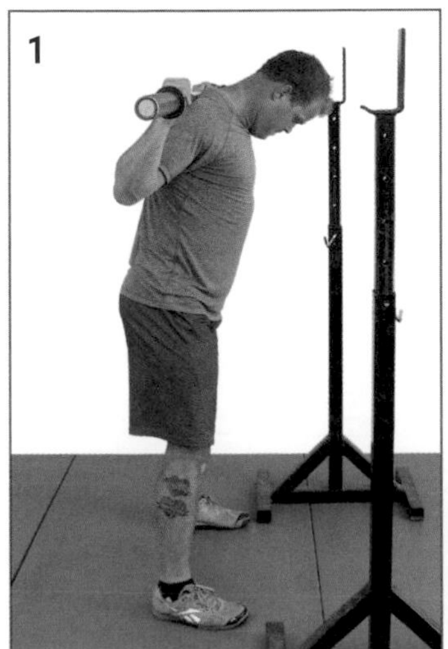
1

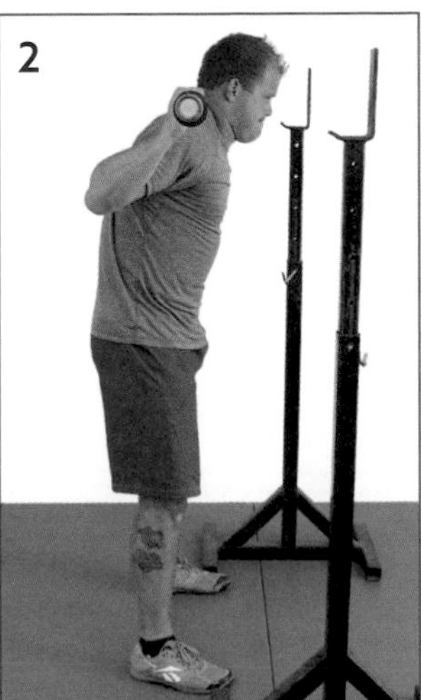
2

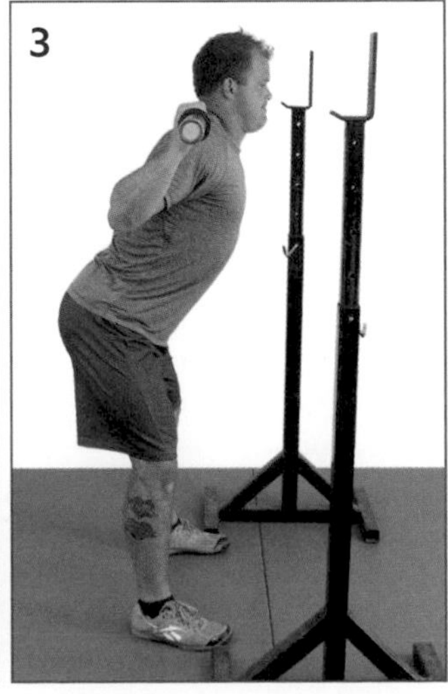
3

MOTOR CONTROL FIX:

This fault is common in athletes who squat with their feet turned out. Make sure that your feet are straight to allow for maximum torsion force.

Create and maintain torque through the entire movement. Think about screwing your feet into the ground, shoving your knees out, and pulling yourself into the bottom position.

Good Morning Squat Fault

This fault is characterized by shooting your hips up and extending your legs out of the bottom position. It occurs when you don't have enough external rotation torque and you don't feel stable in the bottom position, so you raise your hips and hamstrings as a way to support the load.

Without torque, it's impossible to keep your back and hips connected throughout the movement. As a result, you hinge at the lumbar spine as if it were a hip joint and use the strength of your back to complete the movement.

Again, if you have good motor control patterning and the strength to handle the load, your position won't change: You'll go up the same way you went down. If you start to compensate, stop and have a spotter assist the movement, or bail out from underneath the bar. (*Note:* Dumping weight off a failed lift is a complex task that you should learn before handling large loads.) This is easier to see with the deadlift because there's no change in spinal position if you fail. You don't worm around, collapse forward, or look up; you just stop or drop the weight.

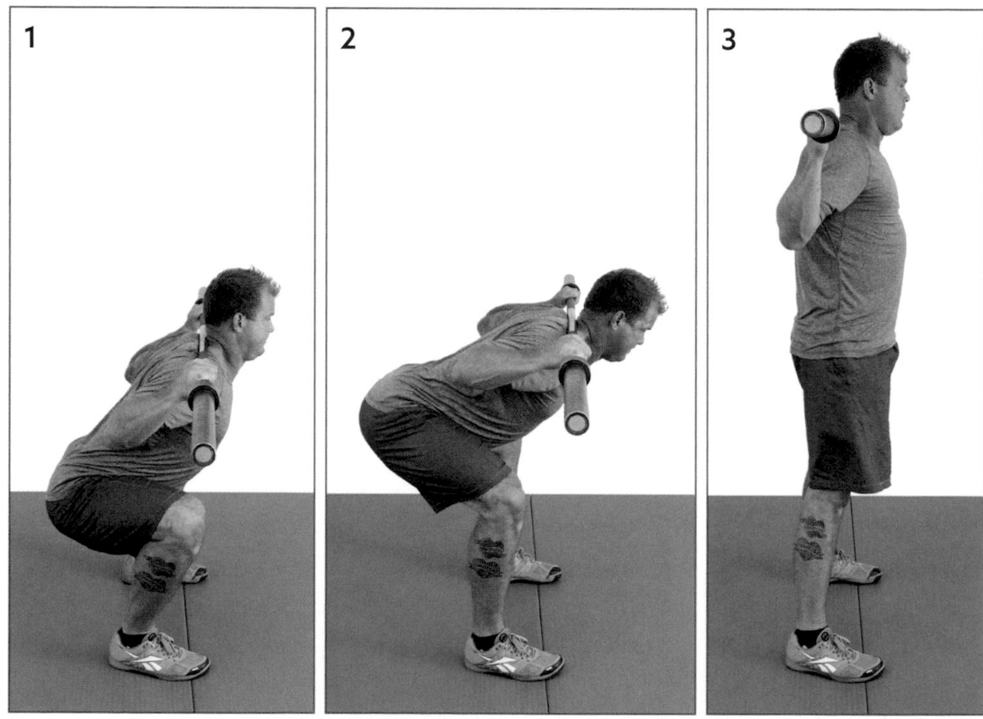

FRONT SQUAT

Squat 1 Archetype

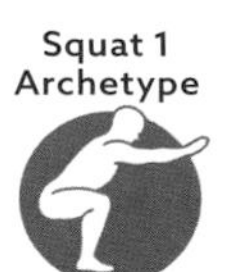

Front Rack 2 Archetype

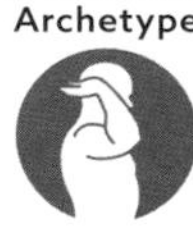

This movement contains the above archetypes. To improve common restrictions associated with this movement, visit the corresponding archetype prescriptions in part 4.

Imagine picking up a keg of beer and lowering it back down to the ground. Can you do that without ripping apart your knees or back? If you know how to front squat, you can.

Lifting a keg, a couch, a bag of charcoal, your kid: Most everyday lifting-related tasks require you to pick something up or lower something to the ground with the load supported in front of your body. What's more, the majority of these tasks require your torso to remain upright. The front squat is a great example of a gym movement that transfers to the tasks of daily life.

The front squat will ferret out shortages in shoulder, hip, quad, and ankle range of motion—weaknesses you may be able to hide while performing the air squat or back squat. In an air squat or back squat, you can tilt your chest forward and reach your hips farther back, giving your hips, hamstrings, and ankles some breathing room. The upright-torso demands of the front squat will reveal these mobility limitations and, once addressed, present opportunities for snagging more performance.

The front squat is a progression to category 3 movements, specifically the clean and jerk—pulling a weight from the ground to shoulder level in one movement and then pressing the weight overhead. It also teaches you how to squat with your shoulders organized in the front rack position—a necessary skill when learning or practicing the clean.

Front Rack Position

Whether you receive the bar in the clean or take it out of a rack, the priority is the same: Organize your shoulders in a stable position by creating external rotation torque with your arms. Failure to do so results in a rounded upper back. Upper back tension and external rotation torque are what you're after. Grip is the place to start.

The conventional method for establishing an ideal grip is to measure a thumb's distance from your hip bone. As you can see in the photos below, raising your arms from this spot can cause your shoulders to internally rotate and your elbows to flare out, leaving you unsecured. A better bet is to align your wrists with your elbows to build a supportive platform.

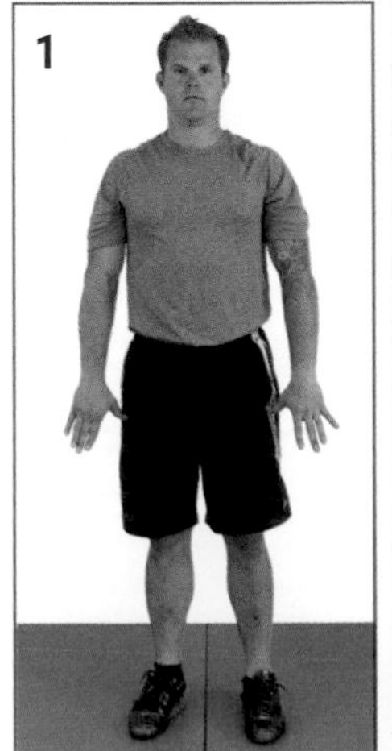

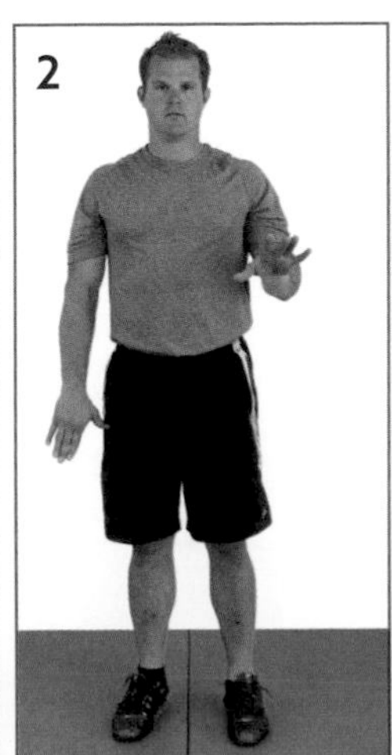

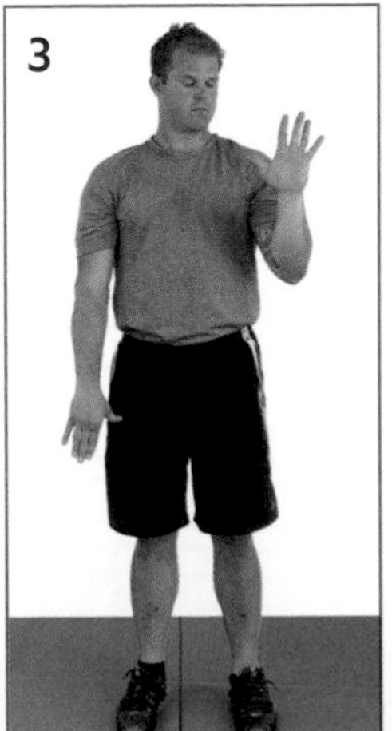

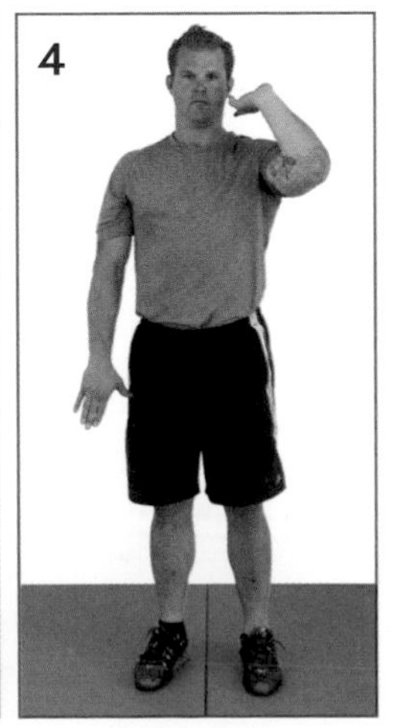

In most cases, using the conventional front rack setup method to find your grip forces you into a compensated position. As you can see, my grip is too narrow, making it impossible to get my elbows in line with my wrists, which is necessary to support the load and create external rotation torque.

This is how you do it. Turn your palm toward the front of your body, curl your hand to your shoulder, raise your elbow to a 90-degree angle, and then flip your palm toward the sky. (Sometimes it's helpful to have a Superfriend give you an assist by manipulating you into this position.) You may need to do a bit of fine-tuning, but this approach will start to get you dialed in on grip width.

If you flex your arm with your palm forward (an externally rotated position), your elbow will deviate out to the side, putting your wrist in line with your elbow. This also sets your shoulders in a stable position, allowing you to maximize torque. As with your squat stance, you may have to tinker around to find the most comfortable and stable position. In most cases, these adjustments are made based on arm length and shoulder mobility. *Note:* For a more detailed description of the lift-out, refer to the back squat section (page 178).

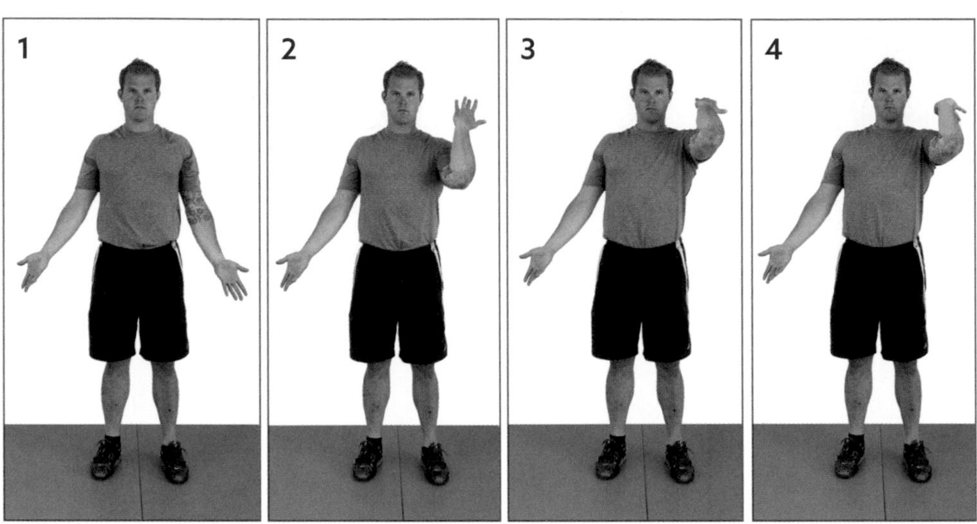

Phase 1: Front Rack Position

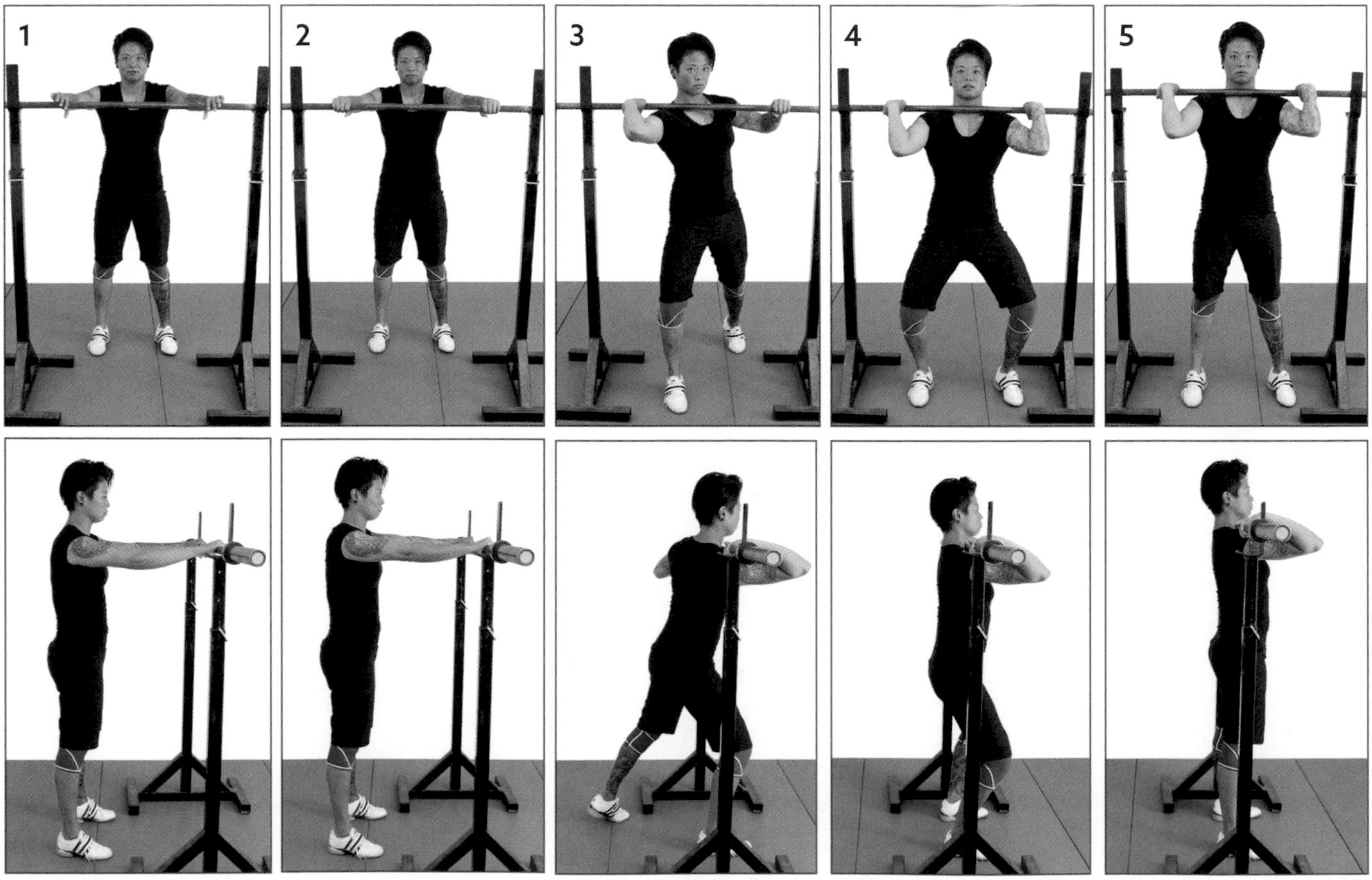

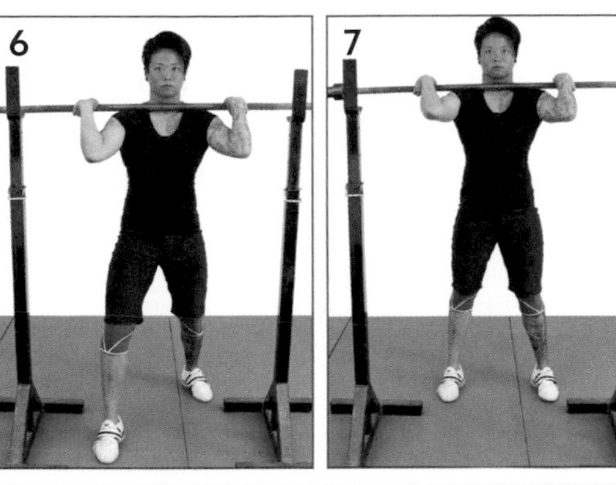

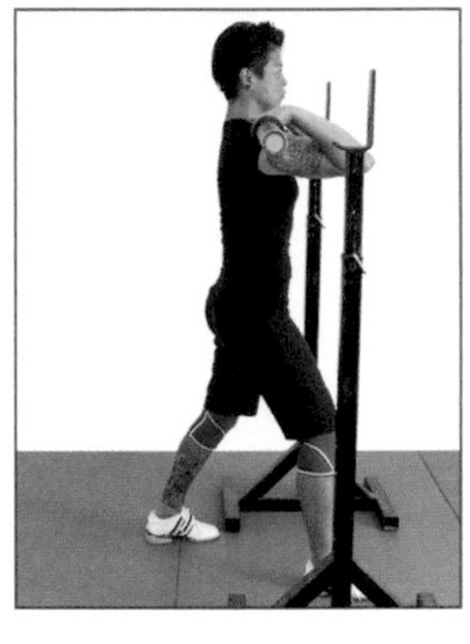

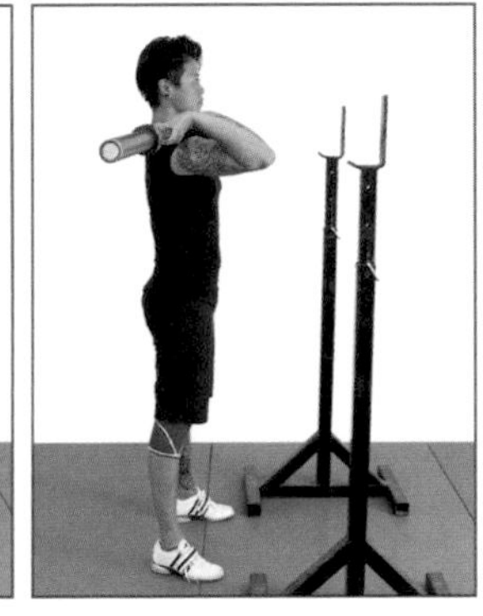

Phase 2: Walk Back

1. Grip the bar with your hands positioned far enough apart that you can create a stable shoulder position.

2. Screw your hands into the bar to light up external rotation torque.

3. Maintaining as much torque as possible, step directly underneath the bar with one foot. Twist the same-side arm underneath the bar so that the plane between your shoulder and arm is parallel to the ground. The idea is to wind up your shoulder to create more tension in your upper back.

4. Step in with your opposite foot. As you assume your squat stance, twist your arm underneath the bar to establish the front rack position. The bar should rest on your shoulders and fingers, but this doesn't mean you want your shoulders forward to support the weight.

5. Keeping your elbows high to maintain torque, screw your feet into the ground, drive your knees out laterally, and lift the bar straight out of the rack.

6. Step straight back. Again, step back with the same foot every single time.

7. Step your opposite foot back and assume your squat stance. Make your steps short and deliberate.

Phase 3: Front Squat

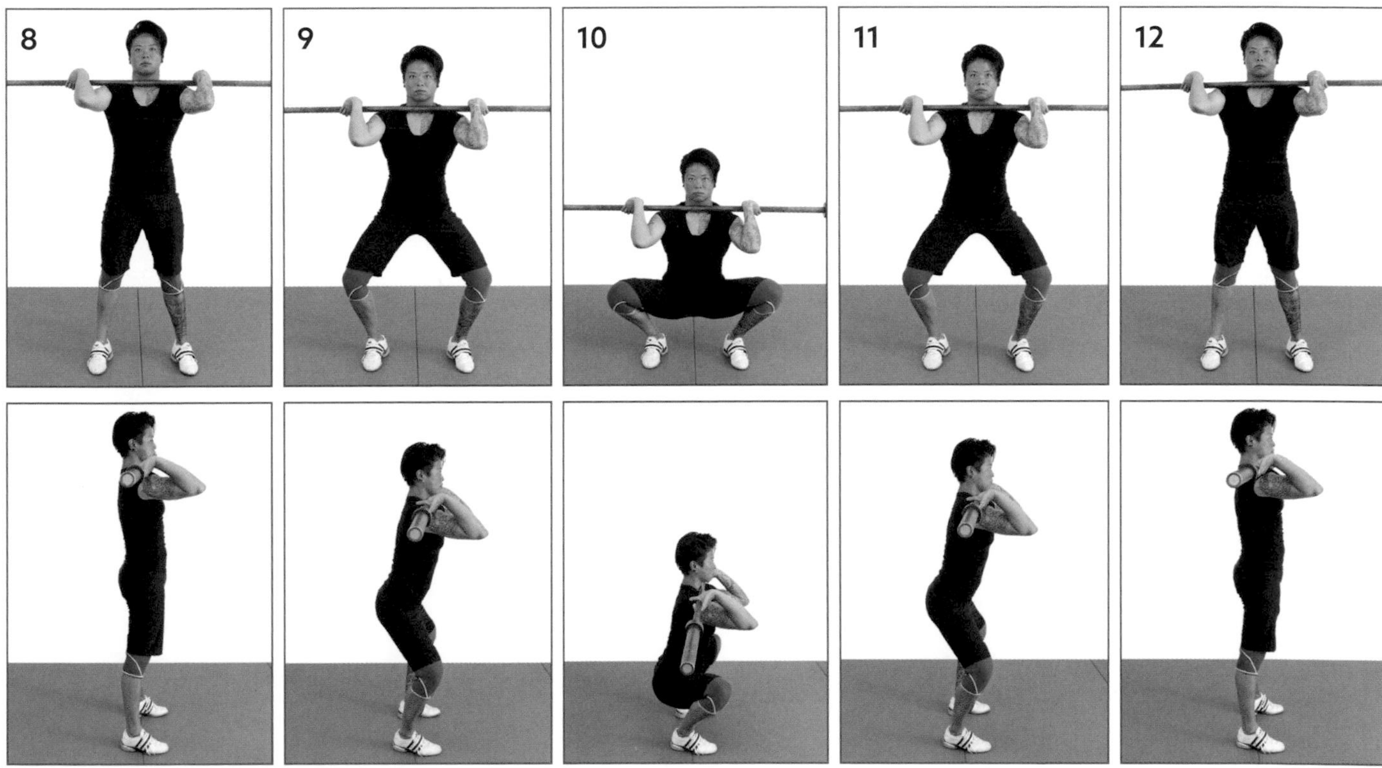

8. Get organized: Squeeze your butt, get your belly tight, and screw your feet into the ground to create tension in your hips.

9. Keeping your elbows up, drive your knees out laterally, draw your hamstrings back slightly, and lower your hips between your feet. Keep your head back and your eyes fixed straight ahead to lock in torque and tension.

10. Pressing your knees out, lower into the bottom of the squat. Keep your elbows high and tension on.

11. With your torso upright, drive out of the bottom position. The ascent should mimic the descent.

12. As you stand up, squeeze your butt and reestablish the top position.

Front Rack 2
Archetype

This fault is associated with the front rack archetype. For a mobility fix, visit the front rack archetype prescription in part 4.

MOTOR CONTROL FIX:

Address front rack mechanics and grip position—see the stable shoulder front rack setup on pages 187–188.

MOBILIZATION TARGET AREAS:

Thoracic spine

Anterior shoulders and chest

Posterior shoulders and lats

Downstream arms (elbows and wrists)

Narrow-Grip Fault (Elbows Out)

If your wrists are positioned to the insides of your shoulders in the front rack, it's a blinding giveaway that your shoulders are in an unstable position. As you can see in the photos below, Diane's elbows flare out to the sides, unloading tons of force on her wrists. That's when it all crumbles. Her shoulders internally rotate, and she can no longer create tension in her upper back. If this is happening to you, don't be surprised when you have to bail on lifts because your wrists feel like they've been chopped with a dull axe.

Moral of the story: It's difficult to manage a heavy load or maintain an upright torso unless your wrists are in line with your elbows.

The motor control fix for this fault is simple: Slide your hands out and address the stable shoulder front rack setup. If the problem can't be solved with motor control, it's possible that you're missing thoracic extension (upper back flat), and flexion and external rotation in your shoulders.

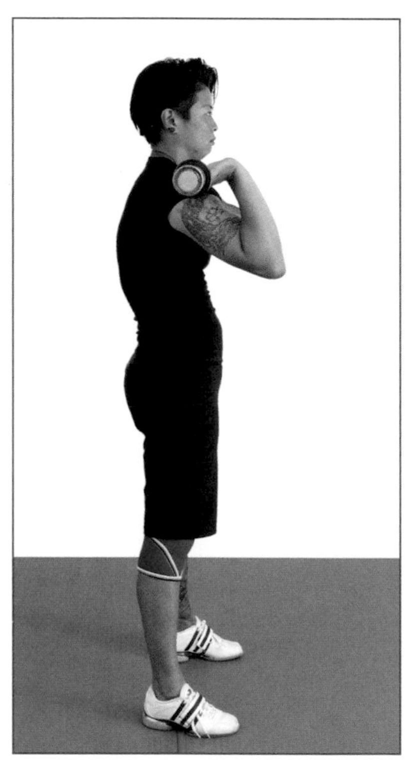

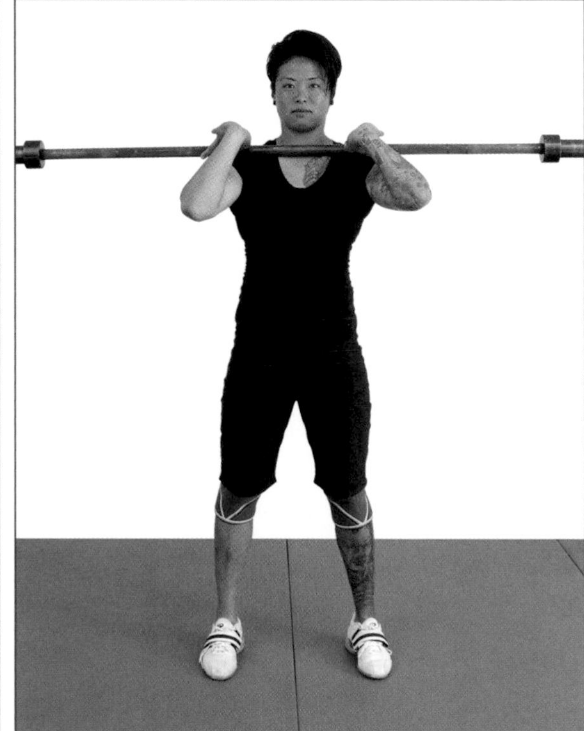

"Elbows Up!"

Being told to get your elbows up during a front squat or clean is not going to fix the position. It might prevent a missed lift, but it will not prevent faults. The only way to correct the problem is to address the issue systematically: Are you creating enough torque to maintain an upright torso? Can you achieve a good front rack position? Can you squat to full depth with your torso upright? If you miss the lift and drop the weight, it's probably a combination of a bad rack and missing range of motion in your hips and ankles. However, if you have a good rack position, you can come forward a little without dropping your weight because you can keep your elbows high and maintain a rigid upper back.

Cross-Arm Fault

The cross-arm front rack position is a classic bodybuilder setup to the front squat. With your arms crossed in front of your body, you can create a platform for the bar without challenging shoulder range of motion. This makes for an easier front rack position. Although this variation still gives you a front squat stimulus, it compromises your shoulder positioning and doesn't transfer to more dynamic lifts. Bodybuilders typically don't perform Olympic lifts, so the fact that it's not a transferable exercise might not matter. However, being unable to create torque off the bar will always present problems. Your shoulders will internally rotate and your upper back will round forward, making it difficult to achieve a neutral position under heavy loads.

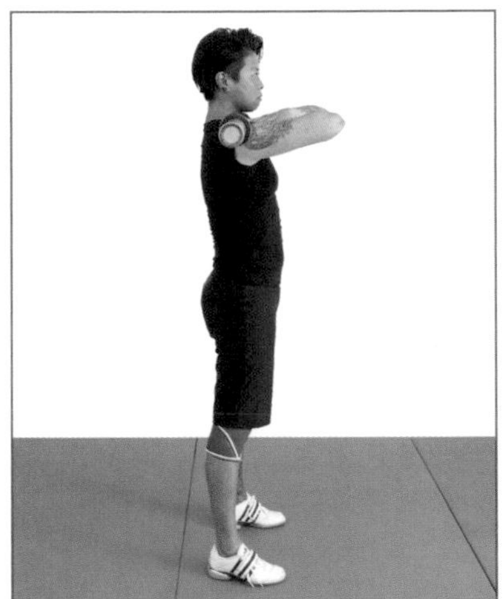

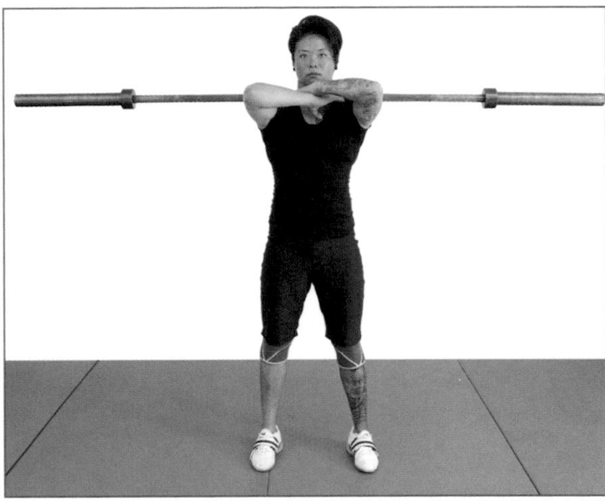

Chest-Forward Fault

When your elbows drop and your chest translates forward in the squat, it's an indication that either you failed to create torque in your hips and shoulders, creating an untenable front rack position, or you are missing range of motion in one or all of the following areas: shoulders (flexion and external rotation), elbows (flexion), wrists (extension), thoracic spine (extension), hips (external rotation), and ankles (dorsiflexion).

Squat 1 Archetype

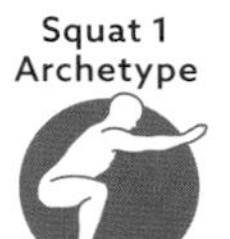

Front Rack 2 Archetype

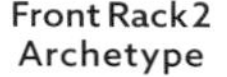

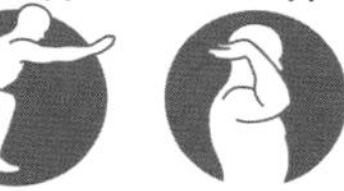

This fault is associated with the above archetypes. For a mobility fix, visit the corresponding archetype prescriptions in part 4.

MOBILIZATION TARGET AREAS:

FRONT RACK

Thoracic spine

Anterior shoulders and chest

Posterior shoulders and lats

Downstream arms (elbows and wrists)

SQUAT

Anterior chain (hips and quads)

Posterior high chain (hamstrings)

Calves and heel cords

Medial chain (adductors)

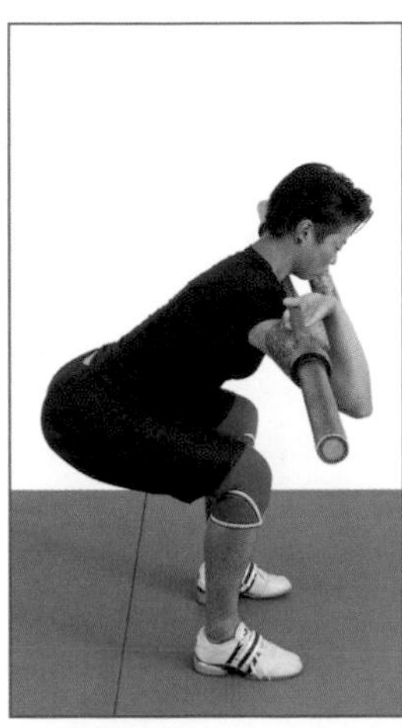

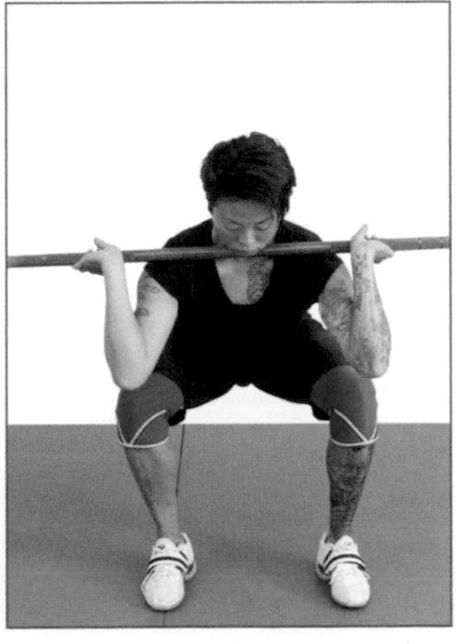

MOTOR CONTROL FIX:

Address front rack mechanics and grip position—see the stable shoulder front rack setup on pages 187–188.

Create and maintain external rotation torque in your shoulders and hips.

Squat 1 Archetype Overhead Archetype

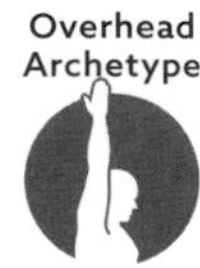

This movement contains the above archetypes. To improve common restrictions associated with this movement, visit the corresponding archetype prescriptions in part 4.

OVERHEAD SQUAT

When it comes to making the invisible visible, the overhead squat will smoke out the truth. It's the most challenging of the squat iterations. In the front squat, you hold the bar in front of your body. In the overhead squat, you stabilize the bar over your head. Nothing tests your ability to create a stable trunk, generate torque, or reveal your range of motion like the overhead squat. In the same way that the front squat reveals weaknesses that can be hidden within the back squat, the overhead squat trumps the front squat as a diagnostic tool. Various disguises of motor control faults or mobility restrictions will be scorched away when you open up the furnace door of the overhead squat.

Say you're missing a bit of external rotation in your hips and dorsiflexion in your ankles. Doing a front squat, you compensate by tilting your torso slightly forward. Your front rack is good, your spine is rigid, and, despite the missing ranges, you can execute the front squat. But things unravel when you take this show down the road to the overhead squat. If you tilt your torso offline in the bottom position of the

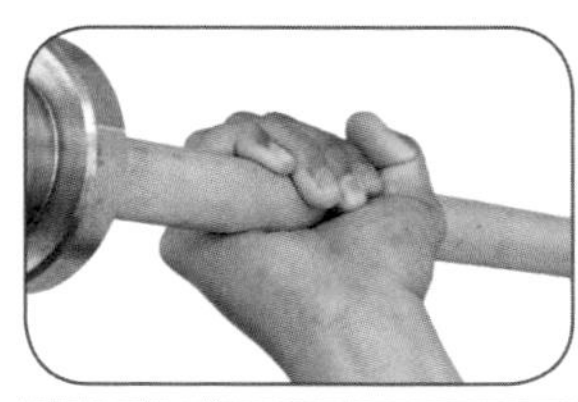

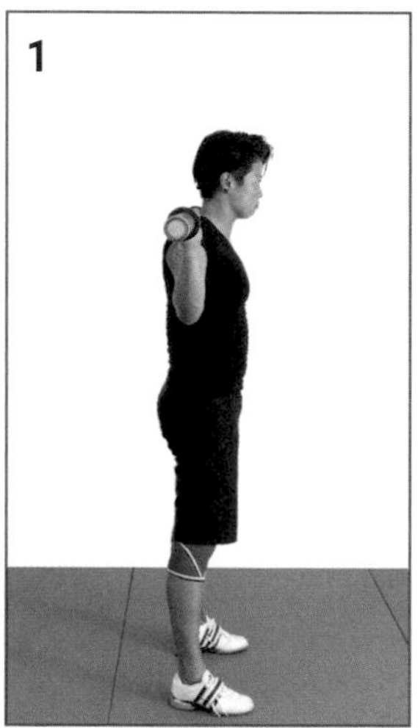

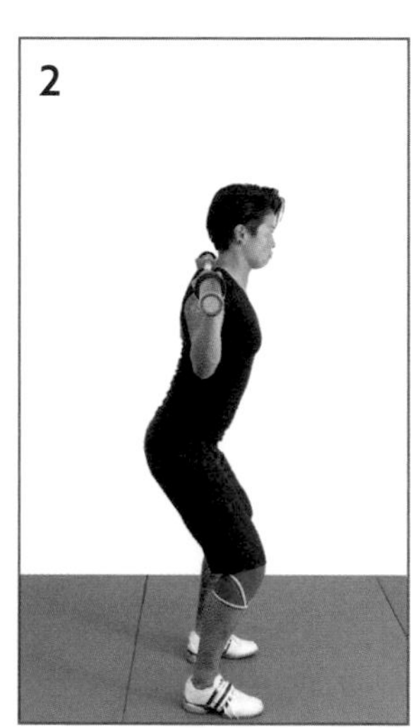

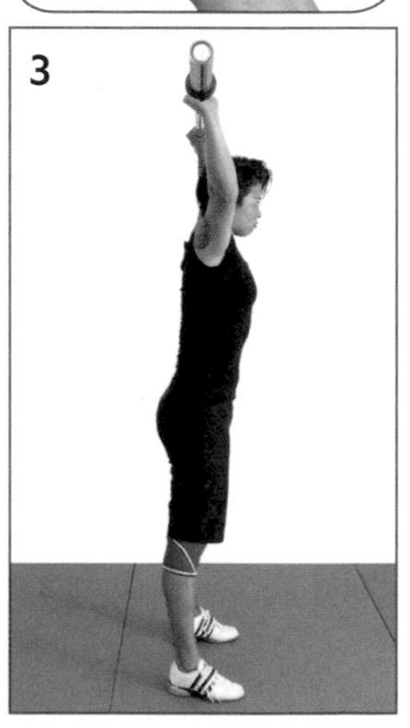

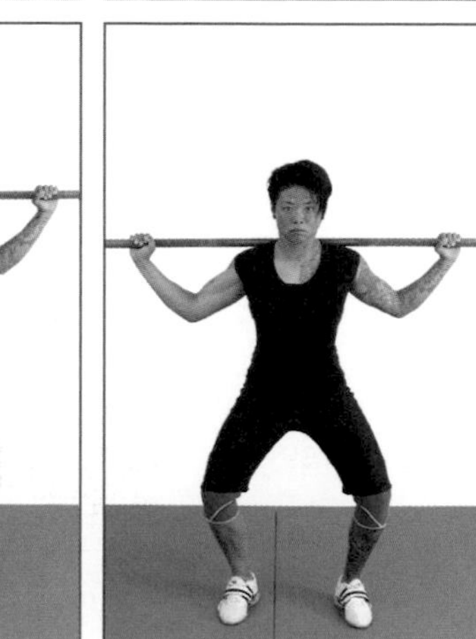

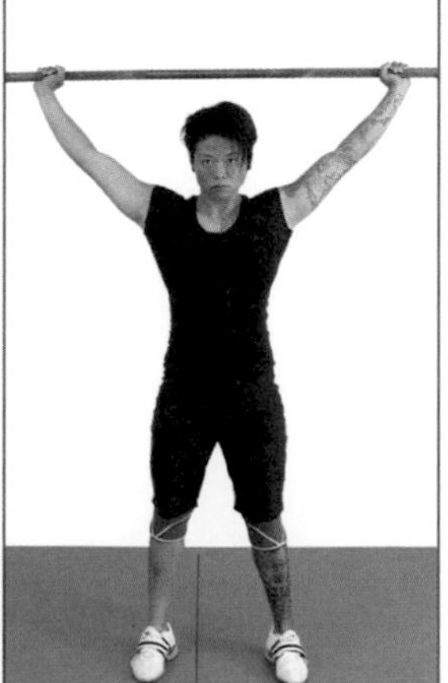

1. Using a snatch grip on the bar, perform the initial movements as you would for the back squat: Create torque (break the bar), perform the lift-out, and walk back. You want the bar positioned on the shelf of your upper back (see "Jesse Burdick's Back Squat Shelf Test" on page 182) and your elbows and wrists on the same vertical plane. To maintain a neutral head position and create tension in your upper back, drive your neck back into the bar, keeping your head level. Then assume your squat stance, squeeze your butt, get your belly tight, and screw your feet into the ground.

2. Shove your knees out, pull your hamstrings back slightly, keeping a rigid spine, and lower your hips between your feet as you would when initiating an upright-torso squat. Remember, your knees are expressed out, not forward.

3. Extend your knees and hips and press the bar overhead. To maintain a stable shoulder position, externally rotate your armpits forward and continue to create torque off the bar. Once the bar is stabilized overhead, readdress the top position sequence (squeeze your butt, get your belly tight, screw your feet into the ground). Notice that the bar is positioned

overhead squat, your shoulders will destabilize and unlock, causing the bar load to sway precariously above you like an anvil in a Wile E. Coyote trap.

If you can overhead squat with exceptional technique, it shows that you not only understand the fundamental principles of bracing and torque, but also have full range of motion in your shoulders, hips, and ankles. This is why the overhead squat with a PVC pipe is such a popular assessment tool. Within two seconds, a good coach can spot motor control problems and mobility restrictions.

As with all movements, the key is to become competent with the overhead squat under light loads (like a PVC pipe or an empty barbell) and then increase the weight or work output to test your ability to maintain good form under greater demand.

Note: Although the overhead squat retains the same preliminary phases of the back squat and front squat—lifting out of the rack and walking the load back—you need to power the load up into the overhead position before you begin the lift. To do so, you can either push-press or push-jerk the weight. The push-press (dip and drive) is fine for lifting light weight, but for more taxing loads or multiple reps, the push-jerk is the preferred method because it costs you less energy.

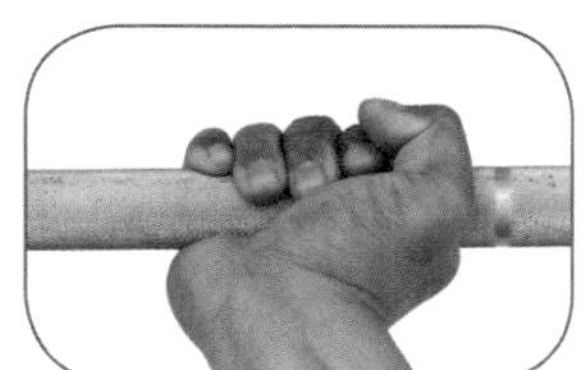

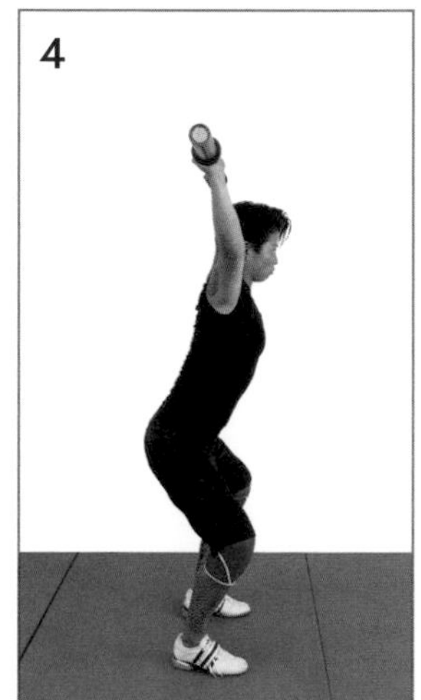

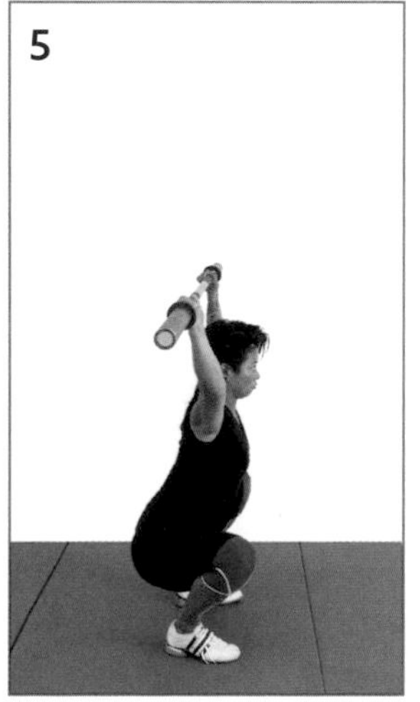

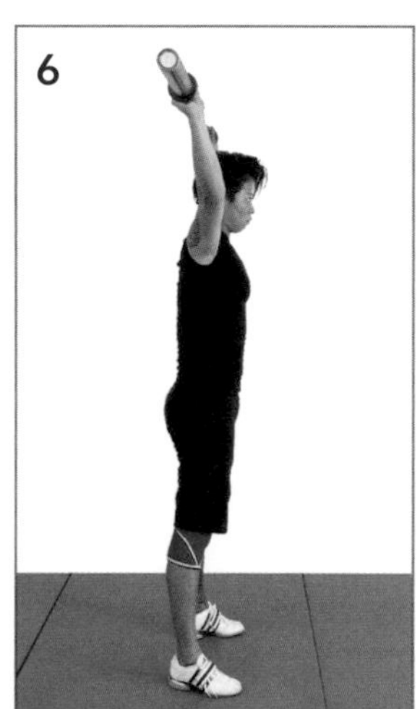

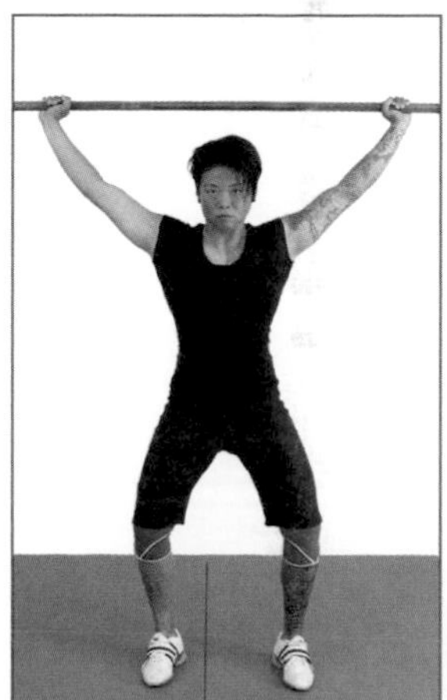

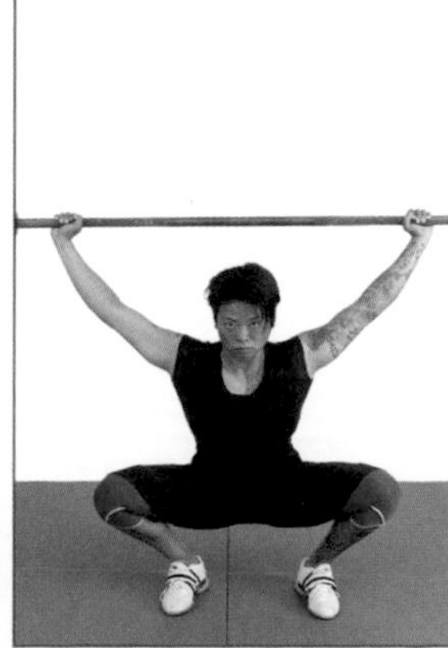

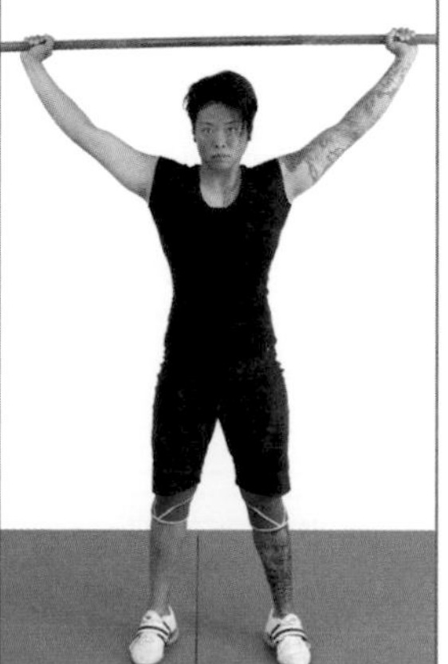

in the center of Diane's palms and her wrists are in line with her forearms (not bent or flexed).

4. Keeping your shoulders in a stable position, draw your hamstrings back slightly, shove your knees out to the limits of your range, and slowly lower your hips between your feet.

5. Still making a conscious effort to drive your knees out, lower into the bottom position. If you have to pause at the bottom to stabilize the weight overhead, that's fine. The key is not to bounce out of the bottom position, tilt your chest forward, or have the bar move behind or in front of your center of mass.

6. Extend your knees and hips and reestablish the top position. *Note:* If you're executing another repetition, go through the top position load order sequence. If you've completed the set, you can lower the weight to your neck or guide it out in front of you. The former should be done only when you're lifting extremely light loads, like the bar. If you're handling anything heavier than that, dump the weight out in front of your body. Don't try to receive 300 pounds on your cervical spine.

Shoulder Shrug Fault

MOTOR CONTROL FIX:

Create torque off the bar, keeping your wrists in a neutral position, and externally rotate your armpits forward.

Make sure that the bar is aligned directly over your center of mass.

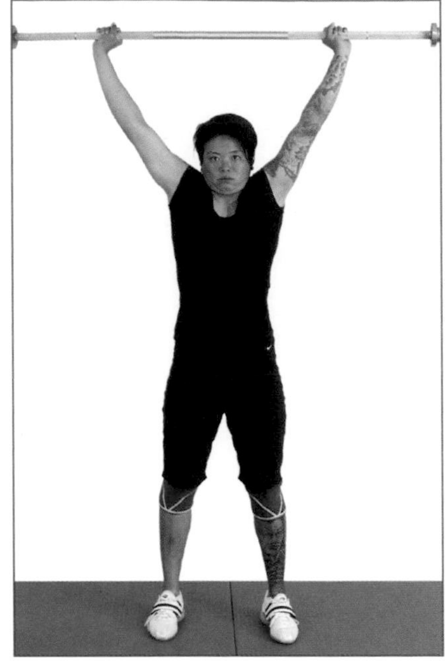

A lot of people mistakenly shrug their shoulders to their ears in an attempt to create a stable position. "Shrug your shoulders" is another of the pointless cues that coaches have been giving athletes for years. The only way to stabilize your shoulders in a good position is to create external rotation torque, which is cued with armpits forward. It's that simple. Telling someone to press her shoulders up to her ears will cause her to internally rotate into an unstable position.

Unstable Shoulders Fault (Bent Elbows)

MOTOR CONTROL FIX:

Create torque off the bar, keeping your wrists in a neutral position, externally rotate your armpits forward, and lock out your elbows.

MOBILIZATION TARGET AREAS:

Thoracic spine

Posterior shoulders and lats

Anterior shoulders and chest

If you can't lock out your arms overhead, either you don't understand how to create a stable shoulder position or you are missing internal rotation in your shoulders. Bending your elbows internally rotates your arms, which unloads tension in your shoulders, lats, and upper back. While this compensation allows you to get overhead, it puts your shoulders in an unstable position, creating a toxic motor pattern that will leak poison into pulling movements like the pull-up, press, and deadlift. You lose power by the metric ton and open the door to elbow injury and pain.

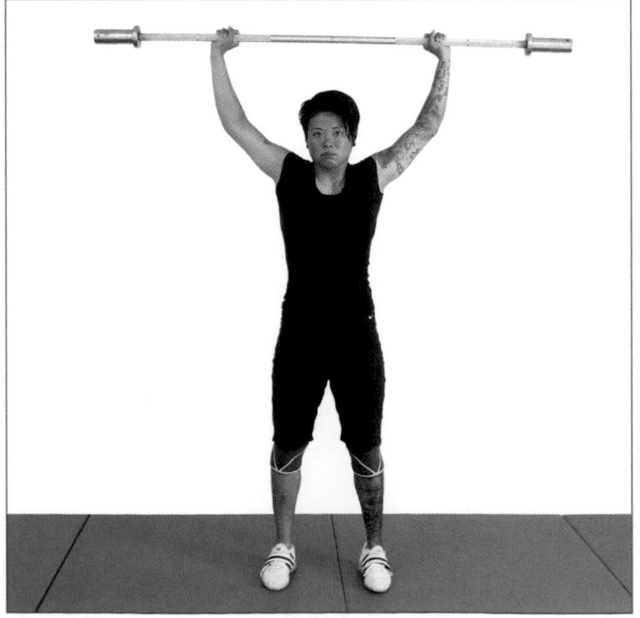

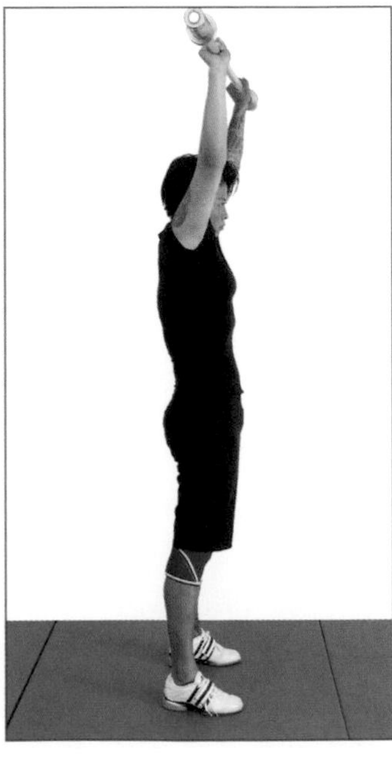

Grip Fault

Wrist pain is a commonly associated with the overhead squat. This is due to a faulty grip. As you can see in the photo below, when your hands are bent back, your fingers have to support the load, placing severe stress on your wrists. In most cases, athletes default to this grip position because they are missing shoulder range of motion. Unable to pull their shoulders into an ideal position as they press overhead, they throw their wrists back to balance the bar over the center of their body. In addition to inviting wrist pain, this broken-wrist grip makes it difficult to generate torque off the bar, compromising power and stability.

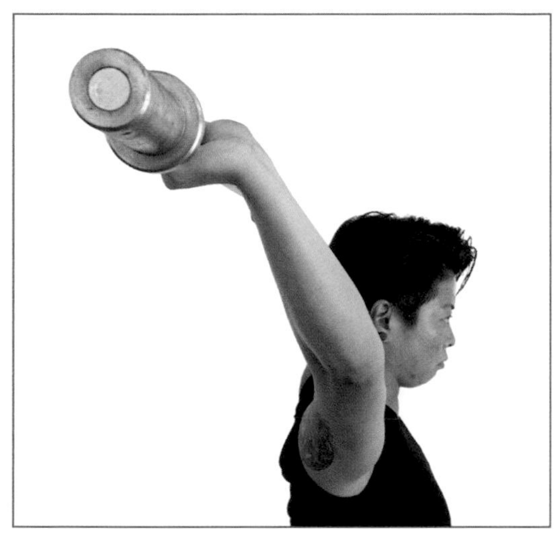

Overhead Archetype

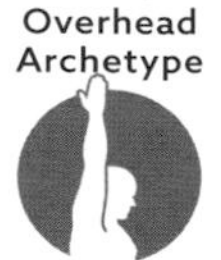

This fault is associated with the overhead archetype. For a mobility fix, visit the overhead archetype prescription in part 4.

MOTOR CONTROL FIX:

Position the bar in the center of your palms and keep your wrists in a neutral (straight) position.

Make sure that the bar is centered over your hips and shoulders.

MOBILIZATION TARGET AREAS:

Thoracic spine

Posterior shoulders and lats

Anterior shoulders and chest

First rib

Chest-Forward Fault

If your chest drifts forward—whether you're missing range of motion or you failed to set your shoulders in a good position—your shoulders will unlock so that you can maintain balance overhead. This is an untenable position. If you feel your shoulders go soft, stop the movement and reset your position. The farther you descend, the higher the likelihood of injury.

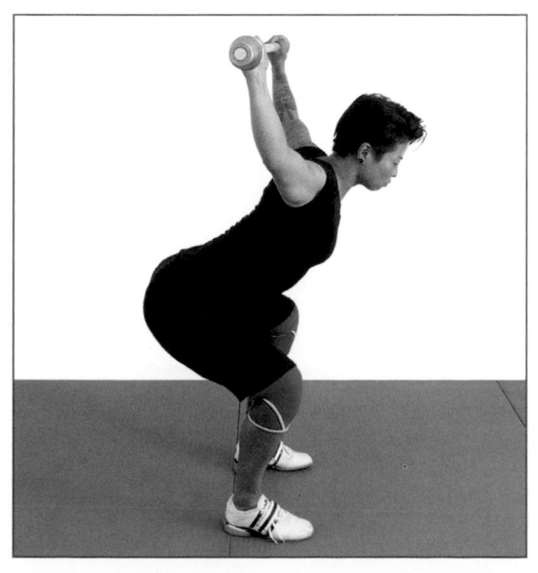

Squat 1 Archetype

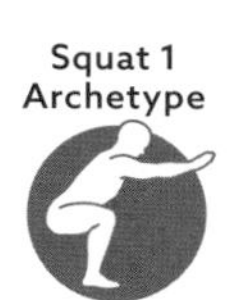

Overhead Archetype

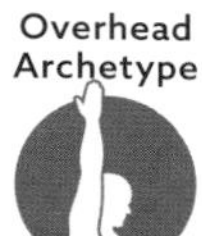

This fault is associated with the above archetypes. For a mobility fix, visit the corresponding archetype prescriptions in part 4.

MOTOR CONTROL FIX:

Create torque early and maintain that force through the full range of motion.

Stabilize your shoulders in a good position by locking out your arms, creating torque off the bar, and getting your armpits forward.

MOBILIZATION TARGET AREAS:

Anterior chain (hips and quads)

Posterior high chain (glutes)

Medial chain (adductors)

Posterior low chain (hamstrings)

Calves and heel cords

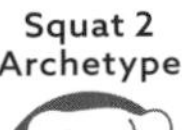

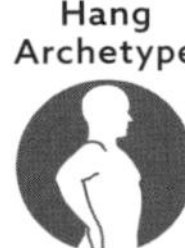

This movement contains the above archetypes. To improve common restrictions associated with this movement, visit the corresponding archetype prescriptions in part 4.

DEADLIFT

The deadlift is both common and crucial to the world of work: Think of a firefighter hoisting someone onto a stretcher, a soldier in the field bending over to grab an ammo box, or a construction worker picking up an electric saw.

Each time you bend over to pick something up off the ground, you're essentially executing a deadlift. Yet few people understand how to do it correctly. The fact that so many people round their back when they bend over to pick things up may explain why millions suffer from low back pain.

People who understand how to deadlift with good form—meaning that they know how to brace and create torque, and never sacrifice form for range of motion—typically have fewer back problems. They have a model for picking something up that is universally applicable: If you know how to set up for a deadlift, you know how to pick up something heavy off the ground without compromising your back.

Deadlift Range of Motion Test

STRAIGHT-LEG DEADLIFT TEST

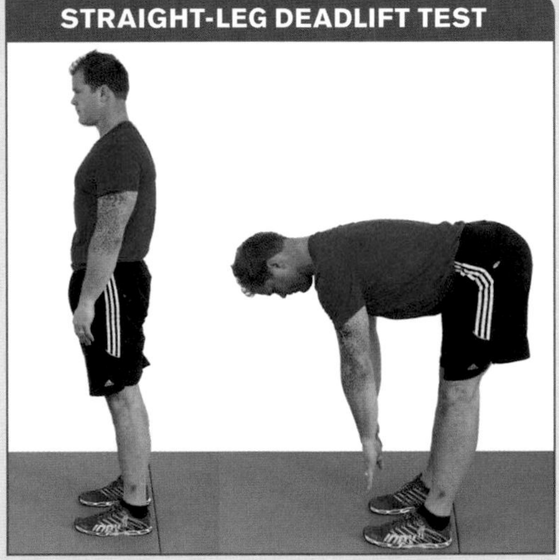

LONG SIT TEST

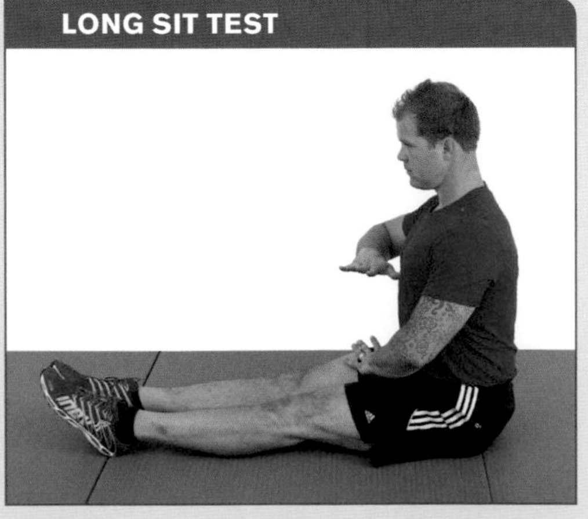

To get a read on your mobility in regard to good deadlifting technique, it's important to assess your posterior chain range of motion—specifically in your hips, hamstrings, and back.

One of the best ways to do so is to hinge forward at your hips with your back flat and legs straight. If you can touch the barbell (which would be slightly above ground level) without rounding your back or internally rotating your shoulders (essentially a straight-leg deadlift setup with your body forked at a 90-degree angle), you have full range of motion and are good to go. If you come up short, you may need to use the knees-forward setup on page 200.

Here's another way to assess posterior range of motion: To start, sit on the ground with your legs out in front of you. With your belly tight, you should be able to sit tall with your back and legs straight. If you bend your knees, round your back, or break from the upright-seated position, it's a dead giveaway that your posterior chain range of motion is wanting or you have a motor control issue.

This is not to be confused with the classic sit and reach test, where in gym class you sat with your feet flush against a box, clenched your teeth, and reached your hands as far past your toes as possible. Once you acknowledge the laws of bracing, this test becomes comical because it reveals nothing about functional range of motion or motor control. It does, however, tell you how good you are at rounding your back into a horrible, broken position.

The straight-leg deadlift is the preferred measuring tool. You don't do a lot of movements from a seated position unless you're a kayaker or rower. So adding a weight-bearing element—the torso—makes it more realistic.

To protect your back and maximize force production, you need to bring consciousness to this fundamental movement pattern so that you can maintain a good position in all situations. You need to optimize and ingrain the deadlift setup so that the movement outcome is the same every single time. Whether you're tired or stressed out or both, you have a blueprint that will enable you to produce maximum power with minimal risk.

The deadlift shares the same load order sequence and universal laws as the squat: Brace, create torque, load your hips and hamstrings, keep your shins as vertical as possible, and distribute your weight in the center of your feet. (For an overview of these principles, review the air squat section beginning on page 162.) These similarities make the deadlift an easy movement to learn. As with all category 1 movements, the deadlift serves as a diagnostic tool for assessing range of motion restrictions and motor control errors. (You can really see spinal errors and posterior chain restriction with this movement.) But before you start down that path, you need to learn how to optimize the setup.

Top-Down Setup

The top-down setup is the easiest and most effective model for lifting something off the ground. By organizing your spine in the top position, you minimize the load on your spine and optimize trunk stability prior to forming your grip on the bar, dumbbells, or other heavy object. Again, it's the same bracing sequence as the air squat. One of the mistakes people make is to bend over, establish their grip, and then try to organize their spine and put their hips in a good position. If you set up for the deadlift by rounding forward, you have to recapture a flat back from the bottom position, which is difficult. It's no different than trying to brace your spine in the bottom of the squat. While you can get your back flat, you likely will end up in a compromised position because you can't create tension in your upper back or stabilize your spine.

To execute the deadlift correctly, you have to take all the slack out of the system by creating as much tension as possible prior to lifting the weight off the ground. You need to actively seek tension. If you lose tension in the setup, specifically in your upper back, hips, or hamstrings, you have to adjust your knees to reload the area (see "Knees-Forward Setup" on page 200).

Bottom line: The more tension you create, the more force you can apply to the movement and the less likely you are to get injured. Set your shoulders in a stable position, load your hips and hamstrings, and then pull on the bar once you've formed your grip (see caption 7 on page 199). You almost want the bar to float before you initiate the lift. If you have 135 pounds on the bar, for example, you should be thinking about putting 130 pounds of tension into the bar. You should hear and feel the bar clink against the inner ring of the weight as you create tension. This is a sign that you're creating tension and that you're ready to initiate the movement by lifting the weight off the ground.

TOP-DOWN SETUP

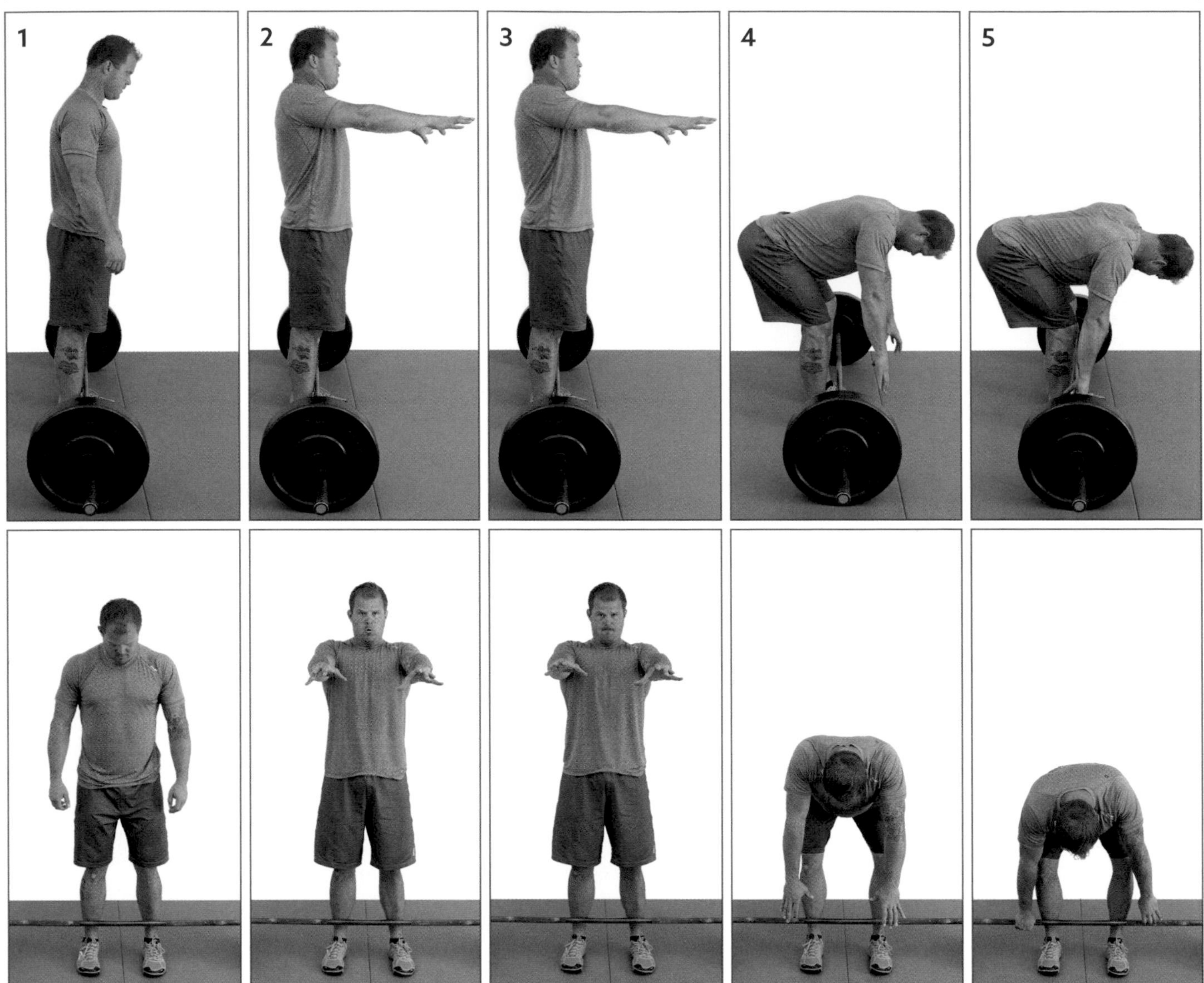

1. To establish a deadlift stance, walk your shins up to the bar and position your feet directly underneath your hips. The bar should bisect the center of your feet. Notice that my feet are pointed straight and positioned slightly narrower than my squat stance. This is a close iteration of my jumping or running stance.

2. Go through the same load order sequence as the air squat: Squeeze your butt to set your pelvis in a neutral position, screw your feet into the ground, raise your arms, pull your shoulders back while externally rotating your arms, and inhale.

3. After setting your shoulders in a stable position, pull your ribcage down over your pelvis, letting out air as you brace your midline.

4. Keeping your back flat, reach your hamstrings back and hinge forward at the hips until you can touch the bar or you reach end range. *Note:* If you can't reach the bar without compromising spinal position due to a lack of hip and hamstring mobility, use the knees-forward setup on page 200 instead.

5. Grip the bar with one hand at a time, forming your grip just outside your shins with your palms facing you. This allows you to form a hook grip on the bar (see page 201) while maintaining tension in your hips, hamstrings, and upper back. For most people, a thumb's distance from your leg is a good start. The key is to have enough room to press your knees out. Before you start your lift, get into position, shove your knees out as far as possible, and make sure that your arms are not in the way.

6. Form a hook grip with your other hand in the exact same fashion. *Note:* I prefer the double overhand (pronated) grip, as shown. It enables me to maximize torque and tension in my upper back. While the mix grip (see page 201) is certainly a viable option,

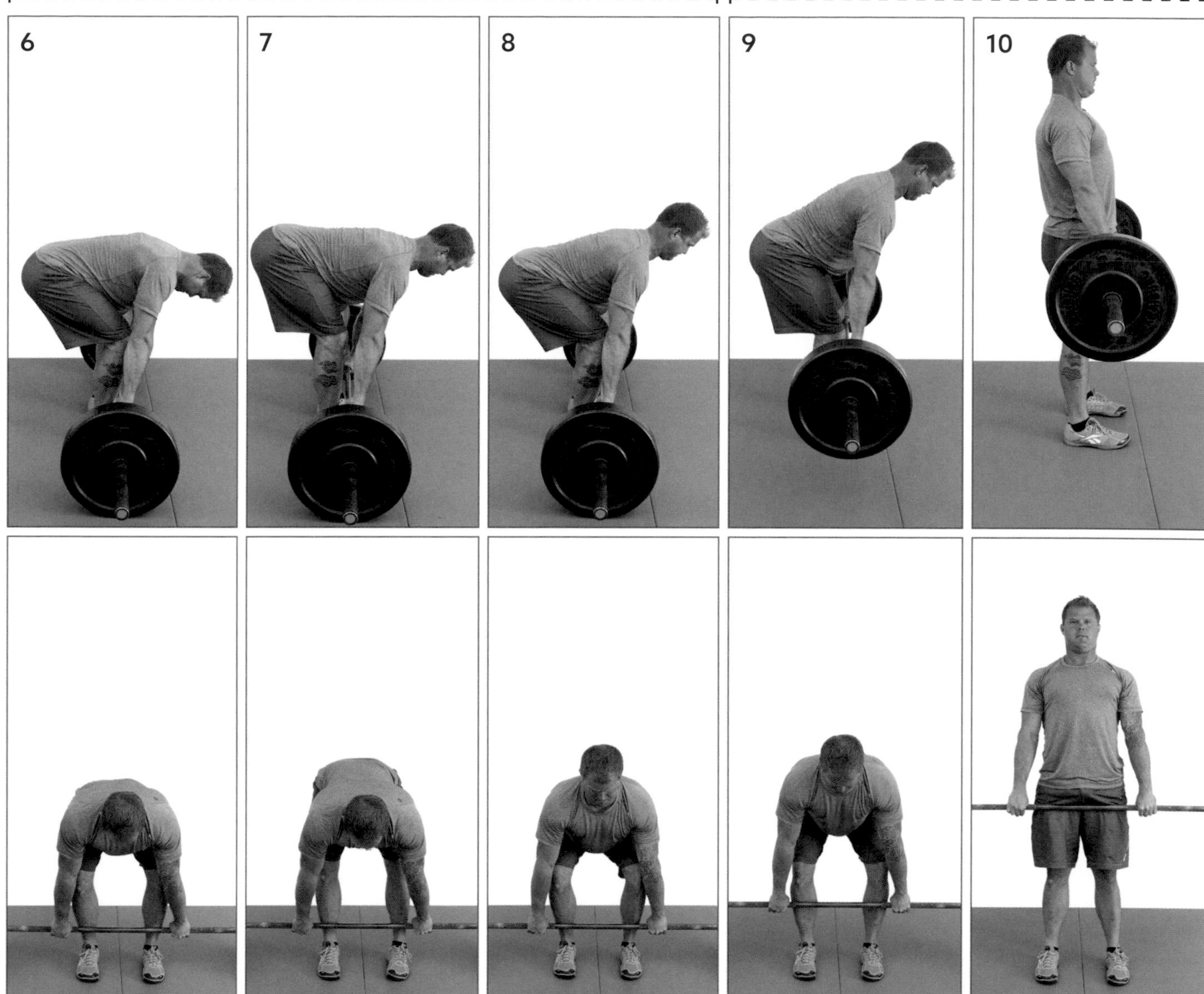

it does not allow you to create torque and stabilize your shoulders to the same degree.

7. As you form your grip, you'll probably notice that there isn't as much tension in the system—meaning that your back is not as tight and your hips and hamstrings are not loaded to the same degree. To reclaim tension, screw your hands into the bar and pull on the bar slightly as if you were trying to lift the weight off of the ground. As you do, raise your hips and pull your knees back, creating as much tension in your hips, hamstrings, and back as possible. Again, there should be no change in spinal position.

8. After reloading your hips, hamstrings, and back, lower your butt slightly while pulling on the bar, keeping your shins as vertical as possible. Imagine pulling yourself into position. Notice that the bar is positioned underneath my scapula. If your shoulders are too far over the bar, it's usually an indication that your shins are not vertical, and you will lose some capacity to generate force.

9. Still screwing your feet into the ground and your hands into the bar, lift the weight straight off the ground. As you start the pull, the position of your spine should remain unchanged.

10. Keeping the bar as close to your body as possible, stand up, squeezing your glutes as you extend your hips into the top position. Don't lean back or try to shrug your shoulders. To lower the bar to the ground, simply reverse the movement: Keep your back flat and head neutral, load your hips and hamstrings, and maintain as much tension in the system as possible.

Knees-Forward Setup

Some people can't quite reach the bar while keeping their hips loaded and shins vertical using the top-down setup. This is generally due to tight hamstrings and hips. If tightness is a problem for you, use this variation instead (or, simply lift from an elevated platform). You carry it out in the same fashion as the top-down setup, in that you stabilize your trunk in the top position and hinge forward from your hips while keeping your shins vertical. But the moment you run out of range of motion in your posterior chain—meaning that you can't hinge forward or push your hips back any farther without compromising your spinal position—bring your knees forward. This allows you to adjust for position while keeping your back flat and your hips and hamstrings loaded. After you establish your grip on the bar, pull your shins back to vertical to reclaim tension. It's the same model: Brace, load your hips and hamstrings, and use your knees to adjust your position.

Some people's ankles (missing dorsiflexion/knees-forward range), hamstrings, and hips are so tight that they can't set up from the ground without rounding their back, even when using this setup. In such a situation, scale the setup by setting the bar to a higher position using blocks, bumper weights, or a rack.

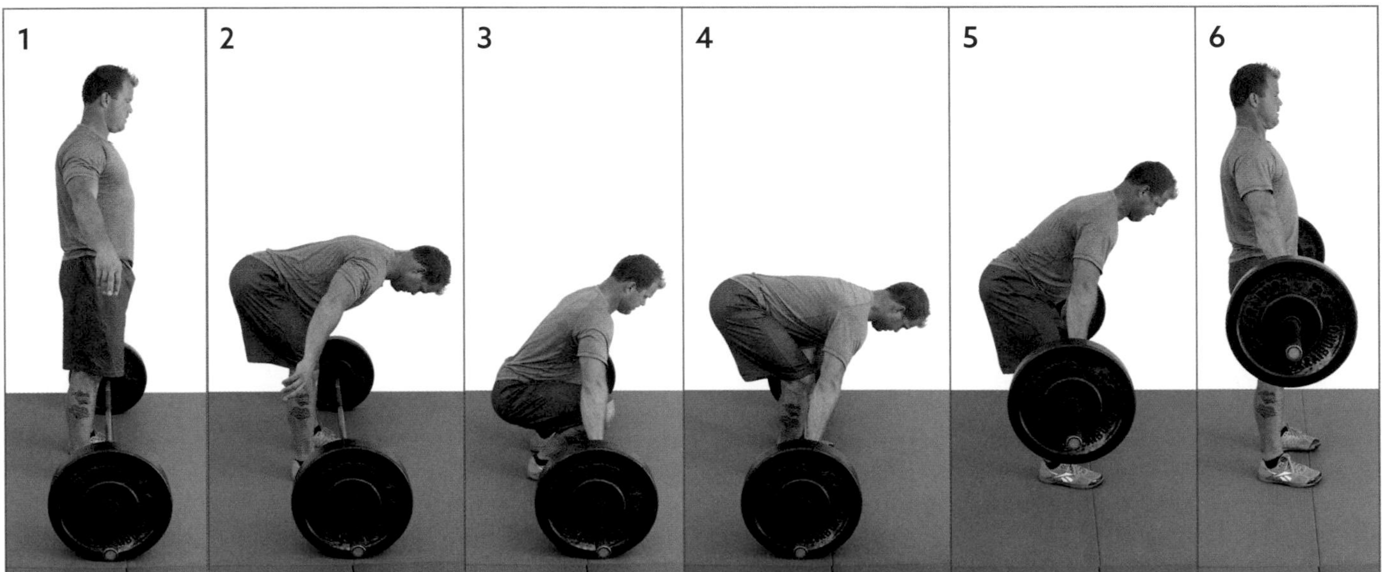

1. Establish your squat stance and stabilize your trunk—see caption 1 in the previous setup.

2. Hinge forward from your hips and drive your hamstrings back.

3. The moment you run out of hamstring and hip range of motion, bring your knees forward and establish your deadlift grip. The key is to keep your heels in contact with the ground and your spine rigid.

4. Reload your hips and hamstrings by pulling your knees and hamstrings back. Get your shins as vertical as possible.

5. Pull the weight off the ground by extending your hips and knees. There should be no change in spinal position.

6. Keeping the bar as close to your body as possible, stand up, squeezing your glutes as you extend your hips in the top position.

Hook Grip

The hook grip is a technique commonly taught to Olympic lifters. As you can see in the photos below, instead of clasping your thumb over your fingers as in a conventional grip, you wrap your thumb around the bar and then wrap your fingers around your thumb. This lock prevents the bar from rolling out of your hand and puts your wrist in a good position for creating external rotation torque. I like to teach this grip for the deadlift because it enables you to handle larger loads and transfers to other lifts, like the clean and snatch.

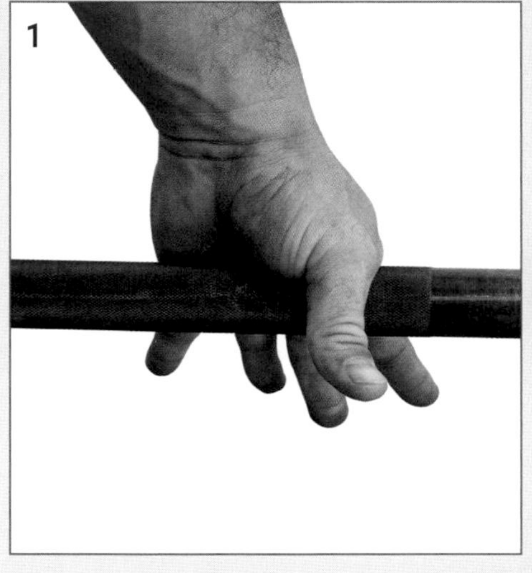

1

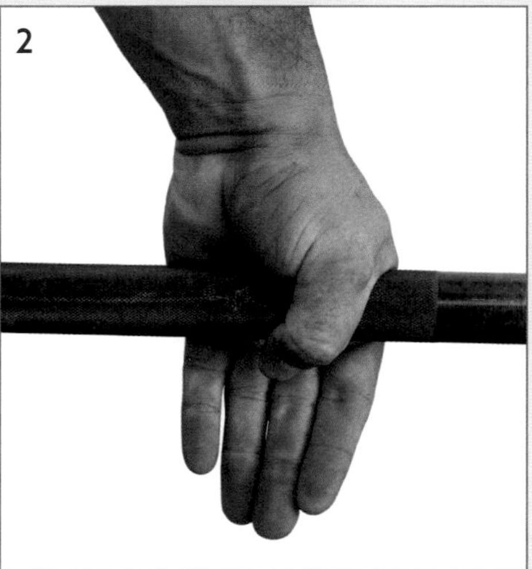

2

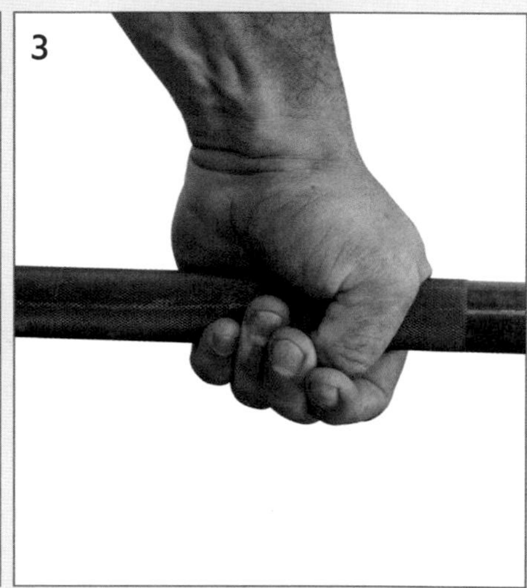

3

Mix Grip

As I mentioned, I generally prefer the double overhand grip because it enables you to maximize external rotation force and builds grip strength. It also transfers to other pull-based exercises (pull-up, clean, snatch, etc.). The mix grip—commonly referred to as the flip grip—doesn't allow for ideal shoulder positioning. As you can see in the photo at right, my left palm is facing forward and my right palm is facing back. The problem here is that I'll never be able to create the same amount of external rotation torque with my left hand as my right, leaving my left arm vulnerable to injury. Not only that, but it is a dead-end grip, meaning that it applies only to the deadlift and doesn't transfer to other movements.

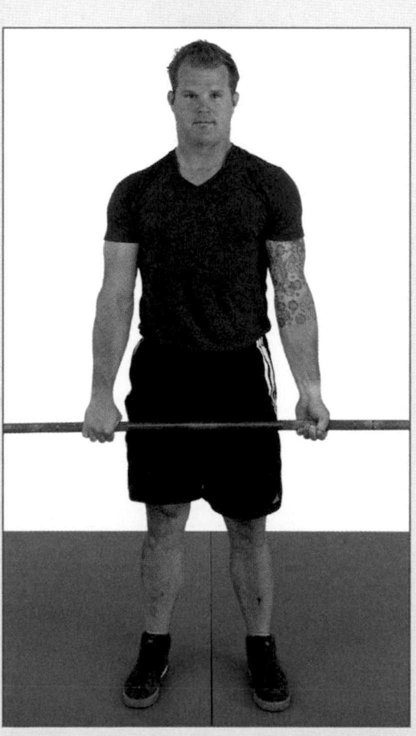

For some people, the mix grip is more comfortable and enables them to lift more weight, so it does have a place in your arsenal of techniques. But does that mean you should use it all the time? Not exactly. Here's what I generally recommend: Use the overhand hook grip until your grip starts to fail, which for most people is at around 90 percent of a one-rep max. Then implement the flip grip.

MOTOR CONTROL FIX:

Address the top-down setup and the knees-forward setup.

Bottom-Up Setup Fault

A lot of people set up for the deadlift by rounding forward, establishing their grip on the bar, and then trying to set their spine and hips in a good position. Don't get me wrong, I've seen people pick up enormous loads setting up in this manner, but they almost always round forward into a compromised position. Here's why: When you hinge forward from your hips without stabilizing your spine, you rely on the anterior musculature of your pelvis to pull your back into a flat position, shortening the fronts of your hips. You can pull your back into a neutral position, but you can't lock in or stabilize the position. If you're deadlifting heavy, you will usually round forward. If the weight is light, you might be able to maintain a flat back, but because your hips are in a shortened state, standing up into a neutral position is difficult. You will usually overextend to get your torso upright. To put it another way, the bottom-up setup loads your back instead of your hips and hamstrings. So if your low back hurts after you deadlift, there's a good chance that you're committing this fault.

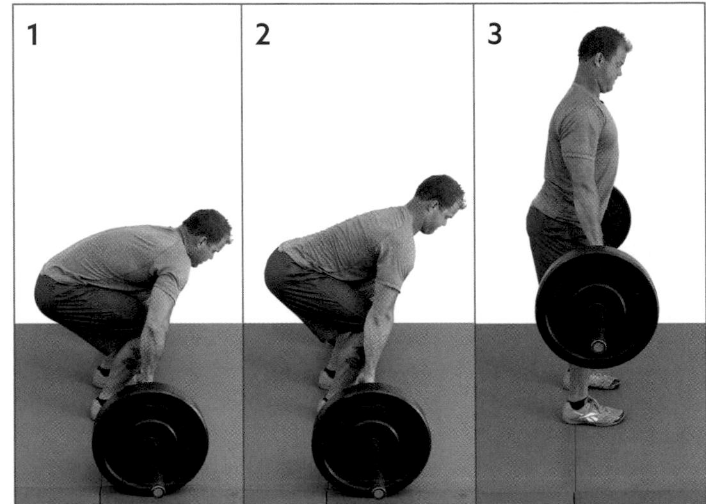

MOTOR CONTROL FIX:

After setting your grip, pull your knees back and raise your hips to load your posterior chain before initiating the pull.

Create sufficient external rotation torque in your shoulders by screwing your hands into the bar, and preload the bar by loading your hips and hamstrings.

Tension-Hunting Fault

Setting up from the bottom position predisposes you to a rounded back. However, this fault is not limited to the setup. Even if you set up from the top position, you will always default into a bad position if you fail to take all the slack out of the system. This is what I call tension hunting. If your hips, hamstrings, and back are not tight, your body will take up the slack, which is expressed by a rounded back. The key to avoiding this fault is to maximize the tension in your body by pulling on the bar. Remember, the deadlift is a slow movement. You never go from 0 to 60; rather, you go from 40 to 60.

Note: Failure to preload the bar will express itself with a definitive click, which is the bar hitting the bumper weight. Again, the weight should feel like it's floating before you lift it from the ground.

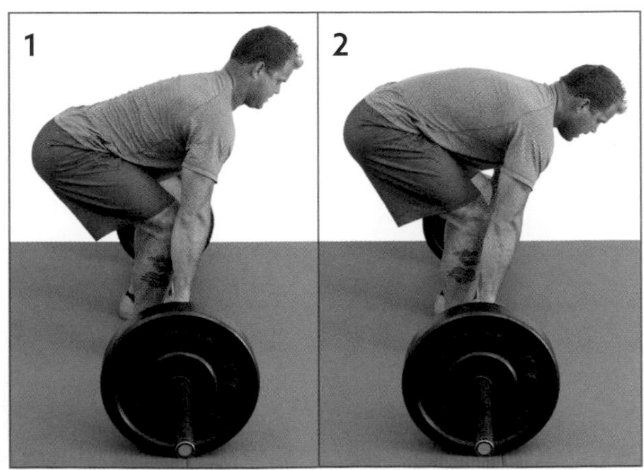

Powerlifters Rounding Their Backs

A lot of powerlifters pull with a rounded upper back—while keeping their low back flat—because it shortens the distance they have to pull the weight to the lockout position of the hips. This is where people often get confused. The upper back is in fixed flexion, meaning that the powerlifters round forward and then create tension and torque in that position.

What you have to remember is that rounding the upper back is a conscious decision that professional powerlifters make. And they understand the consequences. A classic case is Donny Thompson, a professional powerlifter and world record holder. He was practicing deficit deadlifts with a rounded back and suffered a disc injury. His reaction was: "I knew better. I was pulling with a rounded back and it got me." At no point will a professional powerlifter ever round his low back when performing a deadlift. It would be like a bomb going off. However, to get a slight edge, a powerlifter will sometimes sacrifice the safety of his position if it means being able to lift more weight.

That said, a beginner or fitness lifter should never round her upper back as a means of lifting more weight. Why? Because it increases susceptibility to injury, ingrains a dysfunctional movement pattern into daily life, and does not translate to other athletic movements, like dynamic pulling and jumping.

I like Jesse Burdick's rule for pulling heavy with a rounded upper back. When you can deadlift 600 pounds, then you can start to entertain thoughts of rounding your thoracic spine. In fact, many of the best Olympic lifting coaches in the world, like Mike Burgener and Glenn Pendlay, won't let their athletes pull heavy deadlift singles because they don't want to ingrain a pulling pattern with an upper back and shoulder position that won't translate to Olympic-style weightlifting.

Tension Fault

A properly executed deadlift is expressed as a single movement, meaning that everything goes up at the same time (hips and knees extend simultaneously). If, when you start to lift the weight off the floor, your hips come up first and your torso follows, it's an indication that you didn't take up all the slack in the system. You are tension hunting. Although you can still maintain a flat back, which is great, you compromise your ability to generate maximum force.

MOTOR CONTROL FIX:

Before lifting the weight off the ground, raise your butt and bring your knees back. This loads tension into your posterior chain. With your hips and hamstrings fully engaged, lower your hips and shove your knees out, pulling on the bar as you lower into position.

1

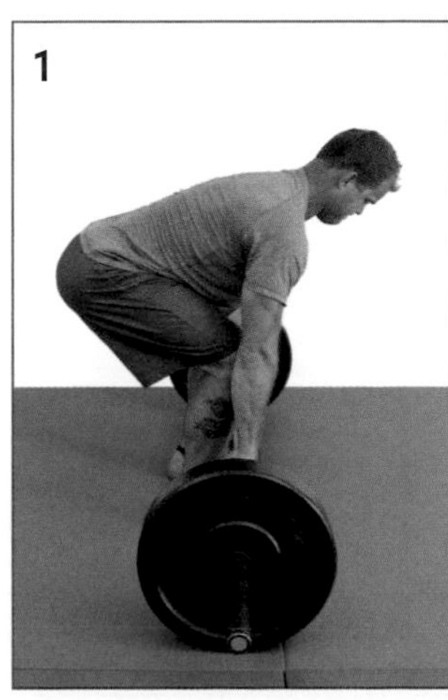

2

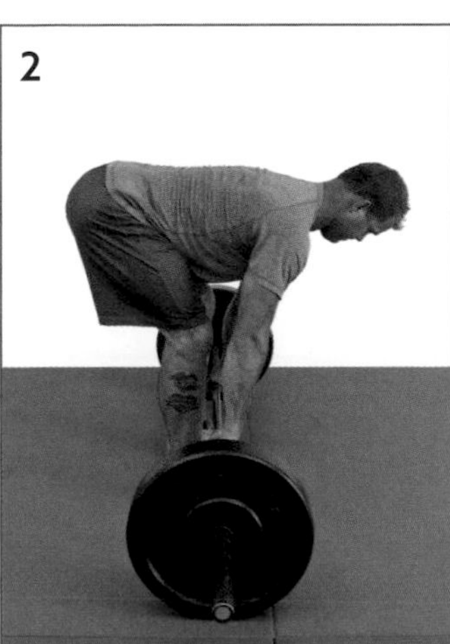

3

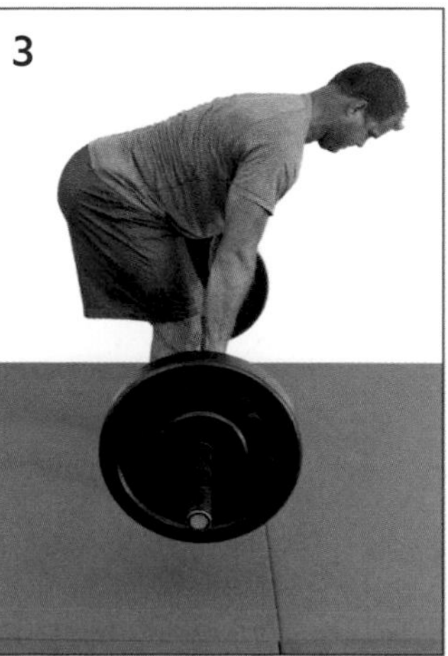

Press Archetype Front Rack 1 Archetype

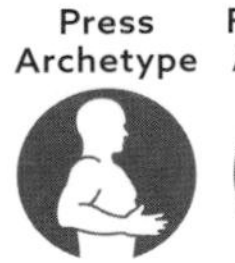
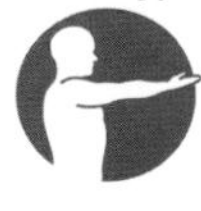

This movement contains the above archetypes. To improve common restrictions associated with this movement, visit the corresponding archetype prescriptions in part 4.

PUSHUP

Most upper-body movements that are conducive to sport and life are performed at midrange and out in front of your body: feeding, grabbing, carrying, pushing, and pulling, to name a few. To operate effectively within this domain, you need a model that teaches you how to create a stable shoulder position.

Enter the pushup.

As with the air squat, you can use the pushup to start layering the principles of bracing and torque. The pushup also serves as a diagnostic tool for assessing motor control and range of motion. But instead of illuminating what's happening at your hips, the pushup tells you what's going on at your shoulders, elbows, and wrists. You go through the same checklist: Do you understand how to brace your spine in a neutral position? Or create external rotational torque by screwing your hands into the ground (setting your shoulders in a good position)? Do you have the range of motion and motor control to keep your hands straight and your elbows close to your body as you perform the movement? Without having to use any equipment, you can see how well you understand the fundamental principles of bracing and torque, as well as identify restrictions in your mobility.

In addition, the pushup serves as a launch pad to more complex pressing motions—the bench press, dip, and overhead press—and to more complex motor patterns. If you understand these basic concepts and can apply them to the pushup, you are less likely to default into bad positions when you're training with more complicated movements.

It's no wonder so many athletes suffer from torn rotator cuffs and dislocated shoulder injuries and experience anterior shoulder pain every time they press. They don't understand the principles that govern good positions as they relate to the shoulders, elbows, and wrists. The pushup teaches and ingrains those fundamental movement patterns and gives athletes and coaches a template for solving problems at the shoulders, elbows, and wrists.

Athletes, coaches, and physical therapists often relate shoulder issues to a weak rotator cuff or weak shoulders. Although this is a contributing factor, it's not necessarily the root cause. It's about position: If you don't have a model for creating a stable position, it's difficult to generate spontaneous torque and force. Once you understand how to perform a pushup correctly, it doesn't matter where your hands are or what you are grabbing, pushing, or pulling. Nor does the orientation of your arms matter. You can still create a stable and mechanically powerful position.

Note: The pushup shares a lot of the same principles with the squat and the deadlift, but instead of loading your hips and hamstrings, keeping your shins as vertical as possible, and distributing your weight over the center of your feet, you load your pecs and triceps, keep your forearms as vertical as possible, and distribute your weight over the center of your hands (in front of your wrists). The concept of stance is also transferable. As with your squat and deadlift stance, you should find a comfortable position that transfers to other pressing motions. Positioning your hands shoulder width apart is a good start. The goal is to establish a position that allows you to perform the movement with good technique. Once you're proficient, start switching up the width of your hands from time to time to create a new stimulus.

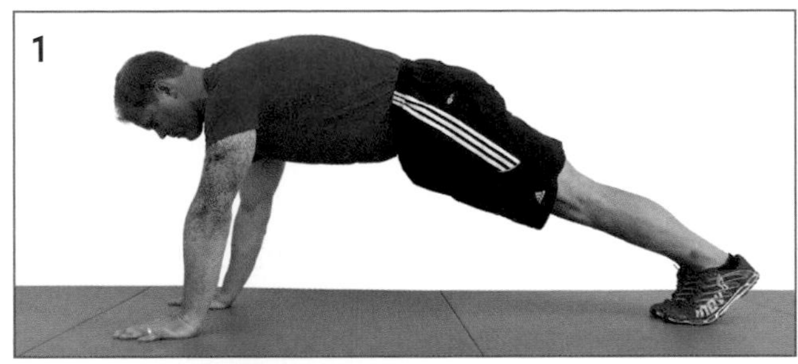

To set up for the pushup, kneel down and situate your hands at about shoulder width with your fingers pointing straight ahead. Then sprawl your legs back, position your feet together, and squeeze your glutes. *Note:* Keeping your legs together maximizes glute activation and tension in your trunk. Notice that I start with my hands out in front of my body. Keeping your weight slightly back takes load off your shoulders, making it easier to screw your hands into the floor and create an external rotation force.

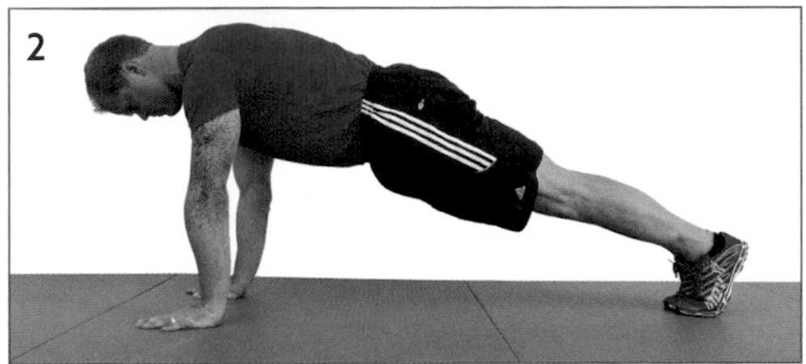

Still actively screwing your hands into the floor, lever forward, positioning your shoulders over your hands. To maximize torque, think about getting the pits of your elbows forward.

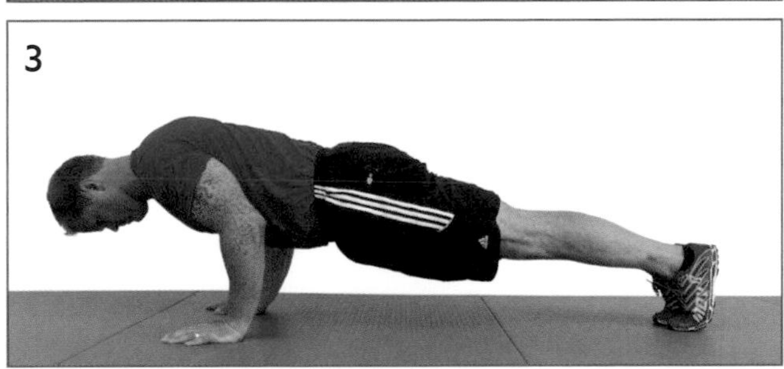

Keeping your weight centered over the center of your hands (just in front of your wrists) and your forearms vertical (elbows in line with your wrists), start lowering into the bottom position. This is the equivalent of keeping your shins vertical in the squat in that it maximizes force production and protects your elbows. Remember, you load your triceps and pecs for the same reason you load your hamstrings and glutes in the squat. Your pecs help stabilize your shoulders in a good position so that your triceps can do their job, which is to extend your elbows.

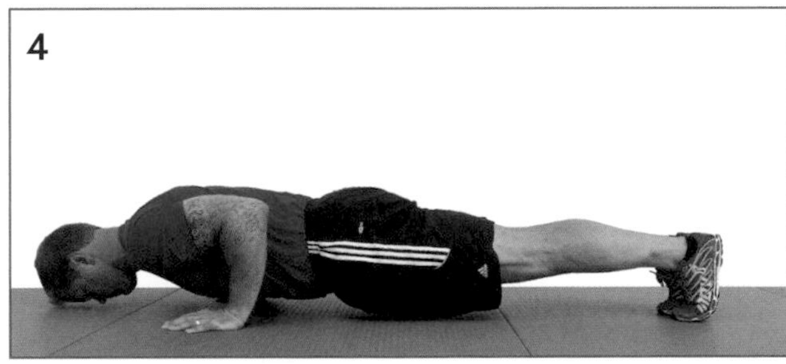

Lower into the bottom position. Keep your butt squeezed, belly tight, and forearms as vertical as possible.

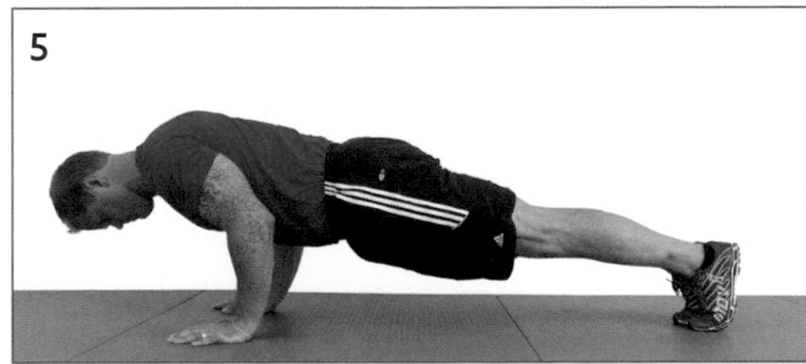

As you press out of the bottom position, there should be no change in your spinal or shoulder position. Your back should be flat and your shoulders pulled back.

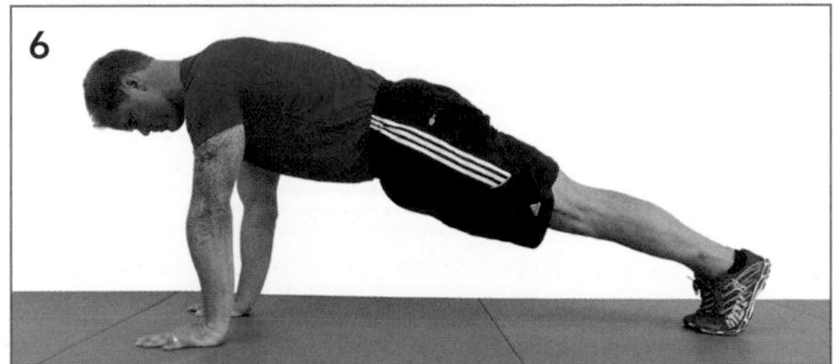

Still screwing your hands into the ground, extend your arms and reestablish the top position.

Elbows-Out Fault

Press Archetype

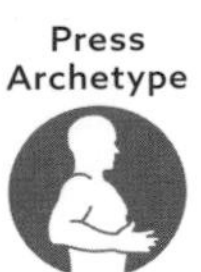

This fault is associated with the press archetype. For a mobility fix, visit the press archetype prescription in part 4.

MOTOR CONTROL FIX:

Address the setup in the top position: squeeze your butt, screw your hands into the ground (elbow pits forward), and keep your forearms vertical as you descend and rise out of the bottom position.

MOBILIZATION TARGET AREAS:

Anterior shoulders and lats

Posterior shoulders and chest

Downstream arms (elbows and wrists)

The majority of people can set up for the pushup in a good position, meaning that they can create torque and get their back flat. But as in the squat, the moment they start lowering into the bottom position, errors become easy to spot. For example, a lot of athletes flare their elbows out and compensate with a shoulders-forward position as they lower their chest to the ground. When I see this happen—whether in the first few inches or in the bottom position—the first thing that comes to mind is a lack of internal or external rotation at the shoulders. While a poor setup and weak triceps can contribute to this fault, it's almost always a shoulder range of motion issue.

As you can see in the photos below, once my elbows fly out to the sides, my shoulders get loaded in a bad position. This is why people experience wrist, elbow, and anterior shoulder pain. Whether they are bench pressing a heavy load, stabilizing a weight overhead as with the overhead squat, or performing bodyweight movements like pushups or dips, they have no choice but to adopt an elbows-out, shoulders-forward position to execute the movement. It's no surprise that people feel burning pain in the fronts of their shoulders when they press. They are missing 100 percent of their internal rotation range of motion.

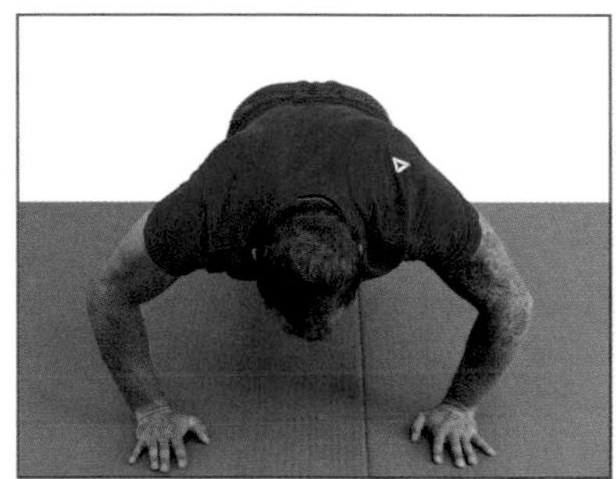

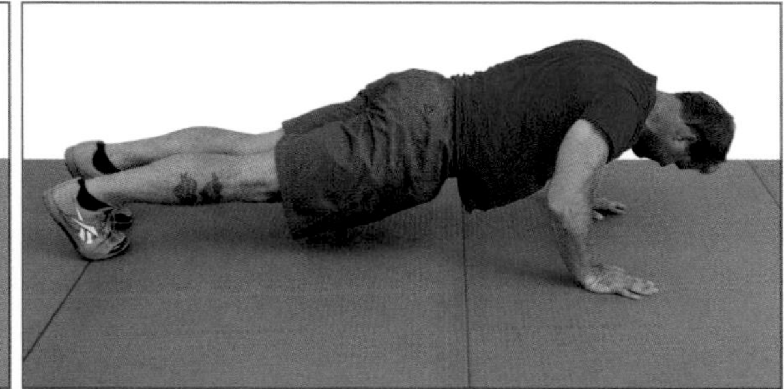

Open-Hand Fault

Press Archetype

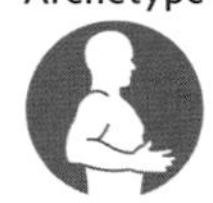

This fault is associated with the press archetype. For a mobility fix, visit the press archetype prescription in part 4.

MOTOR CONTROL FIX:

Focus on the top position of the pushup. Position your hands straight—with your right hand between 12 and 1 o'clock and your left hand between 12 and 11 o'clock.

Screw your hands into the ground, creating an external rotation force, and try to get the pits of your elbows forward.

As I explained in chapter 3 on torque and in the squatting techniques, an athlete who is missing ankle or hip range of motion will generally turn his feet out to increase his range of motion. The same thing happens in the pushup. If an athlete is missing internal or external rotation in his shoulders or flexion in his wrists, he will usually compensate into an open-hands forward-shoulders position. As with the open-foot fault, the open-hand fault causes a landslide of mechanical problems up and down the chain and opens the door to a lot of injuries and pain.

MOBILIZATION TARGET AREAS:

Anterior shoulders and lats

Posterior shoulders and chest

Downstream arms (elbows and wrists)

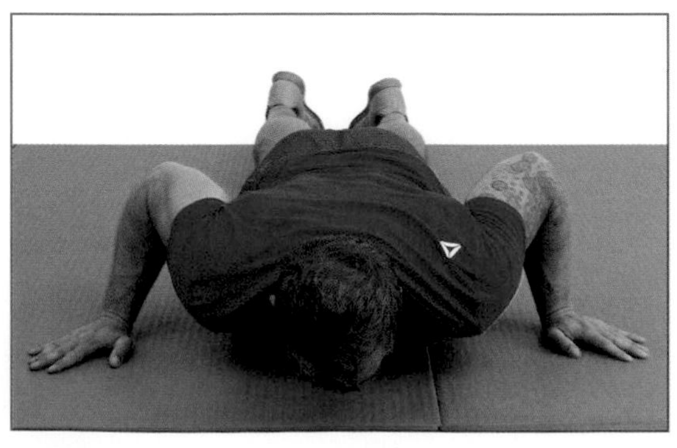

Scaling the Pushup

If you aren't strong enough to perform a full-range pushup with good form, you can do one of two things: place your hands on a higher surface (such as a chair, box, or wall) or make the movement easier by using Mark Bell's Sling Shot. If you don't have access to a Sling Shot (and you should), you can loop a Rogue Monster band around your elbows. Both tools lower the demand, making the movement easier while still allowing you to adopt a neutral spinal position. What's particularly great about the Sling Shot, however, is that it prevents your elbows from flaring out to the sides and supports your weight in the bottom position. So in addition to removing some of the load, it encourages good mechanics. This is the equivalent of doing a pull-up with a Rogue Monster band hooked around your feet. You can mimic the movement without compromising form.

A lot of people mistakenly scale the pushup by dropping their knees to the ground. While this modification reduces the load and makes the pushup easier, it compromises your ability to squeeze your butt and create tension in your trunk. Doing a pushup from your knees encourages poor mechanics. In order to create a rigid, flat back, you need to set your pelvis in a neutral position by keeping your butt squeezed. If you perform a pushup from your knees, it's impossible to accomplish this task.

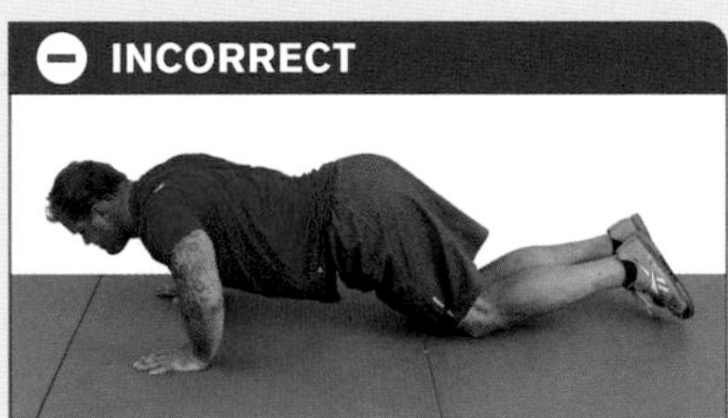

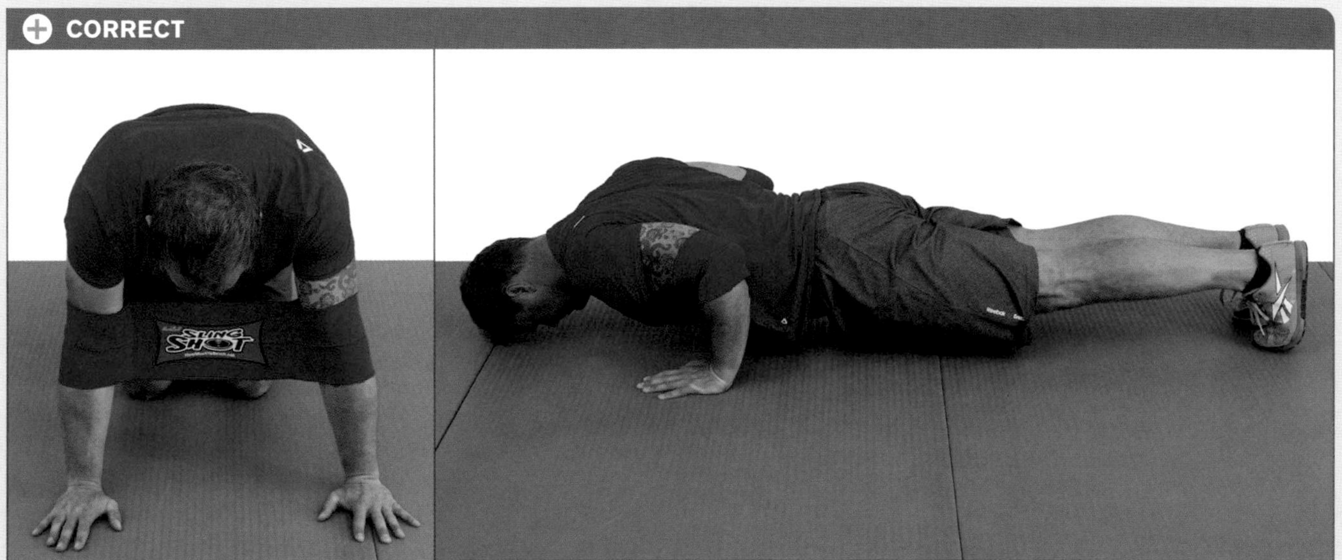

Ring Pushup

Adding rings to an exercise is like injecting the movement with truth serum. Many people can perform a pushup in a low-torque environment and get away with it. When it comes to the rings, though, forget it. The moment you climb on the rings, you have no choice but to generate torque. You have to screw your hands into the rings and keep your elbows over your wrists. This is why athletes sometimes experience pain in the fronts of their shoulders when performing pushups and bench presses, but don't feel pain when doing ring pushups. The instability of the rings makes it difficult to move with bad mechanics. You need to provide the stability.

Also, the rings will show you the light in terms of the position of your hands and the path of your arms—a position and path that should be applied to the pushup and bench press.

The ring pushup offers at least two benefits: It challenges you with increased stabilization demands while also ingraining proper pressing mechanics. Here's why: When you perform pushups on the rings, your hands automatically orient themselves underneath your shoulders. You turn your hands out to create an external rotation force and your forearms remain vertical, allowing your elbows to stay tight to your body. In other words, you instinctively create a more stable trunk and adopt an externally rotated shoulder position because it's the easiest way to stay balanced over the rings. If your hands rotate internally or your elbows deviate back or drift out to the sides, your arms will start to shake, making it impossible to stabilize the position.

Note: Don't feel like the ring pushup is just for advanced athletes. Novices can benefit from learning how to stabilize in the top position.

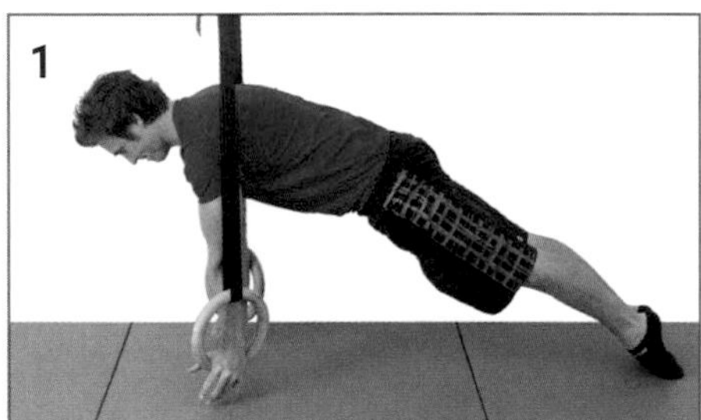

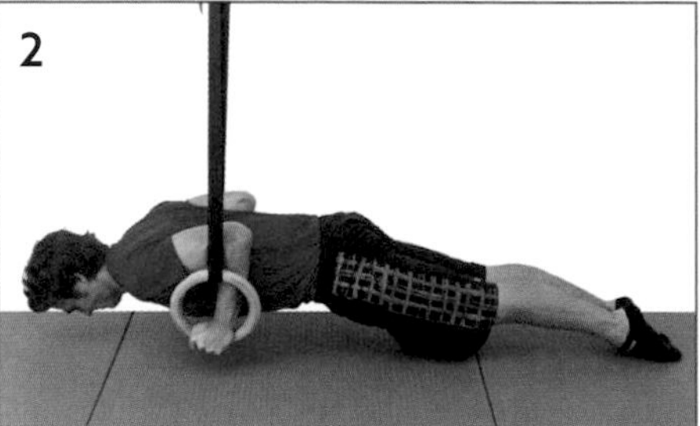

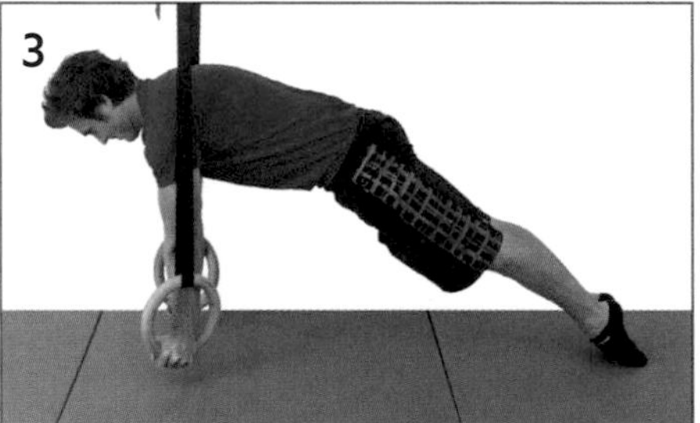

1. Position the rings so they hang at roughly shoulder width. Kneel on the ground, form your grip, and then walk your legs back. Notice that Carl's feet are together and he's balancing on the fronts of his toes (not the balls of his feet). Remember, the ring pushup requires more trunk control than the classic pushup. Balancing on the fronts of your toes maximizes glute activation, which helps you create and maintain a stable trunk. To create stable shoulders, externally rotate your hands so your thumbs are pointing away from your body. Your left hand should be at about 11 o'clock and your right hand at about 1 o'clock.

2. Keeping your butt squeezed, belly tight, and hands turned out, lower into the bottom position. Your wrists should be in line with your elbows (forearms vertical), and your elbows should be tight to your body. Even if you're missing shoulder range of motion, the rings force your arms into an ideal position. However, if you're missing internal rotation in your shoulders, your hands will start to rotate inward. Fight this force and try to reclaim a thumbs-out position as you rise out of the bottom position.

3. Still turning your hands out and keeping your back flat, press out of the bottom position and reestablish the top position.

BENCH PRESS

Press Archetype Front Rack 1 Archetype

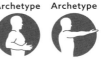

This movement contains the above archetypes. To improve common restrictions associated with this movement, visit the corresponding archetype prescriptions in part 4.

Here's the problem with the bench press: Athletes and coaches generally put more stock in how much weight was lifted than in how well the movement was performed. It begins with a 300-pound bench press club at the high school gym and the status associated with earning a club T-shirt. The question "How much do ya bench?" is the de facto joke within the free weight gym culture. While you should know the answer, the question you should be obsessed with if you're hell-bent on pursuing hot, nasty, high-level athletic performance is this: How good is your bench press form?

Very few athletes understand the variables involved in a proper bench press. It seems so simple: You lie down on the bench, take the bar out of the rack, guide it down to your chest, and then extend your elbows. What's the big deal? But, like the squat or the deadlift, you have to account for a lot of variables. Setting your shoulders in a good position, bracing while lying on your back, and maintaining an ideal bar path takes a lot of practice and technical ability.

A good bench press comes down to using good movement practices. For instance, you should know how to set your shoulders in a stable position and create torque off the bar. You should know how to brace in a globally arched position. Your wrists need to be in line with your elbows. If one of these steps isn't carried out correctly or you are missing key ranges of motion, you will see horrific movement errors: elbows flying out, shoulders rolling forward, head bobbling into crazy positions, and back overextending. Because people can bench press insanely large loads without paying any attention to technique, this movement is probably responsible for more shoulder injuries than any other exercise movement in history.

Teaching people how to bench with good form can save millions of shoulders. The bench press doesn't just teach you how to press through midrange; it also gives you a blueprint for creating torque with your shoulders retracted to the backs of their sockets. The bench press is also a diagnostic tool: You can disguise movement and mobility dysfunction in low-torque environments like the pushup, but you can't hide them once the torque demands are increased with load.

Note: As with the squat and strict press, taking the bar out of the rack is a skill in and of itself. To ensure a successful and safe lift-out, you need to do several things: arch your back, retract your shoulders, create torque off the bar, screw your feet into the ground, take a breath, and get your belly tight. Performing these tasks correctly is predicated on a good bench press setup. If something goes wrong in the lift-out phase, it's difficult to complete the movement with good form. To improve your understanding, I've broken down the setup into categories.

Grip

The best way to figure out your grip distance is to establish the pushup position on the rings with your hands turned out. For most athletes, this is just outside shoulder width, which is much narrower than people typically prefer. The fact is, you need a grip that enables you to keep your shoulder blades pulled back, generate sufficient torque off the bar, keep your elbows in a 30- to 45-degree plane from your body, and maintain vertical forearms. You also want to keep the bar positioned in the center of your palms, aligned with your wrists. While this may seem intuitive, I've seen people adopt some crazy grips, like centering the bar across their fingers. Not only is this grip dangerous—imagine a barbell rolling off your hands onto your neck or face—but it also causes a lot of wrist and thumb pain.

CORRECT GRIP

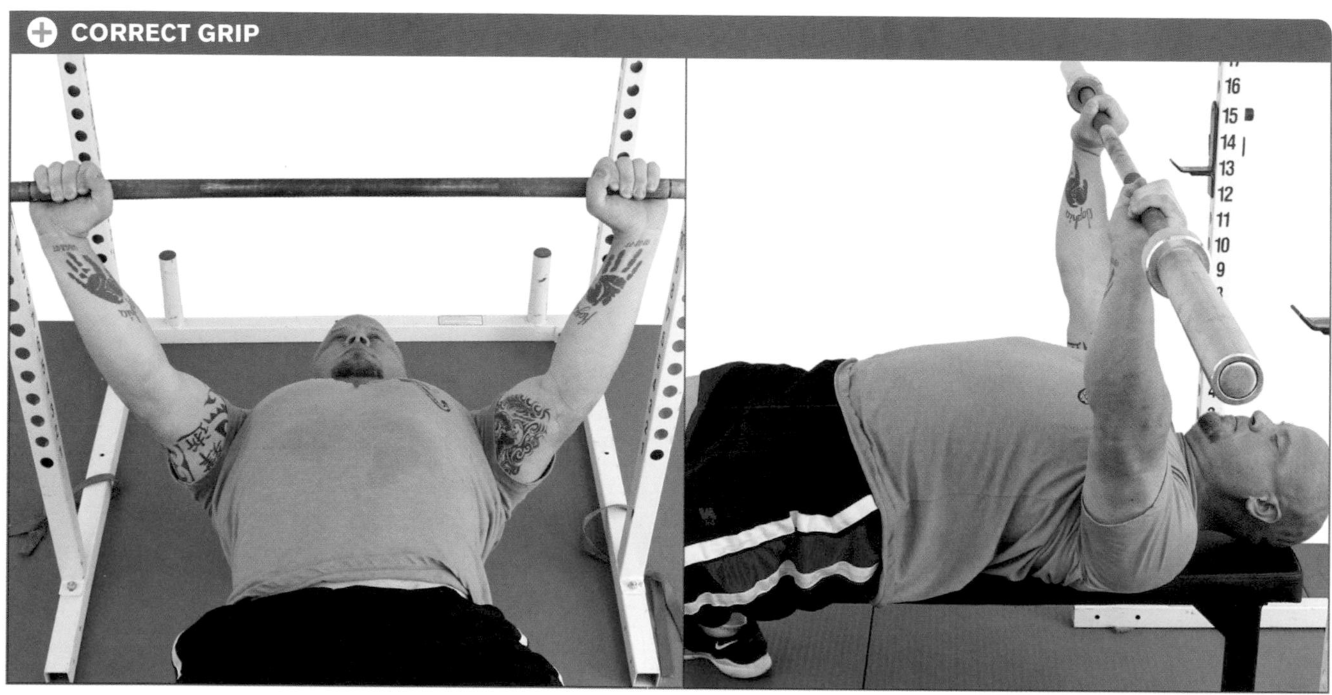

INCORRECT GRIPS

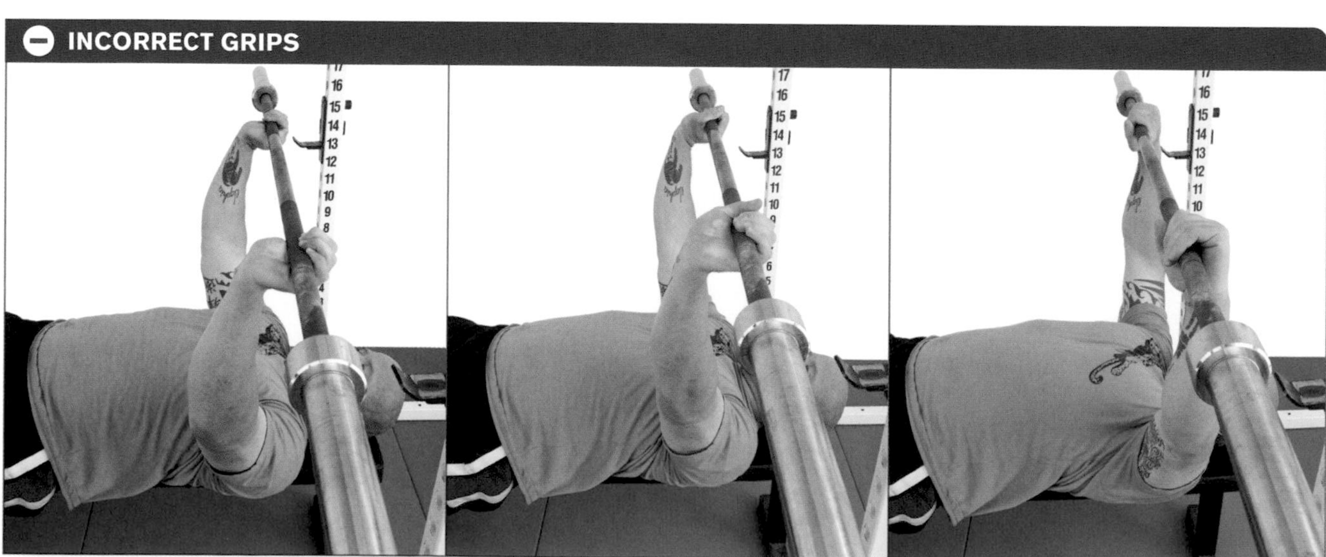

Stance

Just as poorly organized shoulders compromise the efficiency of the squat, poorly organized hips affect your ability to bench press. To maintain a rigid trunk, you need a stance that enables you to create sufficient torque. It should look a lot like your squat stance. All the same rules apply: Keep your shins vertical, screw your feet into the ground, drive your knees out, and distribute your weight over the center of your feet. People adopt untenable stances that make it impossible to create torque or get into a braced position.

CORRECT STANCE

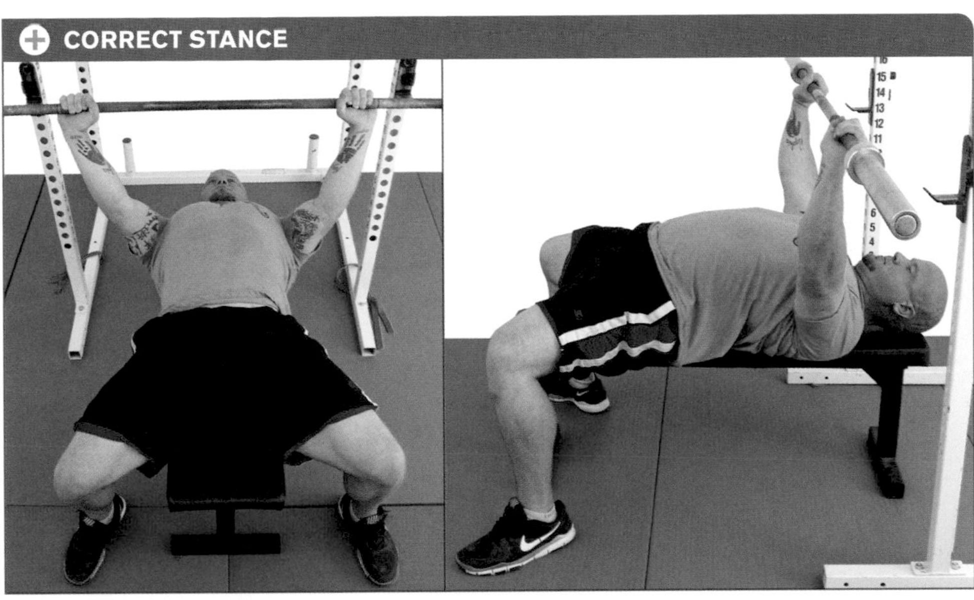

INCORRECT STANCES

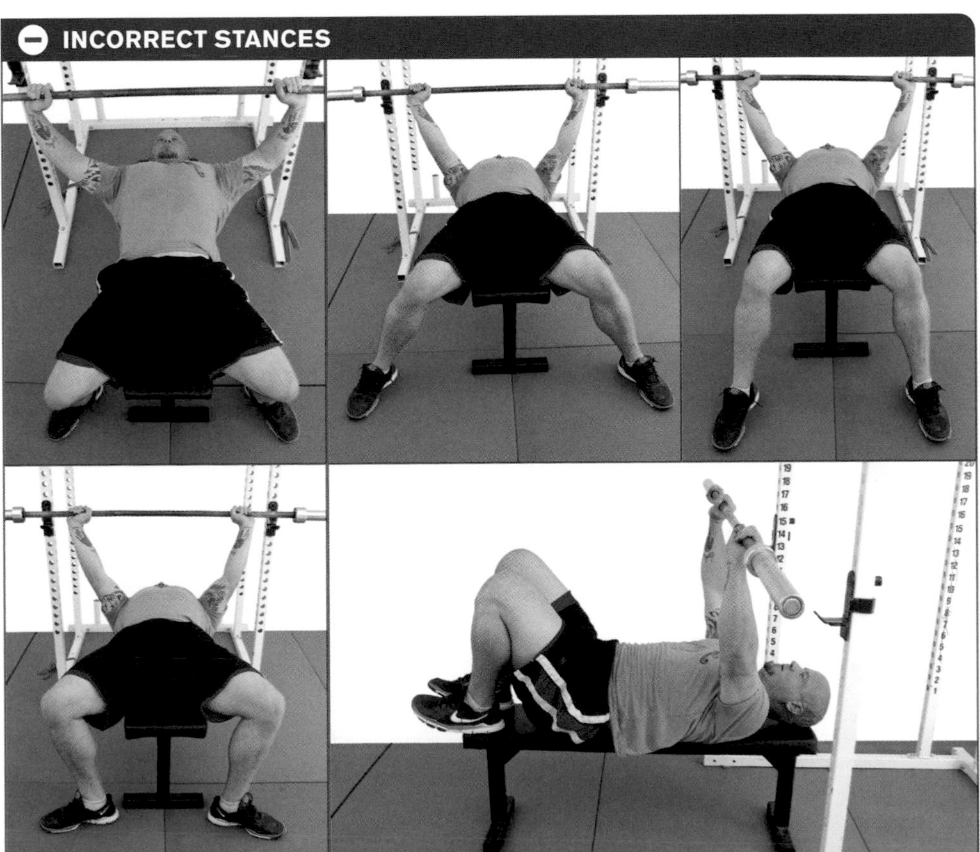

Braced Extension

To perform the bench press correctly, you need to create an arch and keep your shoulders pulled back. However, this does not mean that you're overextended. The key is to arch back to set your shoulders, brace your abs, and then lower your hips to the bench. If you drop your ribcage or keep your back flat to the bench, it's difficult to keep your shoulder blades retracted. This position is not easy and takes time to master. Having a tight thoracic spine can also make it tough to create a good arch.

CORRECT

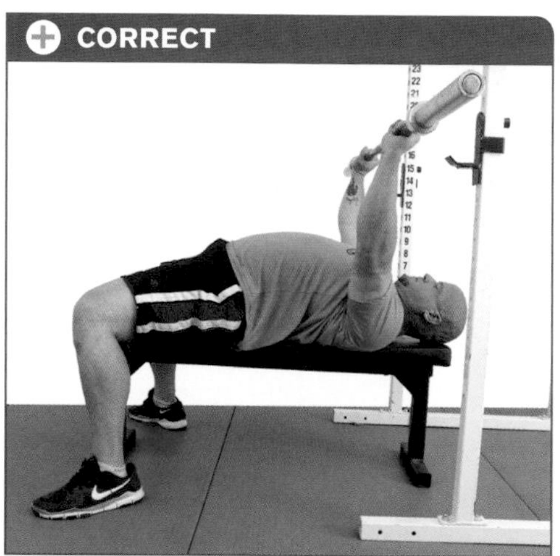

INCORRECT

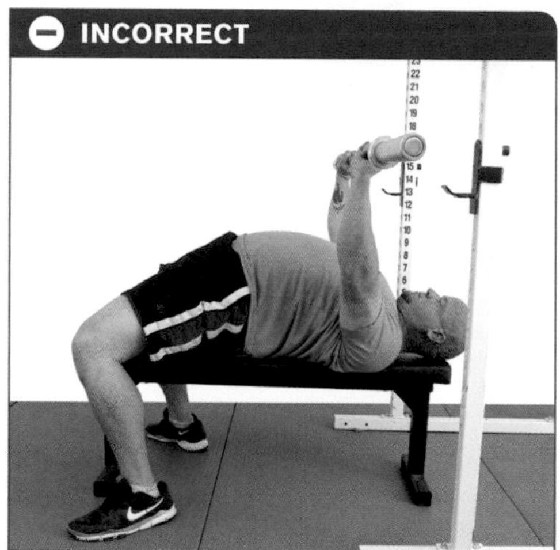

Height of the Rack

Although it seems ridiculous to tell you that it's important to set the rack to the right level, I'll say it anyway: Set the rack to a height that allows for a slight bend in your arms. For an ideal lift-out, you should be able to extend your arms and press the weight out of the rack while keeping your shoulder blades pulled back. If the rack is too high, you will have to protract your shoulders, which is a huge setup error.

Bench Press Sequence

1

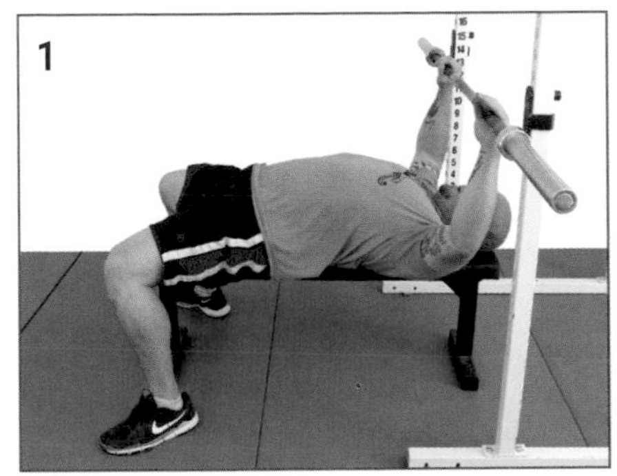

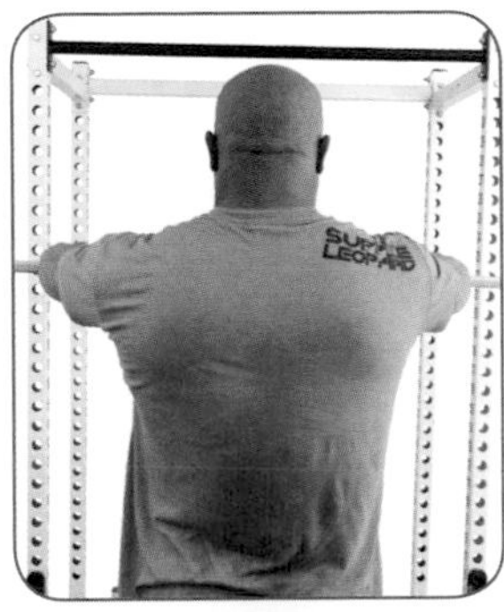

To set up for the bench press, lie underneath the bar so that it bisects your collarbone or neck and assume your stance.

2

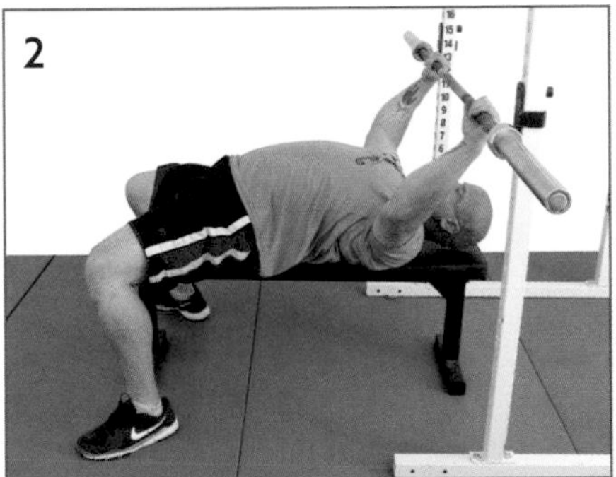

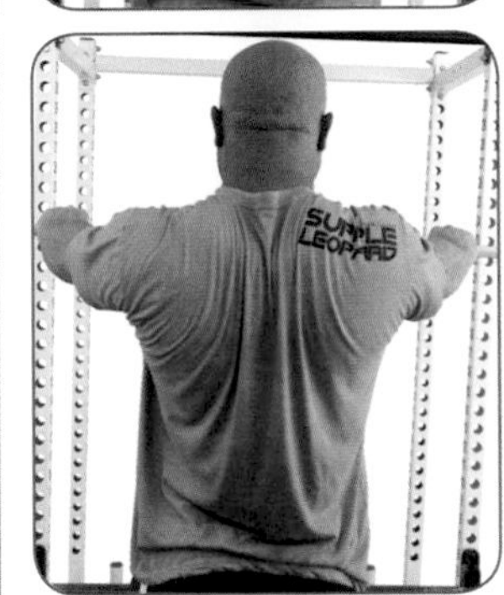

Before lifting the weight out of the rack, pull your shoulder blades back and create torque off the bar. Imagine trying to break or bend the bar with your hands. This tightens your upper back and sets your shoulders in a stable position. As you do this, screw your feet into the ground, drive your knees out, squeeze your butt, and elevate your hips. You will maintain these actions through every step.

3

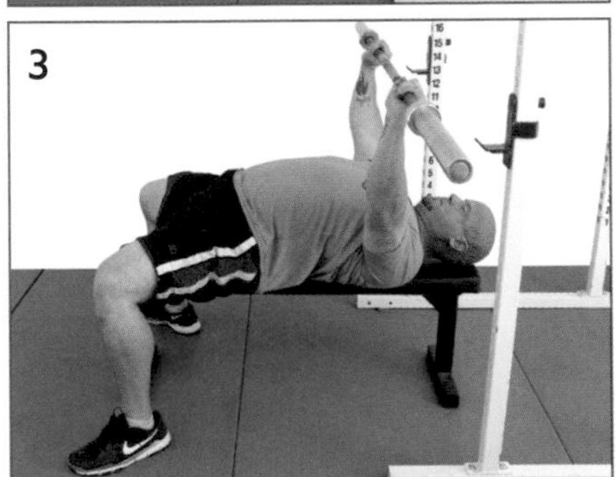

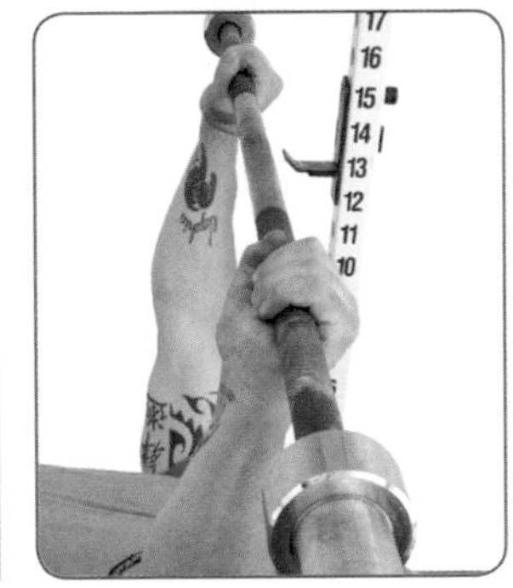

Lift the weight out of the rack and align the bar over your shoulders. Notice that the bar is resting in the center of Jesse's palms, directly over his wrists.

4

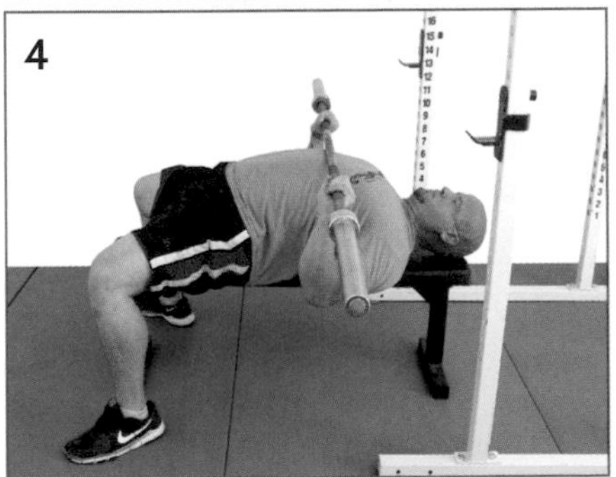

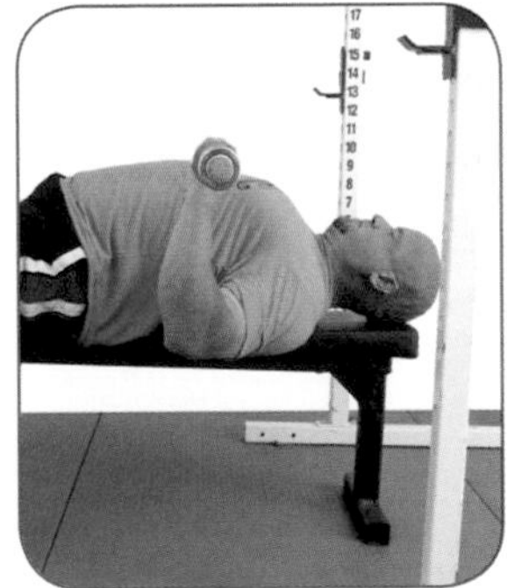

Keeping your shoulder blades pulled back, lower the weight to your chest. Think about loading your triceps and chest by pulling your elbows down and keeping your forearms as vertical as possible.

5

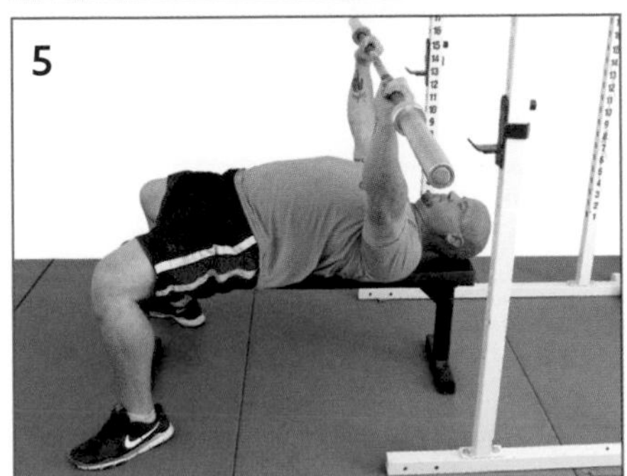

Extend your elbows and reestablish the start position.

Press
Archetype

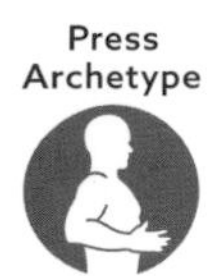

This fault is associated with the press archetype. For a mobility fix, visit the press archetype prescription in part 4.

MOTOR CONTROL FIX:

Focus on trying to bend the bar with your hands and pull your shoulder blades back. Maintain high levels of torque during the movement.

Keep your wrists aligned with your elbows.

MOBILIZATION TARGET AREAS:

Thoracic spine

Anterior shoulders and lats

Posterior shoulders and chest

Downstream arms (elbows and wrists)

Elbows-Out Fault

As with the pushup, a lot of athletes flare their elbows out to the sides because they are missing internal rotation in their shoulders or they failed to create and maintain sufficient torque in the setup. This also happens when you don't keep your shoulders screwed into the backs of the sockets: If there is slack in your shoulders, your elbows will fly out to the sides to take up the tension. If you're missing range of motion, you may want to consider implementing the floor press on the next page as an alternative.

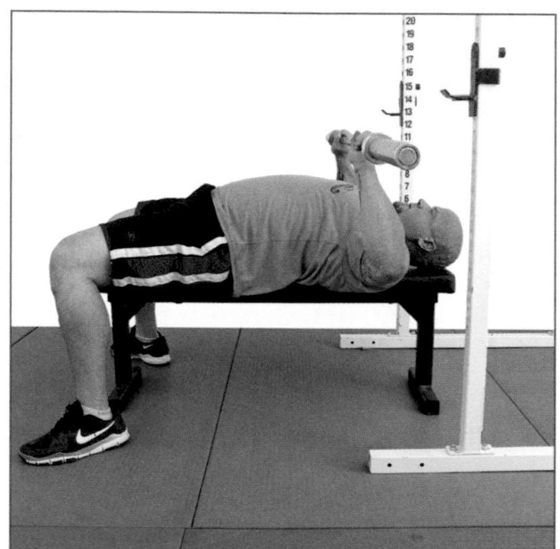

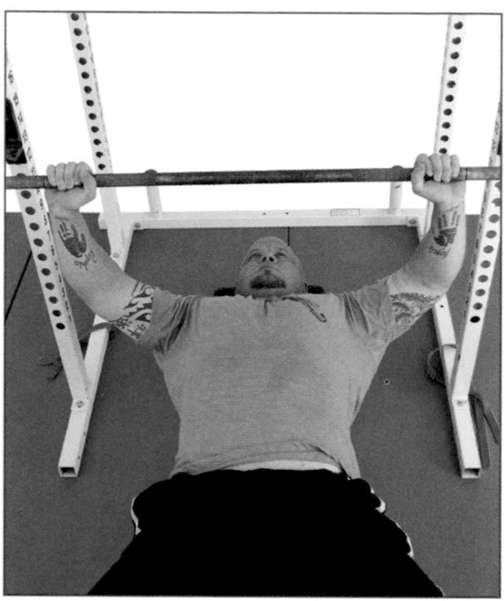

Press
Archetype

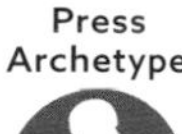

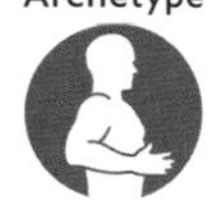

This fault is associated with the press archetype. For a mobility fix, visit the press archetype prescription in part 4.

MOTOR CONTROL FIX:

Create and maintain torque by consciously trying to bend the bar.

Focus on keeping your wrists in line with your elbows while keeping your shoulders back.

Practice the ideal bar path. You can use the ring pushup as a tool to practice good bench press form.

MOBILIZATION TARGET AREAS:

Thoracic spine

Anterior shoulders and lats

Posterior shoulders and chest

Downstream arms (elbows and wrists)

Elbows-Back Fault

The setup is without question the most complex aspect of the bench press. Once your shoulders are set and the bar is aligned over your shoulders, the bench press is largely a function of just bending and extending your elbows. The goal is to bend your elbows, keeping them in a 30- to 45-degree plane from your body, while maintaining vertical forearms. The problem is that a lot of people don't feel comfortable lowering the bar to their sternum because it requires a higher degree of mobility, strength, and control. To circumvent their mobility restrictions and lack of triceps strength, they load their shoulders instead of their triceps and chest. As you can see in the photo below, this puts an incredible amount of shear force on your wrists and elbows.

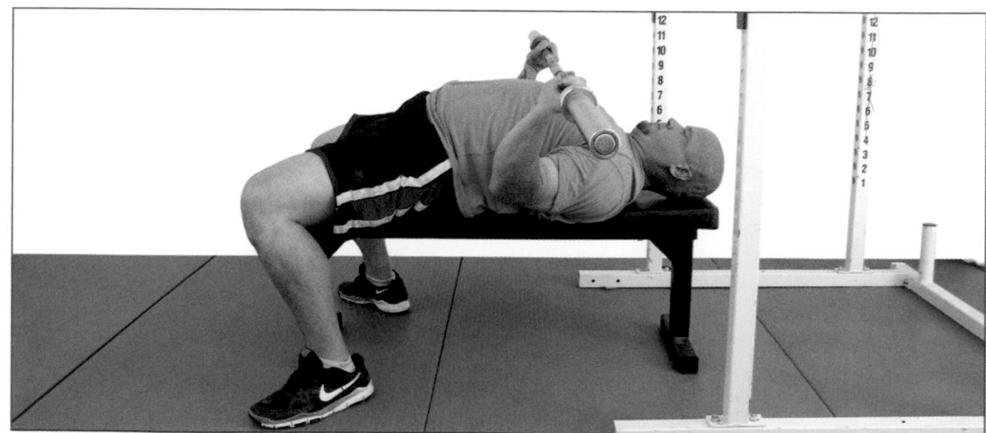

Floor Press

Although the bench press is a fantastic movement, it poses problems for a lot of people. It expresses a high degree of extension and internal rotation of the shoulders—elbows tracking behind your body—and requires triceps strength, which a lot of people don't have. If you are missing internal rotation range of motion in your shoulders or you have underdeveloped triceps, the bench press will exaggerate a lot of faults: Your elbows will fly out, your shoulders will roll forward, and you will squirm underneath the bar in search of stability and power. If this is you, know that you are ripe for ingraining a toxic movement pattern. Make a good decision and scale back to the floor press.

The floor press restricts the bench pressing range of motion action but provides you with the same stimulus—meaning that you can still mobilize your shoulders to the backs of the sockets, load your triceps, and practice a loaded midrange press without having to work around your mobility issues. To put it in simple terms, the floor press is a valuable tool that protects your shoulders while still teaching you how to press through midrange. It is also a great exercise to throw into a large group without worrying about having to correct a lot of faults.

Note: All the same rules apply here. Your grip, stance, and load order sequence are exactly the same as in the bench press.

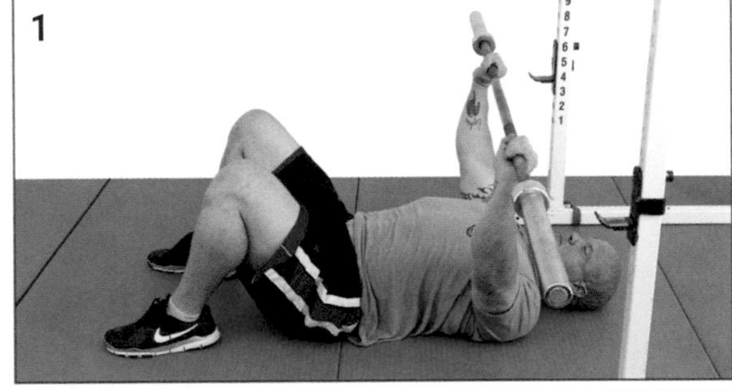

1 The lift-out is carried out in the same manner as the bench press. To see the load order sequence, refer to the bench press sequence on page 213.

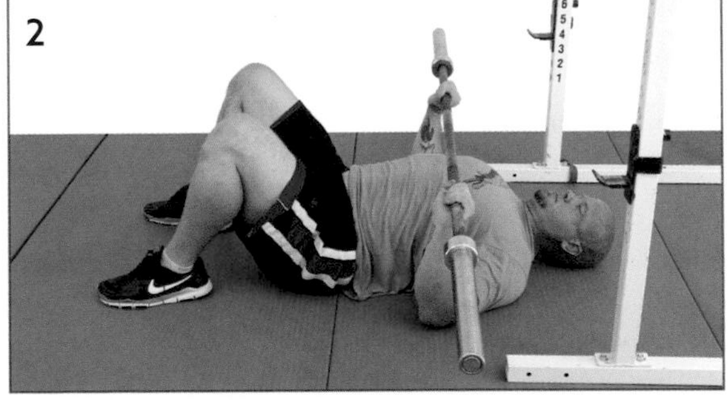

2 Keeping your forearms vertical, shoulders back, and belly tight, lower your triceps to the floor. The key is to load your chest and triceps by keeping your forearms vertical.

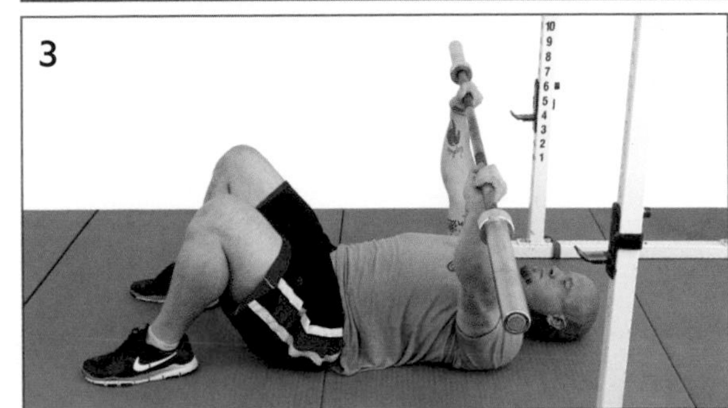

3 The moment your triceps touch down, press the weight back to the start position by extending your elbows.

DIP

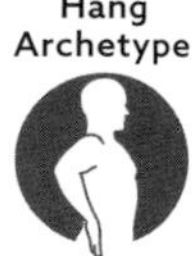

This movement contains the above archetypes. To improve common restrictions associated with this movement, visit the corresponding archetype prescriptions in part 4.

Here's the path to developing optimal power output from the shoulders: Perform a wide swath of exercises that stabilize the shoulders from a variety of ranges.

The pushup and bench press teach you how to stabilize your shoulders out in front of your body (press archetype). The strict press and push-press teach you how to stabilize a load overhead (overhead archetype). And the dip teaches you how to generate stability while your arms are at your sides (hang archetype).

Even though the dip is technically a pressing element, it forces the same stabilization demands as carrying a heavy object. The dip transfers to daily life tasks like carrying a suitcase or getting up out of an armchair.

Although the underlying principles of the dip are the same as those for the midrange and overhead movements—create external rotation torque and pull your shoulder blades back—it represents a new stimulus for the shoulders. If you don't spend time working in these extension ranges, you are more likely to compensate forward into a bad position when carrying or performing basic tasks with your arms at your sides or behind your body.

Plus, being able to perform a full-range quality dip is a prerequisite for more dynamic movements like the muscle-up: If you can't stay in control in the bottom position of the dip, creating spontaneous torque as you transition into a muscle-up is hopeless.

The dip is a complex exercise that requires enormous amounts of strength, control, and shoulder range of motion. For these reasons, you need to understand how to scale the movement.

To scale the dip, start in the top position and make sure that you can stabilize your shoulders in a good position with your arms locked out. If you don't have the strength or range of motion to lower into the bottom position, you can use a band or Mark Bell's Sling Shot to make the movement easier. If you have access to parallel bars, you can walk back and forth with your arms locked out to develop positional strength.

Just because you have the strength to perform the movement doesn't mean that you're doing it right. A lot can go wrong. For example, people often struggle to keep their forearms vertical and load their chest and triceps because they are missing shoulder range of motion or don't follow the proper load order sequence. Instead, they drive their elbows back, overextend, and keep their chest upright and then wiggle around in the bottom position in search of a mechanical advantage. This is where a lot of shoulder damage occurs and is why people experience sternum pain when they dip.

Setup

To perform the dip correctly, you need to make sure your dip station is high enough that you can straighten your legs. If the apparatus is too short, you will be forced to bend your knees and cross your ankles behind your body, resulting in an overextension spinal fault (opposite).

The width of your grip is also important. The conventional method is to use your forearm (elbow to fingertips) to measure your grip distance, which doesn't really tell you anything about your start and finish position. The best way to figure out how far apart you need to position your hands is to stand straight with your arms at your sides and then rotate your hands so that your palms are facing away from your body. You want the bars positioned just inside your pinky fingers. As in the ring pushup, you can also use the rings to determine proper grip width.

While these methods are not perfect, they will put you in a position to maximize torque and shoulder stability. If your grip distance works out to be the same length as your forearm, that's great: You have an easy model for measuring.

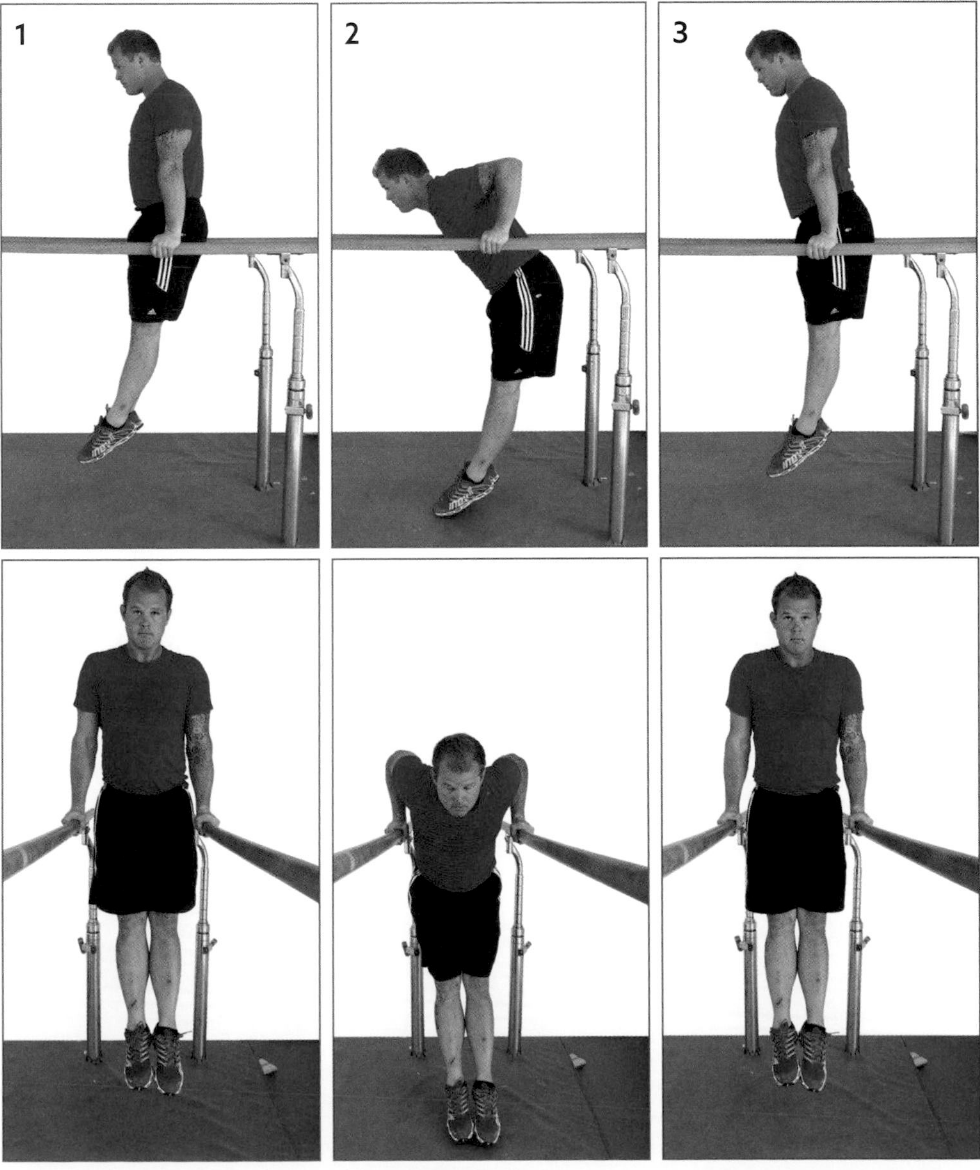

1. The start position shares a lot of the same cues as the pushup and press: Screw your hands into the bars, get the pits of your elbows forward, and externally rotate your shoulders into the backs of the sockets. Keep your feet together, toes pointed, and butt squeezed to support your pelvis in a neutral position. Your feet should be positioned just in front of your body.

2. Keeping your legs straight, toes pointed, butt squeezed, and belly tight, lower into the bottom position by allowing your chest to drop forward. This loads your pecs and triceps. As in the squat, imagine pulling yourself down while screwing your hands into the bars. The key is to focus on keeping your shoulders back (think about squeezing your shoulder blades together as you lever forward), spine rigid, and forearms vertical.

3. Still screwing your hands into the bars, extend your elbows and reestablish the top position. There should be no change in the position of your torso.

Shrug Fault

Hang Archetype

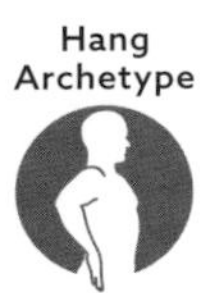

This fault is associated with the hang archetype. For a mobility fix, visit the hang archetype prescription in part 4.

MOTOR CONTROL FIX:

Use the pushup as a model to ingrain proper shoulder stabilization mechanics before progressing to the dip.

Isolate the top position: Focus on squeezing your butt with your legs straight and together, screwing your hands into the bars, getting your elbow pits forward, and pulling your shoulders back.

MOBILIZATION TARGET AREAS:

Thoracic spine

Anterior shoulders and lats

Posterior shoulders and chest

Downstream arms (elbows and wrists)

If you are missing shoulder range of motion, it's impossible to pull your shoulders back into a good position and lock out your elbows. While the same is true for the pushup and bench press, it's easier to disguise. This is what makes the dip such a great diagnostic tool. With your shoulders supporting the full weight of your body, you can't mask limited shoulder mobility.

If you start in an organized position but compensate into a bad position as you lower into the bottom of the dip, it's a good indication that you're missing extension and internal rotation in your shoulders or you lack the strength to perform the movement correctly.

Your pecs are responsible for stabilizing your shoulders in an externally rotated position. Because the dip requires a high level of shoulder stability, your pecs have to work extra hard to keep your shoulders locked in a stable, externally rotated position. If your shoulders roll forward or shrug, your pecs will pull off-axis, which pulls the sternum apart—the reason some people experience intense sternum pain when they dip.

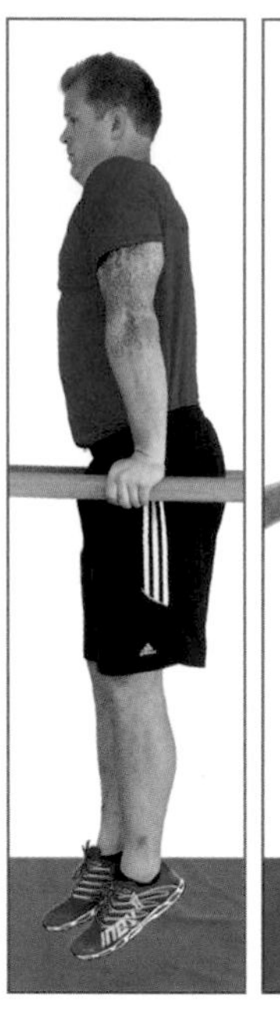

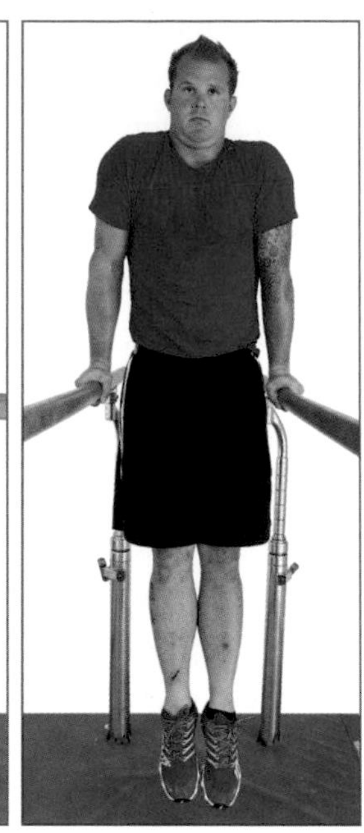

Overextension Spinal Fault

MOTOR CONTROL FIX:

Keep your legs straight and pinned together, pointing your toes. Your feet should be positioned underneath or slightly in front of your body.

Squeeze your glutes and establish a neutral spinal position.

Pull your shoulders back and create torque off the bar.

Bending your knees and crossing your ankles behind your body is a setup error that can cause an overextension fault. It's difficult to engage your glutes and stabilize your pelvis in a neutral position unless your legs are straight and positioned together.

In the photos below, notice that as I press out of the bottom position, I throw my head back and arch into an overextended position. In this example, I've surrendered my spinal position and the stability of my shoulders so that I can generate upward momentum. Arching back, elbows deviating outward, and shoulders compensating forward are my body's ways of finding stability so that I can complete the movement. Not good!

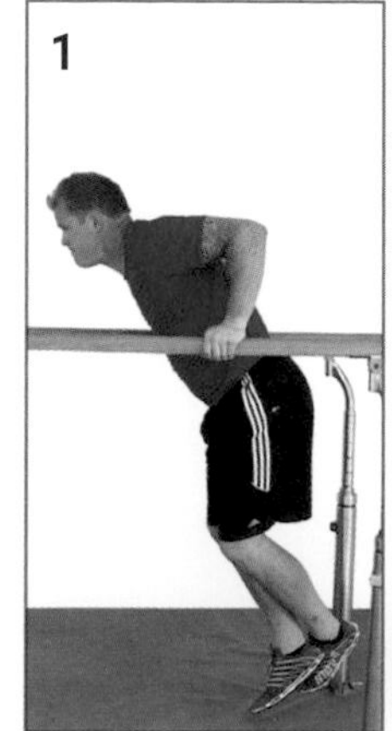
1

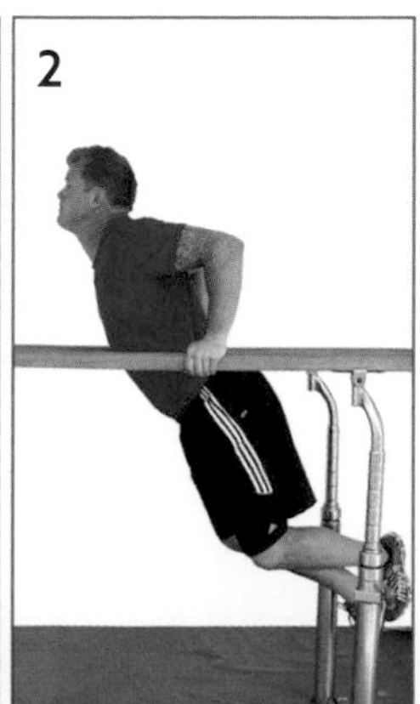
2

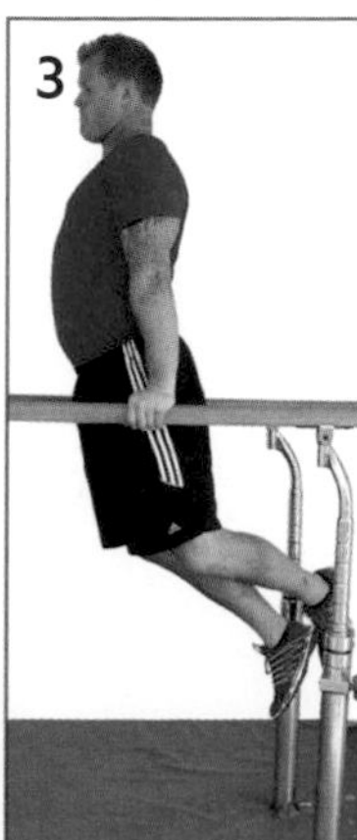
3

Ring Dip

One of the primary functions of the Movement and Mobility System is to teach and progress movements that transfer learning to other movements. The ring dip is a star example. In addition to providing a more challenging stimulus, it preps you for more dynamic movements like the muscle-up.

As with the ring pushup, the ring dip requires an additional dose of problem solving. Mobility issues are forced out of hiding. You can tell when someone is missing internal rotation in her shoulders because she struggles to achieve an externally rotated position and can't lock out her elbows.

The ring dip also promotes good movement practices and automatically corrects common faults. For example, a common fault with the classic dip is to pull your elbows back as you lower into the bottom position. Doing so internally rotates your shoulders, sucking you into a compromised position. However, in order to remain balanced and stable over the rings, you have to keep your forearms vertical. You physically can't press with your elbows behind your wrists.

Although the ring dip is a fantastic diagnostic tool, I rarely program the movement into high-intensity or high-repetition workouts; it's simply too difficult to perform multiple reps correctly when you're fatigued. The same is true with the muscle-up (see page 280). This is not to say that you shouldn't perform ring dips as a strength exercise, though. The key is to stop the moment your shoulder or spinal position starts to deteriorate.

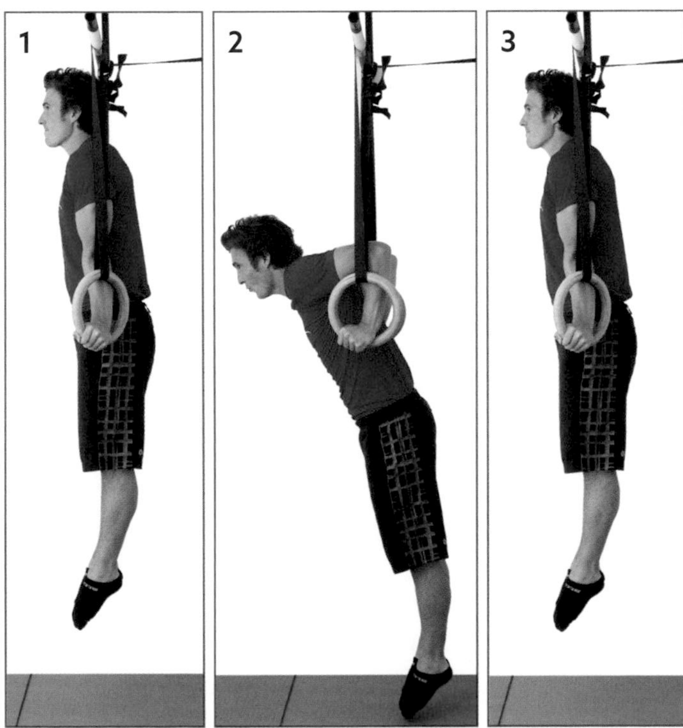

1. To stabilize your shoulders, externally rotate your hands so that your thumbs are pointing away from your body. Now pull your shoulders back. Your left hand should be at about 11 o'clock and your right hand at about 1 o'clock. Position your feet together, point your toes, squeeze your glutes, and then tighten your core.

2. Keeping your butt squeezed, belly tight, and hands turned out, lower into the bottom position. Notice that Carl levers forward, keeping his feet out in front of his body. This loads his triceps and chest and keeps his shoulders and trunk in a good position. Also note the position of his arms: His wrists are in line with his elbows (his forearms are vertical) and his elbows are in tight to his body. It's important to mention that as you lower your hands, you will rotate to about 12 o'clock. If you're missing internal rotation in your shoulders, your hands will continue to rotate inward. Fight this force and try to reclaim a thumbs-out position as you rise out of the bottom.

3. Still turning your hands out and keeping your back flat, extend your elbows and reestablish the top position.

Overhead Archetype

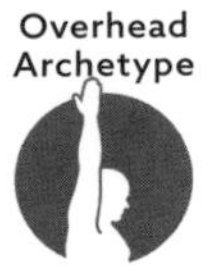

Front Rack 2 Archetype

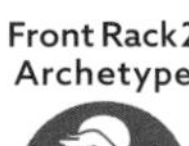

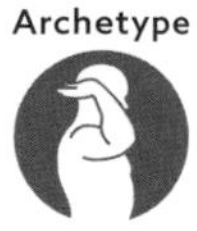

This movement contains the above archetypes. To improve common restrictions associated with this movement, visit the corresponding archetype prescriptions in part 4.

STRICT PRESS

The strict press is a move that offers you a golden opportunity to practice the rules of bracing and torque with your arms overhead. It's also a magnifying glass for assessing motor control trouble spots and mobility restrictions.

For example, say someone can't get her shoulders into the proper position when pressing a bar overhead. What does that tell you about her motor control and shoulder range of motion? And what do you think will happen when she tries to receive a heavy load in the jerk, or rattle off any overhead movement while burning with met-con fatigue? If you don't understand the ideal start and finish position or you lack the range of motion to perform the task, you can't apply these fundamental concepts to more complex overhead actions.

Can you keep your back flat with your ribcage and pelvis neutral? Can you get your shoulders into end-range flexion with your elbows straight? Can you express a stable shoulder position by getting your armpits forward? It's that simple.

The strict press is also a useful rehabilitation tool. For example, if I'm coaching someone who's coming off a knee injury or rehabbing after ACL surgery, this is one of the first weight-bearing exercises that I introduce. It still requires a low level of external rotation torque—the athlete has to shove his knees out and screw his feet into the ground—so it helps strengthen the injured joint and the surrounding musculature, as well as reingrain functional movement patterns.

Stabilizing the Shoulders

In our gym, there is no such thing as a shoulder stabilization exercise. Every shoulder movement has a stabilization component. This is where coaches and physical therapists often miss the mark.

Doing accessory exercises like externally rotating your arm back and forth with a cable machine or light dumbbell is not going to teach you how to pull, push, press, carry, or lift with stable shoulders. You need to incorporate movements that force you to stabilize your shoulders in a good position. That's why it's so important to learn how to perform midrange movements like the pushup, overhead movements like the strict press, and by-your-side or behind-your-back movements like the dip.

A lot of coaches still dismiss exercises like the press for swimmers, baseball pitchers, and volleyball players—athletes who perform a lot of overhead-type movements—because they believe that overhead exercises are dangerous. This is a valid point if you don't understand what a stable shoulder position looks and feels like. Say an athlete has already put in gazillions of overhead repetitions. If he's doing it with crappy form, the last thing his coach wants him to do is more overhead work with bad technique.

What should his coach do, then? Teach him the stable position for the shoulder, then teach him how to do the strict press with good technique. This will not only improve the effectiveness of his overhead position, but also allow the coach to assess his end-range position. He doesn't have to press a lot of weight or perform a ridiculous number of repetitions. However, a responsible coach needs to instill fundamental stabilization principles and highlight mobility and motor control dysfunction.

Barbell versus Dumbbell

People ask me: "Why do you encourage pressing with a barbell? Isn't it safer and easier to learn to press with dumbbells?"

Before I answer, it's important to note that the closer you can position the weight to your center line (general center of mass), the easier it is to press from that position with good form.

If you have limited shoulder range of motion or your technique is off, the dumbbell press is a great option because it allows you to keep your shoulders organized in a good position without compromising your form.

So if you have shoulder pain when you raise your arms overhead with a barbell, pressing with dumbbells will help reduce that pain due to improved setup positioning and more rotational options of your arms when the dumbbells are overhead.

There's no arguing the fact that pressing with dumbbells offers distinct advantages. The same goes for kettlebells. In fact, I encourage all my athletes to do it. However, the dumbbell press will ultimately limit the maximum load you can press overhead.

Additionally, one of the problems we perennially see as athletes move toward more complex lifts like the push-jerk and split-jerk is that they don't have a model for creating torque off a fixed object (barbell) and lack the strength to perform these movements under load. That's why it's so important to get people pressing with a barbell in their developmental stages—because it ingrains fundamental movement patterns that translate to these more complex movements, even as it builds the pressing strength needed to move heavier weight.

However, a barbell does present certain challenges: You have to clear your face as you press the weight overhead; you have to support the load out in front of your body; you have to balance the bar on your chest while keeping your forearms vertical; and you have to generate force from a dead-start position. But, like all the movements described in this book, it teaches you a load order sequence that transfers to other movements and objects.

The objective is to learn movements that express stability in your joints and core through full ranges of motion. While a barbell is by no means a natural implement, it's the easiest tool for challenging your competency overhead. There comes a point where lifting heavy dumbbells simply becomes untenable.

Strict Press Setup

Setting up for the strict press is very similar to establishing the front rack position out of the rack (see front squat, page 187). You still create torque off the bar (breaking the bar and twisting your elbows underneath) one arm at a time, lift the weight out of the rack as if it were a front squat, and walk back. But instead of lifting your elbows to a 90-degree angle and balancing the bar on your fingertips and shoulders, you position the bar on your chest and in the center of your palms.

A couple of nuances worth mentioning are the width of your stance and grip. Determining your stance is easy; it's the same as your jumping or deadlift stance. Your feet are straight and positioned underneath your hips, roughly shoulder width apart. Figuring out your grip is a little trickier. You can use a few different methods: implement the front rack setup demonstrated on page 188, get into the top position of the ring pushup (see page 208), or execute the band press test (see page 226). The keys are to keep your shoulders screwed into the backs of the sockets, your forearms vertical, your wrists aligned with your elbows, and the bar resting in the center of your palms.

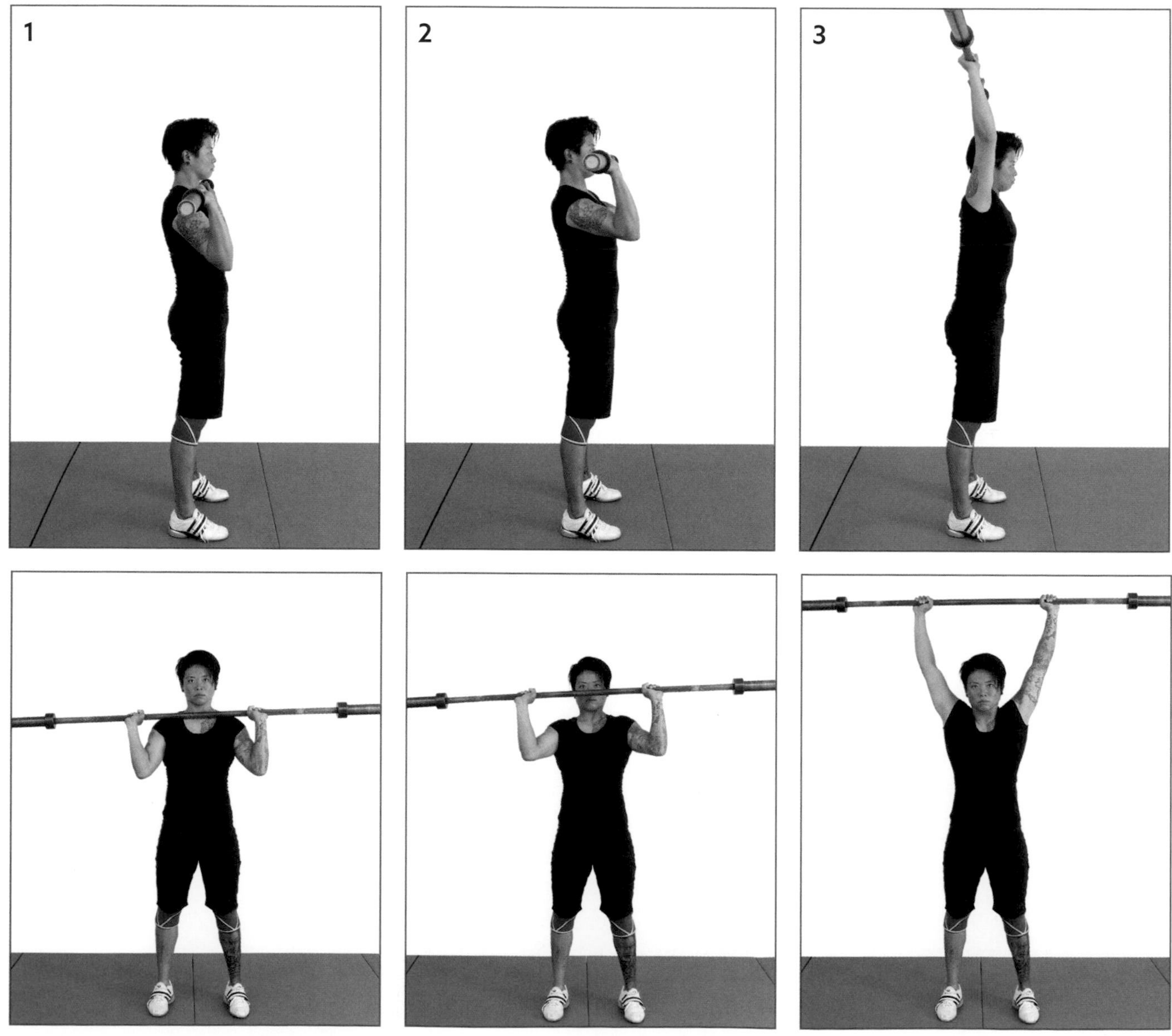

1. Take the weight out of the rack and walk back as you would when performing a front squat (see "Front Rack Position" on page 187). The key is to create torque off the bar, wind your shoulders into the backs of the sockets, and brace your trunk. Your forearms are vertical, with the bar balancing in the center of your palms and chest, and your shoulders are wound tight. The biggest mistake athletes make is to take the weight out of the rack and then try to get tight. This is the equivalent of loading a bar onto your back for a back squat without bracing your midline. Once you establish your stance, screw your feet into the ground and squeeze your glutes.

2. Keeping your shoulders pulled back, butt squeezed, and belly tight, pull your head back slightly and press the weight straight overhead. You want to move your head around the bar, not the bar around your head. Also focus on keeping your elbows in tight and your armpits forward. Don't shrug your shoulders, flare your elbows out, or lean back. There should be no change in spinal position.

3. As you lock out your elbows, push your head through your arms into a neutral position. Think about positioning your armpits forward to maximize torque. Notice that Diane's arm bisects her ears. A lot of athletes mistakenly push their head through or keep their head back, both of which compromise trunk and shoulder stability.

4. As you lower the bar, pull your head back slightly to maintain a vertical bar path. Again, the way down should look exactly the same as the way up. Keep your elbows tight, shoulders back, and butt squeezed as you lower the bar.

5. Maintaining the same level of torque, lower the weight into the start position.

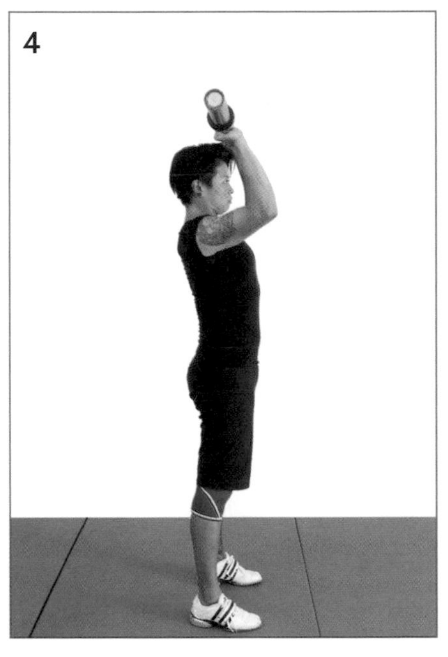

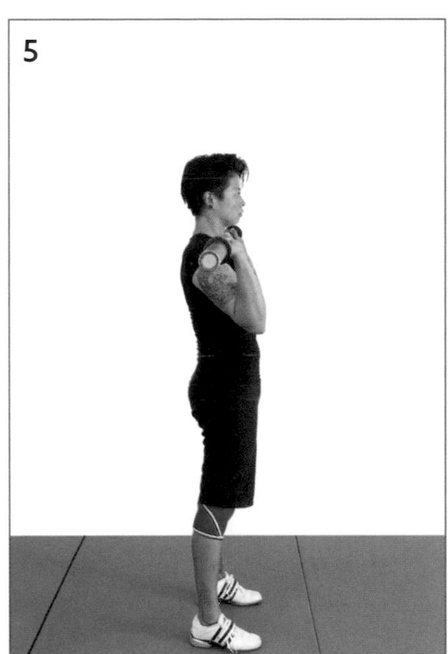

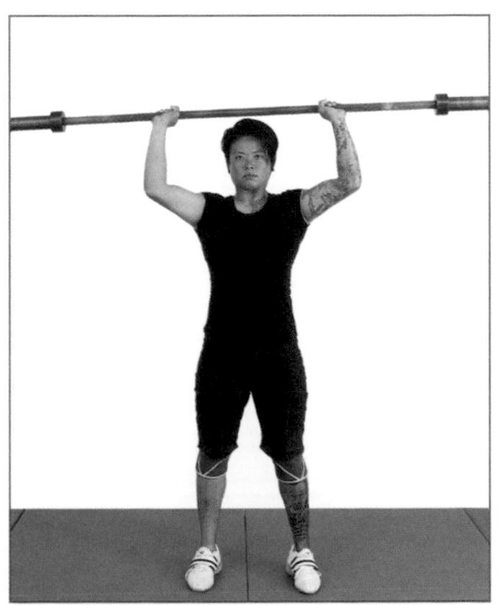

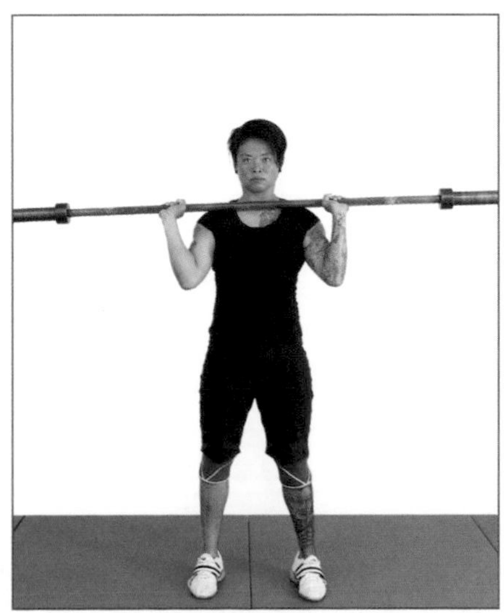

Front Rack Fault

Front Rack 2 Archetype

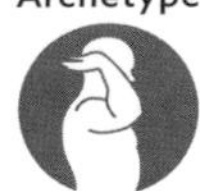

This fault is associated with the front rack archetype. For a mobility fix, visit the front rack archetype prescription in part 4.

MOTOR CONTROL FIX:

Set up for the press out of the rack. Position the bar in the center of your palms and make sure your elbows are aligned with your wrists (and the bar).

Keep your shoulders screwed to the backs of the sockets by generating torque off the bar.

Perform the band press test (page 226).

MOBILIZATION TARGET AREAS:

Thoracic spine

Anterior shoulders and lats

Posterior shoulders and chest

Downstream arms (elbows and wrists)`

A common mistake is to initiate the press from the front rack position. While you can get away with this fault when executing the push-press and push-jerk, it doesn't work with the strict press. With the bar balancing on your fingertips, you can't generate enough force from the start position to lift the weight off your chest. People do this because they don't have a model for pressing with vertical forearms, or they are missing range of motion in their shoulders, or their thoracic spine is brutally tight—or all those things.

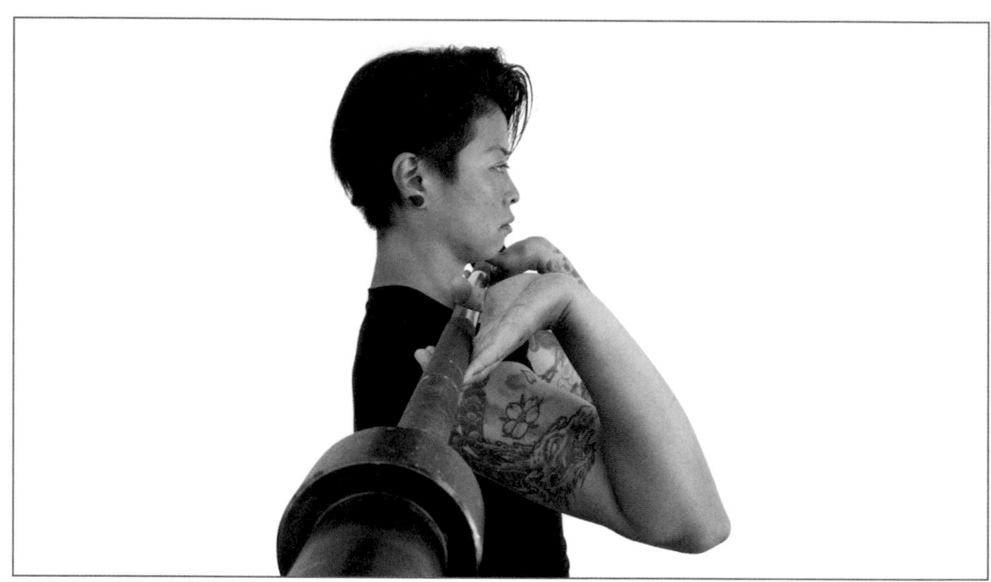

Elbows-Out Fault

Overhead Archetype

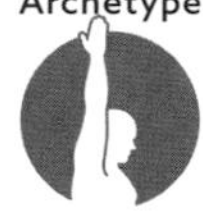

This fault is associated with the overhead archetype. For a mobility fix, visit the overhead archetype prescription in part 4.

MOTOR CONTROL FIX:

Generate sufficient torque in the setup and keep your elbows in as you press overhead.

MOBILIZATION TARGET AREAS:

Thoracic spine

Anterior shoulders and lats

Posterior shoulders and chest

Downstream arms (elbows and wrists)

If your elbows flare out to the sides as you extend your arms overhead, it's an indication that you're not generating enough torque or you failed to set your shoulders in a good position during the setup. However, if you're unable to lock out your arms overhead, which is common, chances are good that you're missing range of motion in your shoulders. This detrimental mechanical pattern will become a real problem when the weight gets heavy or you graduate to more complex lifts, like the push-press and push-jerk.

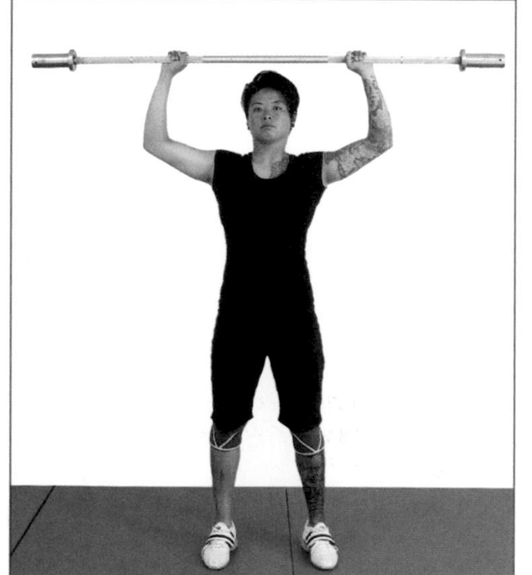

Arch Fault

Trunk stabilization demands are high in the strict press. Unlike the push-press and push-jerk, which harness the power of your legs and hips, the strict press requires you to press using the strength of your shoulders and arms. This dead-start phase is what makes the strict press such a tricky movement. As the weight gets heavier, you might search for a mechanical advantage by arching back and pressing the weight out in front of your body, like a bench press. While this makes it easier to get the weight off your chest, it destabilizes your primary engines, causing your elbows to fly out and your shoulders to roll forward. This fault is also common in people who try to move the bar around their face instead of pulling their head back.

In most cases, you can address this fault simply by lowering the weight, keeping your butt squeezed, and maintaining a vertical bar path by moving your head back. However, if you have a tight thoracic spine and are missing rotation in your shoulders, you might not be able to set your shoulders in a good position. In that case, you might err by pressing the weight out in front of your body.

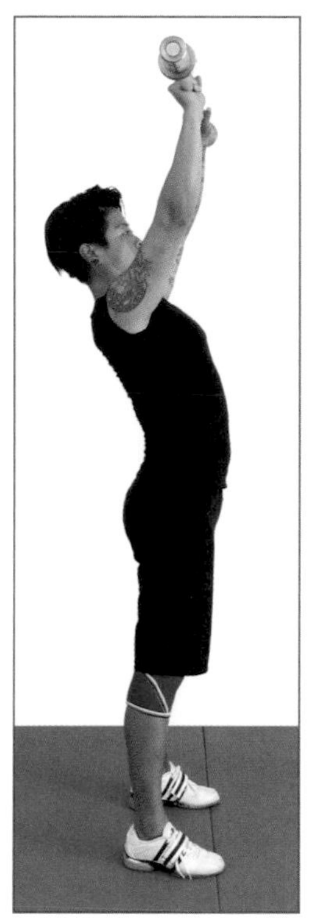

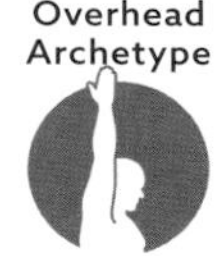

This fault is associated with the overhead archetype. For a mobility fix, visit the overhead archetype prescription in part 4.

MOTOR CONTROL FIX:

Squeeze your glutes and keep your belly tight.

Prioritize the setup out of the rack by screwing your shoulders into the backs of the sockets.

MOBILIZATION TARGET AREAS:

Thoracic spine

Anterior shoulders and lats

Posterior shoulders and chest

Downstream arms (elbows and wrists)

Head-Forward Fault

Another common fault is to push your head through your arms as you extend your elbows overhead. Coaches often cue athletes to push their head through because athletes mistakenly pull their head back to clear their face and then leave it there as they lock out their arms overhead, causing an arch fault. Telling them to push their head through aims to correct this fault by reminding them to move underneath the barbell as it passes their face.

The problem is that a lot of people overcompensate by pushing the barbell backward and driving their head forward. In addition to unlocking the shoulders and compromising spinal position, this error puts an enormous amount of shear on the cervical segments of the neck. So if your head penetrates through your arms and the barbell moves behind your body when you are pressing, you have a recipe for a quick neck injury. The correct technique is to bring your head back just enough to clear your face and then move underneath the bar as you press the weight overhead, keeping your torso and head in alignment.

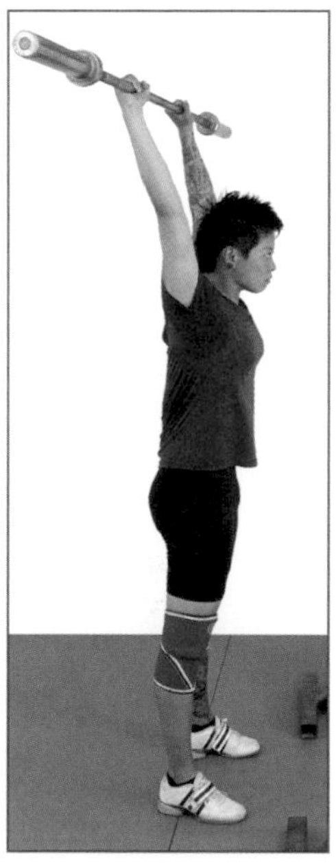

MOTOR CONTROL FIX:

Keep your head in line with your torso.

Think about maintaining a vertical bar path and moving your head just enough to clear your face.

Practice with lighter weights until you're proficient with the technique.

HANDSTAND PUSHUP

Overhead Archetype Front Rack 2 Archetype

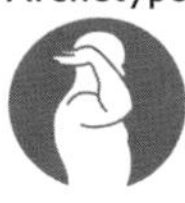

This movement contains the above archetypes. To improve common restrictions associated with this movement, visit the corresponding archetype prescriptions in part 4.

The handstand pushup is not a natural movement. I mean, aside from gymnastics, break-dancing, and CrossFit, people rarely do anything inverted. That said, it is an excellent movement to infuse into your training program. In fact, the handstand pushup is one of the best movements for driving home the relationship between ribcage and pelvis alignment. You have to balance your pelvis and legs on your ribcage, which exposes a lot of holes in midline stabilization and shoulder organization strategy.

Unlike most training movements, the handstand pushup requires you to organize your trunk through your shoulders via your hands, instead of your hips via your feet. For example, when you set up for a squat, you create torque (stability) in your hips by screwing your feet into the ground and then balancing your ribcage over your pelvis. But with the handstand pushup, you do the exact opposite, which is very challenging. You're basically getting organized in the finish position of a press. From a motor learning and trunk stabilization perspective, the handstand pushup is unparalleled.

Band Press Test

The band press test is great for a couple of reasons. For starters, it illuminates the importance and efficiency of a stable shoulder. Second, it shows people that their lovely push-jerk front rack position doesn't translate to the press.

Here's how it works: Hook a band around your foot and adopt a pressing position that is similar to the front rack. Then try to extend your arm overhead from that position. You'll find that your shoulder immediately translates forward into an unstable position and you struggle to raise your arm overhead. Next, pull your shoulder back into a good position and press. Right away, you will see that it's much easier to lock out your arm. As soon as you bring your shoulder back and get your elbow tight to your body, it's much easier. You're able to harness all the stability of your shoulder and transmit energy to the band effectively.

In a nutshell, the band press test is a great way to challenge the efficiency of your press and sheds light on what an effective press should look and feel like.

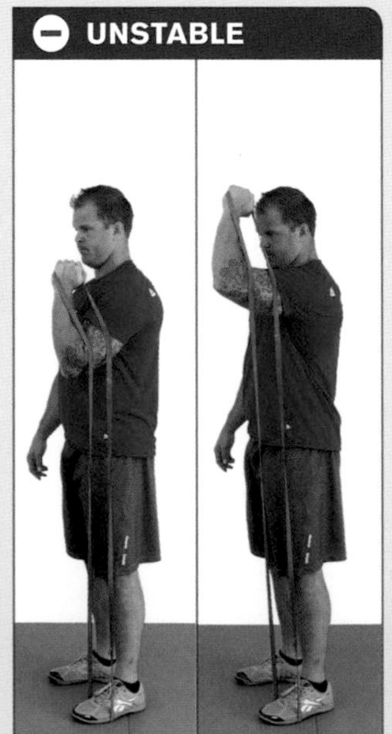

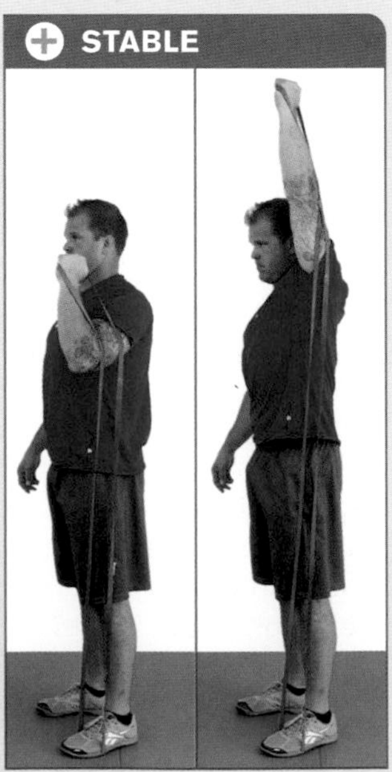

Again, to improve as an athlete, you have to find different ways to challenge your motor control. The more training tools you have in your movement arsenal, the better and more stable you will be. Does this movement belong in the repertoire of all athletes? No. Powerlifters or Olympic lifters are certainly not going to do handstand pushups. They have plenty of other skill-transfer exercises that teach good shoulder positioning and trunk stabilization. But if you're an average person, the handstand pushup is a fundamental skill that will improve your athleticism and, more important, will tell you a lot about your ability to organize your shoulders and trunk in an unfamiliar position.

Note: If you'd like to learn more about the handstand pushup, I highly recommend coach Carl Paoli's blog GymnasticsWOD.com and his bestselling book, *Free+Style: Maximize Sport and Life Performance with Four Basic Movements.*

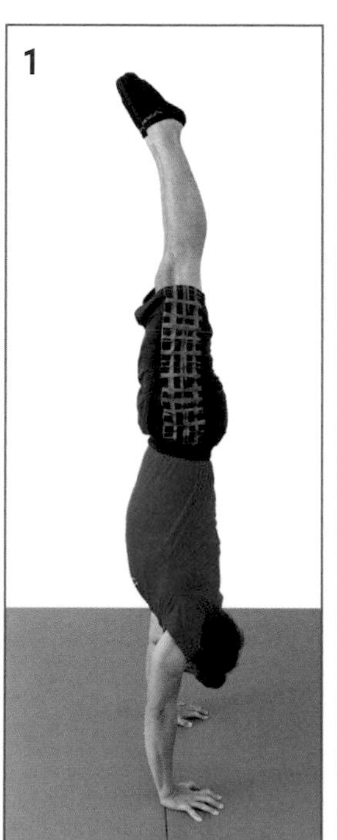

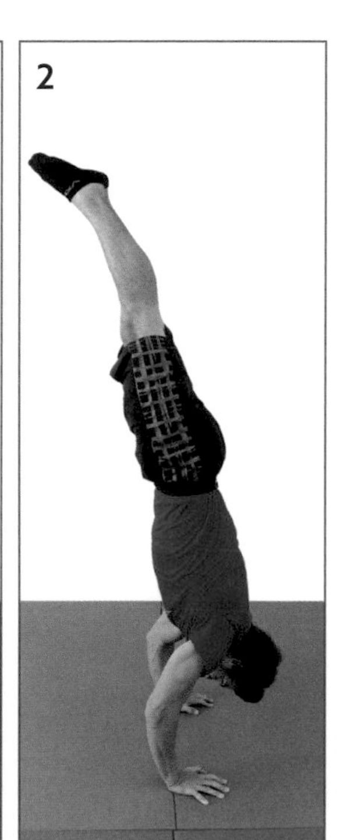

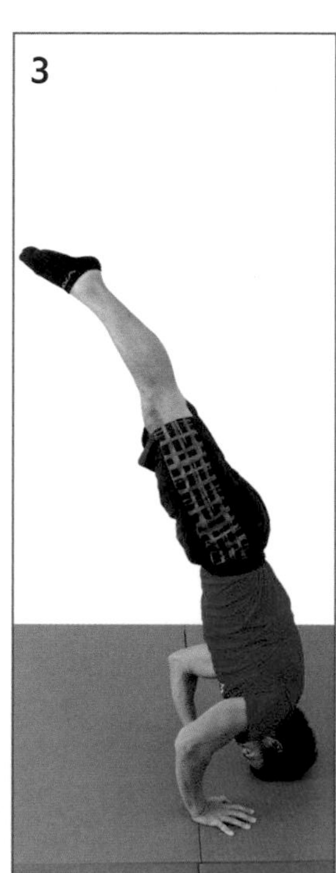

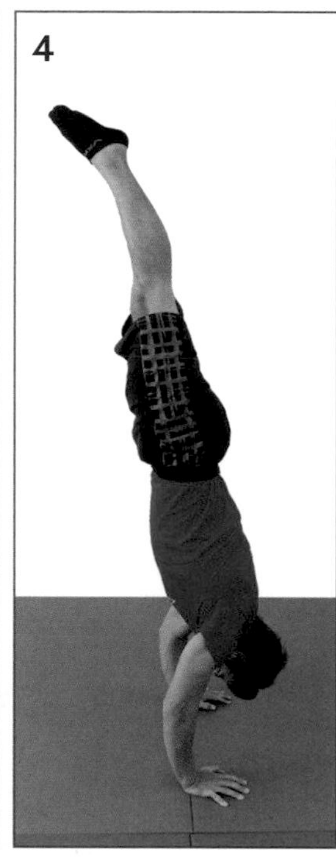

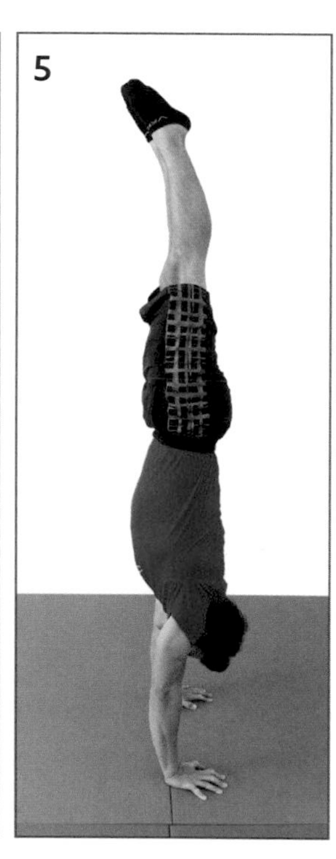

1. To set up, go through the bracing sequence and hinge forward from your hips as if you were executing a single-leg deadlift. Using your free leg as a pendulum, place your hands on the ground at your pushup distance and kick up to a handstand by swinging your legs over your body. Keep your legs straight and create an external rotation force by screwing your hands into the ground as you transition into the handstand. The key is to keep your legs together and your toes pointed to maximize glute activation and stability. Focus on keeping your butt squeezed, belly tight, and armpits forward.

2. Still screwing your hands into the ground, break at your elbows and let your entire body tilt back, keeping your body rigid. One of the compromises of doing a handstand is that you can't leave your head in a perfect position. Notice that Carl tilts his head back just slightly so he can see the ground.

3. Lower your body until your head touches the ground.

4. As you press out of the bottom position, think about keeping your body rigid and your elbows in tight to your body.

5. As you lock out your arms, get your head through your arms and underneath your body to level out. At the same time, try to get your armpits forward to maintain external rotation torque.

Handstand Pushup (Supported)

A freestanding handstand or freestanding handstand pushup—that's the goal. But it takes an extreme amount of strength, stability, and motor control to pull off. The stepping-stone to such a skill is to use a support, like a wall. This is the equivalent of squatting or benching on a Smith machine in that you can move up and down in a straight line. Another option is to have a Superfriend support your feet. This requires a higher level of stability and is great for finding your balance while inverted.

You don't even need to perform the actual movement; just get into the start position and work on locking out your elbows, getting your armpits forward, and organizing your trunk. It's a great way to learn about shoulder and trunk stability. Like I said, nothing challenges the ribcage-to-pelvis relationship like the handstand pushup.

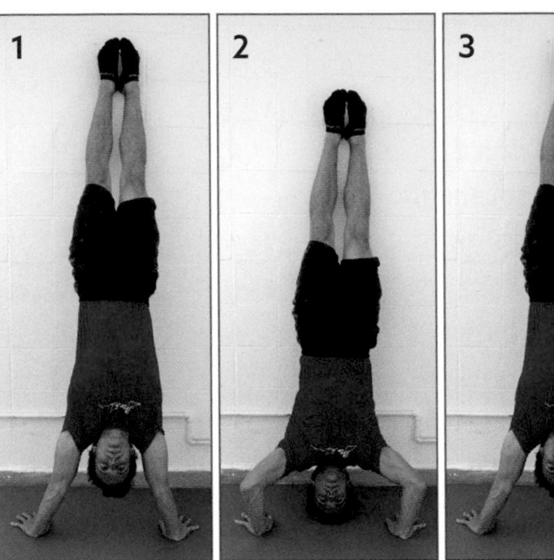

1. Positioning your hands roughly 6 inches from a wall, go through the bracing sequence and then kick up into a handstand. Keep your hands straight, butt squeezed, legs together, toes pointed, pelvis balanced over your ribcage, and armpits forward.

2. Screwing your hands into the ground, break at the elbows and lower your head to the ground. As you descend, try to keep your forearms vertical, elbows in tight to your body, and back and legs aligned.

3. As you press out of the bottom position and lock out your arms, get your armpits forward.

Scorpion Handstand Pushup Fault

The faults for the handstand pushup are the same as those for the strict press: ribcage tilt, head up, elbows out, and shoulders forward. And just like the pushup, some people spread their legs, which puts their butt offline, causing a gross overextension spinal fault. It's a disaster.

Interestingly, this is what most people look like when they try to walk on their hands. I see it all the time, and I think to myself: "Congratulations, you're walking on your hands…and you're wrecking your motor patterning for all your pressing motions and destroying your back and shoulders." Seriously, there are so many things wrong with this picture, I don't even know where to begin.

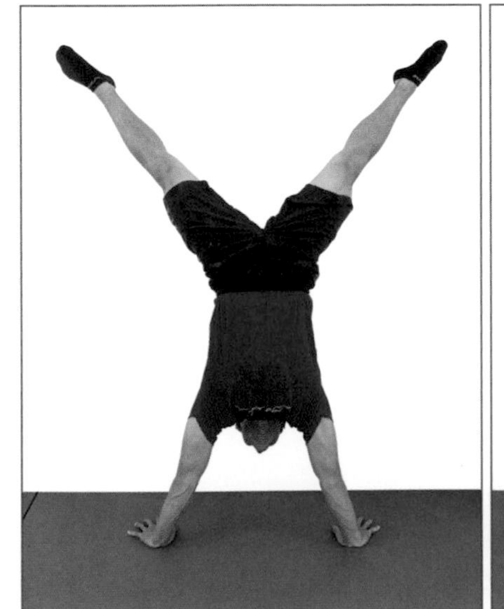

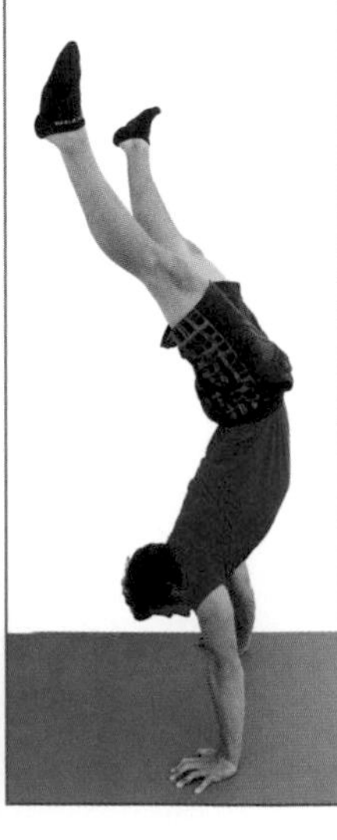

The fact is, you would never press in this position. If I flipped the photos of Carl upside down, put a barbell in his hand, and told you to evaluate his position, what would you say? I suspect nothing good.

Here's the deal: You have to get organized at the trunk and work on setting your shoulders in the correct position—armpits forward. Keep your hands straight so that you can maximize torque, keep your feet together, and point your toes to maximize glute activation. If you have to look down to see the ground, try not to exaggerate the movement. Aside from that, the motor control solution and mobility prescription are the same as those for the strict press faults.

PULL-UP

As I've said, if you view athletic movement through the lenses of "how much" and "how fast," your odds of defaulting into bad positions skyrocket. The pull-up is a sizzling example. In most cases, little or no attention is paid to how an athlete sacrifices his spine, neck, and shoulder position. The quality of a pull-up gets reduced to "Was he able to get his chin over the bar? Yes or no?"

It's not about whether a movement was completed, but rather whether the movement was completed *with good form.*

Imagine if I told you that rounding your back when you deadlift heavy is acceptable as long as you complete the lift. That wouldn't make sense, right? It contradicts the underlying theme of this book. Well, it's the same thing with the pull-up. If you can't perform the movement correctly without compensating into a bad position, it's damaging. You can get away with it for a while, but eventually hanging with bent elbows and overextending your lumbar spine is going to catch up to you.

At our gym, we teach athletes the strict pull-up for the same reason we teach the strict press: It allows us to teach and ingrain good mechanics in a low-risk environment. We can then progress our athletes to more dynamic movements like the kipping pull-up with less risk of defaulting into poor positions. The idea is for the athletes to develop physical competency with the movement from a dead start at end range before being challenged with a speed element.

Once we can get athletes to create and maintain a rigid spine and stable shoulders, it becomes an issue of strength. If an athlete can't initiate the movement with good form, we simply scale the movement by hooking a band around his feet or positioning a box underneath the bar so that he can use his legs to assist in the movement. In addition to building strength, the band reduces the torque demands and allows him to move through a full range of motion.

Overhead Archetype | Front Rack 2 Archetype

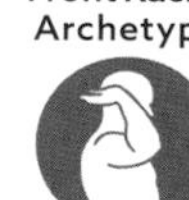

This movement contains the above archetypes. To improve common restrictions associated with this movement, visit the corresponding archetype prescriptions in part 4.

Hook Grip

Just as the position of your feet dictates your ability to generate torque in your hips and maintain a neutral spine, your grip dictates your ability to generate torque in your shoulders and keep your ribcage down when performing a pull-up. For most people, positioning the hands at roughly shoulder width or adopting the same grip distance as their pushup or strict press is a good start.

The next step is to learn how to grip the bar. In the photos at right, notice that Carl implements a unique grip. Instead of hooking his thumb over the top of the bar, he wraps his thumb over his index or middle finger. He also positions his pinky finger over the top of the bar, creating a slight bend in his wrist. This grip is superior because it locks his hand to the bar and allows him to create torque, which sets his shoulders in a stable position.

This modified false grip offers a couple of distinct advantages. For starters, it winds up his shoulders into an externally rotated position. In other words, he doesn't have to think about breaking the bar because he's already torqued. When your wrists are positioned directly underneath the bar, you have to work a lot harder to create torque in your shoulders. Second, this hook grip dead-hang position is a great diagnostic

⊕ PULL-UP HOOK GRIP

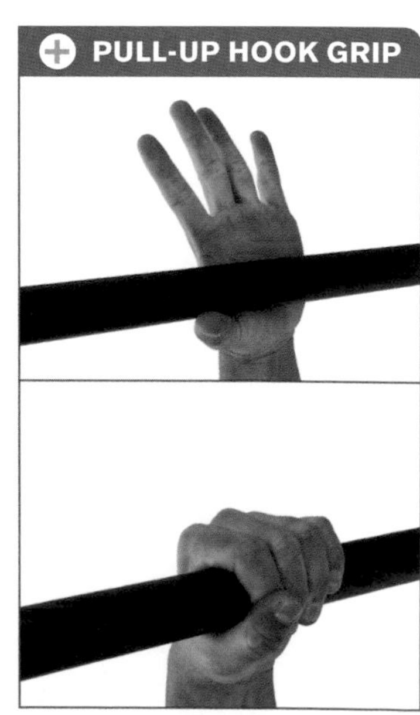

tool for assessing overhead range of motion: If you can keep your torso integrated while hanging with the pull-up hook grip, it's an indication that you have full range of motion overhead.

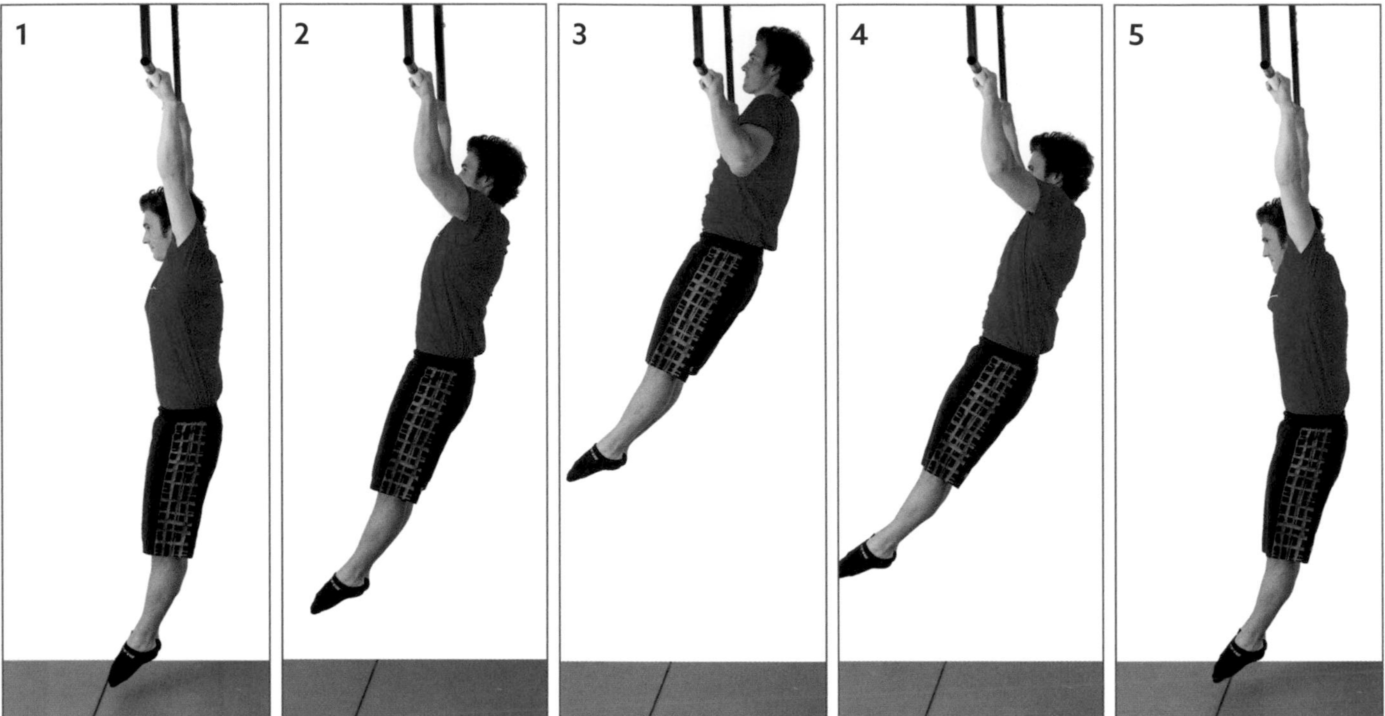

1. Establish a pull-up hook grip. Then brace your trunk by squeezing your glutes and pulling your ribcage down. Position your legs together with your toes pointed. This allows you to maximize tension in your glutes and core. Notice that Carl's back is flat, his ribcage is balanced perfectly over his pelvis, and his shoulders are screwed into the backs of the sockets (armpits forward).

2. Keeping your belly tight and butt squeezed, pull yourself up. To keep your torso and shoulders integrated, imagine pushing your feet forward as you initiate the pull. Don't make the mistake of disengaging your core as your torso deviates back.

3. With your pinkies still positioned over the bar, pull your chest to the bar—keeping your head in a neutral position. *Note:* If you can't raise your chin over the bar with your head neutral, stop. Don't try to throw your head back to complete the movement.

4. As you lower yourself to the start position, nothing should change: Your back is still flat, butt squeezed, belly tight, pinkies over the bar, head neutral, legs together, and toes pointed. As long as you maintain a braced neutral trunk and your grip stays intact, you don't have to think about breaking the bar—you will remain in a state of high torque.

5. Finish the movement the same way you started, in a good position.

Upper Back Flinch Fault

As mentioned, very few people are strong enough or have the necessary motor control to initiate a strict pull-up. To gain a mechanical advantage, athletes often tilt their ribcage back, unlocking their shoulders, and overextend their lumbar spine. This is also common with people who are missing internal rotation in their shoulders or are not comfortable with the hook grip. Rather than create torque, they keep their shoulders soft, which feeds slack downstream to the torso, making it easier to initiate the pull.

If your back, shoulders, and trunk are not on tension as you enter the movement, your body will hunt for stability. This is characterized by your ribcage tilting, elbows flaring out, shoulders rolling forward, and head cranking back—all the same faults you see with the strict press. Coincidence? I think not.

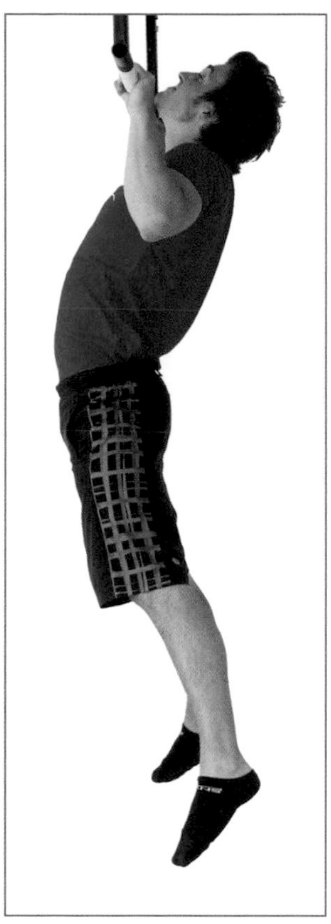

Overhead Archetype

This fault is associated with the overhead archetype. For a mobility fix, visit the overhead archetype prescription in part 4.

MOTOR CONTROL FIX:

Address grip mechanics: Make sure that your pinkies are positioned over the bar.

Squeeze your butt, pull your ribcage over your pelvis, position your legs together, and point your toes.

MOBILIZATION TARGET AREAS:

Thoracic spine

Posterior shoulders and lats

Anterior shoulders and chest

Downstream arms (elbows and wrists)

Cross-Leg Fault

As with the dip, a lot of people mistakenly set up for the pull-up by hooking their feet behind their body and bending their legs. This prevents your legs from flying apart, which happens when you're not strong enough to perform a strict pull-up, and allows you to pump your knees up to your chest to generate momentum.

This also occurs if you set up on a bar that is too low to the ground. Regardless of why you do it, this fault makes it impossible to engage your glutes and set your ribcage over your pelvis, putting you in an overextended position. If you start from an overextended position, there is no way to create torque and stability in your shoulders. So in addition to moving with a disorganized spine, your shoulders move up to your ears and your lats turn off. Put simply, you're hanging from unstable shoulder joints.

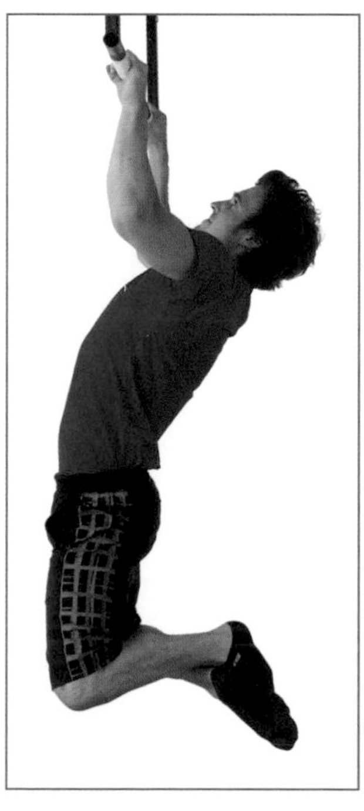

MOTOR CONTROL FIX:

Address grip mechanics: Make sure that your pinkies are positioned over the bar.

Straighten your legs, position your feet together, and point your toes. Squeeze your butt and balance your ribcage over your pelvis.

Chin-Up

The goal is to be able to create torque from any hand position and express a full range of motion with every movement. In fact, performing pull-ups with your hands in different positions is a nice way to test your understanding of the movement. However, you don't want to adopt a position that undermines your technique. For that reason, I recommend you start by learning the conventional palms-forward pull-up. It teaches you how to create torque, puts your shoulders in a stable position, and makes it easier to maintain a braced neutral spine. Once you're competent with a full range of motion overhead, test your position by implementing the chin-up.

If you're unable to lock out your arms and keep your ribcage down with a chin-up grip, there's a good chance that you're missing range of motion overhead.

Putting your arms in a position of full external rotation provides more stability because you don't have to actively hunt for tension. The problem is that externally rotating your hands makes it difficult to create torque at end range. Not only that, but if you can't get into an end-range start position, your elbows bend and your ribcage tilts, which is less than ideal. In addition to pulling from a compensated position, you're not expressing a full range of motion. (No wonder they're easier!)

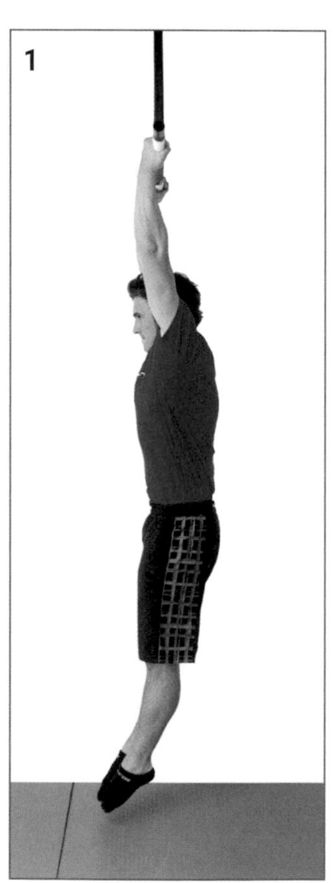

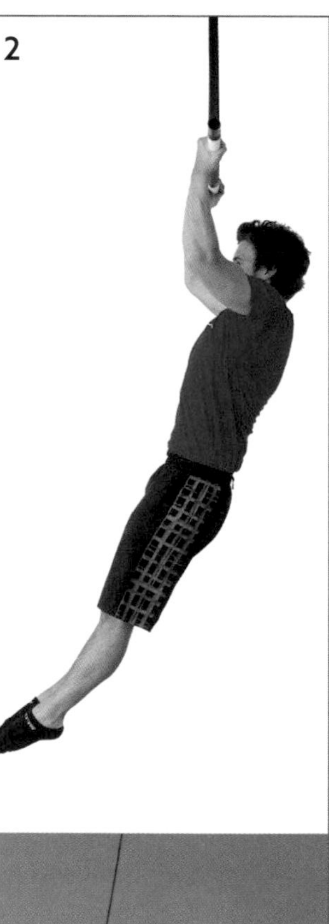

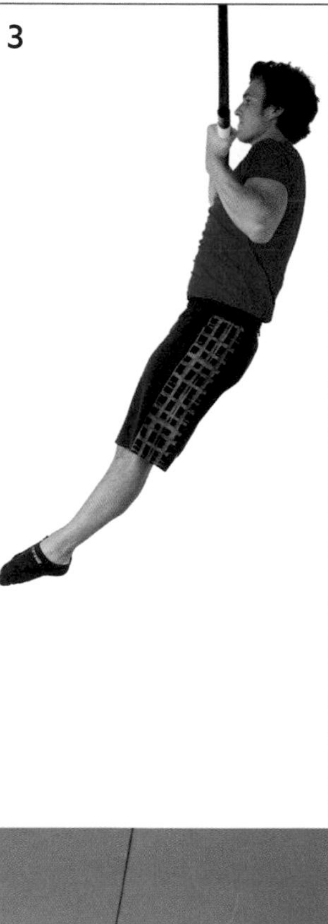

1. The setup is the same as for the pull-up: Squeeze your butt, position your legs together and out in front of your body, point your toes, pull your ribcage down, and keep your head neutral. Notice how Carl's shoulders are fully externally rotated. While this sets his shoulders in a good position, he will have to work extra hard to keep his ribcage down and his spine neutral as he initiates the pull.

2. Keeping your elbows tight, ribcage down, head neutral, and butt squeezed, pull yourself toward the bar. Think about keeping your legs out in front of your body as you lever back.

3. Pull your chin up over the bar. Keep your head neutral and avoid reaching for the bar with your chin.

POSITION OF HIGH STABILITY (PHS) → REMOVE CONNECTION → POSITION OF HIGH STABILITY (PHS)

CATEGORY 2 MOVEMENTS

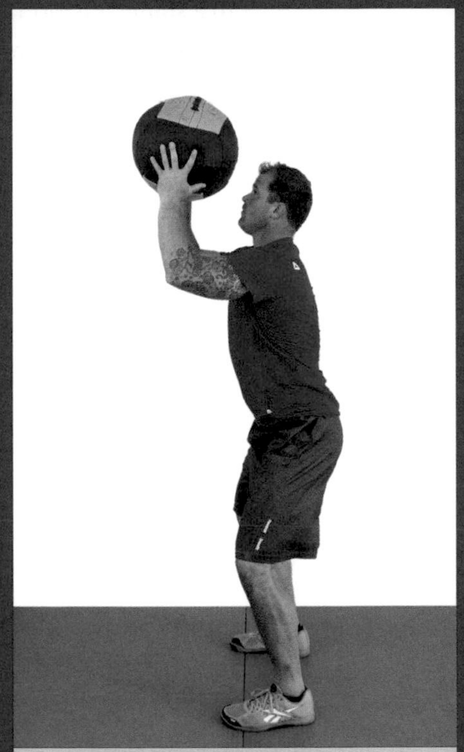

WALL BALL (P 234)

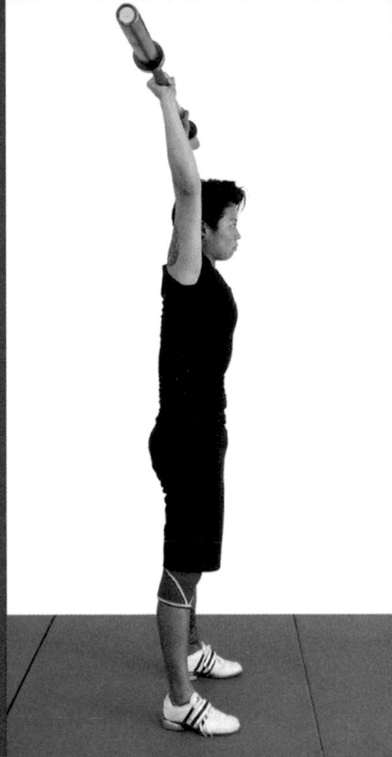

PUSH-PRESS (P 236)

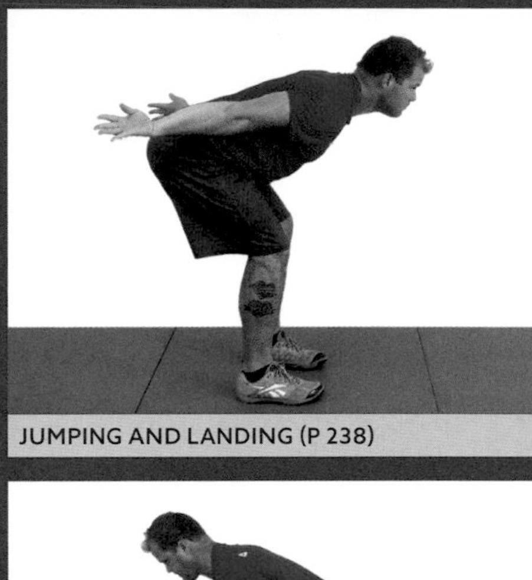

JUMPING AND LANDING (P 238)

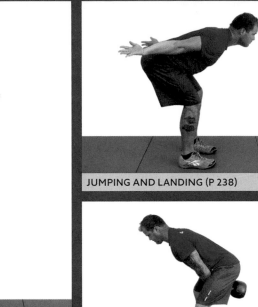

KETTLEBELL SWING (P 240)

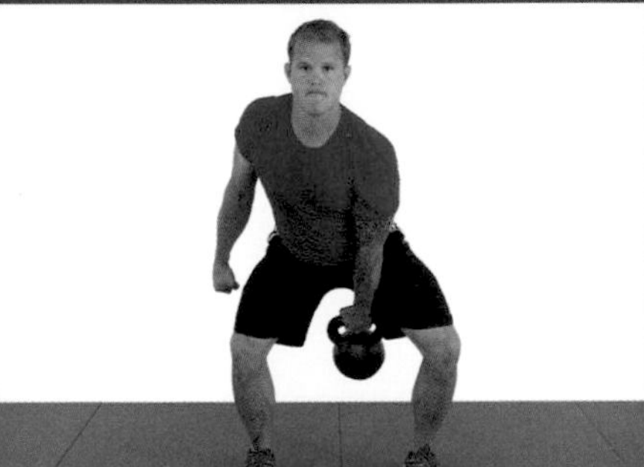

ONE-ARM SWING (P 246)

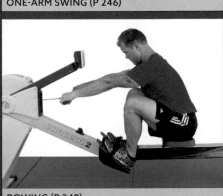

ROWING (P 249)

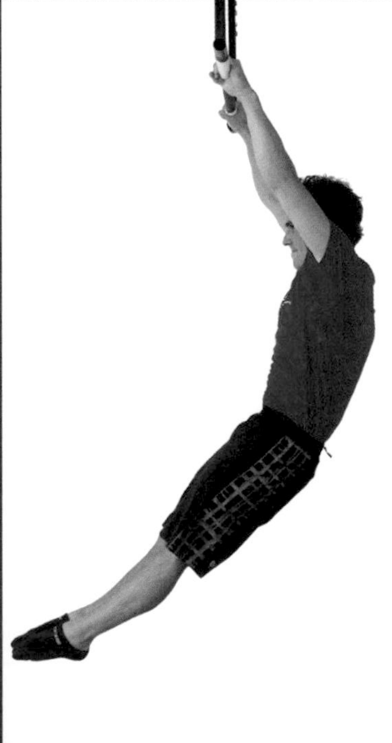

KIPPING PULL-UP (P 252)

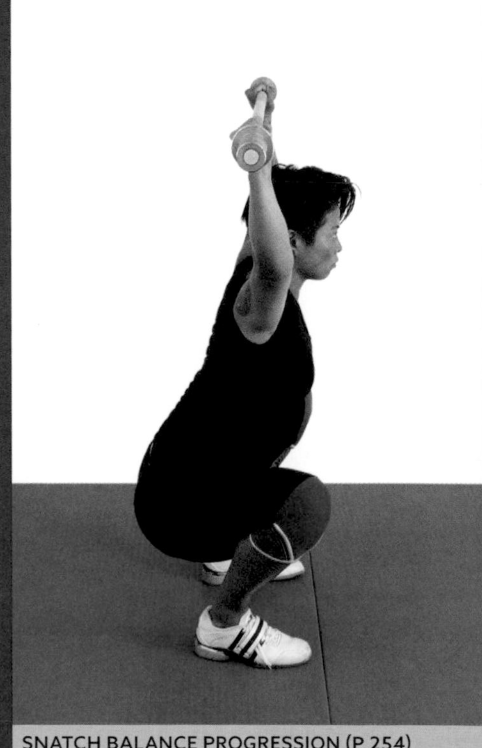

SNATCH BALANCE PROGRESSION (P 254)

Overhead Archetype	Front Rack 2 Archetype	Squat 1 Archetype
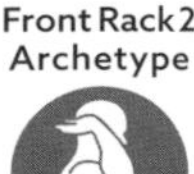	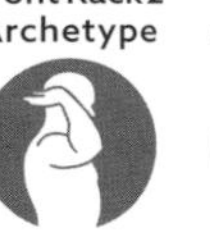	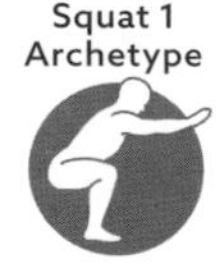

This movement contains the above archetypes. To improve common restrictions associated with this movement, visit the corresponding archetype prescriptions in part 4.

WALL BALL

As a quick recap, category 2 movements are similar to category 1 movements in that you start and finish in a position that allows you to cultivate trunk stiffness and torque. But instead of staying connected to the movement—meaning that you maintain torque and tension through the entire range of motion—you add a speed element and momentarily remove the connection.

The wall ball is one of the first category 2 movements that I introduce to novice athletes or to someone coming off an injury. It's a simple squat that adds a dynamic stimulus—throwing and receiving a medicine ball—while challenging the ability to maintain a vertical torso. It's a great way to assess motor control patterns and deficiencies.

Here's an example: Say you're training a novice athlete. He's now competent with the fundamental movement principles and category 1 movements. You've also challenged him under load with an upright torso. The next step is to introduce category 2 movements such as the wall ball. What you will find is that the moment he's asked to spontaneously create torque off an object that is not a barbell, everything falls apart. He will start overextending his lumbar spine, rounding his upper back, and driving

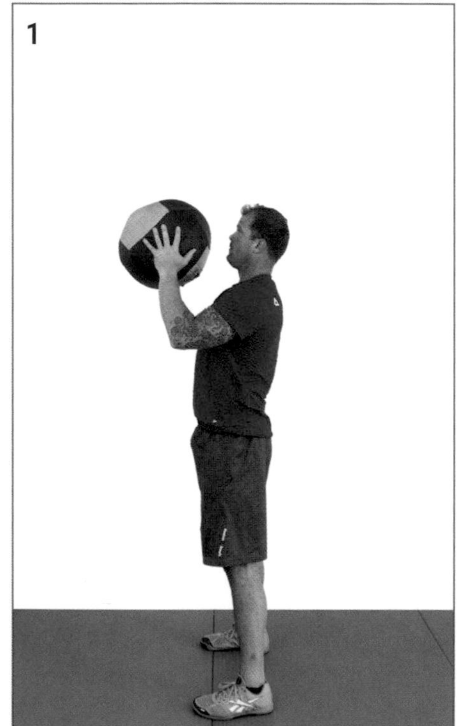

1. To set up for the wall ball, assume your squat stance with the medicine ball positioned at head level, screwing your hands into the ball to create a stable shoulder position. Stand far enough away from your target that you can receive the ball in the start position. In other words, you don't want the ball to fall in front of or behind you, but right at head level.

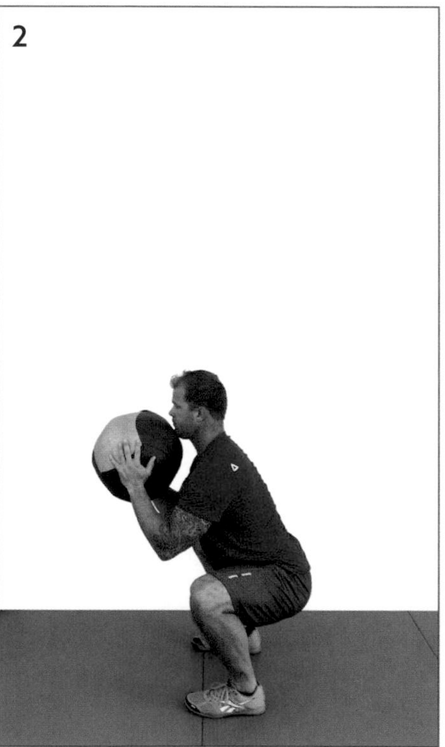

2. Keeping your torso upright, lower yourself into the bottom position just as you would when performing a front squat—see page 187. Keep your head neutral and focus on keeping your back flat. Don't try to crane your neck so you can see your target.

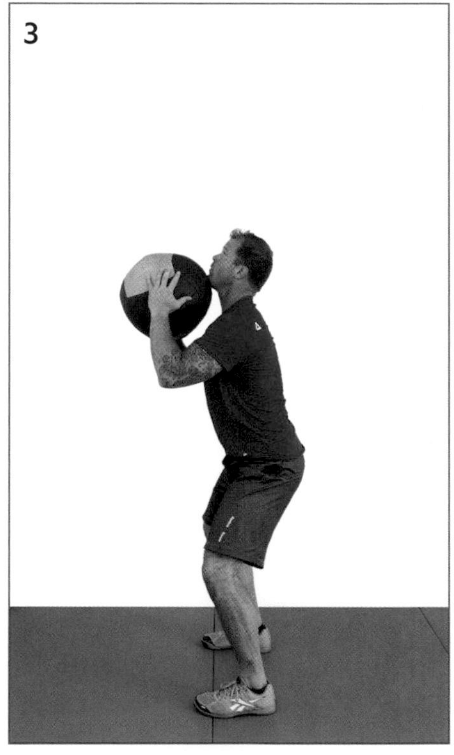

3. As you increase your elevation, focus your gaze on your target. Again, you don't need to throw your head back to do so. If you set up correctly, you'll be standing far enough away that you can see your target without craning your neck.

his knees forward. And the only thing you asked him to do was squat with a medicine ball, throw it toward a target, and receive it in a stable position.

Now, should the wall ball be part of every elite-level athlete's training program? Not necessarily.

This is the idea: By adding a speed element, you expose weaknesses in the athlete's profile in an environment where the chances of getting injured are very low. (You can also add a metabolic demand to the equation, making it even harder for him to disguise his poor movement patterns and mobility restrictions.) This is extremely useful for you as a coach because now you have a simple model for teaching the athlete how to transmit force from his hips to his shoulders. You can teach him how to spontaneously create torque in the bottom position of the squat as a progression to the Olympic lifts: If he can't receive an 8-pound ball in a good position, what do you think will happen with a 95-pound barbell? This is what makes the wall ball such a rich and useful movement.

Note: The common faults associated with the wall ball include forward inclination of the torso, internal rotation of the shoulders, overextension of the low back, and valgus knee collapse. Revisit the air squat (page 162) and front squat (page 187) for motor control and mobility solutions.

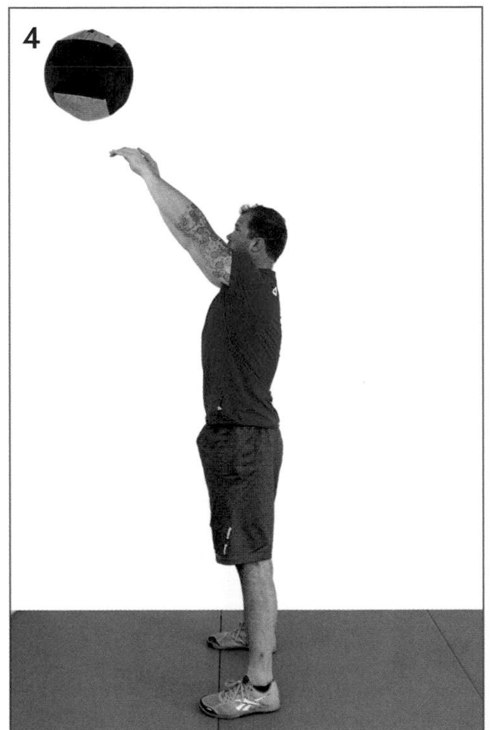

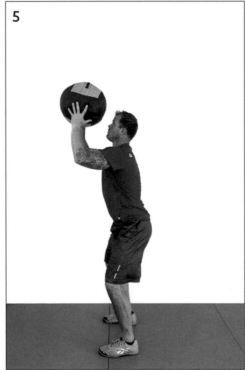

4. As you stand tall, extend your arms and throw the ball to the target. The key is to extend your arms equally. In other words, don't try to throw the ball like you're shooting a free-throw. A lot of people overcompensate with their dominant arm, which compromises their ability to receive the ball in a good position. Be sure to squeeze your glutes as you stand tall and reestablish a strong upright position before receiving the ball.

5. Receive the ball out in front of you in the exact same position in which you started. The idea is to receive the ball overhead and move down with the ball, screwing your hands into the ball to set your shoulders in a good position as you descend.

PUSH-PRESS

Overhead Archetype Front Rack 2 Archetype

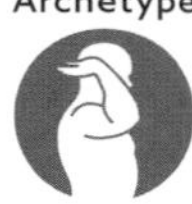

This movement contains the above archetypes. To improve common restrictions associated with this movement, visit the corresponding archetype prescriptions in part 4.

You set up for the push-press as you would for the strict press (see page 220). But instead of pressing the weight off your chest from a dead start, you bend and extend your knees to accelerate the weight overhead. The "dip and drive" addition of power enables you to handle larger loads. It also teaches you how to transmit force from your hips to your shoulders, a pattern that transfers to more complex movements, like the clean and jerk.

In the push-press, you don't have to generate as much torque in the start position because you're using the power of your legs and hips to press the weight off your chest. So if you have mobility issues that make the strict press rack position untenable, the push-press rack position will give you some breathing room and still allow you to go overhead.

Think of the push-press as a weighted vertical jump. In fact, the push-press is a great way to layer and teach upright-torso jumping and landing mechanics: If you understand how to dip and drive by shoving your knees out and keeping your back flat, you have a model for jumping and landing with a vertical posture that doesn't trash your back or your knees.

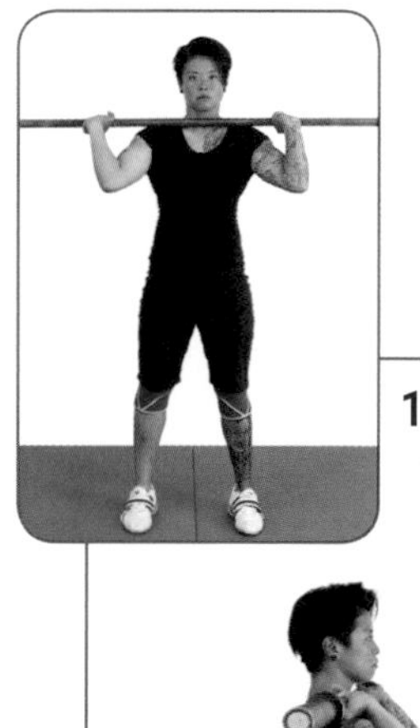

1

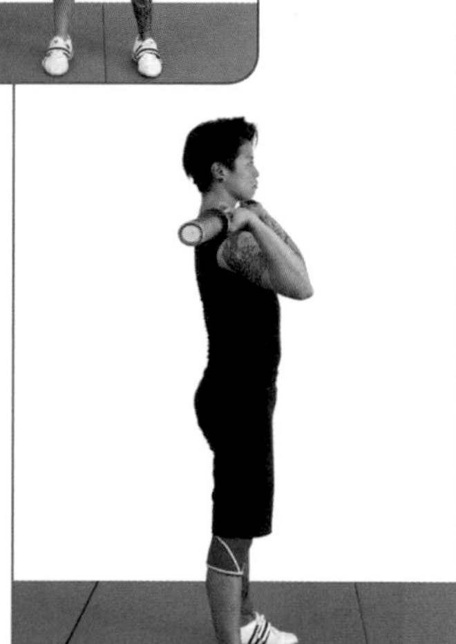

2

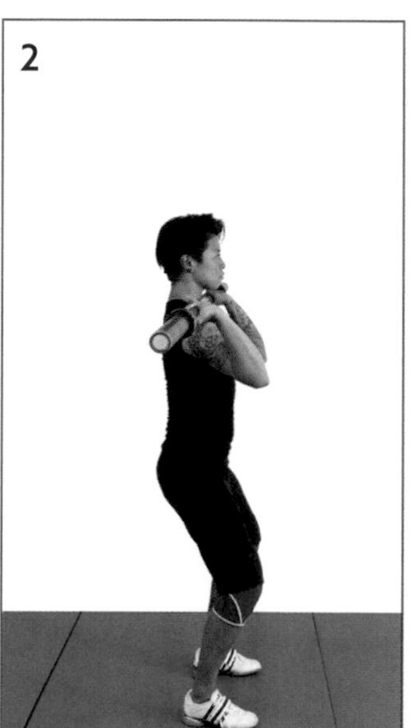

3

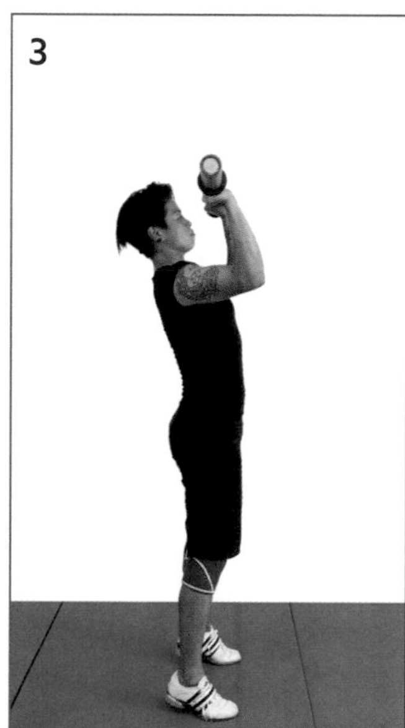

4

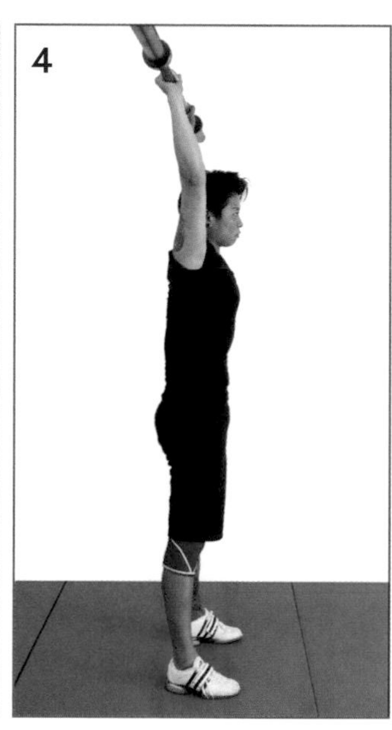

1. The setup is similar to the setup for the strict press: Establish your grip (same grip distance as the strict press), break the bar to set your shoulders in a good position, assume the front rack position, lift the weight out, walk back, and establish your stance. The same rules apply: Squeeze your glutes, get your belly tight, take a breath, and then go. As you can see in the photo, the push-press rack position is halfway between the strict press and front squat rack positions. Notice that Diane's elbows are positioned at roughly a 45-degree angle. The bar is positioned in the center of her palms, supported by her chest and shoulders. By keeping your elbows up, you can maintain enough torque to keep your shoulders in a stable position without the bar sliding down your chest as you dip.

2. Keeping your torso upright, drive your knees out laterally—screwing your feet into the ground—and lower your hips between your feet.

3. In one explosive movement, extend your knees and hips, move your head back slightly (just enough to clear your face while maintaining a vertical bar path), and press the weight overhead. The goal is to keep your posture as vertical as possible and keep your weight centered over your feet. If you roll up onto your toes, you will fall forward, and if you're on your heels, you'll roll backward. As the bar accelerates upward, maintain torque by keeping your elbows in and your shoulders back.

To help with your understanding, think of the dip and drive as the jump and lowering the weight as the landing. Most people have not been taught how to jump and land with good form.

Imagine jumping up for a rebound, spiking a volleyball, or performing a strength-and-conditioning circuit that calls for high-repetition box jumps and push-presses, like CrossFit's Fight Gone Bad workout. What happens when you don't have a model for shoving your knees out or keeping your back flat? You drive your knees forward and overextend. No wonder so many people suffer from insidious knee pain—commonly referred to as jumper's knee (patellar tendonitis)—after engaging in such activities.

Note: The most common faults associated with the push-press include driving your knees forward, overextending your lumbar spine, pressing the barbell out in front or behind your body, flaring your elbows out, and internally rotating your shoulders. To address the knee forward and overextension faults related to the dip and drive, revisit the air squat (page 162) and front squat (page 187). To address the pressing faults, flip back to the pushup (page 204) and strict press (page 220).

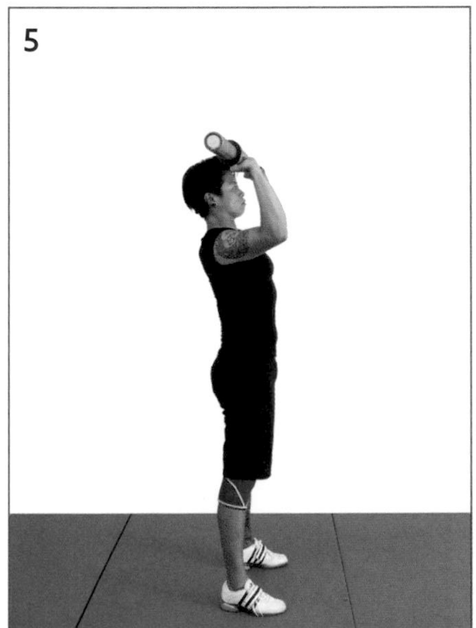

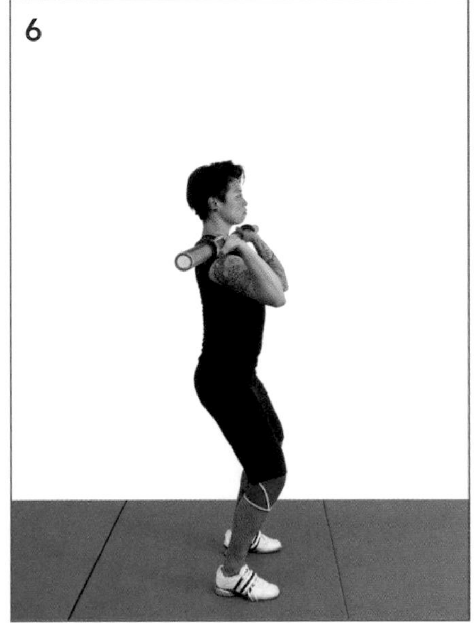

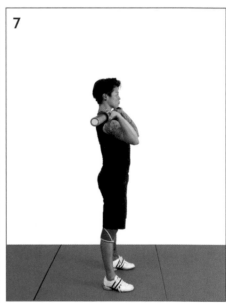

4. As you lock out your arms overhead, pull your torso and head underneath the bar. Continue to squeeze your glutes, maintain tension in your core, and generate torque in your hips and shoulders.

5. To lower the weight, pull your head and torso back slightly, keeping your butt squeezed to support your back. It's imperative that you continue to generate torque by keeping your elbows in and shoulders back.

6. Receive the weight onto your chest by dipping into a quarter squat. Shove your knees out, drop your hips between your feet, and reestablish the push-press rack position. It's extremely important that you consciously cultivate torque into the receiving position because it sets you up for the next rep. If you dump torque by letting your elbows flare out or your shoulders roll forward as you lower the weight onto your chest, you will start the next rep in a bad position. This is why it's important to perform high-repetition elements: because it teaches you how to create and maintain torque. Say you're doing a workout that calls for 15 push-presses. If you take the weight out perfectly, press one time, but fail to maintain torque on the way down, the next 14 repetitions will be done from a bad position.

7. Extend your hips and knees and reestablish the top position.

Squat 2 Archetype

Squat 1 Archetype

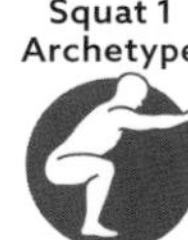

Overhead Archetype

Press Archetype

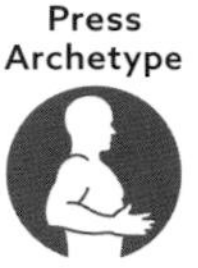

This movement contains the above archetypes. To improve common restrictions associated with this movement, visit the corresponding archetype prescriptions in part 4.

JUMPING AND LANDING

Jumping straight up and down, or even bounding forward from a square, stationary stance, is essentially an unloaded dynamic squat: You hinge forward from your hips, loading your posterior chain, create external rotation torque through your hips, and keep your shins as vertical as possible. We also see the same faults.

Some people drive their knees forward. If their feet are angled out, their ankles collapse, they commit valgus knee faults, they overextend at the lumbar spine, etc. The only difference with jumping and landing is that the consequences are much higher, especially if you're coming down from an elevated platform or combining a ton of jumping and landing sequences in a single workout.

Consider a sport like basketball or volleyball, where athletes put in countless jumping and landing cycles. Now imagine what will happen if they develop a knees-forward or open-foot or -knee error in their movement pattern. They're doomed. The insidious load on their knees is insane, and it's the mechanism for how they get jumper's knee. (*Note:* Jumper's knee is caused by an irritation of the patellar tendon, which connects the kneecap to the shinbone, due to forward and valgus translation of the knee during jumping and squatting movements.) It also invites ACL and MCL injuries.

Mobilizing and smashing the upstream and downstream tissues will certainly alleviate a lot of the irritation caused by jumper's knee and help you get into a better position. But the only way to fix this issue is to address the technique. With jumping and landing from a stationary stance, it's easy: Adhere to the movement principles and focus on keeping your knees neutral, shins vertical, and feet straight. And remember, squatting, pulling, and push-pressing movements are all great ways to build good jumping and landing movement patterns.

Note: If you are executing an upright-torso jump—rebounding a basketball, for example—remember that you have to drive your knees out (externally rotate from your hips) and create higher levels of torque to minimize the compression forces on your knees.

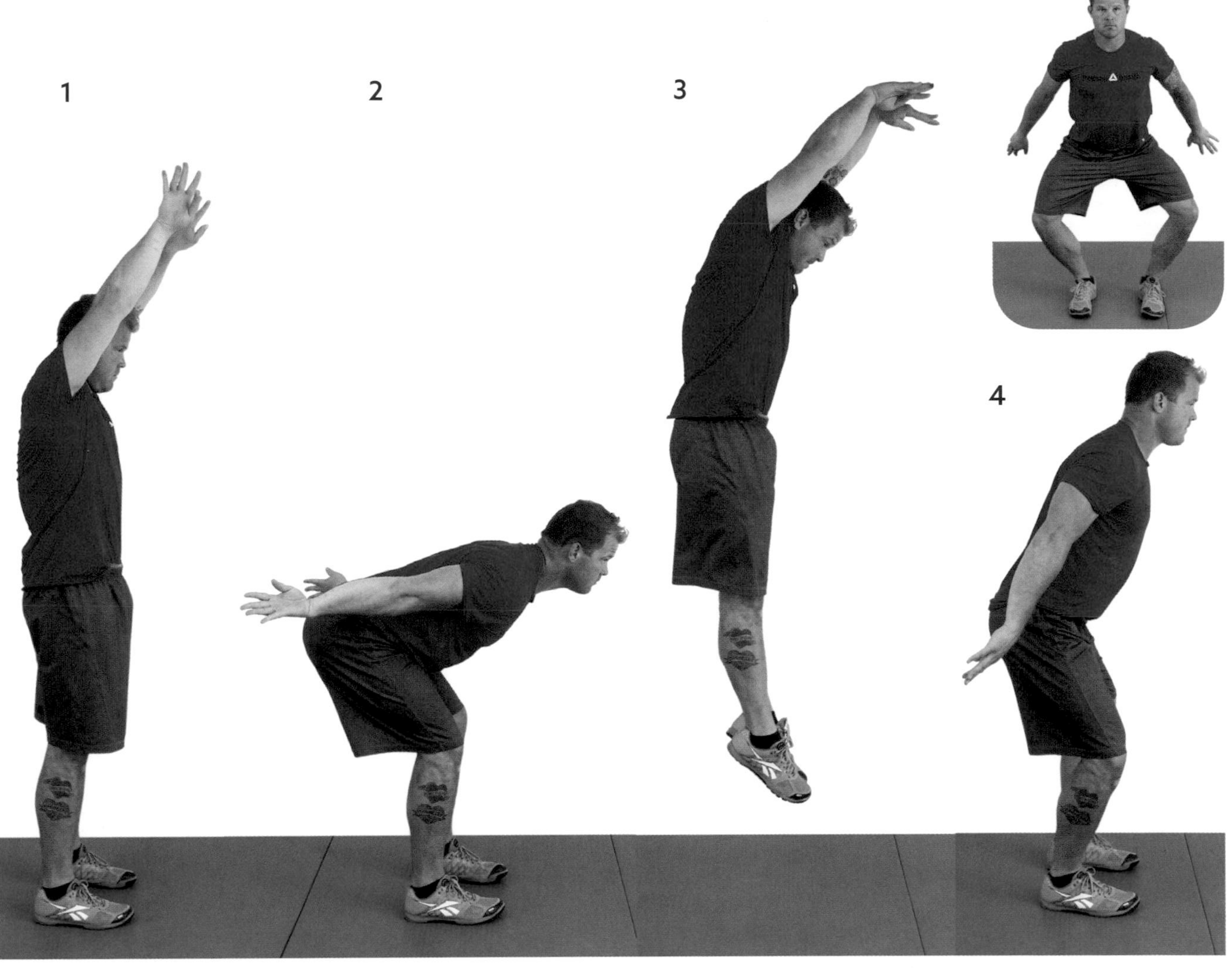

1. If you're trying to jump as high as possible from a stationary stance, position your feet underneath your hips, keeping your feet straight. Then go through the bracing sequence and raise your arms just overhead. Notice in the photo how my arms are internally rotated. This leaves my shoulders in a stable position, helping me keep my back flat as I tilt my torso forward and swing my arms back.

2. To load up for the jump, tilt your torso forward, loading your hips and hamstrings, screw your feet into the ground, and drive your knees out. Keep your shins as vertical as possible.

3. Swing your arms overhead while simultaneously extending your hips and knees. Notice that my legs are together and my feet are pointed. This allows me to activate my glutes and keep my spine organized while airborne. Pointing your toes also sets you up for landing on the balls of your feet, which is ideal.

4. As your feet touch down, create an external rotation force by driving your knees out and screwing your feet into the ground. Let your torso translate forward as you drive your hips and hamstrings back.

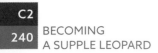

KETTLEBELL SWING

Squat 1 Archetype

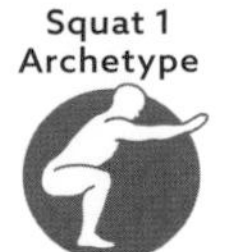

Squat 2 Archetype

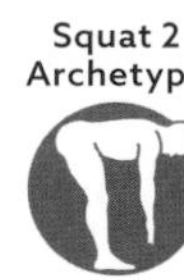

Hang Archetype

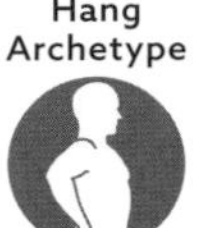

Overhead Archetype

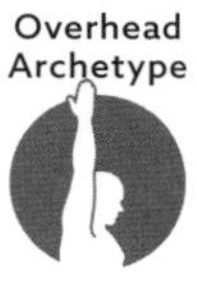

This movement contains the above archetypes. To improve common restrictions associated with this movement, visit the corresponding archetype prescriptions in part 4.

When it comes to learning complicated movements, the key is to make them uncomplicated. We do so by breaking them down into precise, manageable steps. Then we emphatically encourage like-your-life-depends-on-it focus in performing each step. This is the path to a tight learning curve. It's the foundation required for optimal performance. It also reduces the risk of injury.

Consider the back squat. Instead of teaching it as one movement, we break up the back squat into three distinct phases: the lift-out, the walk back, and the squat. This not only simplifies the movement and brings consciousness to each step, but also serves as a diagnostic tool. Right away, we can see if an athlete understands how to brace and create torque in the setup. If he fails to create torque off the bar and doesn't set his pelvis in a neutral position during the lift-out, we can work to correct that fault before he loads his spine. This is an extremely useful tool for us as coaches because we can start to correct faults before an athlete initiates a full-range movement.

The kettlebell swing is another example. In order to perform the actual swing, which is the focus of the movement, you first have to lift the kettlebell off the ground. This phase of the movement is no different from the beginning phase of a deadlift: brace, hinge forward at the hips with a flat back, create torque in the shoulders, and then stand up. It's telling that people fail to make this connection and immediately begin from a bad position by bending over with a rounded back, drive their knees forward, and lift the weight up with unstable shoulders. No wonder so many people struggle with the kettlebell swing. It's not that they lack the motor control or range of motion to perform the movement correctly; they just set up in a bad position.

This is why layering category 2 movements is so important: It allows you to see an athlete's default motor patterns when there is a dynamic stimulus. If you want to highlight why an athlete has jumper's knee, have him perform a kettlebell swing as a diagnostic test. In two seconds, you will see him drive his knees forward instead of pulling his hamstrings back, a fault that may have gone unnoticed in category 1 but gets lit up in category 2.

Russian Swing versus American Swing

Two different kettlebell swings commonly used in strength and conditioning circles are worth mentioning here: the American swing and the Russian swing. The former requires you to swing the kettlebell overhead, while the latter requires you to swing the kettlebell to chest or head level. Both iterations are extremely helpful in terms of assessing motor control and mobility, but they serve slightly different purposes.

The American swing obviously requires greater shoulder, trunk, and hip control, so it illuminates more faults than its Russian counterpart due to the increased range of motion demands. But you can't handle as much weight. And if you don't have a full range of motion overhead, the American swing will exaggerate bracing and torque faults (overextension in the top position, internal rotation in the shoulders). If you don't have a full range of motion, performing the American swing just to reach some arbitrary range is not a particularly brainy move.

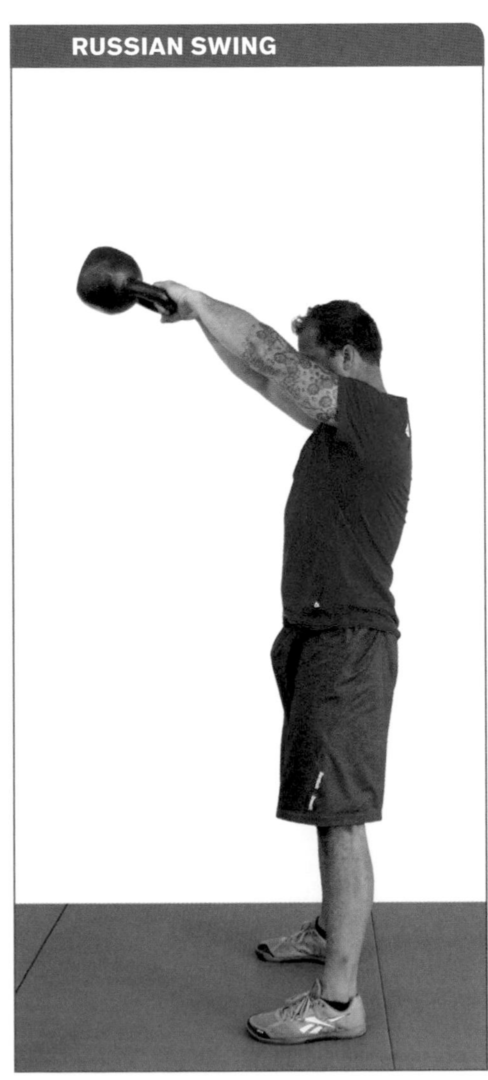
RUSSIAN SWING

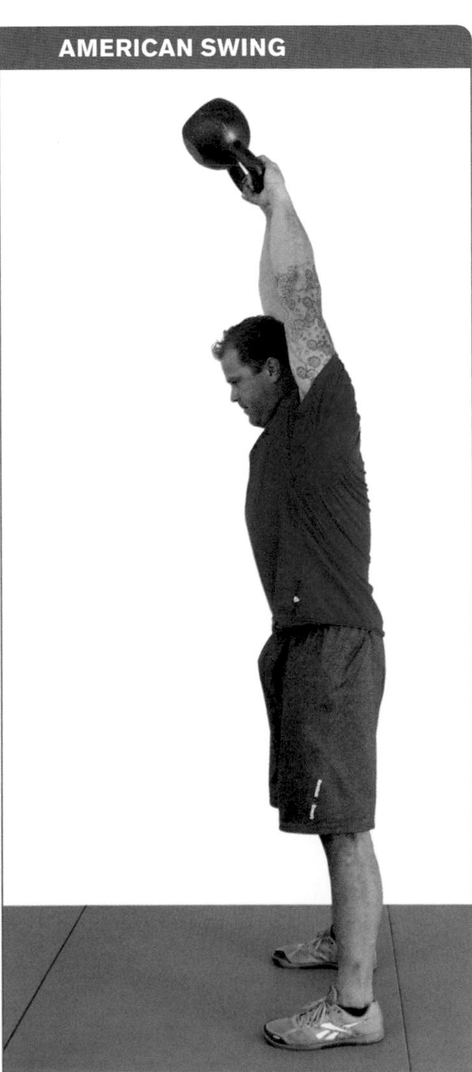
AMERICAN SWING

TOP-DOWN SETUP

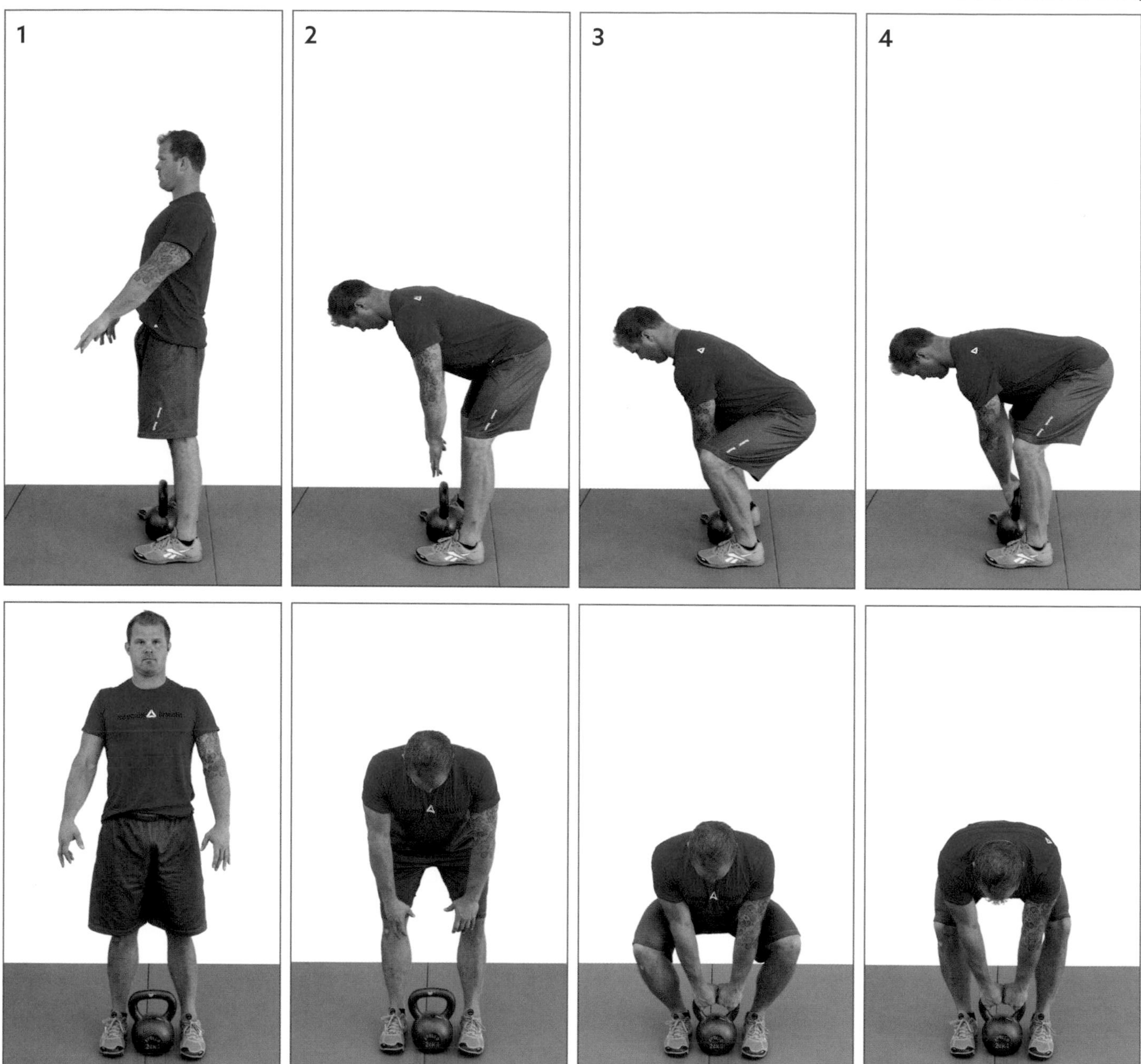

1. To set up for the kettlebell swing, follow the same top-down approach you would when performing a deadlift. Notice that my feet are straight at about shoulder width, my trunk is in a braced neutral position, and my shoulders are externally rotated.

2. Keeping your shoulders pulled back, shins vertical, and head neutral, drive your hamstrings back and bend over with a flat back.

3. As you reach end range, bend your knees and lower your hips—keeping your belly tight, shins as vertical as possible, and back flat—so you can assume your grip on the kettlebell. To set your shoulders in a stable position, create an external rotation force by screwing your hands into the handle. If you can't keep your shoulders pulled back because you're missing internal rotation, you can grip the outside of the kettlebell. (Keep reading to see this variation.)

4. To maintain a good position, you need to take out all the slack in your body and put tension back into the system. To do so, continue to drive your knees out, raise your hips, and get your shins as vertical as possible.

THE SWING

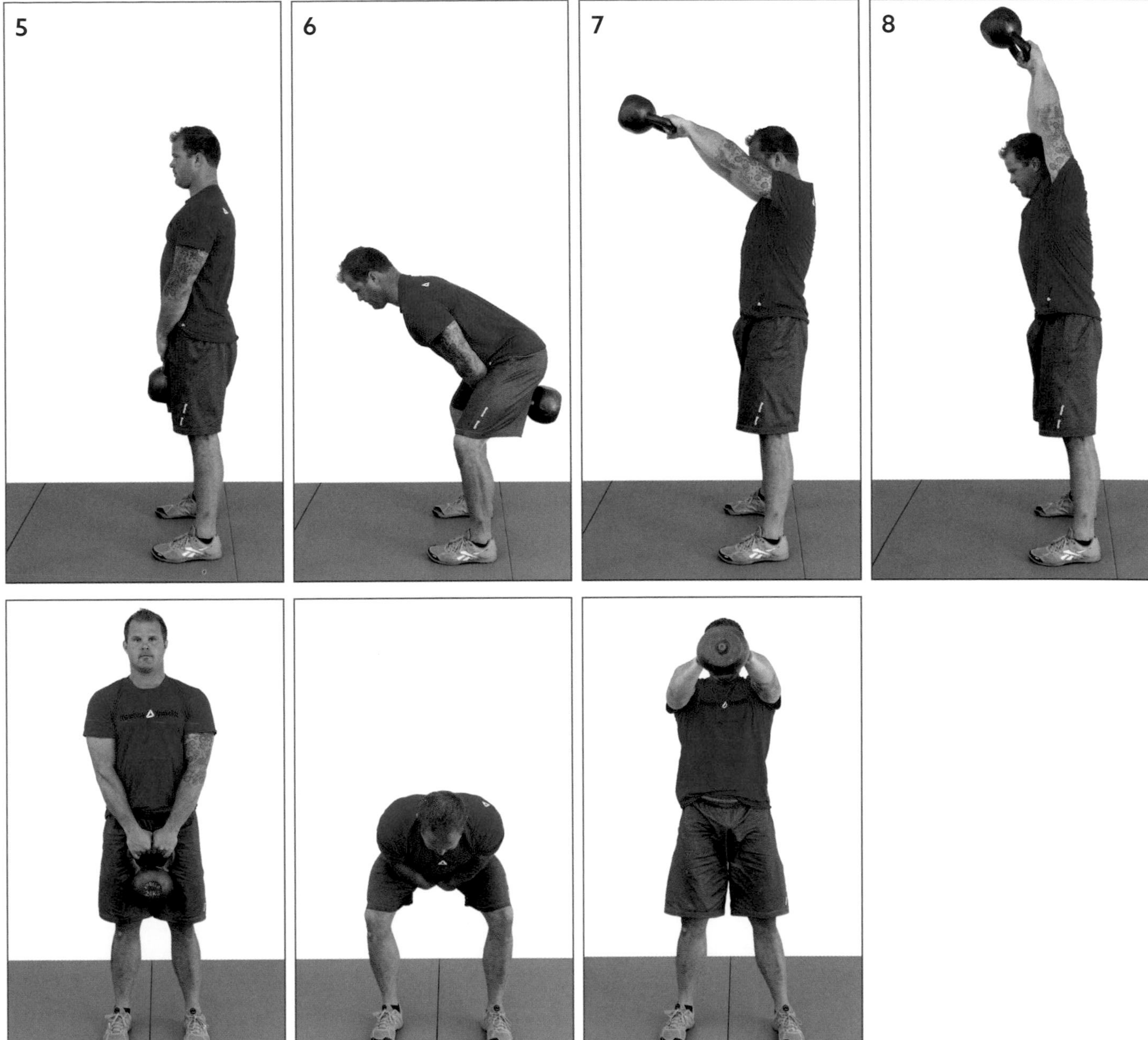

5. Deadlift the kettlebell into the standing position. As you extend your hips and lock out your knees, squeeze your butt in the top position, keep your shoulders pulled back, and screw your feet into the ground.

6. To initiate the swing, drive your knees out, sit your hamstrings back, and hinge forward at the hips. It's the same movement sequence as the first 6 inches of a low-bar back squat (see page 178). As you do this, hike the kettlebell between your legs. The key is to keep your head in a neutral position, shins vertical, and shoulders pulled back.

7. Keeping your weight distributed over the center of your feet, extend your hips and knees simultaneously, squeezing your glutes as you reach full hip extension. The idea is to drive your hips into your forearms and use this explosive hip extension to power the swing. Your arms should not deviate away from your body until your hips reach full extension.

8. Harnessing the power generated by your hips, raise your arms overhead. There is a moment of weightlessness, so take advantage of it by squeezing your glutes and organizing your position. From here, receive the weight the same way you initiated the swing, by pulling your hamstrings back—keeping your shins vertical and head neutral—and maintaining a rigid spine.

Torque Fault

Hang Archetype

This fault is associated with the hang archetype. For a mobility fix, visit the hang archetype prescription in part 4.

MOTOR CONTROL FIX:

Use the top-down deadlift setup to pick the kettlebell off the ground.

Screw your hands into the handle and pull your shoulder blades back.

MOBILIZATION TARGET AREAS:

Posterior shoulders and lats

Anterior shoulders and chest

If you fail to create torque off the kettlebell handle, your shoulders will compensate into an internally rotated position. This fault is easily fixed by addressing the top-down setup. However, if you're missing internal rotation in your shoulders, it's difficult to establish a stable position with a narrow grip. In that case, scale your grip by grabbing the outside of the kettlebell handle. This gives your shoulders some breathing room so that you can get into a good position. But remember, this is not normal. You shouldn't have to circumvent your poor mobility by scaling movements. Get to work on improving shoulder range of motion like it's your job.

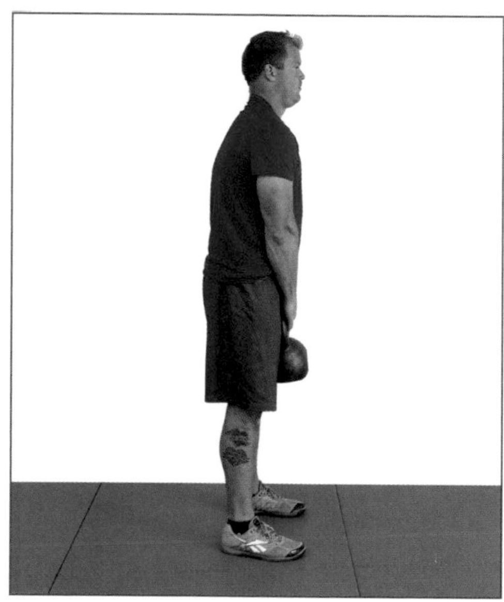

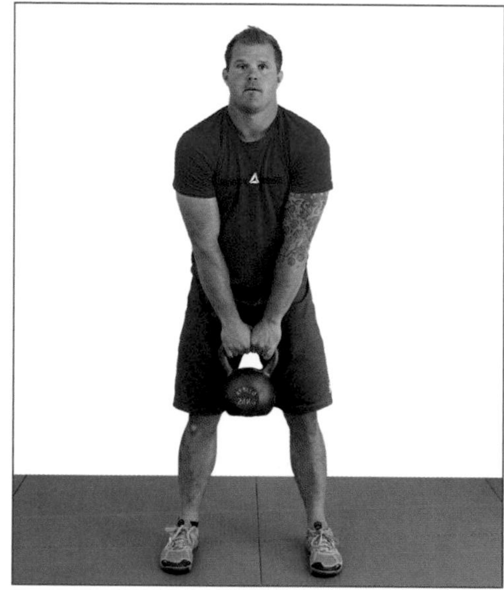

Scaling Your Grip

If you can't get your shoulders into a good position because you're missing internal rotation, you can buy yourself some breathing room by grabbing the outside of the kettlebell handle.

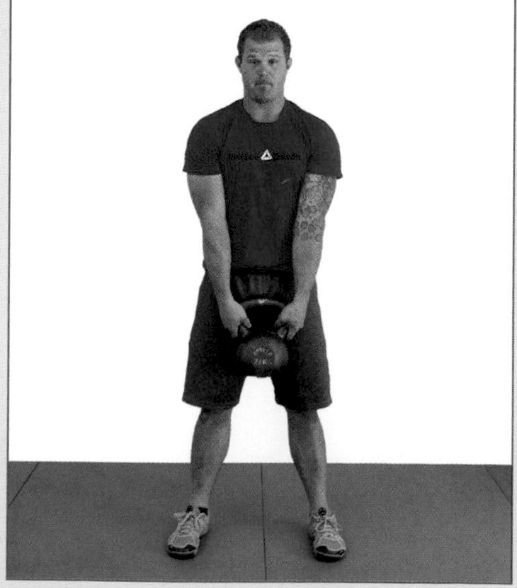

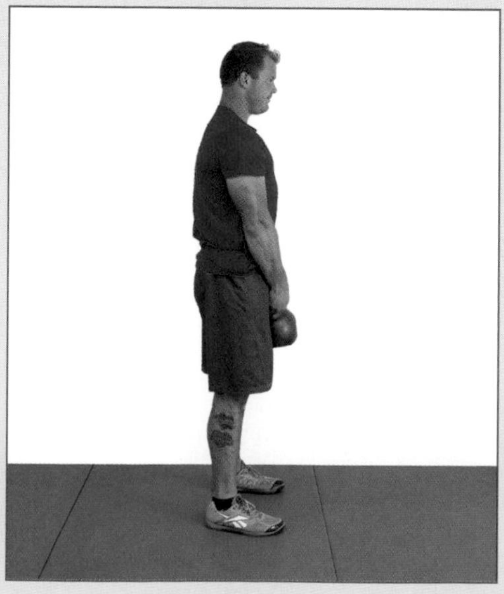

Head Fault

MOTOR CONTROL FIX:

Keep your head neutral and focus your gaze about 6 feet in front of your body.

Here's a common scenario: You set up perfectly for the kettlebell swing, but as you load your hips and hamstrings to initiate the movement (or receive the weight from the top position), you sacrifice your neutral spinal position by throwing your head back. In most cases, this fault occurs because you are fighting against the downswing, which pulls your torso forward. Throwing your head back is a way to counterbalance that force and avoid falling forward—see the hip hinge fault below.

Think about it like this: The kettlebell swing shares the same movement pattern as the first 6 inches of a low-bar back squat. The key is to keep your head neutral and focus your gaze on the ground about 6 feet in front of you. If you're looking straight ahead, you're more likely to commit this fault.

Hip Fault

MOTOR CONTROL FIX:

Don't chase the kettlebell with your torso, look down, or release tension after completing your last repetition. Control the weight down to the ground as you would with a heavy deadlift.

Another common fault is to follow the weight between your legs as if you were hiking a football. This happens when you fail to create torque or brace, or if you have a weak low back. In the photos below, I am demonstrating a grossly exaggerated version of this fault. However, it does happen, especially after the last rep. Instead of controlling the weight down, an athlete will count her last rep at the top position, release all tension in her shoulders and hips, and let the momentum of the weight pull her forward. This little gem is a great way to finish a workout with a tweaked low back. Remember, injuries often occur at the beginning or end of an exercise. Make the right decision and start and finish the movement in a good position.

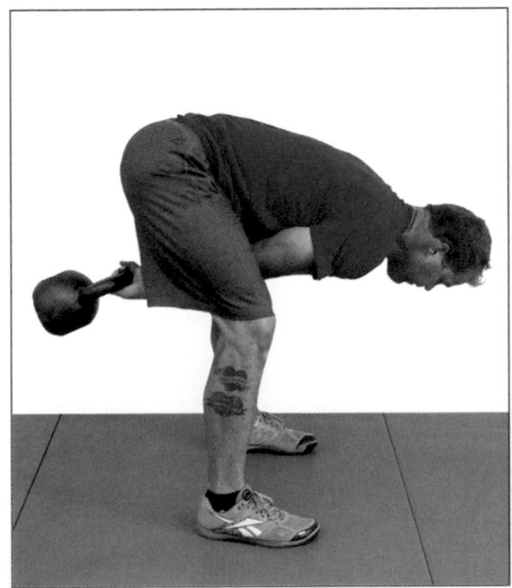

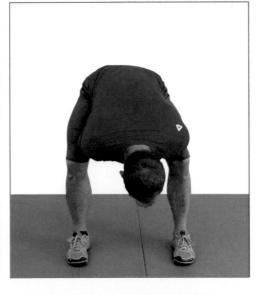

ONE-ARM SWING

In my opinion, the kettlebell is better suited to the one-arm swing than the classic kettlebell swing. The one-arm swing is a surprisingly challenging movement because there's a rotational element that makes stabilizing your shoulders and trunk difficult. For example, on the downswing, with the kettlebell swinging between your legs, the momentum of the weight pulls your shoulder into an internally rotated position. You have to resist that force to keep your shoulder back.

The one-arm swing also highlights your strategy for stabilizing your non-swinging hand. I know this is a mantra that I've been harping on throughout this book, but I'll say it again: If you don't create a stable position by bracing your spine and creating torque in your primary engines, your body will find stability

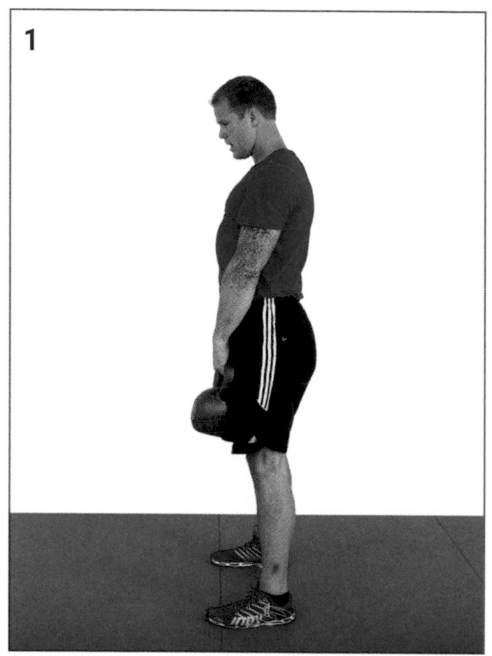

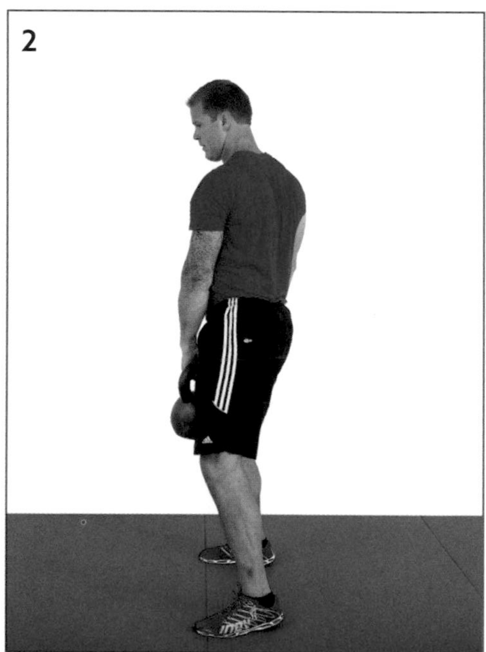

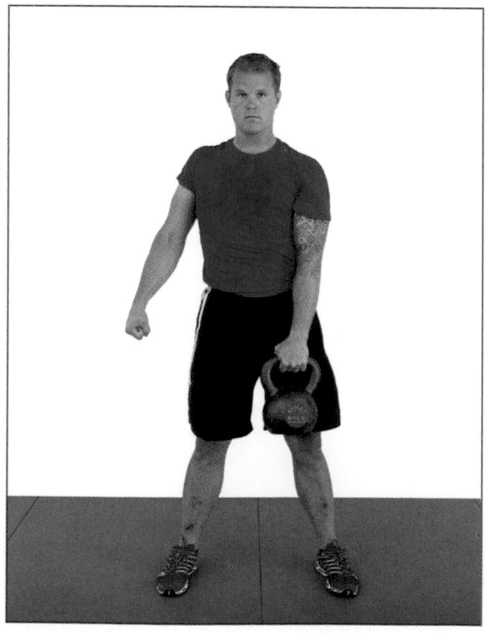

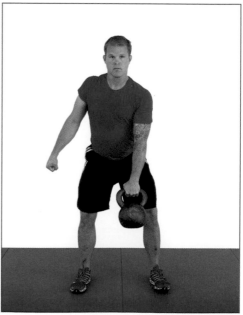

1. Follow the top-down setup as demonstrated in the kettlebell swing (page 242). But instead of gripping the kettlebell with both hands, grab the center or far end of the handle. Be sure to set your shoulder back and wind up your opposite arm to keep tension in the system.

2. Keeping your shoulder back and your torso upright, rotate your body toward your free arm and maneuver the kettlebell toward your center line. If you're holding the kettlebell with your left hand, turn toward your right side. If you're holding the kettlebell with your right hand, turn toward your left side.

somewhere else. You have to organize your opposite hand by making a fist or splaying your fingers, and wind your shoulder into the back of the socket. This idea carries over to all single-arm, unilateral movements, like one-arm dumbbell pressing, dumbbell snatches, and the Turkish getup.

The bottom line is this: It's much harder to create stability in a single shoulder than in two shoulders, especially when there's a dynamic element. You can't create torque off the implement, so it really highlights your understanding of fundamental movement patterns.

Note: The setup is exactly the same as the double-arm swing in that you use a top-down setup approach.

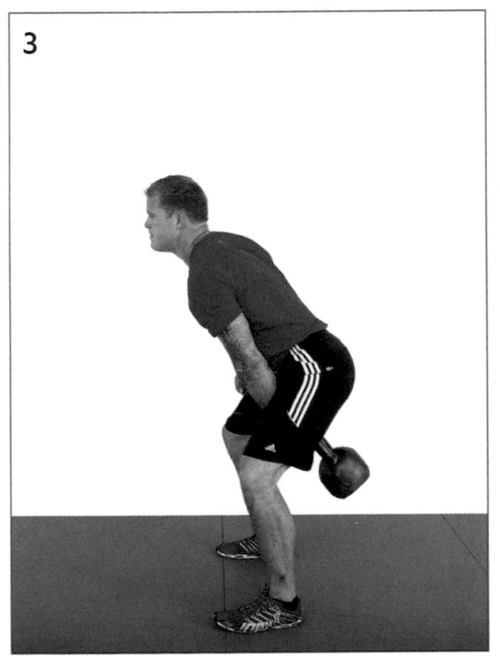

3

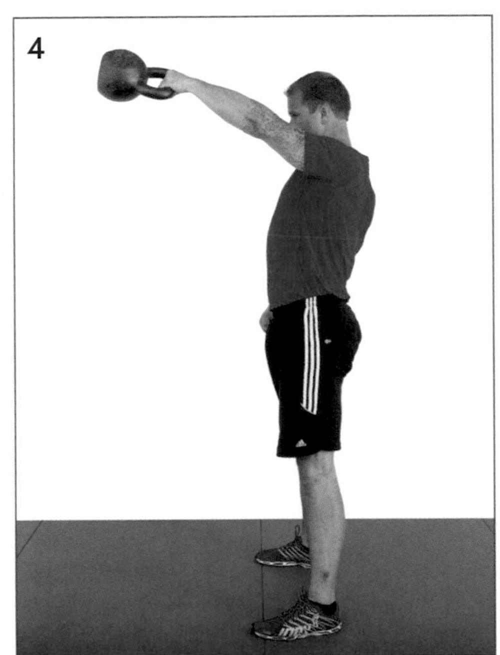

4

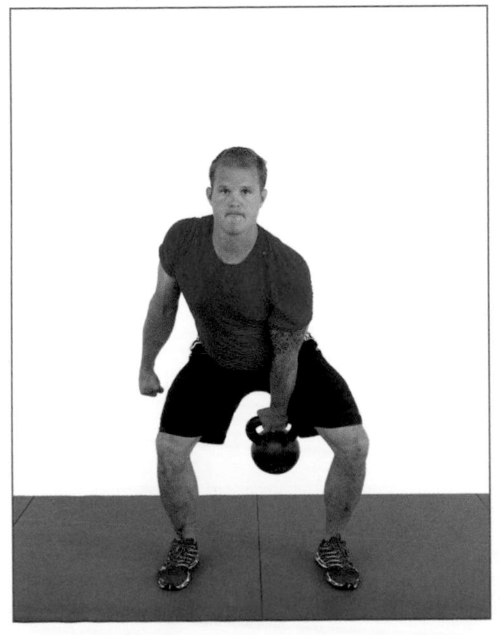

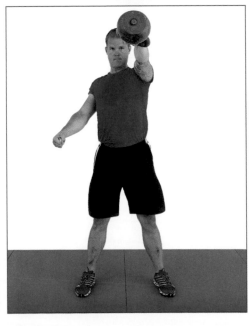

3. As you maneuver the kettlebell toward your center line, pull your hamstrings back—keeping your back flat, head neutral, and shins vertical—and hike the kettlebell between your legs. *Note:* Some coaches will tell you to internally rotate your hand in this step. Personally, I focus on keeping my knuckles forward because it allows me to clear my leg while still maintaining a stable shoulder position. If you internally rotate your hand, it's harder to keep your shoulder back.

4. In one explosive movement, extend your hips and knees. As with the classic double-arm swing, think about driving your hips into your arm so you can effectively transmit force from your hips to your shoulder.

MOTOR CONTROL FIX:

Keep your head neutral and focus your gaze about 6 feet in front of your body.

Unstable-Shoulder Fault (Hook-Hand Fault)

As I just mentioned, if you don't organize your free arm, it will contort into some strange positions—often characterized by a hook hand and grossly internally rotated shoulder. In addition to looking really weird, it creates an open circuit fault, which travels through the kinetic chain and makes it difficult to create and maintain stability.

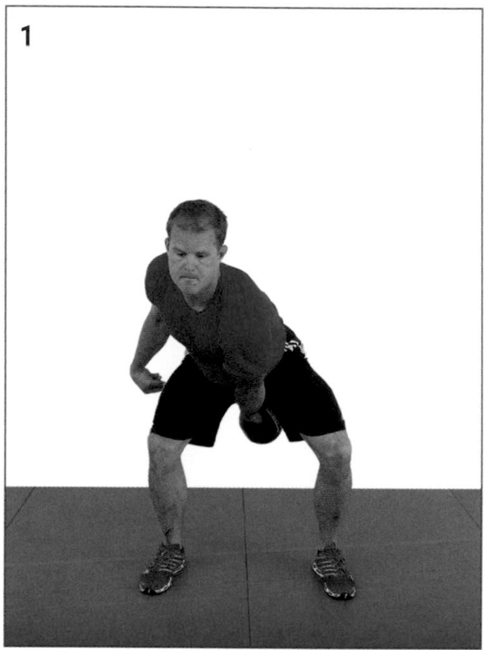
1

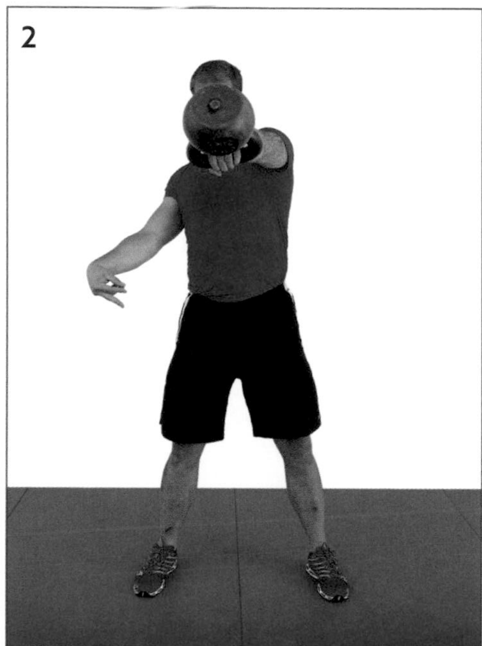
2

ROWING

If you know how to deadlift with good form, rowing is simple. The two movements share the same load order sequence and start position. So if I tell you to row 1,000 meters, I want you to think 60 to 80 deadlifts. This not only makes it easier to sequence the right movement patterns, but also brings consciousness to each stroke.

Unlike the deadlift, however, rowing is a low-resistance, high-repetition exercise. In addition to adding speed, timing, and a metabolic stimulus, you have to reconstitute the same start and finish position over and over again. This is what makes rowing a minefield.

Introduce speed and people start falling apart. Although the consequences of rowing in a bad position are not as immediate as deadlifting with bad form, there's a cumulative effect. For example, say your ankles collapse every time you pull and return the handle to the start position. If you're rowing at 30 strokes a minute for 20 minutes, that's 600 collapsed ankle compressions. You may get away with it for a while, but injuries will result over the long haul. It also ingrains poor movement patterns.

Here are the key takeaways of rowing:

1. Rowing highlights ankle, posterior chain, and hip flexion range of motion.
2. You can identify load-sequencing errors. It's easy to see if someone is loading his low back and rounding forward instead of keeping his spine rigid and assigning tension into his hips and hamstrings.
3. It helps strengthen your understanding of this principle—namely, if the positioning of your head, shoulders, or spine is off, it's impossible to perform the movement with good form.
4. It tests your coordination and ability to repetitively generate force from the same position.

Note: A lot can be said about the technical aspect of rowing, especially the timing, but breaking into the minutiae of things like stroke rate is beyond the scope of this chapter. My intention is to drive home the relationship of bracing, torque, and movement transferability as it relates to functional movements.

Squat 1 Archetype
Squat 2 Archetype

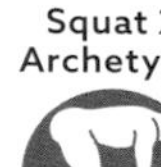

Front Rack 1 Archetype
Press Archetype

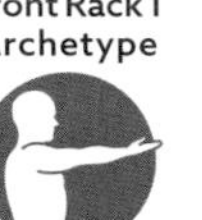

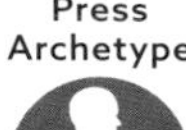

This movement contains the above archetypes. To improve common restrictions associated with this movement, visit the corresponding archetype prescriptions in part 4.

DEADLIFT SETUP

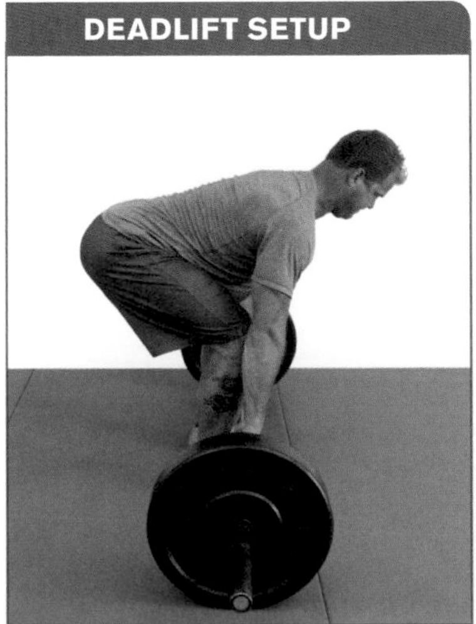

ROW SETUP

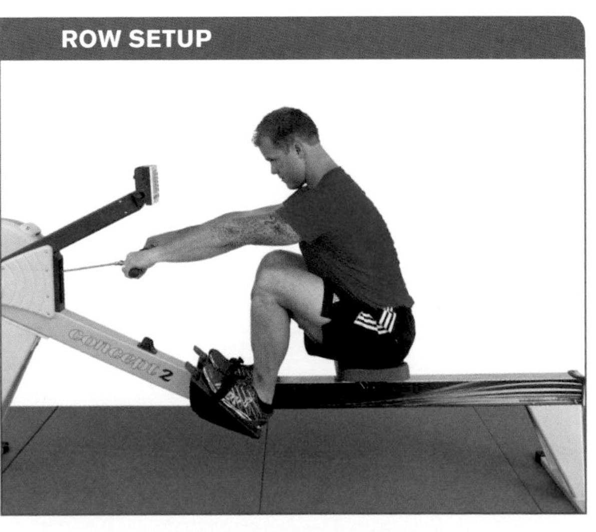

The setup for the row is nearly identical to the deadlift.

To set up for rowing, first adjust the footboards so the straps wrap around the base of your toes. Tighten the straps around your feet, grab the oar handle with both hands, straighten your legs, and slide your seat back on the monorail. (The idea is to take some of the compression forces off your pelvis so you can flatten your back.) With your legs straight, sit tall, flatten your back, and then pull your shoulder blades together and screw your hands into the handle. To maximize torque, hook your thumbs around the handle. Keeping your back flat, head neutral, and shoulders back, drive your knees out and slide your hips and seat forward, allowing your torso to deviate forward slightly. As with the deadlift, you want your shins vertical and hips loaded.

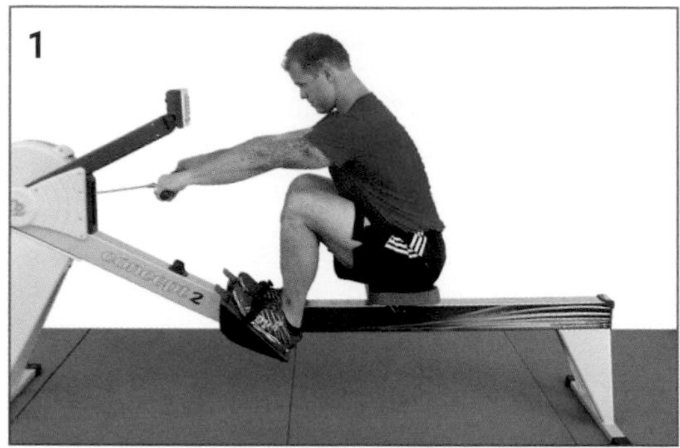
1

Keeping your arms straight while still creating torque off the handle, extend your knees, lean back slightly, and drive your hips back. To help maintain a neutral head position, focus your gaze on the chain.

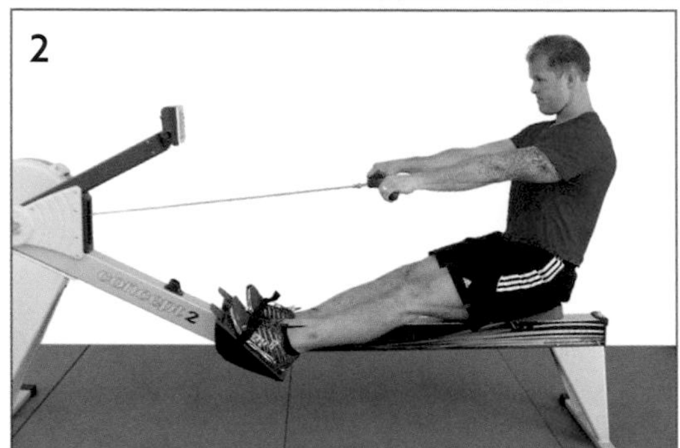
2

As you extend your knees, pull the oar handle to your sternum. Notice that my forearms are nearly horizontal and my shoulders are pulled back. If you flipped the photo 90 degrees counterclockwise, it would look a lot like the bottom of a dip. Many of the same rules apply. You want to keep your shoulders back, head neutral, and wrists aligned with your elbows.

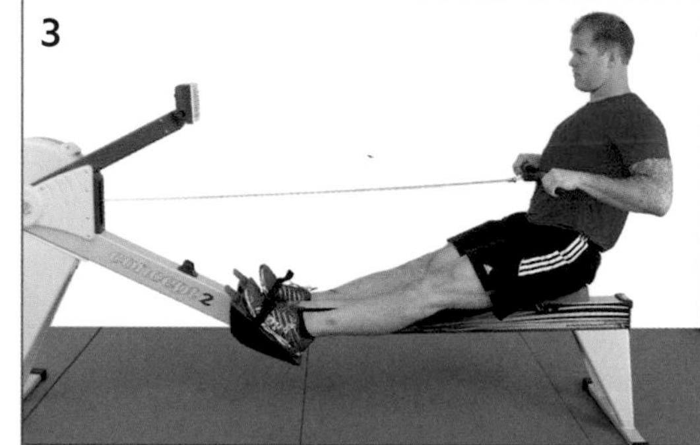
3

After a momentary pause, straighten your arms. Although this is technically referred to as the recovery phase, you still want to create torque off the handle and keep your shoulder blades pulled back.

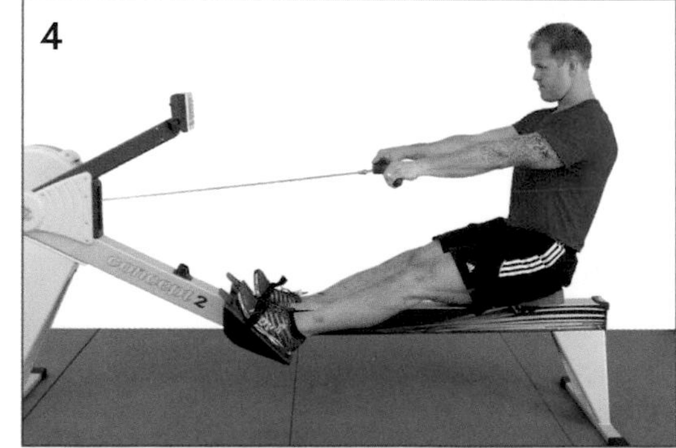
4

As your hands track over your knees, hinge forward at your hips, allowing your torso to tilt forward, and slide your hips toward your heels. You should arrive in the same position in which you started.

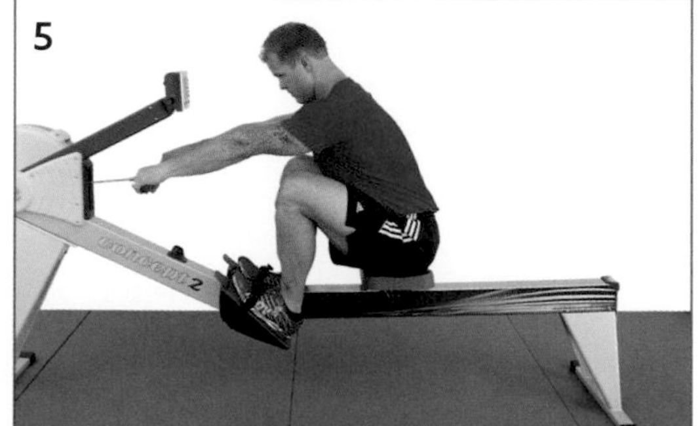
5

Head, Spine, and Shoulder Fault

Once you surrender your head position, your back will round and your shoulders will go soft. If that happens, force transmits to your back instead of your hips and your shoulders internally rotate, affecting the power of your pull. Other factors that can contribute to this fault include missing shoulder range of motion and a tight thoracic spine.

Press Archetype

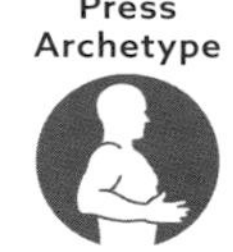

This fault is associated with the press archetype. For a mobility fix, visit the press archetype prescription in part 4.

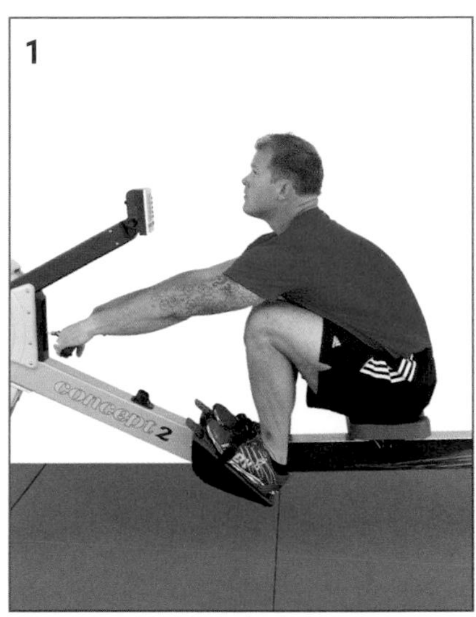

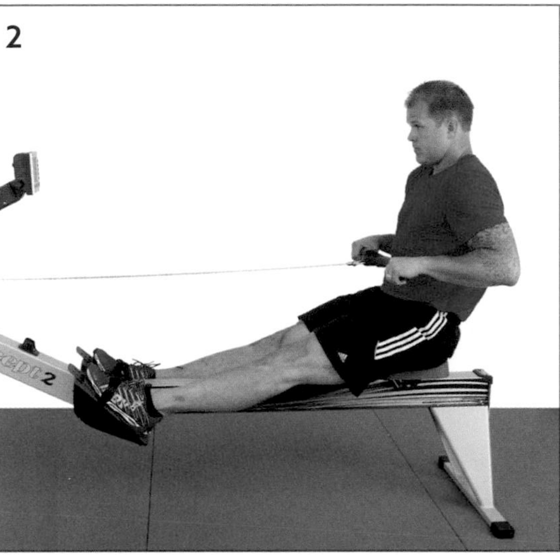

MOTOR CONTROL FIX:

Pull your shoulder blades together and screw your hands into the oar handle to generate torque.

To maintain a neutral head position, focus your gaze on the chain.

Keep your back as flat as possible and your shins vertical.

MOBILIZATION TARGET AREAS:

Anterior shoulders and chest

Posterior shoulders and lats

Thoracic spine

Sequencing Faults

The start position and initial pull phase of the row are similar to the deadlift in that you simultaneously extend your knees and hips. However, due to the speed and timing element of rowing, a lot of athletes struggle with this sequence. Rather than move the body as a single unit, they either drive their hips back, leaving their torso forward, and pull with their back, or they lean back, leaving their knees bent, and pull with their arms.

This also happens during the recovery phase—when they return the oar handle to the start position—but in the opposite order. They leave their hips back and lean their chest forward, or they bend their knees before they straighten their arms, forcing them to move the oar handle over their legs. Regardless of the order or phase at which these sequencing faults occur, they disrupt rhythm, compromise force, and can cause a ton of problems up and down the athletic chain.

MOTOR CONTROL FIX:

Move your body as a single unit and focus on extending your knees and hips at the same time.

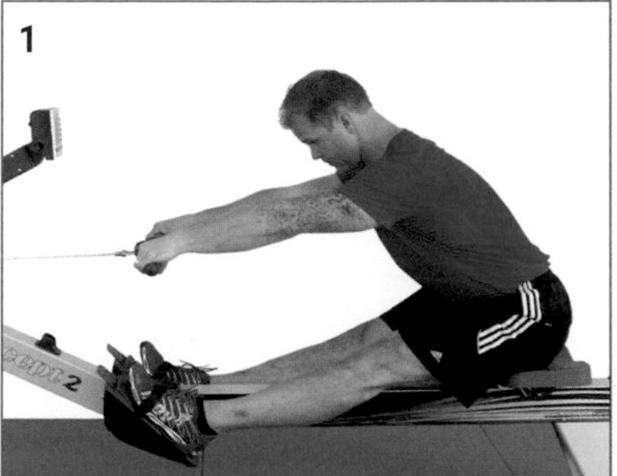

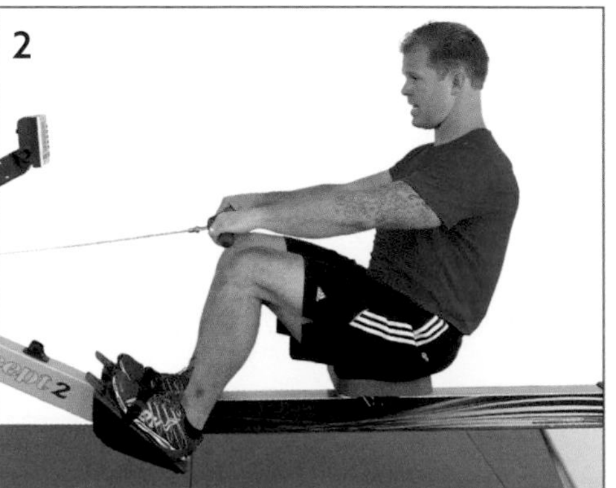

Overhead Archetype   Front Rack 2 Archetype

This movement contains the above archetypes. To improve common restrictions associated with this movement, visit the corresponding archetype prescriptions in part 4.

KIPPING PULL-UP

The kipping pull-up is a gymnastics-based technique that combines a back-and-forth horizontal swing with a pull. The swing is powered by a leg kick and hip drive. The idea is to harness momentum along a horizontal plane to make it easier to raise your chin over the bar.

A lot of strength and conditioning pundits criticize the kipping pull-up as being unsafe. And they're right, but only if it's done incorrectly. The simple fact is, kipping allows you to execute more repetitions in a shorter span of time, but it will wreak havoc on your shoulders, elbows, and low back if performed improperly.

So how do you kip without inviting injury?

First, you need to have full range of motion in your shoulders, meaning that you can hang from the bar with your elbows straight, armpits forward, and spine in a braced neutral position—see the overhead archetype Basic Quick Test on page 100.

Second, you need to start with the strict pull-up (see page 229) and address the basics before you start swinging from the bar. Once you have a fundamental

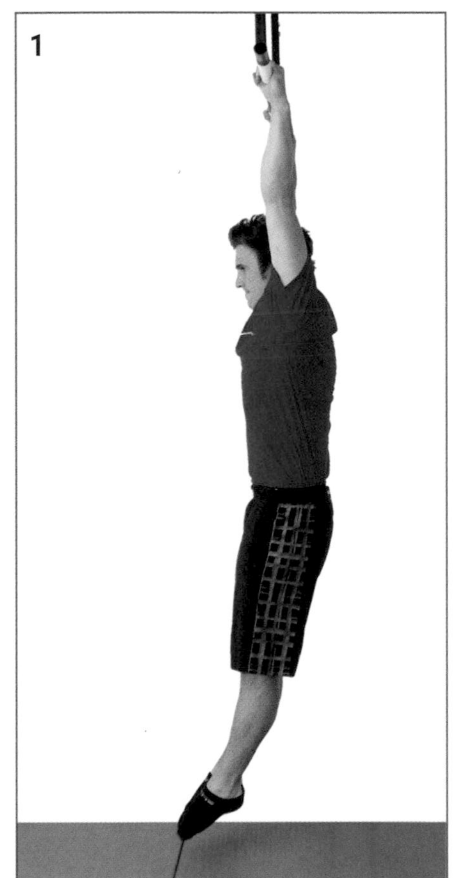

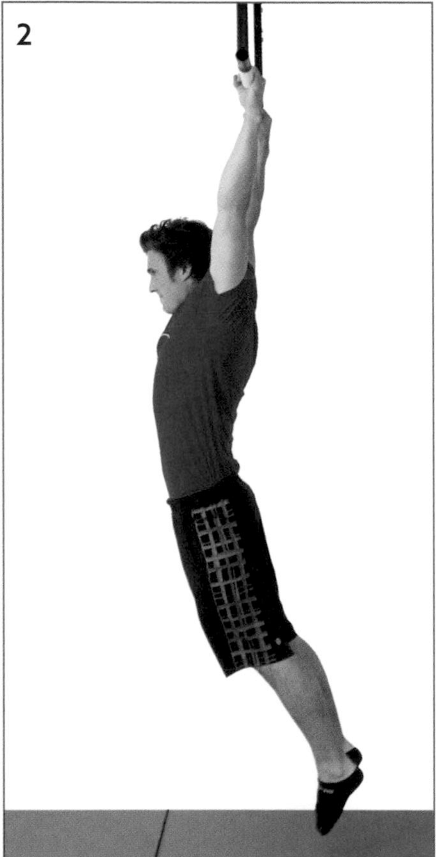

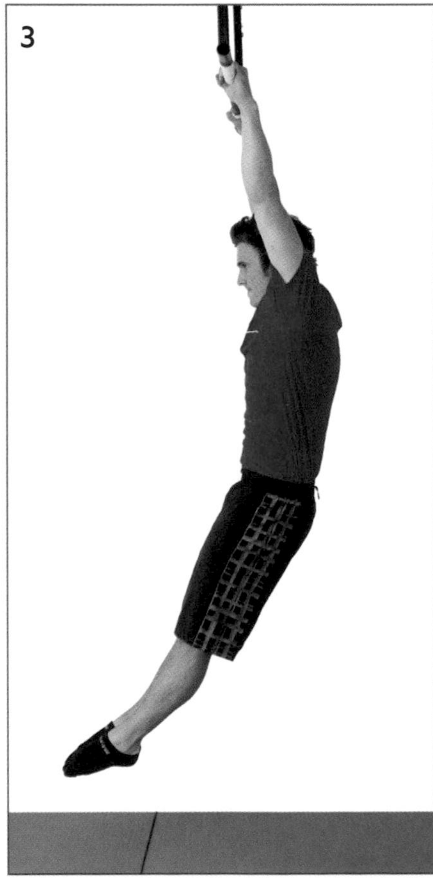

1. Jump up to the bar and establish a pull-up hook grip (see page 229). With your elbows straight and your armpits forward, squeeze your glutes, pull your ribcage down, and get your belly tight. Position your legs together and point your toes.

2. Keeping your butt squeezed, armpits forward, and legs together, kick your legs back and pull your head and chest underneath the bar. Squeezing your glutes prevents you from overextending your low back. Notice that Carl is in a globally arched position. Although his back is in extension, his spine is protected.

3. With your armpits forward and your elbows locked out, swing your legs forward and push away from the bar.

understanding of how to form your grip and organize your body in a good position, you can start to layer the kip not only as an exercise, but also as a way of assessing shoulder mobility and motor control. Say your elbows bend and shoulders roll forward while swinging from the bar. That's a good sign that either you don't understand how to set up and swing, or you're missing end-range shoulder flexion, internal rotation, or thoracic extension.

Another reason the kip is such a useful movement is that it fits into our model of movement transfer exercises. In the photos below, notice that the back swing exaggerates a movement pattern that is expressed in a lot of sports, specifically throwing motions. For example, a tennis player's serve, a volleyball player's spike, and a baseball player's pitch all mirror the action of the kipping pull-up. In addition, the dynamic opening and closing of the hips used in the kip is similar to Olympic lifting techniques, like the clean and snatch. The hip action of the kip is also a building block to other gymnastic movements, like the muscle-up (see page 280).

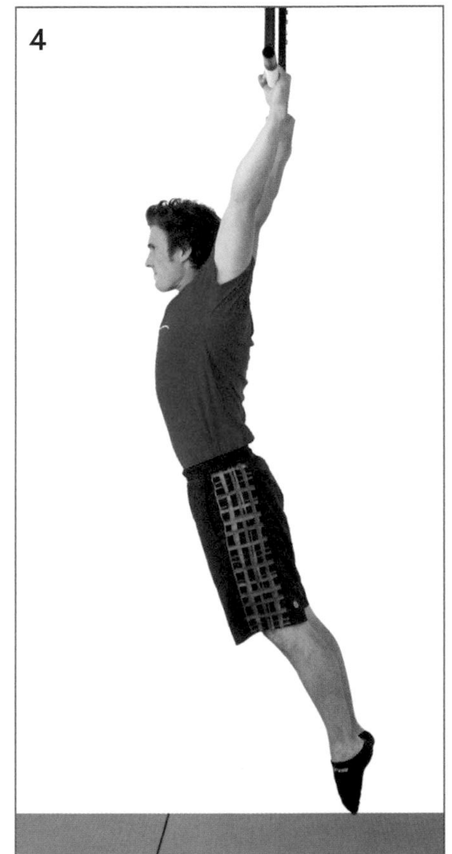

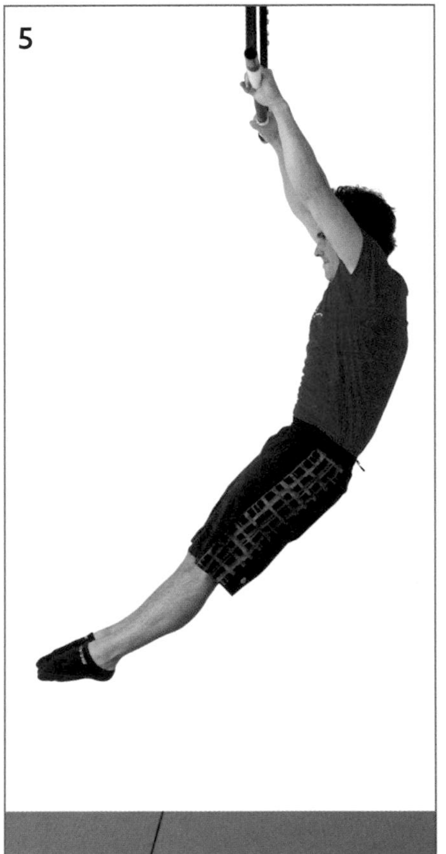

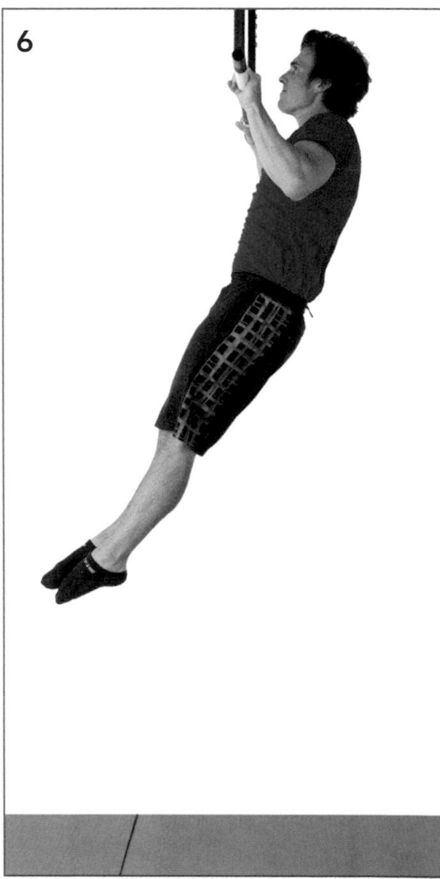

4. Pull your hips back and push your shoulders forward.

5. Still squeezing your glutes and keeping your belly tight, swing your feet forward and push your body away from the bar.

6. As you swing back, pull your chin over the bar, keeping your elbows in tight and your spine neutral. Again, the idea is to harness the energy of your backswing to help raise your chin over the bar. To seamlessly transition into your next rep, push yourself away from the bar and then, as you extend your arms, pull yourself under the bar as demonstrated in steps 2 and 4. As with all category 1 and category 2 movements, the way down should look exactly like the way up.

Squat 1 Archetype

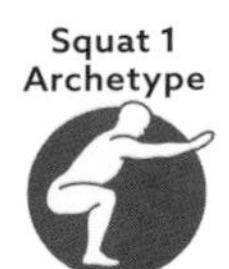

Overhead Archetype

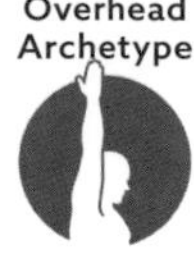

This movement contains the above archetypes. To improve common restrictions associated with this movement, visit the corresponding archetype prescriptions in part 4.

SNATCH BALANCE PROGRESSION

The snatch balance is an Olympic lifting exercise that isolates the catch phase of the snatch. Specifically, it's a movement that requires you to transition from the top position of the back squat with your snatch grip and quickly drop underneath the bar into the full overhead squat position. The purpose of this exercise is to get comfortable receiving weight in the bottom of the overhead squat, which is the most challenging and intimidating phase of the snatch. You have to organize your hips and shoulders in a good position while maintaining a rigid spine and upright torso.

There are three versions of the snatch balance technique, the first of which falls into a different category within the movement hierarchy. Because these techniques follow a specific progression and are typically layered as such, I thought it best to present all three in sequential order. By lumping these movements together, I hope to illustrate the small differences between the variations, as well as illuminate why going from a category 1 movement (the pressing snatch balance) to a category 2 movement (the heaving snatch balance and snatch balance) is so difficult.

Note: Although it's shown here with a barbell, the snatch balance progression can also be done using a PVC pipe. This makes it appropriate for athletes of all ages and ability levels. For the common faults associated with the snatch balance, revisit the overhead squat on page 192.

Pressing Snatch Balance

The first progression in this series is the pressing snatch balance. To execute this technique, you assume your overhead squat stance and, without moving the bar, press yourself into the bottom of the overhead squat. As you can see in the photos on the opposite page, Diane does not press the bar over her head. Rather, she presses her body underneath the bar. This is without question the most difficult category 1 movement because it synchronizes two techniques: the press and the overhead squat.

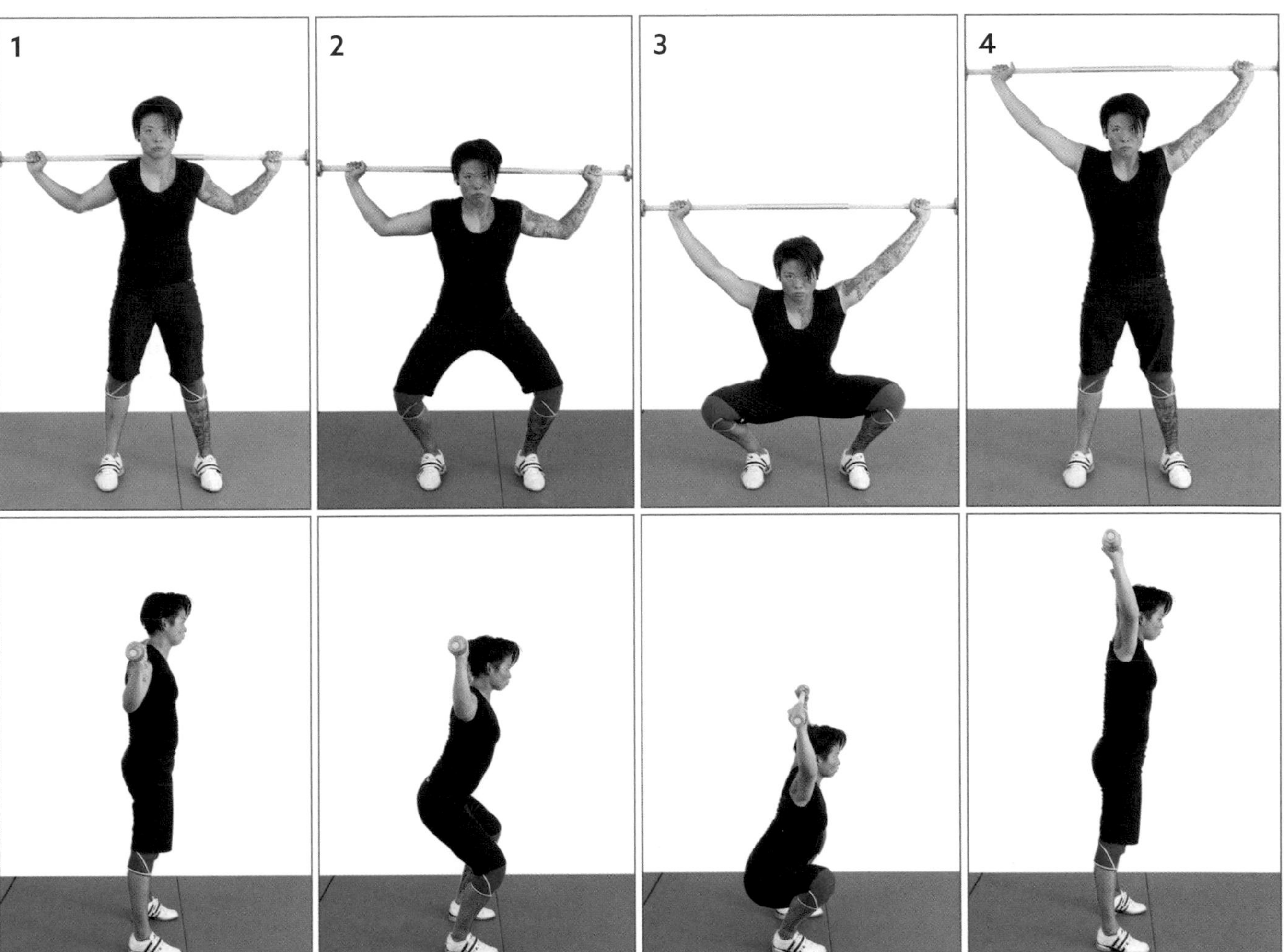

1. Assume your snatch grip and take the bar out of the rack just as you would when performing a back squat (page 178).

2. With your torso upright and spine neutral, sit your hamstrings back and sink your hips between your feet. At the same time, apply just enough upward force to the bar so it stays in the exact same position. Imagine pressing yourself underneath the bar as if it were an unmovable object.

3. Keeping the bar in the same position, press yourself down into the bottom position. Your elbows should lock out overhead as your hips drop below knee level. The key is to maintain torque in your hips and shoulders by shoving your knees out, pulling your shoulder blades back, and positioning your armpits forward.

4. Overhead squat the weight into the standing position.

Heaving Snatch Balance

The heaving snatch balance is similar to the pressing snatch balance in that you drop underneath the bar into an overhead squat without changing your stance (foot position). But instead of pressing yourself underneath the bar from a dead start, you add a dip and a drive—the exact same technique you use when performing a push-press or push-jerk. The idea to harness the energy from your hips in order to bump the weight off your back, and then drop underneath the bar into a full squat with your arms locked out. Here your focus is speed, unlike the pressing snatch balance, which you perform slowly.

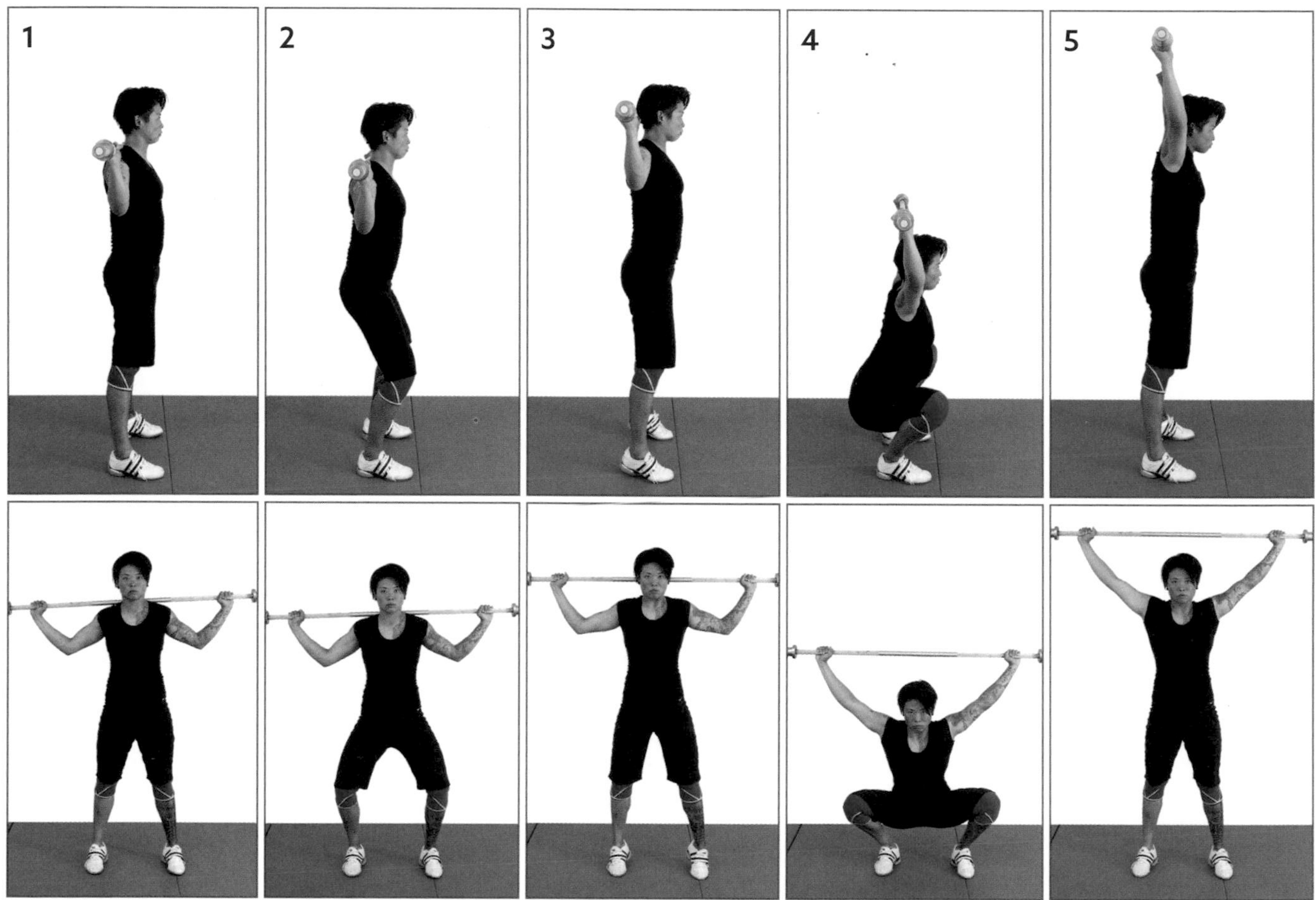

1. Establish your snatch grip and then take the bar out of the rack just as you would when performing a back squat (page 178).

2. Driving your knees out and keeping your torso as vertical as possible, sit your hips between your feet.

3. In one explosive motion, simultaneously extend your knees and hips. The idea is to harness the energy generated from your dip and drive to accelerate the weight off your upper back, just enough to drop underneath the bar.

4. As the bar travels upward, drop into the overhead squat position. The goal is to arrive in the bottom position with your knees out, elbows straight, and armpits forward.

5. Overhead squat the weight into the standing position.

Snatch Balance

The snatch balance adds one more piece. Unlike the pressing and heaving snatch balance iterations, which start and end in an overhead squat stance, the snatch balance requires you to change the position of your feet as you drop underneath the weight. Instead of remaining in your overhead squat stance, you assume your pulling stance (deadlift, clean, and snatch stance). Another way to think of it is that you start in your jumping stance (deadlift) and finish in your landing stance (squat). This uncovers another set of faults because people often default into an open foot position as they drop into the full squat to compensate for their lack of mobility or their inability to create spontaneous torque. Put simply, it's a quick and dirty way to highlight range of motion issues and assess an athlete's understanding of torque and bracing.

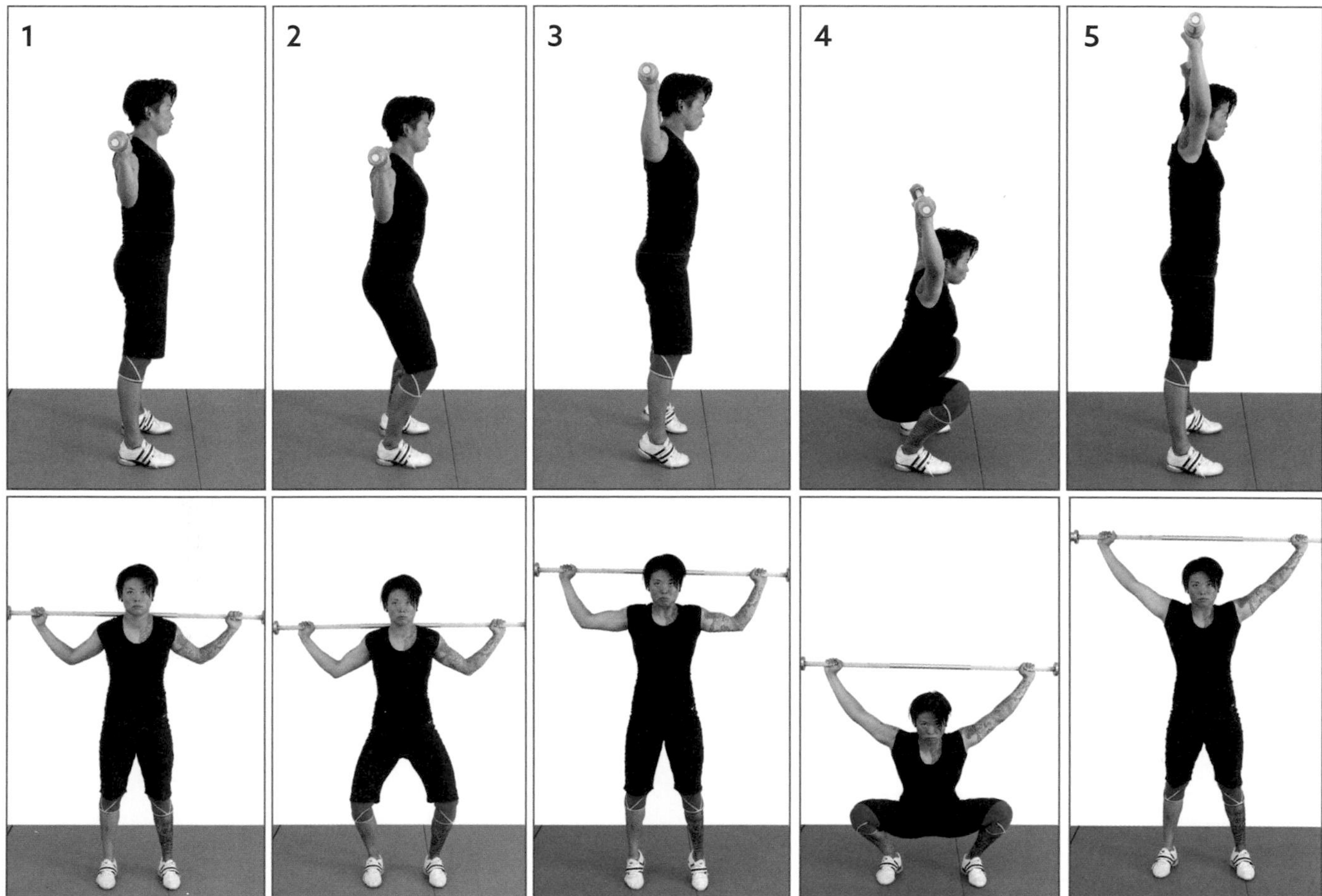

1. Establish your snatch grip and then take the bar out of the rack just as you would when performing a back squat (see page 178). Position your feet in your pulling (snatch, clean, deadlift) stance.

2. Keeping your torso as vertical as possible, drive your knees out and lower your hips between your feet.

3. Extend your knees and hips simultaneously as if you were performing a vertical jump. The idea is to transmit power from your hips to your shoulders and bump the bar off the backs of your shoulders.

4. As the bar accelerates upward, drop into the bottom position of the overhead squat, pressing your body underneath the bar. At the same time, slide your feet out into your landing (squat) stance, immediately screwing your feet into the ground, and receive the bar overhead with your arms locked out. Keep your feet straight, knees neutral, and armpits forward.

5. Stand up as if you were executing an overhead squat.

CATEGORY 3 MOVEMENTS

POSITION OF HIGH STABILITY (PHS) → REMOVE CONNECTION → POSITION OF HIGH STABILITY (PHS)

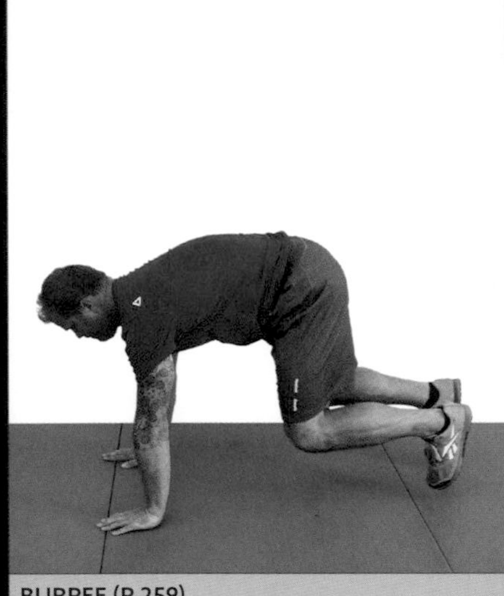
BURPEE (P 259)

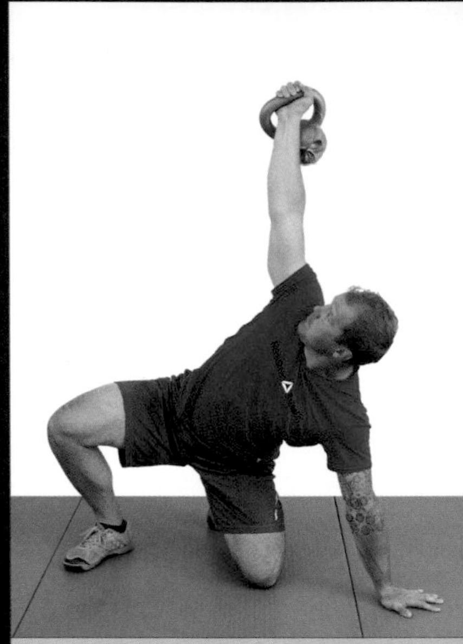
TURKISH GETUP (P 262)

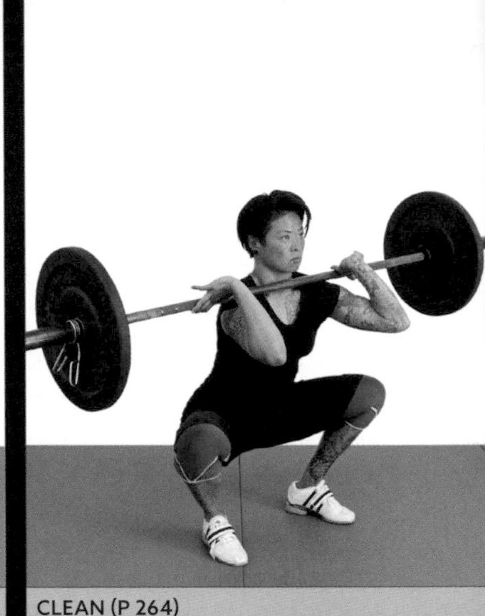
CLEAN (P 264)

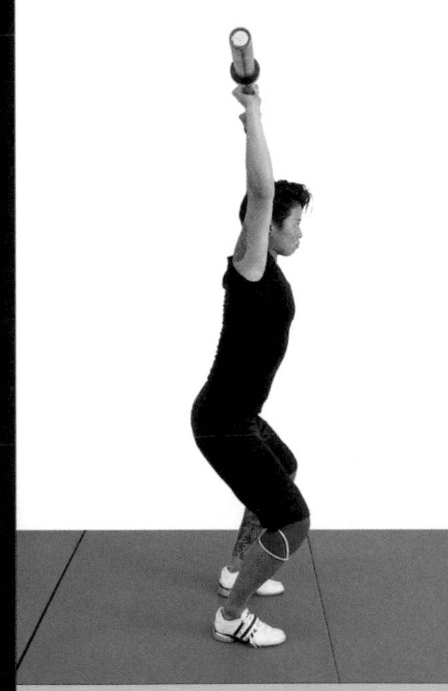
JERK (P 272)

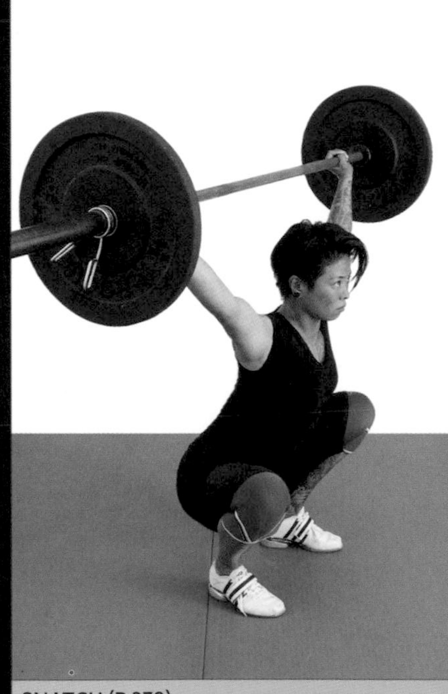
SNATCH (P 278)

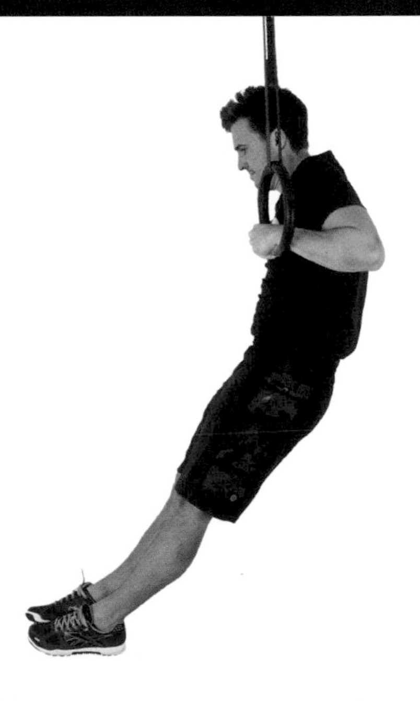
MUSCLE-UP (P 280)

BURPEE

The burpee basically combines a pushup, a squat, and a vertical jump into one seamless movement. This makes it easy to identify where the problems are because you already know what the start and finish positions look like. And by now you should be able to identify the common faults. All you are doing is reconstituting the same basic positions and reinforcing the same movement patterns over and over again. The difference is that you're adding transitions.

Can you drop into a dynamic plank while keeping your trunk stabilized and your shoulders in a good position? Perform a pushup with your forearms vertical? Transition into the bottom of the squat, create spontaneous torque, and then jump with an upright torso?

What's interesting is that people often show proficiency with the pushup, squat, and jumping and landing techniques, but the moment you ask them to arrive in these positions spontaneously, everything falls apart.

Think about it like this: You essentially enter and exit three different tunnels. If you start the pushup in a bad position, you will transition into the squat in a bad position, and by the time you jump you're a broken mess. The faults that occur in each movement compound the faults that occur in the subsequent movement. Make it a fast, high-repetition workout testing stamina, and the injury risk rises as form degrades.

You have to be able to reproduce the same stable positions with accuracy and speed in every single repetition. It's not a matter of how much work you can get done, but rather how many quality repetitions you can complete. So if you do burpees often (and you should), you need to organize your workouts so that you approach the exercise with care.

I'll use a CrossFit group class as an example. Say you're coaching a group of athletes through a workout that calls for 25 consecutive burpees. Rather than have the class rip through 25 burpees in a row as fast as possible—which will inevitably result in some burpees that bring to mind dying animals—reconstruct the workout so that it rewards athletes for their movement quality, not for finishing with the fastest time. For example, you could pair them up and have one person perform a set number of burpees in a row while her partner silently counts a point for every fault she commits. The goal is to get the lowest score possible.

By simply changing the game of the workout, you change the athlete's mindset. Now she's thinking about the quality of her movement and reproducing the same good position over and over again, which is what it's all about!

Another point worth mentioning is the universality of the burpee. Following the theme of using strength and conditioning movements that transfer to sport and life, the burpee is seen a lot in martial arts and fighting sports (think of an MMA fighter or a wrestler defending a takedown by sprawling his legs back and jumping back up to his fighting stance). We also see it in sports like surfing and in collision sports like football.

Squat 2 Archetype

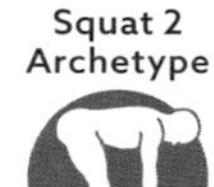

Squat 1 Archetype

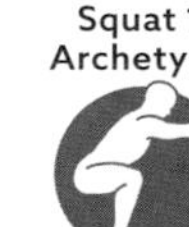

Press Archetype

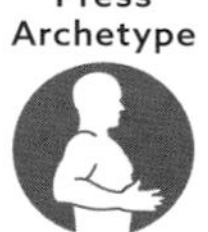

Front Rack 1 Archetype

Overhead Archetype

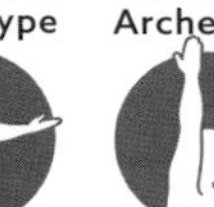

This movement contains the above archetypes. To improve common restrictions associated with this movement, visit the corresponding archetype prescriptions in part 4.

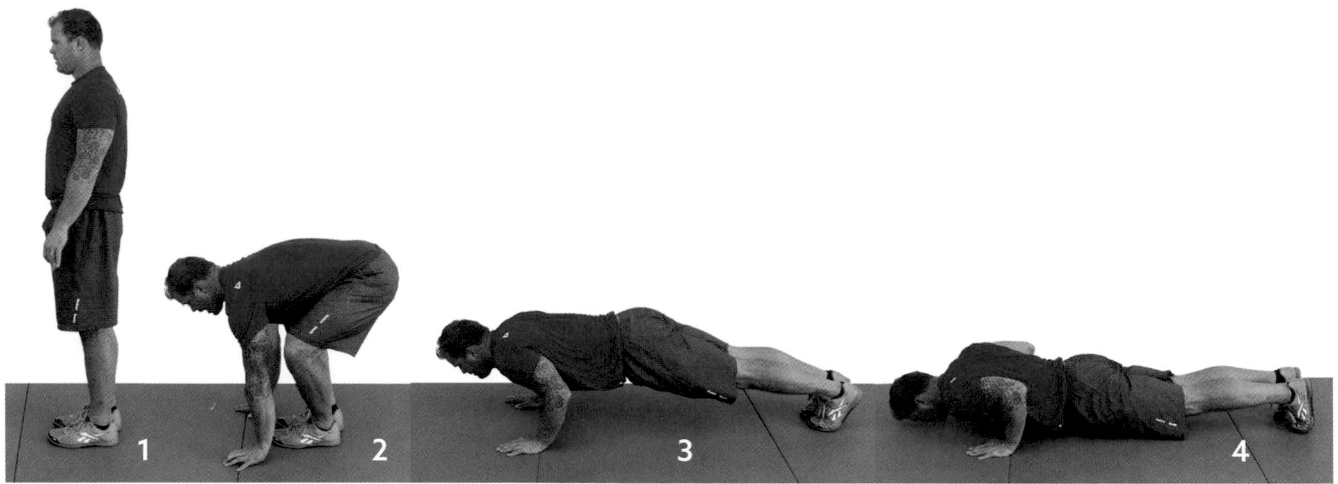

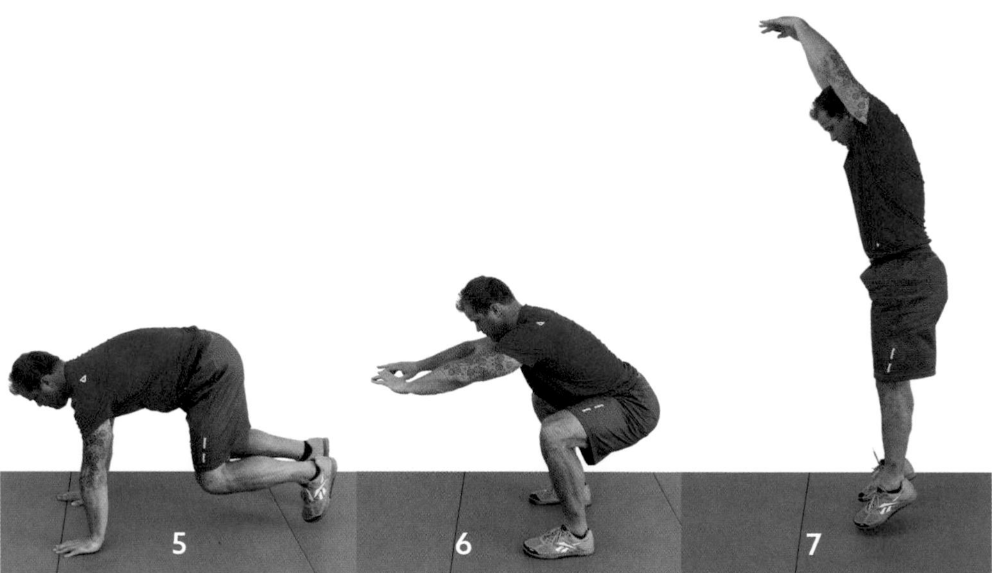

1. Start in your jumping stance and go through the bracing sequence.

2. Reach your hamstrings back—keeping your shins as vertical as possible and your knees neutral—hinge forward at the hips, and place your palms on the ground with your fingers facing straight forward. The key is to keep your low back flat and sprawl or slide your feet back as your hands touch down.

3. Slide your feet back and establish the top of the pushup. Remember to screw your hands into the ground, squeeze your butt, and keep your belly tight.

4. As you lower your chest to the ground, keep your elbows in tight to your body and your shoulders aligned over your wrists.

5. In one explosive motion, extend your elbows, drive your hips up as you reach full extension, and pull your knees toward your chest.

6. As you pull your legs underneath your body, try to replace your hands with your feet. The idea is to land in the bottom of the squat with your feet as straight as possible and your back flat.

7. Drive out of the bottom position of the squat and perform a vertical jump. Notice that my legs are together, my shoulders are back (armpits forward), and my toes are pointed. From here, I will land in my stance and transition right into another burpee. To see how to land, revisit the jumping and landing technique (page 238).

Burpee Fail

Because the burpee combines so many movements into one seamless, coordinated action, a ton of faults can occur. For example, people will bend over with a rounded back, flop on the ground in a broken mess, jump up into the dreaded dog poop position, burn their knees standing up, and then donkey-kick their legs back as they jump. It's as if you combined all the deadlift, pushup, squat, and jumping faults into one movement. Like I said, it's a disaster. If your burpees look anything like the photo sequence below, take a step back and isolate each movement until you achieve competency.

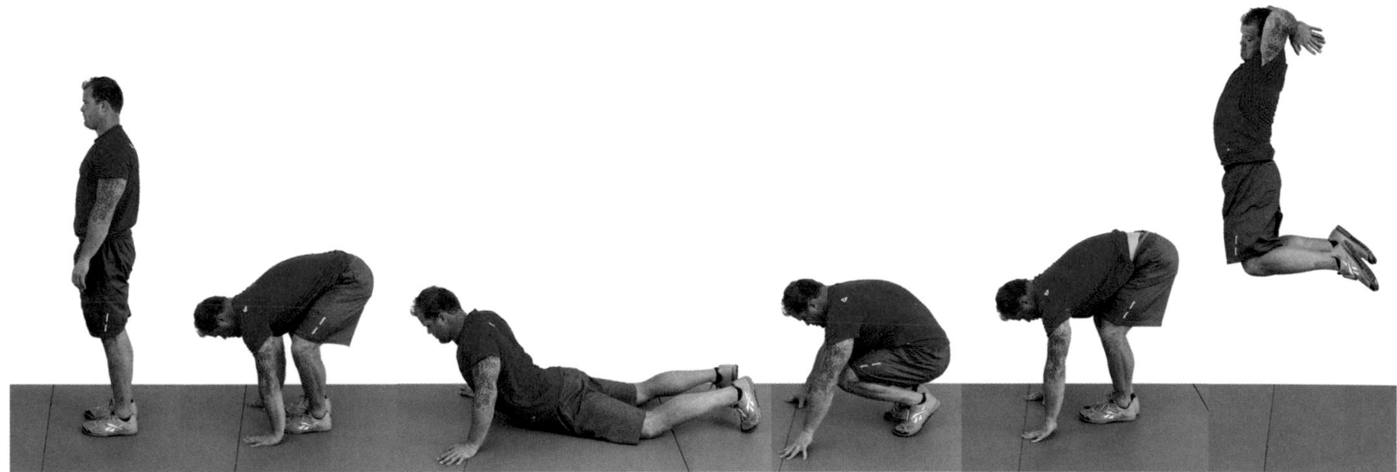

Scaling the Burpee

Consider a soldier lying on the ground wearing an 80-pound pack. What's the most efficient way to stand up? It's not that different from a burpee. Get into the bottom of the pushup, get your forearms as vertical as possible, press up into a globally arched position, and then bring one leg up at a time and stand up. You can also lunge into the standing position. The goal is to get your foot flat on the ground and your shin vertical, and stand up with your spine in a well-organized, stable position. We use this same model in the gym for folks who can't transition from the pushup to the bottom of the squat with good form.

Think of the scaled burpee as the formal expression of getting up off the ground from your stomach.

TURKISH GETUP

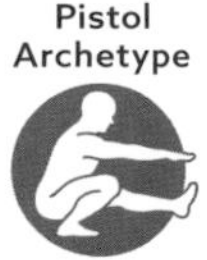

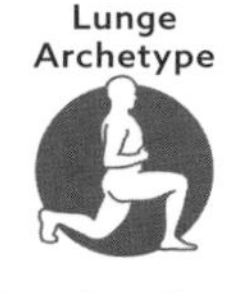

This movement contains the above archetypes. To improve common restrictions associated with this movement, visit the corresponding archetype prescriptions in part 4.

Martial artists—specifically Brazilian jiu-jitsu practitioners—refer to the Turkish getup as the "technical getup." It allows them to get up to their feet using the least amount of energy possible while giving them options in terms of other movements they can employ.

So that's the critical everyday-life application for the Turkish getup. It teaches you how to get up off the ground in the most efficient way possible. Imagine the value this has for an elderly person needing to get to his feet, for example.

The Turkish getup is also an invaluable diagnostic tool. When I am working with an athlete who is rehabbing from a shoulder injury, or if I simply want to test his understanding of a stable shoulder, the Turkish getup is one of the first category 3 exercises I introduce. It forces him to lock his shoulder in a stable position without the benefit of generating torque off a fixed object like a barbell or the ground and to move through a full range of motion. And unlike other category 3 movements, it's performed slowly, making it a safe and useful tool for driving home these concepts of stability.

At any point during the movement, you can stop and make corrections to your shoulder position—not just with the arm overhead, but with your supporting arm as well. The arm holding the dumbbell is expressed with armpit forward, and the arm supporting your body is expressed with shoulder back—screwing your hand into the ground. So it's a nice two-for-one shoulder diagnostic. In addition, you can start to see how loss of shoulder position translates to other problems in the athletic chain: If your shoulder is unlocked, chances are good that your ankles will collapse, your knees will track inward, your lumbar spine will overextend, and so forth.

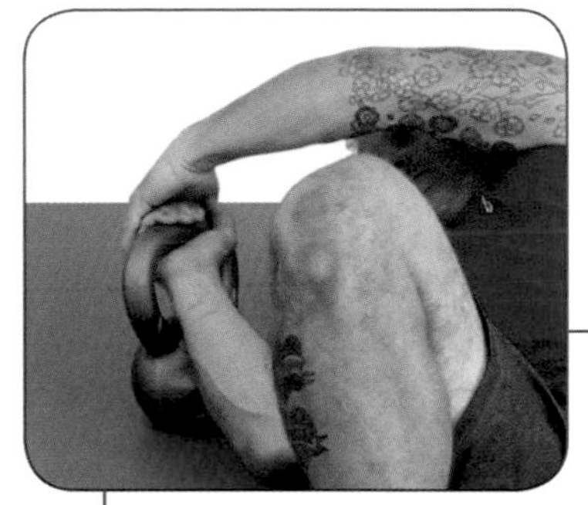

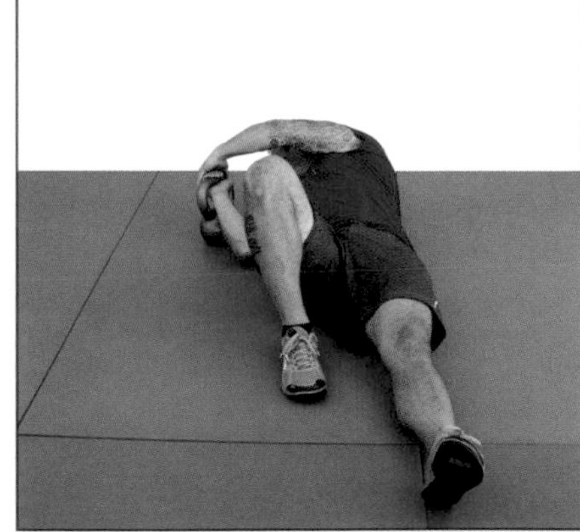

1

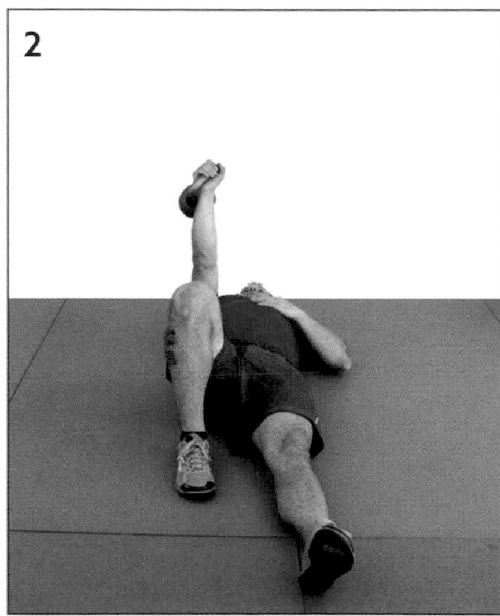

2

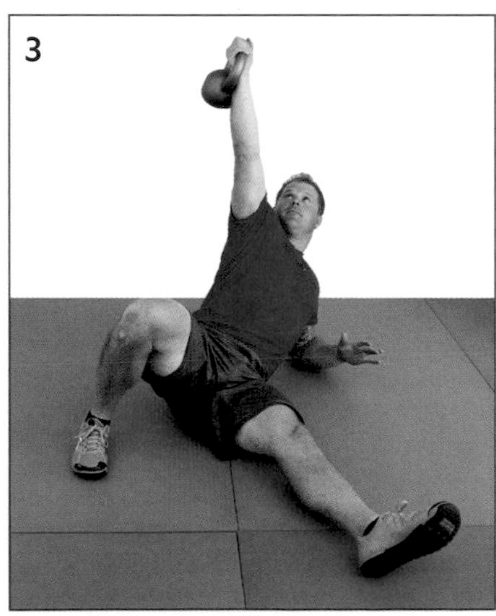

3

1. Lie on your back, position a kettlebell next to your right (or left) shoulder, and grip the handle. Notice how I've posted up on my right foot and reached over my body with my left arm and grabbed the kettlebell. Squeeze your glutes and keep your belly tight. Keep your foot straight so you're in a good position as you transition into the lunge and stand up.

2. Pulling the kettlebell toward the center of your body with your left hand, extend your right elbow. Keep your elbow in tight to your body and your thumb facing your head.

Once your arm is locked out, allow your shoulder to drop to the back of the socket and wind up your left arm to create a stable position. Keep your eyes locked on the kettlebell throughout the movement.

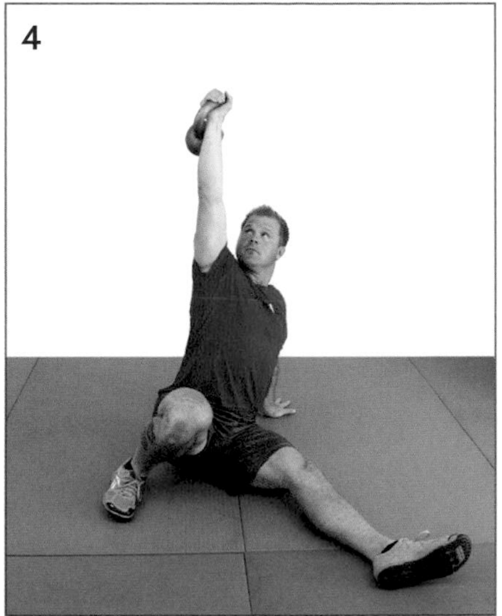
4

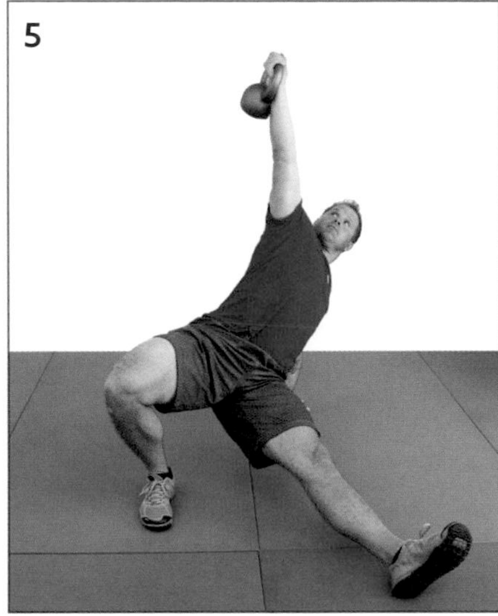
5

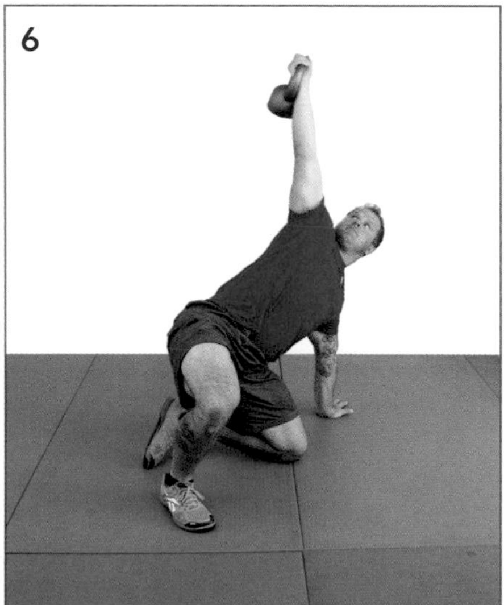
6

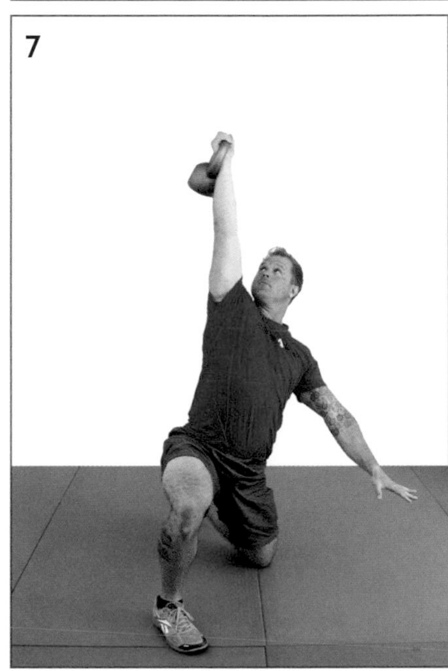
7

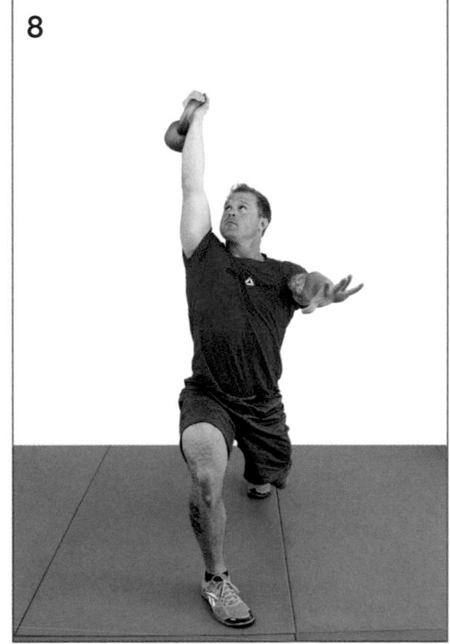
8

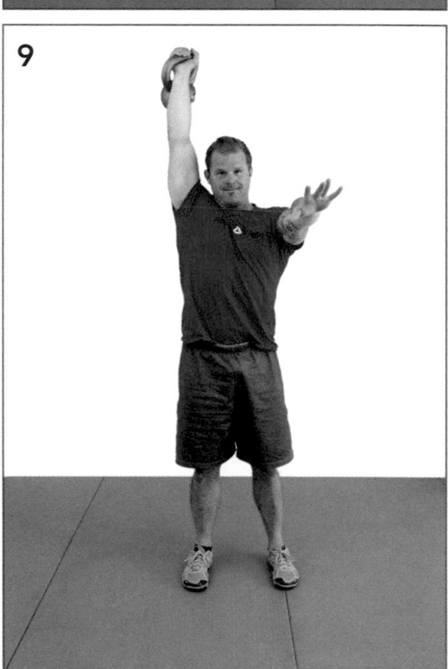
9

3. Keeping your right arm straight and actively driving your thumb away from your body, drive off the ground with your right leg and come up onto your left elbow. The goal is to get your elbow aligned with your shoulder. It's important to keep your shoulder blades pulled back and your trunk braced.

4. Sit up and plant your left hand on the ground. You want your hand aligned with your left shoulder. As you transition into the overhead position, think about getting your armpit forward.

5. Still squeezing your glutes, push off the ground with your right foot and extend your hips.

6. Supporting the weight of your body with your left arm and right leg, pull your left leg underneath your hips, then plant your knee underneath your center of mass (aligned with the kettlebell).

7. Keeping your eyes locked on the kettlebell, shift your weight toward your right side and get your torso vertical. The moment your left hand leaves the ground, pull your shoulder back and externally rotate your arm. Make sure that your left leg is internally rotated.

8. Keeping your right knee neutral, push off your right leg and stand tall, keeping the weight positioned over your center of mass. Use your left arm for balance and maintain stability in that shoulder.

9. As you stand tall, step your left foot forward, squeeze your glutes, and establish the finish position.

Squat 1 Archetype

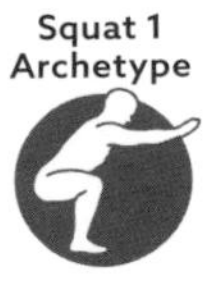

Hang Archetype

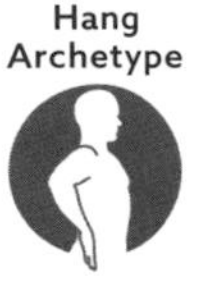

Front Rack 2 Archetype

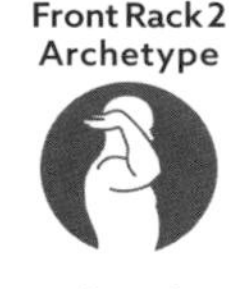

This movement contains the above archetypes. To improve common restrictions associated with this movement, visit the corresponding archetype prescriptions in part 4.

CLEAN

The clean tells you a lot. Can you pull dynamically off the floor with speed while maintaining a neutral spine? Can you reproduce the same load order sequence with every rep? Can you keep your trunk, hips, and shoulders stable while transitioning from one position to another?

With all this additional complexity, the possibility of making a technique error increases. But it's also an opportunity to improve performance and highlight potential weaknesses in your athletic profile. This is the mindset that you need to cultivate as you start to introduce, layer, and train category 3 movements.

It's like this: You can deadlift and front squat. That's fantastic. Now show me that you can pull with speed and create torque off a fixed object while it's in motion. Show me that you have the motor control and mobility to drop into the bottom of a front squat with speed and accuracy.

If you want to pick something up off the ground and receive it onto your shoulders, you need a model for learning and teaching that skill. The clean is the formal blueprint for layering this movement pattern.

A Bad Mix

The top-down approach is without question the best setup for the deadlift, but it doesn't necessarily transfer as well to Olympic lifting. In fact, Glen Pendlay—world-renowned Olympic lifting coach—doesn't allow his Olympic lifters to deadlift heavy singles because he believes that the loss of upper back extension and "deadlift shoulders" wrecks their movement patterns for Olympic lifting.

Although this is a sport-specific approach, it fits with our "practice makes permanent" philosophy. If you pull from a bent-over position, you have to get your torso vertical as you pull the bar past your thighs, resulting in a forward hip thrust kettlebell-like action. This transfers your hip energy forward instead of upward. What happens is that you either miss the lift or have to jump forward in order to receive the weight.

DEADLIFT SETUP

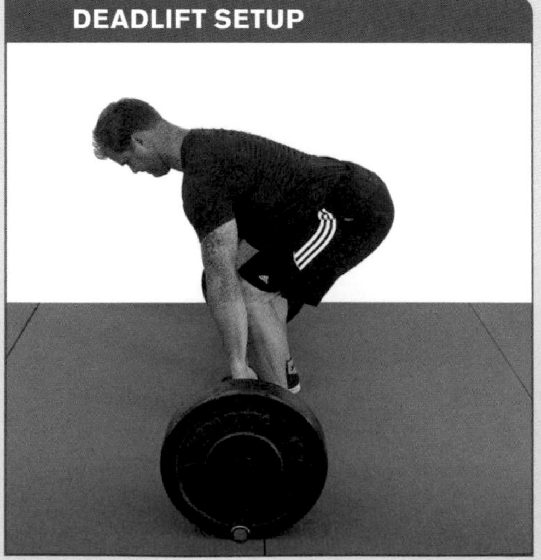

CLEAN SETUP

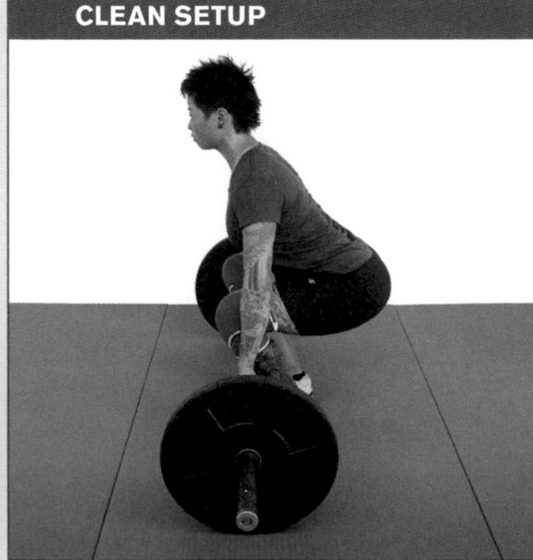

Bottom-Up Setup

Unlike setting up for the deadlift, which works from the top down (see page 197), you set up for the clean from the bottom up. There are some similarities in the load order sequence: With your back flat and shoulders pulled back, you load your hips and hamstrings and use your knees to adjust for position. But instead of bending over and forming your grip with your hips and hamstrings on tension, you drop into the bottom of the squat and set up from there.

Here's why: First, the bottom-up setup is used for Olympic lifts, as it allows you to optimize thoracic extension. By lowering into the bottom of the squat, you can effectively pull your shoulder blades back—using the bar as an anchor—and maximize tension in your upper back. Why is this important? Simple: You're setting yourself up to receive the load in a good front rack position.

You have to consider your finish position as you formulate your setup strategy. It's not just about entering the tunnel in a good position, but also about exiting in a good position. By setting up in the same position in which you finish (bottom of the squat), you improve the stability of your receiving position.

Second, the bottom-up approach allows you to prioritize an upright torso position, which is critical in both the pull (lifting the weight from the ground to hip and chest level) and catching phase (dropping into the bottom of the squat while receiving the weight in the front rack).

Most important, the bottom-up setup gives you a template that will yield the same reproducible results every time you approach the movement.

Note: A lot of people don't have the mobility to implement the bottom-up setup. In that case, the top-down approach is the better option, and still quite functional—just ask some of the best weightlifters in America. But it's less than ideal because your upper back and shoulders aren't in the most mechanically optimal position. Figure out what's holding you back and address the issue.

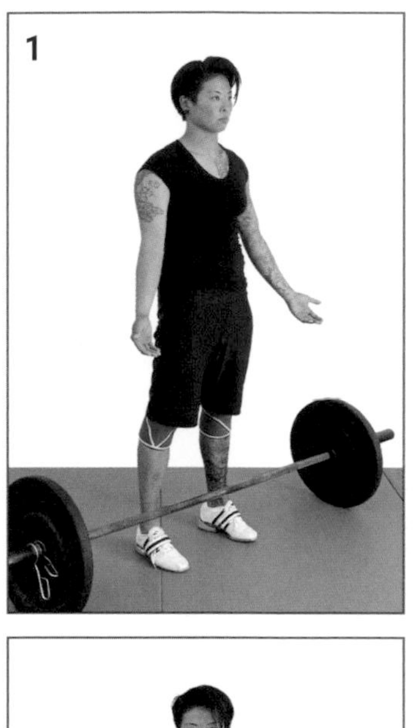

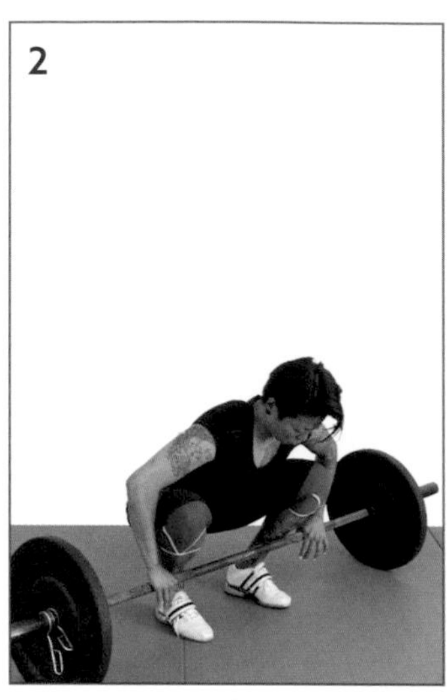

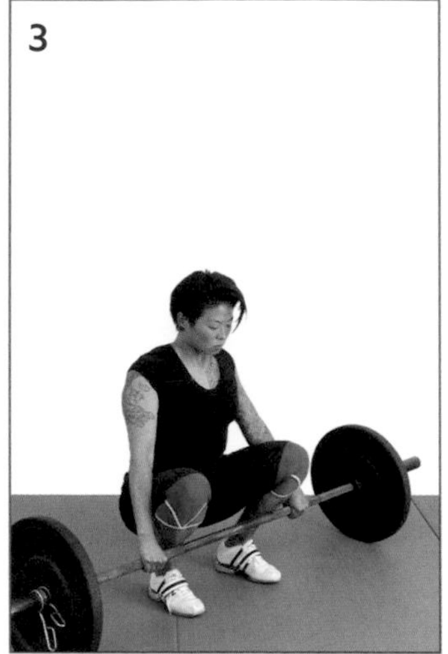

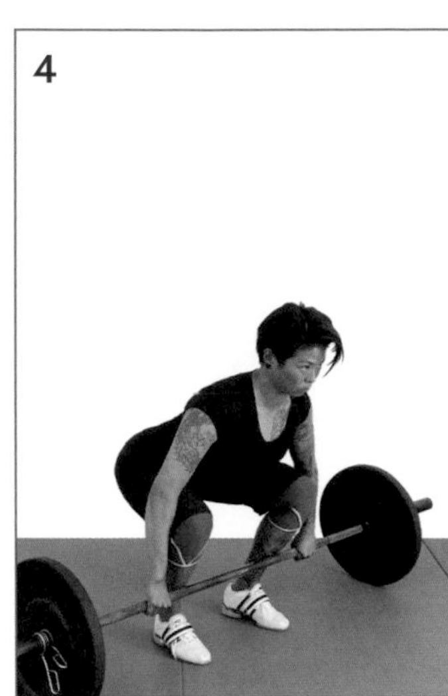

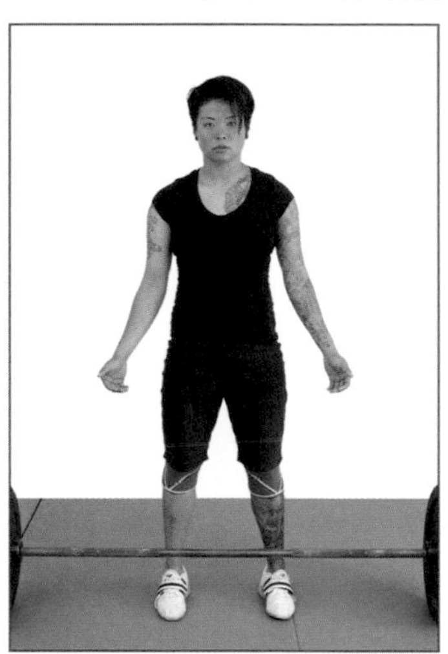

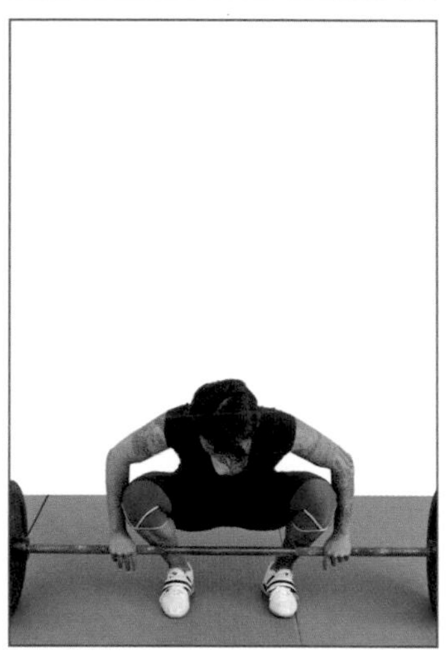

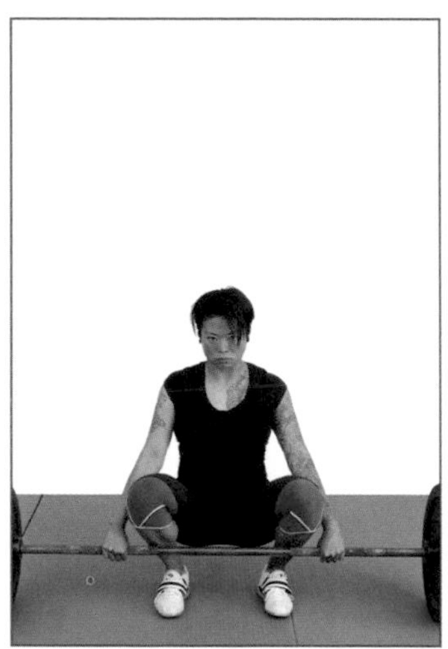

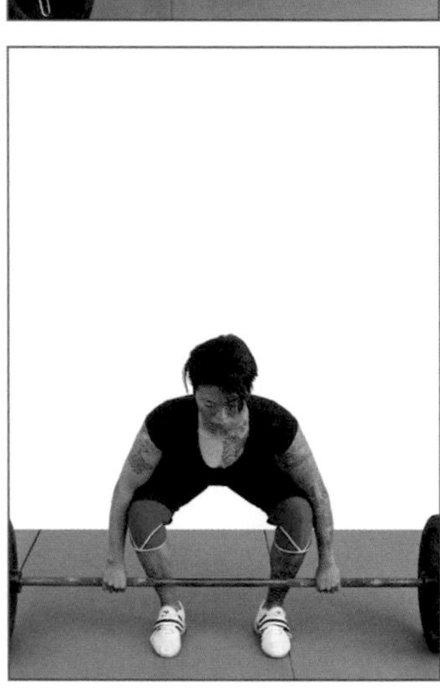

1. Assume your clean stance (same as your jumping and deadlift stance), retract your shoulders, and go through the bracing sequence.

2. Lower into the bottom of the squat—keeping your back flat, shoulders upright and tight—and establish a hook grip (see page 201). *Note:* Your clean grip should be the same as your front rack grip. To see how to set up for the front rack, flip back to page 187.

3. Driving your knees out, drop your butt, pull your torso vertical, retract your shoulders, and screw your hands into the bar. This maximizes tension in your upper back and sets your shoulders in a stable position.

4. Still creating tension off the bar, take a breath and get your belly tight. Then load your hips and hamstrings by raising your hips.

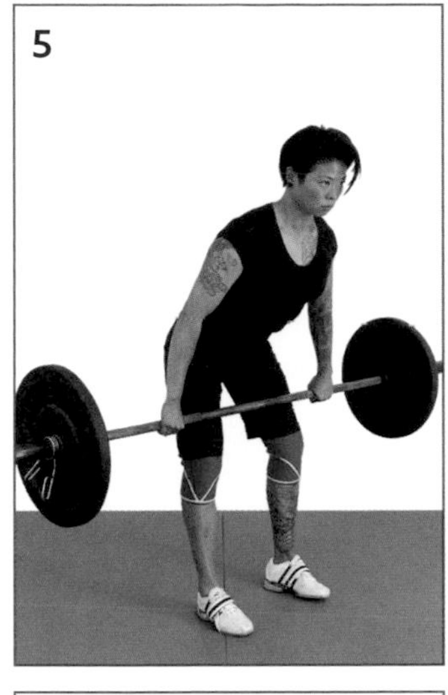
5

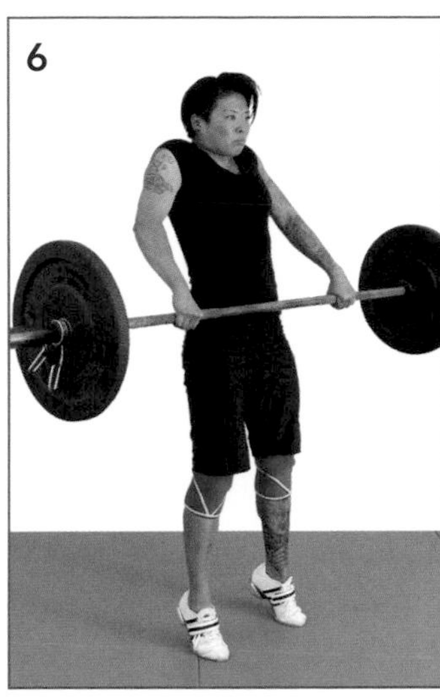
6

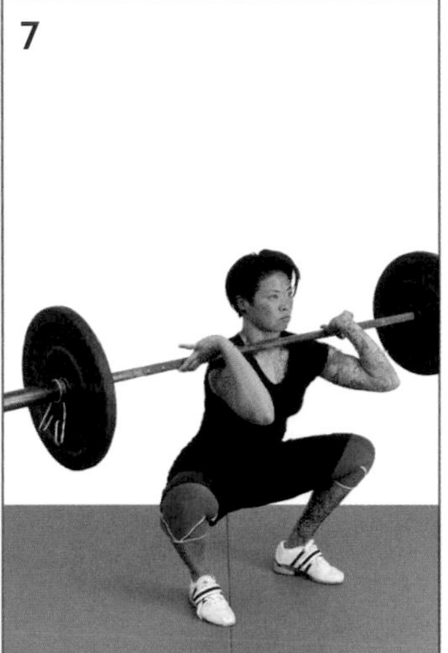
7

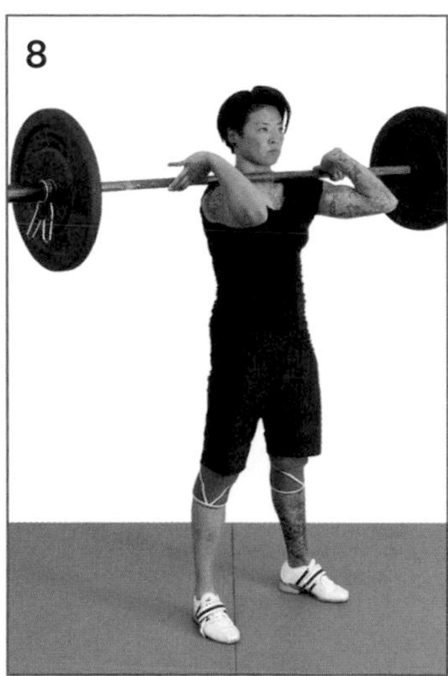
8

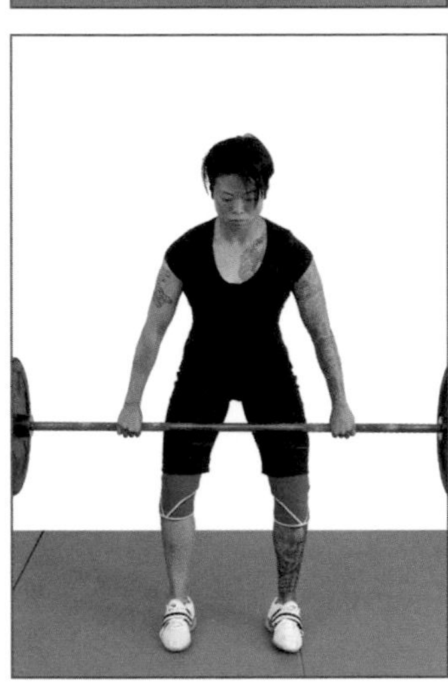

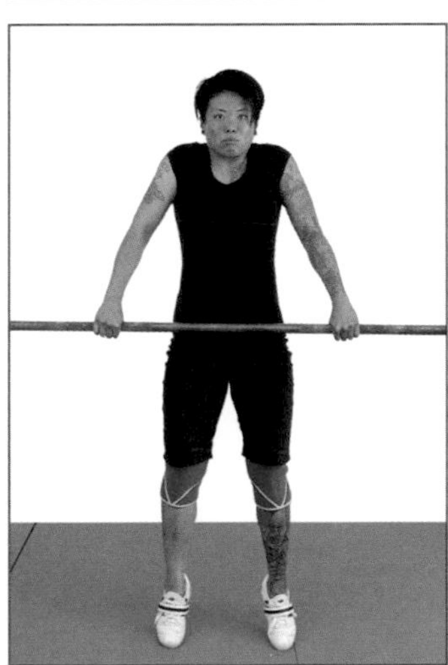

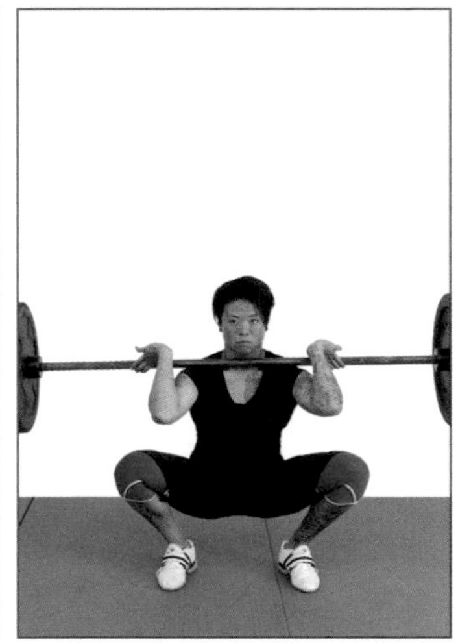

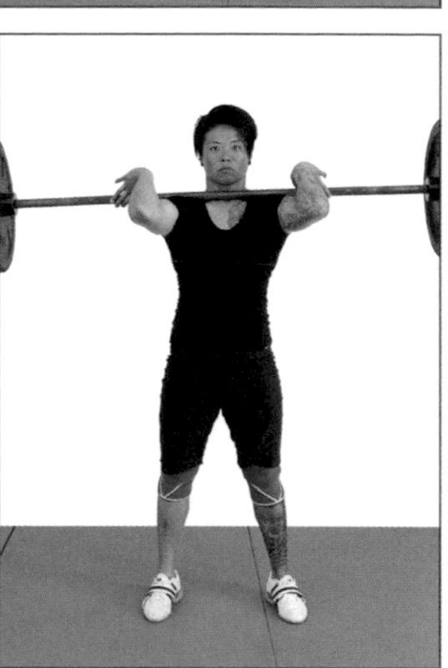

5. Keeping your back flat, knees neutral, and shoulders tight, extend your hips and knees simultaneously. Again, there should be no change in your spinal position as you pull the bar off the ground. If your butt comes up first, there's a click on the bar, or your knees come in—those are all errors.

6. As the bar passes your knees, scoop your hips forward, keeping the bar as close to your body as possible. As you reach triple extension (ankles, knees, and hips in extension), shrug your shoulders. Notice that Diane's arms are straight and that 100 percent of the energy generated from her legs and hips is being transferred to the bar.

7. As the bar travels upward, slide your feet out into your landing stance and pull yourself underneath the weight. A common fault is to kick your heels back and stomp your feet—commonly referred to as a donkey kick. Although stomping your feet fires your posterior chain and optimizes your landing position, you want to avoid the dreaded donkey kick. The idea is to slide your feet out and screw your feet into the ground as you land.

8. Front squat the weight up to the top position.

Power Clean

If you're an NFL lineman, you need to know how to go from a four-point stance to a vertical torso with organized shoulders and ready to hit. You have to do so at near light speed. Learning how to power clean helps train this motor pattern.

The power clean is a scaled-down iteration of the clean. Instead of receiving the weight in the bottom of the squat, you receive the weight in a quarter squat or in the top position. A lot of people don't have the mobility to clean, so the power and hang variants are great ways to dial in good motor patterns.

That said, there's no excuse to avoid the full clean and snatch. If you can't drop into a clean or a snatch, you need to figure out what is holding you back and address the problem.

The goal is to develop motor control through a full range of motion. If you're consistently hiding the deficits of your motor control and mobility through shortened ranges, you'll end up compensating into bad positions when you're forced into end-range positions. You'll end up failing at the margins of your experience. To put it simply, you need develop the motor control at end ranges.

Don't hide your weaknesses. Park your ego, get hungry, and go after them.

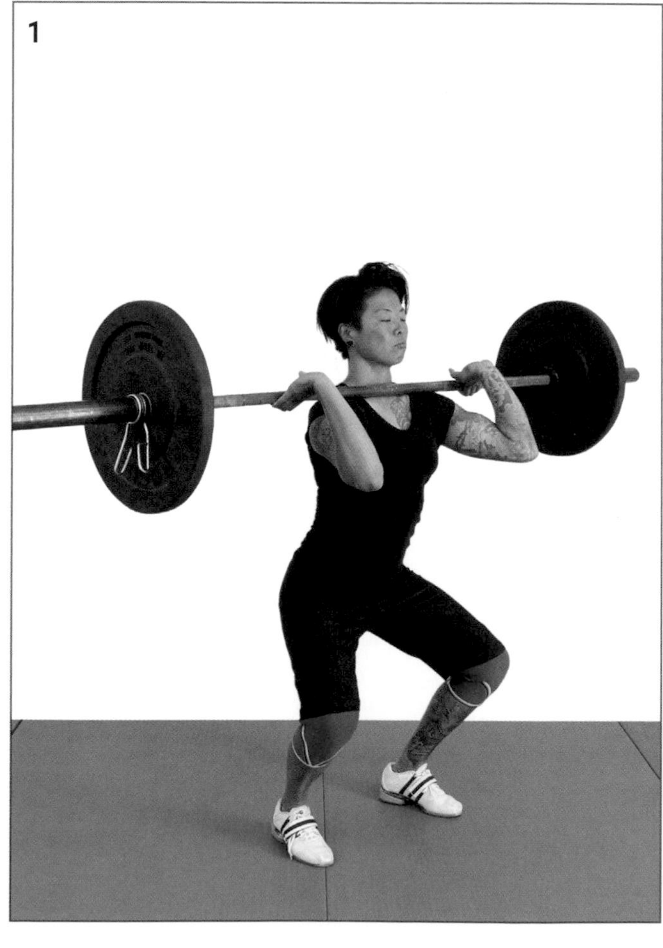

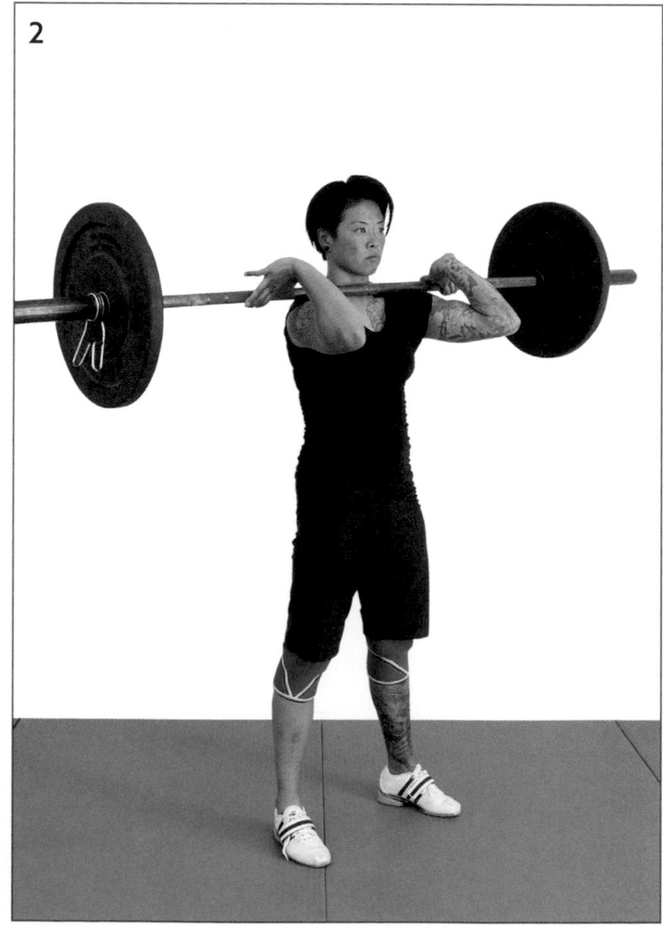

Hang Clean

Complex movements like the clean and snatch must be layered accordingly. If you plan on taking the Olympic lifts seriously, you need to isolate and practice each phase. For example, the hang variants—starting from the standing position—allow you to focus on the second phase of the pull (triple extension), the catch phase of the lift (front rack), and the landing.

This is great for a few reasons:

1. Breaking down the movement to a defined phase shortens the learning curve.
2. It allows you to highlight areas that are giving you trouble.
3. You can get around mobility issues (such as being unable to set up or receive weight in the bottom position) while working on other aspects of the movement.

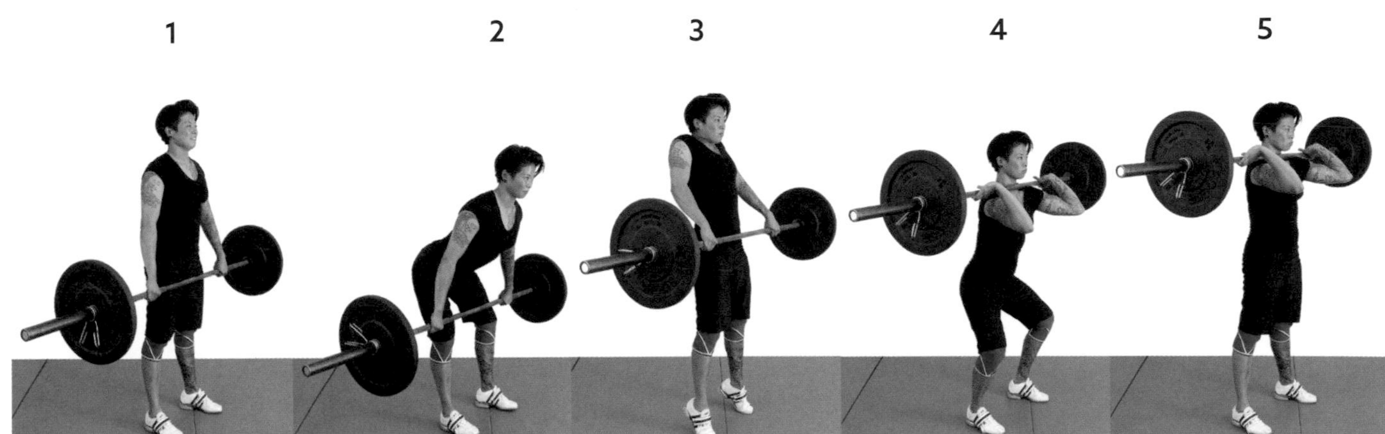

1. Deadlift the weight into the standing position.

2. Sitting your hamstrings back, lower the bar to the tops of your knees. Keep your shoulders back, torso as vertical as possible, and knees neutral.

3. In one explosive movement, extend your hips and knees as if you were jumping straight up and shrug your shoulders.

4. As the bar travels upward, drop underneath the weight, receiving it in the front rack position.

5. Front squat the weight into the top position.

Tension-Hunting Fault

Squat 2 Archetype Squat 1 Archetype

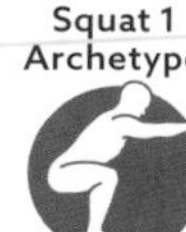

This fault is associated with the above archetypes. For a mobility fix, visit the corresponding archetype prescriptions in part 4.

MOTOR CONTROL FIX:

Drive your knees out in the bottom position and load your hips and hamstrings before you initiate the pull.

MOBILIZATION TARGET AREAS:

Anterior hips and quads

Posterior high chain (glutes)

Posterior low chain (hamstrings)

Calves and heel cords

If you fail to shove your knees out or you're missing flexion and external rotation range of motion, your butt will shoot up as you initiate the pull, causing an overextension spinal fault. This is your body's way of putting tension in the system. Take up the slack by driving your knees out in the bottom position.

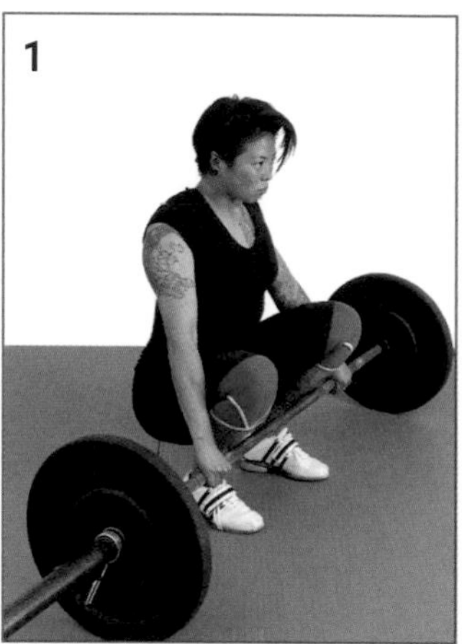

1

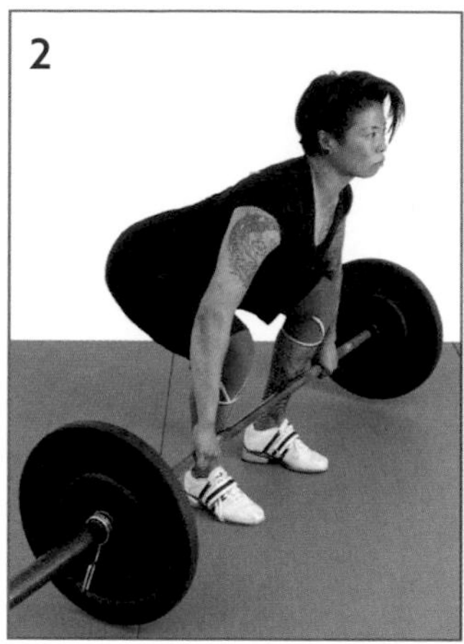

2

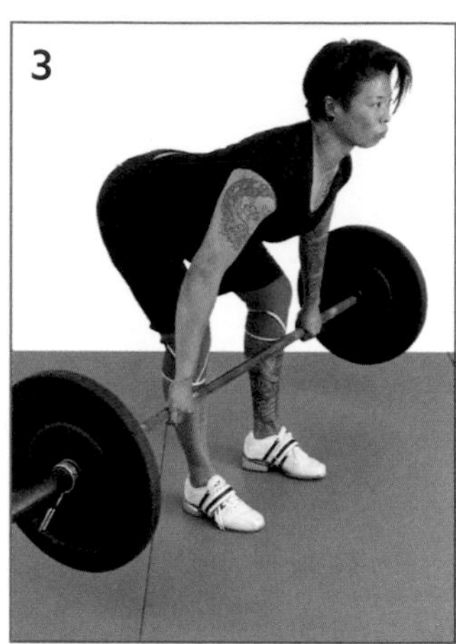

3

Early-Pull Fault

MOTOR CONTROL FIX:

Isolate the phase of the pull that is giving you the most trouble by implementing a clean pull or hang clean variant.

Think about getting your elbows high after locking out your hips and shrugging your shoulders.

MOBILIZATION TARGET AREAS:

Anterior hips and quads

Once the bar moves past your knees, the goal is to get your torso as vertical as possible so that you can open your hips into full extension. This is what enables you to transmit upward energy from your hips to the bar. If you're bent over (you've implemented the top-down setup) or you're missing extension range of motion in your anterior chain (hip flexors and quads), reaching full hip extension is difficult. What happens? You end up pulling with your arms instead of harnessing the power of your hips.

To correct this fault, implement the hang clean variant—deadlift the weight to the standing position, lower to your thighs, and then pull—or just work on extending your hips without transitioning into the receiving position (clean pull). If tight hips or quads are holding you back, pony up and get to work on those stiffened tissues.

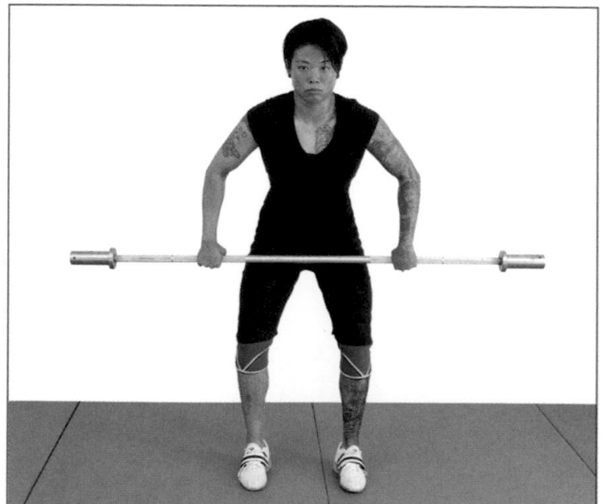

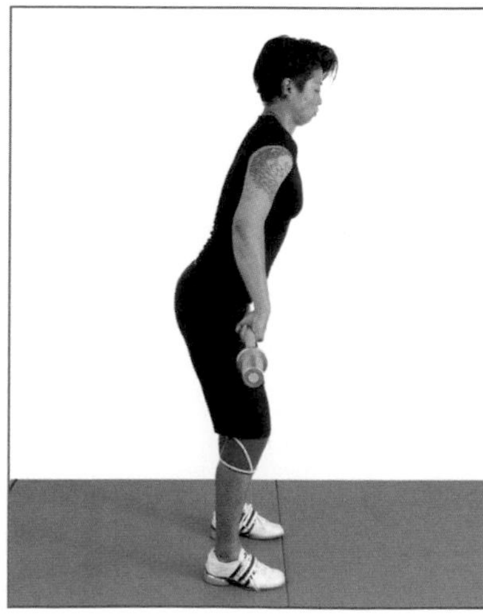

Next Rep Transition

If you're stringing together multiple repetitions, you need to be conscious of your shoulder position as you lower the weight to the ground. Think about keeping your shoulders back, screwing your hands into the bar, and lowering into your start position. This will allow you to seamlessly transition into your next rep without defaulting into a poor position.

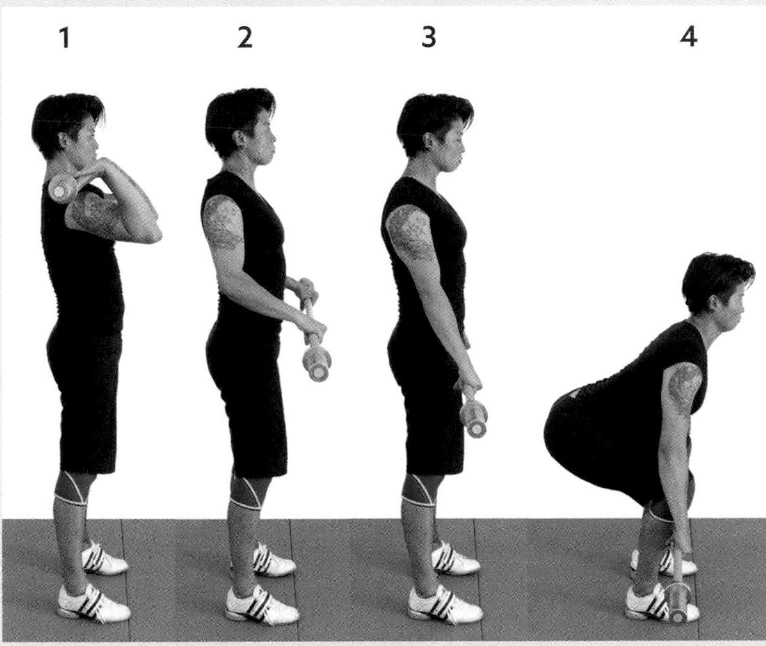

Soft Shoulders Fault

A lot of people mistakenly unlock their shoulders as they lower the bar to the ground. As you can see in the photos below, this compromises the integrity of your spine and puts your shoulders in a bad position.

MOTOR CONTROL FIX:

Keep your shoulders back and screw your hands into the bar as you lower it to your thighs.

Think about keeping your back flat and driving your knees out as if you were initiating a hang clean.

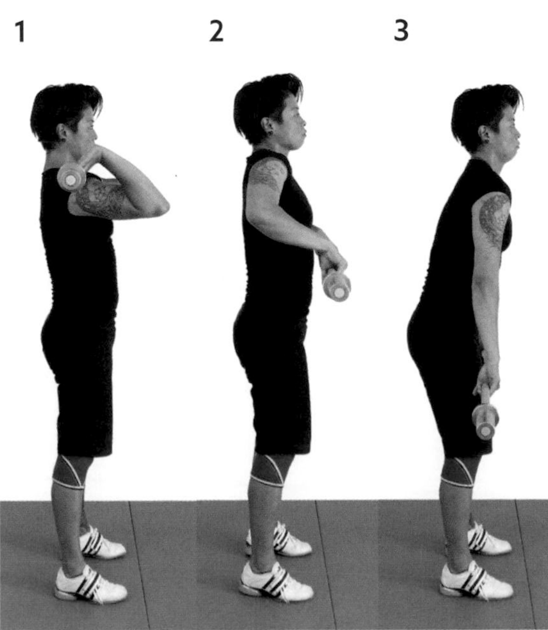

JERK

We have a saying around our gym: Your shoulders are abnormal unless you can jerk.

While it's important to learn the basic, stable overhead positions, it's not enough to say that you have full range of motion overhead or that you can press and push-press. To fully express the stability and effectiveness of your overhead position, you need to be able to lock out your arms, as well as spontaneously generate a stable shoulder position (armpits forward) with speed and accuracy. In other words, you need to be able to jerk.

If you can do that—lengthen and stabilize both shoulders simultaneously—it shows that you understand the stabilization concepts repeated throughout this book and have a model that translates to dynamic overhead actions like swimming, throwing, and blocking. And, like all category 3 movements, the jerk highlights torque dumps and force bleeds, as well as spotlights shoulder mobility issues that may go unnoticed when implementing the basic overhead pressing elements.

If you're just learning how to jerk, it's helpful to get the bar from a rack. This allows you to optimize the setup and isolate the movement. (To see how to take the bar out of the rack, check out the front squat on page 187.) However, if you plan on Olympic weightlifting, you have to learn how to transition from a clean to a jerk. To do so, reset your feet into your pulling stance and adjust your front rack position by lowering your elbows. You want your elbows to be at about a 45-degree angle (halfway between a front squat rack position and a strict press rack position).

As with the push-press, you use a dip and drive (bend and extend your knees) to accelerate the weight upward. But instead of staying in your jumping stance, you drop underneath the weight, catching it in either a squat (landing) or split squat position. Regardless of which variation you implement, the goal is to receive the weight in a strong, stable position at the apex bar height. For the average athlete, pausing for a second in the lockout position is a valuable stimulus and allows the coach to evaluate the quality of the athlete's position.

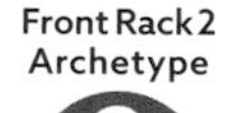
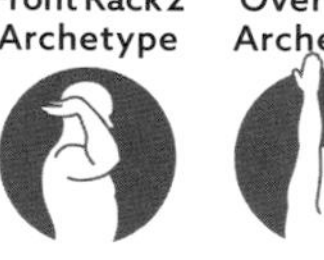
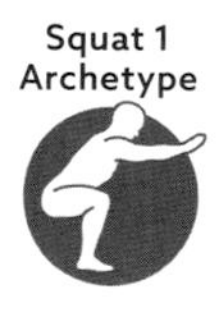

This movement contains the above archetypes. To improve common restrictions associated with this movement, visit the corresponding archetype prescriptions in part 4.

Push-Jerk

The push-jerk variation allows you to evaluate vertical jumping and landing mechanics with a dynamic overhead stimulus. The key to performing the push-jerk is to keep your torso upright, drive your knees out as you dip and catch, and position your feet straight as you go from a jumping to a landing stance. The faults to look out for include lumbar spine overextension, knees forward, bent elbows and internally rotated shoulders, and the dreaded donkey kick.

Note: The push-jerk is often implemented in low-weight, high-repetition workouts because it allows for a quick recovery and setup. The split-jerk enables most people to press more weight.

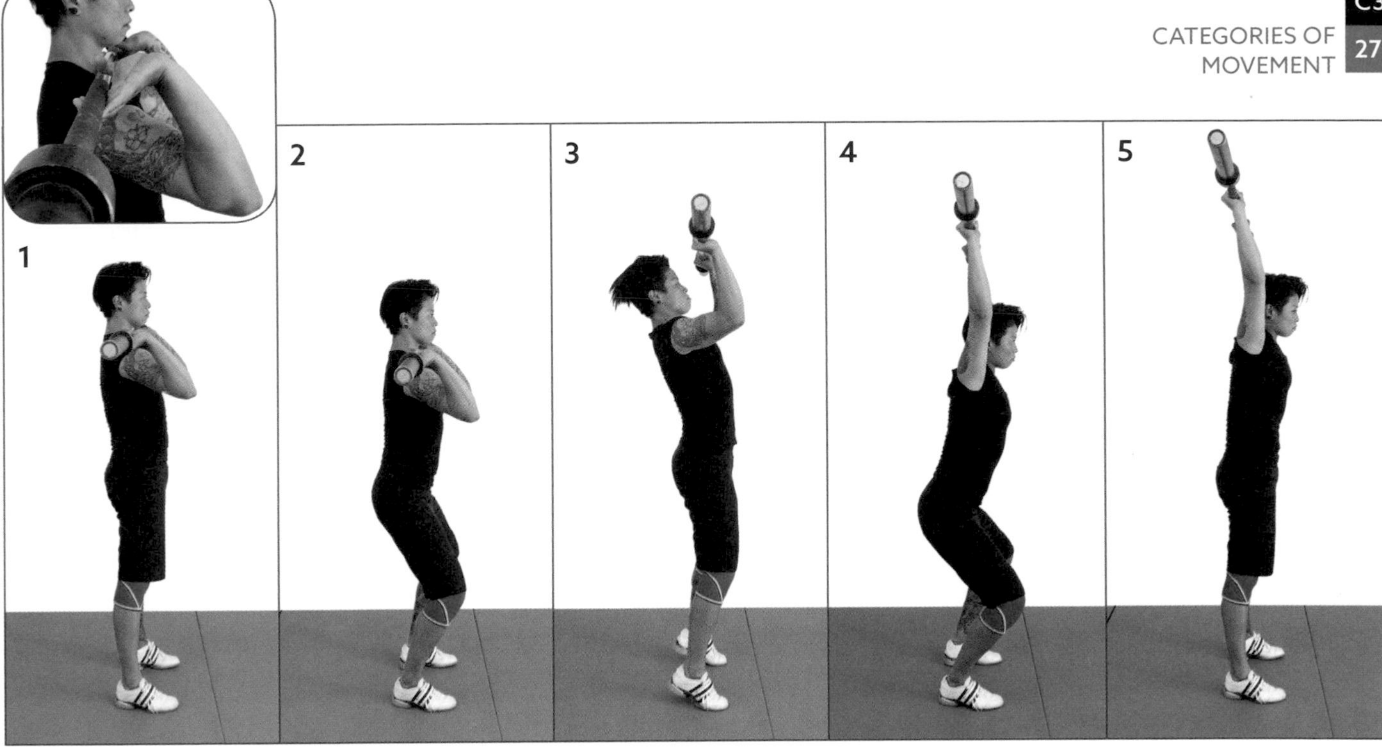

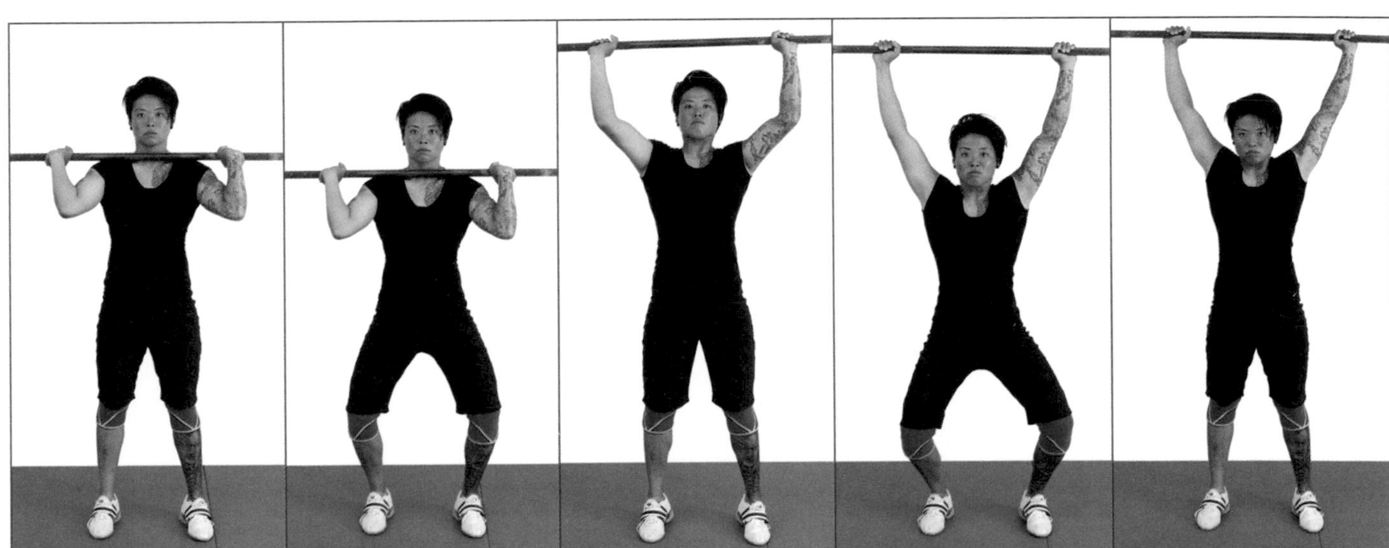

1. Whether you take the bar out of the rack or clean the weight to your shoulders, the setup is the same: butt squeezed, belly tight, feet straight, and shoulders back. Notice that Diane is in her pulling or jumping stance and has the bar balanced on her fingertips and deltoids. Her elbows are halfway between a strict press and front rack position, at about a 45-degree angle. *Note:* Your jerk grip width should be close to your front squat rack position.

2. Keeping your torso as upright as possible, sit your hamstrings back slightly, drive your knees out, and lower your hips between your feet. The dip should look no different than the first 6 inches of a front squat.

3. In one explosive motion, extend your knees and hips into triple extension. As the bar jumps off your shoulders, pull your head back slightly, just far enough to clear your face and maintain a vertical bar path.

4. As the bar accelerates upward, slide your feet out into your landing stance—screwing your feet into the ground and shoving your knees out—and press yourself under the bar. Catch the weight with your elbows straight, shoulders back, and armpits forward.

5. Overhead squat the weight into the top position.

Lunge Archetype | Overhead Archetype | Front Rack 2 Archetype

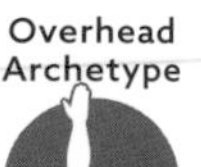
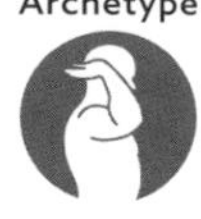

This movement contains the lunge archetype. To improve common restrictions associated with this movement, visit the lunge archetype prescription in part 4.

Split-Jerk

It's a lot easier to maintain an upright torso and stabilize your shoulders in the split stance. This is why you likely can move more weight with the split variation of the jerk (unless you happen to be a very competent Chinese Olympic lifter). That's wonderful, but the real magic with the split-jerk is that it gives you a model for creating a stable hip position when one leg is in extension—behind you—and the other leg is in flexion, which is what it looks like when you cut, run, or lunge.

There are a few key points to keep in mind when performing the split-jerk:

1. Create a stable foot position. To do so, land with both feet slightly internally rotated—your front foot turned toward the inside of your body with your weight centered just in front of your ankle, and your rear leg internally rotated with your weight centered over the ball of your foot. The front-foot position allows you to create external rotation without

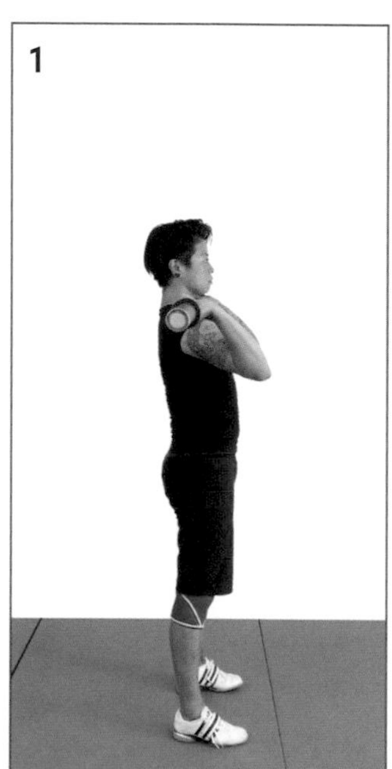

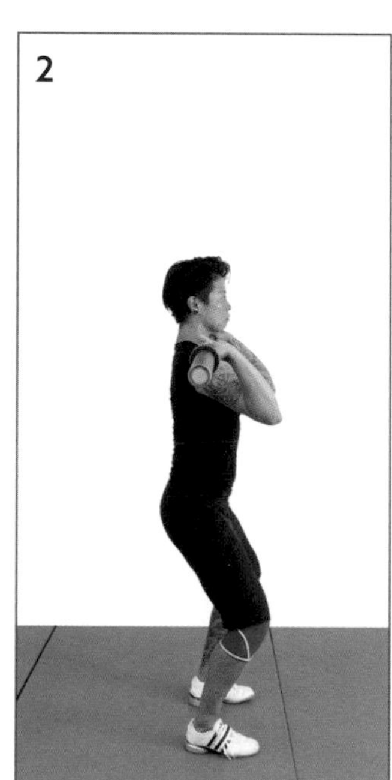

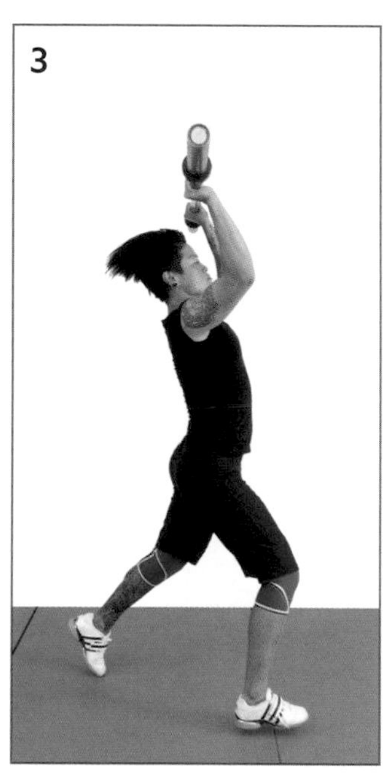

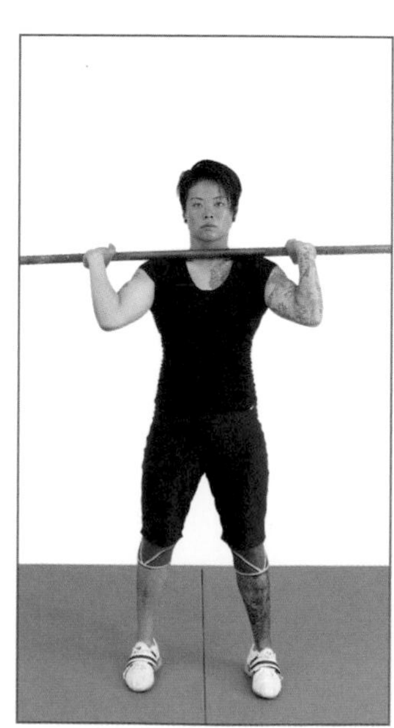
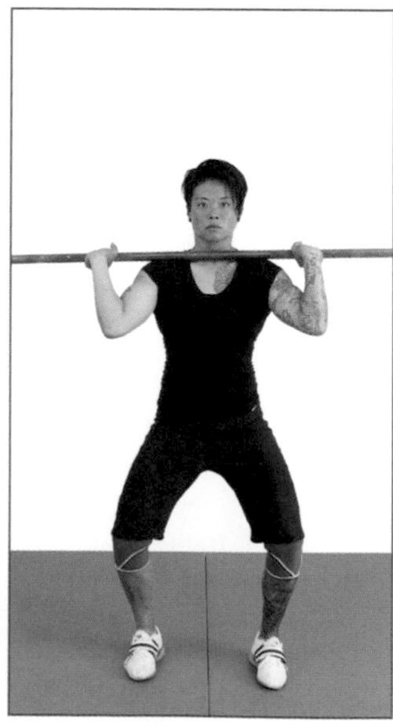
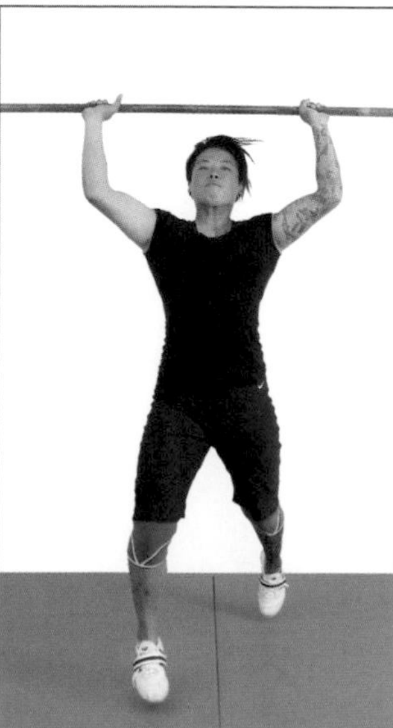

1. Assume the jerk front rack position. To see how to take the bar out of the rack, flip back to the front squat on page 187. To transition into the jerk from the clean, adjust your feet into your pulling stance and lower your elbows into the jerk front rack position.

2. Drive your knees out, sit your hamstrings back slightly, and lower your hips between your feet. Keep your shoulders back, back flat, and torso as vertical as possible.

3. Jump the weight off your chest by extending your knees and hips simultaneously. As you do so, pull your head back slightly to clear your face from the vertical path of the bar, slide one foot straight back, and slide your opposite foot forward.

your knee tracking too far outward, and the rear-foot position stabilizes your hip, allowing you to support an upright torso with a neutral pelvis.

2. Always draw your feet together at the finish of the lift by moving your front leg first. Don't rush it. Slide your lead foot back and then step your rear foot into your squat stance. Master the habit of this sequence in the same way you walk out the bar when performing a squat.

3. Unless you're a competitive Olympic lifter, alternate your stance. Become a switch-hitter of sorts. Sometimes jerk with your left leg forward, and other times jerk with your right leg forward. It's natural for one side to be stronger than the other, but just as a good fighter practices from both a southpaw and an orthodox stance and a good skateboarder switches between standard and goofy, a well-rounded athlete should practice jerking from both stances.

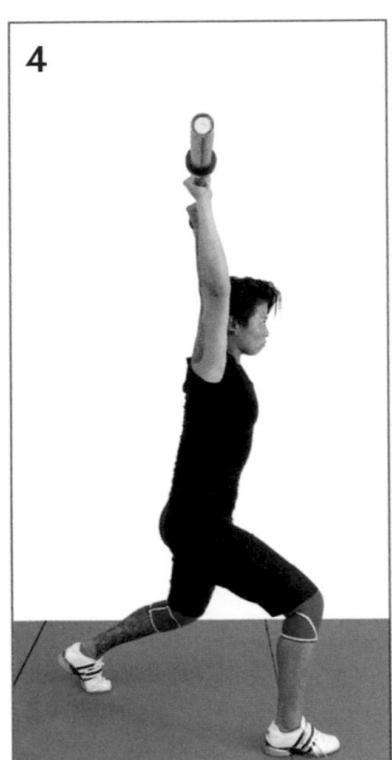

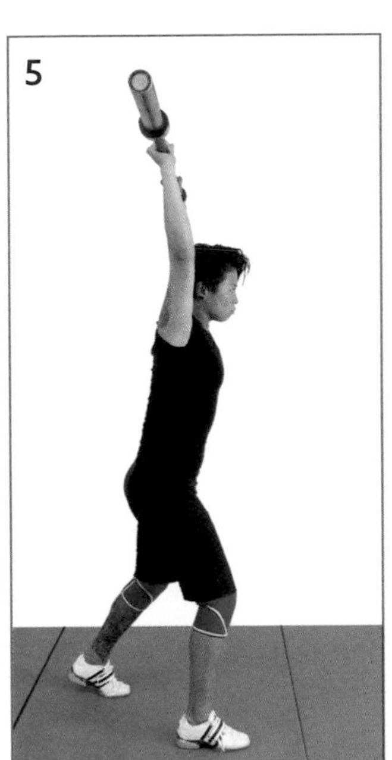

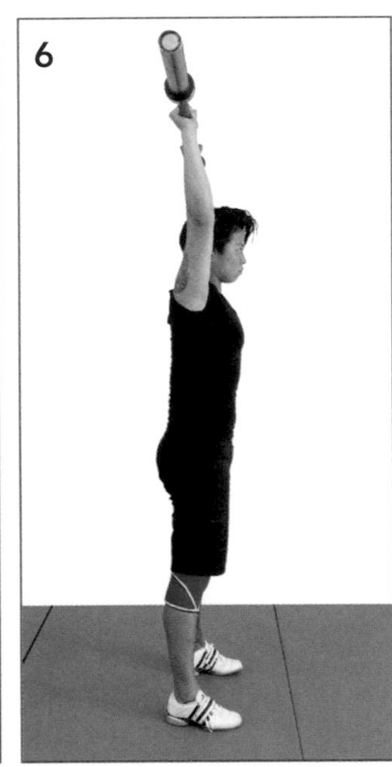

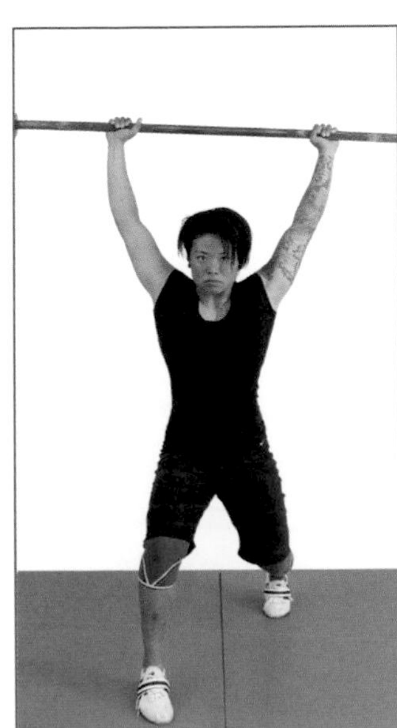

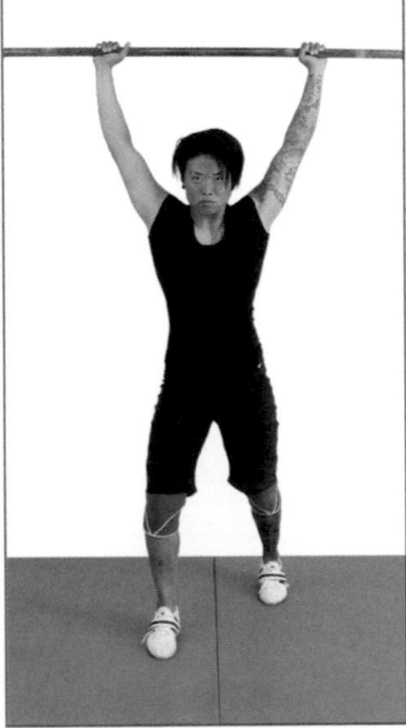

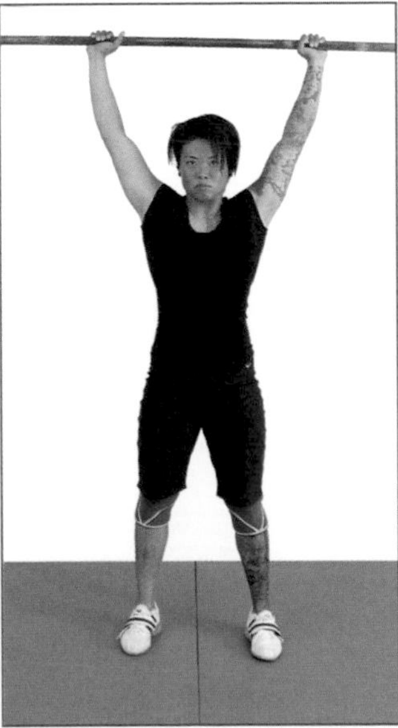

4. Push your head through your arms (but not too far) as the bar passes your face. Lock out your elbows and get your armpits forward, catching the bar at its apex. Notice that Diane is on the ball of her rear foot and her leg is slightly internally rotated. Her lead foot is turned slightly inward and her shin is vertical. Both legs have roughly a 45-degree bend. This is the most stable position for your ankles, knees, and hips. The key is to think about driving your lead knee out and your rear knee in—squeezing your rear glute—while keeping your hips square.

5. Keeping your belly tight, armpits forward, and elbows locked out, slide your lead foot back.

6. Step your left foot into your start position stance.

Lunge Archetype

This fault is associated with the lunge archetype. For a mobility fix, visit the lunge archetype prescription in part 4.

MOTOR CONTROL FIX:

Focus on internally rotating your back leg with a slight knee bend.

MOBILIZATION TARGET AREAS:

Posterior high chain (glutes)
Anterior hips and quads
Posterior low chain (hamstrings)

Open-Foot Fault

A lot of athletes, especially novices, turn their back leg out as they drop into the lunge position. This is a huge blow to force production, and, as you can see in the photos below, it puts your back leg in an awful position. Like all movements, start out using a PVC pipe or light weight and drill the proper mechanics. If you can't get into a good position because you're missing internal rotation of the hip, you know what to do: Flip to the mobility section devoted to hip internal rotation (starting on page 381) and get to work.

Note: We see this same open-foot movement pattern in running. The mobility prescription is the same: Start at the hip and work your way down.

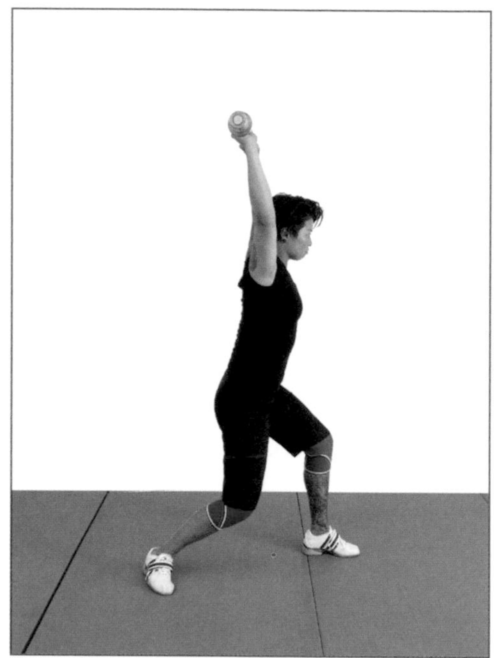

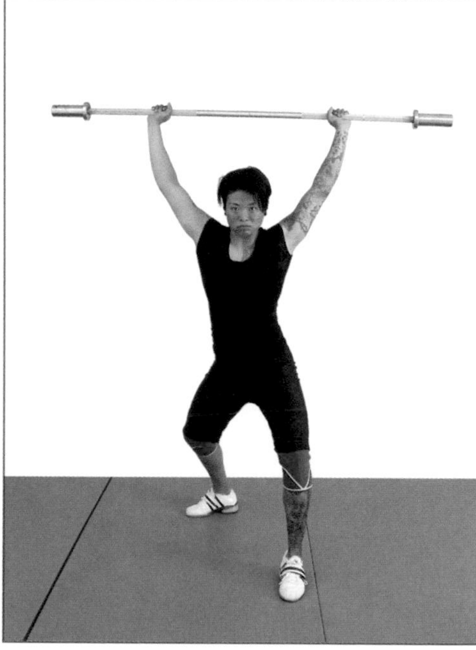

Knee Fault

Dropping into the lunge position feels unstable to a lot of people, especially when they're first learning how to jerk. To avoid dropping to depth, athletes often keep their back leg straight and overextend to keep their torso vertical. As with most motor control faults, you need to take a step back and drill the movement using a PVC pipe, empty bar, or bar with a light amount of weight. It's that simple. If, while working on your technique, you realize that the position is unattainable due to limited mobility, figure out what's holding you back and fix the problem. For this particular fault, tight anterior structures surrounding the hip are usually to blame.

MOTOR CONTROL FIX:

Think about bending your right knee and turning it toward the inside of your body. Remember, you want about a 45-degree bend in your legs.

MOBILIZATION TARGET AREAS:

Anterior hips and quads

Trunk

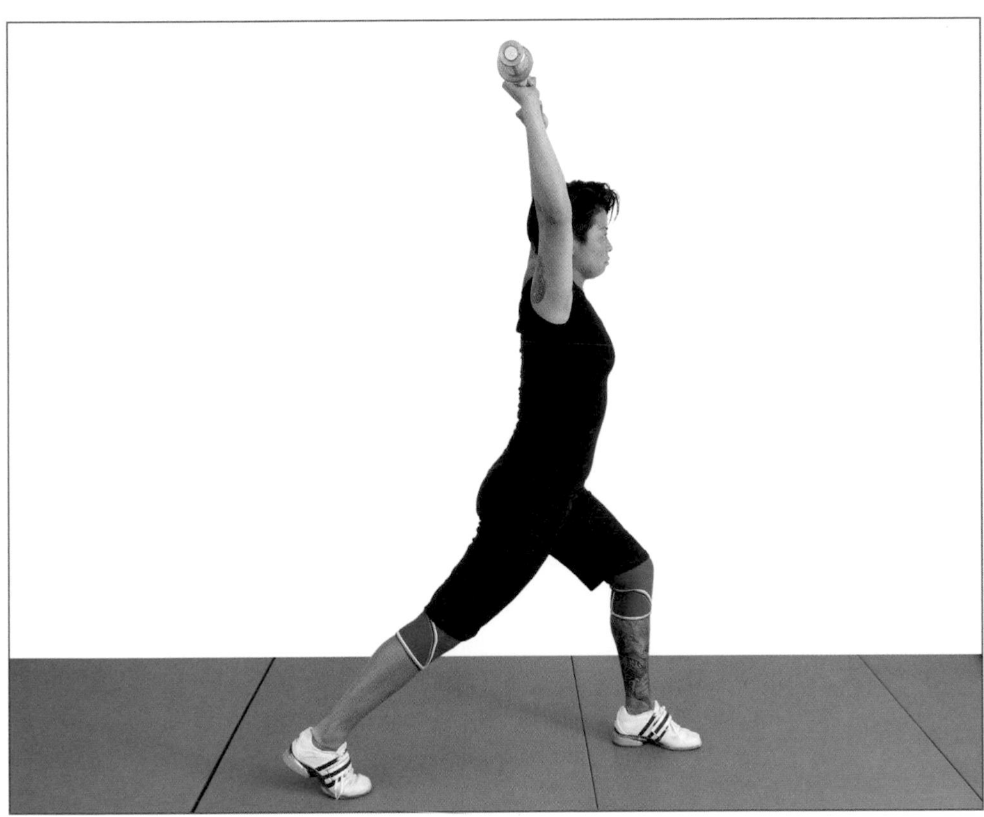

SNATCH

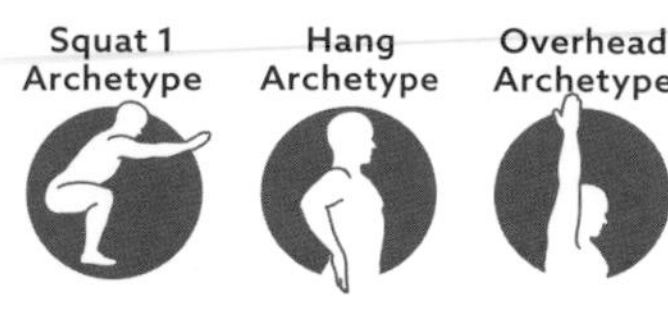

This movement contains the above archetypes. To improve common restrictions associated with this movement, visit the corresponding archetype prescriptions in part 4.

Nothing will tell you more about an athlete's range of motion and understanding of the midline stabilization and torque principles than the snatch. It's the ultimate assessment tool for a coach and consequently the most challenging category 3 movement for an athlete.

The snatch shares the same bottom-up setup as the clean, but requires a higher degree of motor control and mobility. You have to pull with a wider grip and receive the weight in an overhead position. In other words, you have to get into a deeper squat and create torque off a wider grip, adding another level of difficulty—screwing

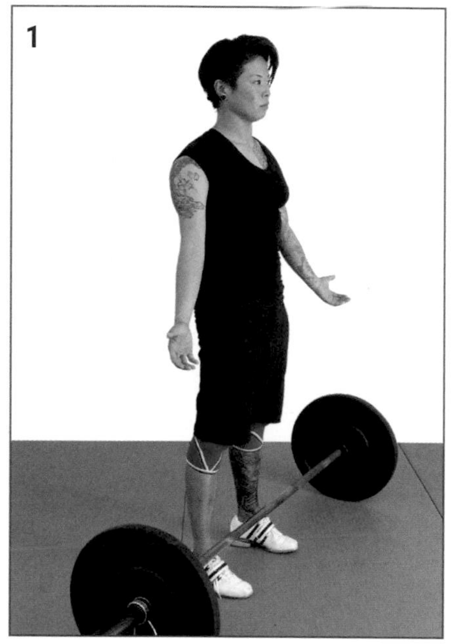

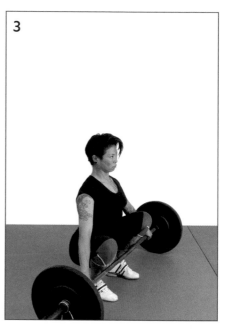

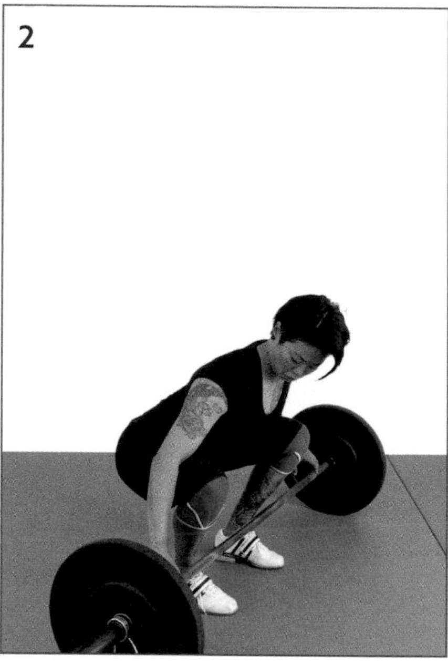

1. Assume your snatch stance (which is the same as your jumping and deadlift stance), pull your shoulders back into external rotation, and go through the bracing sequence.

2. Lower into the bottom of the squat—keeping your back flat, shoulders upright and tight, and knees out—and establish a hook grip (see page 201).

3. To maximize tension in your upper back and get your torso vertical, screw your hands into the bar—creating an external rotation force—pull your shoulders back, and sit your butt to your heels.

4. Load your hips and hamstrings by elevating your hips. As you do, be sure to keep your back flat, shoulders retracted, shins vertical, and knees out. Remember to take all the slack out of the system before you pull.

5. Extend your hips and knees simultaneously. There should be no change in your spinal position as you pull the bar off the ground.

6. As the bar passes your knees, scoop your hips forward, keeping the bar as close to your body as possible. As you reach triple extension, shrug your shoulders. Notice that Diane's arms are straight and that 100 percent of the upward energy generated from her legs and hips is being transferred to the bar.

7. As the bar travels upward, slide your feet out into your landing stance (screwing your feet into the ground), lower into the squat position, and pull yourself underneath the weight.

8. Catch the weight in the bottom of the overhead squat. Keep your shoulders retracted, elbows straight, and armpits forward.

9. Stand up from the overhead squat position.

your hands into the bar with a hook grip and maintaining that external rotation force as you go from a pull to a stable overhead position is extremely tough. This is why so many people struggle to stabilize their shoulders in a good position, keep their torso vertical, and keep their spine rigid. If you make the slightest error or you are missing the smallest corner in your mobility, everything will fall apart.

Note: For the proper width of the snatch grip, I suggest this rather critical notion: Grip the bar so that if things get sketchy, you can dump the weight behind your back and keep it from smashing into your skull. Shoulder flexibility is typically an issue when it comes to the snatch grip; ideally you can work with a coach to figure out what's best and safest.

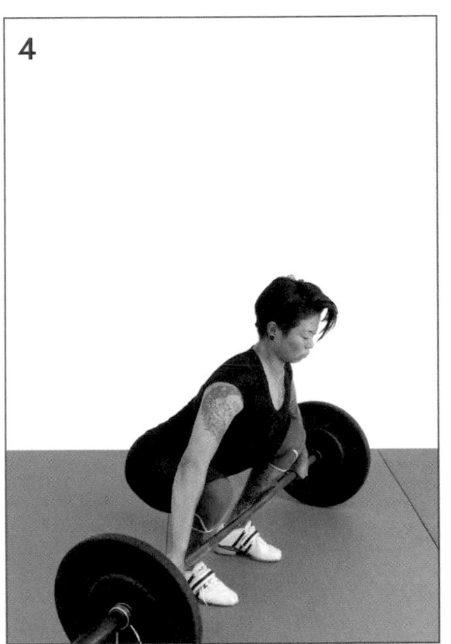

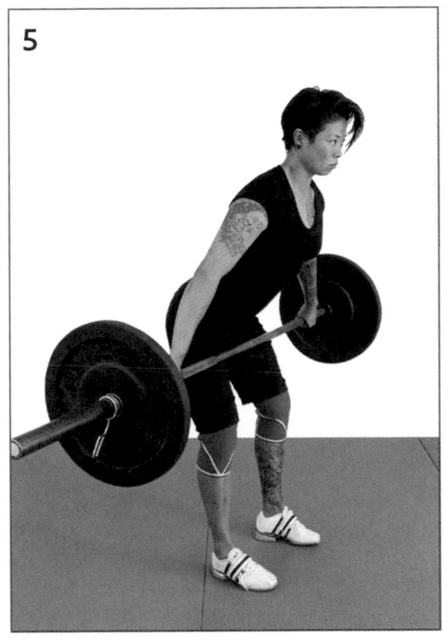

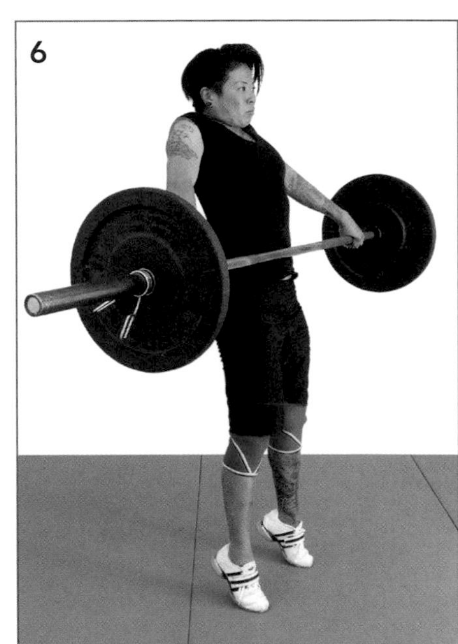

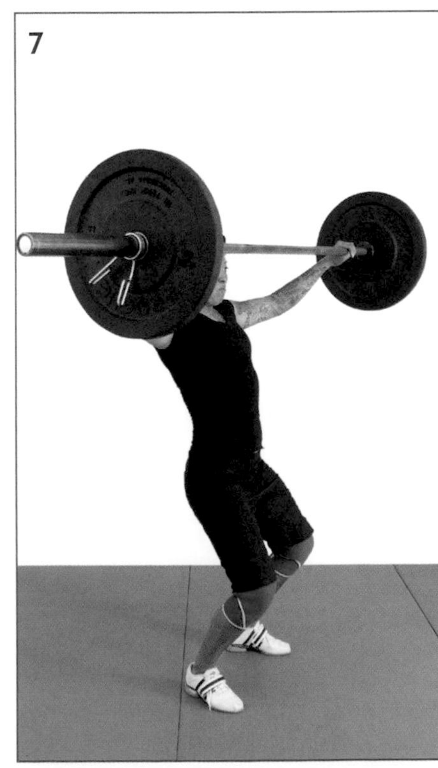

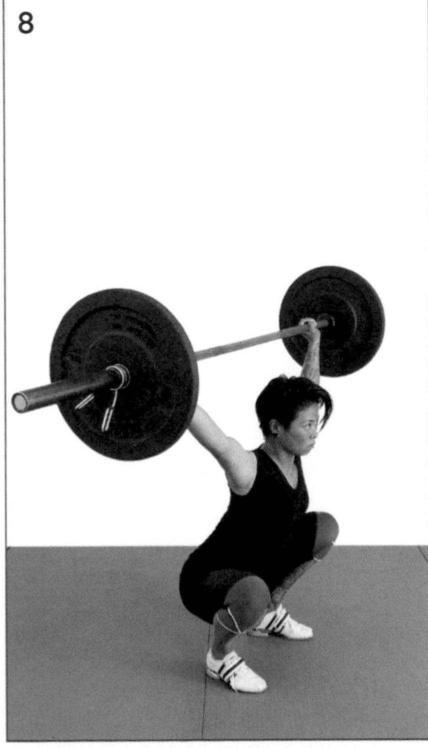

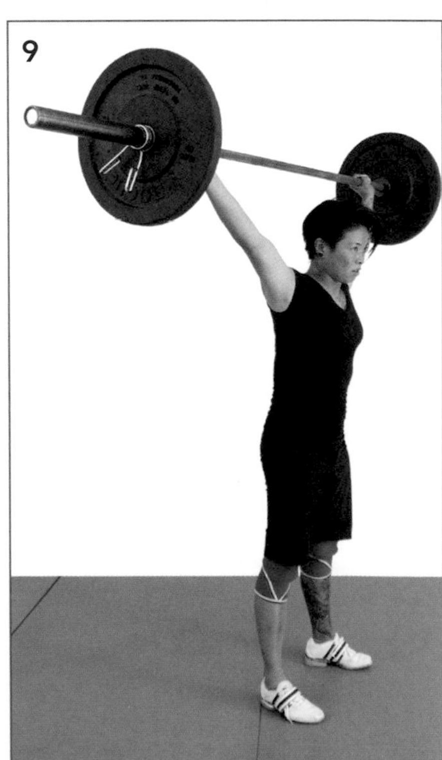

Overhead Archetype

Front Rack 2 Archetype

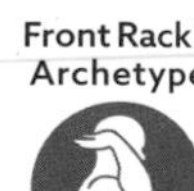

Press Archetype

Hang Archetype

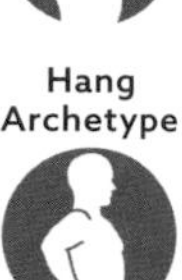

This movement contains the above archetypes. To improve common restrictions associated with this movement, visit the corresponding archetype prescriptions in part 4.

MUSCLE-UP

So you can do a strict pull-up and a ring dip without struggle. That's great! But can you combine the two movements into one seamless, coordinated action? Can you do it while keeping your back flat and your shoulders organized?

The level of trunk and shoulder control required to perform a strict muscle-up is insane. Add a dynamic element like a kip, add a dose of fatigue, or string together multiple reps, and you will reveal any and all crappy motor control habits.

By the way, the rings don't do you any favors. You have to cultivate torque and maintain stability as you go from a pull to a press, a sort of motor control highwire act. It's the equivalent of attempting a snatch while balancing on a pair of rotating, shaking plates. The point is that if you don't have a model for generating torque off an unstable object, you're going to bleed force and get sucked into poor positions that leave you prone to injury.

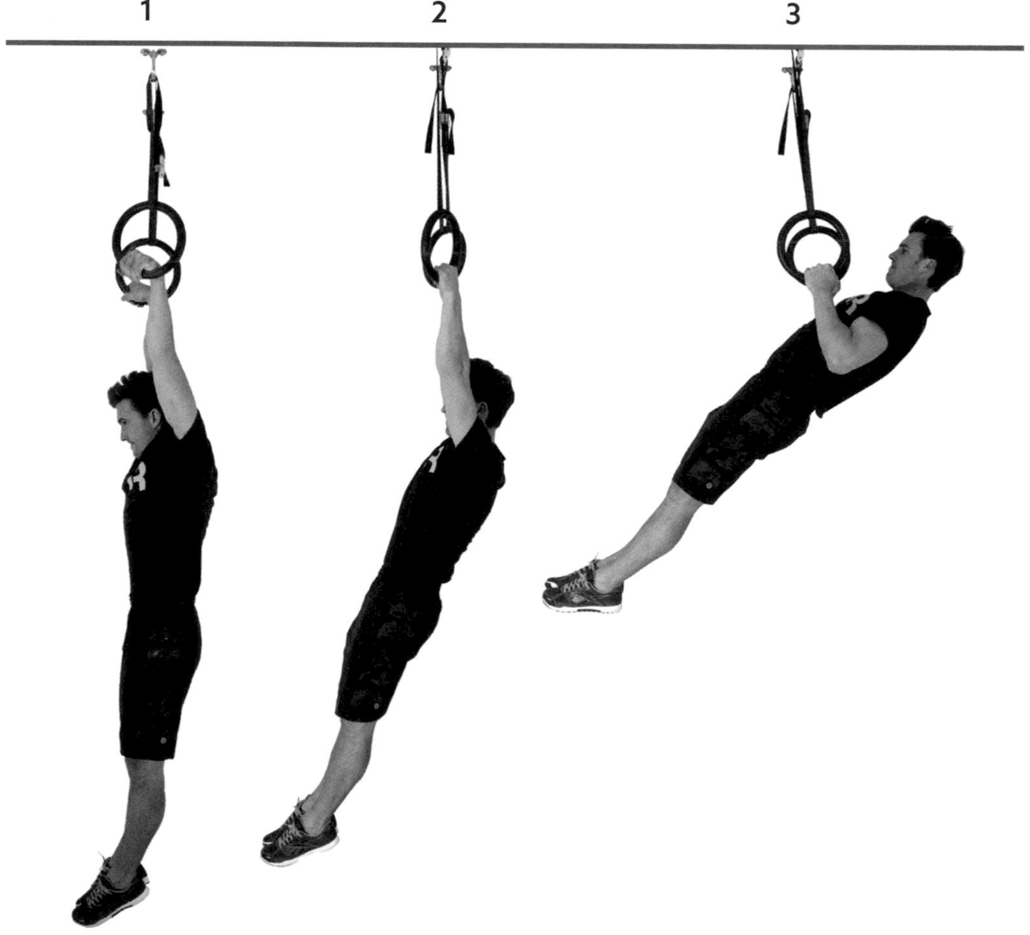

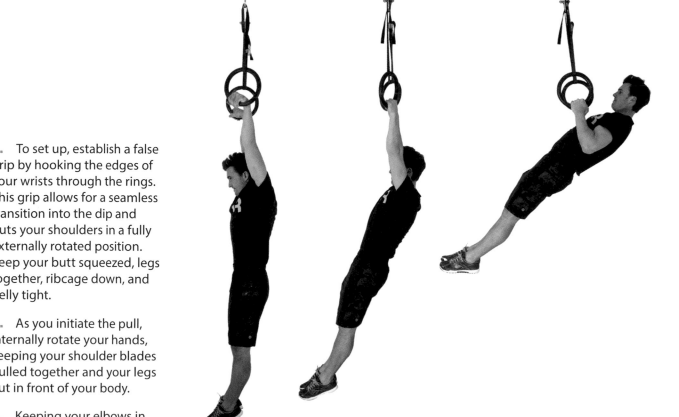

1. To set up, establish a false grip by hooking the edges of your wrists through the rings. This grip allows for a seamless transition into the dip and puts your shoulders in a fully externally rotated position. Keep your butt squeezed, legs together, ribcage down, and belly tight.

2. As you initiate the pull, internally rotate your hands, keeping your shoulder blades pulled together and your legs out in front of your body.

3. Keeping your elbows in tight to your body, pull yourself up. To keep your torso and shoulders integrated, imagine pushing your feet forward as you initiate the pull.

Just because you have the strict pull-up and the full-range ring dip doesn't guarantee that you will be able to do a muscle-up. As with all category 3 movements, the challenge lies in the transition. To shorten the learning curve, we often have athletes practice the transition with the rings low to the ground so that they can use their legs to support their body weight. We also layer in the heaving dip balance, which requires athletes to remove connection with tension and drop from the top to the bottom of the dip. This teaches the athletes how to create spontaneous torque in the bottom of the dip and prepares them for the muscle-up transition. In the meantime, we make it a mission to develop shoulder rotation range of motion.

Note: The kipping muscle-up is performed in much the same way as the kipping pull-up. (To see how to kip, revisit the kipping pull-up on pages 252–253.)

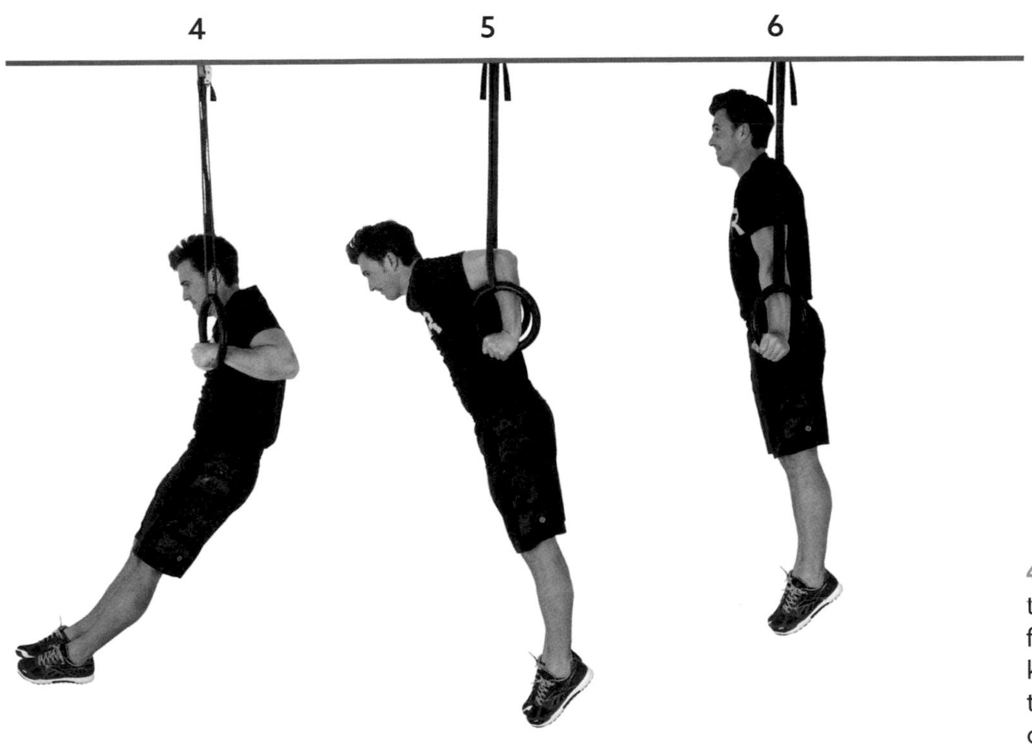

4. As you pull your chest to the rings, punch your torso forward. Again, think about keeping your toes pointed, legs together, and feet positioned out in front of your body.

5. The moment you arrive at the bottom of the dip, actively spin your thumbs toward the outside of your body to create torque in your shoulders.

6. Still turning your hands out, extend your elbows and establish the top of the dip position.

PART 3 MOBILIZATION TECHNIQUES

Are you missing range of motion in one or more areas of your body? Do you have an achy joint that's causing you pain? If you've read part 1, you know what you need to do to fix the problem: Correct the dysfunctional position or movement pattern and get to work mobilizing. You have the knowledge; now it's time to execute.

In this part, you will learn how to perform all the mobilization techniques used in my system. These techniques will help you address short and tight muscles, soft tissue and joint capsule restriction, motor control problems, and joint range of motion limitations. This section, in a nutshell, will equip you with the tools you need to resolve pain, improve position and movement mechanics, and perform basic maintenance on your body.

To help you navigate this section, I've divided the mobilizations into body areas. You can browse by area (upper back, posterior shoulder, etc.) or use the mobility prescriptions in part 4 as your guide. I've also included archetype icons next to the techniques. They tell you which archetype(s) each mobilization will improve. For example, if you see the overhead archetype icon next to the technique you're going to perform, you know that it will improve the overhead archetype. So if you're missing range of motion in a specific position, you can use that archetype icon to help you select specific techniques.

Each mobilization is presented as its own sequence, but most of the techniques can and should be used in combination. For example, you can combine the Quad Smash with the Adductor Smash, or pool all the T-spine mobilization techniques into one long sequence. There are no rules when it comes to combining techniques.

Remember, knowledge is power, but execution is how you make change. Resolve to spend at least 10 to 15 minutes every day working on your position and mobility. The time is now. No excuses!

AREA MAP

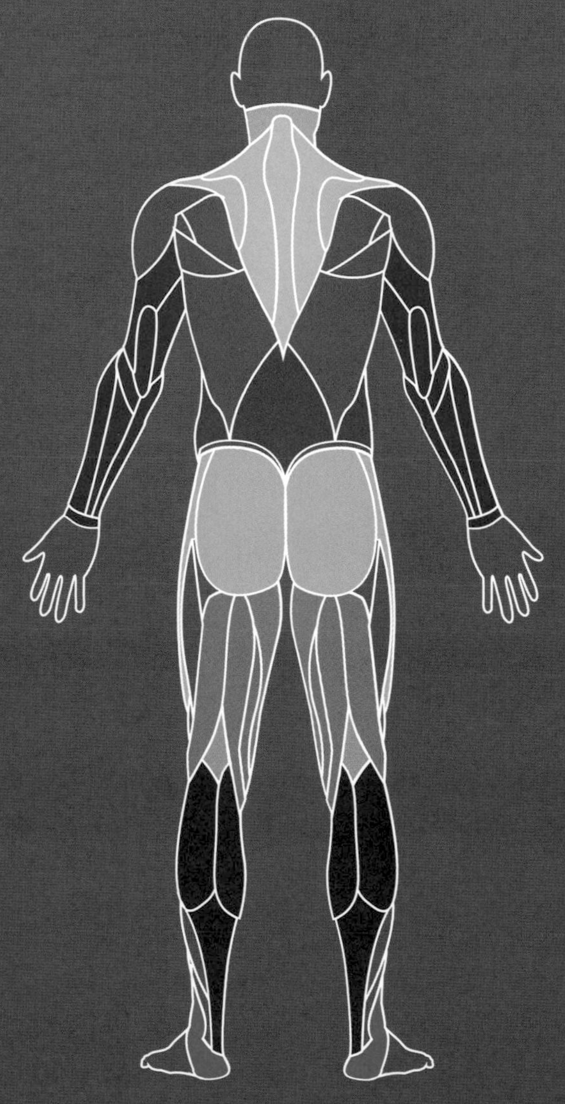

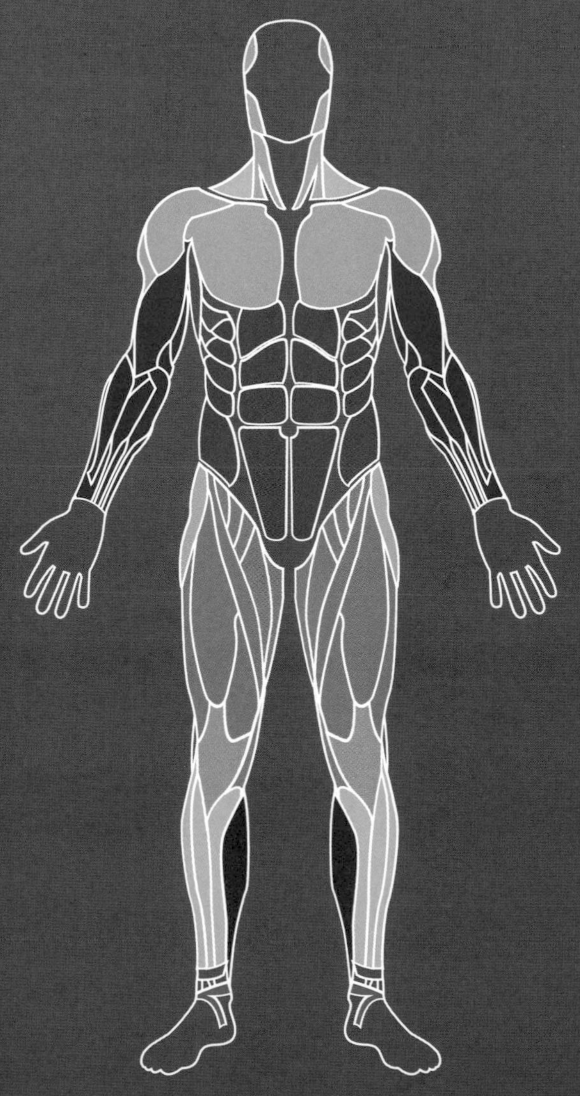

MOBILIZATION TARGET AREAS:

- **AREA 1:** Jaw, Head, and Neck (p. 287)
- **AREA 2:** Upper Back *(Thoracic Spine, Ribs, Trapezius, Scapula)* (p. 292)
- **AREA 3:** Posterior Shoulder, Lat, Serratus (p. 309)
- **AREA 4:** Anterior Shoulder and Chest (p. 322)
- **AREA 5:** Arm *(Triceps, Elbow, Forearm, Wrist)* (p. 335)
- **AREA 6:** Trunk *(Psoas, Low Back, Obliques)* (p. 348)
- **AREA 7:** Glutes, Hip Capsules (p. 367)
- **AREA 8:** Hip Flexors, Quadriceps (p. 384)
- **AREA 9:** Adductors (p. 397)
- **AREA 10:** Hamstrings (p. 403)
- **AREA 11:** Knee (p. 412)
- **AREA 12:** Shin (p. 419)
- **AREA 13:** Calf (p. 424)
- **AREA 14:** Ankle, Foot, and Toes (p. 431)

Mobility Tools

To perform the techniques demonstrated in this section, you will need a few pieces of equipment. If you don't have the exact tools listed, you can improvise by using whatever you have lying around the house: wine bottles, rolling pins, dog toys, sports equipment—the list goes on and on. For example, if you don't have a VooDoo Floss Band, cut a bicycle tire tube in half and you have yourself a functional compression band. I never want to hear the excuse, "I don't have a lacrosse ball or pipe to roll on, so I can't do it." Use your imagination and make use of what's in reach. It's all fair game.

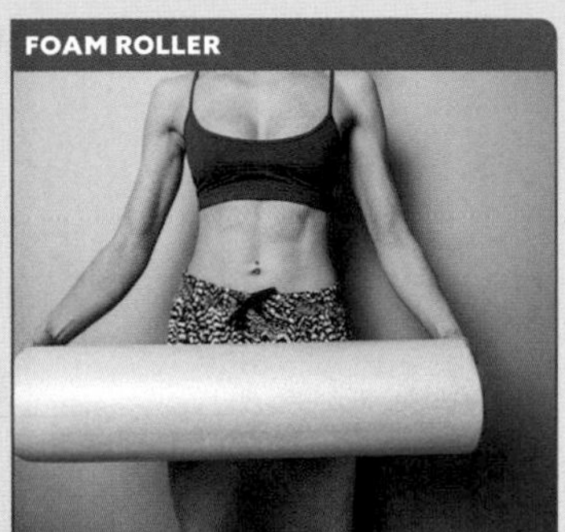
FOAM ROLLER

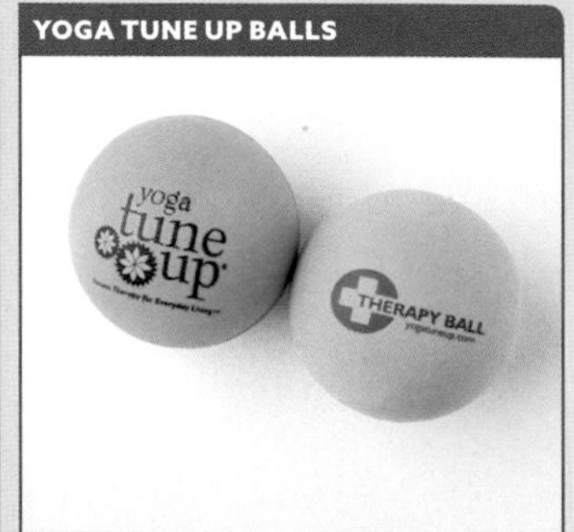

YOGA TUNE UP BALLS

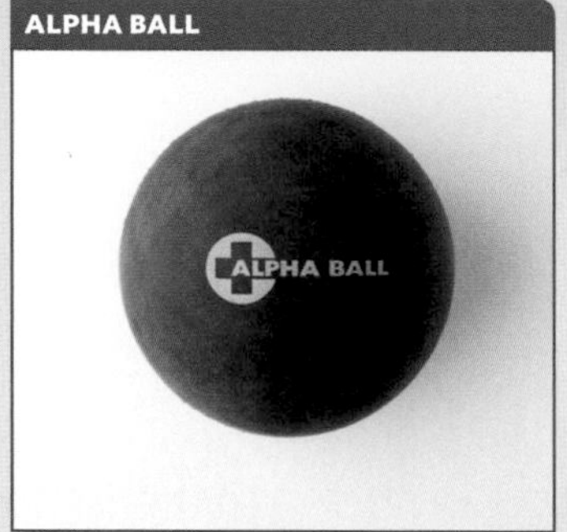

ALPHA BALL

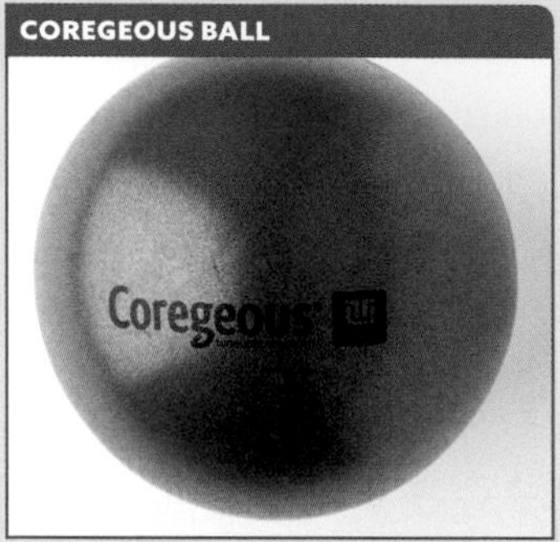

COREGEOUS BALL

LEVEL 1 MOBILIZATION TOOLS

These are the easiest and least painful mobilization tools. If you're super sore or new to mobilization exercises, stick with these tools. But hear this: You will never make significant change if you implement only the level 1 tools. Use these as a warm-up and try to progress to level 2 and 3 mobilization tools.

FOAM ROLLER

Good for: contract and relax, pressure wave, smash and floss

To be blunt, I think foam rollers are fine for beginners and children, but to effect the kind of change an athlete needs for top performance, you need a tool that can penetrate deeper into your tissues and create more shear. But you do need some type of roller. Opt for something with a little bite to it, like the Battlestar, a pipe, or a barbell.

YOGA TUNE UP BALLS

Good for: contract and relax, pressure wave, smash and floss, tack and twist

From fascia and pain relief expert Jill Miller, these balls are about the same size as lacrosse balls, but are softer and have a stickier surface. They give you a different spin on the techniques for which you could also use a lacrosse ball, but they're especially useful for tacking and twisting tissues, such as those on the top of your foot, and breathing some life into your fascias. (Available at www.yogatuneup.com)

ALPHA BALL

Good for: contract and relax, pressure wave, smash and floss, tack and twist

Another of Jill Miller's tools, this ball is 3.5 inches in diameter, a bit soft, and a bit sticky, so it's good for hotspot work when you're trying to unglue stuck sliding surface tissue. (Available at www.yogatuneup.com)

COREGEOUS BALL

Good for: smash and floss, contract and relax

Jill Miller's inflatable 9-inch ball is used primarily for global gut smashing. It's a little bit sticky, so you can tack the ball into a spot and work on the dreaded psoas. (Available at www.yogatuneup.com)

LACROSSE BALLS

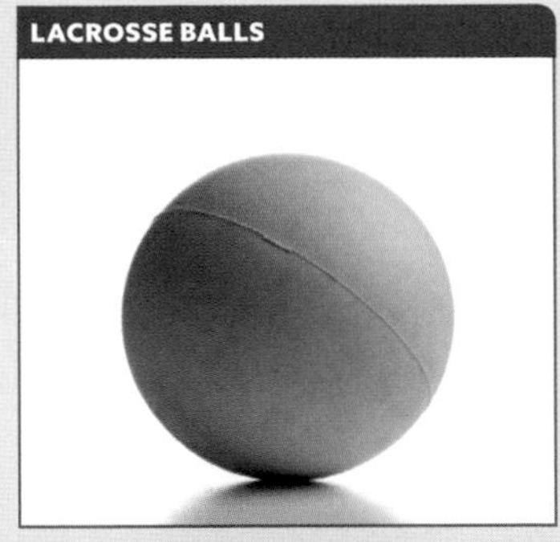

BARBELL

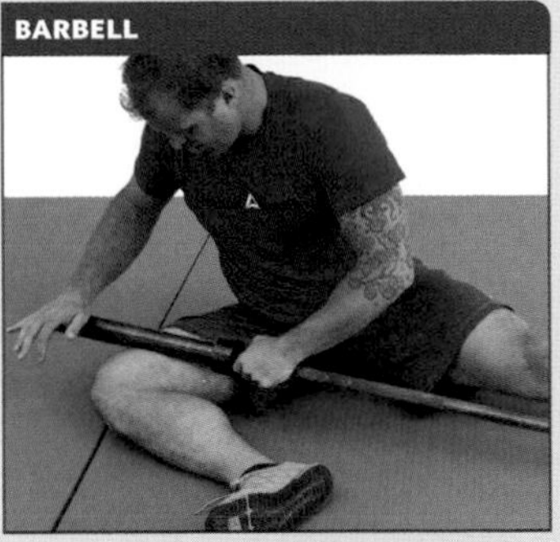

KETTLEBELL

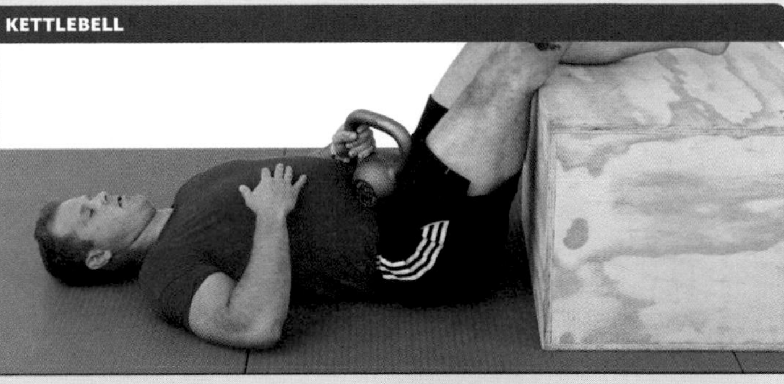

SOFTBALL

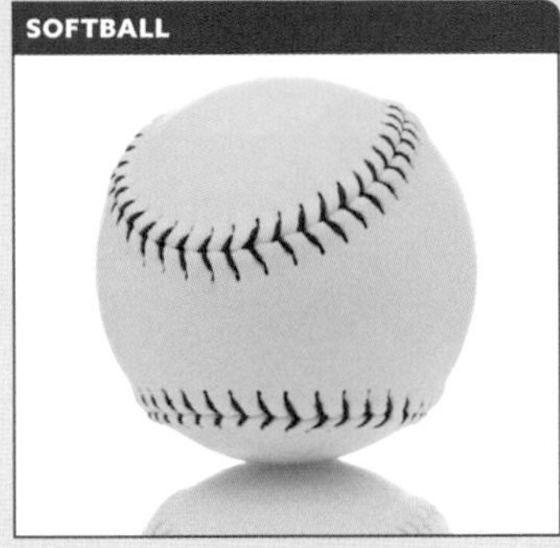

SOCCER BALL

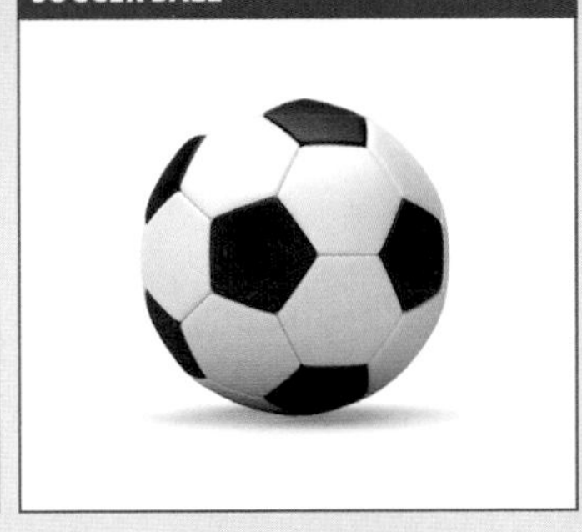

ROGUE MONSTER BAND

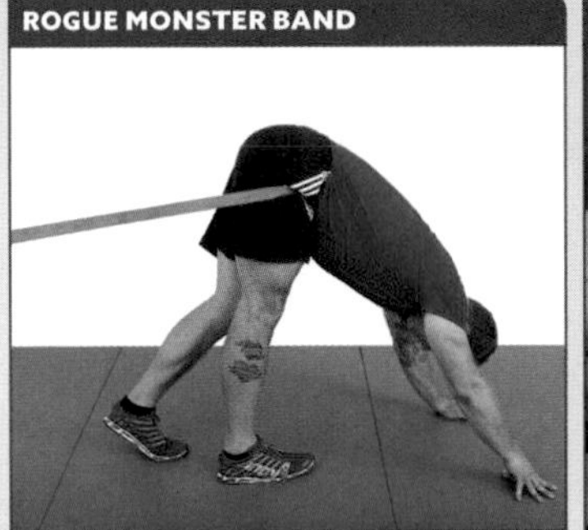

DOUBLE LACROSSE BALLS

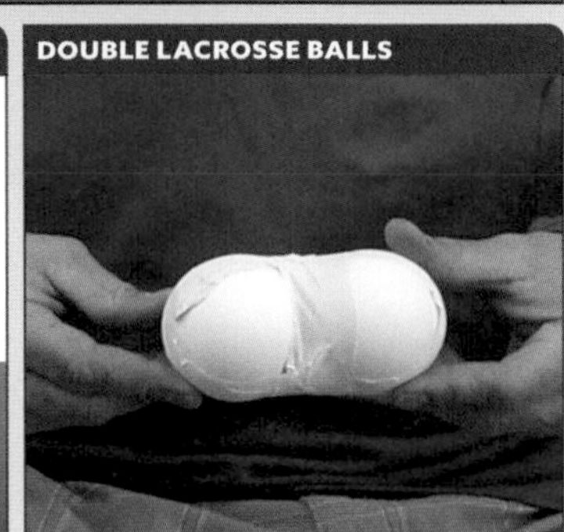

LEVEL 2 MOBILIZATION TOOLS

Using a band or tools that are smooth yet hard (think PVC pipe, lacrosse ball, and softball) falls into the level 2 category. These tools are more painful but also more effective than level 1 tools, and they serve as a progression into the level 3 tools.

LACROSSE BALLS

Good for: contract and relax, pressure wave, smash and floss, flexion gapping, tack and twist

Lacrosse balls are firm enough to sink deep into your tissues. You can do some incredible mobility work with lacrosse balls alone. Tape two lacrosse balls together (see below) for mobilizations that target the thoracic spine.

BARBELL AND KETTLEBELL

Good for: smash and floss, contract and relax, pressure wave

A barbell is a crude yet highly effective smashing implement. Almost every gym has one lying on the floor, so if you don't have access to a roller or double lacrosse ball, a barbell is a great option.

SOFTBALL

Good for: contract and relax, smash and floss, pressure wave

Sometimes you need an object larger than a lacrosse ball to get where you need to go with a smash. A softball is especially good for smashing into the large glute muscles.

SOCCER BALL

Good for: contract and relax, smash and floss, pressure wave

In athletes, the psoas gets incredibly tight, setting off a wide range of mobility troubles. Smashing your gut with a deflated soccer ball is a great way to restore suppleness to the area.

ROGUE MONSTER BAND

Good for: contract and relax, banded flossing

This robust rubber band is used primarily for banded flossing. It helps put your joint into a good position and helps with joint capsule restriction. (Available at www.roguefitness.com)

How to build a double lacrosse ball

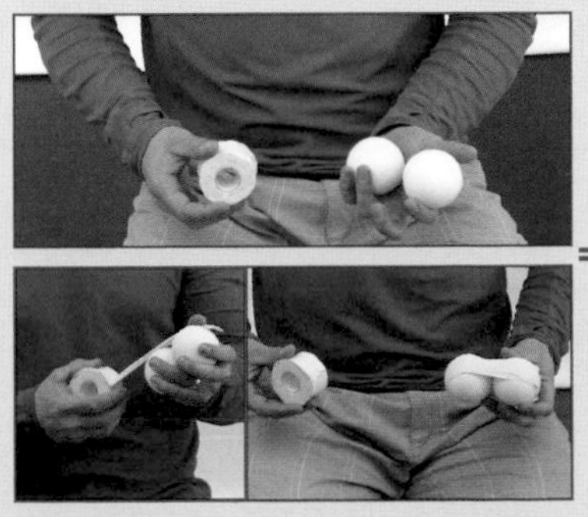

=

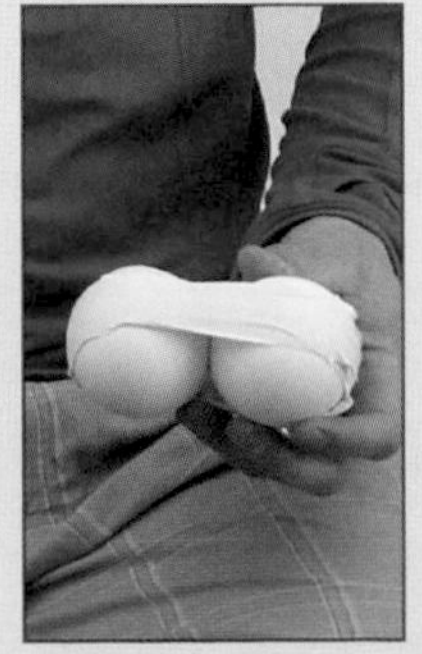

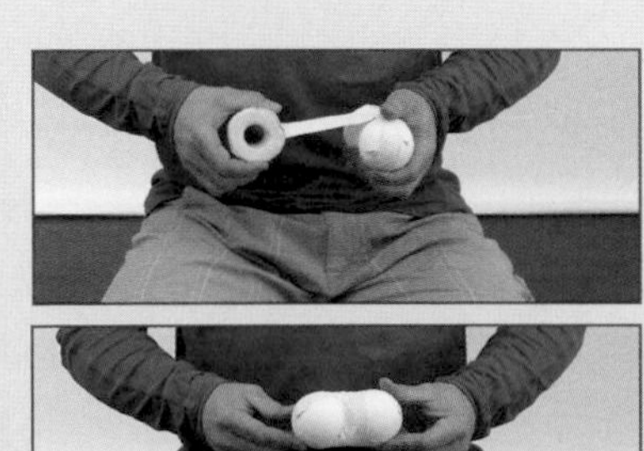

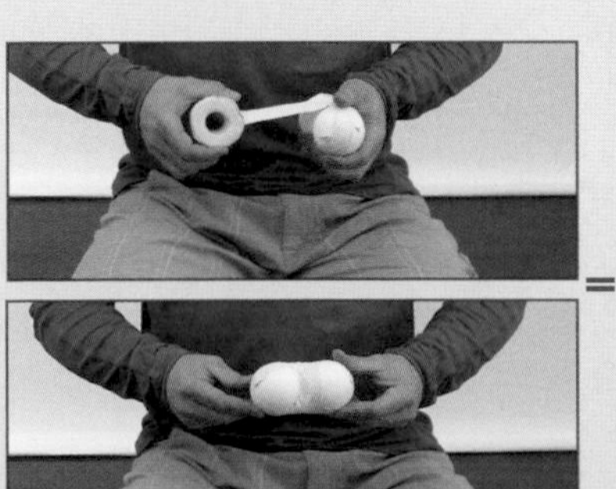

=

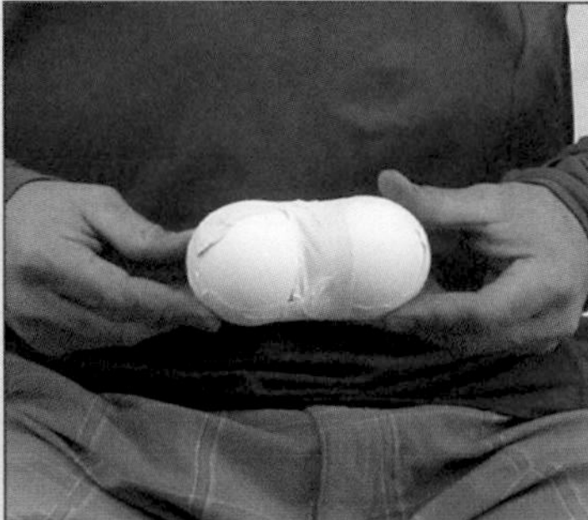

BATTLESTAR & LITTLE BATTLESTAR

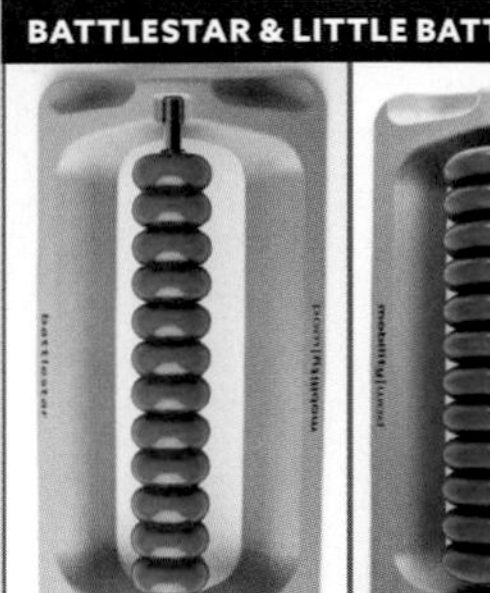

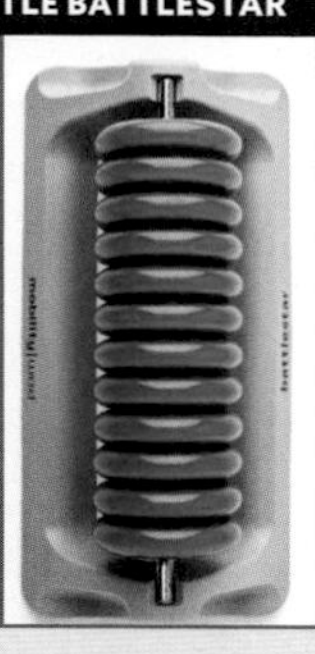

SUPERNOVA AND SUPERNOVITO

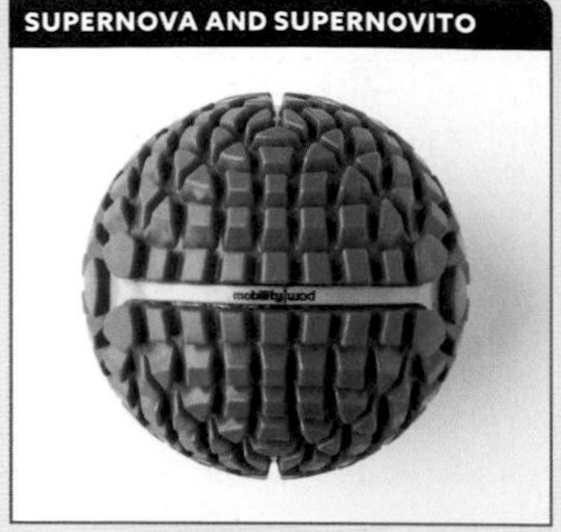

GEMINI

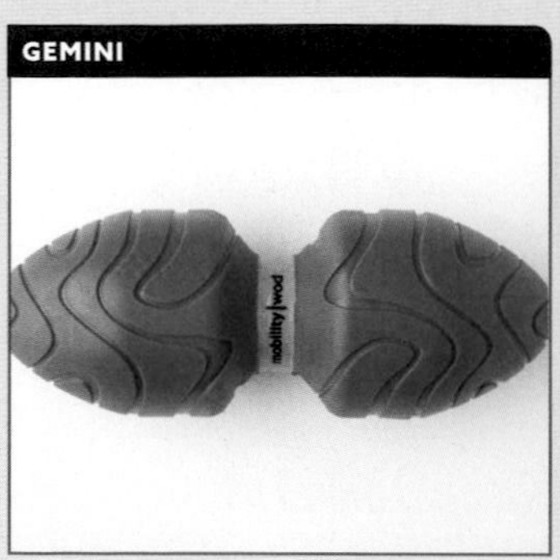

VOODOO FLOSS BAND

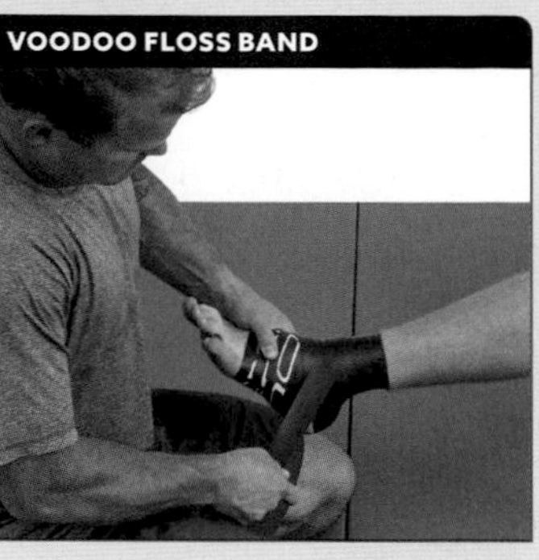

LEVEL 3 MOBILIZATION TOOLS

These harder, uncompromising mobilization tools are often associated with technique variations that increase pressure and range of motion. These tools are likely to send you into deep crevices of the pain cave, but don't be scared. They are also the most effective and give you the biggest bang for your buck.

BATTLESTAR AND LITTLE BATTLESTAR

Good for: contract and relax, pressure wave, stripping, smash and floss, global shear

An extreme upgrade to the standard foam roller. I like to equate the Battlestar with what you'd get if you combined a chainsaw, a wolverine, and a steamroller. I designed this tool to execute both the global shearing of a hard foam roller and acute, detailed raking work. (Available at www.roguefitness.com)

SUPERNOVA AND SUPERNOVITO

Good for: smash, contract and relax, pressure wave, stripping, smash and floss

An upgrade on the softball, the Supernova was invented to dole out a much higher percentage of grip and shear when working into a deep pocket of tissue, like the hip or hamstring. The teeth of the Supernova are designed to separate the many layers of tissue that you need to penetrate for optimal mobility work. (Available at www.roguefitness.com)

GEMINI

Good for: smash, contract and relax, stripping, smash and floss

I started with the double lacrosse ball setup for work on the T-spine, where it's ideal for blocking off the facet joints, but this tool provides more detail and grip to get a little more out of targeted trigger point work. (Available at www.roguefitness.com)

VOODOO FLOSS BAND

Good for: VooDoo Floss Band compression

The VooDoo Floss Band is engineered for therapeutic compression on hotspots and swollen joints. A household alternative is to splice a bike tire tube lengthwise. (Available at www.roguefitness.com)

AREA 1 JAW, HEAD, AND NECK

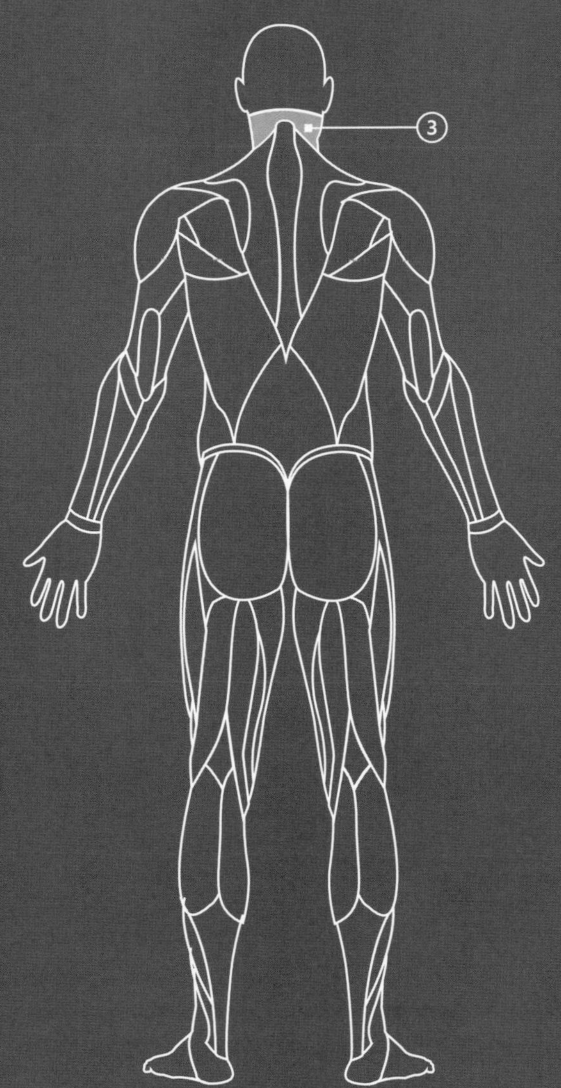

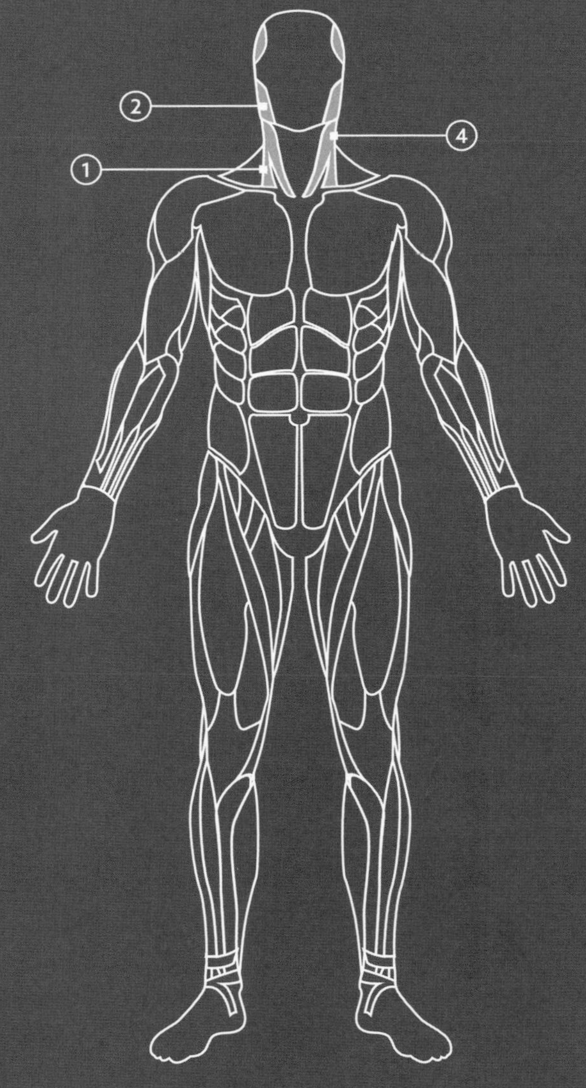

MOBILIZATION TARGET AREAS:

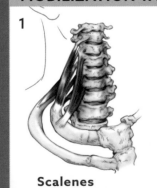

1 Scalenes

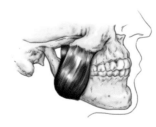

2 Masseter

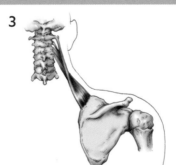

3 Levator Scapula

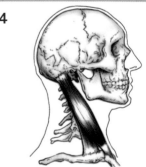

4 Sternocleidomastoid

IMPROVES:
Headaches
Jaw function
Jaw pain (TMJD)

METHODS:
Tack and twist
Contract and relax

JAW AND HEAD

If you grind your teeth at night, clench your jaw, hang out with your mouth open, or adopt funky jaw positions when you lift, then these mobilizations are for you. But don't use these mobs as a crutch. You need to get these habits under control. Your mouth is an open circuit that can leak power and stability from your system—not to mention the insidious tightness that aggregates when combined with eating, grinding, and clenching.

Just like everything else, the musculature of your jaw and head gets tight, which can cause a lot of problems. In fact, if you're prone to exertion or tension headaches, then this mob should be high on your list.

The truth is, we don't talk to these tissues as much as we should. Use these mobs to get in there and clean up some of the funky head and jaw stiffness that tends to cause problems downstream.

Note: To effectively treat a tension or exertion headache, open up your thoracic spine by using one of the techniques in the next section, and then combine all the mobilization techniques contained in this section—see the Tension and Exertion Headache prescription on page 467.

Jaw Mob

1. Position a ball at the corner of your jaw with your palm facing away from your body.
2. Pressing the ball firmly into your jaw, twist your hand. This captures all the fascia and surrounding musculature underneath and around the ball.
3. Move your jaw around in all directions.

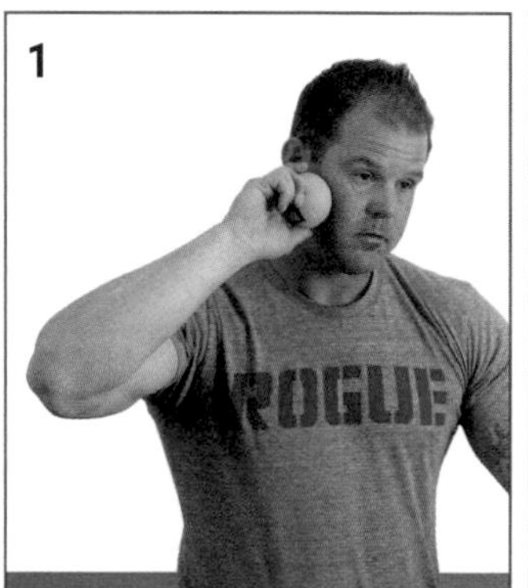

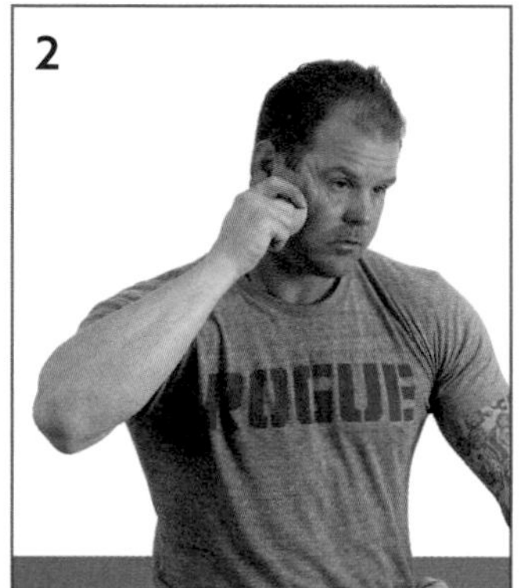

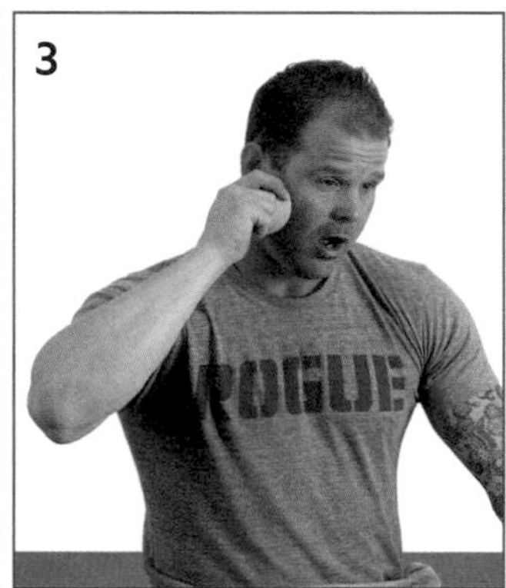

Head Mob

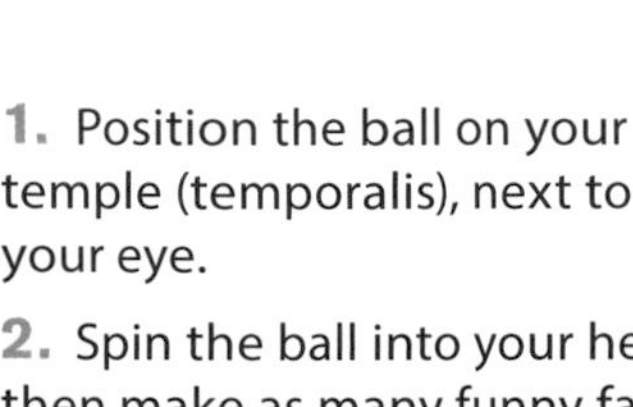
1. Position the ball on your temple (temporalis), next to your eye.
2. Spin the ball into your head, then make as many funny faces as possible—make circles with your eyes, raise your eyebrows, open your mouth, etc.

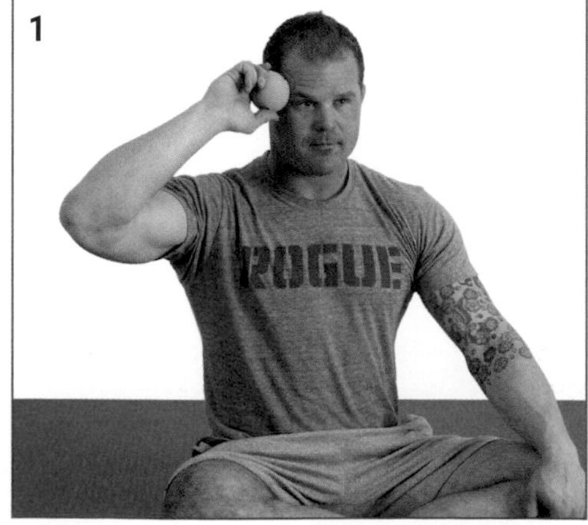

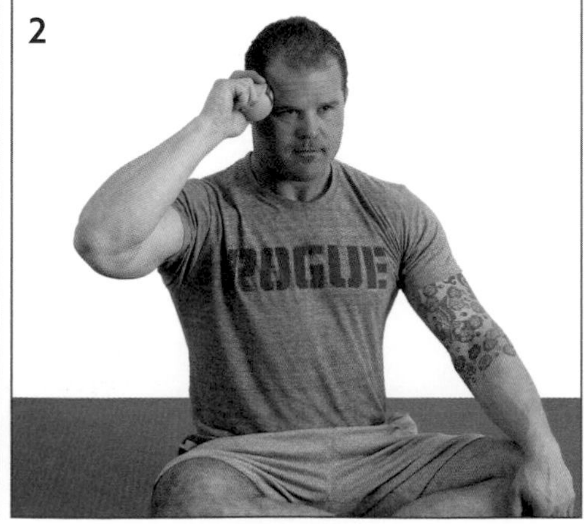

Anterior Neck Mob

IMPROVES:

Tension or exertion headaches
Forward head on neck position
Neck mobility
Neck pain

METHOD:

Tack and twist

Have you ever fallen asleep in an airplane seat with your head down? It's no fun. The sleep is poor, and your short neck flexors get screwed. Slouching produces a similar result. When you slouch—meaning that you round forward, internally rotate your shoulders, and assume the dreaded forward-head-on-neck position—the muscles in the front of your neck get short and stiff. Whether the front of your neck is tight from sleeping in a bad position, slouching, or exercising, you need to get in there with a ball and clean up the area. Failure to do so can compromise your breathing, wreck your posture, and even cause headaches.

This mob restores sliding surfaces and range of motion to your neck flexors, which run from your jaw down to your clavicles and around the front of your neck. The tack and twist technique is key here. Conventional methods for dealing with tight neck flexors tell you to anchor your head and pull it to the side (imagine grabbing the left side of your head with your right hand and pulling your right ear down to your right shoulder). I was taught this method in PT school, and I'm still not a fan. In order to unglue the nerves that are tacked down and stiff, you need to bind up the matted-down tissue with a ball and create movement.

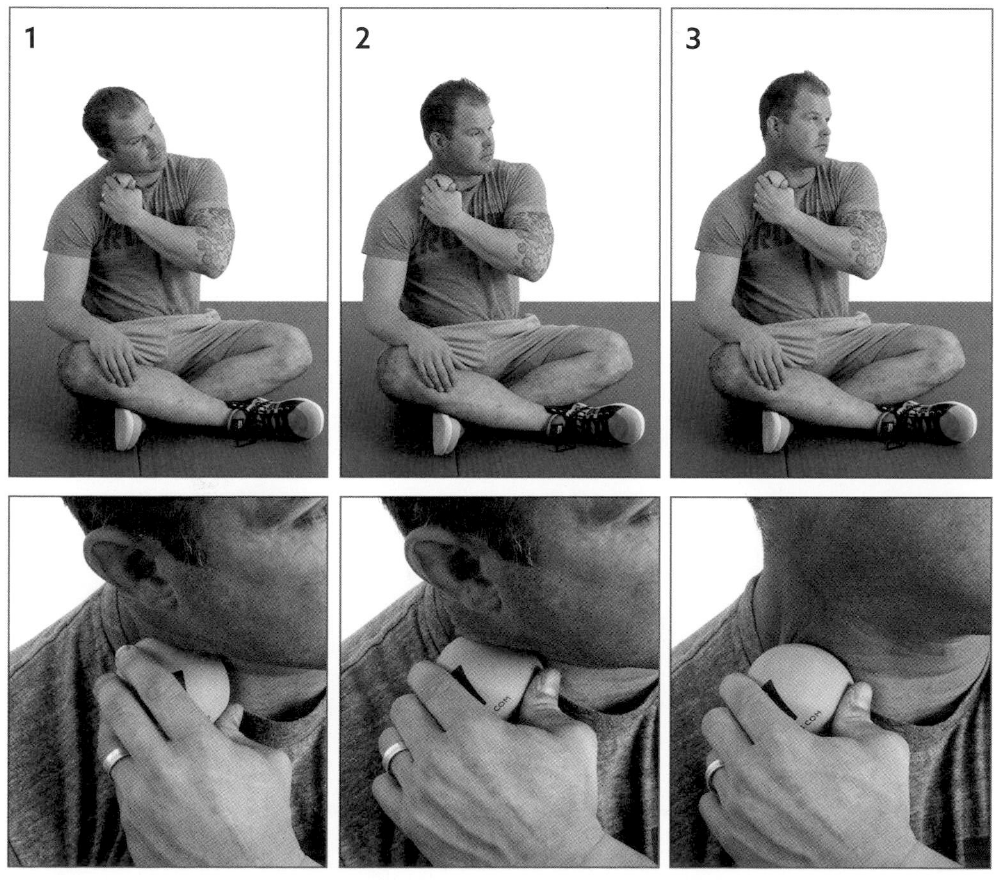

1. Tilting your head to the side, pin the ball on the side of your neck, just above your clavicle. *Note:* You can use this mob to target the entire front and side region of your neck, from your ear to the outline of your collarbone.

2. Maintaining pressure, bind up the tissue by twisting the ball in place.

3. Look away from the ball and move your head in different directions. You can also slide the ball around as a way of breaking up tacked-down tissue. If you feel like you need more tension in the system, maneuver your arm behind your back on the same side as the area you're mobilizing.

IMPROVES:

Tension and exertion headaches

Forward-head-on-neck position

Neck strain or neck extensor stiffness

Neck mobility

METHODS:

Pressure wave

Contract and relax

Posterior Neck Mob

Consider a lifter who throws his head back as he performs a deadlift, swings a kettlebell, or squats. Or a deskbound weekend warrior who can't help but default into a slouched position while working. Anytime you throw your head back or slouch, you're putting your neck in an overextended, compressed position, which can cause the back of your neck to get brutally tight. When your neck extensors get locked down, it tends to cause a lot grief. Neck pain, neck strains, and tension headaches are common.

There's no doubt that keeping your head in a neutral position is difficult to manage, especially given its weight. (A human head can weigh up to 10 pounds.) Neck strains happen. You need a template for cleaning up the back of your neck because this area gets tight in everyone. And it's easy to do. You can do this mob while watching TV or between sets during a workout.

Take whatever ball you have—you can use an Alpha ball, use the Supernova, or even put a lacrosse ball on an ab mat (small mat)—and scour the outline of your skull, from the base of your skull to your ears. If you find a tight spot, try scrubbing back and forth across the knotted-up tissue. You can also add more pressure by loading your head into the ball or by positioning your hands on your head (see option 2).

This is the best mob for cleaning up the back of your neck near the base of your skull, specifically your neck extensors. To address your cervical spine, however, consider using a double lacrosse ball, pair of Yoga Tune Up balls, or Gemini. Position the tool at the base of your head. The idea is to target the vertebrae segments of your cervical spine, stopping at each segment, and then floss by moving your head around in all directions. You can also place the tool on an ab mat and work on loading your weight into it, effectively tacking down the tissue, and then curling your head by dropping your chin to your chest. The last option is to roll up a hand towel, place it around your cervical spine between your vertebrae, and move your head from side to side and backward and forward.

TARGET AREA

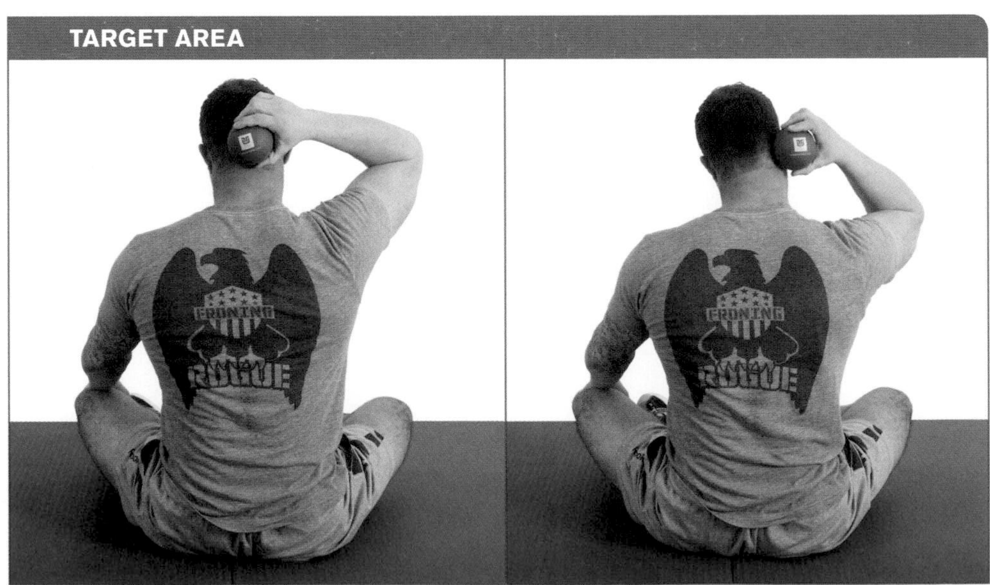

Start at the base of your neck and skull (occiput) and trace the outline of your head to the back of your ear.

Posterior Neck Mob: Option 1

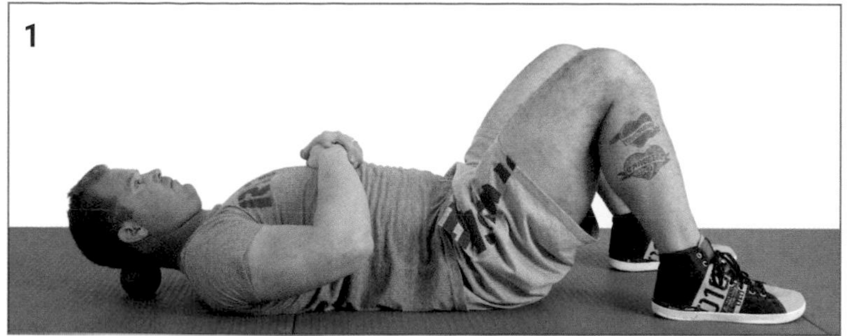
1

Lying on your back, position a ball in the center of your skull. You will feel a small pocket.

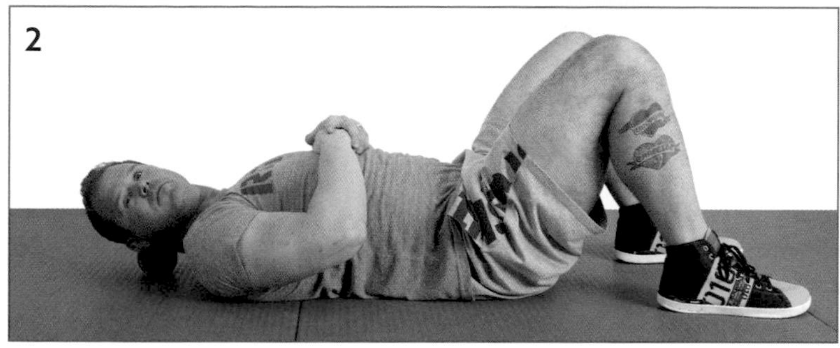
2

Slowly rotate your head to the side, rolling the ball along the base of your skull to the corner of your ear.

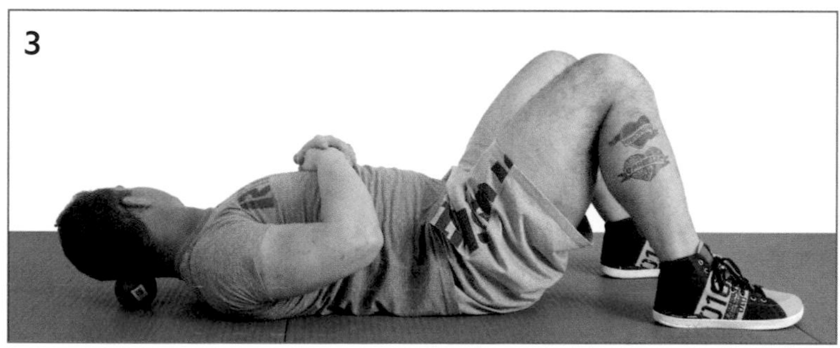
3

Turn your head to the opposite side, scouring the entire base of your skull.

Posterior Neck Mob: Option 2

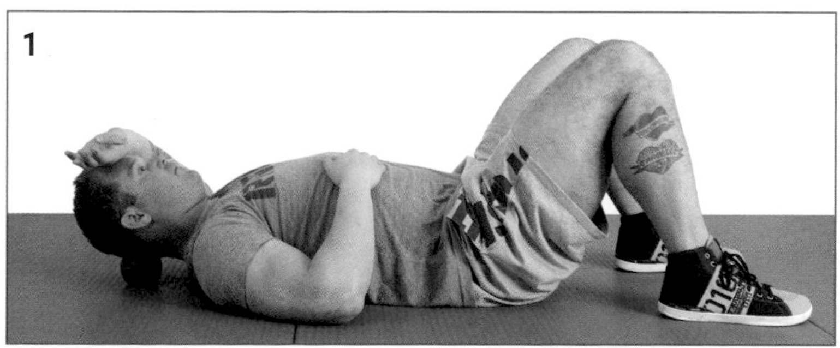
1

To increase the downward pressure, place your wrist over your forehead with your palm facing the ceiling.

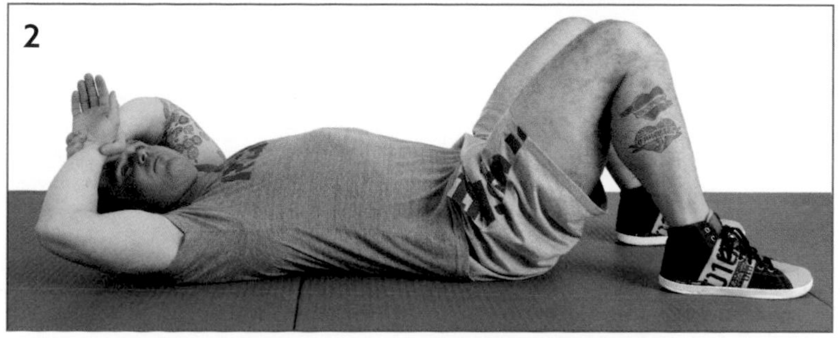
2

Grab the wrist of your opposite arm and slowly scrub along the base of your skull using slow, back-and-forth movements.

AREA 2 UPPER BACK (THORACIC SPINE, RIBS, TRAPEZIUS, SCAPULA)

MOBILIZATION TARGET AREAS:

Trapezius

Erector Spinae

Rhomboids

Supraspinatus

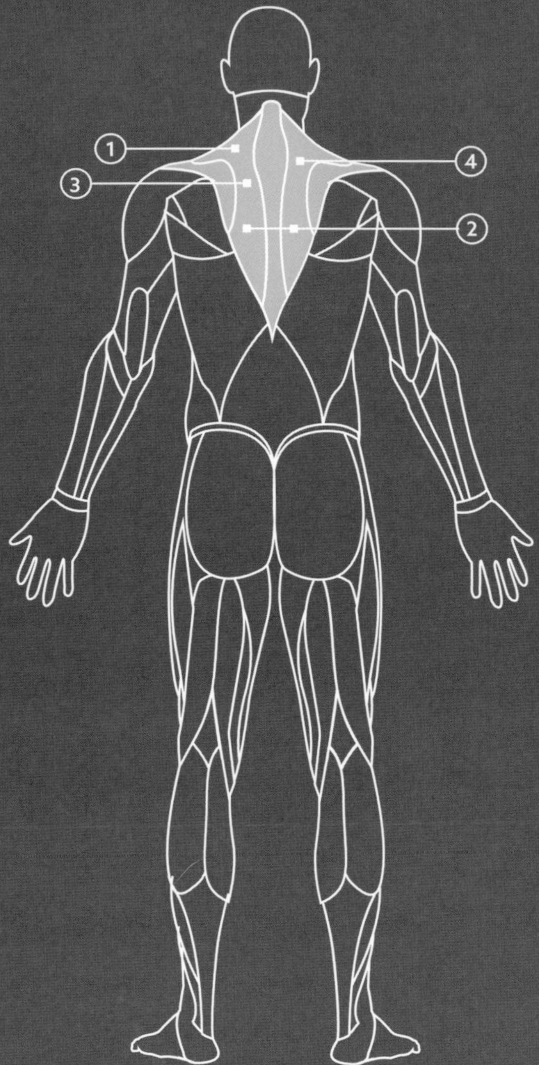

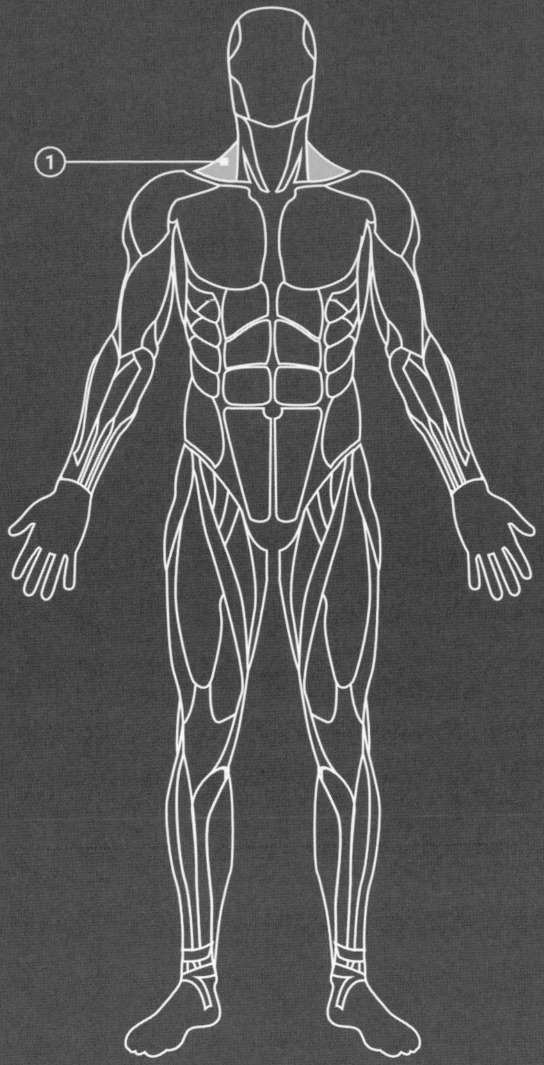

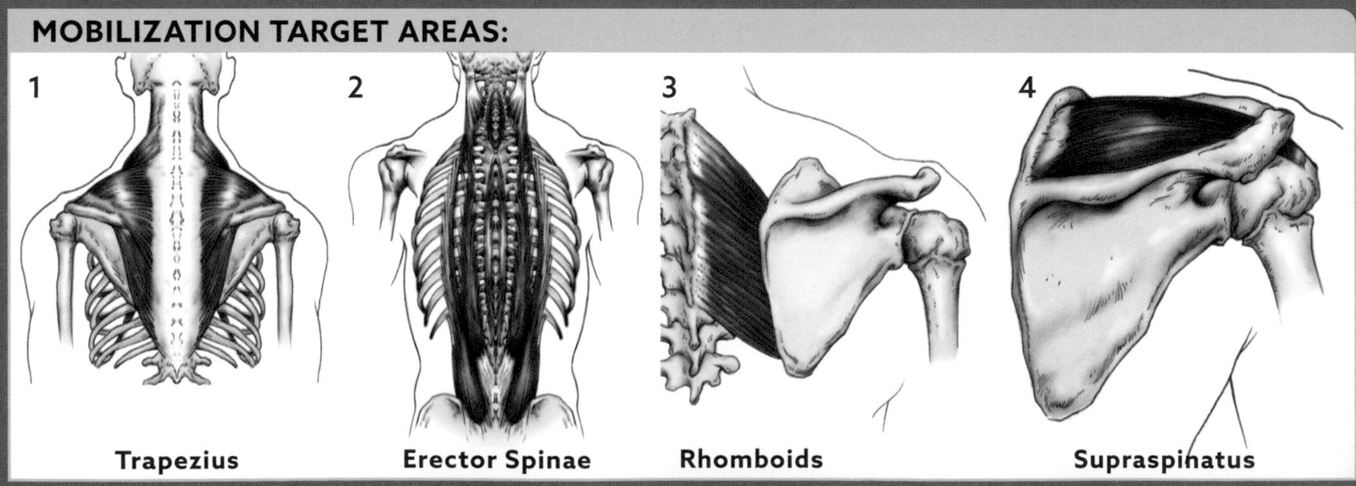

T-Spine Roller Smash Mobilizations

When your thoracic spine gets stiff, it's difficult to stabilize your shoulders and head in a good position. It can also result in neck and shoulder pain. The T-Spine Roller Smash Mobilizations are your first stop on the road to better thoracic mobility.

These mobilizations are what we call global extension exercises. You're not trying to target any single tissue or motion segment as you would when using a double lacrosse ball. Instead, the goal is to open up your entire thoracic system. While a ball is more precise at digging into tight, nasty spots, a foam roller or Battlestar can tackle two or three motion segments of your back, your rib facet joints, and some of the soft tissues in your upper back.

Overhead Archetype

Press Archetype

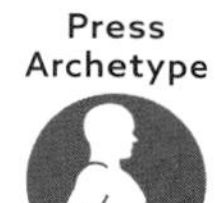

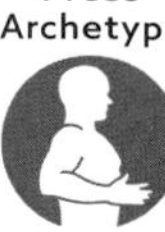

Front Rack 2 Archetype

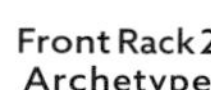

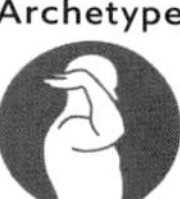

Front Rack 1 Archetype

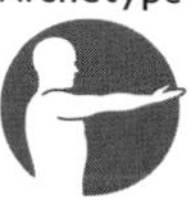

Hang Archetype

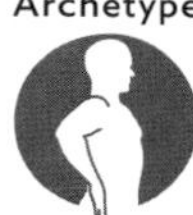

This mobilization will help improve the above archetypes.

IMPROVES:

Neutral spinal position
Shoulder function
Thoracic mobility (global flexion and extension)
Neck, upper back, & shoulder pain

NOTE ON THE BATTLESTAR:
A foam roller is the most basic of the mobility tools that we use. Anytime you see the Battlestar pictured, remember that you can always substitute a foam roller.

Option 1: Extension Smash

The key to this mobilization is to focus on creating large extension forces over the roller by arching back. A common mistake is to mindlessly roll back and forth with zero intention. At the gym, you often see people foam rolling aimlessly in the name of warming up—while catching up on a new *Game of Thrones* episode. This does nothing. To make real and lasting change, you have to create as much of a teeter-totter effect and extension force over those tissues as possible.

When you find a tight area, use the roller as a fulcrum by arching your back. Think about letting the roller break you into extension. You can take a big breath and try to snake your way around, extend back and forth, elevate your hips to add pressure, and then lower your butt to the ground. Explore the area, find where your back is tight, and stay on that area until you've made some change.

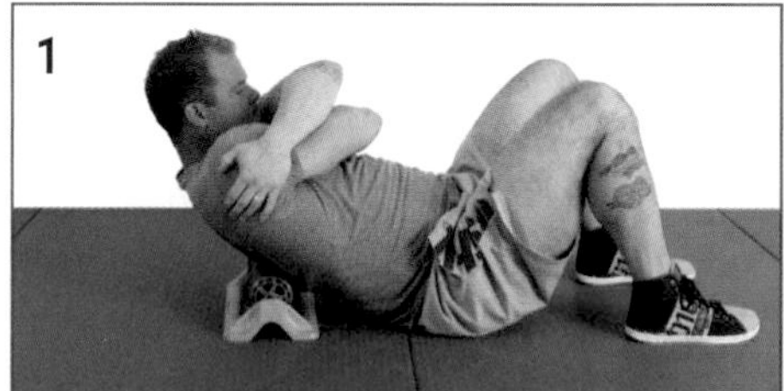

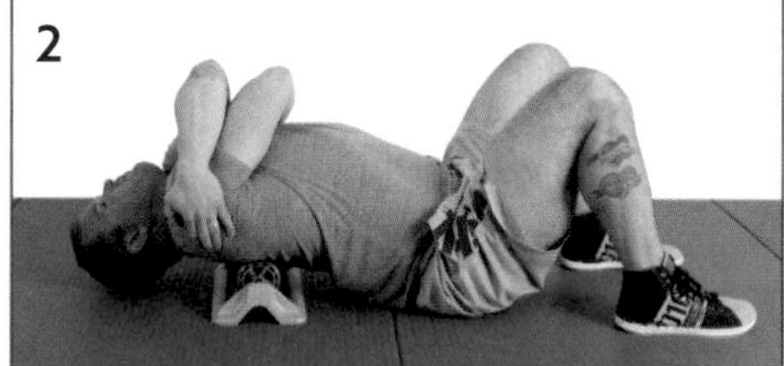

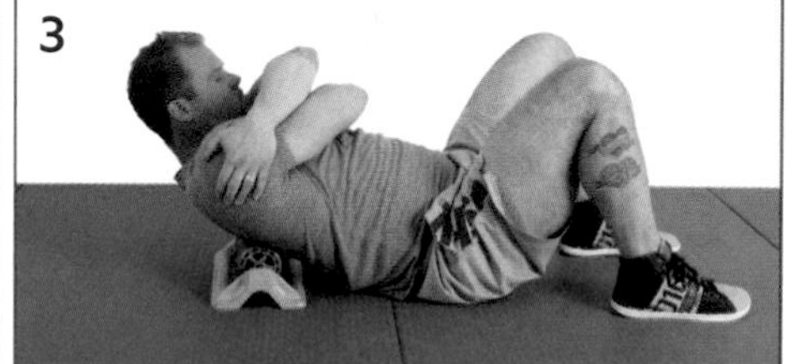

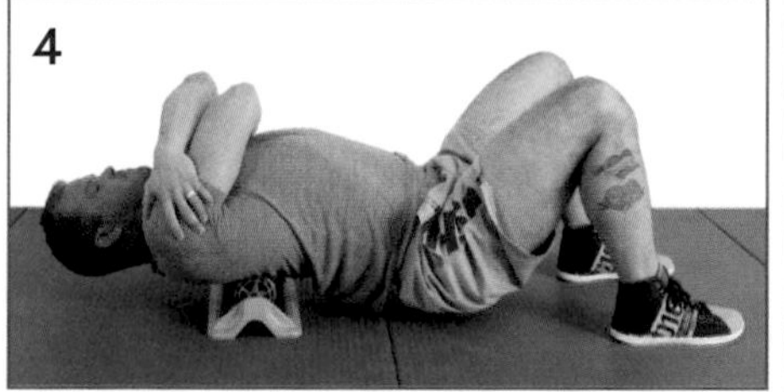

5

1. Wrap your arms around your chest and position the roller at the base of your ribcage. Wrap your arms into a big hug, sucking up the slack in your back, pulling all the soft tissue and the scapula out of the way so you can target the motion segments of your back.

2. With the tissues of your upper back wound up tight, create an extension force over the roller by arching back. From this position, spend as much time as necessary extending over the roller until you feel change in the area.

3. Keeping your arms wrapped tightly around your body, sit up as if you were doing a crunch. Keeping the majority of your weight positioned over the roller, scoot your butt toward your feet, slide your back down the roller, and move on to a new area.

4. Having positioned the roller in the middle of your upper back, arch back and extend over the roller, creating as much extension as possible.

5. When you've experienced enough change, progress up your spine to the base of your neck. To create more extension over the roller, squeeze your butt and elevate your hips as you arch back.

Option 2: Side-to-Side Smash

Simply arching over a roller isn't always enough to challenge what's most resistant in your signature brand of tightness. If you stumble across a stiff area that is not responding to the large extension forces, try rolling from side to side across the tissue. This side-to-side smashing enables you to seesaw through some of the soft tissues adjacent to your spine that can limit extension and rotation. If you play golf, tennis, or baseball or engage in any activity that requires you to twist, lock the Side-to-Side Smash into your mobility routine.

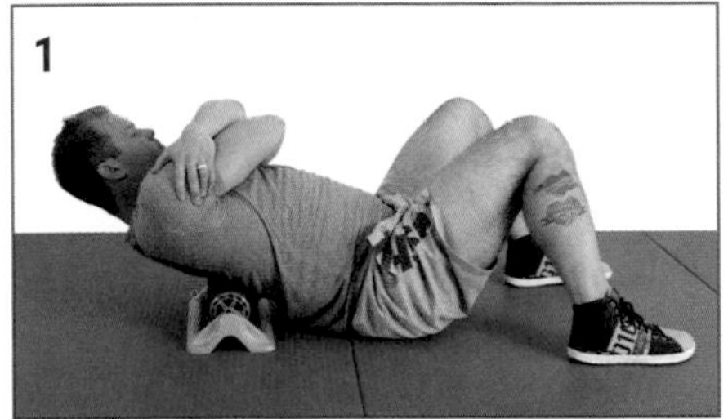

1 Wind up the tissues of your upper back by wrapping your arms around your body, and position the roller at the base of your ribcage.

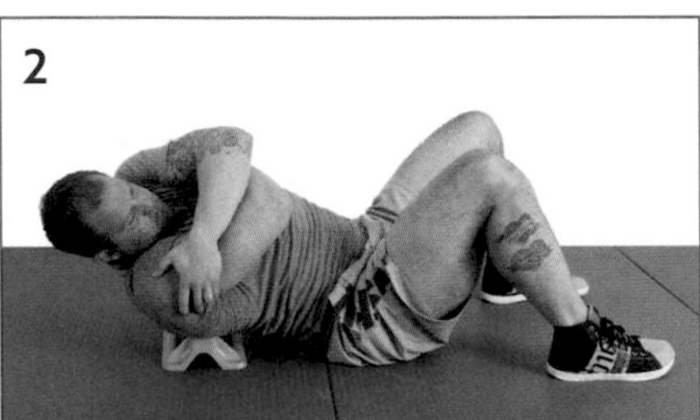

2 After hunting down a stiff area, roll back and forth, keeping your upper back tight. You can twist from your hips or rotate your entire body. There is no wrong way.

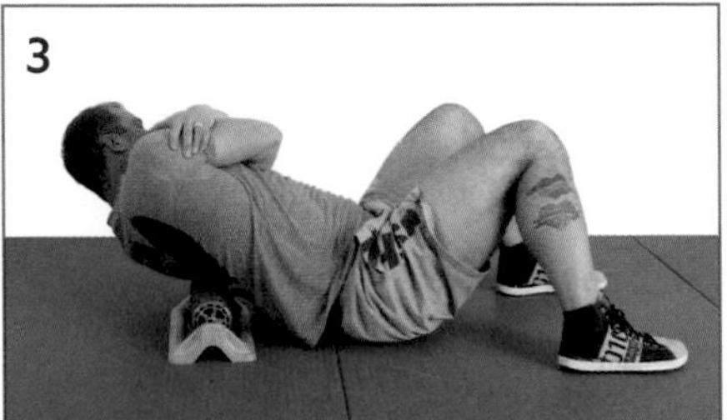

3 Roll across the roller onto your left side. Seesaw back and forth like this until you've experienced enough change. If you notice that one side is tighter than the other, remain on that side and implement the Side Roll smash (option 3).

Option 3: Side Roll

If you notice that one side of your spine is tighter than the other, consider it an alarm that requires an urgent response. The stiffer side of your back will impair your ability to rotate on that side. Failure to attack the issue will trigger problems upstream and downstream of the area.

If you notice that the left side of your upper back is tighter than the right side, for example, one way to address the issue is to turn onto your left side and smash that area. Don't overthink the situation by trying to diagnose the root cause. Just know that the left side should feel like the right side. It's that simple.

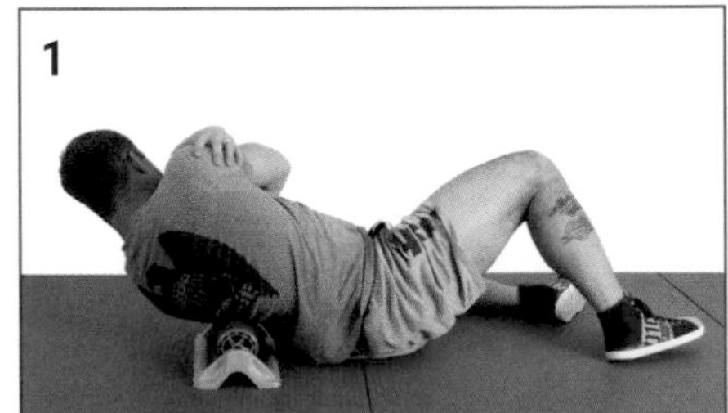

1 Roll onto the side of your upper back that is tighter than the other and slowly roll up and down the tight area.

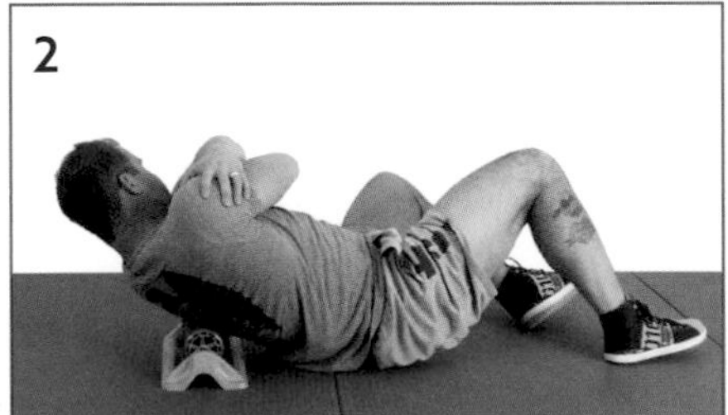

2 Roll up and down the side of your back, pressure waving into the tight area.

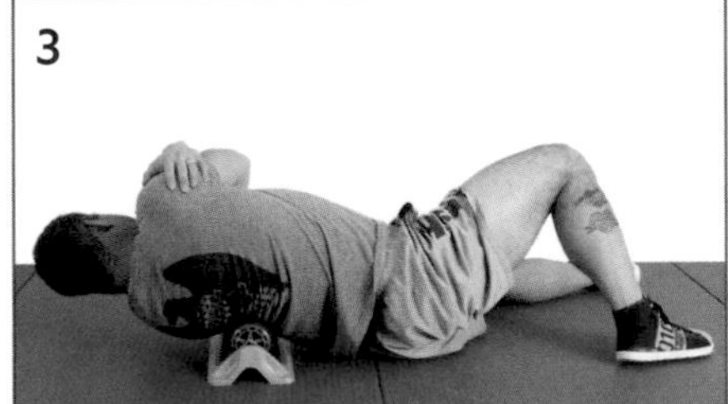

3 Remember, you're not limited to rolling up and down. You can also pressure wave into the stiffness or side bend over the area.

T-Spine Ball Smash Mobilizations

Working on your upper back with a roller works your thoracic system in a global way. Working on your upper back with a double lacrosse ball or Gemini, on the other hand, enables you to localize the target and zero in on one segment at a time. This makes for a more acute thoracic mobilization. You'll usually find that one or two segments of vertebrae are responsible for restrictions that are riddling your entire back.

There are multiple variations of this technique, as there are with the roller. You can arch your back, elevate your hips and lower them to the ground while arching back, rotate from side to side, raise your arms overhead, or use a combination of these methods. As with all the mobilization techniques that I demonstrate, you're not limited to what's shown in the photos.

Overhead Archetype | Press Archetype | Front Rack 2 Archetype

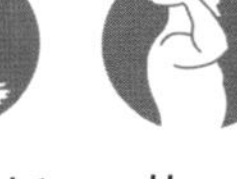

Front Rack 1 Archetype | Hang Archetype

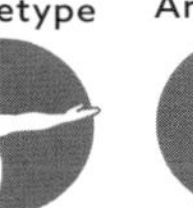

This mobilization will help improve the above archetypes.

IMPROVES:

Neutral spinal position

Localized thoracic mobility (targeting one motion segment at a time)

Option 1: Smash Extension

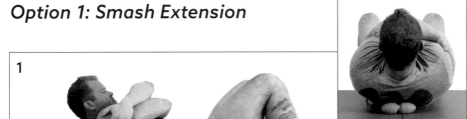

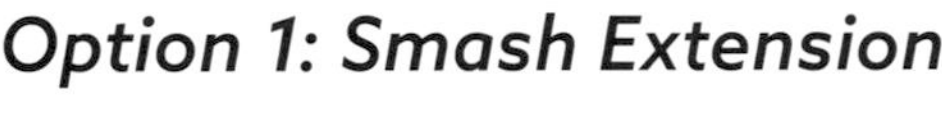

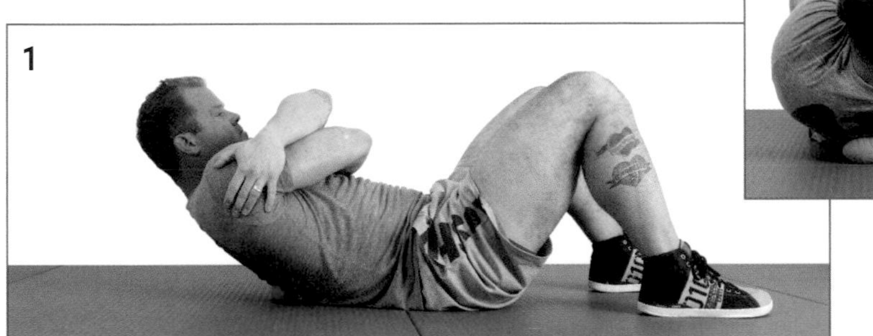

Hug your arms around your body to take up slack and move your scapula out of the way. As you mobilize the length of your thoracic spine, nestle the points of the double lacrosse ball or Gemini between vertebral segments.

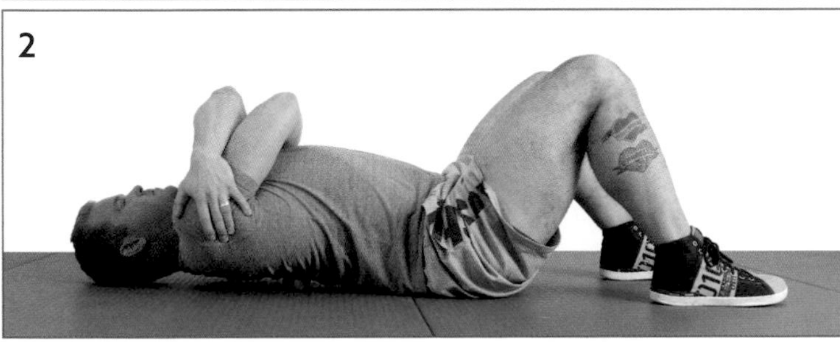

After creating tension in your upper back, slowly extend over the double lacrosse ball or Gemini. Because these tools provide a more acute fulcrum, you have to keep the base of your ribcage anchored to your pelvis. To avoid overextending your lumbar spine, keep your core engaged. From here, you can sit up and then continue to arch over the balls or Gemini. If you need more pressure, elevate your hips while continuing to arch.

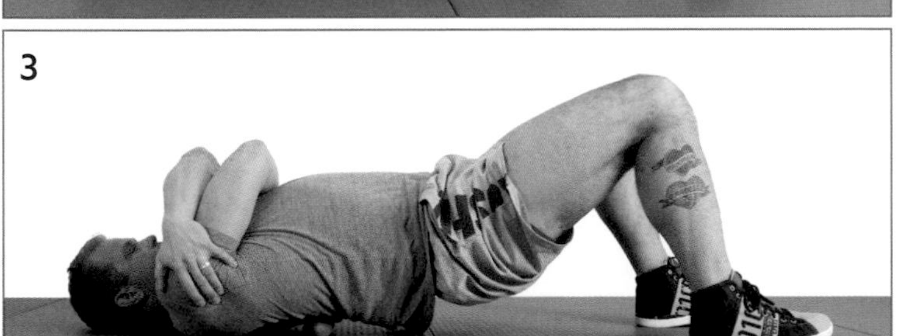

To add more pressure, drive your heels into the mat and elevate your hips. To effect change, you can roll from side to side, rotate from your shoulders, and snake around.

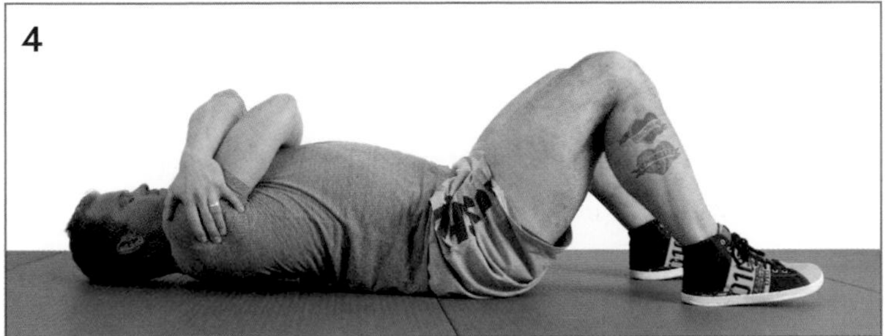

Still in extension, slowly lower your butt to the mat. *Note:* You can combine the arch with the hip lift as demonstrated in this sequence, or isolate the technique. In other words, you can arch, sit up, and repeat, or arch, elevate your hips, drop your hips, and repeat. The former biases the tissues upstream of the target area, and the latter biases the tissues downstream of the target area.

IMPROVES:

Acute thoracic spine stiffness in athletes

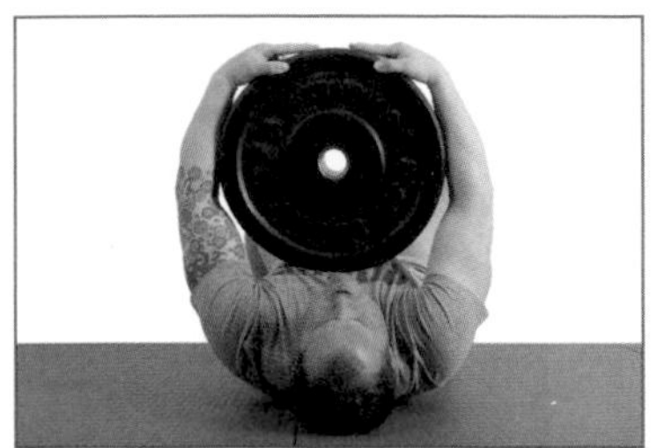

1. Position a 45-pound bumper plate over your chest and hug your arms around it. Hugging the weight pulls the soft tissue out of the way, allowing you to focus on the motion segments of your vertebrae. With the weight in place and a double lacrosse ball positioned into the motion segments you want to change, arch backward over the balls.

2. Slowly roll onto your side. The weight is going to pull you onto your side, so you have to go slowly and fight that force. For the best results, focus on the motion segments you're trying to change.

3. Keeping your arms wrapped tightly around the weight, roll toward your right side.

4. For another stimulus, tuck your chin to your chest and sit up as if you were doing a poorly executed ab crunch.

5. To create additional pressure, tilt the weight toward your face and elevate your hips.

6. To improve overhead range of motion, arch back and raise one arm overhead, keeping your elevated arm externally rotated and stable while using your opposite arm to support the weight.

Option 2: Plate Smash

Hard-training athletes are stiff in a more layered and labyrinthine way than your average Joe. If you're a big, strong athlete, you probably need to add weight to the double lacrosse ball smash to spur some change. The best way to accomplish this is to position a plate, ideally a 45-pound bumper plate or heavy med ball (see option 3), over your chest and wrap your arms around the weight. Adding pressure to your chest gets your ribs involved, which play a role in T-spine and overhead shoulder mobility. It also forces more downward pressure into the weight, allowing for a more acute and aggressive thoracic mobilization.

1
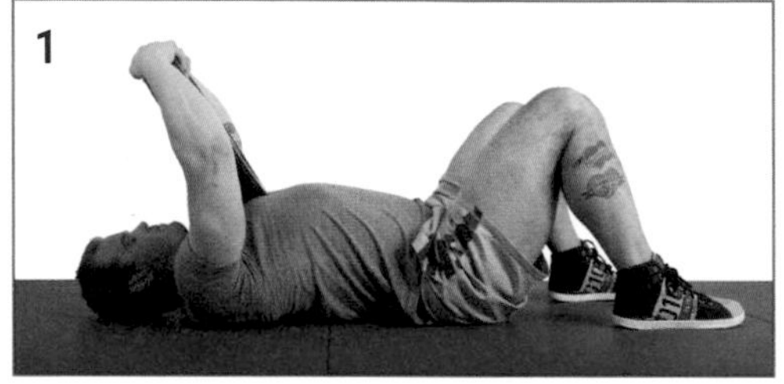

2
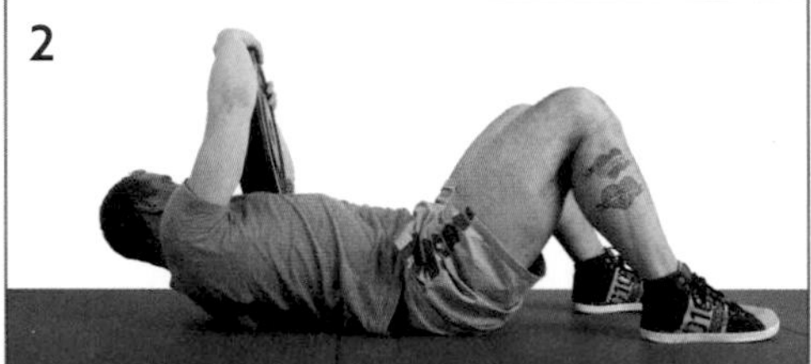

3
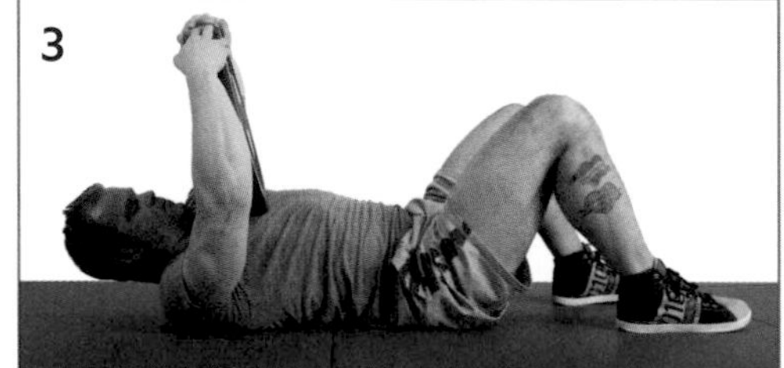

4
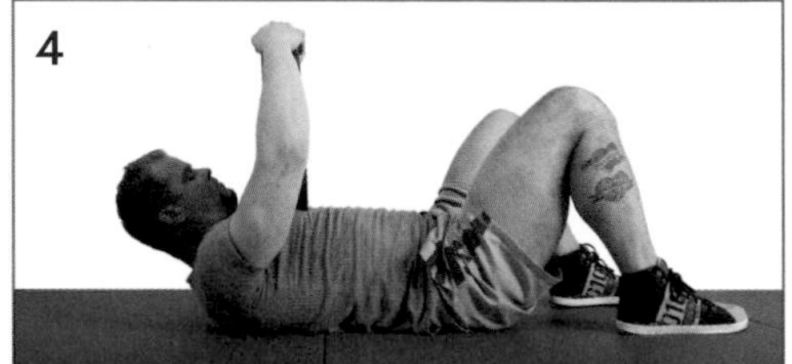

5
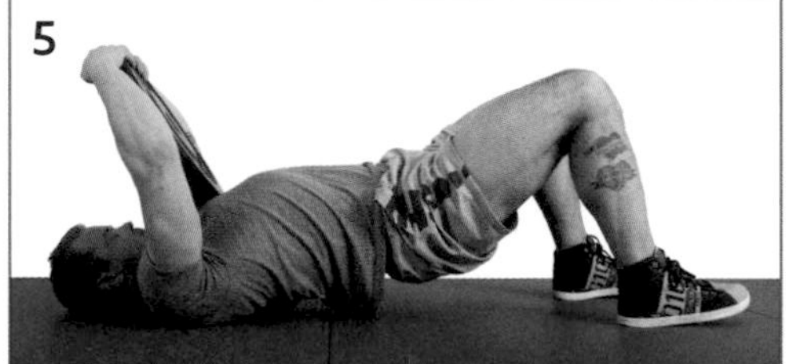

6
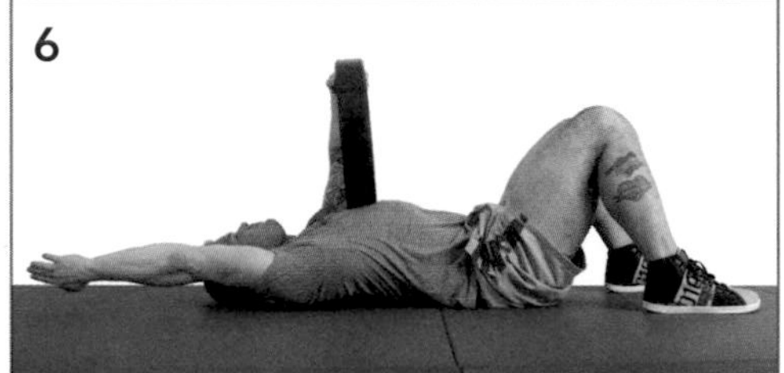

Option 3: Med Ball Smash

You can also use a med ball for a similar stimulus. Although a med ball doesn't give you the same acute pressure as a bumper plate, it's easier to load onto your chest and gives you greater control while mobilizing. A med ball is particularly useful when targeting your upper thoracic spine because you can load the ball higher on your chest. For the best results, focus your attention on your upper thoracic spine as you load the ball onto your chest. Breathe into the tight area to increase pressure, and use the contract and relax method to free up tight segments.

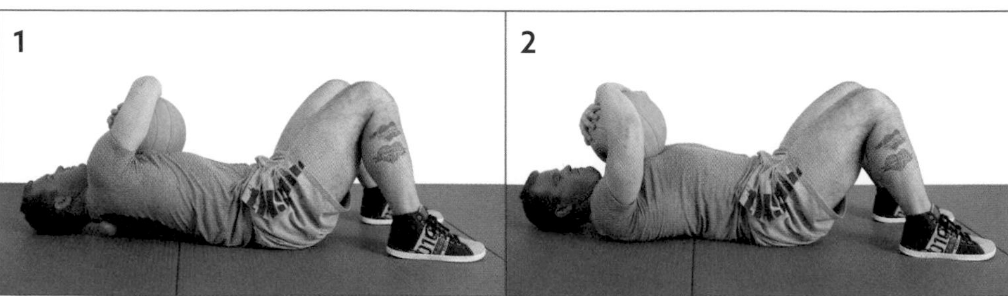
1 2

T-Spine Overhead Extension Smash Mobilizations

Overhead Archetype

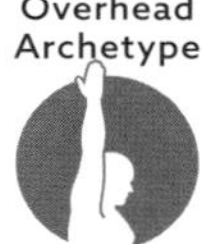

This mobilization will help improve the above archetype.

IMPROVES:

Overhead position
Thoracic extension and upper body rotation
Throwing mechanics

Although wrapping your arms around your body is an effective way to improve thoracic mobility, it's specific to your upper back. Reaching your arms overhead ties in your shoulders and improves the relationship between shoulder flexion, thoracic extension, and rotation. Think of a baseball pitcher's fastball, a tennis serve, or a volleyball spike: All these actions require overhead position, thoracic spine extension, and upper body rotation.

Your upper back is an intricate network of systems that relate, react, and communicate with each other. Garbled systems in your back can make it difficult to stabilize your shoulders or lift your arms overhead. So, if you're trying to improve your overhead position, you need to mobilize around the shape you're trying to change. The T-Spine Overhead Extension Smash is a perfect example of this concept.

Although you can set up for the overhead extension variations from scratch, you don't have to do these mobilizations independently of the previous techniques. In other words, you can go from the hug position to arms overhead, back to the hug, then back into overhead extension. Just make sure to keep your shoulders in a stable position and your midline engaged. Be careful not to bend your elbows or hinge at the base of your thoracic spine. (That's probably the most common error.) Bending your elbows puts your shoulders in an unstable position, while hinging at the base of your thoracic spine causes overextension at your lower back. To avoid these faults, you have to fight against the hinge at the junction of your thoracic and lumbar spines by keeping your abs tight and locking out your elbows overhead while actively positioning your armpits forward.

Option 1: Overhead Extension

1

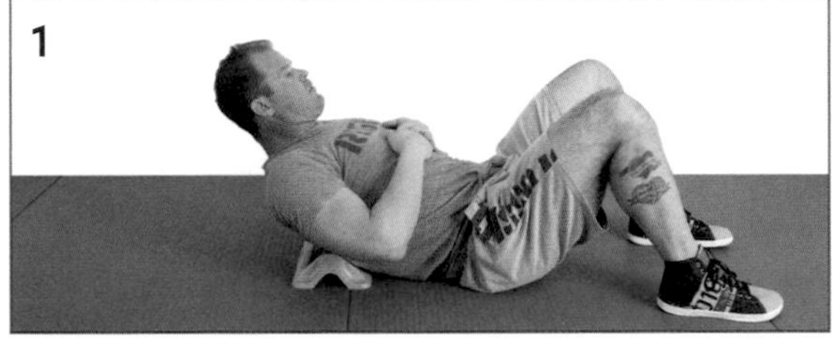

Position the base of your ribcage against a roller or Battlestar. Remember that raising your arms overhead creates an additional extension force, which can cause you to overextend at the lumbar spine. To avoid this fault, maintain a neutral and engaged midline.

2

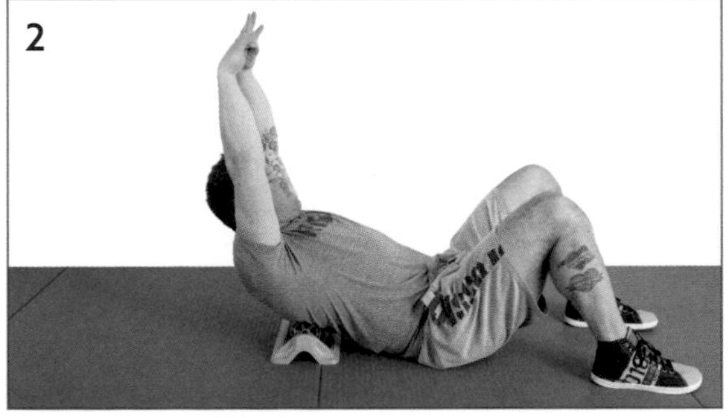

Raise your arms overhead. In the photo, notice that my elbows are locked out, my armpits are forward, and I'm actively reaching toward the ceiling.

3

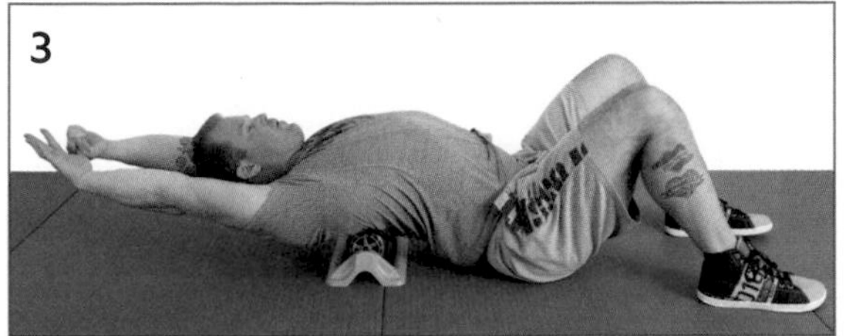

Keeping your midline engaged and your shoulders in a stable position, arch over the roller or Battlestar. To increase the pressure, you can raise your hips off the ground.

Option 2: Overhead Anchor

In the photos below, notice that I anchor my hands to a barbell. (It could just as easily be the frame of a couch.) Then I lower my hips toward the ground to emphasize extension. I'm using my lower body to create an extension force by bracing my shoulders in a fixed position.

Many people, when they're lying over a roller or lacrosse ball, can't move their arms into a good overhead position and press their hands on the ground due to a lack of mobility. This is why I recommend anchoring your hands to the ground. It facilitates better reach and increases the impact of the exercise.

Let's explore an important concept here. Imagine two exercises that are similar in shape but have a different effect on your system—like the handstand pushup versus the strict-press. Both require a good overhead position, yet each one exaggerates a different movement. One begins in the overhead position, while the other finishes in the overhead position. On paper they appear very similar—but you wouldn't restrict yourself to just one exercise, right? Of course not! All self-respecting athletes and coaches understand the importance of balancing exercises as a means of maximizing performance and health. It's intuitive. However—and here's the message that I want you to embrace—people tend to get stuck in one dimension when it comes to mobility.

The point is, you have to address both ends of the spectrum in your mobility work. If your goal is simply to improve thoracic extension and bias arm flexion in the process, the previously demonstrated exercises are great. But if you want to create change across the entire system, you have to approach mobility from both ends—just as you stimulate a multidimensional training effect by using both the strict press and the handstand pushup. For optimal results, you have to balance it out.

1. Wrap your arms around your body and take up all the slack in your upper back. Then extend over the roller with your ribcage in line with your pelvis by elevating your hips. Don't arch back into extension.

2. With your hips elevated, anchor your hands to the bar, keeping your elbows locked out and your armpits forward, and then slowly lower your hips toward the ground. The closer together you can get your hands, the better. Notice how this variation enables you to prioritize your overhead position and then exaggerate extension with your lower body.

3. Continue to lower your hips toward the ground.

4. As your butt touches down, straighten your legs, anchoring your hips to the ground. You can hang out here until you experience change, or move on to another area. The key is to maintain a good overhead position, keep your midline engaged, and elevate and lower your hips over the fulcrum or hang out in a globally extended position until you effect change.

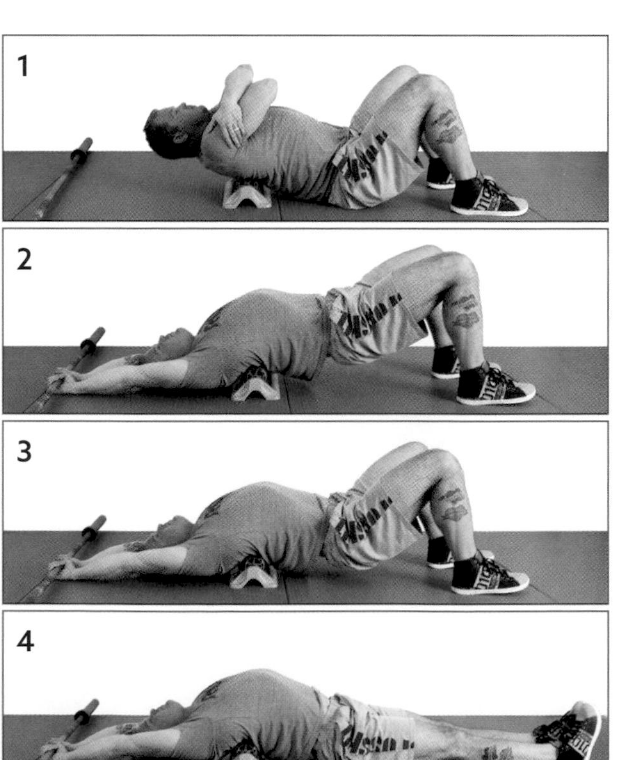

Option 3: Double Lacrosse Ball

This is the same idea in that you're tying in some end-range shoulder flexion with thoracic extension. Instead of mobilizing around multiple motion segments, however, you're isolating individual vertebra segments.

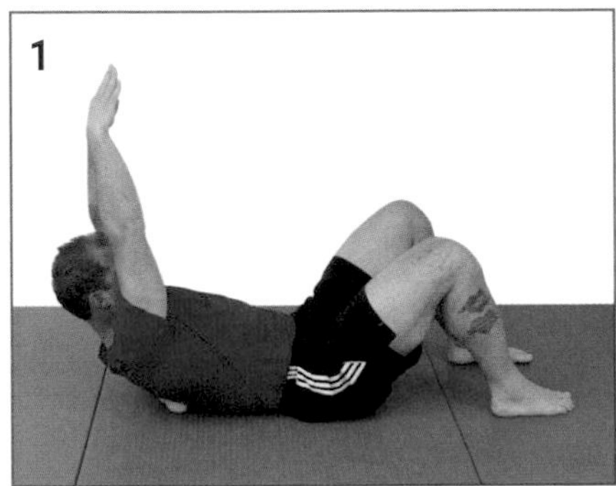

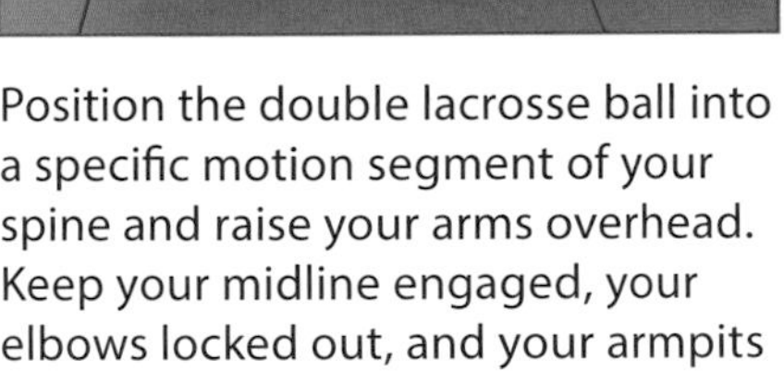

Position the double lacrosse ball into a specific motion segment of your spine and raise your arms overhead. Keep your midline engaged, your elbows locked out, and your armpits facing forward.

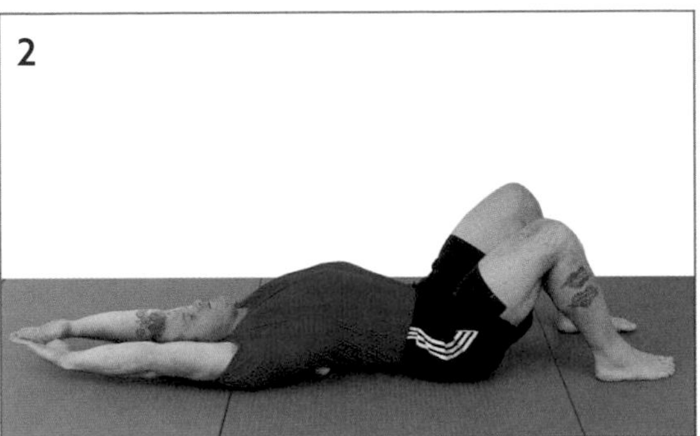

Still reaching your arms overhead, extend over the balls. From here, you can roll from side to side or elevate your hips to create additional pressure.

Option 4: Double Lacrosse Ball Overhead Anchor

This is the exactly the same as option 2, but it uses a double lacrosse ball instead of a roller to attack specific spots. For the best results, position the double lacrosse ball on your upper back around the base of your neck.

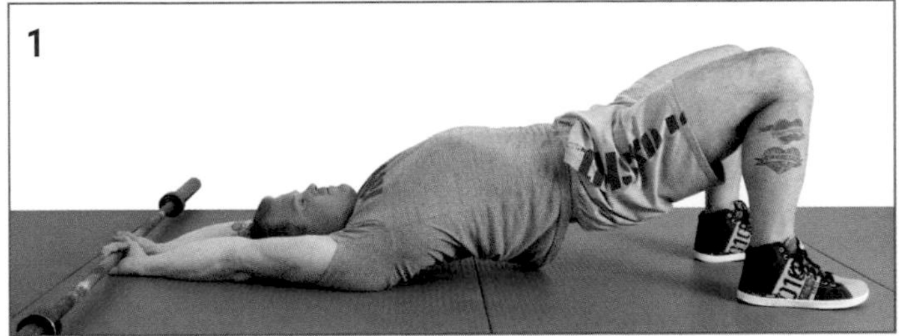

Position the double lacrosse ball near the base of your neck, elevate your hips, and anchor your hands to the barbell with your elbows locked out and your armpits facing forward.

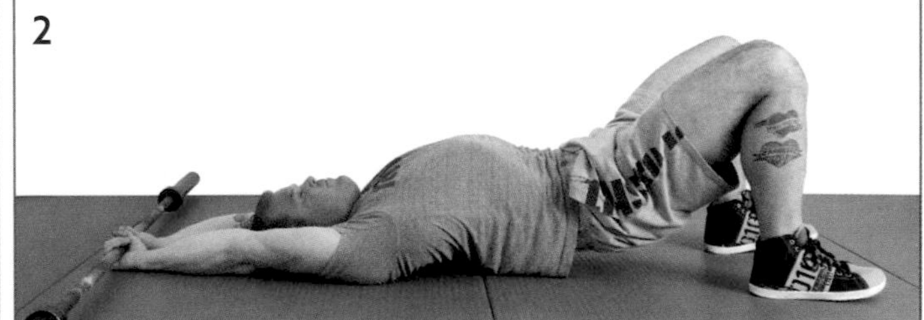

Keeping your midline engaged to avoid overextending your lumbar spine, slowly lower your hips to the ground.

Overhead Archetype

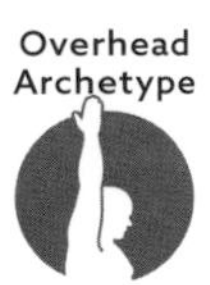

This mobilization will help improve the above archetype.

IMPROVES:

Thoracic mobility (global flexion and extension)

T-Spine Global Extension Mobilizations

Most members of the Supple Legion have a keg lying around the house or gym, which I can appreciate because it serves multiple purposes. You can fill it up with the obvious or use it as a tool to improve performance: an indisputable double win. For the purposes of this section, you can use it to create a large global extension of your spine, which is good for two reasons.

First, it allows you to explore global positions that tie in all the motion segments of your vertebrae. For example, if you're arching over a foam roller or pipe, you're in global extension, but you're probably getting only two or three motion segments of your spine. When you extend over a keg, you're able to explore the relationship of all the motion segments and create a global impact on your spine. A lot of people try to exaggerate this motion in the form of a bridge, which is characterized by sloppy shoulder, back, and hip extension. The keg allows you to focus on the extension without having to strain to maintain a good position.

The second benefit of using a keg is that it opens up the playing field. Often, when you're extending over a roller or double lacrosse ball, the ground restricts your reach. When you're on a keg or other large, round surface—like a medicine ball stacked on top of a couple of plates—you can get a much larger arch in the tissues you're trying to change.

Option 1: Overhead Extension

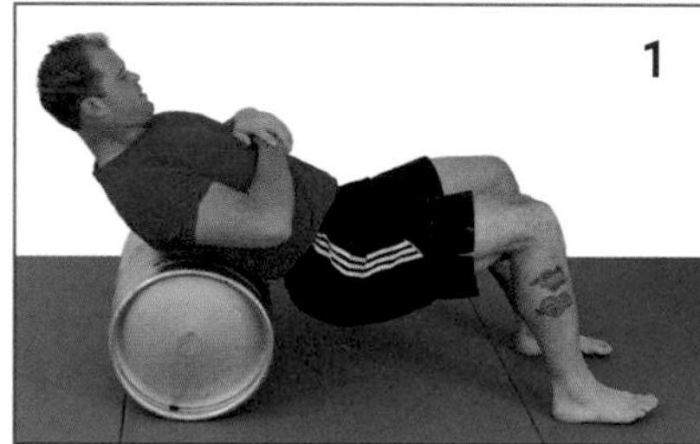

1 Position your back over a keg. Keep your ribcage in line with your pelvis, your midline engaged, and your shoulders in a good position.

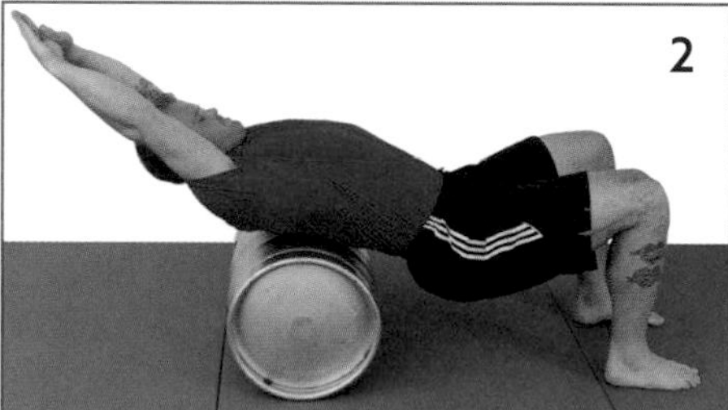

2 Reach your arms overhead. Notice that I keep my hands close together, lock out my elbows, and position my armpits forward.

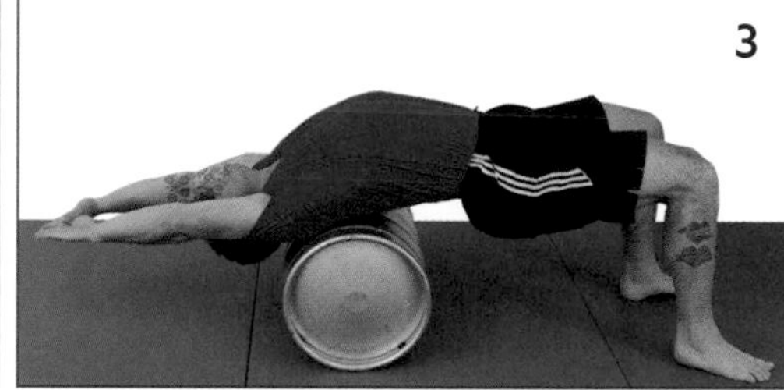

3 Keeping your shoulders in a stable position with your hands reaching overhead, elevate your hips and extend over the keg.

Option 2: Kettlebell or Barbell Anchor

You can treat a keg just like a foam roller and implement all the variations previously demonstrated. In this sequence, I demonstrate the opposite version of the previous technique, which you accomplish by gripping a kettlebell to anchor your hands to the ground and then lowering your hips. Again, because you're a little higher up and not restricted by the ground, you can get a lot more global extension through your spine and shoulders.

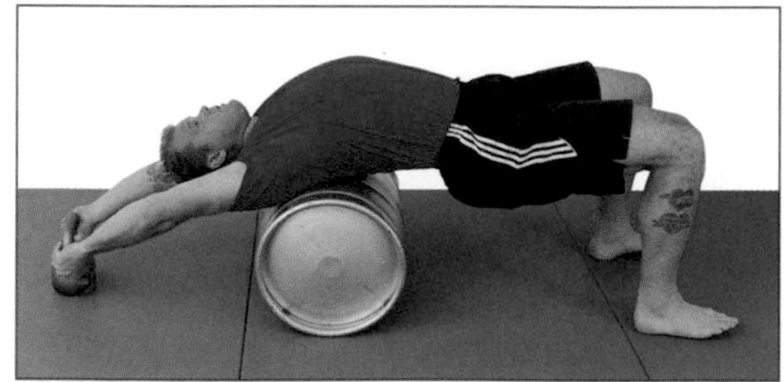

Option 3: Overhead Banded Distraction

This is the same idea as option 1, but you're adding a little bit of a distraction to the shoulder joint. Although this variation is more advanced and it takes some tinkering to get into the right position, it works wonders. As with all the techniques that require large global extension forces, you have to remain engaged and active.

I was working with the Navy, and one of the head instructors said it best. Pointing to a group of Navy ninjas hanging from a bar with their midlines disengaged, he said, "Look at those guys just hanging on their meat." That statement paints a perfect picture of what you don't want to do. You never want to hang on your meat. Respect yourself.

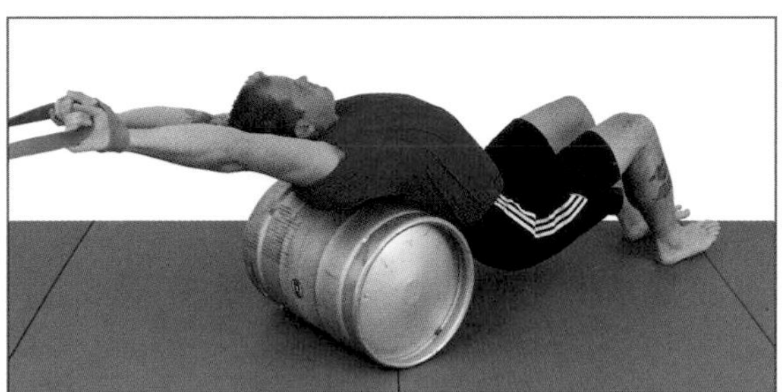

Overhead Rib Mobilization

Overhead Archetype | Front Rack 2 Archetype | Front Rack 1 Archetype

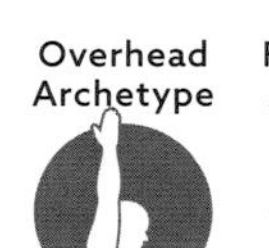

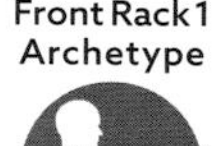

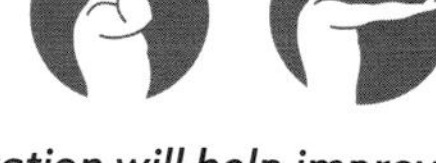

This mobilization will help improve the above archetypes.

IMPROVES:

Shoulder range of motion
Shoulder, upper back, & neck pain
Rib stiffness
Thoracic mobility

METHODS:

Pressure wave
Contract and relax
Smash and floss

TARGET AREA

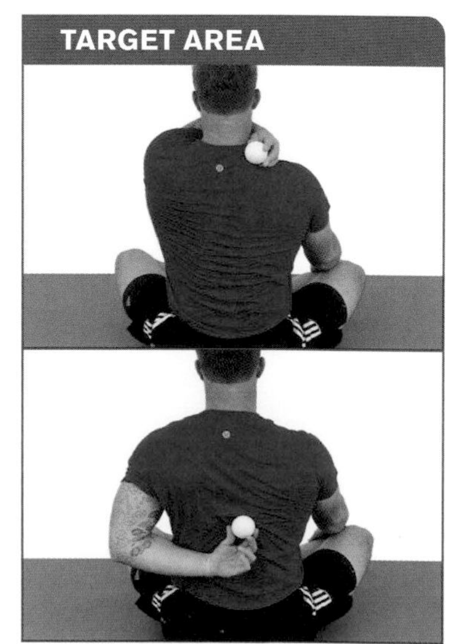

In addition to restoring motion through your vertebrae, you want to be sure that your ribs are mobile and supple. It's easy to forget is that your ribs attach on your spine and can have a profound effect on the joint mechanics of the system. Having stiff ribs not only blocks key motion segments of your thoracic spine, but also restricts the resting relationship of your scapula, which dampens your ability to stabilize your shoulders. You can use these simple mobilizations to restore suppleness to your ribs.

The sequence on the next page is one of the most basic and effective techniques for fixing stiff ribs. As you can see in the photos below, the mobilization target area is from the second rib up. It extends from the median trap (top photo) and tracks down the areas bordering the scapula (bottom photo). The general prescription is to spend at least 30 seconds on each rib and accumulate 15 to 20 slow arm swings.

As a rule, you want to spend your time mobilizing the areas that are stiff and restricting movement. However, sometimes you just don't have time to address all your issues before a workout—maybe your entire back is a matted-down mess, but you have only a minute to warm up and improve your position for the upcoming workout. In such a situation, it helps to know where you need to focus your time and energy so that you can make the biggest impact on the movement you're going to perform. Naturally, it would be great if you could deal with all your issues, but you have only so much time to fix yourself. That's why you have to break it up into calculated chunks. Here's what I suggest:

If you're going to do anything overhead, focus your attention on your upper ribs. If you're doing anything that requires extension or internal rotation, like dips, bench presses, or pushups, focus your attention on your lower ribs. The reasons are simple: If you have a shoulder impingement that's preventing you from getting your arm into a stable overhead position, chances are good that your scapula is locked in place, blocking the path of your moving arm. Although all the ribs that border the scapula are implicated, the upper ribs tend to impede upward elevation to a higher degree. In such a situation, starting in the median trap and working your way down is probably your best bet.

Conversely, if you're doing a workout that requires a lot of extension and internal rotation of your shoulders, you may want to start lower on your ribcage, because stiff lower ribs can act like a strut that limits good scapular positioning.

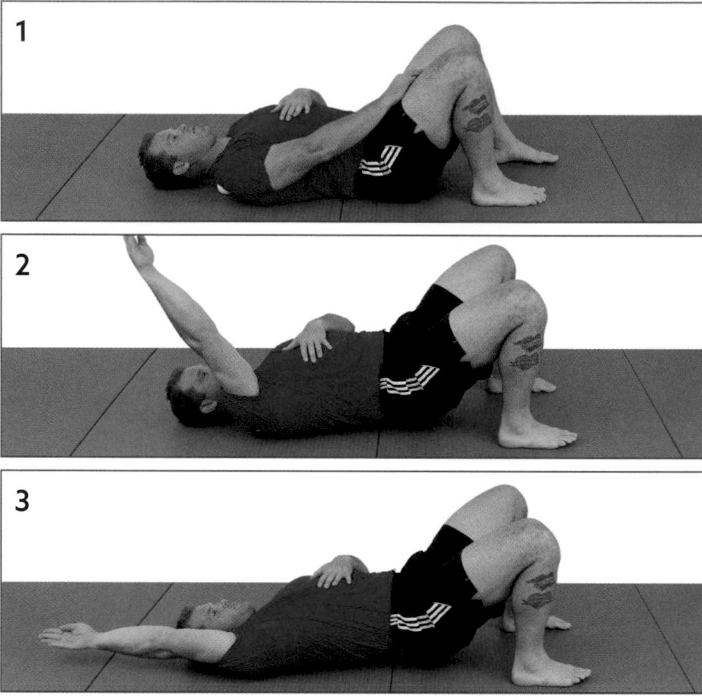

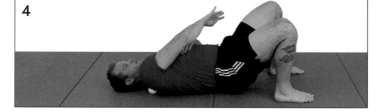

1. Position a lacrosse ball in the area bordering your scapula, between your right shoulder blade and spine.

2. To create additional pressure, drive your heels into the mat and elevate your hips. As you do so, reach your hand toward the ceiling, lock out your elbow, and pull your arm overhead. Remember, you want to keep your shoulder in a stable position, so don't bend your elbow or internally rotate your arm as you go overhead. If you default into a bent-arm, internally rotated position, stop. That's your end range. Bending your elbow is a cue that you're missing internal rotation of the shoulder.

3. Keeping your elbow locked out, push your arm overhead.

4. With your hips still elevated, bring your right arm across your body and try to touch your left hip. Bringing your hand across your body with a straight arm takes up the soft tissue slack and biases further excursion (more movement) of your shoulder blade. The idea is to have that shoulder come as far off your scapula as possible so you can get maximum range in the tissues.

Organizing the Scapula

A lot of athletes, coaches, and physical therapists seem to think that an impingement of the shoulder automatically means a rotator cuff issue. Here's what's really happening: When your scapula is in a disorganized position, it turns off your rotator cuff. So if someone tells you that your rotator cuff isn't working correctly, you probably need to restore the scapula position so that your rotator cuff turns back on.

If you start at the top of the scapula, place the ball between your shoulder blade and spine. Bridge your butt up as high as possible, driving the ball deep into your soul, and reach your arm overhead. Keep your elbow locked out. Now draw your arm across your body and try to touch your opposite hip. Those rhomboids, traps, and paraspinals get really tight. Bringing your arm across your body is a great way to unglue them. As you work your way down the border of your scapula, continue to swing your arm overhead as illustrated in the photos above. If you're trying to bias extension and internal rotation, on the other hand, the next technique will have a more beneficial impact on the tissues you're looking to change.

Lower Rib Smash: Internal Rotation

Stiff lower ribs have a profound impact on your ability to stabilize your scapula in moments of extension and internal rotation. Think about it like this: If your lower ribs are stiff, the tissues between your lower rhomboids are trapped, and the tissues between your scapula and spine are not relating well with each other. As a result, you experience a diminished capacity to maintain a stable shoulder when doing anything that requires extension and internal rotation of the shoulder. For example, if you're bench pressing, dipping, or Olympic lifting (I'm referring specifically to the high-hang position) with stiff lower ribs, you'll find it extremely difficult to maintain control of your scapula. Once you lose scapular control, you automatically default into an internally rotated, shoulders-rolled-forward position. You lose power and bleed torque, and your susceptibility to injury increases. Not good! To ensure that you can maintain control of that scapula to stabilize your shoulders through movement, you have to restore suppleness to those stiff ribs and tissues surrounding the base of your scapula, which is exactly what this mobilization aims to do.

Press Archetype
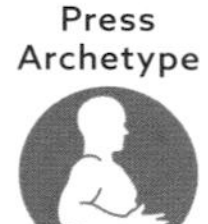
Hang Archetype
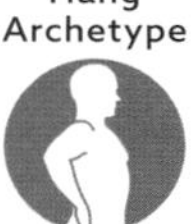

This mobilization will help improve the above archetypes.

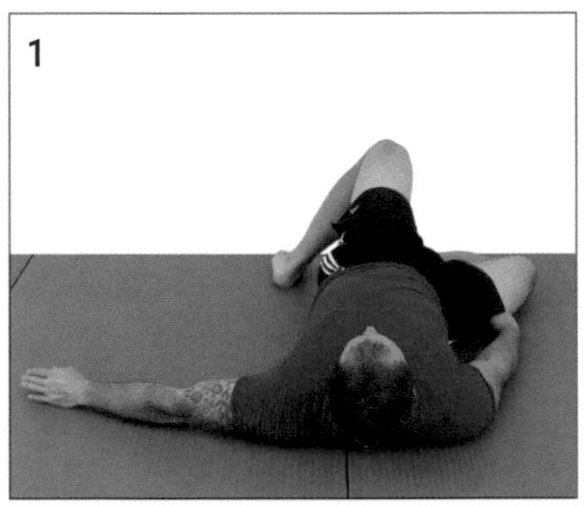

1. Position a lacrosse ball in your lower ribs between the base of your scapula and spine. Base out on your left hand and rotate your hips toward your right side.
2. Keeping the ball in place, slide your left hand underneath your lower back and drop your left hip to the mat.
3. With your arm pinned behind your back, rotate toward your right side, focusing on driving the ball into the border of your scapula.
4. Rotate toward your left side. From here, you can hunt around for tight corners by moving your body up and down, driving the ball into the border of your depressed scapula. Really work on restoring sliding surfaces to the stiff tissues surrounding your ribs.

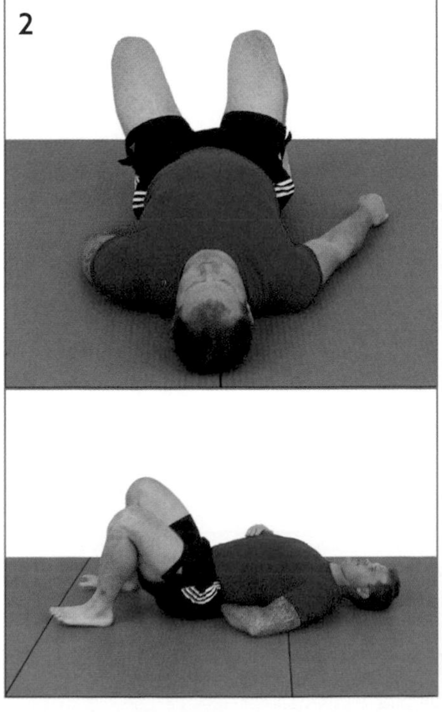

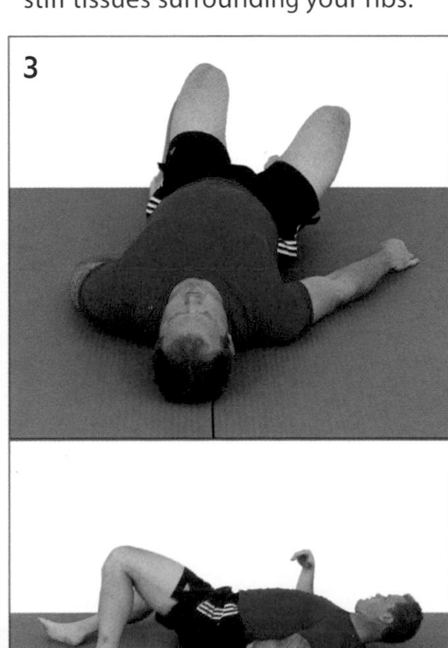

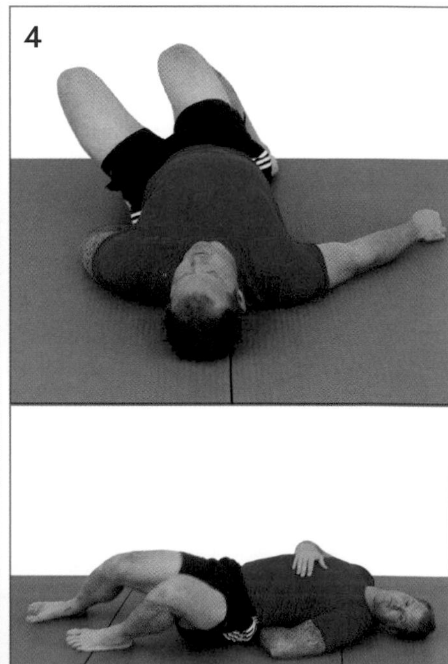

Front Rack 2 Archetype · Front Rack 1 Archetype · Overhead Archetype

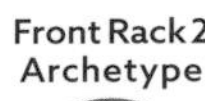
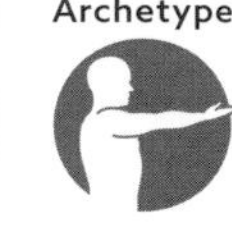
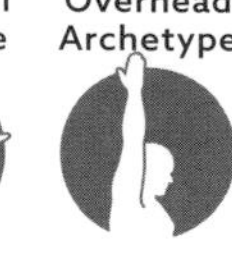

Hang Archetype · Press Archetype

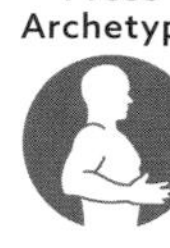

This mobilization will help improve the above archetypes.

IMPROVES:

Upper trap tweaks

Pain and stiffness in the neck, thoracic spine, & shoulder complex

Sliding surfaces to the fascia and musculature of the trapezius

Neck and shoulder stability

METHODS:

Pressure wave

Contract and relax

Trap Scrub

Sometimes a tight thoracic spine is really just a gummed-up trapezius (trap) that is restricting your movement. Remember, you are a system of systems. To get the most out of your mobility work, always think about what's connected to the tissue or area you're trying to change. For example, if you're trying to free up your thoracic spine or improve shoulder range of motion—rotation, extension, and elevation—you need to hit your trap, which ties these two systems together.

Because your trapezius is responsible for stabilizing your shoulders and neck, it has a ton of connective tissue that binds the shoulder, neck, and back complex. It's no surprise that this area tends to get really stiff and cause a lot of problems upstream and downstream. Most notably, it opens the door to the dreaded upper trap tweak. To prevent and treat this common training setback, you need to hammer this tissue like you're tenderizing meat. It's robust and probably very stiff, so get to work.

To perform this mobilization correctly, you want to nestle a ball (either a lacrosse ball or a large ball such as the Supernova) in your trapezius and levator scapulae, get as much weight as you can into the ball, and then scrub from side to side. For an easy two-for-one, position two equal-sized balls in the same target area. The goal is to get some transverse, cross-friction movement into the ball. If you hit an ugly spot, contract and relax until the ball enters your soul.

Warning: If you've been doing a lot of heavy pulling (such as Olympic lifting), this mob will be intense. You'll immediately notice just how junky and ropy these tissues are.

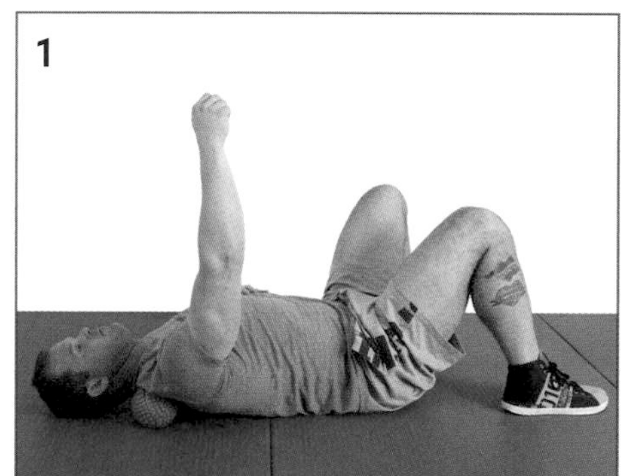

Position a ball in your trapezius—the area above your scapula, between your neck and shoulder—and elevate your arms.

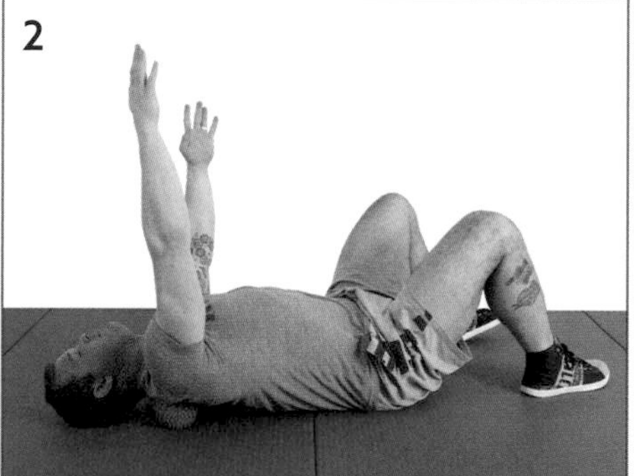

Keeping your arms outstretched, create some transverse, cross-friction pressure by worming your body from side to side. Jill Miller uses this analogy, which I find helpful: Imagine that you're driving a school bus with a big steering wheel. The idea is to move slowly so that you can take the full pressure of your weight.

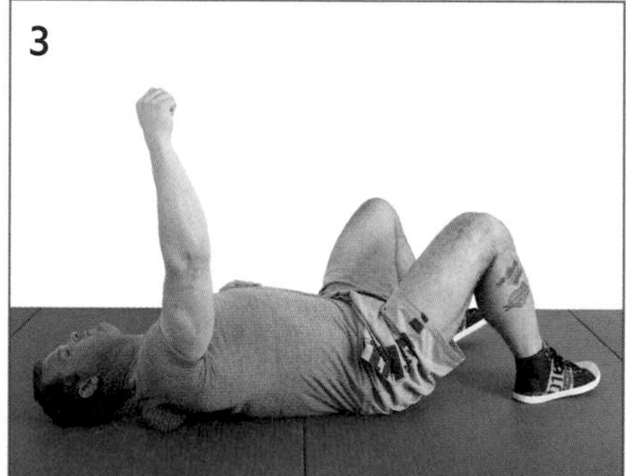

If you find a particularly tight spot, stop there, then contract and relax to sink deeper into the ball. You can also move your arm around in all directions for a flossing effect. To create additional pressure, drive your heels into the mat and elevate your hips.

Barbell Trap Mob

Overhead Archetype

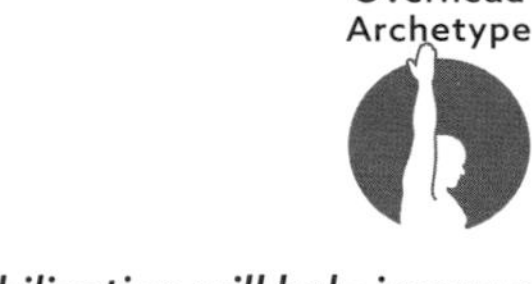

This mobilization will help improve the above archetype.

Capturing the top of your trapezius is tricky. I've found that one of the best ways to target this area is to set up underneath a barbell. You can position yourself underneath a squat rack and drive your trap upward into the weighted barbell, or simply position an unloaded barbell over your shoulder. The former gives you a bit more control, allowing you to target specific areas. If you're smaller person, stick with this one, because you can control the pressure and avoid banging your collarbone. Balancing it on your trap also has its advantages. You can teeter-totter the barbell over your trap and neck and use your supporting hand to twist and oscillate the bar, creating a scrubbing effect.

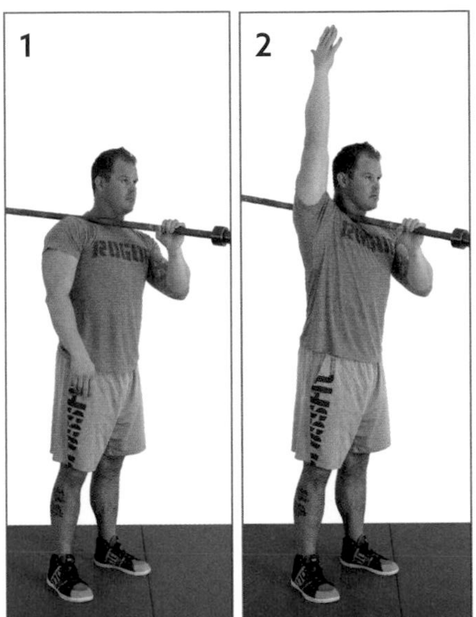

1. Either position a barbell over your trap and neck as shown, or set up underneath a squat rack. If you opt for the latter, make sure to position the barbell high on your trap at the base of your neck.

2. Raise your arm overhead and externally and internally rotate your shoulder. This will capture not only your trap and neck, but also your first rib. You can also play with teeter-tottering the bar over your trap, controlling the up-and-down movement with your opposite hand. Twisting the barbell and oscillating it forward and backward are also good techniques to play with.

First Rib Mobilizations

Overhead Archetype

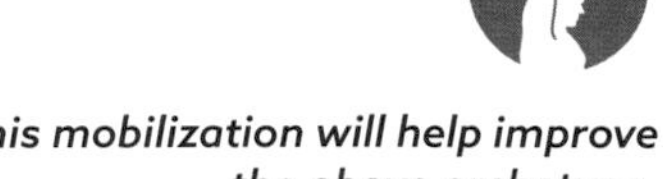

This mobilization will help improve the above archetype.

IMPROVES:

Overhead range of motion—specifically elevation of the shoulder

Shoulder function

Pain and stiffness in the shoulder and neck

METHODS:

Flossing (arm movement)

Contract and relax

Let's say you work at a computer all day with poor posture. Or maybe you've been doing some overhead movement in less than optimal positions. What can happen is that your shoulder and the surrounding tissues will shorten, causing your first rib to stiffen.

The first rib functions like a pump handle. To go overhead, you need that first rib to glide down as you elevate your arm. If that first rib is stiff, an impingement is created that undermines shoulder stability, making you look like a zombie when you reach upward.

To address this issue, you have to locate the first rib, which is the bony structure between your collarbone and the base of your trapezius and neck. Do so by sliding your hand down the base of your neck and pressing straight down into your trap. If you do this, you'll always hit the first rib. Once you've located the target area, you can implement a few mobilization options. The most practical tools for compressing the area are a band or barbell and a ball. Regardless of which option you choose to employ, the goal is to restore suppleness by moving your arm overhead, oscillating your arm back and forth, or taking a big breath in and driving your body into the ball. The key is not to just hang out and suffer, but to get as much motion at the first rib as possible.

If you're a tactical athlete who has to pack 50 to 100 pounds of gear, put a gold star next to this mobilization and place it near the center of your mobility target.

Think about it: The weight of your pack is bearing down on your neck and shoulder, pressing into your first rib. In addition to getting brutally tight, the motion segment gets jammed into the nerves coming out of your neck. No wonder your hands are numb and you can barely raise your arm overhead. By attacking the first rib, you can restore normal function to the scapula. *Note:* A lot of nerves exit your neck in this area, so respect your numbness and tingling. If it feels sketchy, reduce the pressure and back off a little bit.

Option 1: Basic First Rib Smash and Floss

This is one of my favorite first rib mobilizations due to its simplicity and effectiveness. You can do it in a doorway, on a corner of a wall, or on a square post or beam. I like to use a squat rack because I have room to move my head and arm around in all directions and use the pole to pull myself into the ball, creating more pressure. The key is to use the contract and relax technique and direct your breath into the area to create additional motion through your shoulder and first rib complex. As you relax into the ball, you can let your arm dangle or move your arm into end-range positions as shown in the photos. You can also move your head to the side to tie in your neck. And don't feel like you're limited to your first rib. This is an excellent mobilization for targeting your trapezius and neck regions.

1. Locate your first rib, which is between your clavicle and the base of your trap and neck, and nestle a lacrosse ball or Yoga Tune Up ball in the area.

2. Keeping the ball pinned in place, drive your body forward into the ball. Notice that I'm using my arms to pull myself into the ball. This creates more pressure.

3. After a few contractions, raise your arm overhead, rotating externally.

4. Pull your arm back, internally rotating your shoulder as you extend.

5. To complete a full range of motion with your arm, move your hand behind your back.

6. Passively move your head away from the ball to tie in your neck and trap. Combine all these movements with the contract and relax method and you will experience big results in a very short period.

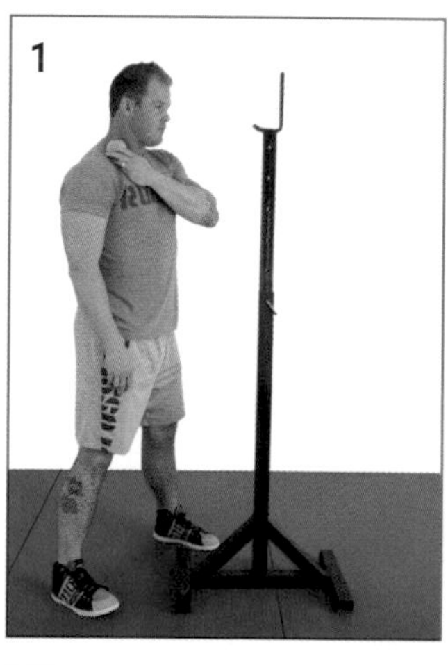

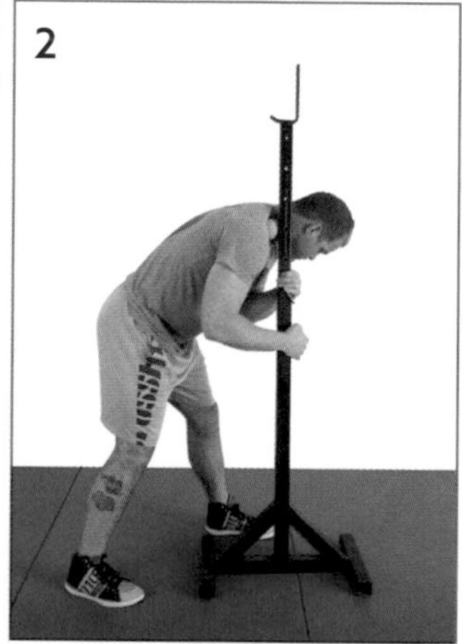

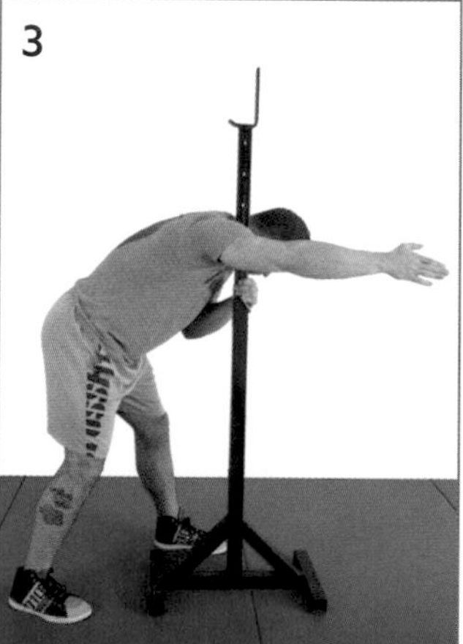

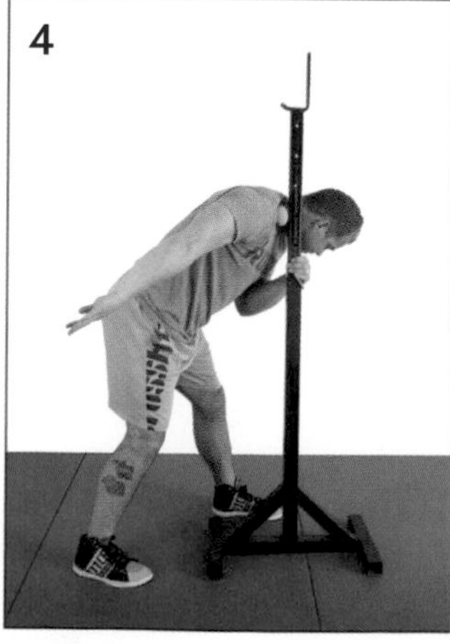

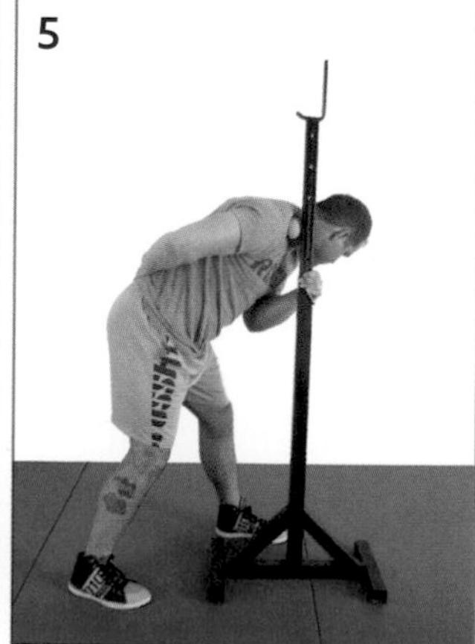

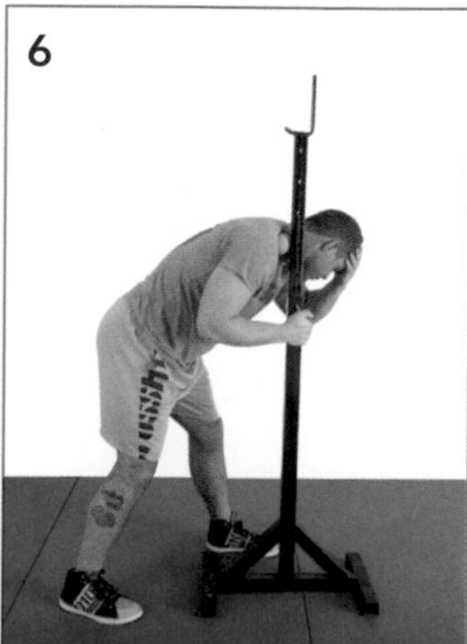

Option 2: Barbell Bubo First Rib

When you're responsible for maintaining your own body, you have to find clever ways to mobilize areas that are difficult to target. For example, getting pressure into your first rib or trying to smash your pec minor or psoas complex is no joke. To penetrate these areas, you need a special kind of mobility tool. Enter the barbell bubo. The barbell bubo makes use of two very functional mobility tools: a barbell and a lacrosse ball. This unique concoction has many purposes and a ton of functionality. In our gym, we have balls taped to old barbells, poles, and dip stations. You'd be surprised at how much they get used. I find that more people mobilize between sets and actually target areas that need attention but otherwise would have been skipped. For a temporary setup, you can use a VooDoo Floss Band to attach the ball, as shown.

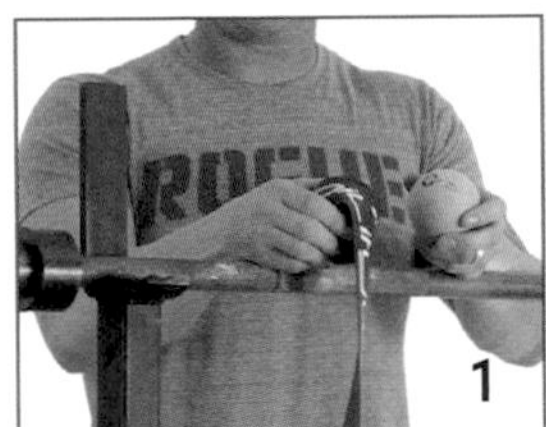

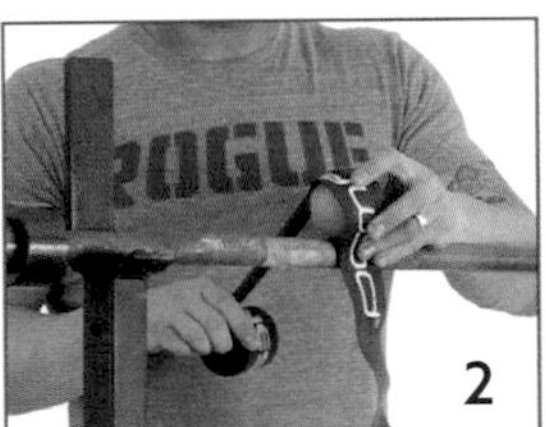

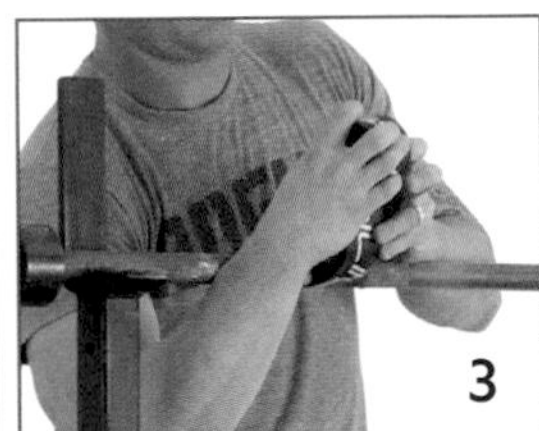

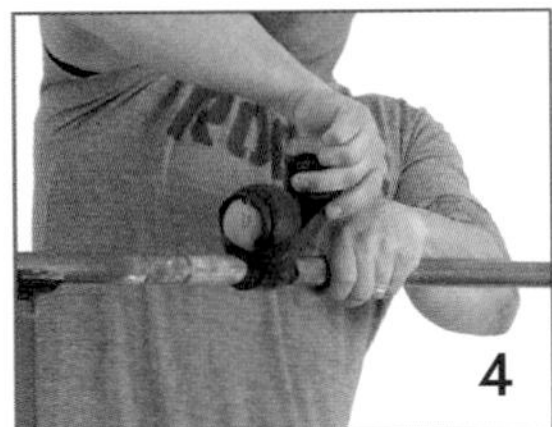

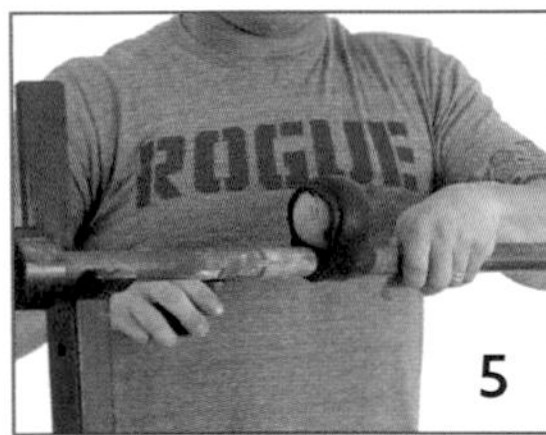

If you have an old barbell lying around, I recommend permanently taping a lacrosse ball or Yoga Tune Up ball to it. This ensures continual and easy use. If you have only one barbell or you're looking for a temporary setup, you can use a VooDoo Floss Band to get the job done, as shown above.

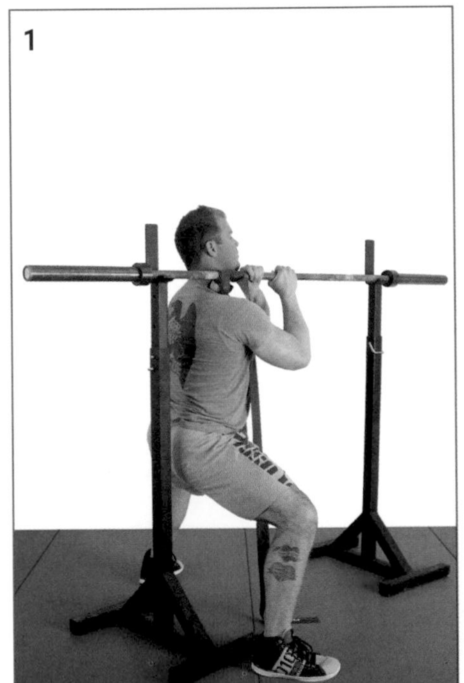

After attaching a ball to a barbell, set up underneath the bar with the ball nestled between your trap and collarbone. You can camp out here and drive your weight upward into the barbell.

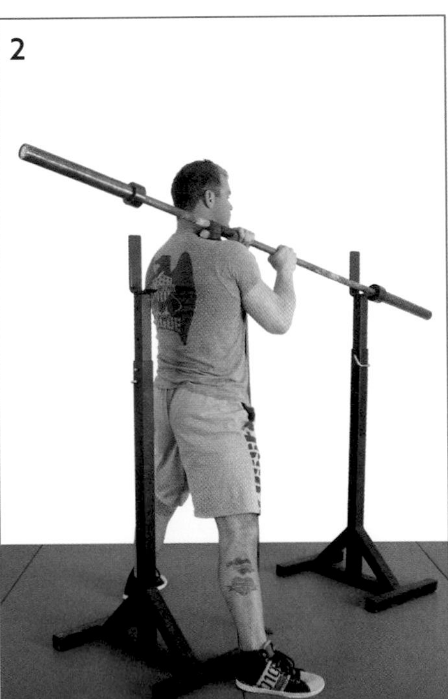

Standing up with the barbell is another option. You can contract and relax and get movement through the first rib area by tilting your head to the side.

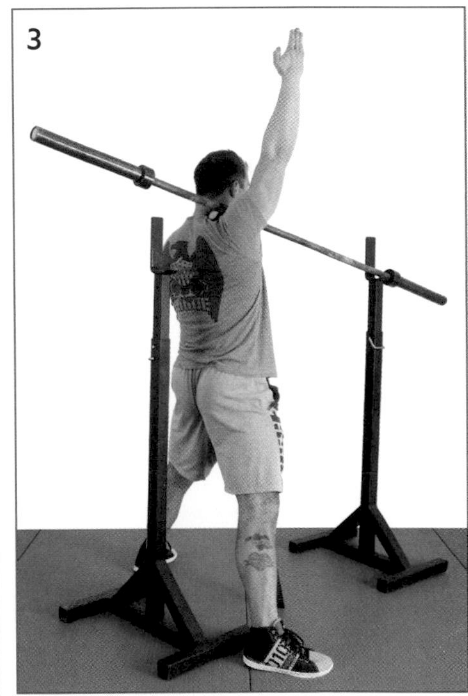

Raise your arm overhead while externally rotating your shoulder. From this position, try elevating your shoulder. You can also contract and relax from the overhead position. To complete a full range of motion with your shoulder, move your arm behind your back.

Option 3: Banded First Rib

Using a band to pin a ball into your first rib is another creative way to mobilize the area. Setting up for this mob is a bit tricky, but once you have the ball in place, it's easy to get work done. As with the barbell bubo variation, the idea is to get movement through your shoulder and neck while using the contract and relax method. The best part is that you don't need to hang out inside the band for very long to make change. A minute or two will produce big results, especially when it comes to your overhead position.

Note: You don't have to use a ball to get results. The band alone will tack down your trap, capturing the first rib. It's not nearly as potent, but it's enough to make change.

1. The idea is to pin the ball between your trap and collarbone by using a band.
2. To set up, grip the ball and band in one hand and throw it over your shoulder as if you were putting on a camera bag or purse.
3. Holding the ball and band with your right hand, bend over and hook the band underneath your left foot.
4. As you stand up and create tension in the band, adjust the ball so that it's nestled into your first rib.
5. Raise your banded arm overhead—externally rotating your shoulder to end range—and turn your head away. From here, you can contract and relax by elevating and dropping your shoulder (engaging and relaxing your trap) and create movement by doing arm circles, moving your arm behind your back, and tilting your head to the side.

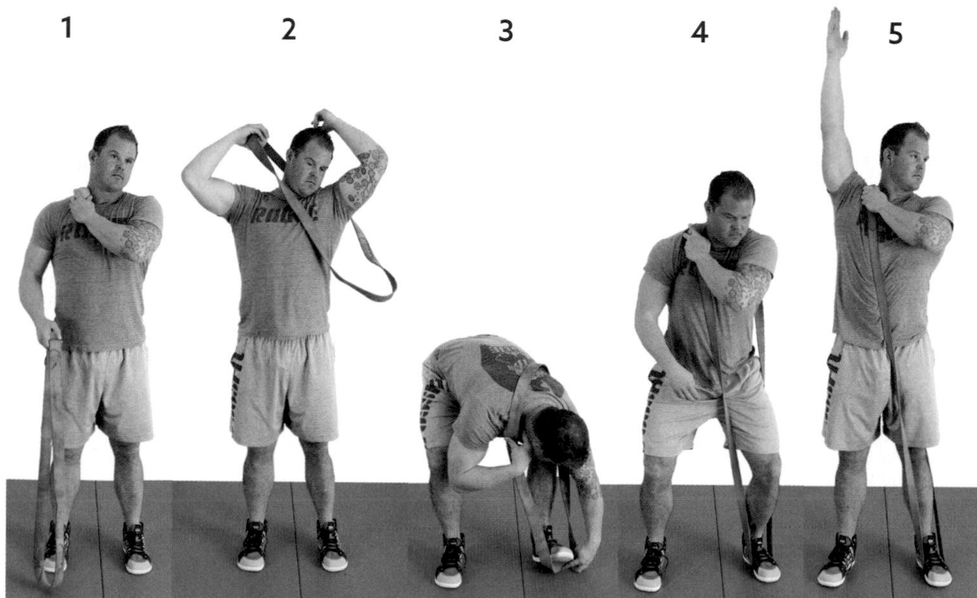

Option 4: Classic First Rib

This is the original first rib mobilization. Although the previous techniques are a bit more practical, especially in a gym environment, this option is still a useful and effective way to mobilize your first rib.

1. Jam a wooden dowel into a corner and position it on your first rib. Take a big breath in, drive your heels into the ground, and slide your body toward the wall.
2. With the dowel pinned in place, straighten your arm over your head. If you run into a barrier, oscillate back and forth and try to get as much movement through the tissues as possible.
3. With your elbow locked out, reach your arm straight overhead. From here, you can lower and raise your arm, work to elevate your shoulder, or bring your arm underneath your body.
4. To hit additional corners, position your hand underneath your body.

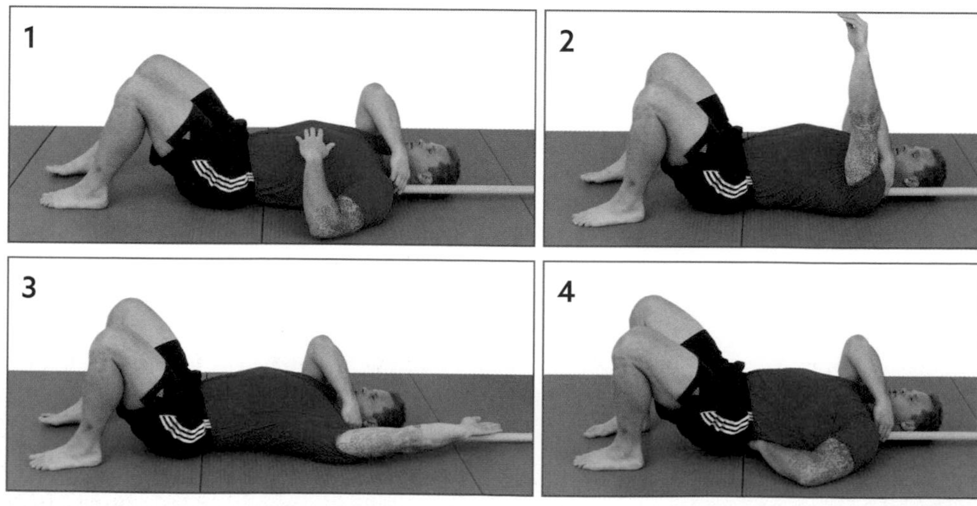

AREA 3 POSTERIOR SHOULDER, LAT, SERRATUS

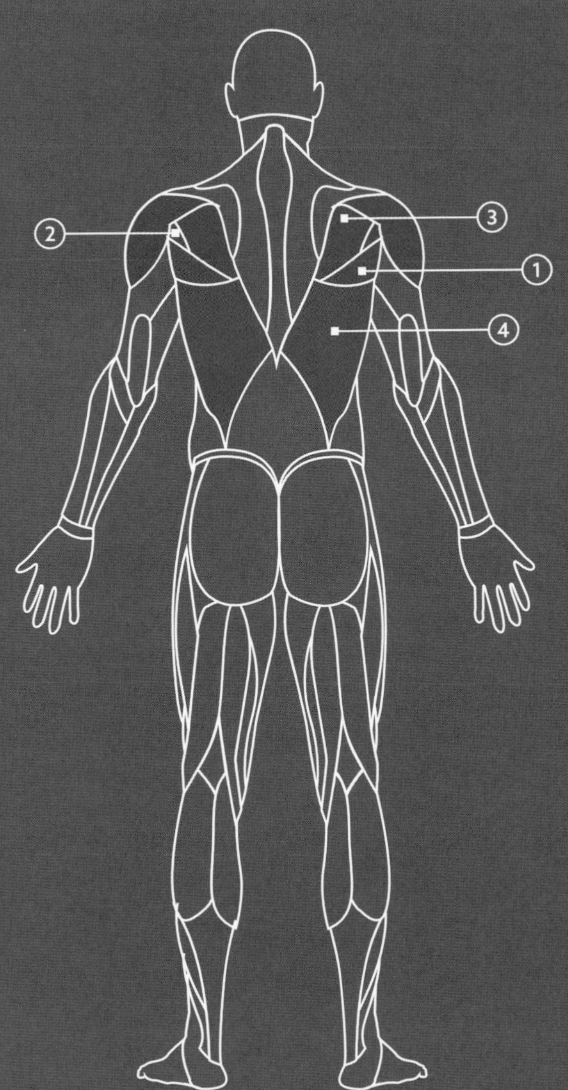

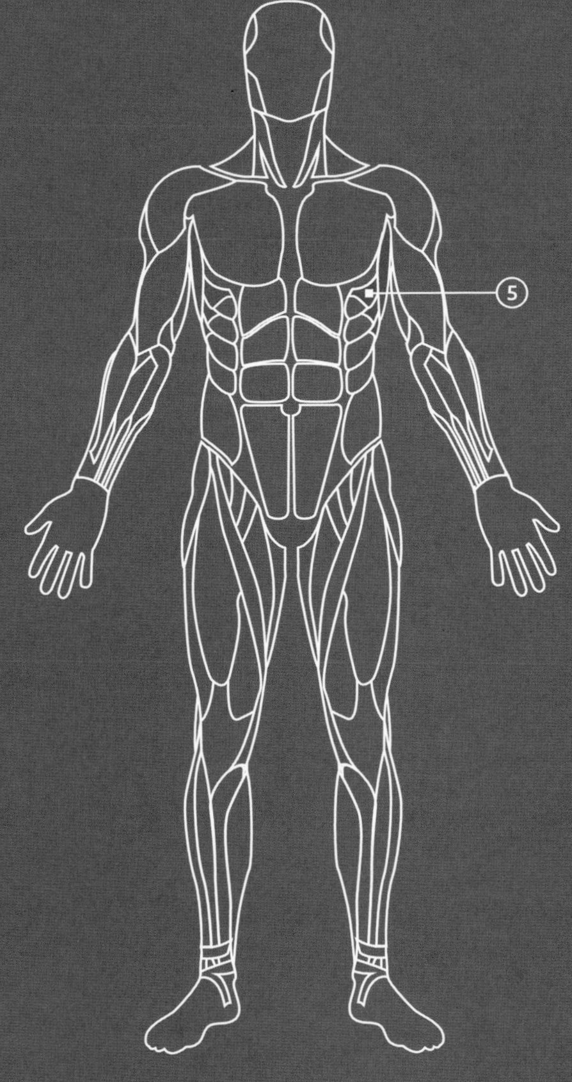

MOBILIZATION TARGET AREAS:

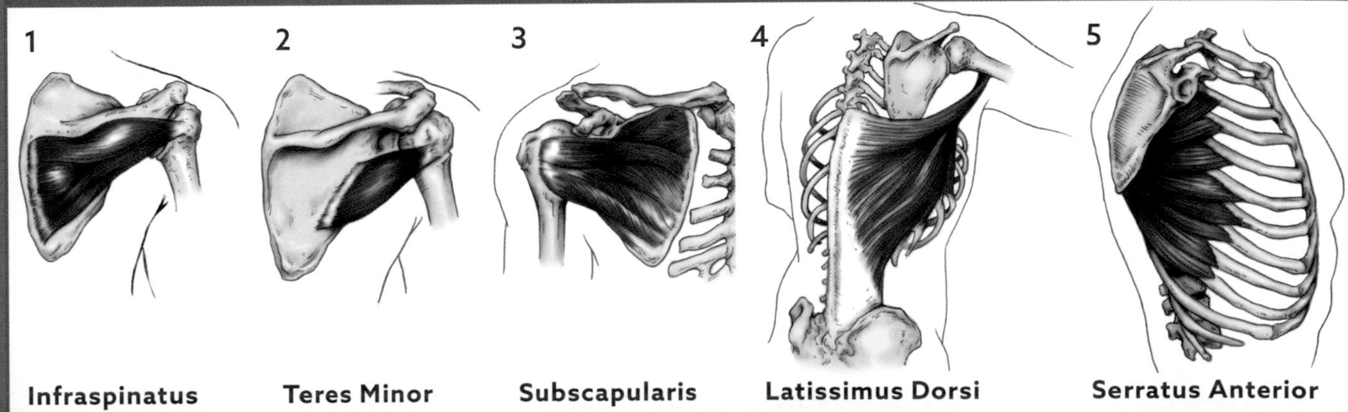

Overhead Archetype | Press Archetype | Front Rack 2 Archetype

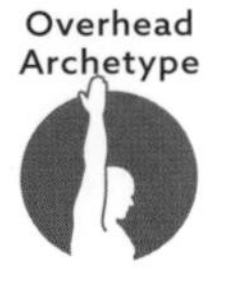
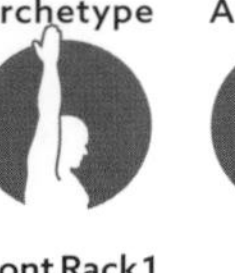

Front Rack 1 Archetype | Hang Archetype

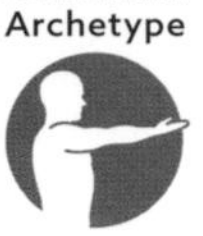
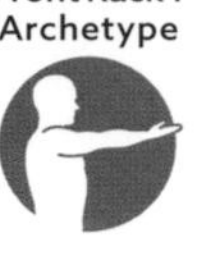
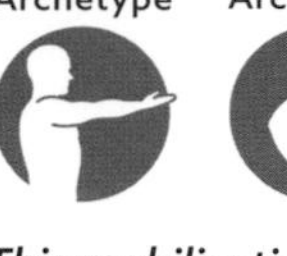

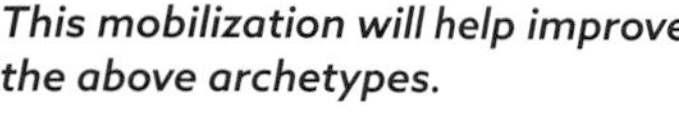

This mobilization will help improve the above archetypes.

IMPROVES:

Shoulder position and function
Recovery after a shoulder tweak
Shoulder pain

Shoulder Capsule Mobilization

One of the issues of being a modern human is that you end up living in the front of your shoulder capsule. If you spend any amount of time driving or working at a computer, chances are good that your shoulders have been resting in the fronts of the capsules to such an extent that your posterior shoulder capsules are extremely tight. This not only makes it difficult to pull your shoulders to the backs of the sockets, but also causes you to lose the capacity to generate effective rotation in your shoulders. To fix this issue, you have to set your shoulders to the backs of their sockets so that you can effectively mobilize your posterior capsules.

People have been trying to solve this issue of posterior stiffness for some time. Athletes do the classic shoulder stretch, where they pull their arm across their body, almost instinctively as a way to mobilize the posterior shoulder capsule. They're really just causing an impingement in the shoulder, which leads to more problems. Do you really think that rolling your shoulder forward into a crappy position and then pulling it across your body is going to help you? Of course not! Mobilizing in a compensated position is never okay. If you want to make change in your posterior capsule, you have to set your shoulder in a good position and then pull across.

The problem is this: If you've been hanging out in the front of your capsule, or you have strained or tweaked your shoulder, there's a good chance that your posterior capsule is tight. In such a situation, setting your shoulder to the back of the socket, which is the stable position for the joint, is difficult. This is where the Shoulder Capsule Mobilization comes into play. By using a heavy kettlebell, you can effectively drive that shoulder to the back of the socket and then bias or encourage the tissues into external rotation. This resets your shoulder into a good position, stretches the posterior capsule, and accounts for the passive accessory motion of the joint. In addition, the act of externally rotating gives you some neuromuscular cueing (think breaking the bar), which transfers to many midrange pressing skills, such as the bench press and pushup.

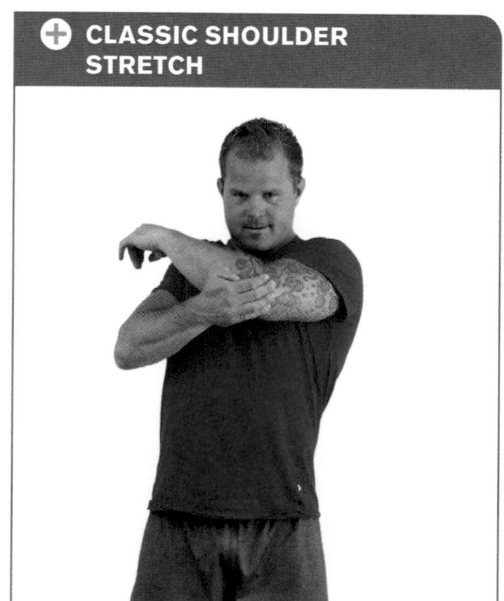

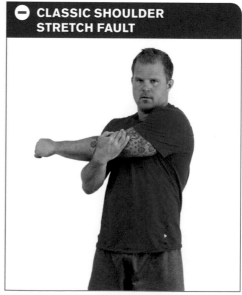
+ CLASSIC SHOULDER STRETCH

− CLASSIC SHOULDER STRETCH FAULT

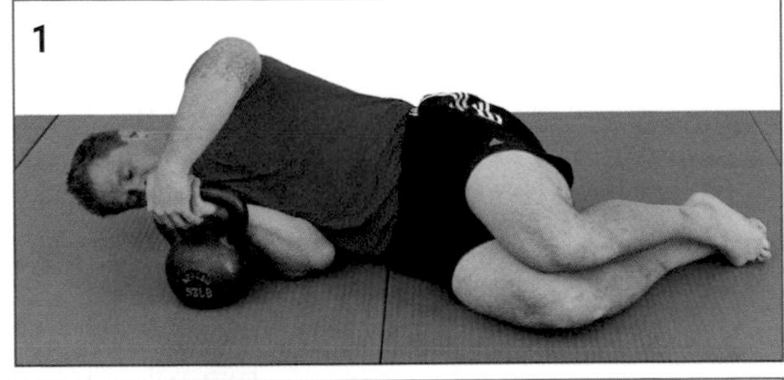

Position a kettlebell next to your right shoulder and latch onto the handle with your knuckles facing the ground. Notice that I'm gripping the top of the handle with my left hand.

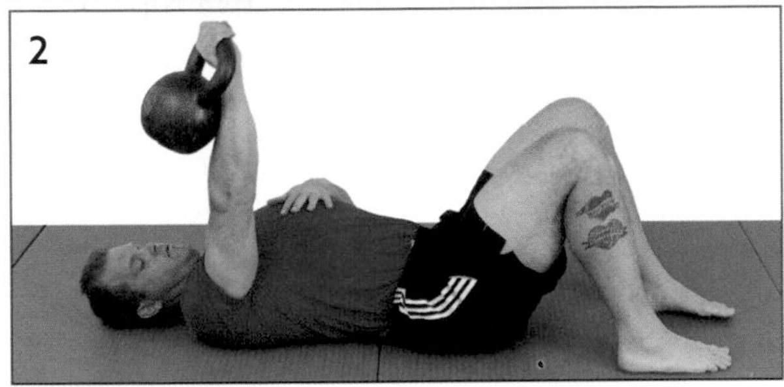

Roll onto your back and pull the kettlebell over your right shoulder while pressing it into extension.

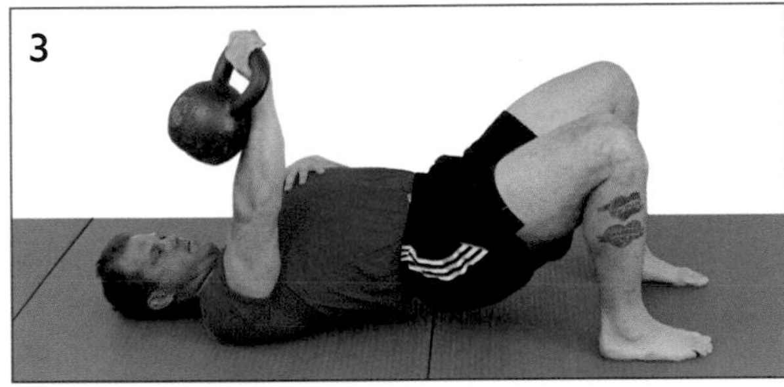

To set your shoulder to the back of the socket, elevate your hips, move your shoulder blades out of the way, and pull your right shoulder to the mat. This is very similar to, if the not the same as, the setup for a bench press or floor press.

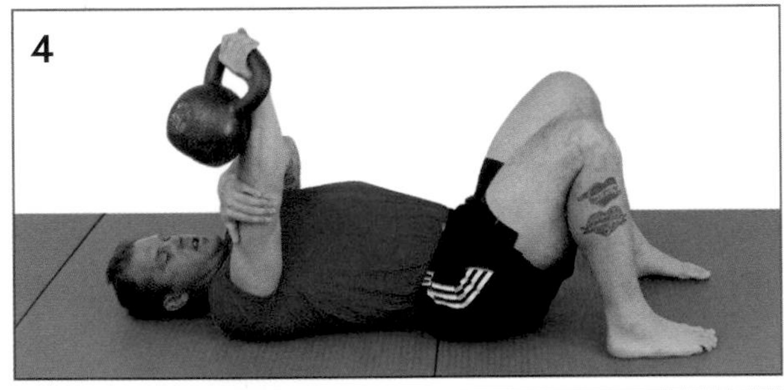

Keeping your midline engaged and your shoulder positioned to the back of the socket, lower your hips to the ground. There should be no space between your shoulder and the mat. To keep your elbow locked out and your arm straight, reach your left arm across your chest and cup the front of your elbow.

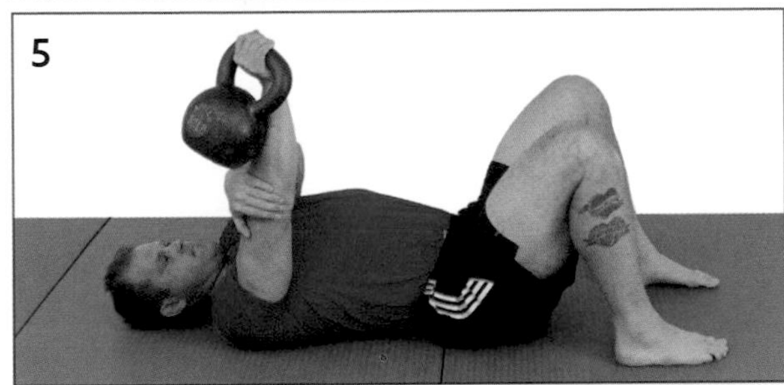

With your shoulder pulled to the back of the capsule, externally rotate your hand. Continue to internally and externally rotate your arm to restore normal function to your shoulder.

DISTRACTION VARIATION

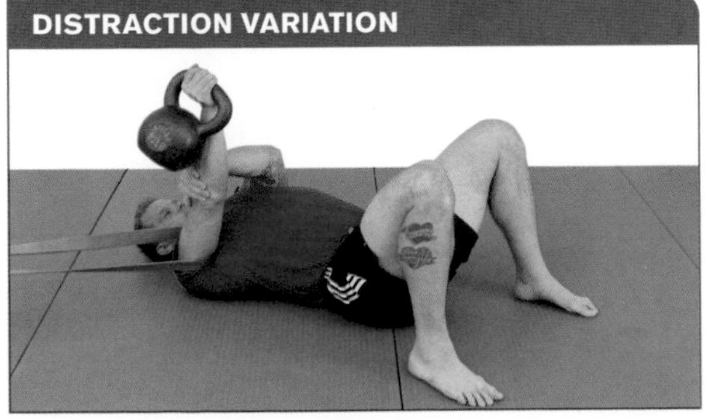

If your posterior capsule is extremely tight, it can be difficult to fully reset your shoulder into a good position by using the classic mobilization. In such a situation, add a lateral distraction to open up the tissues so that you can let your shoulder sink into the back of the capsule.

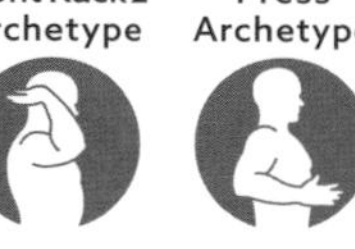

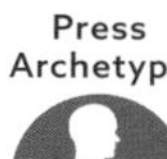

This mobilization will help improve the above archetypes.

IMPROVES:
Shoulder function
Shoulder pain

METHODS:
Smash and floss
Contract and relax

TARGET AREA

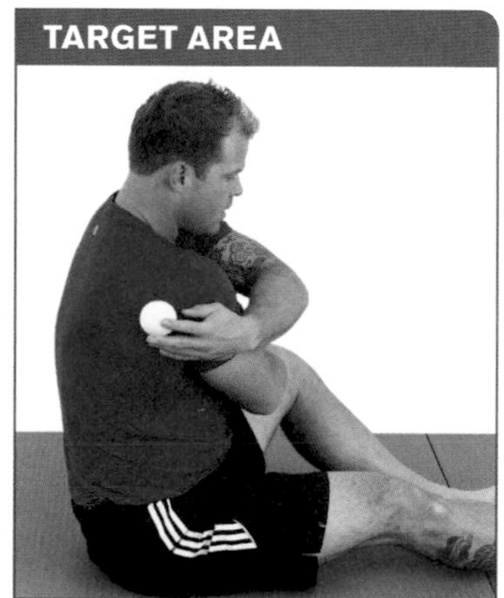

1. Position a lacrosse ball right above the insertion of your lat near your armpit. This is where the external rotators insert behind your shoulder. It's important to note that there's no right or wrong way. The goal is to get some pressure on the ball. If you want something a little more aggressive, roll onto your side to get some additional weight over your shoulder.

2. With the tissue behind your shoulder tacked down, rotate your hand toward the ground.

3. Internally rotate your arm until you reach your end range. From here, you can continue to move your hand back and forth.

Shoulder Rotator Smash and Floss

If you've tuned in to MobilityWOD.com or attended one of my seminars, you've inevitably heard me refer to rolled-forward shoulders as the dreaded douchebag shoulder position. Why? Have you ever seen "that guy" walking around with his shoulders forward and his chest puffed out in an attempt to look jacked and tough? Of course you have. And I'd be willing to bet that the first thing that ran through your mind was something along the lines of, "Damn, that guy looks like a giant douchebag." Hence "douchebag shoulders."

If your shoulders are rolled forward because you sit at a desk all day with bad posture, or you're a cyclist who's constantly stuck in a rounded position, it doesn't mean you're a douchebag; it just means that you have douchebag shoulders. The problem with douchebag shoulder syndrome is that a rolled-forward shoulder is an unstable position that limits your capacity to create external rotation torque, which, as you know, is a mechanism for dysfunctional movement patterns, force dumps, torque bleeds, etc. Not only that, but when you hang out in an internally rotated position, the external rotators of your shoulders get overstretched, brittle, and extremely stiff, which can lead to acute shoulder pain.

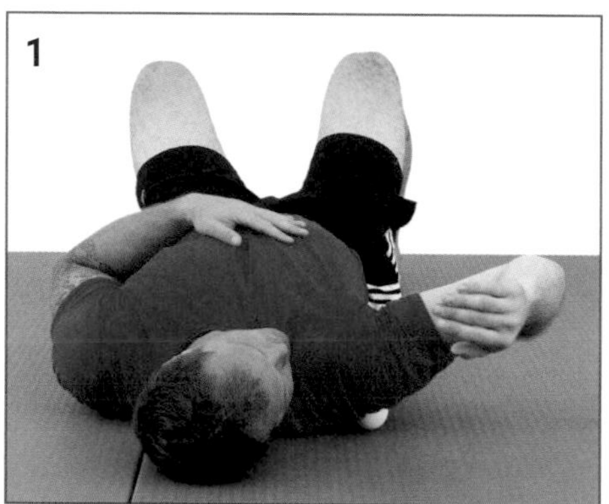

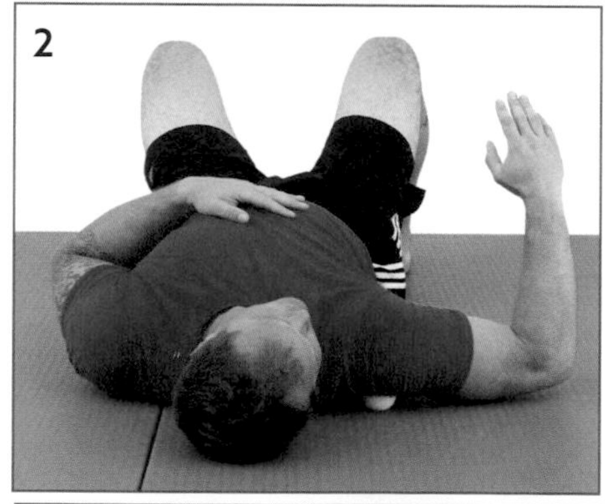

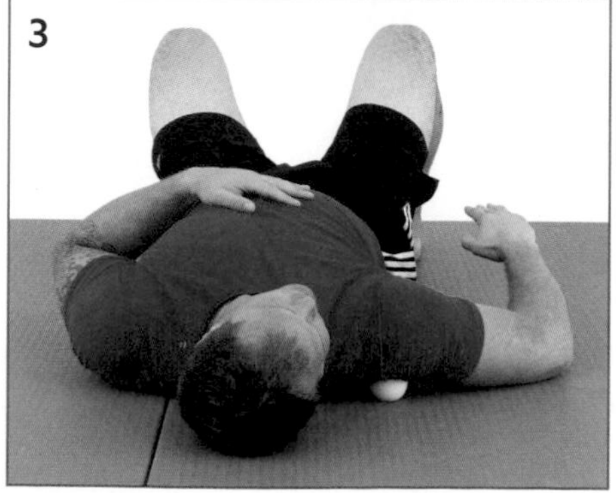

Fortunately, restoring suppleness to the area and relieving pain is simple. All you need is a hard ball (ideally a lacrosse ball), and you can effectively unglue the tissues that are compromising your mechanics, causing you pain, and making you look douchey.

Remember that the human body has a lot of big muscles that have an internal rotation effect. Very few have an external rotation effect. You can't afford to put those external rotators in a position where they become ineffective. Put another way, if you've rendered your external rotators impotent by your douchebag shoulder position, you're going to have shoulder pain and probably injure your rotator cuff. This is why, when someone comes up to me and says, "I have shoulder pain," I immediately ask him if he's smashed the backs of his rotators yet. If the answer is no, I tell him, "Go hit this mobilization and then tell me how you feel." In most cases, just a few minutes of smashing will relieve shoulder pain and reduce the douche-ness of your shoulder position. It makes a huge difference.

Overhead Tissue Smash Mobilizations

Whenever possible, you want to mobilize in a position that is similar in shape to the movement or position you're trying to change. For example, if you're trying to improve your overhead position, it makes sense to put your arm overhead and mobilize anything that might be limiting your range. In most cases, you'll find that your underarm region, which is where your lat and rotator cuff insert into your armpit, is really stiff and grotty. The approach is simple. If you can't get your arm overhead or you're having overhead pain, just ask yourself: Which tissues are limiting that overhead position? Put your arm overhead, lie on a ball or roller, and start hunting for tight corners. Chances are you'll find something that is really stiff and painful.

In this sequence, I provide a few options for mobilizing the lateral seam of your upper body, specifically the underarm region and latissimus (lat) muscle. Your lat plays a key role in stabilizing your shoulder, so if you're experiencing shoulder pain overhead or you're having trouble stabilizing your shoulder in a good position, get on a ball or roller and get to work.

Overhead Archetype | Front Rack 2 Archetype

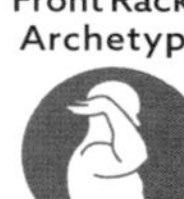

This mobilization will help improve the above archetypes.

IMPROVES:

Shoulder function
Shoulder pain

METHODS:

Contract and relax
Pressure wave
Smash and floss

TARGET AREA

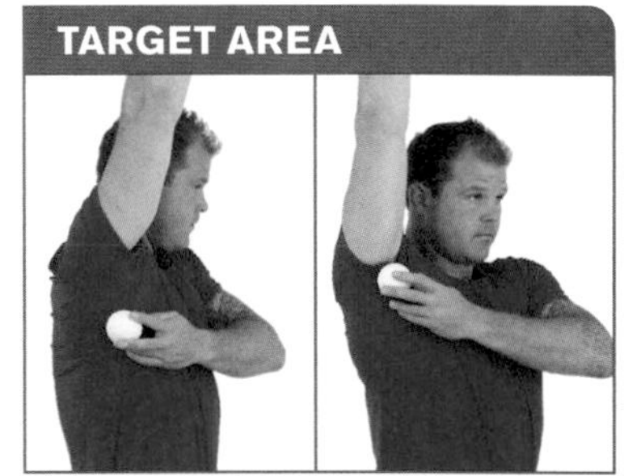

Option 1: Lacrosse Ball Smash

A tight lat compromises your ability to stabilize your shoulder and is a mechanism for shoulder pain. Spend some time scrubbing back and forth across your ropy bits and restore order to your shoulder. And remember, you are responsible for mobilizing your entire lat, which runs from your armpit to your lower back.

1

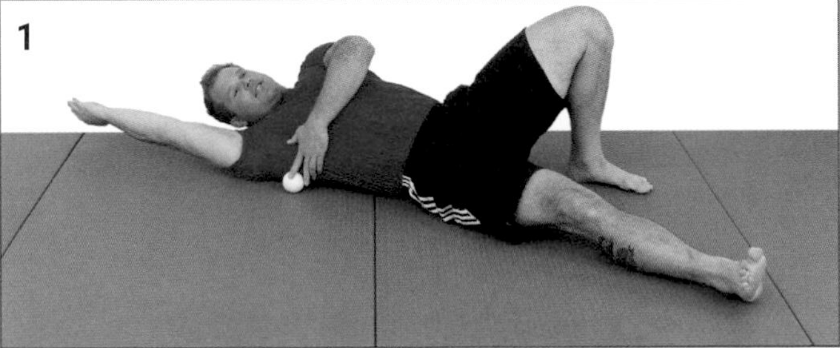

2

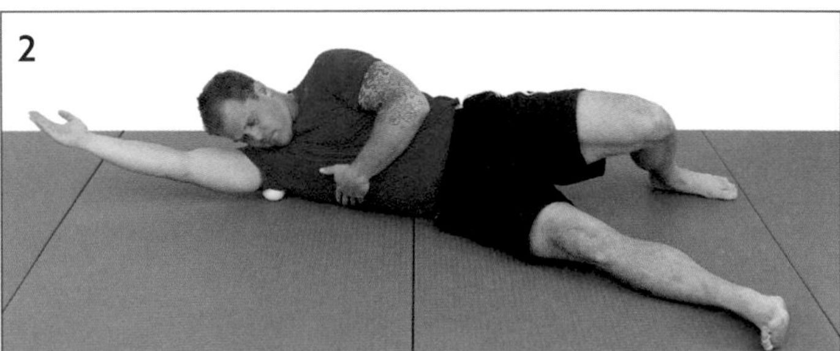

3

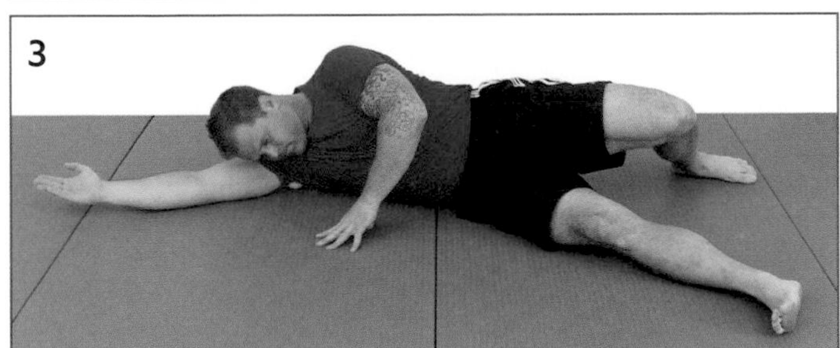

1. Position a lacrosse ball in your armpit near the insertion of your lat and rotator cuff.

2. Roll slowly onto your right side, smashing the underlying tissues.

3. Pressure more weight into the ball and slowly oscillate around your armpit area.

VARIATION: SUPERNOVA BALL SMASH

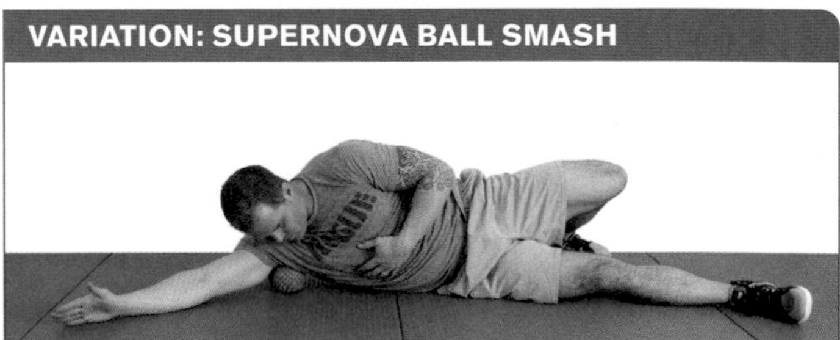

VARIATION: LITTLE BATTLESTAR SMASH

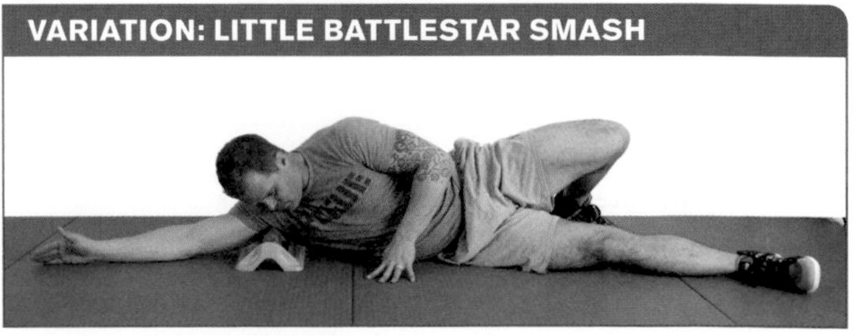

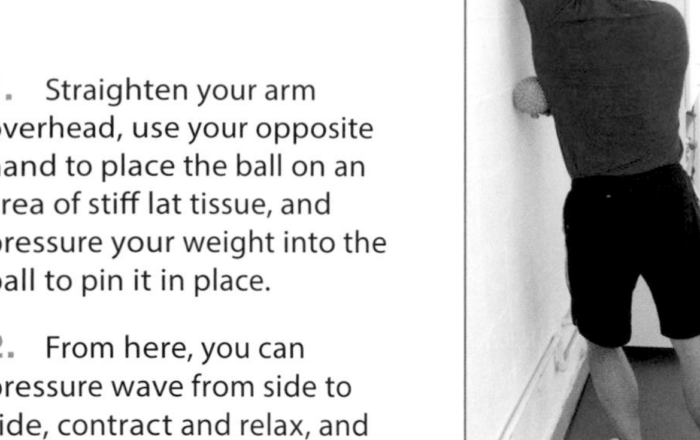

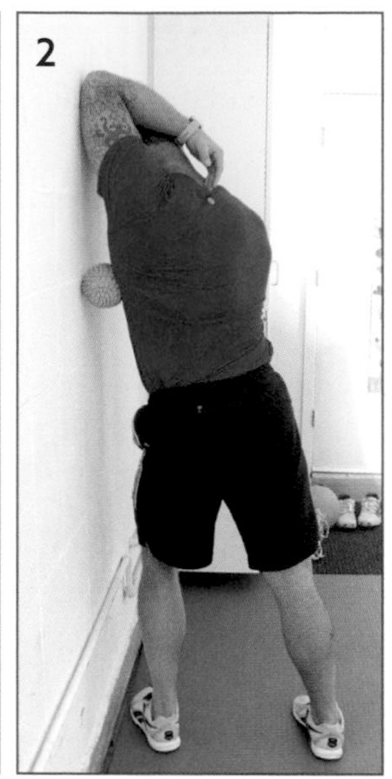

1. Straighten your arm overhead, use your opposite hand to place the ball on an area of stiff lat tissue, and pressure your weight into the ball to pin it in place.

2. From here, you can pressure wave from side to side, contract and relax, and smash and floss by bending your arm.

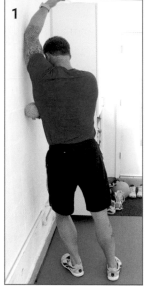

Option 2: Wall Smash

Another way to bias the Overhead Tissue Smash is to pin a lacrosse ball or softball against a wall. The target area is the same, but executing the mobilization from a standing position enables you to get deeper into the tight tissues of the lat. In addition, standing gives you a little more range to flex your arm, which not only takes up soft tissue slack but also allows for a different flossing stimulus.

Option 3: Superfriend Overhead Tissue Smash

Employing a Superfriend to smash your underarm region is another excellent option. The Superfriend's job is simple: Block your arm in an overhead position with his rear foot and then apply slow, steady downward pressure across your armpit and lat region using his opposite foot. The idea is to peel across the fascia and tacked-down tissue using his heel and the outside of his foot. There are two different yet equally effective approaches: Your Superfriend can rotate his foot back and forth as he pressure waves across the tissue as if he were trying to put out a cigarette on your arm, or he can wind up the tissue (tack and twist) by spinning his heel into the meat and then pressure waving through.

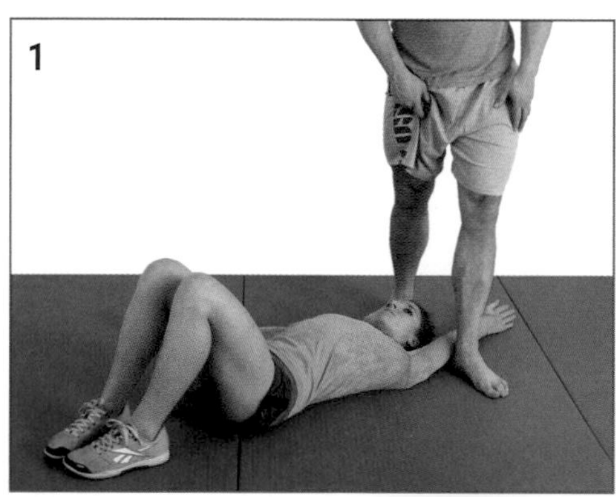

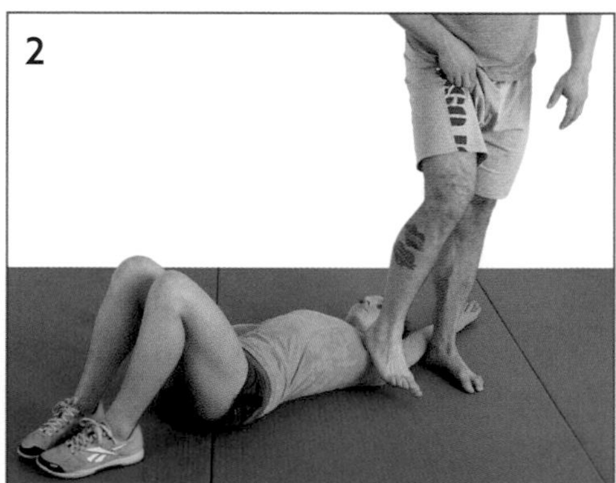

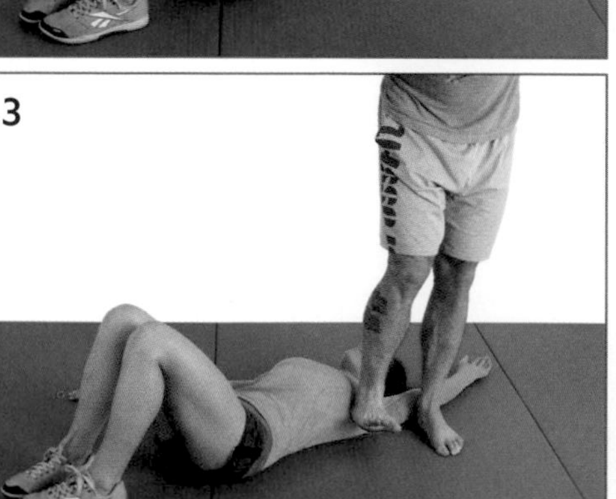

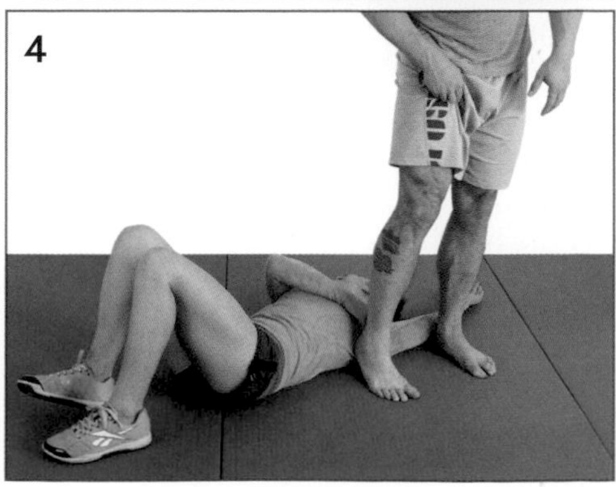

1. Lie on the ground with your arm raised overhead. Have your training partner pin your arm in the overhead position by posting his heel next to your elbow.

2. Have your Superfriend slowly apply pressure into your lat using his heel and the outside of his foot.

3. If he finds a stiff spot or you want him to apply more pressure, he can flex his foot and rotate it from side to side.

4. The idea is to smear across your lat as he drives his foot to the ground. From here, he can even keep the ball of his foot on the ground to support his weight while smearing his heel into your lat.

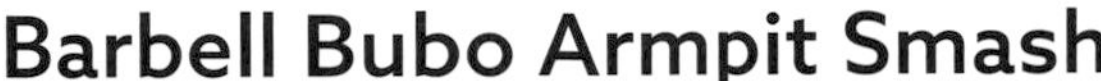

Barbell Bubo Armpit Smash

Overhead Archetype Front Rack 2 Archetype

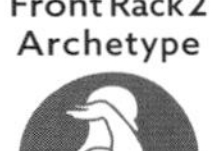

This mobilization will help improve the above archetypes.

IMPROVES:

Shoulder function
Shoulder pain

METHODS:

Contract and relax
Pressure wave
Smash and floss

Your armpit houses a lot of converging musculature that serves your arm and shoulder: the deltoid, triceps, biceps, pec, lat, and rotator cuff tendons (to mention a few) all insert into this area. Most of the movements seen in sports and weightlifting employ strenuous use of these muscles. When these insertion points get hot—meaning tight and inflamed—pulled muscle damage, shoulder pain, and arm strains generally follow.

While the previous techniques captured the posterior and lateral seam, it's difficult to tap into the muscles and insertion points underneath the arm, specifically the coracobrachialis and subscapularis. To do that, you need a barbell bubo. What's great about the barbell bubo setup is that you can hang over the bar and swing your arm back and forth to create movement through the area, which helps break apart tacked-down muscles and matted-down connective tissue.

Note: Although attaching a ball to a barbell is ideal for targeting the small, hard-to-reach muscles underneath your shoulder, you can still perform this mob on a clean barbell to mobilize your lats and the surrounding musculature.

TARGET AREA

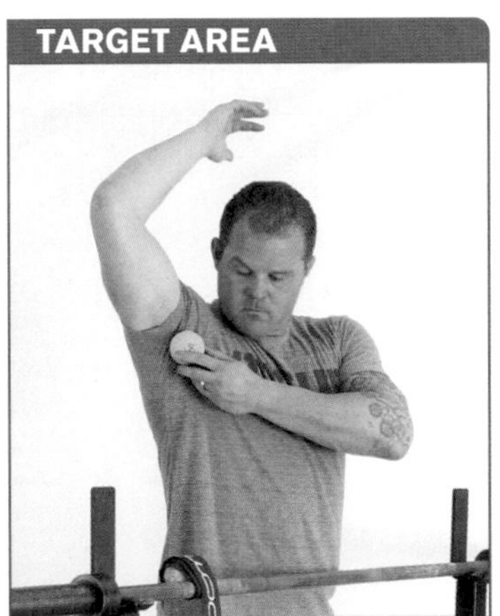

1

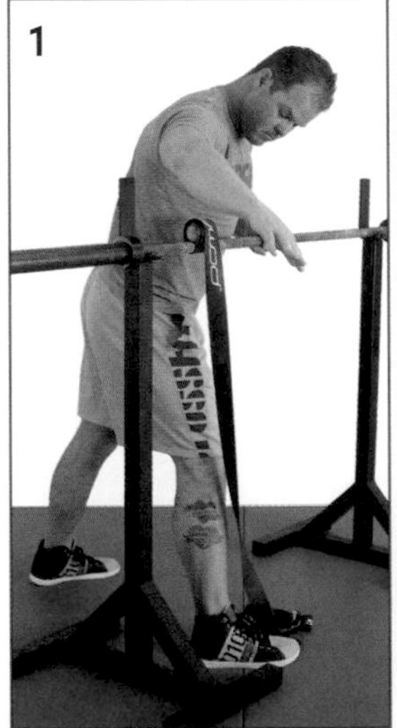

2

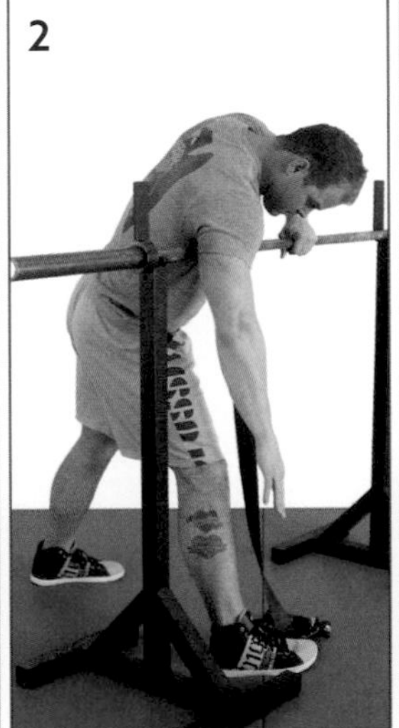

3

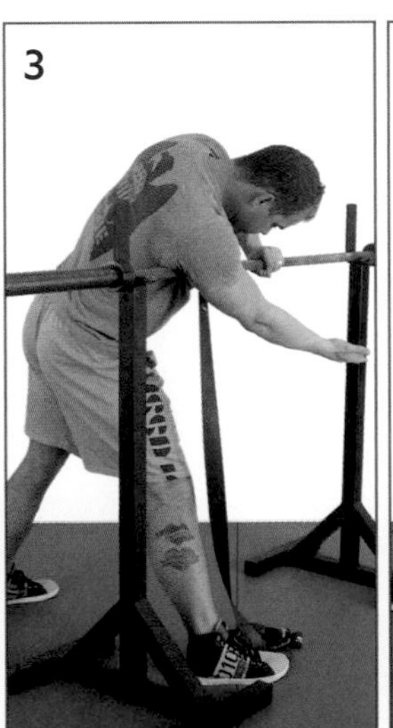

4

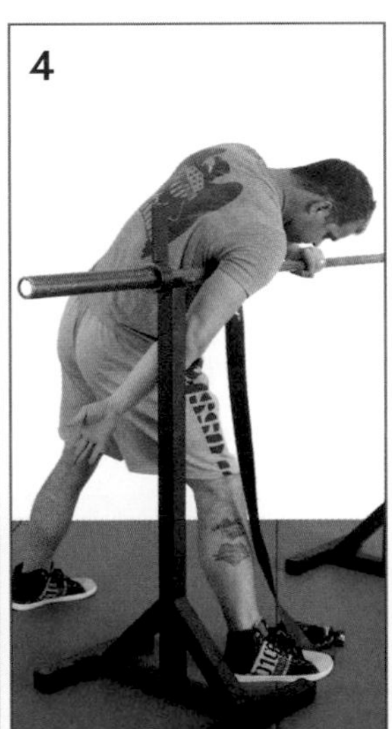

5

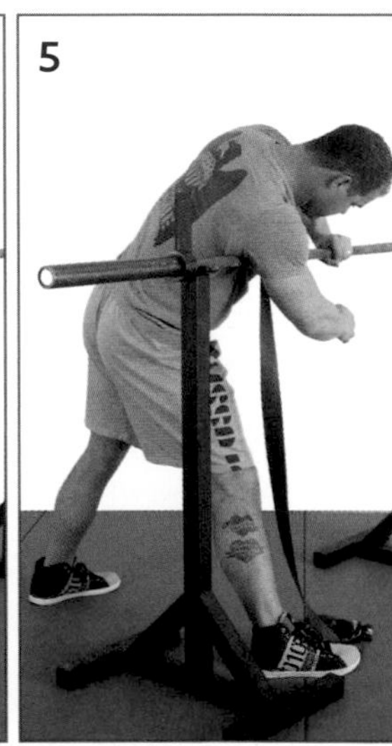

1. Attach a ball to a barbell (you can use a VooDoo Floss Band for a temporary setup; see page 307) and set the height of the rack to hip level.

2. Hang your arm over the barbell, positioning the ball in the center of your armpit—putting as much weight over the ball as you can handle.

3. Keeping your elbow in tight to your body and your weight distributed over the bar, raise your arm toward your head. Externally rotate your shoulder as you perform this motion. From here, contract by curling your arm toward your head, then relax by sinking more of your weight into the ball.

4. Reach your arm behind your body to bias extension and internal rotation.

5. Don't be afraid to explore all vectors: reach your arm under the bar toward your far hip, reach for the ground, and try to get as much rotation through your shoulder as possible.

Serratus Smash

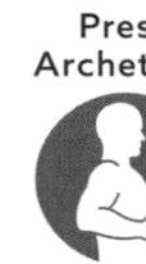

This mobilization will help improve the above archetypes.

IMPROVES:

Throwing, punching, swinging mechanics

Shoulder pain

METHODS:

Smash and floss

Contract and relax

If you're on a ball mobilizing your lats and underarm region, you may as well venture into your serratus anterior muscles, which are located to the inside of your lat. These muscles attach to your ribs and wrap behind the scapula, and they are responsible for protracting and retracting the scapula to make room for your moving arm. This is why the serratus anterior muscles are commonly referred to as the "boxer muscles": The movement pattern of punching and reaching is possible due to scapular protracting and retracting. Common sport movements like throwing, spiking, and swinging employ strenuous use of these muscles. When these tissues get stiff or weak, rotation and shoulder mobility are compromised.

To test the mobility of your serratus, swing your arms to the side as demonstrated in the test and retest photos below. As you swing your arm overhead, there's a moment of loading on the serratus, which gives you immediate feedback. You will instantly feel if this area is tight and tacked down, making this exercise a great model for gauging the effectiveness of the mobilization. In addition, it serves as an excellent warm-up for rotation.

Note: This area can be a bit sensitive, so use a softer ball if necessary. I like to use the Supernova, but a smaller, softer Yoga Tune Up ball is also a great option because it allows you to target your intercostal muscles, which run between your ribs.

1. Lie on the ball with your arm outstretched to the side, positioning the ball between your lat and pec, just underneath your armpit.

2. With as much weight distributed over the ball as you can handle, slide your weight toward your outstretched arm. Scrub across the serratus and intercostal muscles with slow, deliberate movements.

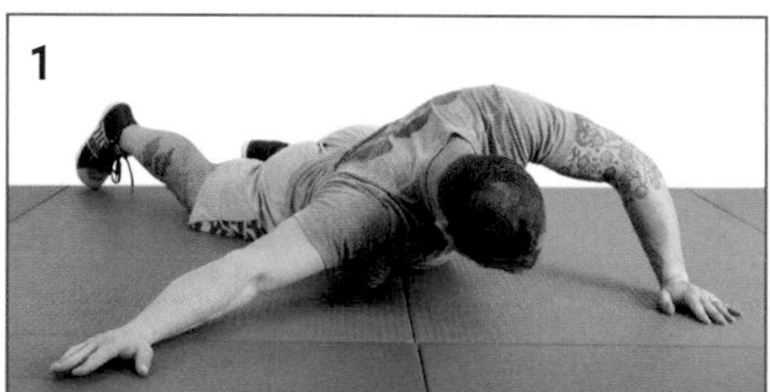

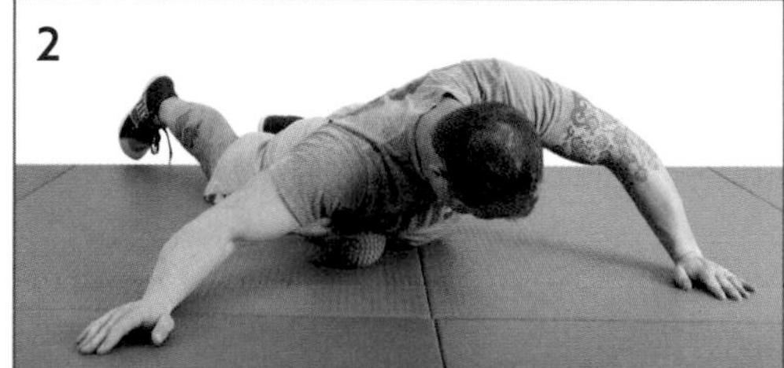

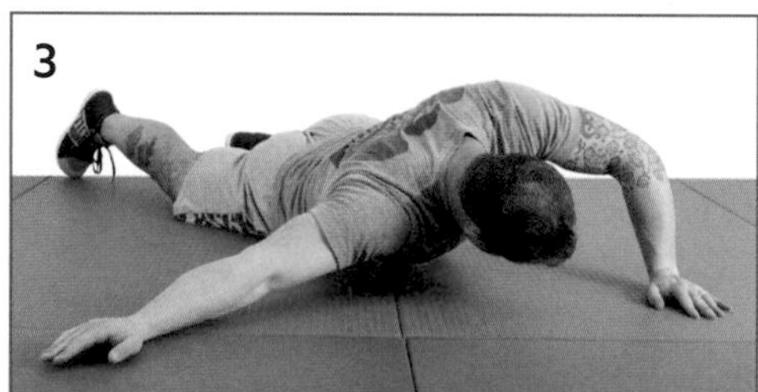

3. Using your arms to control the side-to-side movement, scrub back and forth across the area. You can contract by screwing your hands into the ground—keeping your weight over the ball—and then relax by dropping your outstretched shoulder to the ground. Slide your arm up and down across the mat for a flossing effect.

TEST AND RESET

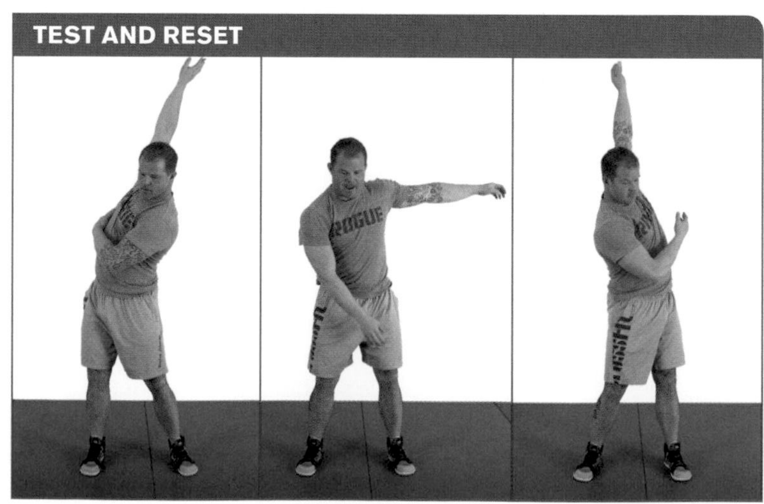

To test and retest the effectiveness of this mob, swing your arms from side to side as if you were warming up for a golf swing. The goal is to keep your arms relaxed, your shoulders externally rotated, and your body straight. Imagine that you're stuck between two panes of glass preventing you from tilting forward or backward.

Banded Overhead Distraction

If you've ruled out motor control as a limiting factor in going overhead, you know that you have a mobility obstacle working against you. The template for improving the overhead position is a no-brainer: Simply mobilize the tissues you're trying to change while practicing the movement. Although this concept is easy enough to grasp, people still seem to get it wrong. If you ask someone who is missing overhead range how much time she's spent mobilizing overhead, she can usually count only the seconds, not the minutes, that she's accumulated in that position.

Here's an example:

Athlete: "Coach! I'm having trouble in the bottom of the squat."

Me: "Did you mobilize in the bottom position?"

Athlete: "Sure, I did some air squats. That counts, right?"

Me: "Your butt only touched the bottom position for 0.1 second for every squat. So, no, that doesn't count. Maybe try this: Drop into the bottom position and spend some real time mobilizing in the position that's giving you trouble."

Although this seems obvious, it's not intuitive. When I see someone who is missing overhead range, this is one of the first mobilizations I prescribe, because it forces her to spend a great deal of time under tension while working at end range.

To perform this mobilization correctly, make sure that you create external rotation torque by turning your palm up prior to loading your shoulder. You can do so either by grabbing your thumb and forcing your palm up or by having a Superfriend do a jiu-jitsu wrist lock on you, putting your wrist into an externally rotated position. Far too many people just grab the band and distract their arm overhead. This does not account for a full range of motion! You're just hanging on your meat. Remember, full range is not putting your arm overhead. That's still an unstable position. Full range of motion means that you can put your arm overhead to its end range with rotational capacity.

Overhead Archetype

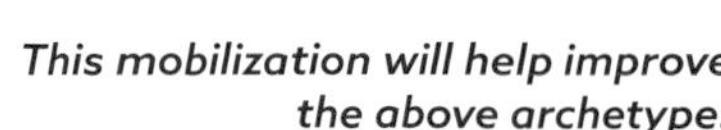

This mobilization will help improve the above archetype.

METHOD:

Contract and relax

1. Hook your wrist through the band and grab both ends. Don't make the mistake of latching onto the end of the band!

2. Use your left hand to bias your right arm into external rotation so your palm is facing up and your thumb is pointing toward the outside of your body.

3. Keep your arm locked in an externally rotated position. Create tension by sinking your hips back and lowering your torso toward the mat. With your arm externally rotated in the overhead position, contract and relax and try to distract your shoulder into new end ranges.

4. Start hunting around for stiff areas. For example, start by throwing your right leg behind you, which lengthens that fascial line, increasing the aggressiveness of the stretch. The key is to keep your right palm up and your thumb out as you explore.

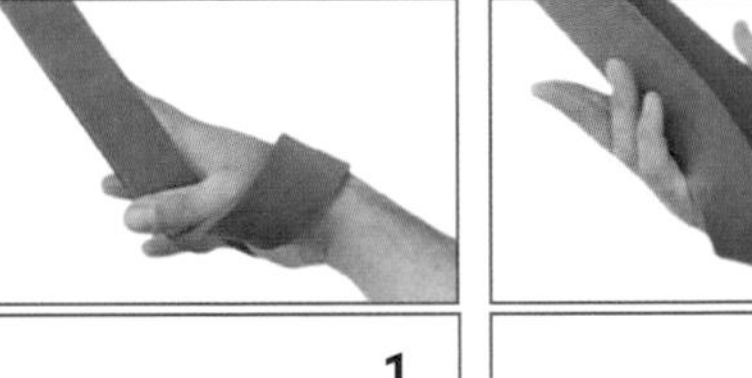

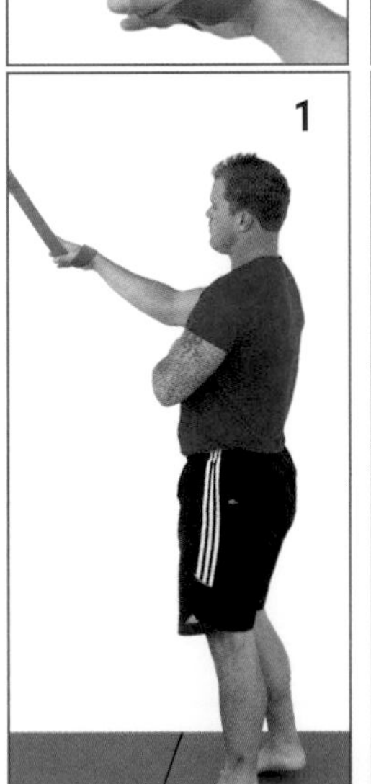

1

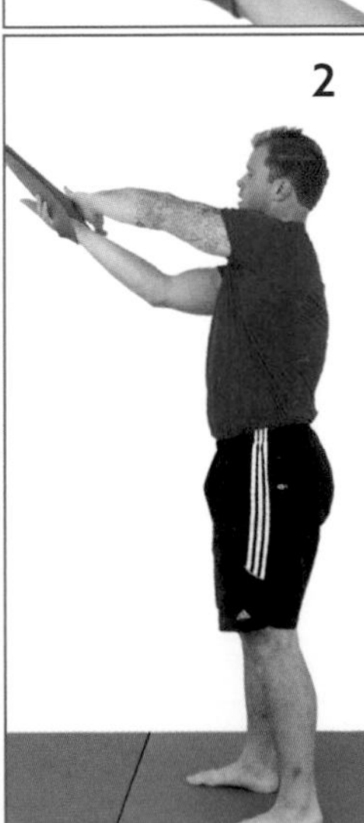

2

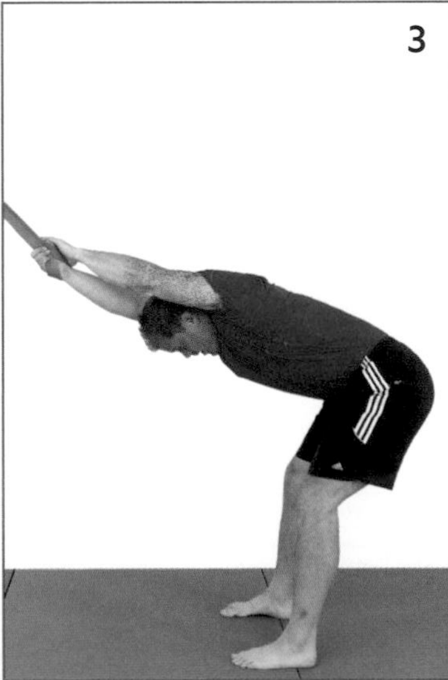

3

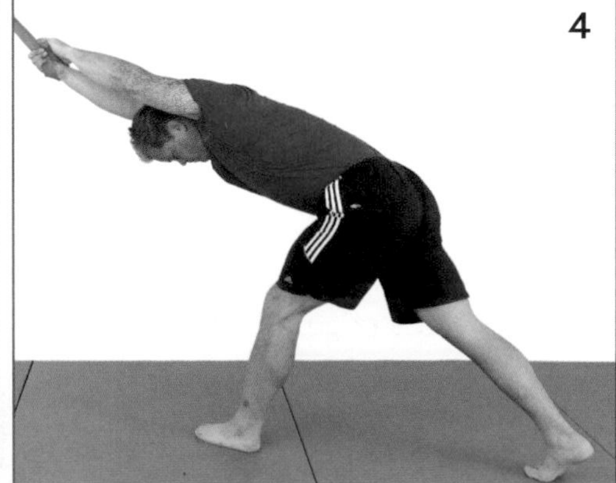

4

Overhead Distraction with External Rotation Bias

Overhead Archetype 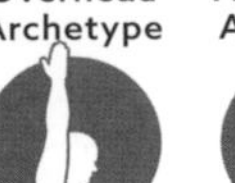 Front Rack 2 Archetype 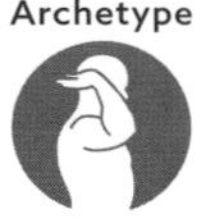

This mobilization will help improve the above archetypes.

METHOD:
Contract and relax

This mobilization is a companion piece to the Banded Overhead Distraction. As you can see in the photos below, your elbow is fixed and being held by the band, allowing you to plumb a deeper range of shoulder flexion. Put simply, you change the dynamics of the shoulder by changing the position. It's like one of them is a barbell push-press and the other is a handstand pushup. They're very similar, but they give you very different stimuli.

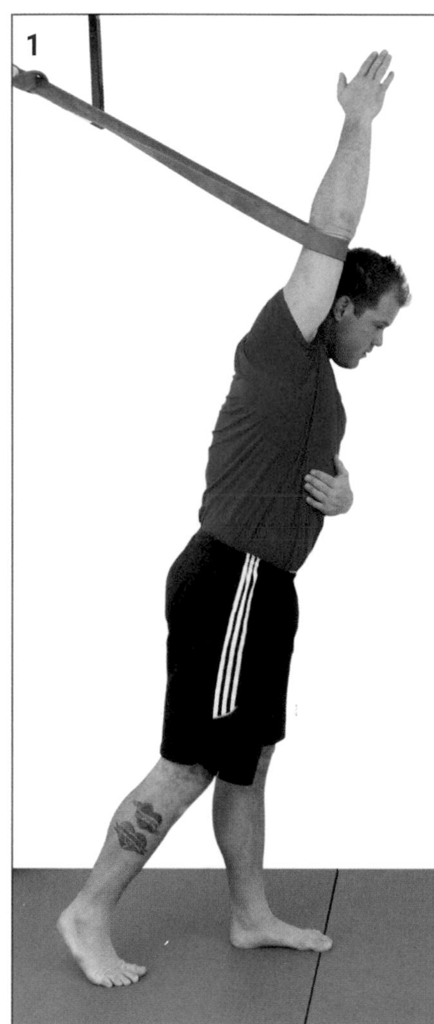

Punch your arm through the band and hook the strap around your elbow.

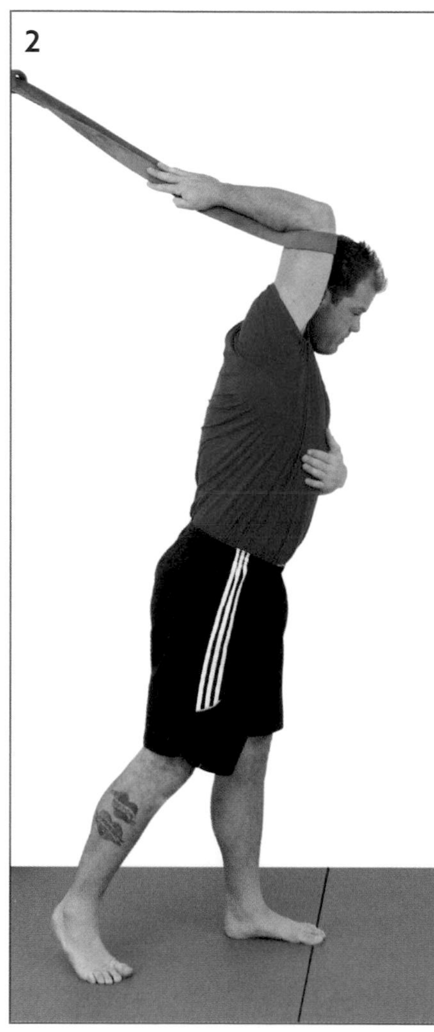

With the band distracting your arm, latch onto the outside of the band with your right hand. The key is to keep your ribcage down and your midline tightly engaged.

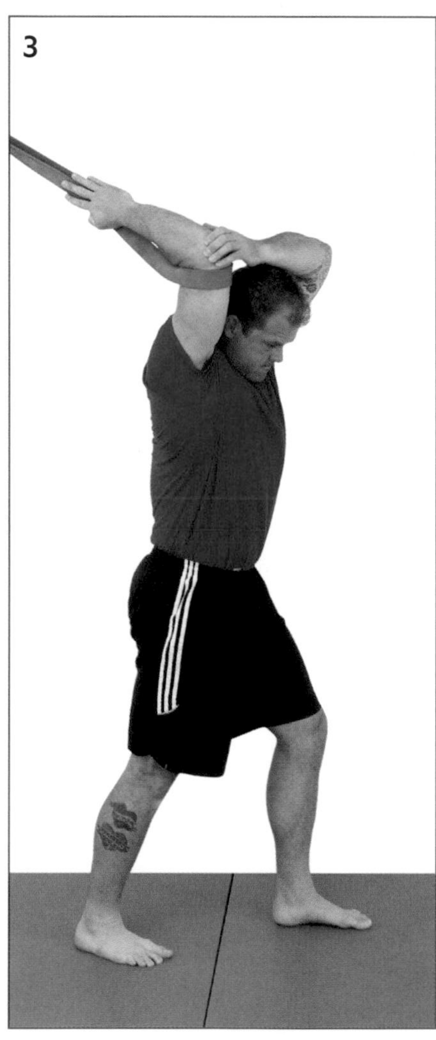

To add tension and increase the aggressiveness of the mob, grab the back of your elbow, pull it toward your head, and lower your elevation. As you do so, fight to maintain external rotation torque.

Bilateral Shoulder Flexion

Overhead Archetype　Front Rack 2 Archetype

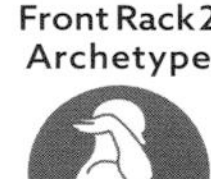

This mobilization will help improve the above archetypes.

METHOD:
Contract and relax

This is another fantastic mobilization that improves overhead position as well as midrange flexion movements like the bench press and pushup. What's different is that you're bringing your arms closer to your center line and then adding external rotation. The rotation helps tie in the posterior shoulder capsule. So, unlike the previous mobilizations, which highlight end-range flexion and then add external rotation, this mob biases end-range external rotation first and then adds flexion as a tensioner.

To hit the ugly corners of your external rotators, you want to create as much torque as possible, which you accomplish by keeping your elbows close together. Here's why: As you apply tension to the load, your elbows spread apart. You can't help it. There is so much torque that when you apply tension to the position, your elbows go wide and torque is lost. To help you make the connection, imagine someone pressing a heavy load overhead with her elbows out. If you've read chapter 3, you know that this is a huge torque dump. The same thing is happening here. As your elbows go wide, you bleed torque and the stretch becomes less intense.

To prevent your elbows from spreading, have a Superfriend block your elbows together or wrap your arms with a band—see the Banded Version below.

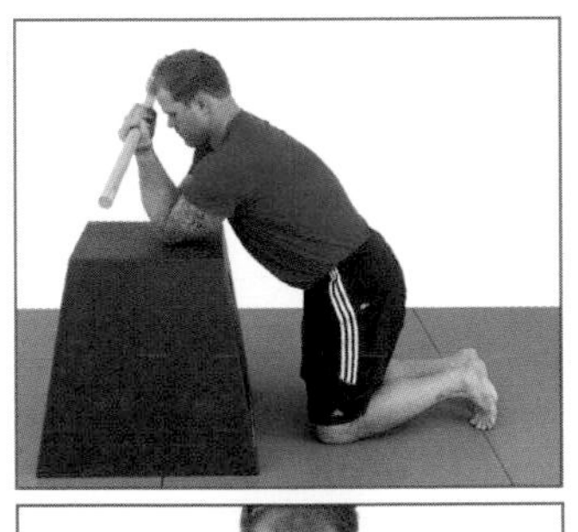

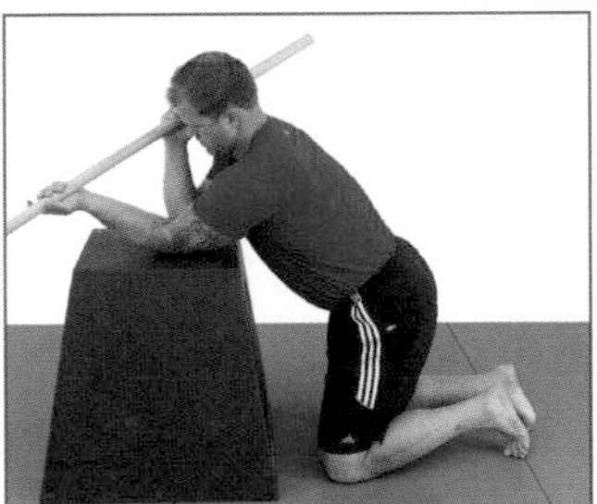

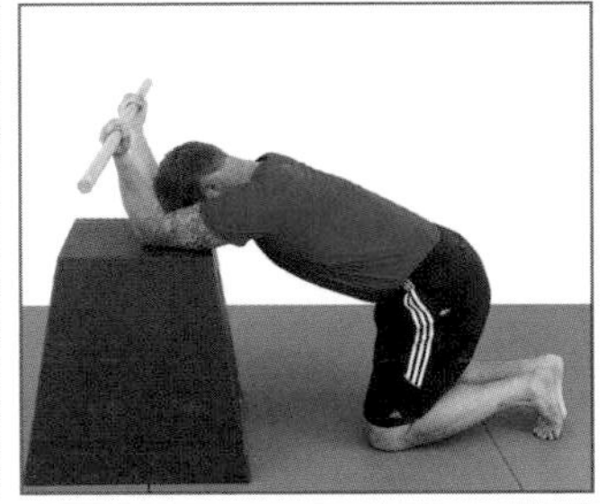

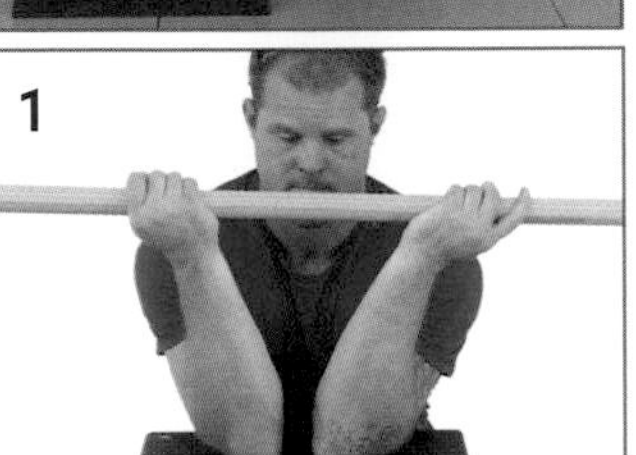

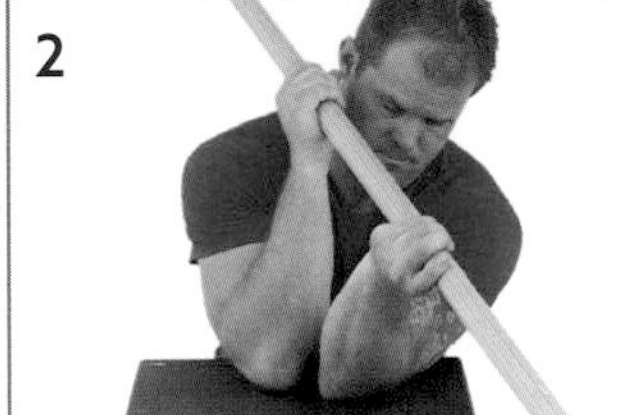

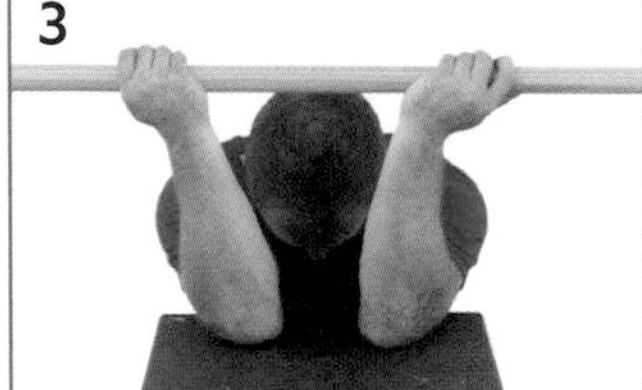

1. Kneel in front of a box and grasp a wooden dowel with your palms facing your body and your elbows together.

2. Keeping your elbows as close together as possible, rotate the dowel and spread your hands apart until you reach end-range external rotation.

3. With your shoulders wound up into an externally rotated position, apply tension to the load by pushing your body back and dropping your elevation. This hits all the big, soft tissues of the lats as well as the external rotation features of your shoulders.

Bilateral Shoulder Flexion: Banded Version

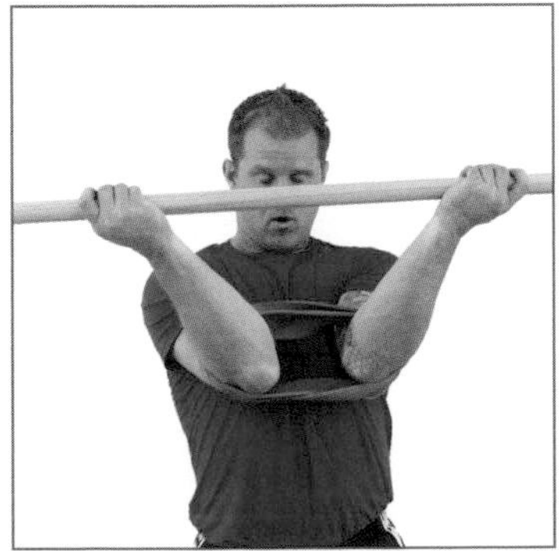

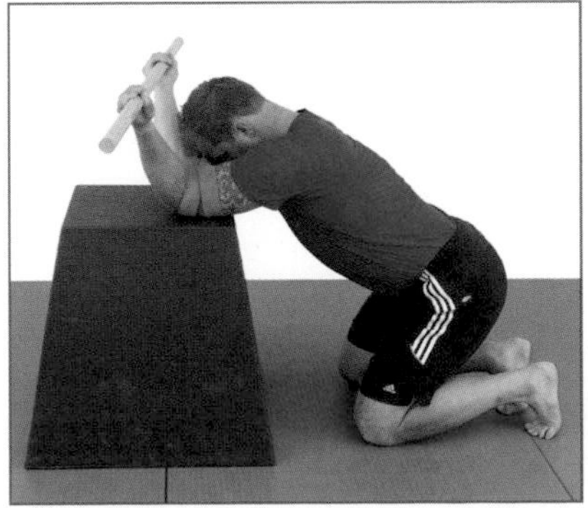

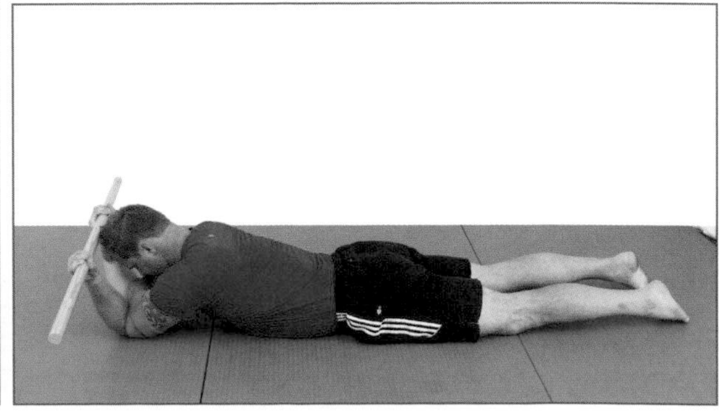

Wrap a band into 3 loops, hook it around your elbows, and then bias external rotation by twisting a dowel and spreading your hands apart. With the band preventing your elbows from spreading, you can implement the same strategy with the box by sinking your hips back and punching your head through your arms. You can do the same mobilization on the ground.

Overhead Archetype

Front Rack 2 Archetype

This mobilization will help improve the above archetypes.

METHOD:

Contract and relax

Super Front Rack

The Super Front Rack is my go-to mobilization for improving the overhead position, more specifically (to state the obvious) the front rack position. The key to this technique is to keep your hand up and your elbow in. You'll find that as you step through and create tension, your hand will turn down and your elbow will fly out to the side—two ways to lose torque. These faults also make it difficult to maintain a neutral position. When you try to create tension off an unstable shoulder, it's much easier to break into overextension. The same thing happens in the front rack position when you fail to create a stable platform. You can't get your elbows up because your shoulders are douched, so you have to overextend to maintain an upright position.

To avoid these faults, try to exaggerate the hand-up position, use your opposite hand to prevent your elbow from flying out, and stay integrated as you walk out to create tension.

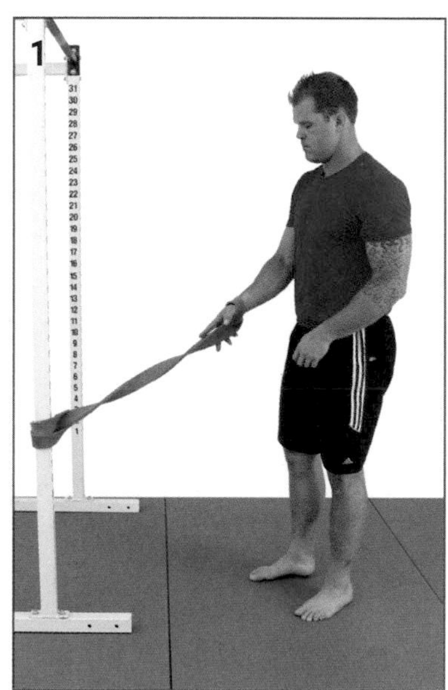

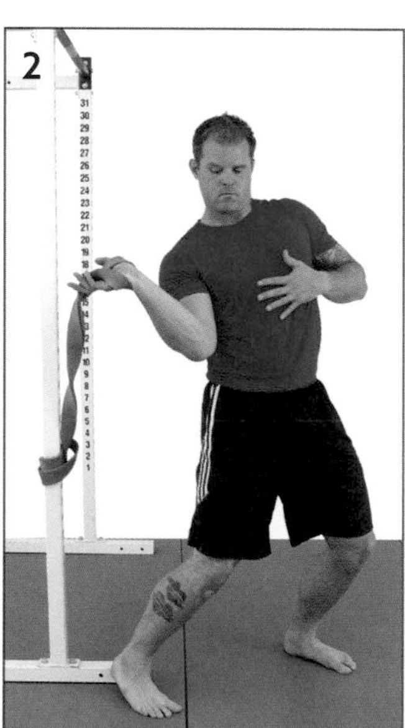

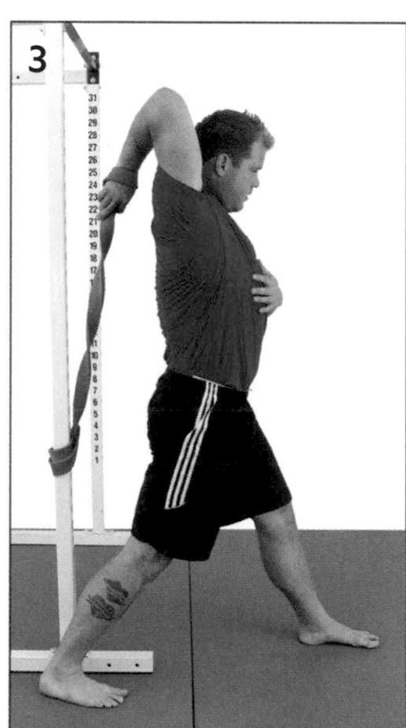

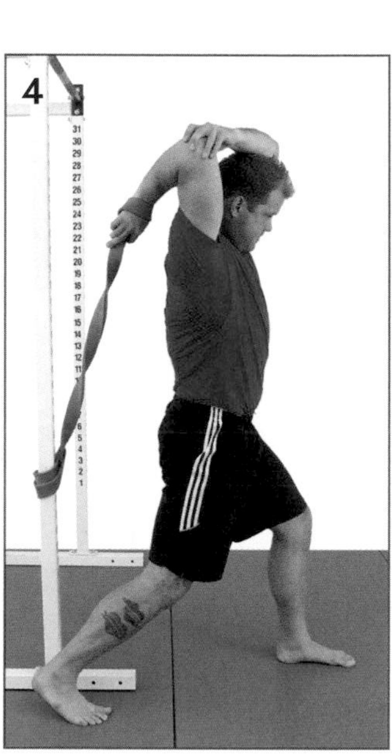

1. Hook your wrist through a band.

2. Turn your palm up and wind your shoulder into external rotation. As you do so, step through, rotating your body underneath the band as if you were setting up for a judo throw.

3. Keeping your palm up, maneuver your shoulder underneath the band and stand upright to create tension. Squeeze your right glute and keep your abs turned on to avoid breaking into overextension.

4. Still fighting to keep your right palm up, grab the outside of your right elbow using your opposite hand (which prevents your arm from flying out to the side) and shift your weight forward.

Classic Triceps and Lat Stretch

When was the last time you spent a significant amount of time smashing and mobilizing your triceps? Wait. I already know the answer. Never.

The Classic Triceps and Lat Stretch hits the long head of the triceps, the lat, and some of the structures that limit overhead movement across the shoulder. To make this mobilization even more effective, wrap a VooDoo Floss Band around your upper arm and floss your triceps. I guarantee that VooDoo Flossing your triceps will bring new life into an area that you've probably neglected your whole life. Doing this mobilization with a VooDoo Floss Band increases its effectiveness by 100 times, or maybe more.

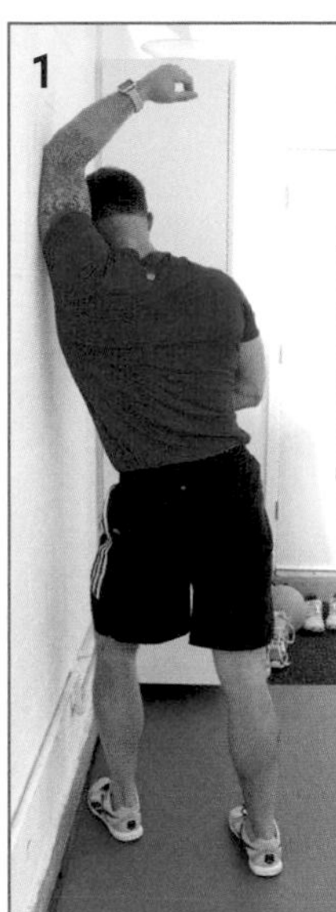
1

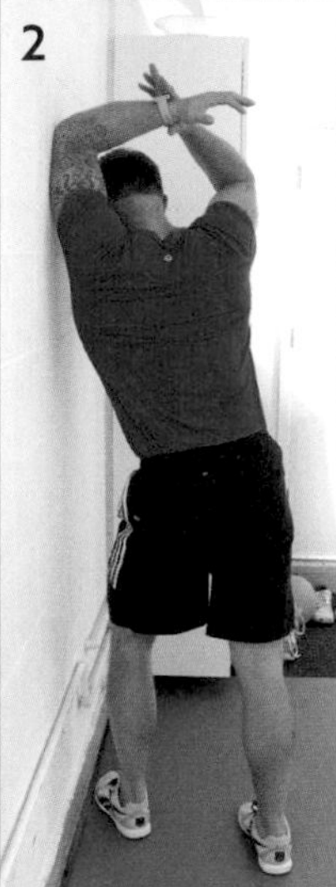
2

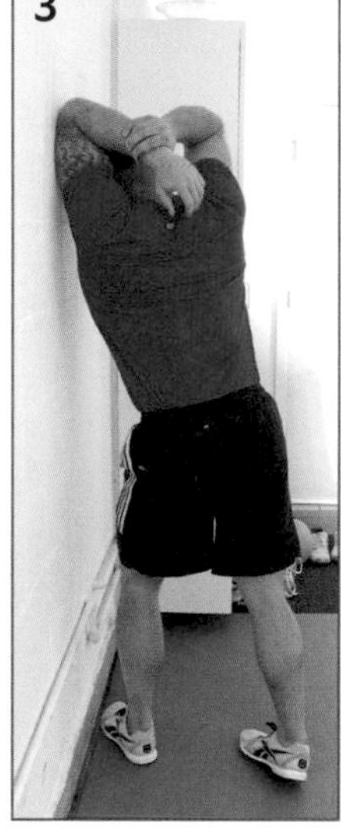
3

Overhead Archetype

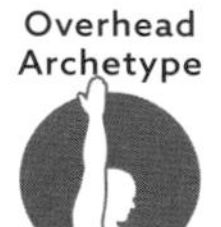

Front Rack 2 Archetype

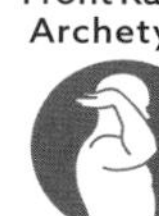

This mobilization will help improve the above archetypes.

METHOD:

Contract and relax

1. Position your distal triceps and elbow against a wall.

2. Drive your weight into the wall, creating a stretch through the long head of your triceps, and latch onto your left wrist with your right hand.

3. Force your left arm into flexion by pushing your left hand toward your left shoulder.

Reverse Sleeper Stretch

We all have busy lives, so we have to find ways to mobilize and improve positions when we're jammed into a 737 window seat, sitting at a desk, etc. This mobilization is a low-tech and highly versatile way to work on the internal rotation of your shoulders. It is my car/airplane/trapped-in-a-chair internal rotation mob. I've done it for a long time and still do it to this day—it's an oldie but a goodie.

Hang Archetype

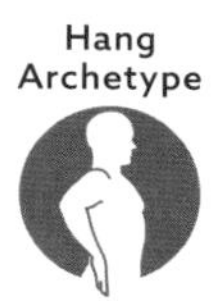

This mobilization will help improve the above archetype.

METHOD:

Contract and relax

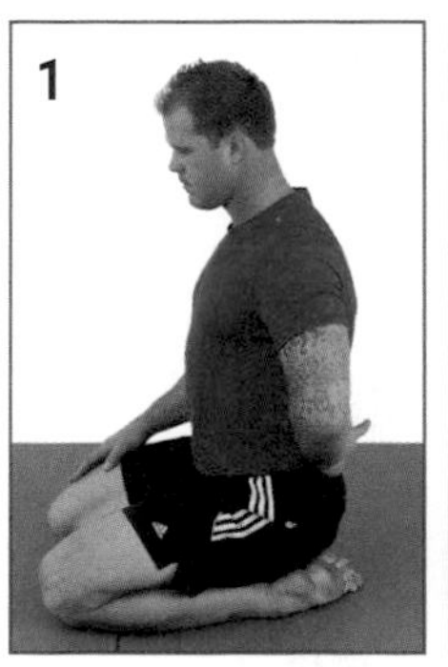
1

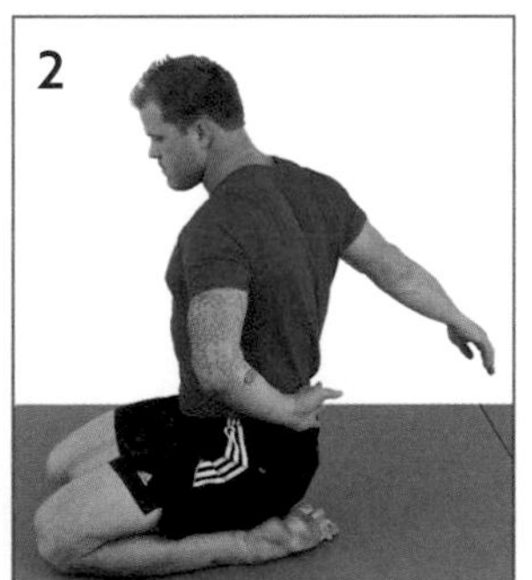
2

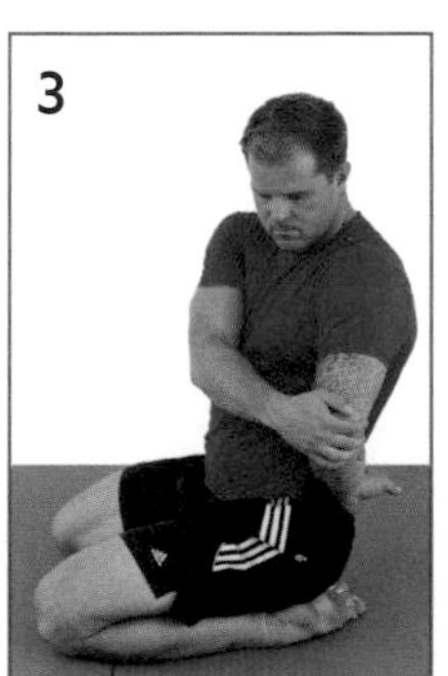
3

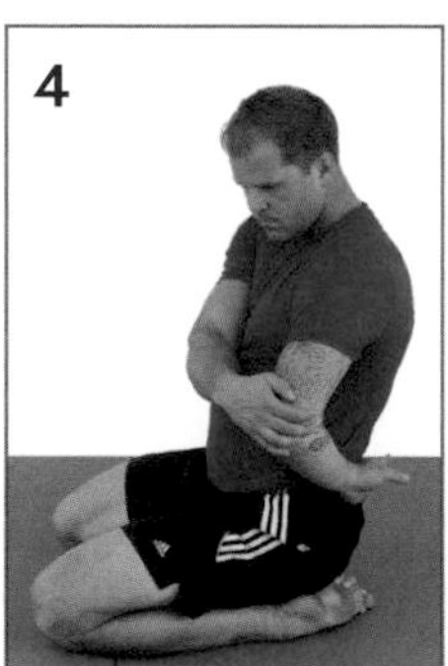
4

1. Pull your left shoulder into a tight position, then place your left hand behind your lower back with your palm facing away from you.

2. Sometimes reaching across your body with your other arm behind your back is difficult. If you feel like you're going to round forward and compromise your posture, cock your arm back before swinging it across your body.

3. Swing your right arm across your body and grab your left elbow with your right hand.

4. Pull your elbow toward your center line to emphasize internal rotation. As you pull your arm across, focus on keeping your shoulder back. If you let your shoulder roll forward into a compensated position, you'll create an impingement and lose the effectiveness of the mob.

AREA 4 ANTERIOR SHOULDER AND CHEST

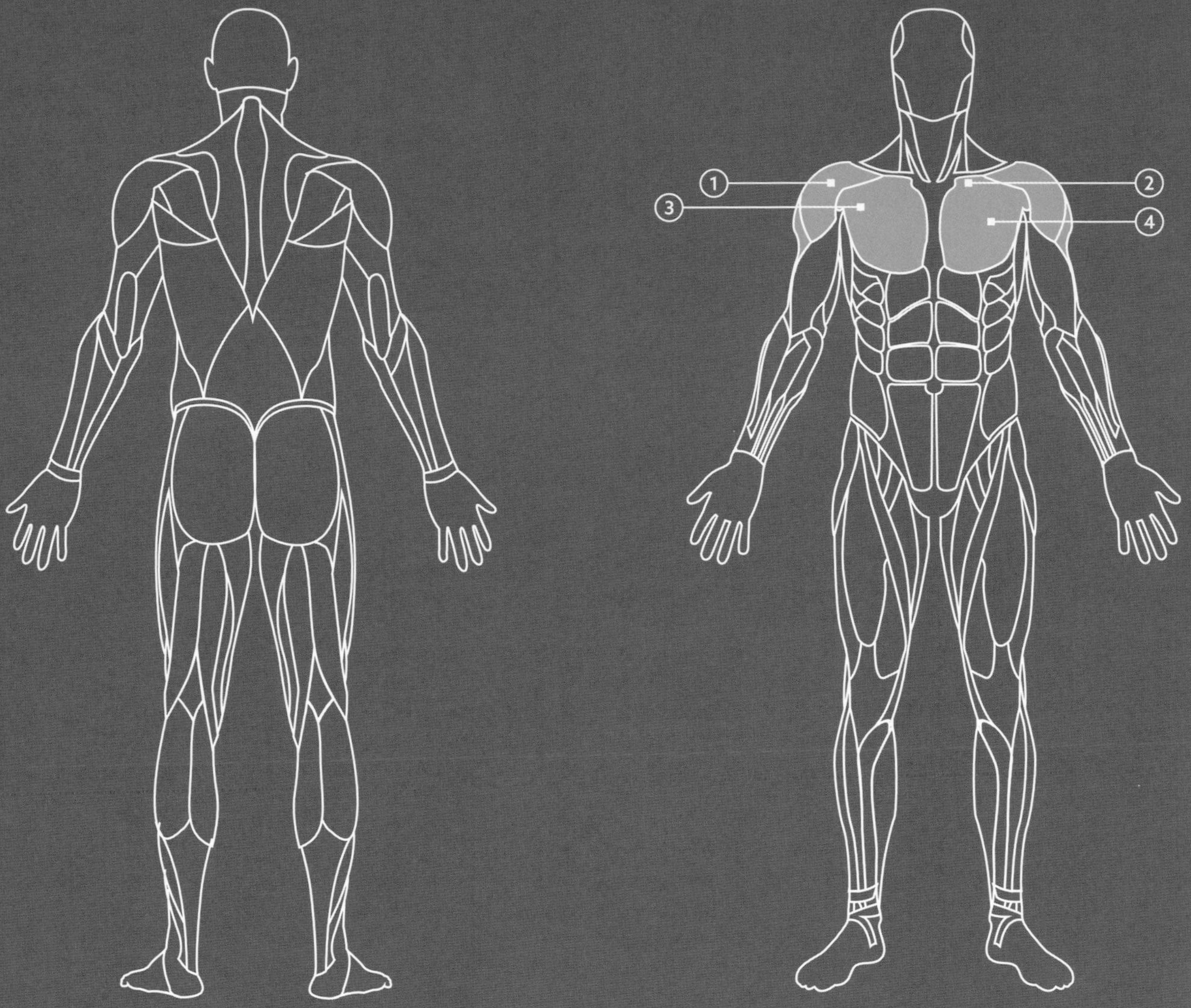

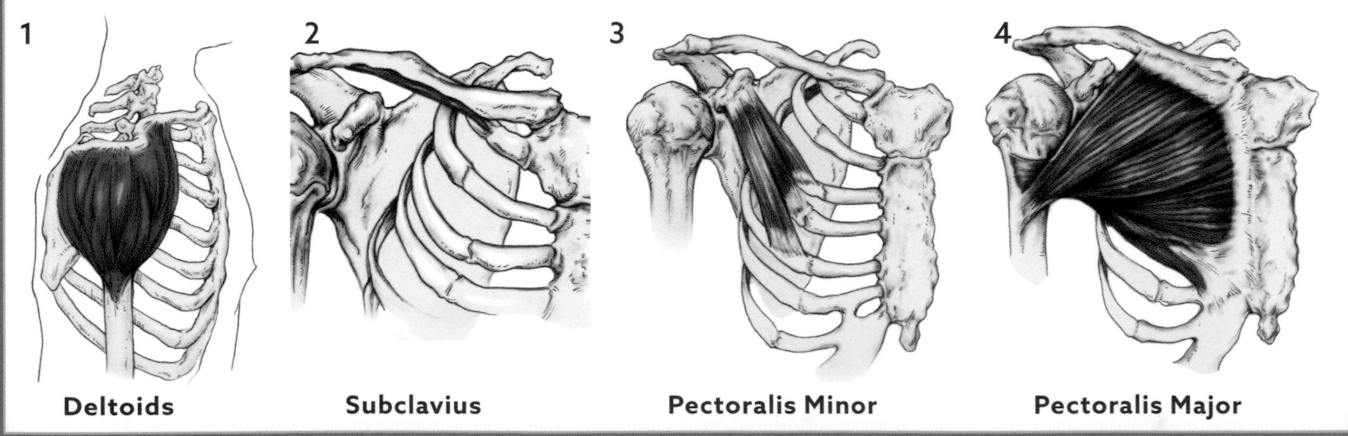

Anterior Compartment Mobilizations

Athletes tell me all the time that they have a hard time getting their shoulders into a good position, even after attacking the thoracic spine and posterior structures. What they forget is that the condition of the anterior compartment can do as much to limit good shoulder position as the condition of the scapula, ribs, and thoracic spine. It's an interconnected system. If any of the tissues that attach to your shoulder blade get tight and short, it will restrict your ability to put your shoulders in a stable position. For example, if you sit at a desk all day, or you spend a lot of time in a car, or you're a cyclist, or you're simply missing internal rotation, chances are good that you spend a lot of time in a forward-shoulders position. While this compensated position wreaks havoc on your thoracic spine, scapula, and ribs, your pec minor, which runs from your shoulder blade to your sternum, gets brutally stiff, effectively locking your shoulders into an unstable position.

This is a huge problem, because now your arms have to internally rotate as a way to stabilize your shoulders and rectify your limited range. It's your body's way of dealing with the open circuit of an unstable shoulder. Internally rotating is less of a liability than having your shoulder flop around in the socket. So if you spend any amount of time under load or tension in that compensated position, your pec minor has to work really hard to keep your shoulder stable, causing it to get chronically tight as a result.

In the subsequent mobilizations, I demonstrate a few methods for restoring suppleness and function to the area.

Overhead Archetype

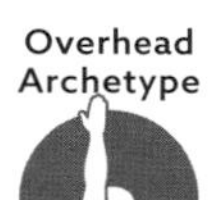

Press Archetype

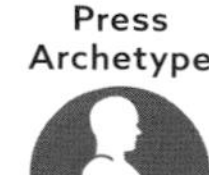

Front Rack 2 Archetype

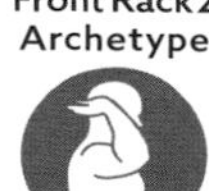

Front Rack 1 Archetype

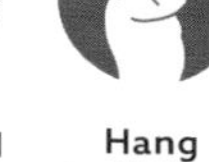

Hang Archetype

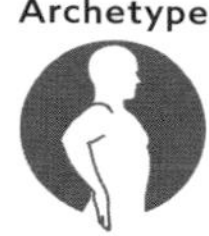

This mobilization will help improve the above archetypes.

IMPROVES:

Shoulder position and function
Flexion fault (rounded shoulders)
Shoulder and neck pain

METHODS:

Pressure wave
Contract and relax
Smash and floss
Tack and spin

TARGET AREA

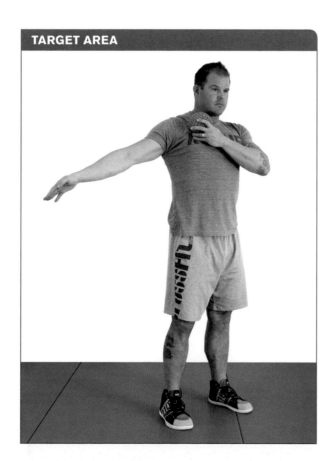

Option 1: Blue Angel

The Blue Angel is my favorite/least favorite mob for addressing the anterior compartment of the chest and shoulder. It's my favorite because you can tie in all the methods—tack and spin, contract and relax, pressure wave, and floss—allowing you to make a ton of change in a very short time. It's also my least favorite because it is so potent and painful. Luckily, you can do it facedown and respectfully hide your ugly pain face.

As you can see in the photos below, the idea is to mimic the motion of making a snow angel with your arms.

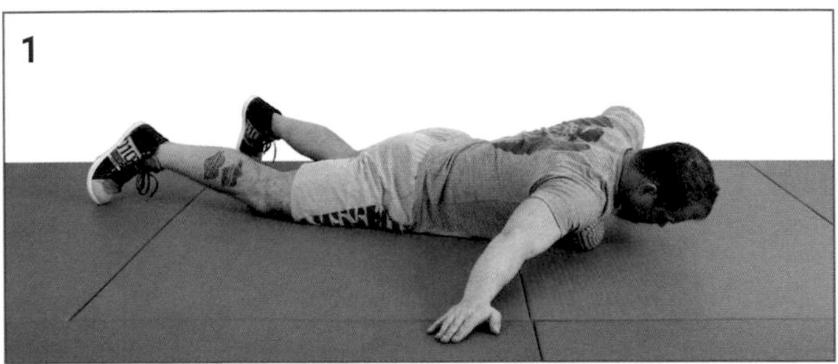

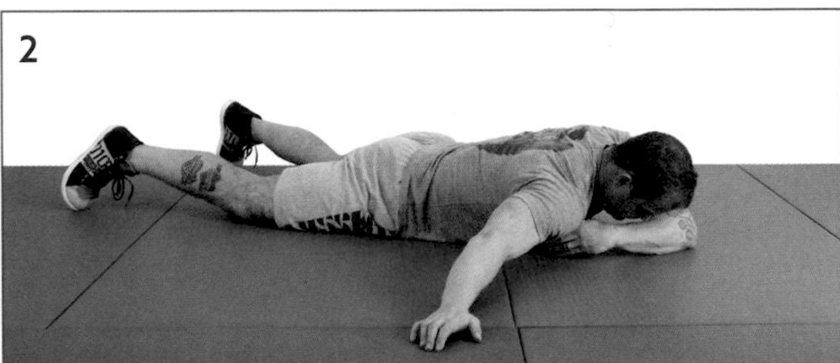

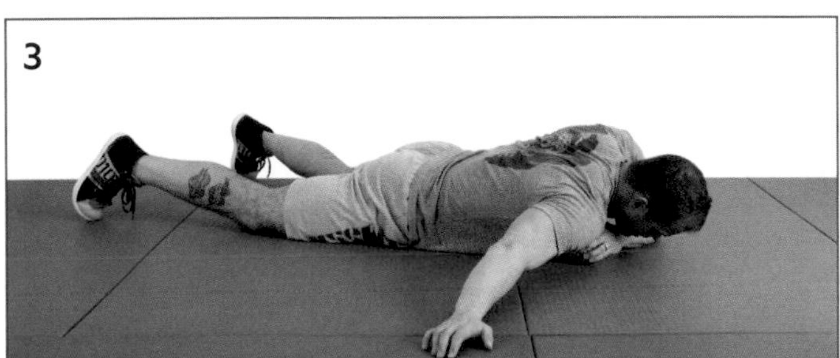

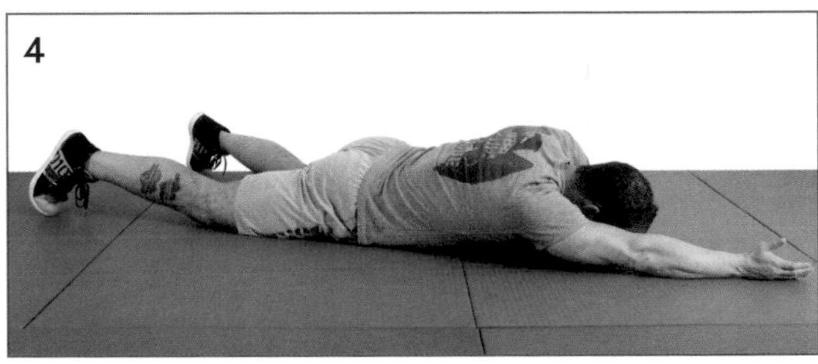

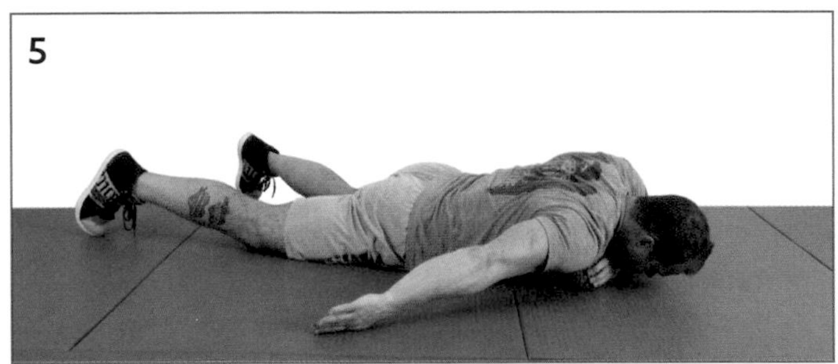

6

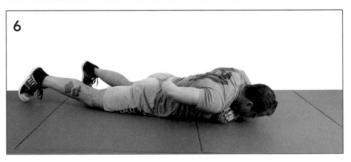

1. Lie on the ground and position a ball underneath your collarbone, between your chest and shoulder. With your arm outstretched to the side, load as much weight as you can handle over the ball. From this position, you can contract by pressing your outstretched arm into the mat as if you were doing a pushup, then relax by letting more of your weight sink into the ball.

2. Grab the ball with your opposite hand.

3. Take up all the soft tissue slack by spinning the ball away from the shoulder you're mobilizing.

4. Keeping your arm outstretched, externally rotate your shoulder while sliding your arm across the ground toward your head.

5. To capture all the vectors in your shoulder, internally rotate your shoulder by maneuvering your arm toward your back.

6. With your arm behind your back, you can reach behind your back with your other hand, grab your wrist, and then use that grip to pull your arm up your back. This not only forces you to explore end ranges, but also loads more of your weight over the ball. I'm not going to lie: It's miserable.

Option 2: Blue Angel Wall Smash

You can also perform the anterior compartment smash against a wall or in a doorway. A doorway is ideal because you're free to move your arm out in front of your body, allowing you to hit some nasty corners that are unavailable to you when you're mobilizing on the ground. The only caveat is that you can't get as much pressure or weight into the ball.

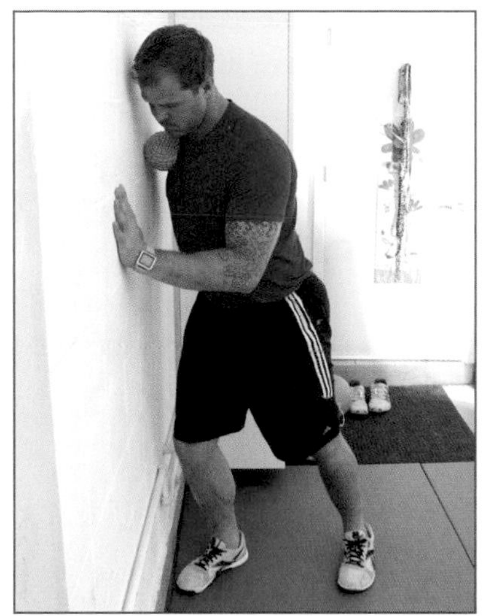

Use the same movements and methods as in the previous technique: Scour your chest and anterior shoulder region, try to get as much motion through your shoulder as possible, and contract and relax on tight spots.

Option 3: Gemini Pec Smash

TARGET AREA

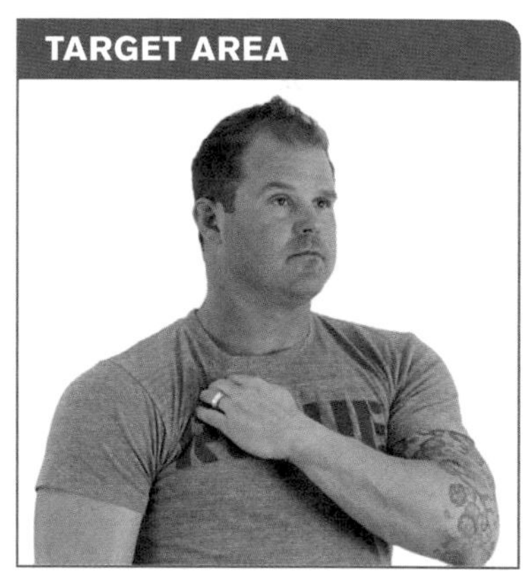

Sometimes it's difficult to tap into the muscle tissue bordering the collarbone and shoulder when using a larger tool like the Supernova. To clean up the hard-to-reach points that remain untouched by a larger ball, you need something that has a point, like a Gemini or small ball. In short, employ the Blue Angel to target the meat or big musculature of your chest (pec major) and shoulder, and use the Gemini Pec Smash to clean up the border of your collarbone and the crevices between your chest (pec minor) and deltoid.

1

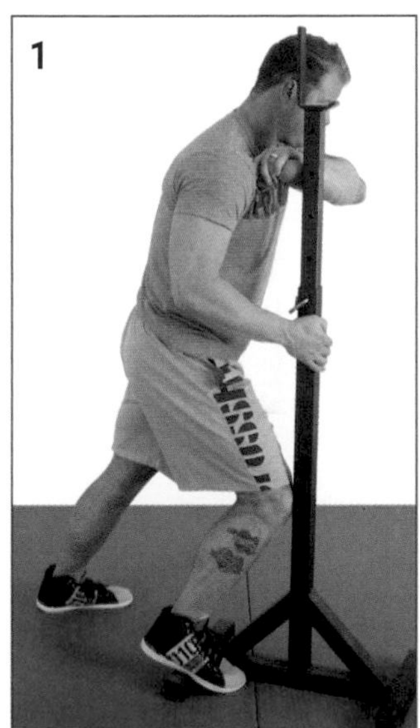

2

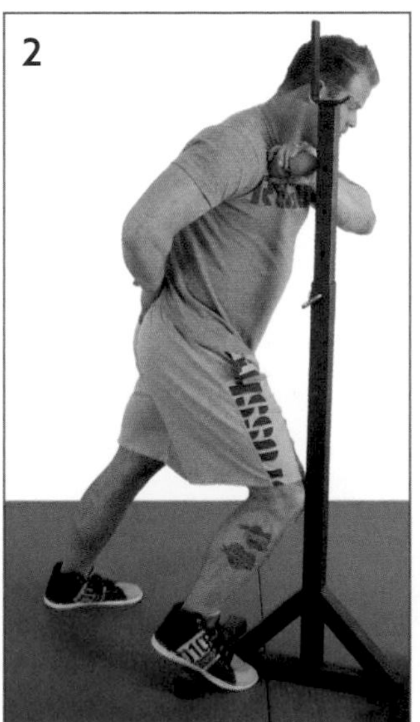

3

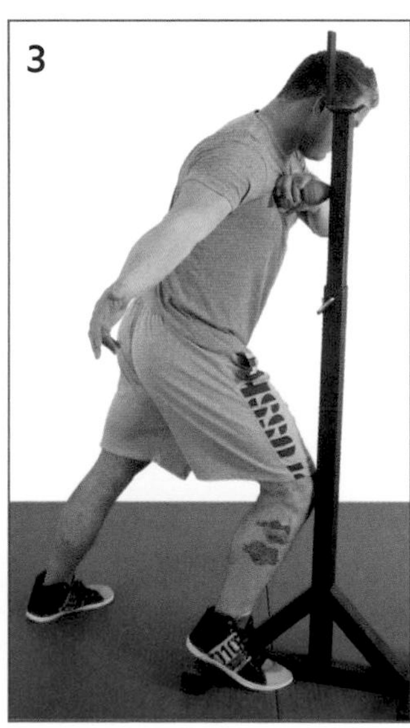

Place the end of the Gemini into the corner of your shoulder, underneath your clavicle, or anywhere that feels tacked down around the border of your deltoid and pec. Before you contract and relax or start flossing, twist the Gemini to wind up the fascia and take up all the soft tissue slack. Then explore the areas of your chest and find your tight bits. You can move your arm behind your back to bias extension and internal rotation, or open up your chest by externally rotating your shoulder and reaching out to the side.

Bubo Barbell Pec Smash

The Bubo Barbell Pec Smash is a variation of the next technique, which was created to restore sliding surfaces to the deltoid. By attaching a lacrosse ball or Yoga Tune Up ball to a bar, you can turn the Barbell Shoulder Shear into an acute pec-smashing technique. As with the previous technique, this allows you to target the insertion points bordering your chest and deltoid, specifically where the pec minor attaches to the shoulder.

Note: To turn this into a two-for-one mobilization, place a lacrosse ball underneath your shoulder—see the Shoulder Rotator Smash and Floss (page 312).

Hang Archetype   Press Archetype

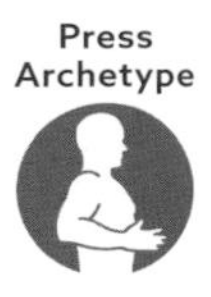

This mobilization will help improve the above archetypes.

IMPROVES:

Shoulder position and function
Flexion fault (rounded shoulders)
Shoulder pain

METHODS:

Contract and relax
Smash and floss

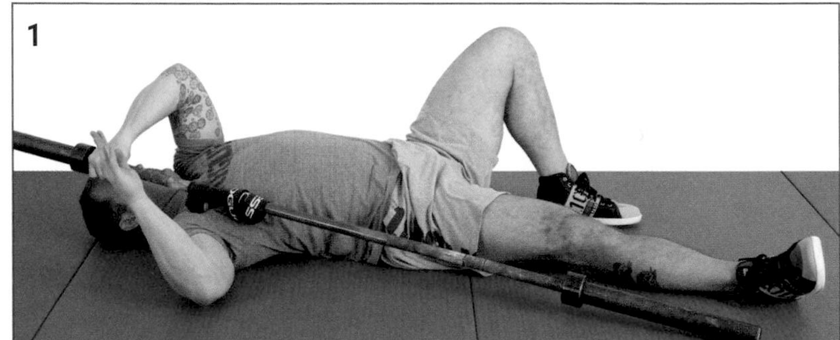
1

Lie on your back and position the ball in the anterior deltoid area, where your pec minor enters your shoulder.

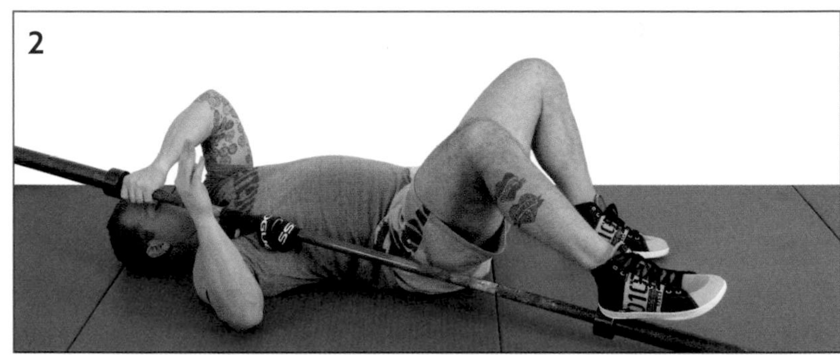
2

Step your right foot on the bar. This not only helps pin the barbell in place and adds pressure, but also helps push your shoulder to the back of the socket.

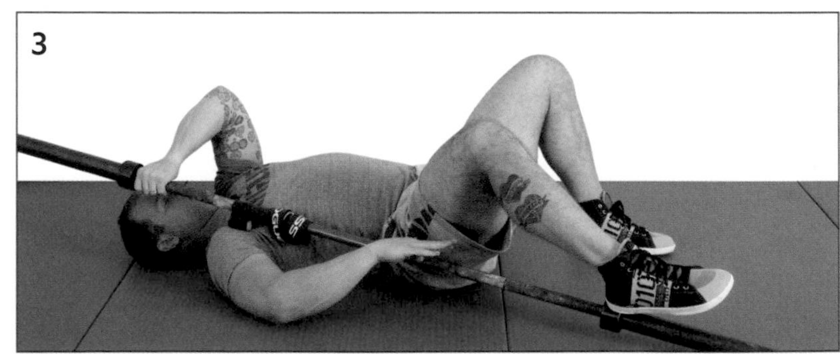
3

After you've tacked down the anterior tissue, internally rotate your shoulder. To maintain top-end pressure, push down on the barbell with your left hand.

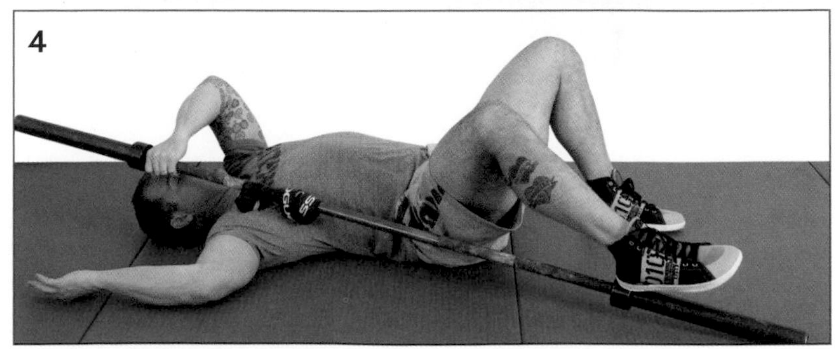
4

To move your arm through a full range of motion, externally rotate your shoulder—keeping your elbow bent—and try to get your arm flush to the ground.

Barbell Shoulder Shear

If you're missing internal rotation, your entire shoulder complex has to compensate. Put in enough duty cycles from an unstable position and you will end up with shoulder pain or, worse, an injury. In my practice, I treat a lot of athletes who are missing critical internal rotation range. One of the first things I clear is the anterior deltoid in the area of the upper shoulder. Cleaning up this area effectively fixes a lot of the dysfunctional shoulder mechanics that are typical in most athletes.

The fact is, most of us live in a shoulders-forward position. And the problem is that most of the demands of daily life and training involve loading up the anterior deltoid complex, causing it to get extremely tight. One of the easiest and most effective methods to unglue matted-down tissues in this area is to employ this smash or Superfriend Internal Rotation Smash. If you perform it correctly often enough, you may feel like you've been blessed with a new shoulder. I've yet to find anything that unglues the ugliness and restores internal rotation faster than these two pieces, specifically the Superfriend variation with a VooDoo Flossed shoulder. It's like magic.

The key to this mob, whether you're implementing the barbell or the Superfriend variation, is to lie on your back and avoid getting into a sleeper stretch position by rolling onto your side. The problem with the sleeper stretch is that it is trying to fix internal rotation from a poor position. You don't need to fix internal rotation with your arm across your body. That doesn't look like anything! What you need to do is mobilize in positions that look like athletic movements: the high hang position, the recovery phase of the swimming stroke, the dip, or jumping. You get the idea.

Note: To turn this into a two-for-one mobilization, place a lacrosse ball underneath your shoulder—see the Shoulder Rotator Smash and Floss (page 312).

Hang Archetype

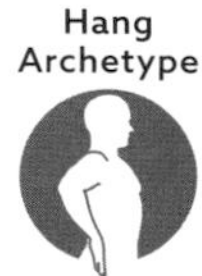

Press Archetype

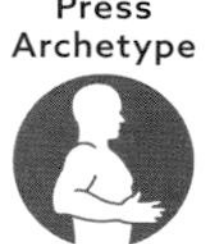

This mobilization will help improve the above archetypes.

IMPROVES:

Shoulder position and function
Flexion fault (rounded shoulders)
Shoulder pain

METHODS:

Contract and relax
Smash and floss

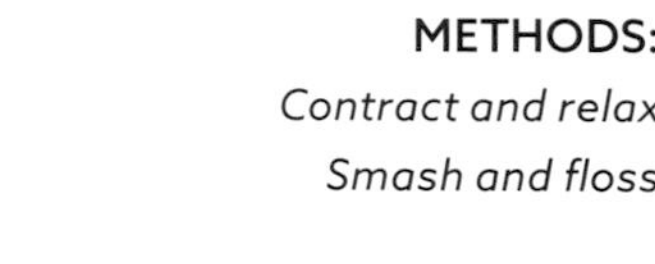

TARGET AREA

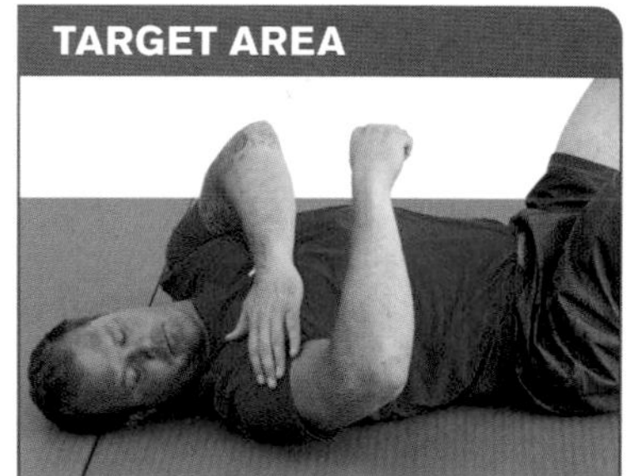

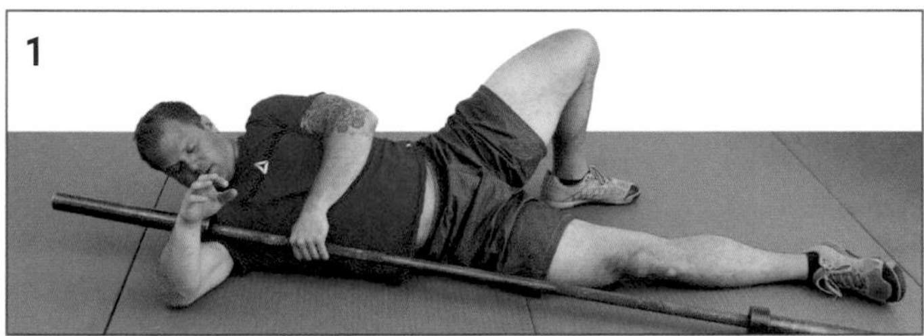

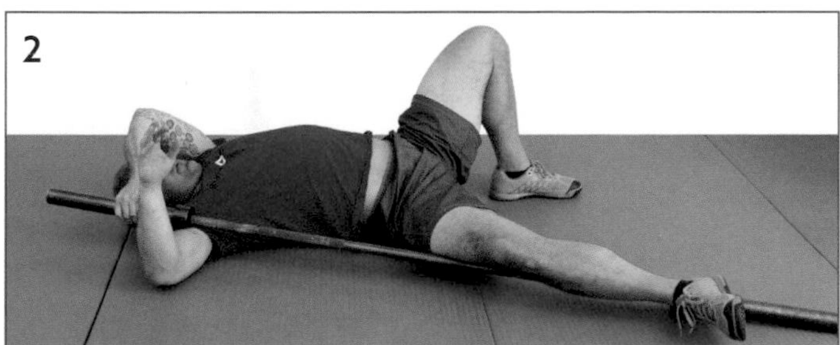

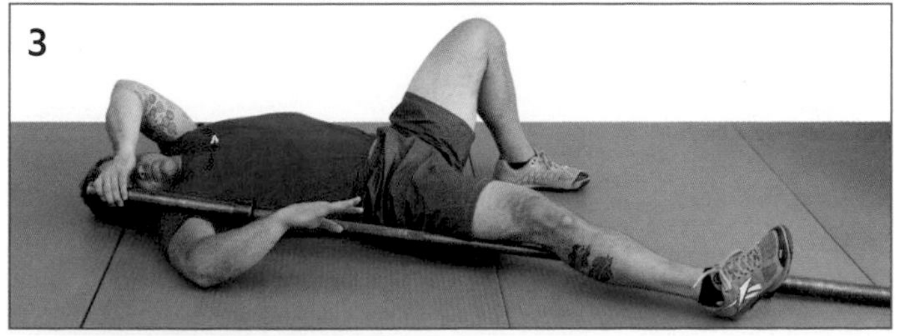

1. Lie on your back and position the notch of the barbell in your anterior deltoid area.

2. Throw your right leg over the bar. This not only helps pin the barbell in place and adds pressure, but also helps push your shoulder to the back of the socket. As you do so, lie back to put your right shoulder in a good position and grab the sleeve of the barbell with your left hand.

3. After you've tacked down the anterior tissue, internally rotate your hand and push down on the barbell with your left hand. This combination of actions creates a lot of shear, which allows you to unlaminate the tissues of your anterior shoulder.

SLEEPER STRETCH FAULT

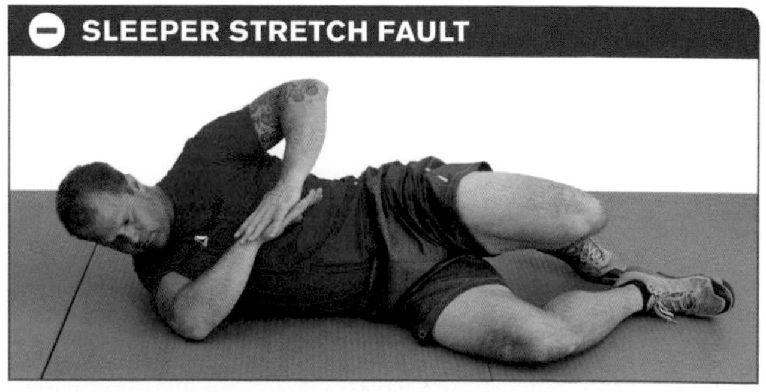

Hang Archetype

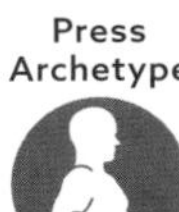

Press Archetype

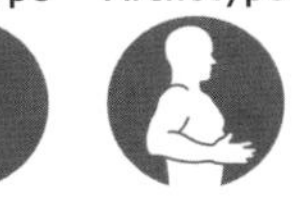

This mobilization will help improve the above archetypes.

IMPROVES:

Shoulder function

Shoulder pain and swelling

METHOD:

VooDoo Floss Band compression

Shoulder VooDoo: Superfriend Internal Rotation Smash

This is an excellent variation to implement if you have a team of athletes. You can have the people in one group wrap the arms of the people in the other group and step on their shoulders, then switch after a couple of minutes. It's literally the fastest and easiest way to improve and restore internal rotation to the shoulder.

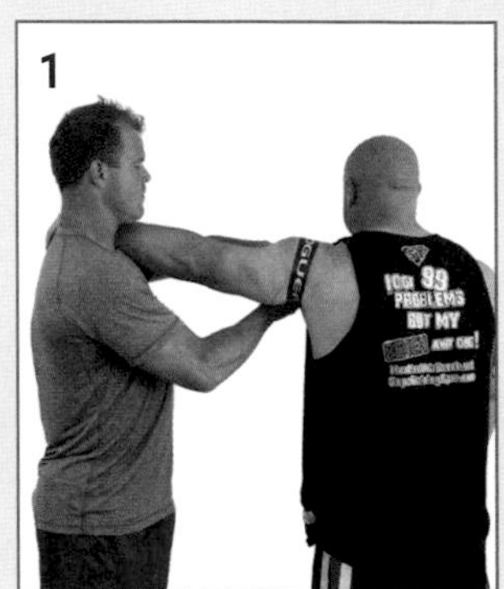

1

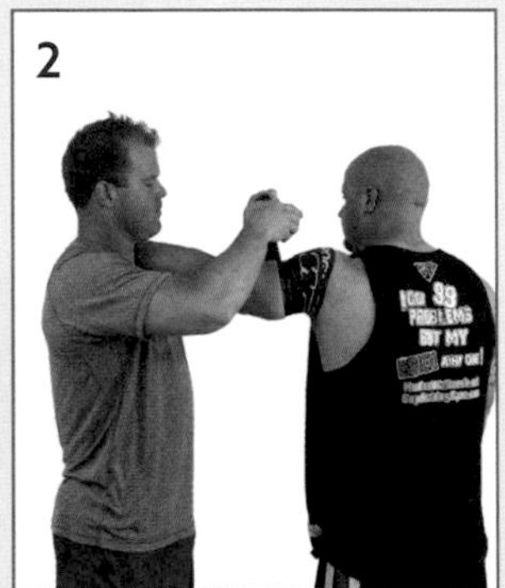

2

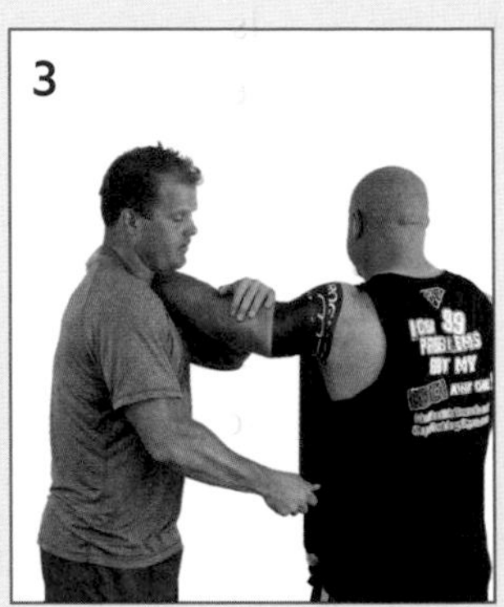

3

Starting from the top of the shoulder, wrap the shoulder with a VooDoo Floss Band to create compression. For more on the wrapping technique, see page 149.

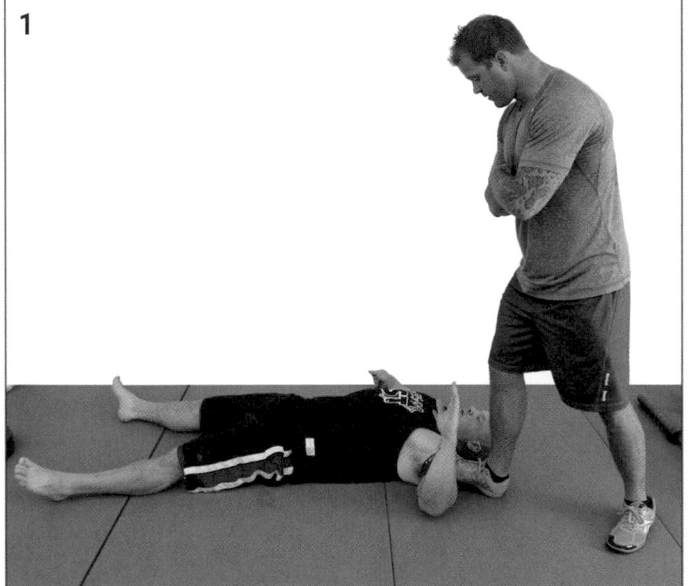

1

With his shoulder wrapped, Jesse lies on his back and positions his arm at a 90-degree angle. To ensure that his shoulder is in a good position and to help tack down his laminated tissues, I step on the front of his shoulder with the ball of my right foot.

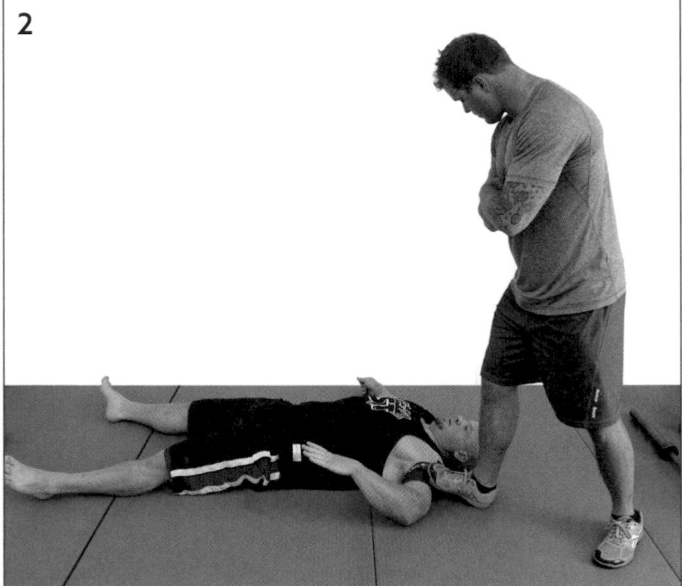

2

With my foot tacking down his shoulder, Jesse internally rotates his arm past my foot, effectively ungluing all the matted-down tissues of his shoulder.

Bilateral Internal Rotation Mobilization

The Bilateral Internal Rotation Mobilization is a quick and dirty way to work on extension and internal rotation. As with the Shoulder VooDoo mob, this is an excellent mobilization to throw into a big group of athletes in a class setting.

It's important to note that you can't relieve truckloads of muscle stiffness or restore a lot of motion to the joint with just a static stretch. For optimal results, you have to tie in the contract and relax method and try to work in and out of end-range tension. In addition, you have to focus on keeping your shoulders pinned to the mat and avoid compensating into a forward-rolled position as you lower your hips into your hands. This can be very difficult to do, especially if you're missing some of these key internal rotation and extension corners. The best way to deal with this issue is to have a training partner press down on your shoulders. This not only ensures that your shoulders remain in a good position, but also allows you to hit more extreme vectors.

I only like doing this mobilization when I have a Superfriend on hand because it's so difficult to keep your shoulders back. However, even if you don't have someone to help you out, this is an excellent mobilization to see just how your body compensates for its lack of range. You can really feel what's happening. Sometimes, when you're descending into a dip, it's less obvious. You can't feel when you compensate. Setting up in this position, on the other hand, will tell you exactly whether it's motor control or a mobility issue. It makes the invisible visible.

Hang Archetype

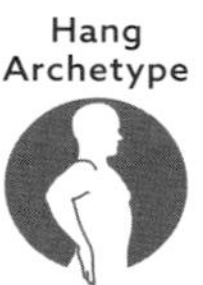

Press Archetype

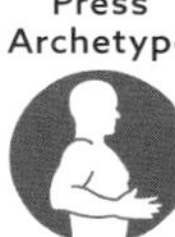

This mobilization will help improve the above archetypes.

METHOD:
Contract and relax

COMMON FAULT

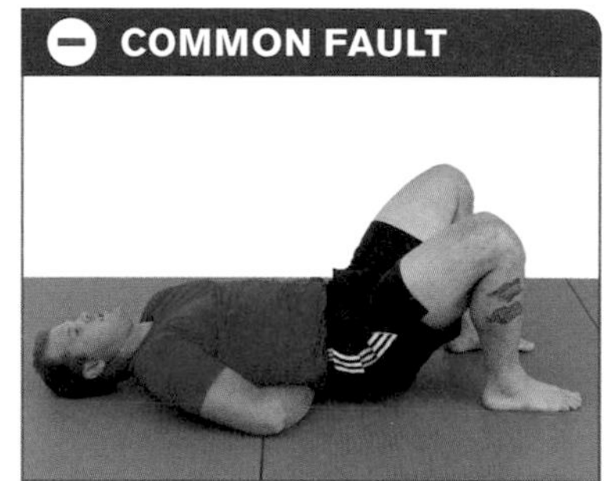

1

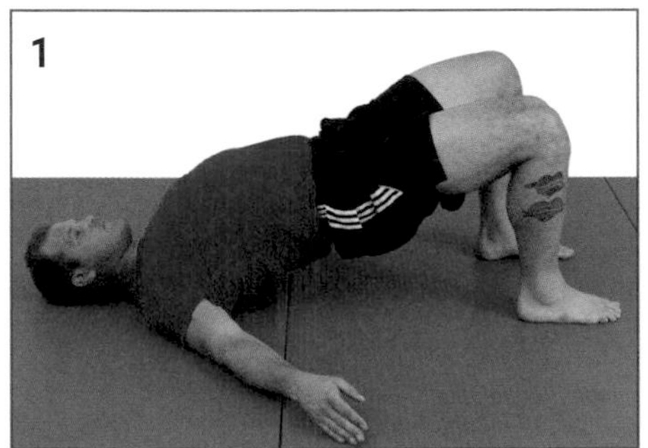

2

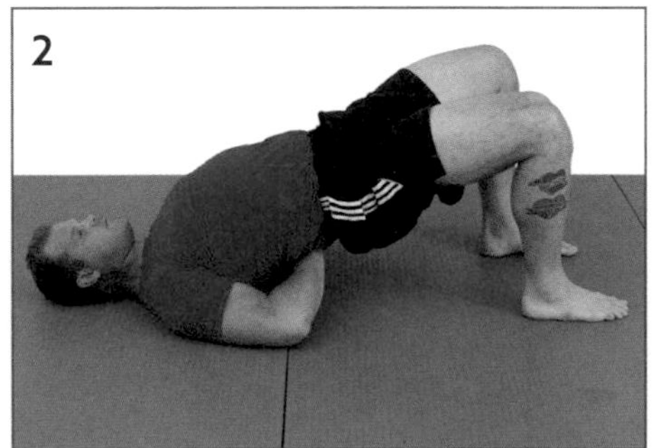

3

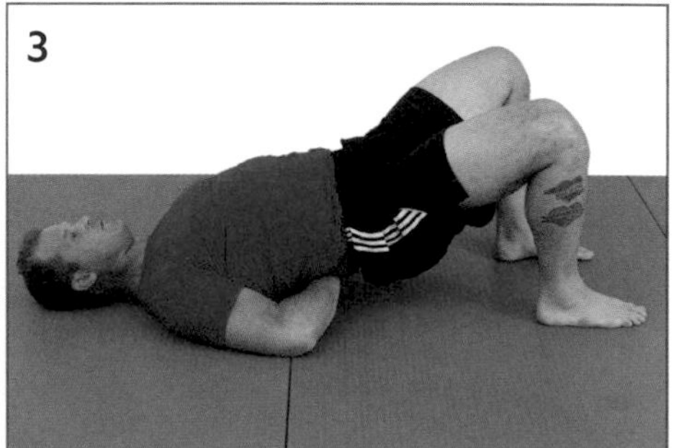

1. Lying on your back, drive your heels into the mat, bridge your hips, and drive your shoulders to the backs of their sockets.

2. Maneuver your hands underneath your lower back.

3. To add a tension force, slowly drop your hips toward the mat and lower your back into your hands. From here, you can contract and relax as well as oscillate in and out of end-range tension. It's important to avoid compensating into a forward-rolled position. Fight this force and control the tension.

SUPERFRIEND VARIATION

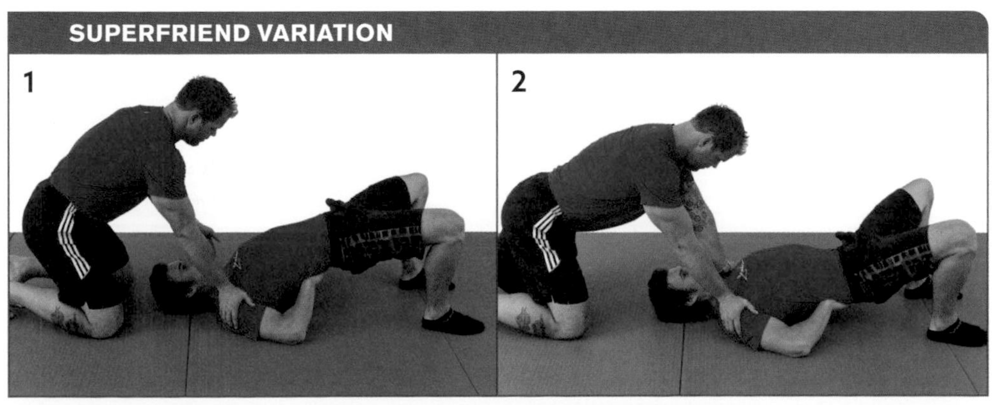

1. As the Superfriend, I position my hands over the fronts of Carl's shoulders. Before Carl starts to lower his hips, I load some pressure into his shoulders.

2. As I keep Carl's shoulders pinned to the ground, he lowers his hips into his hands to apply a tension force.

Banded Bully

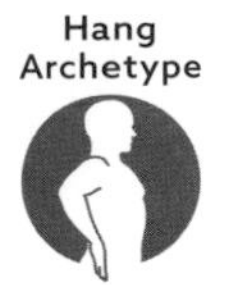
Hang Archetype

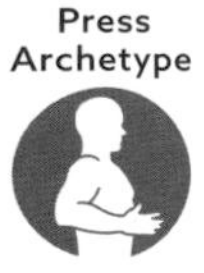
Press Archetype

This mobilization will help improve the above archetypes.

METHOD:

Contract and relax

It's not easy to improve extension and internal rotation without ending up in a weak shoulder position. This is why I recommend the Superfriend variation of the previous technique. It prevents you from blowing off torque, dumping tension, and defaulting into a crappy forward-shoulder position.

If you don't have a Superfriend in range, though, the Banded Bully is good alternative. As you can see in the photos below, the band pulls the shoulder to the back of the socket, which not only enables you to mobilize from a stable position, but also intensifies the work.

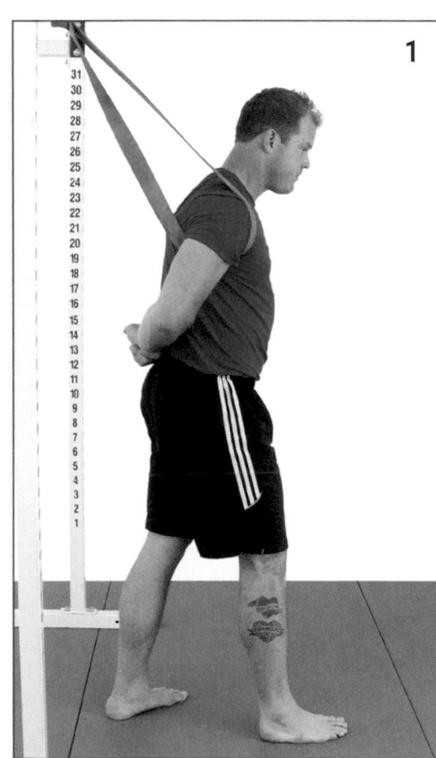

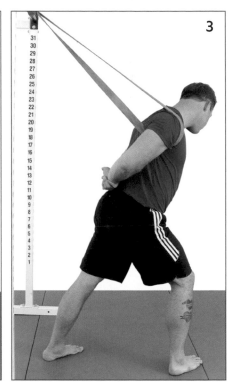

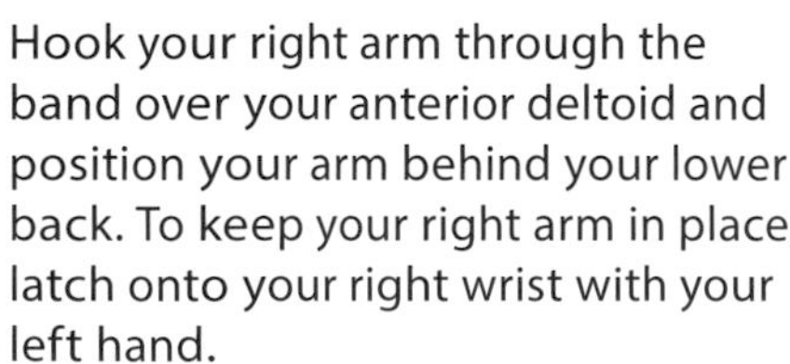
Hook your right arm through the band over your anterior deltoid and position your arm behind your lower back. To keep your right arm in place, latch onto your right wrist with your left hand.

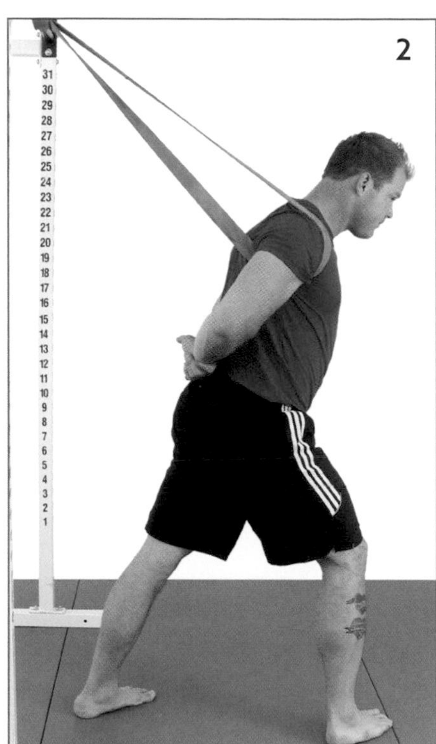

To create tension in the band, lean forward and allow the band to pull your shoulder into the back of the socket.

With your right shoulder locked into an ideal position, start hunting around for stiffness by pulling your right arm up and across your body with your left hand. This helps bias internal rotation with extension. You can also tilt your head to the side to tie your neck into the mobilization.

Triple Bully

The bully mobilizations look a lot like a cop restraining a purse-snatching suspect with a behind-the-back arm lock. If you've ever been winched into this position, you know how much it hurts, especially when applied correctly and with the right amount of force. The lock is effective because it forces your arm into red-hot corners that you never really explore on your own. Not to mention that you're probably missing serious internal rotation. No wonder you submitted so easily!

The Triple Bully is designed to hit these corners using three key motions. With your hand fixed to a pole or rack, first step away to create extension; second, twist away from the arm you're mobilizing to bias a little more adduction (moving toward your center line); and third, drop your elevation and pull your fixed arm up and across your back to add more internal rotation.

As with any mobilization, you have to use a combination of motions to bring about the most change. Thinking in terms of singular motions, like flexing, is a mistake. You're never going to express the true nature of the joint and how it moves. But the Triple Bully—that's another story. The combination of these three motions enables you to wind up your shoulder in a tight position and floss in and out of some really stiff and painful vectors of the joint that rarely get attention. It's an easy way to mobilize your shoulder into some crazy positions without having a cop put you in an arm lock and push you into the back of a squad car.

Hang Archetype

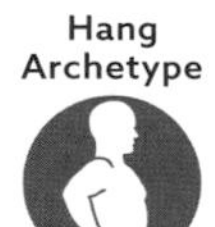

Press Archetype

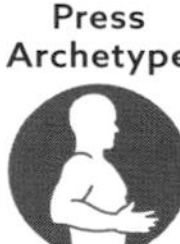

This mobilization will help improve the above archetypes.

METHOD:

Contract and relax

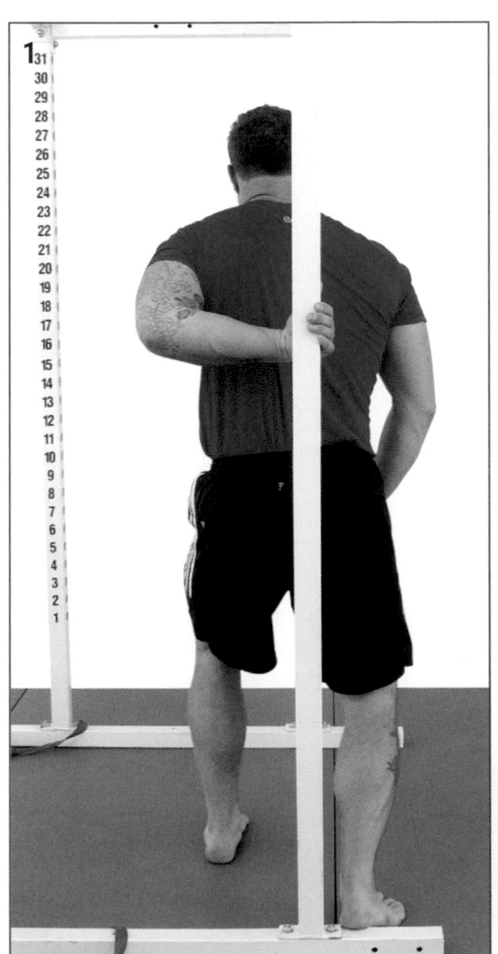

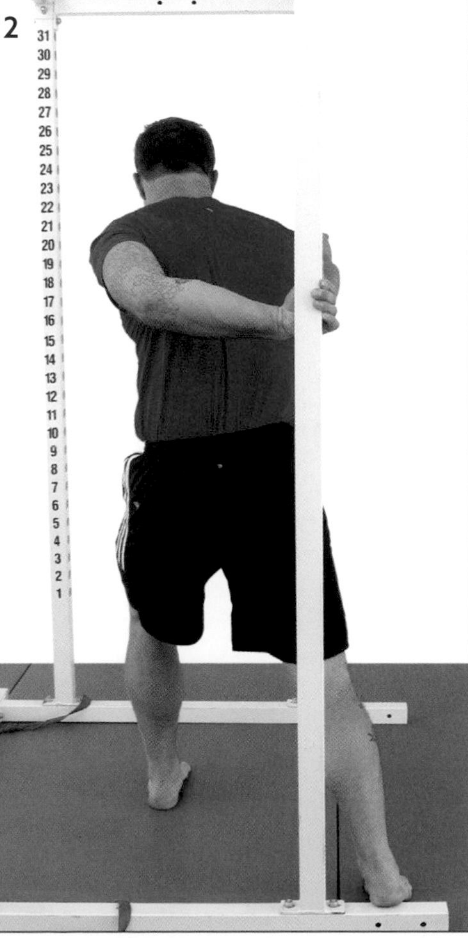

1. Grip the rack with your left hand so that your thumb is pointing up. Actively pull your shoulder into the back of the socket and create extension by stepping forward.

2. Having created tension in your shoulder as well as biased extension of the joint, twist your body counterclockwise and lower your elevation. The former biases adduction, while the latter biases internal rotation. From here, you can keep your hand fixed in the same position while continuing to twist lower and pull your body away in an attempt to find untapped corners of your shoulder. The key is to keep your shoulder in an ideal position as you explore its ugliness. The moment you feel your shoulder dump torque, release the tension and re-establish a stable position.

Bully Extension Bias

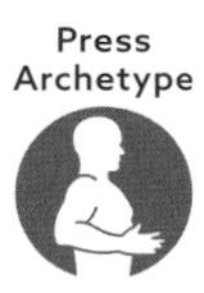

This mobilization will help improve the above archetypes.

METHOD:
Contract and relax

There is considerable overlap among the shoulder mobilizations. That's a good thing, because each one has a slightly different stimulus. I want you to play around and use the mobilizations that give you the best results.

With the Bully Extension Bias, you're still working on internal rotation and extension of your shoulder, but in this particular mobilization you exaggerate extension first and then add internal rotation as a tensioner. In addition, because your hand is fixed to a band, you can distract the joint into the back of the socket, which allows you to put a little more love and attention into the extension of your shoulder. This gives you a slightly different feel than if your hand is fixed in the same position as in the Triple Bully.

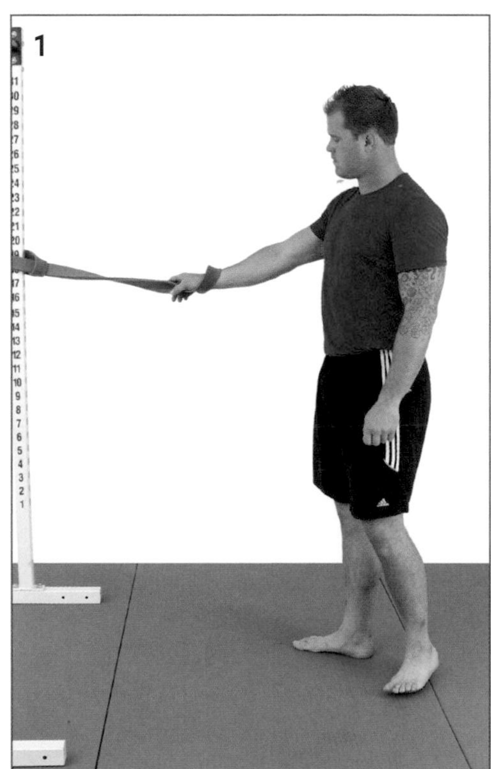

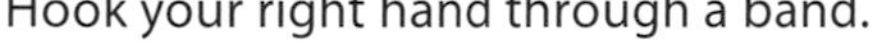

Hook your right hand through a band.

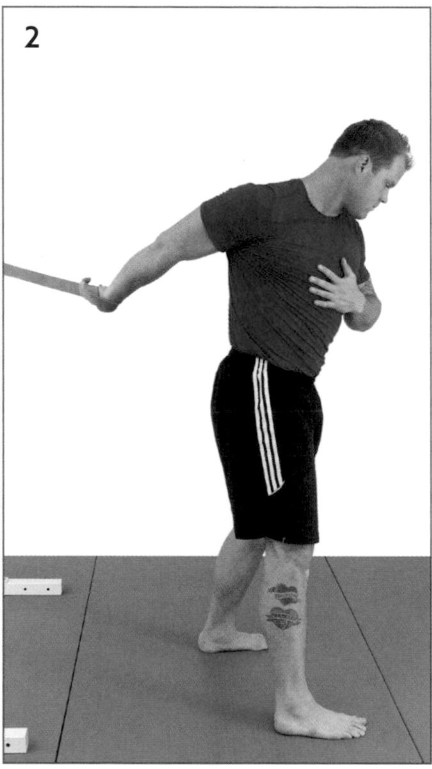

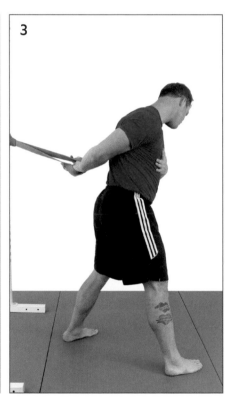

Wind up your right shoulder into extension by turning your body counterclockwise 180 degrees so your back is facing the structure. As you step through with your right foot, rotate your right hand so your palm is positioned toward the ceiling. This helps bias internal rotation of your arm. With your banded hand exaggerated into extension, you can contract, relax, and go hunting for tight corners by lowering your elevation and twisting your upper body.

After spending some time in deep extension, go hunting for new corners by twisting away from your arm as if you were trying to wrap the band around your body. This adds more internal rotation to the mobilization. You can also tilt your head to the side to tie in the components of your neck/shoulder complex.

Sink Mobilization

The Sink Mobilization is nonspecific, meaning that it doesn't really bias the joint, but rather attacks anything that is tight or limiting your shoulders in extension. It's a global mobilization. The fact that it's not very sophisticated means that you can use it just about anywhere, anytime. If there's a fence pole, railing, or sink nearby, you can work on improving your shoulder extension.

The Sink Mobilization is especially useful for runners because it improves pulling the elbow straight back during the running stride. If you're missing extension range, you will hit an extension wall as you pull your arm back during the stride, causing your elbow to fly out, which in turn forces you into a compensated shoulder position. Here's what most people do in that situation: Instead of swinging from front to back, which is the proper technique, they go around the body, which slows them down, accelerates fatigue, and aggravates tissues. That, and it looks really weird. Don't be that person. Learn how to run correctly.

Hang Archetype

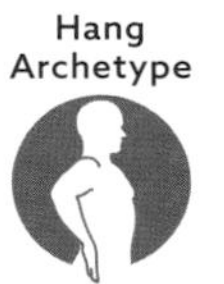

Press Archetype

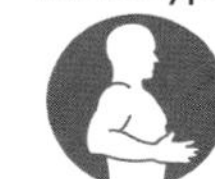

This mobilization will help improve the above archetypes.

METHOD:

Contract and relax

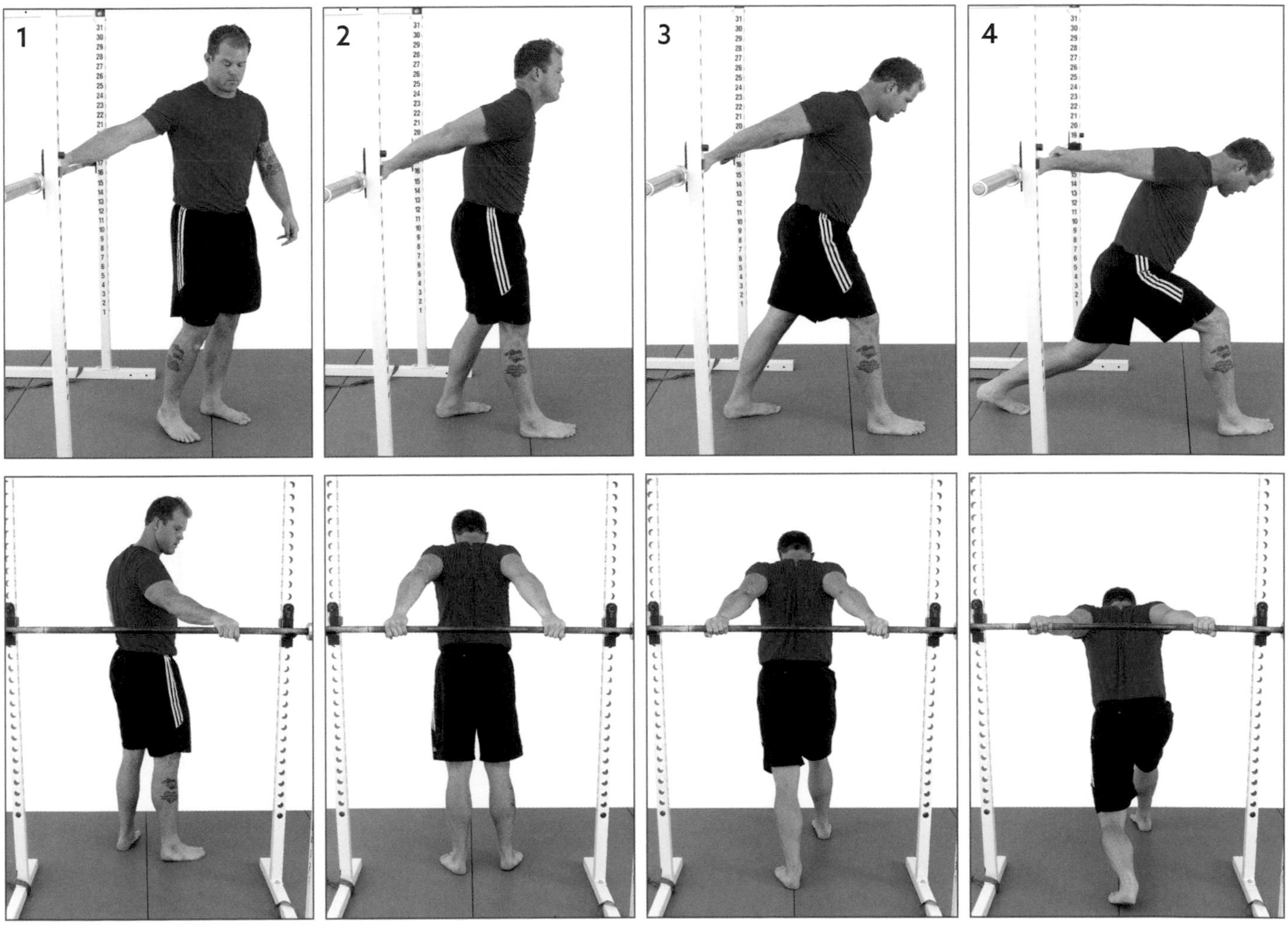

1. Latch onto a barbell with your right palm.

2. Grab the bar with your left hand, positioning your hands as close together as possible without losing shoulder position.

3. Keeping your shoulders back, apply tension by straightening your arms and leaning forward.

4. Still leaning forward, increase the tension by dropping your elevation. The goal is to position your hands on the same horizontal plane as your shoulders without having to compensate.

Front Rack 2 Archetype | Front Rack 1 Archetype | Press Archetype

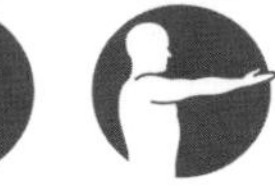

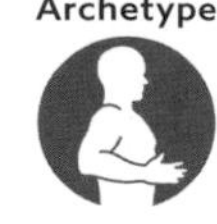

This mobilization will help improve the above archetypes.

METHOD:

Contract and relax

Banded Lateral Opener

The Banded Lateral Opener is another global mobilization that exaggerates arm extension. But instead of opening the shoulder into internal rotation, it distracts the shoulder into external rotation, ties in the front of the chest, and puts the pec into a full stretch. It's a quick, easy, and beautiful prep for any kind of pressing motion, specifically the pushup and bench press.

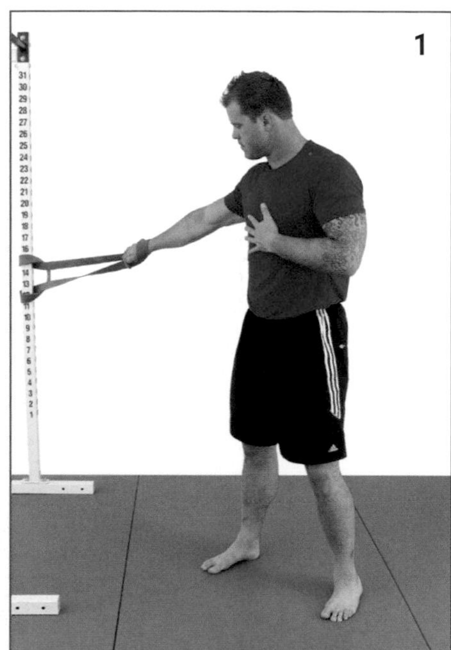

Hook your right hand through a band and create tension.

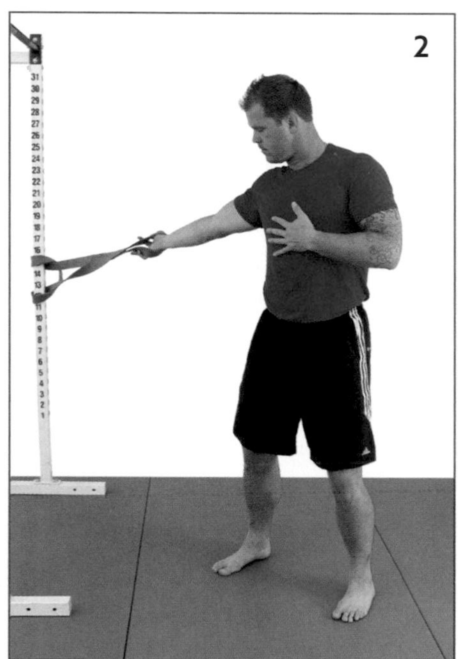

Rotate your palm upward, biasing external rotation of your shoulder.

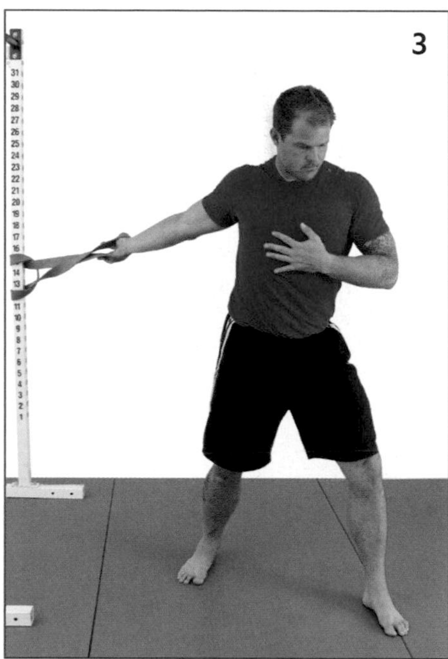

Keeping your arm externally rotated and your shoulder back, turn away from the band and twist your upper body counterclockwise. This opens up your chest and arm and allows you to capture the connective and soft tissues along those fascial planes.

AREA 5 ARM (TRICEPS, ELBOW, FOREARM, WRIST)

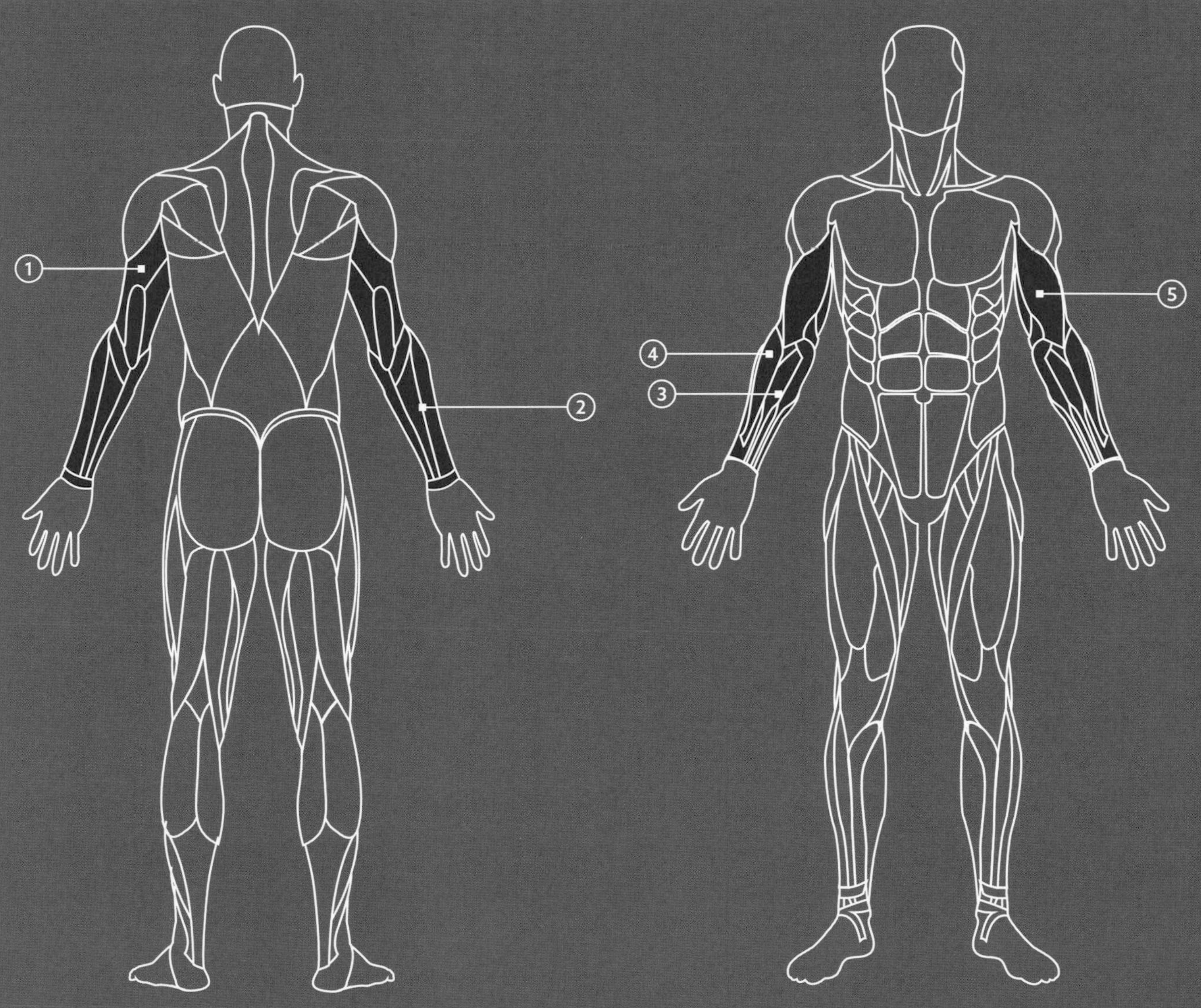

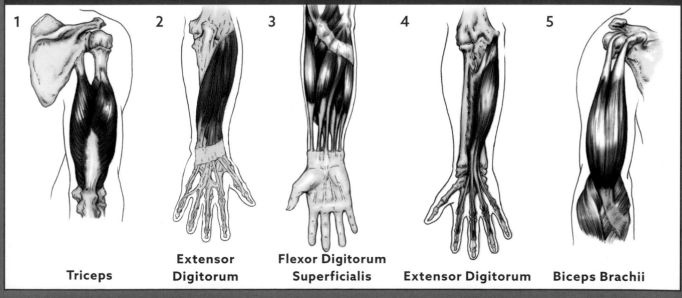

MOBILIZATION TARGET AREAS:

1 Triceps

2 Extensor Digitorum

3 Flexor Digitorum Superficialis

4 Extensor Digitorum

5 Biceps Brachii

Triceps Extension Smash

Overhead Archetype · Front Rack 1 Archetype · Front Rack 2 Archetype

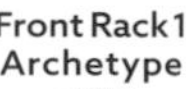

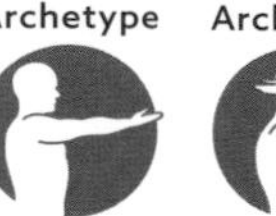

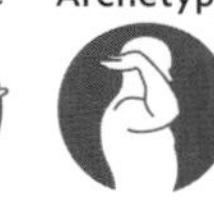

This mobilization will help improve the above archetypes.

IMPROVES:

Triceps suppleness

Elbow and shoulder pain

METHODS:

Contract and relax

Pressure wave

Smash and floss

If the primary movers of your hips (hip flexors, quads, or hamstrings) get tight and restricted, how do you think that will impact your range of motion and overall movement mechanics? Here's what we know: If your anterior hip is tight, limiting extension range of motion, your leg will turn out when you run, walk, or lunge. If you squat with stiff quads, your knees are likely to collapse inward as you reach full depth. We think about the hips a lot and spend a ton of time working on the primary movers connected to the hips, but what about the primary movers of your shoulder and arms? When was the last time you mobilized your triceps? Don't answer that. If you're like most athletes, you spend a ton of time mobilizing your hamstrings and quads, but very little time on your triceps. This is a mistake.

When your triceps get tight and you do nothing about it, they get adaptively short, causing you to lose extension in your arms. If you don't have the full length of your triceps—specifically the long heads of your triceps—creating external rotation torque and locking out your elbows is difficult. Elbows tend to chicken flap out into a compromised position, especially during heavily loaded, high-speed movements (think push-press and snatch). The same thing happens with your legs in the squat when you have stiff quads: You end up missing external rotation and dumping torque by collapsing your knees inward.

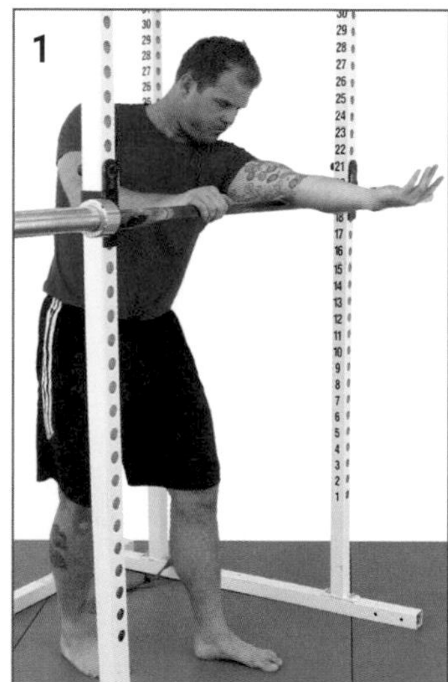

1 Position the head of your triceps (right above your elbow joint) on a barbell with your arm in extension. To take up the skin slack at your elbow, twist the barbell counterclockwise toward your body. Apply downward pressure with your arm to tack down the underlying tissue.

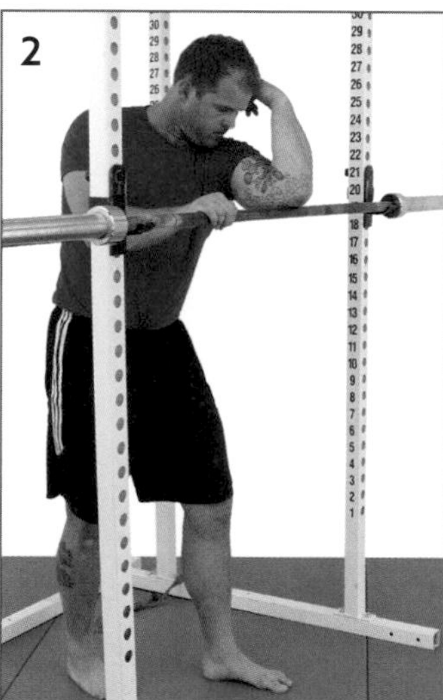

2 Having tacked down a stiff area of tissue at the base of your left elbow, pull your left hand to the left side of your head.

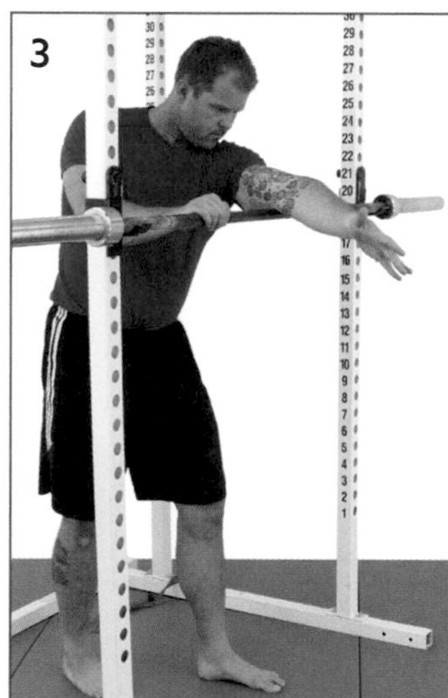

3 Staying on the stiff tissue, straighten your arm. The idea is to find a tight spot and push and pull past it by bending and straightening your arm.

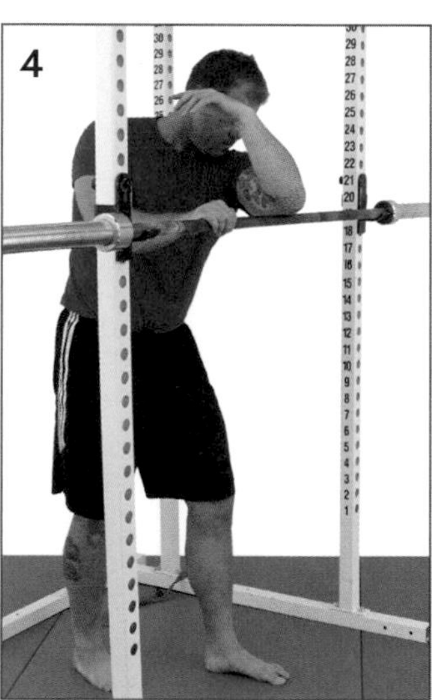

4 To get full excursion of the tissue, bend your left arm to the opposite side of your body.

These big tissues dictate your capacity to generate stability in your primary engines. Your triceps affect your shoulders and your quads affect your hips. If these regions get stiff, it's going to be reflected in your movement mechanics and eventually express itself in the form of pain. That means you have to address the ugliness by smashing away the stiffness so that you can reclaim stable positions. And the Triceps Extension Smash options demonstrated here are the best ways to accomplish that.

Although all the smashing techniques that I demonstrate employ different tools, the technique and methods remain the same: pressure wave across the tissue from side to side, contract and relax on tight spots, and floss by curling and straightening your arm.

Note: When smashing your triceps, consider the archetype and area you're trying to change. If you're working on your overhead position, get on the ground and work on the long head of your triceps with your arm in extension. If you're working on your front rack position, mobilize around your elbow with your arm in flexion. There are a couple different ways to approach smashing from the ground: You can floss by bending and extending your arm, or you can roll your arm from side to side with your arm bent or straight. The key is to emphasize internal and external rotation from your elbow as you flex and extend your arm.

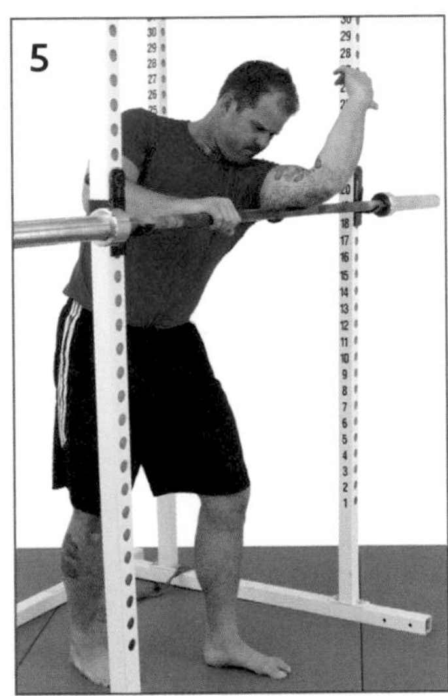

Keeping your arm bent, continue to smash the tissue by moving your arm toward your left side. The idea is to pressure wave back and forth, smashing the tissues laterally.

Variation: Battlestar or Gemini Triceps Smash

If you don't have a rack, don't panic. You can perform the Triceps Extension Smash on the ground using a roller, Gemini, barbell, Little Battlestar, double lacrosse ball, rolling pin, wine bottle, or whatever you have at your disposal.

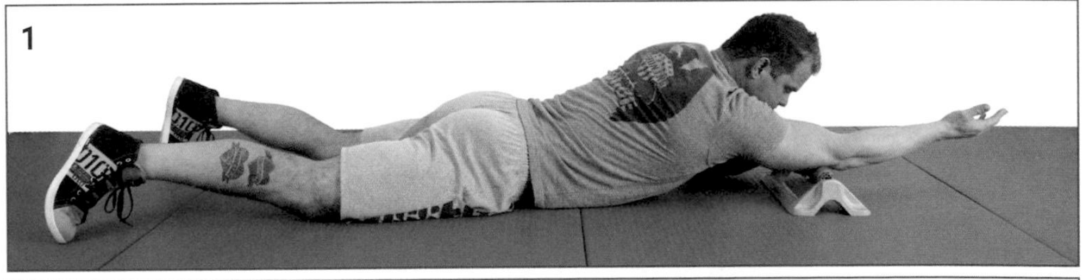

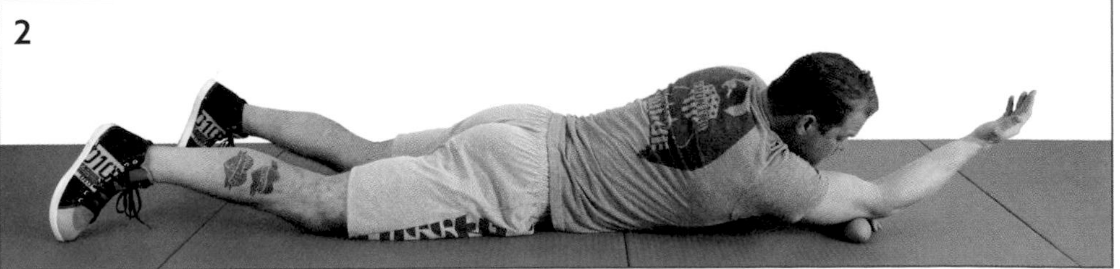

Superfriend Triceps Smash

The Superfriend Triceps Smash offers a slightly different stimulus. Rather than go after the sliding surfaces of the fascia, which is the case with the previous mobs, you target the deep muscle tissue as you scrub across the heads of the triceps. Both the person smashing and the person being smashed will probably feel a definitive clonk as the foot rolls over the arm. Although this clonk is common, it's not normal. You don't have a triceps bone.

Note: You need only a little bit of pressure. It doesn't take a lot of weight before the smashing becomes intolerable. Position an ab mat or some kind of pad under the arm, agree on a safe word, and be careful.

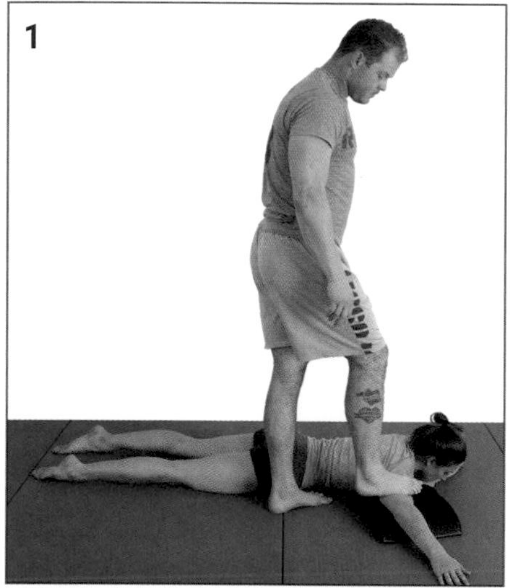

Lie on your belly with your arm stretched out to the side and your palm facing the mat.

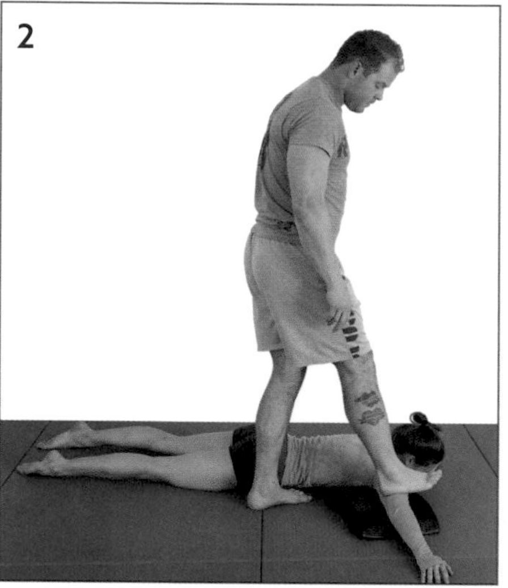

Place an ab mat or pad underneath your arm to protect your elbow. To begin, have your training partner position the middle of his foot over your triceps, being careful not to apply too much pressure, and slowly slide his foot forward.

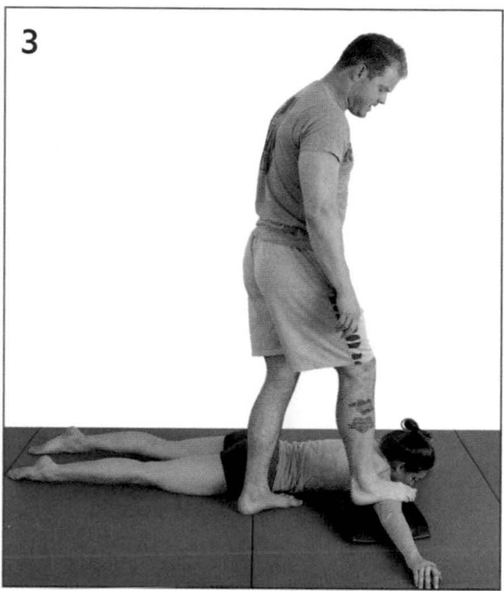

Have your training partner scrub back and forth over the heads of the triceps, keeping his foot flush with your arm and maintaining light pressure.

Elbow VooDoo

Wrapping a VooDoo Floss Band above and below your elbow and then spending a few minutes moving through a full range of motion is one of the fastest and most effective ways to address elbow pain and restore suppleness to your triceps and forearm. If your elbow aches or you're missing key corners in your mobility—elbow extension or flexion—this should be one of your first stops. In fact, if I have an athlete who is suffering from epicondylitis (tennis elbow), this is the first thing I have him do. Seriously, nothing I've seen, experienced, or been taught solves "hot elbow" problems as quickly and effectively as the Elbow VooDoo. To learn more about the proper wrapping technique, see page 149.

Press Archetype

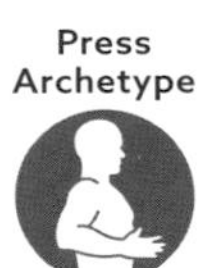

Overhead Archetype

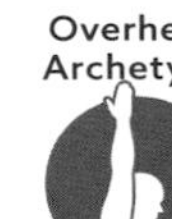

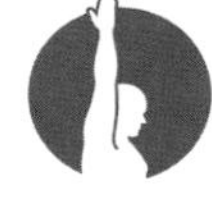

Front Rack 1 Archetype

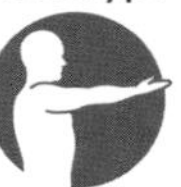

Front Rack 2 Archetype

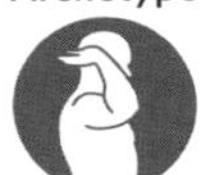

This mobilization will help improve the above archetypes.

IMPROVES:

Elbow pain and swelling
Elbow flexion and extension

METHOD:

VooDoo Floss Band compression

SUPERFRIEND TORTURE

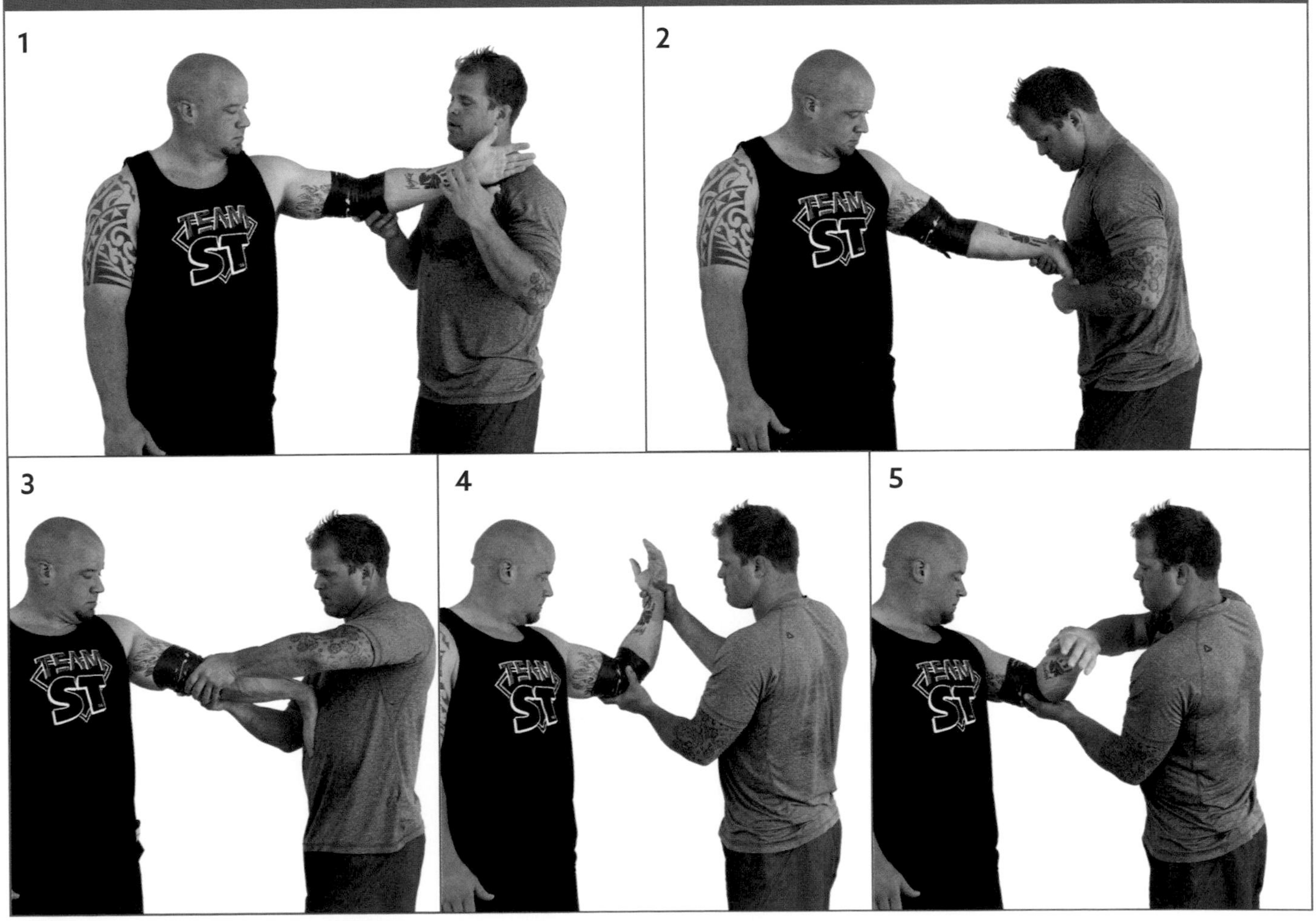

After I wrap Jesse's elbow, the first thing I do is rotate his elbow toward the ground, position his palm flush against my chest, and then pull his arm into full extension. As I do so, I externally rotate his arm to capture all the corners of the joint. My role as a Superfriend is to force his elbow into as much range of motion as possible while making sure that he doesn't pass out. As with most of the highly effective mobilization techniques, VooDoo Flossing your elbow is not a pleasurable experience. This is why having a Superfriend manipulate your arm into key ranges is ideal, because he is not limited by your pain. However, as with all Superfriend mobilizations, you'll probably need to pick and respect the use of a safe word.

FORCED FLEXION AND EXTENSION

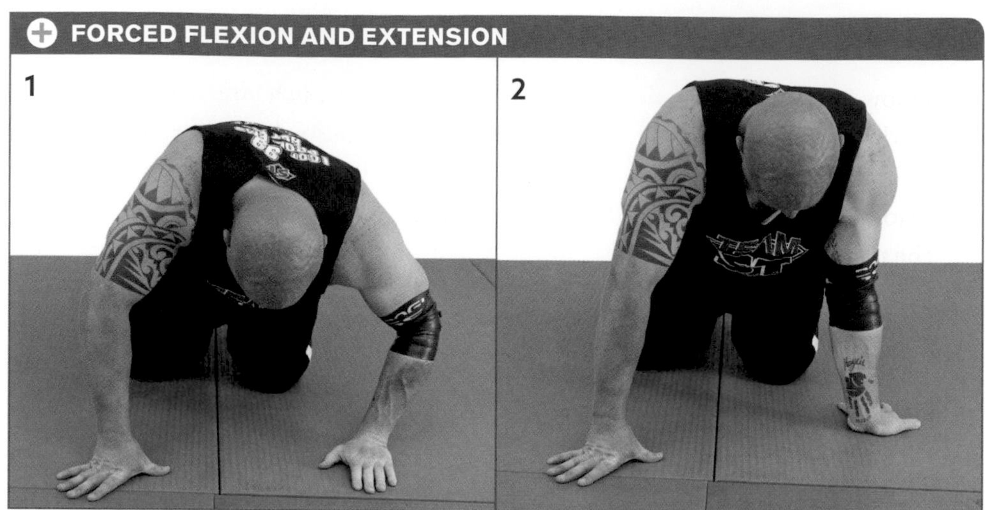

Placing your palm on the ground is a great way to encourage flexion and extension through the elbow. The idea is to explore different positions and accumulate 15 to 20 arm bends.

MOBILIZE IN THE POSITION YOU'RE TRYING TO CHANGE

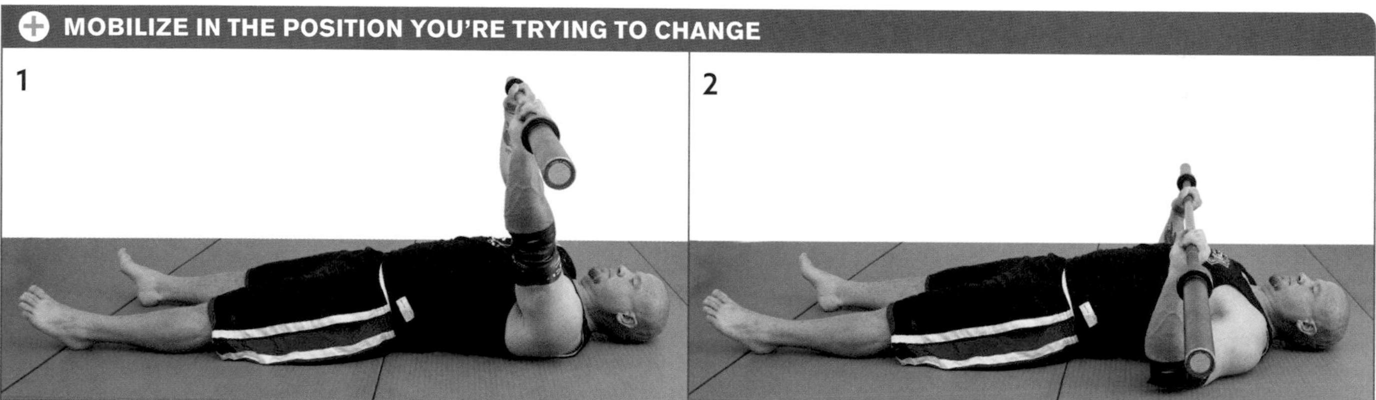

One of the best aspects of VooDoo Flossing is that you can mobilize in the position you're trying to change. For example, if you're benching, pressing, or doing a workout that involves a lot of pushups, wrap your elbow and perform the movement you are about to perform.

HANG FROM A BAR

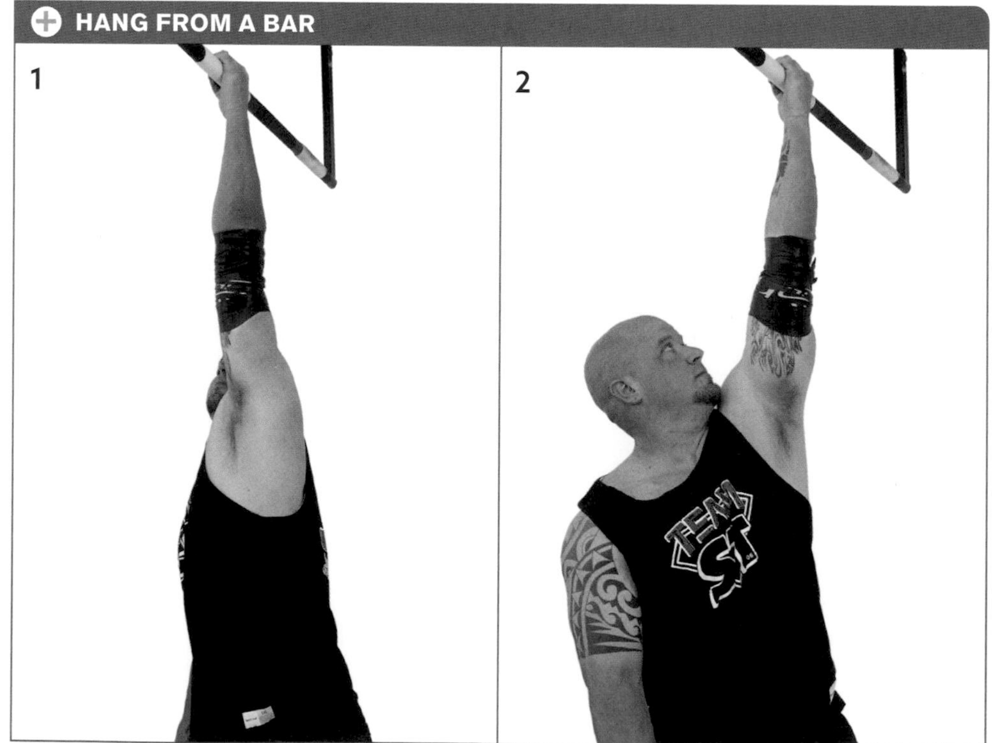

Anchoring your hand to a bar and twisting your body is a great way to tie in the rotational components of your elbow. The key is to spend some time in both hand positions: supinated (chin-up grip) and pronated (pull-up grip).

Banded Elbow Extension

Overhead Archetype

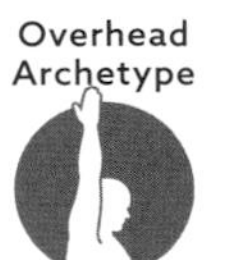

Front Rack 1 Archetype

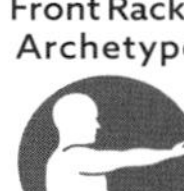

This mobilization will help improve the above archetypes.

IMPROVES:
Elbow extension

METHOD:
Banded flossing

The elbow is a workhorse. It's insane. Think about how much you use and count on the work flowing through your elbows. Flexing and extending your arms is a big part of daily life. So it's no great mystery that elbows get stiff and painful, and full extension of the arm comes with a grimace (if at all).

The trouble tends to spread. Consider an athlete with limited range of motion in his elbows pressing a barbell overhead. As he nears locking out his elbows, he flares his elbows out and rolls his shoulders forward. He's risking more pain and injury to complete the lift.

People tend to think of the elbow as a simple joint that just bends and extends, but there's a rotational component that contributes to shoulder stability. This goes back to the idea that the smaller structures dictate the capacity to create stability in the primary engines. In this case, it's your shoulders.

Think of the front rack position. Being able to externally rotate your shoulders into a good position to create a stable platform is predicated on having full range of motion in your downstream joints, like your elbows and wrists. In other words, missing extension doesn't just affect your ability to lock out your arms; it also messes with your ability to create the rotation in your elbows that helps stabilize your shoulders.

People think they can get away with missing a little bit of extension in their elbows. They can't. To get an idea of what I'm talking about, try this simple test: Get in the pushup position, bend your arms slightly, and then externally rotate your arms to create a stable shoulder position. Then lock out your arms and do the same thing.

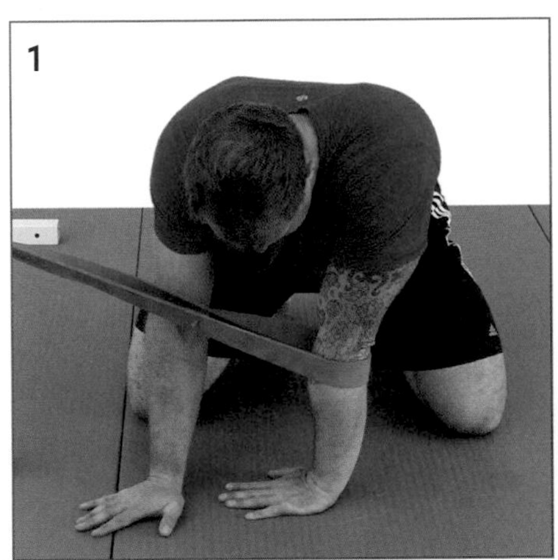

1

Hook a band around your elbow and create tension by sliding your arm back. Notice that my fingers are pointed in the direction of the band.

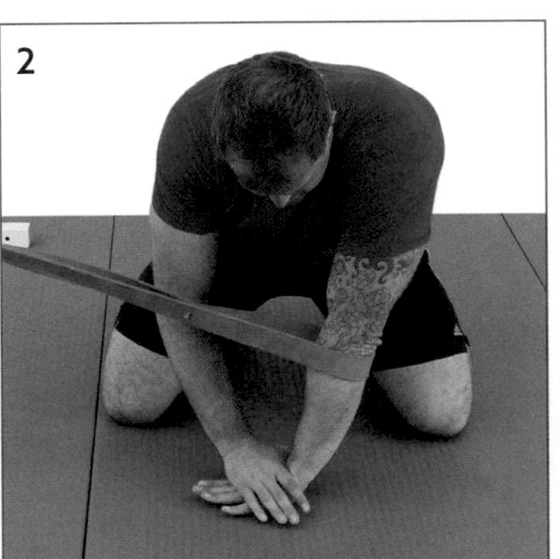

2

Staple your palm to the mat by placing your right hand over your left hand.

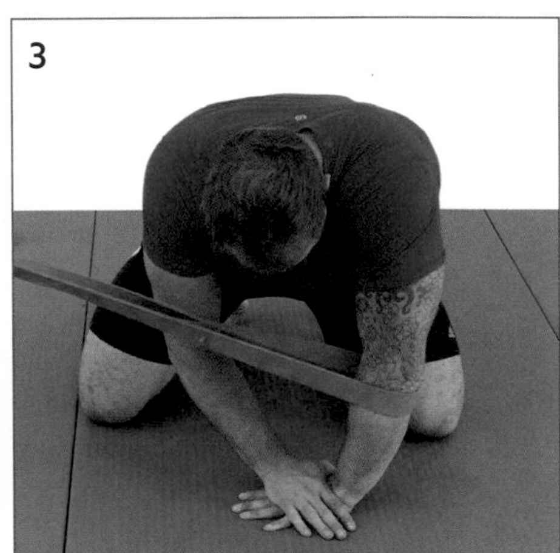

3

Keeping your shoulder in a stable position, flex your elbow into the band.

As you will find, locking out your arms creates a much stronger and more stable position. If you don't have full extension in your elbows, perform this test using the squat. Stand with your knees slightly bent and then create an external rotation force by forcing your knees outward. Then do the same thing with your knees locked out. You'll find that when your knees are locked out, your butt turns on and you can really feel the stability of your position. Per the one-joint rule (refer to chapter 2), the same thing happens in your shoulders.

So let's go after restoring full range of motion to the elbows.

As you can see in the photos, this mobilization works the elbow from two different positions to account for the rotational component. The key is to floss in and out of extension by bending your elbow into a band and then, with control, slowly straighten your arm into extension, really allowing the band to distract the joint to the end range of the capsule.

Note: For the best results, execute the Banded Elbow mobilizations with a VooDoo Flossed elbow. As a case study, Sarah Hopping—All-American hammer thrower and CrossFit phenomenon—came to my practice at San Francisco CrossFit seeking to correct her elbow position and eliminate pain. She had broken the head of her radius, a catastrophic injury, and couldn't lock out or extend her elbow to end range. This dramatically restricted her overhead position. I saw her for one session and essentially focused on VooDoo Flossing her elbow using these techniques. With just a little bit of VooDoo love, we managed to restore full range to her joint. She ended up winning the snatch ladder at the NorCal CrossFit 2012 Regionals shortly afterward. Her physicians were left in disbelief.

The moral of the story is this: If you can wrap a compression band around your elbow and VooDoo Floss using these techniques, do it. It will work miracles!

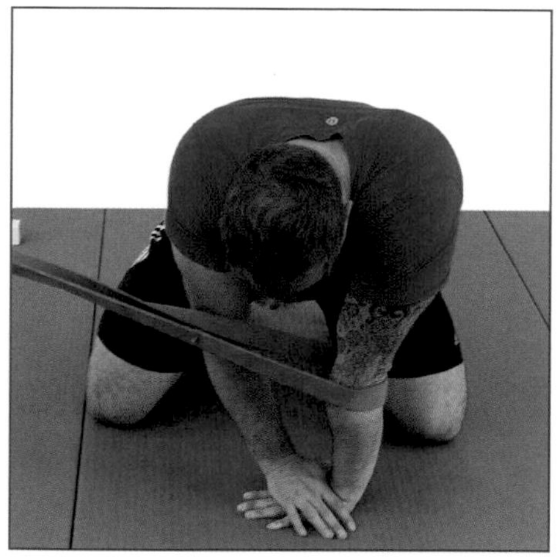

Controlling your arm into extension, allow the band to pull your elbow to its end-range position. From here, flex and extend your elbow until you have full range of motion or you can feel change in the joint capsule.

VARIATION: BANDED ELBOW EXTENSION

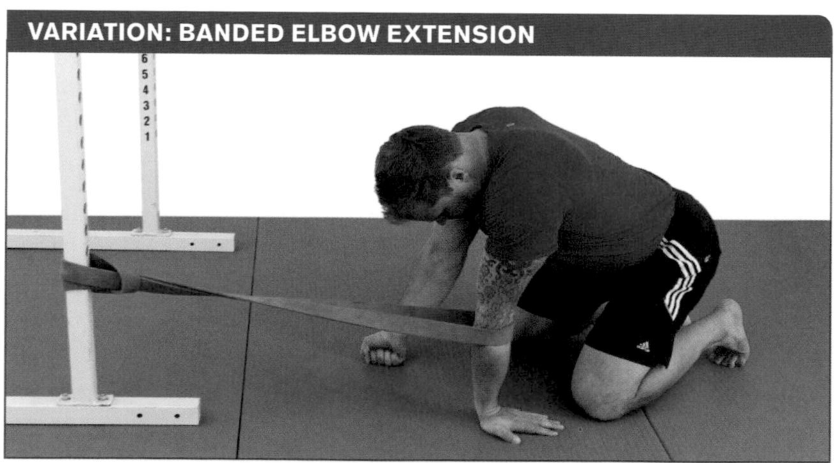

To capture the entire capsule, you have to hit your elbow from both an open-palm position and a closed-palm position. In other words, you're working from full pronation and full supination. This helps account for the rotational components of the elbow and ties in the forearm and wrist structure.

Banded Elbow Distraction

The Banded Elbow Distraction is another way to solve poor mobility in your elbows and treat pain. This technique also works on improving full flexion in your elbows. As you can see in the photos below, the band distracts your elbow joint and creates a gapping force in the crook of your elbow. This distraction force puts your elbow in a good position within the capsule, which clears any impingement in the joint and enables you to floss unrestricted. The key is to focus on moving your arm in different directions. Doing so will account for the rotational component of your elbow structure and accumulate as many bends in your elbow as possible.

Think about the paper clip concept. You aren't going to get anywhere just by bending it back and forth a couple of times. To break the paper clip, you need to bend it anywhere from 30 to 60 times. That is exactly what you want to do here. To make any kind of change, you need to oscillate in and out of end-range flexion, as well as explore the full excursion of your elbow by turning your palm toward you and away from you. It's not a fixed-position mobilization. By turning your hand and scouring all the ranges of your elbow joint, you can completely change the dynamics of how your elbow is mobilized. Not only that, but switching hand positions helps account for common grips such as the chin-up grip (palms in, or supinated) and the rack and pulling position (palms away, or pronated).

Press Archetype | Front Rack 2 Archetype

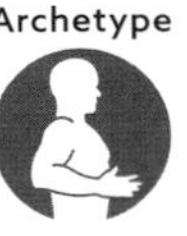

This mobilization will help improve the above archetypes.

IMPROVES:

Elbow flexion
Elbow pain

METHODS:

Distraction with gapping bias
Banded flossing

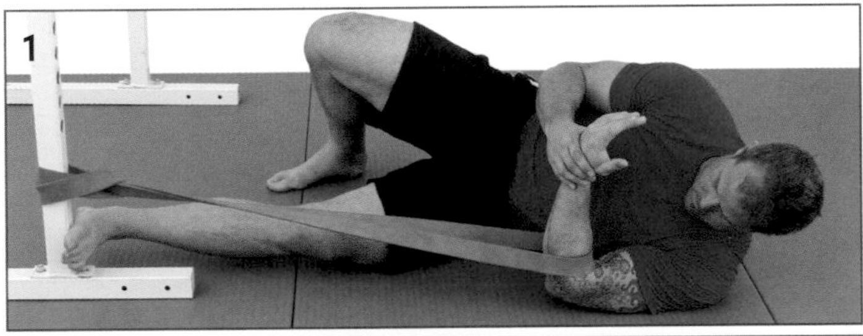

1 Hook a band around your forearm, near the crook of your elbow, and then push yourself away from the rack to create tension in the band.

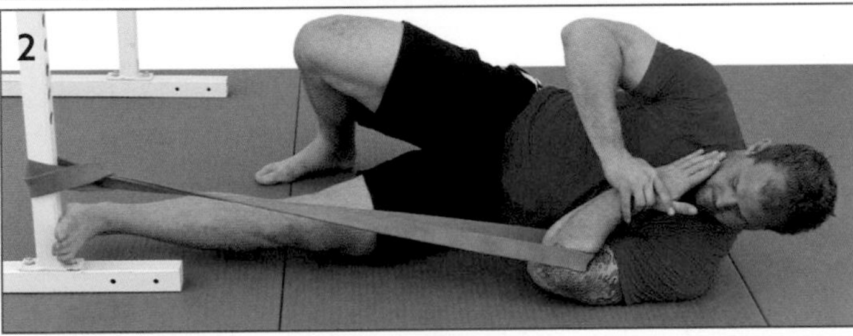

2 Pull your left hand toward your face using your right hand. I'm not going to lie: This hurts. Stay out of the pain cave and break your elbow like a paper clip until you effect change.

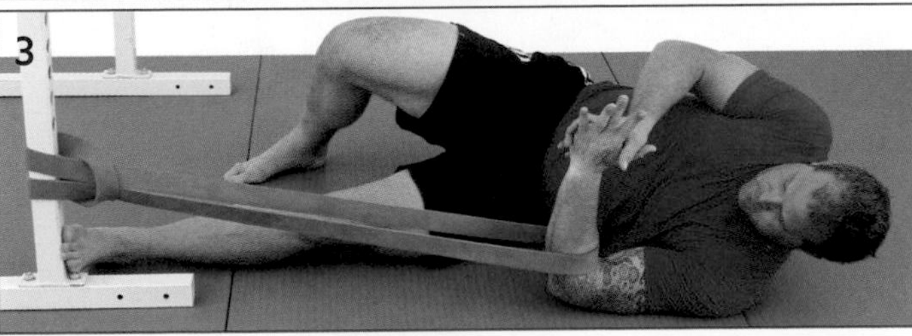

3 To ensure that you hit all corners, reposition your grip on your left hand, this time gripping your palm.

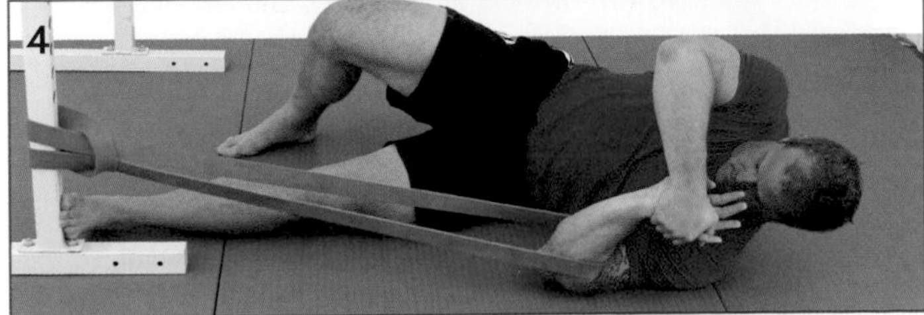

4 Pull your left hand to your face again, keeping your palm facing away from your body.

Press Archetype

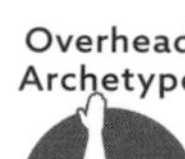

Overhead Archetype

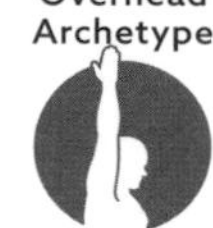

Front Rack 1 Archetype

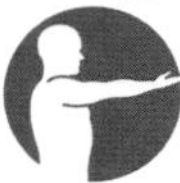

Front Rack 2 Archetype

This mobilization will help improve the above archetype.

IMPROVES:

Wrist and elbow pain

Wrist and elbow joint dynamics (extension, flexion, and rotational capacity)

METHODS:

Smash and floss

Tack and spin

Contract and relax

Forearm Smash Mobilizations

If you're one of those unfortunate souls who are stuck in static positions at work all day, stretching is not going to do that much for you. When your muscles mold and adapt to your positions—meaning that they get adaptively short and stiff—restoring elasticity requires ungluing.

For example, wrist pain is a common problem of deskbound athletes. So what do they do about it? Stretches like flexing and extending the wrist. You need a better plan. To treat the problem, you have to not only address the positions you're in, but also implement a combination of smashing, flossing, and distracted joint mobilizations.

A much better option is to look upstream of your wrist and attack the tissues that are pulling on your elbow and hand. Your forearms do an unbelievable amount of work for your hands, and you probably do nothing for them. No wonder you have tennis elbow or you can't assume a good front rack position. The strings that control your hands have turned into steel cables.

Here's the bottom line: If you have elbow or wrist pain, your forearms probably need some love. Work on those tissues by using these four options.

Option 1: Forearm Tack and Twist

This simple and quick mobilization is great for treating acute elbow pain. Notice in the photos below that I'm targeting my forearm extensors near the bend of my elbow. When this area gets stiff and sore, it tends to cause a lot of discomfort.

If you type all day with your arms stuck in a flexed position, you're an athlete who does a lot of heavy, high-volume pulling exercises (such as pull-ups, rowing, or Olympic lifting), or you're a martial artist who does a lot of punching and grappling, bookmark this mobilization and commit to doing it often.

Note: For most athletes, I recommend VooDoo Flossing the elbow because it captures all the muscles that insert into the elbow. The problem is that wrapping your own arm is difficult and sometimes not an option. This mob is a practical and effective substitute. You can do it by yourself at the office, pre- or post-workout, or anytime the area flares up. All you need is a lacrosse ball or Yoga Tune Up ball and a few minutes of free time.

1. Press a lacrosse ball or Yoga Tune Up ball into the top of your forearm next to the crook of your elbow.

2. To take up all the skin and soft tissue slack, twist the ball while maintaining downward pressure.

3. Flex your wrist and add rotation by internally and externally rotating your wrist and elbow.

4. Extend your wrist and splay your fingers. The idea is to create movement while your hand is in extension (think waving) by internally and externally rotating your wrist and elbow.

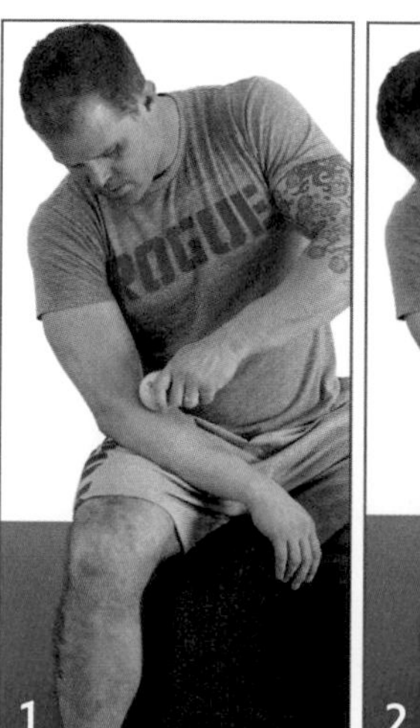

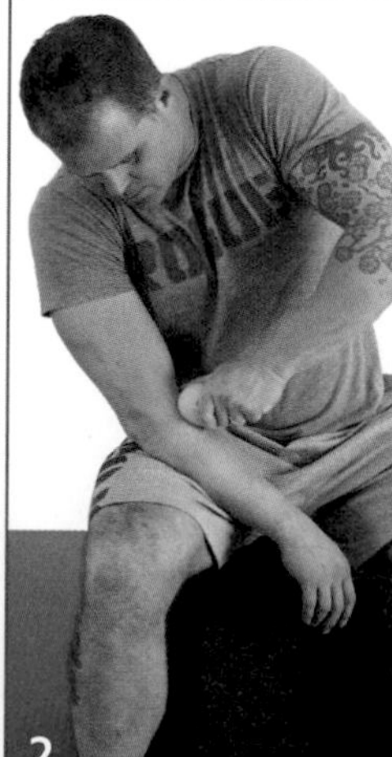

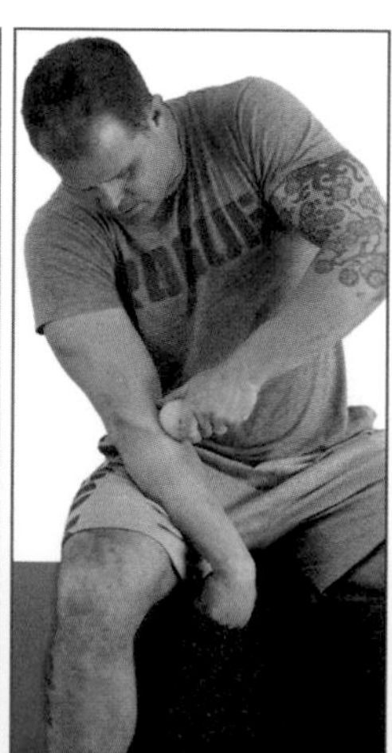

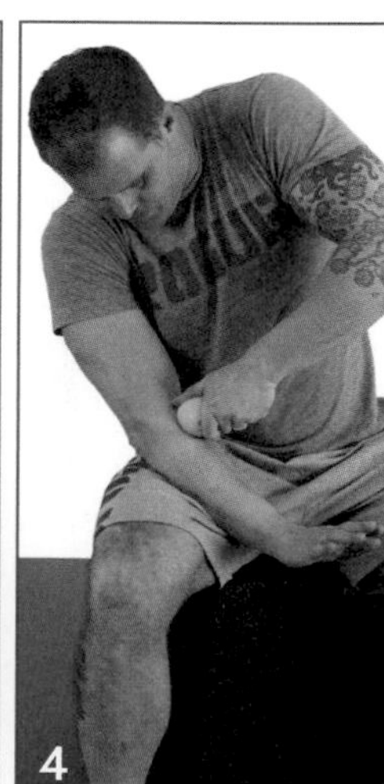

Option 2: Forearm Extensor Smash

As I've said, when the extensors of your forearm get overused and stiff, it can cause a lot of problems at your elbow and wrist. This is another highly effective forearm smashing technique that you can do at the office, at home, or at the gym. Although you can use a double or single lacrosse ball, I prefer Yoga Tune Up balls here. Their pliability and grip allow you to smash across the entire posterior compartment of your forearm, from your elbow down to your wrist.

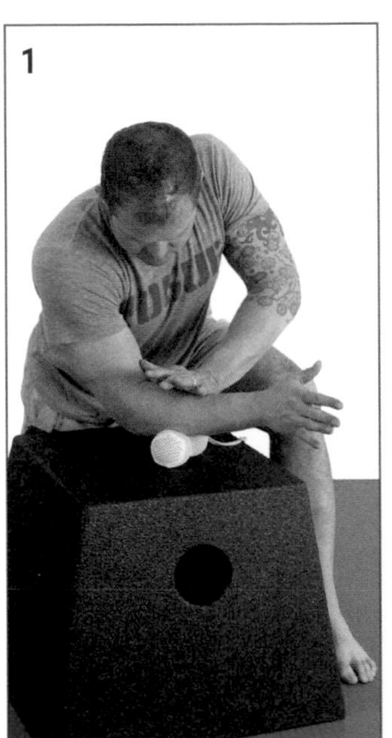

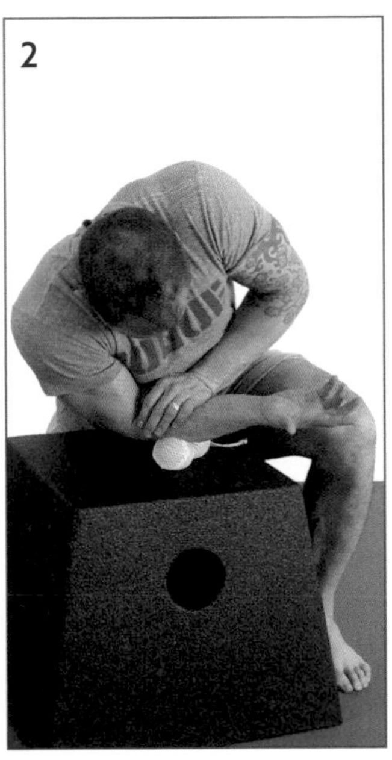

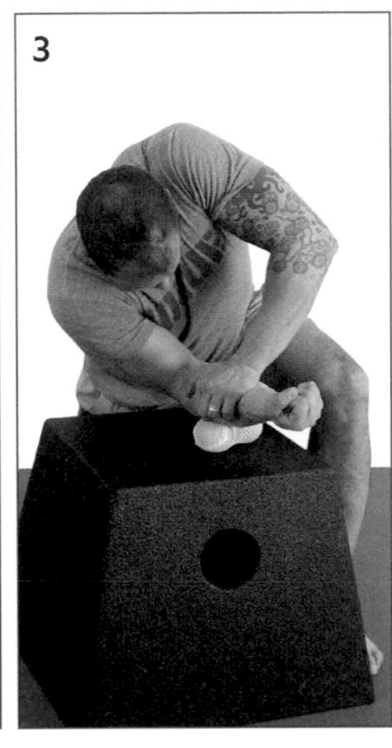

1. With your thumb facing the ceiling, position the outside edge of your forearm between two Yoga Tune Up balls.

2. To get enough pressure into your forearm, shift the weight of your upper body over your arm while simultaneously pressing your opposite hand into your forearm directly over the balls. At the same time, externally rotate your forearm, smashing across the posterior compartment of your forearm. The idea is to use your top hand to aid in the rotation.

3. If you find a painful trigger point, you can contract by making a fist and then relax by opening your hand. Do this until you stop making change or you can handle the full pressure of your weight.

Option 3: Forearm Stack and Smash

This is a two-for-one mobilization in that you can hit both the anterior and the posterior compartment of your forearm. As with the previous options, the key is not only to smash (pressure wave) across the muscle, but also to contract and relax on hotspots and floss by moving your wrist in all directions.

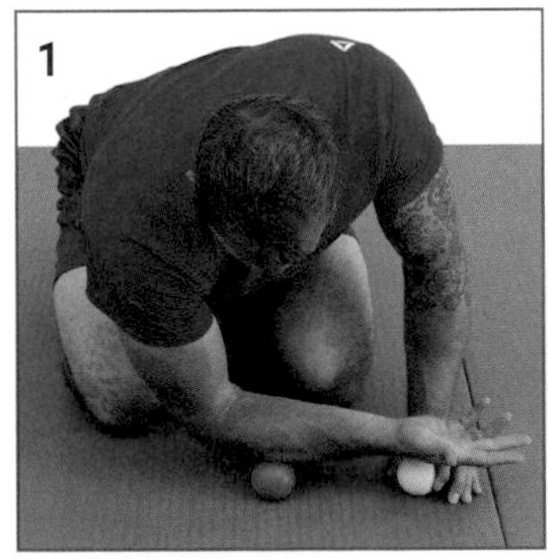

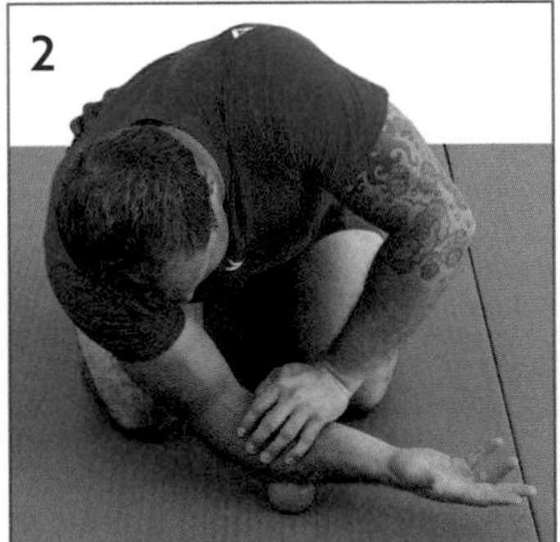

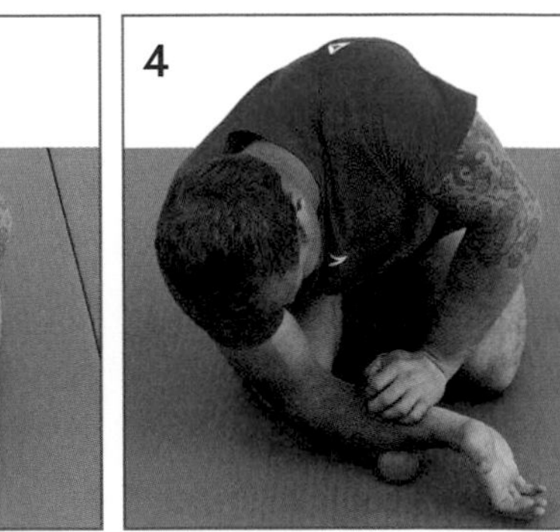

1. Position your forearm over a lacrosse ball with your palm facing the ceiling. You can place this bottom ball anywhere in the meat of your forearm, ideally on a stiff spot.

2. Position another lacrosse ball directly over the bottom lacrosse ball and drive it into your forearm with your opposite hand, effectively sandwiching the tight tissue.

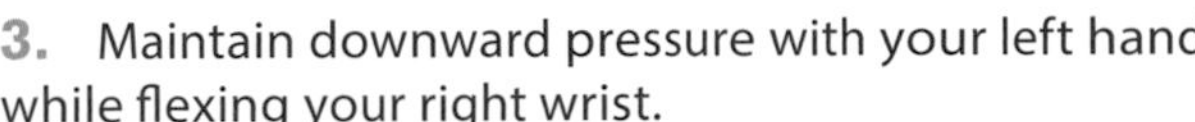

3. Maintain downward pressure with your left hand while flexing your right wrist.

4. Make circles, flex, extend, and move your hand in all directions. Once you feel some change, move on to another tight spot.

Option 4: Superfriend Forearm Smash

After you complete a brutal grip-intensive workout, smashing your own forearms is probably the last thing on your mind. The next time you burn your grip from a workout, employ a Superfriend to smash your forearms for you. As with the Superfriend Triceps Smash, it doesn't take a lot of pressure to smash the forearms, so go easy and be careful.

1. Lie on your belly with your arm internally rotated and your palm facing the ceiling. This exposes the anterior compartment of your forearm. Using the arch of his foot—between the ball of his foot and heel—have your training partner apply light pressure across your forearm. He can use his heel or the ball of his foot for a more acute, trigger-point effect.

2. The same rules and techniques apply to smashing the posterior compartment of the forearm. To set up for this variation, rotate your arm so that your palm is facing the mat. With your arm in extension, it's important to position an ab mat or pad underneath your forearm to protect your wrist and elbow.

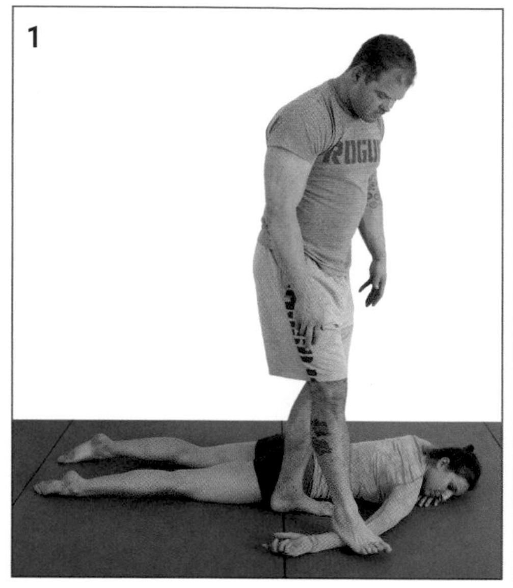
1

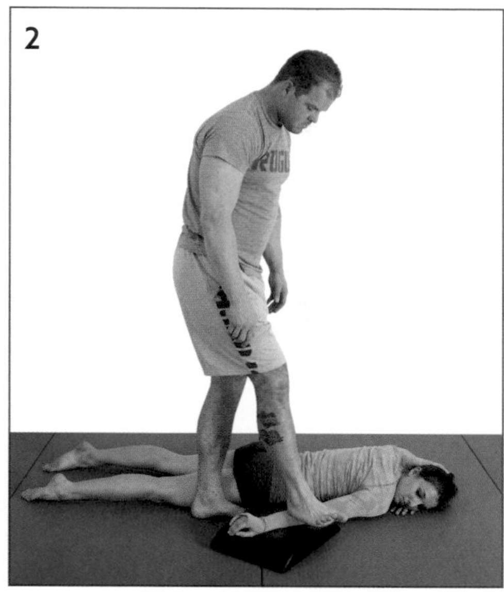
2

Wrist Tack and Spin

If you suffer from carpal tunnel syndrome or wrist and thumb pain, this mobilization is for you. Smartphones—like chairs—set us up to do damage to our bodies. Consider your wrist position and the number of thumb cycles you burn through when using your phone: You use your thumbs to scroll, text, and type with your wrists locked in an untenable position. In addition to causing repetitive stress injury, spending too much time on your phone or keyboard can cause your skin to get tacked down to the underlying tissue and bone, restricting movement and compressing nerves. The next time your thumb or wrist hurts, use this technique in conjunction with the mobilizations demonstrated on the next page.

1. Position a lacrosse ball or Yoga Tune Up ball on the inside corner of your wrist at the base of your thumb.

2. Applying pressure, take up the skin slack by twisting the ball.

3. Flex and extend your wrist for a flossing effect.

4. Target the outside corner of your wrist by using the same technique: pin, spin, and floss. The idea is to cover the entire base of your thumb and both sides of your wrist.

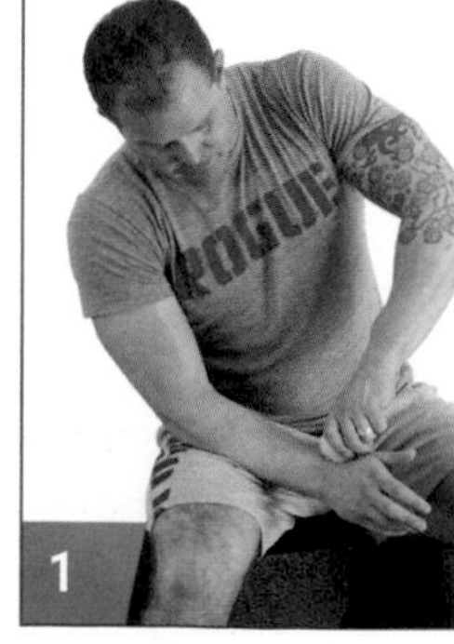
1

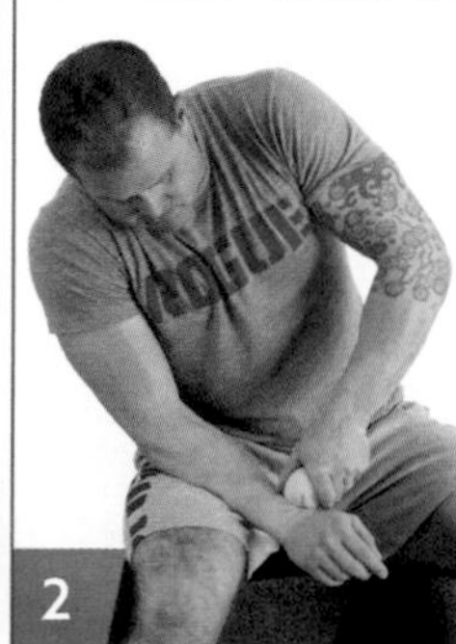
2

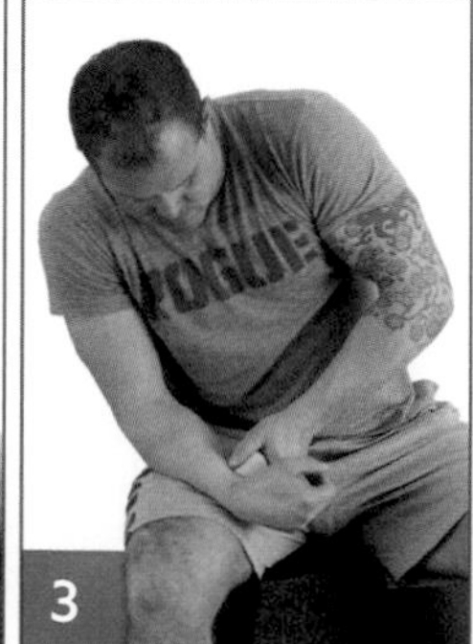
3

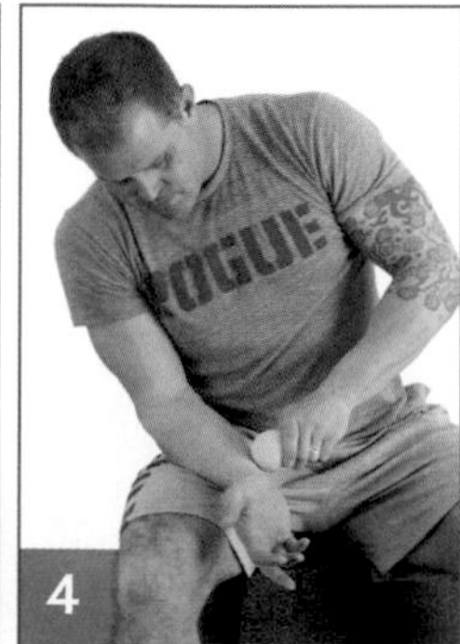
4

Banded Wrist Distraction with VooDoo Wrist Sequence

The Banded Wrist Distraction is similar to the ankle mobilizations in that you oscillate in and out of end range to improve the dynamics of the joint. It's a simple mobilization that is very effective for treating wrist pain. It's also a great way to prep for any demanding front rack exercise. For the best results, wrap your wrist with a VooDoo Floss Band and work your way through the sequence.

Front Rack 2 Archetype

This mobilization will help improve the adjacent archetype.

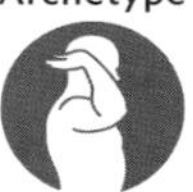

IMPROVES:

Joint mechanics
Wrist pain

METHODS:

Banded flossing
VooDoo Floss Band compression

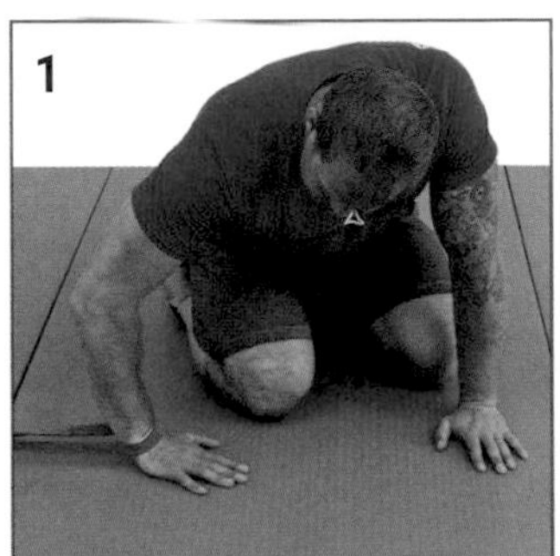

1 Hook a band around your wrist.

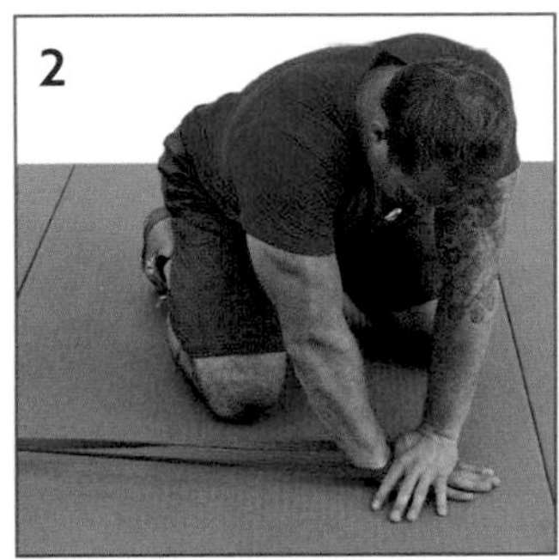

2 Slide your hand to create tension in the band. This distracts your wrist joint into a good position. Then staple the base of your hand to the mat with your left hand.

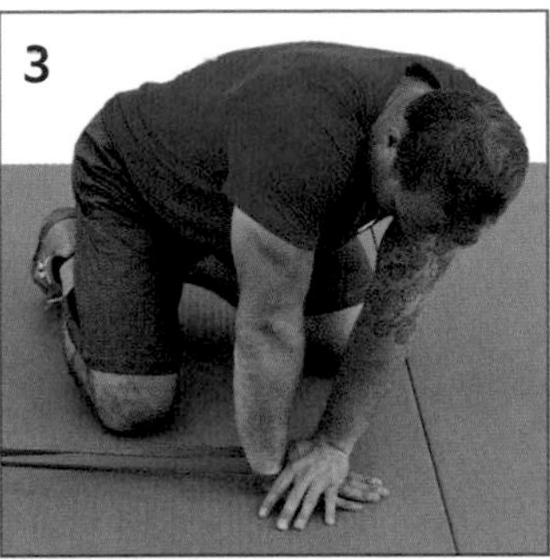

3 Block your right wrist with your left hand, lock out your elbow, and extend your right arm over your right hand. Then floss in and out of end range until you feel change in the joint.

VOODOO BANDED WRIST TARGET AREA

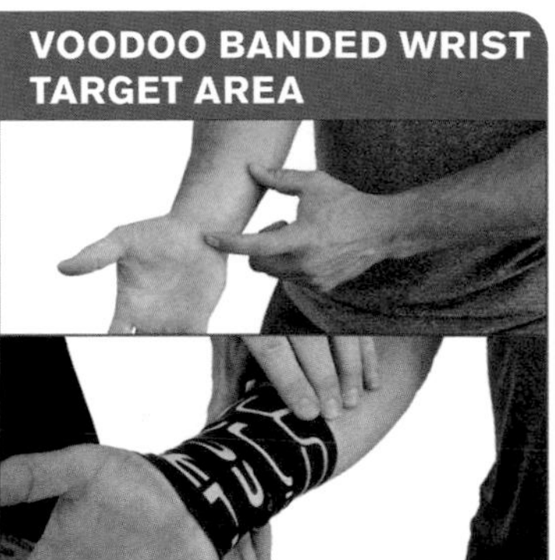

INFORMED FREESTYLE

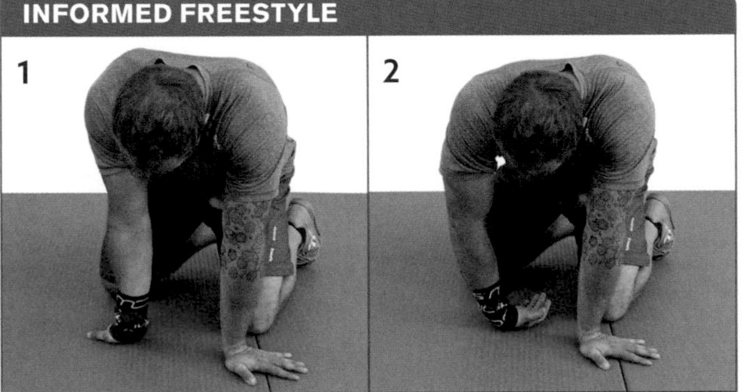

1 2

After you've wrapped your wrist, play around with different mobilizations by forcing your wrist into common positions.

VOODOO BANDED WRIST DISTRACTION

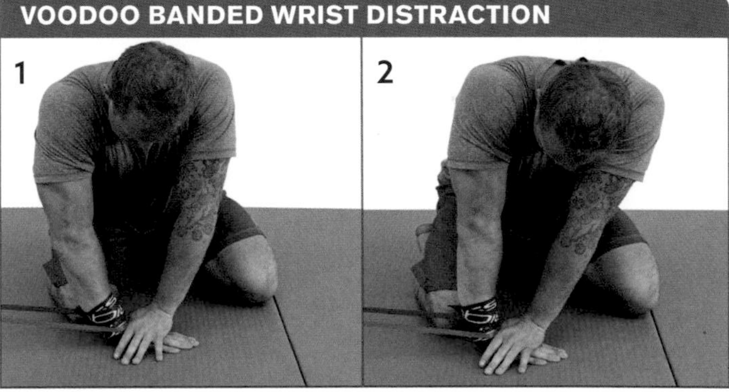

1 2

Combining a distraction with a VooDoo Floss Band is always a good idea. As with the elbow extension, block your wrist, lock out your elbow, and extend your arm over your planted hand, flossing in and out of end range.

VOODOO BANDED WRIST COMPLEX

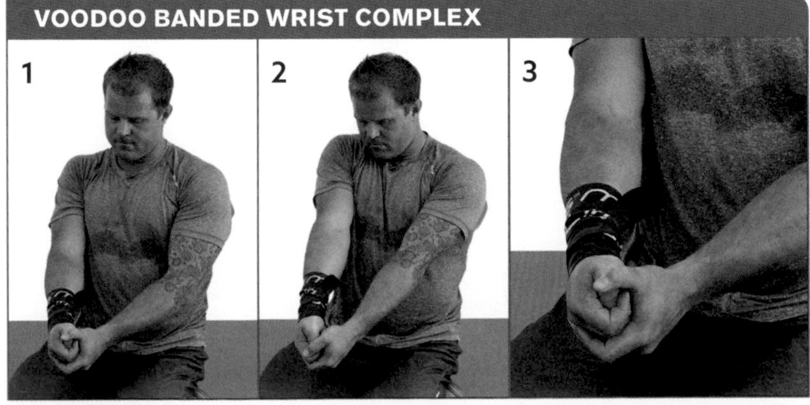

1 2 3

This wrist mobilization gets a gold star for effectiveness. It should be the first stop for keyboard warriors who suffer from stiff thumbs and wrists. Make a fist over your thumb, then lock out your arm while bending your wrist toward the ground. This helps unglue the laminated tissues surrounding your thumb and wrist complex, restoring sliding surfaces to the area.

AREA 6 TRUNK (PSOAS, LOW BACK, OBLIQUES)

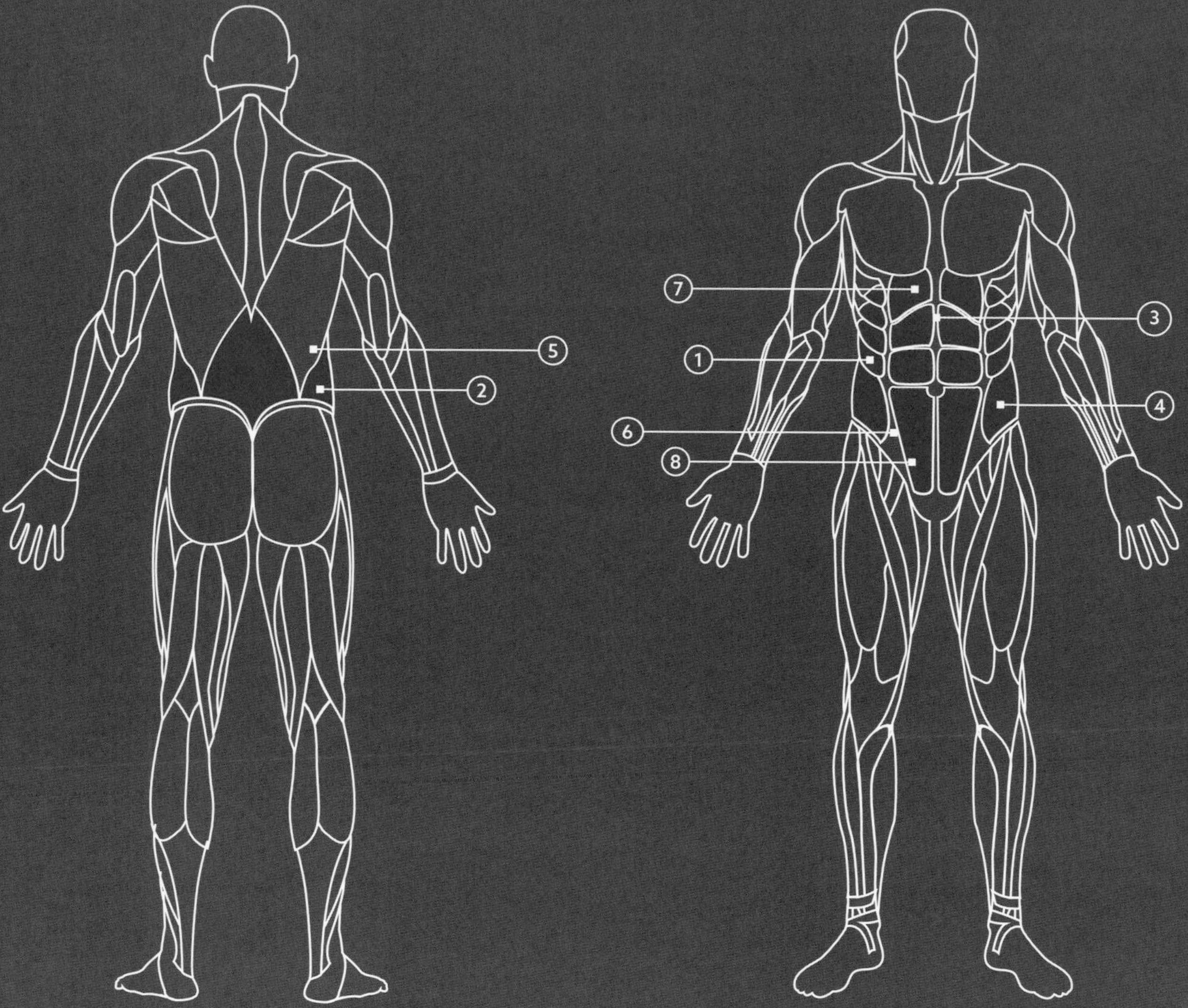

1
2
3
4
5
6
7
8

MOBILIZATION TARGET AREAS:

1
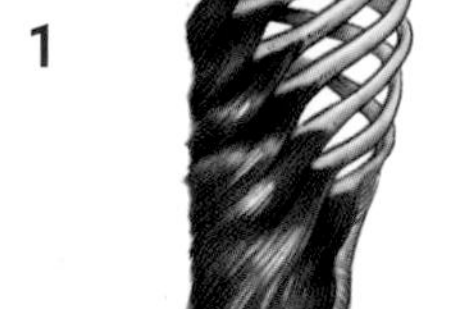
External and Internal Abdominal Obliques

2
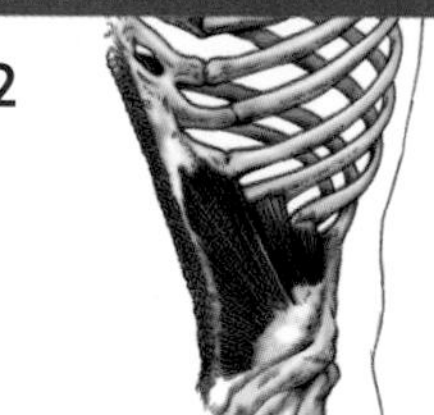
External and Internal Abdominal Obliques

3
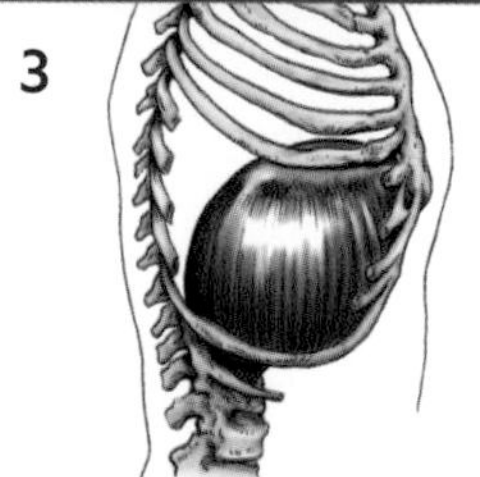
Diaphragm (side view)

4
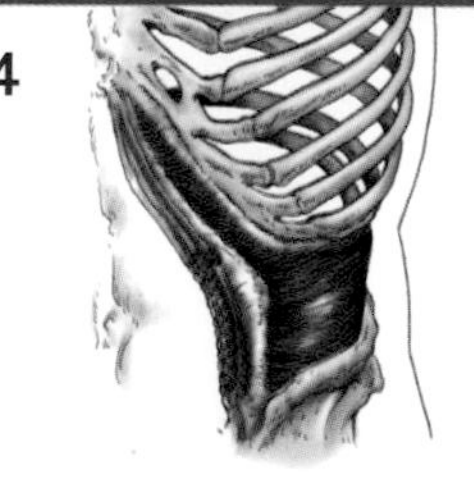
Transverse Abdominis

5
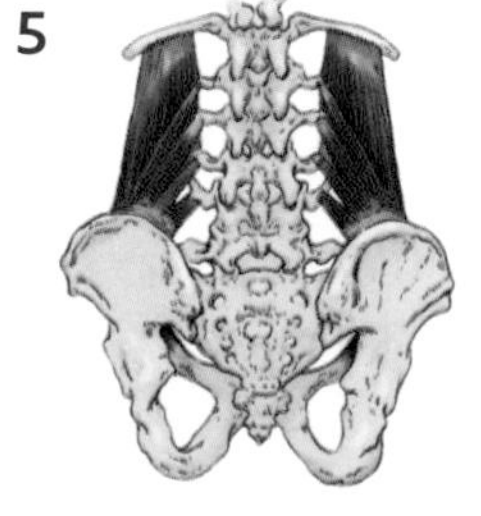
Quadratus Lumborum

6
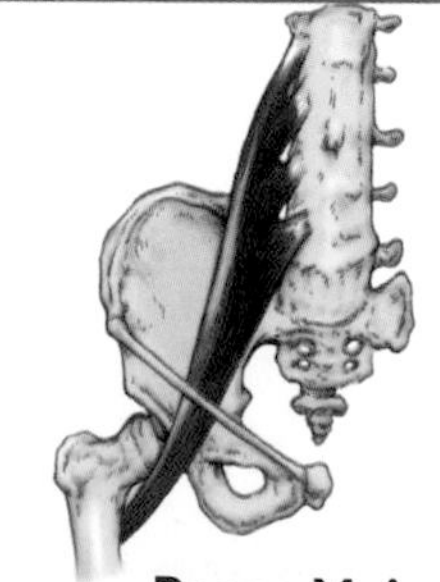
Psoas Major

7
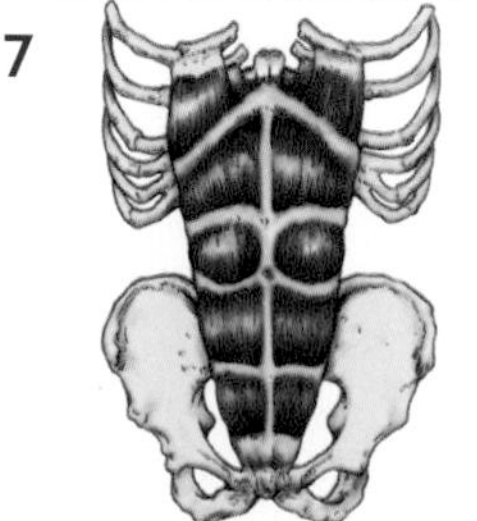
Rectus Abdominis

8
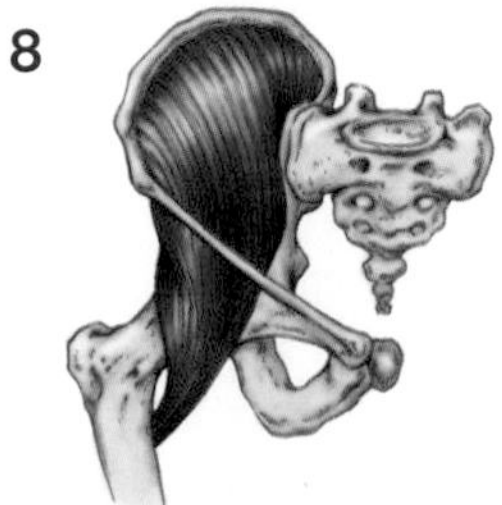
Iliacus

Low Back Smash

Low Back Smash: Option 1

If you have low back pain, put this mobilization at the top of your list. By sticking a lacrosse ball in your low back and upper glute region, you can effectively unglue the matted-down tissues that cause low back pain and restrict movement and positional mechanics.

It's better to perform this mobilization with your feet elevated on a box or chair, for three reasons. First, it's easier to mobilize in a good position without breaking into overextension. Second, you can get more pressure into the ball, which is necessary for effecting change in the tissue. And third, it takes the slack out of the musculature of your trunk and low back, making it easier to maintain a neutral spinal position.

Squat 2 Archetype

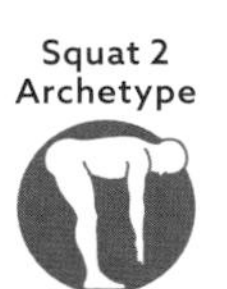

Squat 1 Archetype

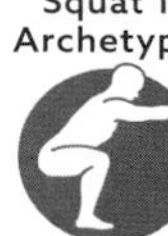

This mobilization will help improve the above archetypes.

IMPROVES:

Low back pain and stiffness
Lumbar joint mechanics
Global rotation

METHODS:

Pressure wave
Contract and relax

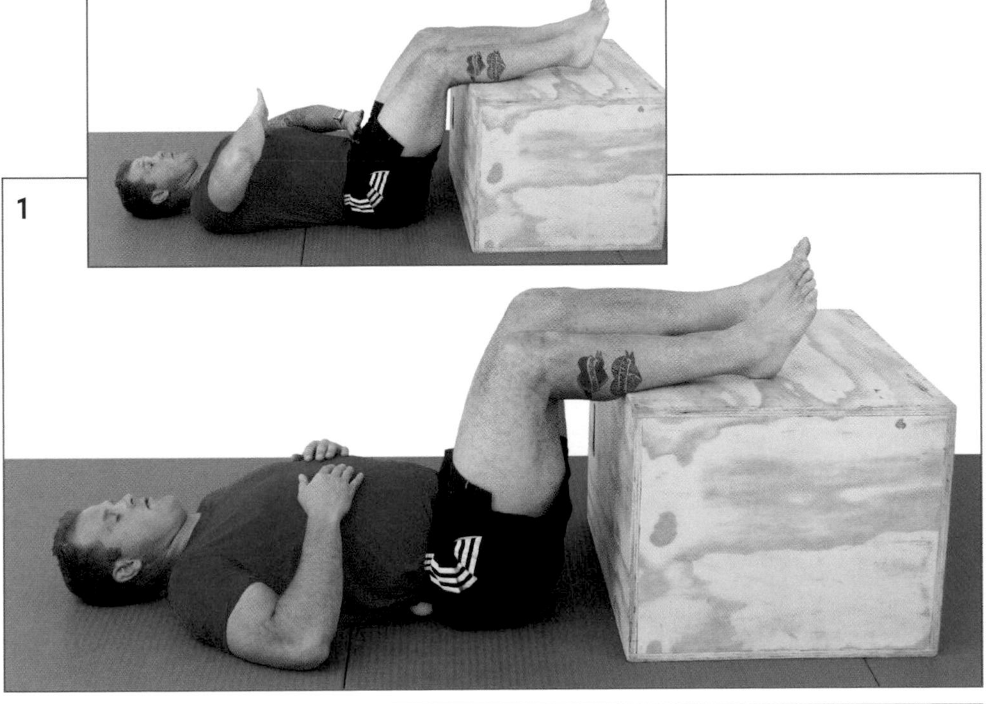

1

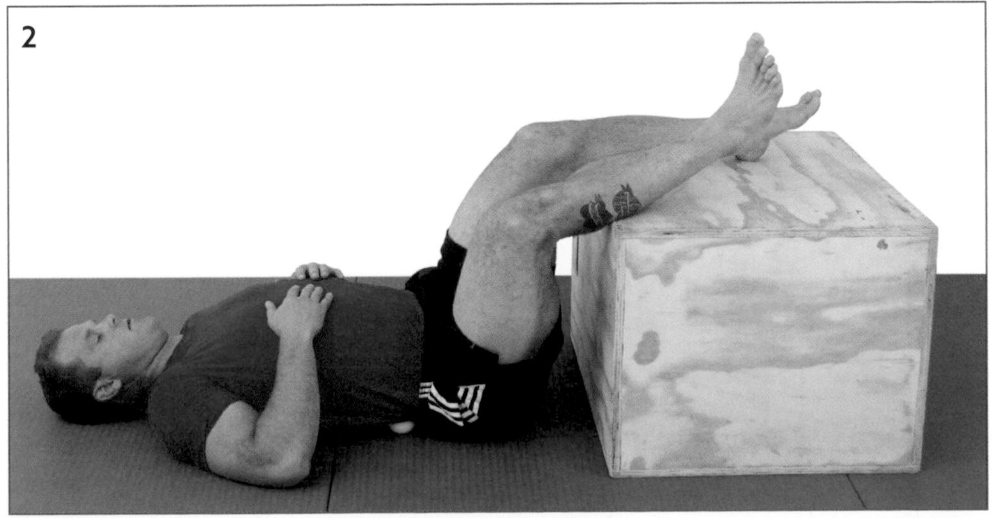

2

TARGET AREA

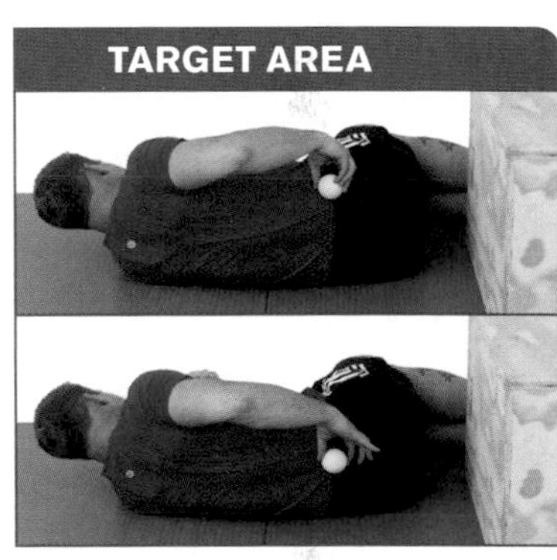

The goal is to work back and forth from the side of your hip to your spine, trying to stay on the crest of your pelvis and superior glute.

1. Place a lacrosse ball on your low back just above your pelvis and position your feet up on a box. Focus on keeping your midline engaged so you can maintain a neutral spinal position. If you overextend by tilting your pelvis, which is a common fault, you will only make your low back pain worse.

2. Slowly shift your hips toward your left. The goal is to grind back and forth against the grain of the muscle and slowly smash the tissue using the pressure wave technique.

Back Tweak? Reset Your Pelvis!

Typically, low back pain stems from either sitting for long hours with poor posture or moving and lifting in a compromised position. Once you ingrain dysfunctional movement patterns or adopt a poor position while seated, low back pain turns into a real problem. You can treat the issue by using mobilization techniques, but the moment you default into your bad positions, it flares up again. That is why I say things like, "The number one predictor for low back pain is a previous history of low back pain." Once you burn out your duty cycles, the issue persists. Unless you address your position and perform constant maintenance on the problem areas, it's always an issue.

If you don't have a history of low back pain, on the other hand, the number two predictor of low back pain is having a pelvic rotation obliquity stemming from a back tweak. For example, if you have tweaked your back playing sports or doing whatever, chances are good that one side of your pelvis has rotated out of position, creating side-to-side differences in your mobility. So if you have one hamstring that is a lot tighter than the other hamstring pulling down on one side of your pelvis and you try to lift a large load, it creates a rotational shear on your hips and pulls your pelvis into a bad position, which in turn tweaks your low back. You don't even have to be lifting a heavy load for this to occur. Sometimes low back tweaks happen when you're not braced and you rotate or move the wrong way. Regardless of how it happens, you can use a simple technique to reset your pelvis into a neutral position.

The idea here is to use rotation and counter-rotation by pushing on one knee and pulling on the other. This action fires your hamstring and hip flexor at the same time for the purpose of resetting your pelvic position. The general prescription is to hold both positions for 5 seconds while resisting the pressure with your legs, switch sides 3 or 4 times, and then finish by squeezing a ball between your knees as hard as you can. This last step helps reset your pubic symphysis.

To put it in simple terms, you're using your muscles to restore a normal pelvic position. Often, you'll hear a pop or feel your pelvis "clunk" into position.

1. Push on your right knee with your right hand while countering the pressure with your right leg, which fires your right hip flexor. At the same time, pull on your left knee with your left hand while countering the pressure with your left leg, which activates your left hamstring.

2. After holding the position for 5 seconds, switch hands and apply the same push-pull pressure, counter-pressure to your knees. Repeat this sequence, going back and forth between positions and resisting for 5 seconds.

3. Once you've completed a few rotations and then a few counter-rotation cycles, position a medicine ball between your knees and squeeze as hard as you can for 5 seconds. Repeat this process for 3 to 5 sets until you feel or hear a clunk.

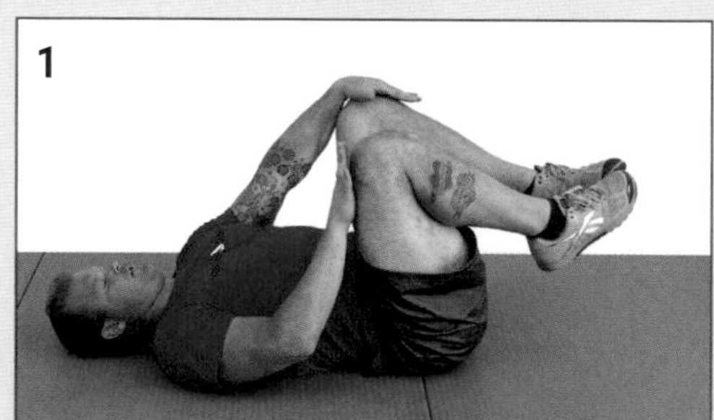

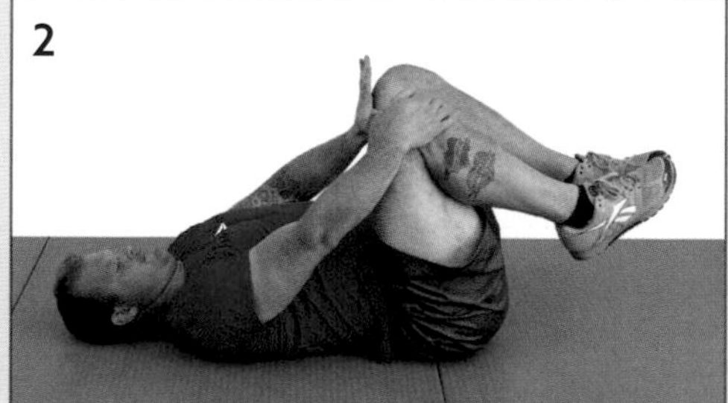

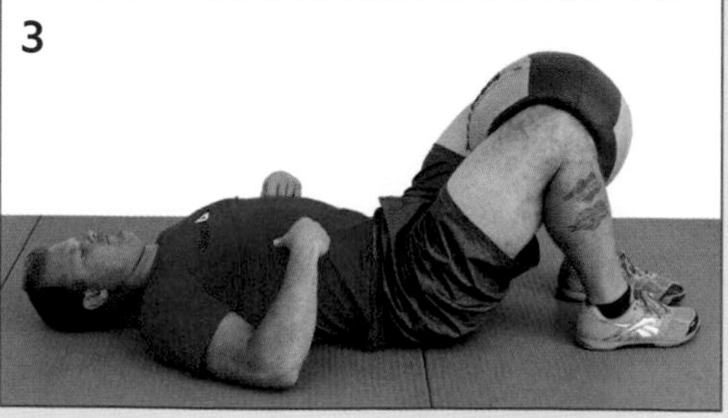

Low Back Smash: Option 2

If you have a stiff low back, chances are good that you're missing range of motion in your lumbar spine. This makes you highly vulnerable to back tweaks. This simple mobilization restores basic spinal motion and relieves stiffness in your low back. It's very similar to option 1, but instead of working on the muscles that tie into the area, you're targeting the motion segment vertebrae of your lumbar spine. The former deals with muscle stiffness, while the latter addresses joint mechanics. But unlike using a single lacrosse ball, you don't have to worry as much about overextending because the ball supports both sides of your spine. However, that doesn't mean you can put your abs to sleep. You want to keep enough tension to maintain a neutral position and avoid tilting your pelvis as you drop your knees from side to side.

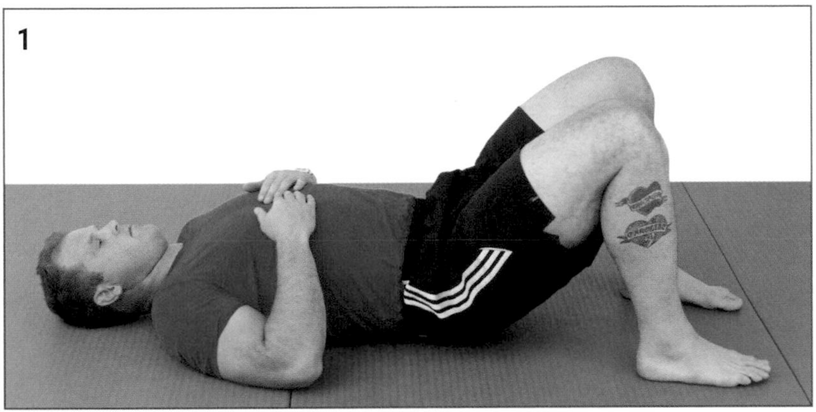

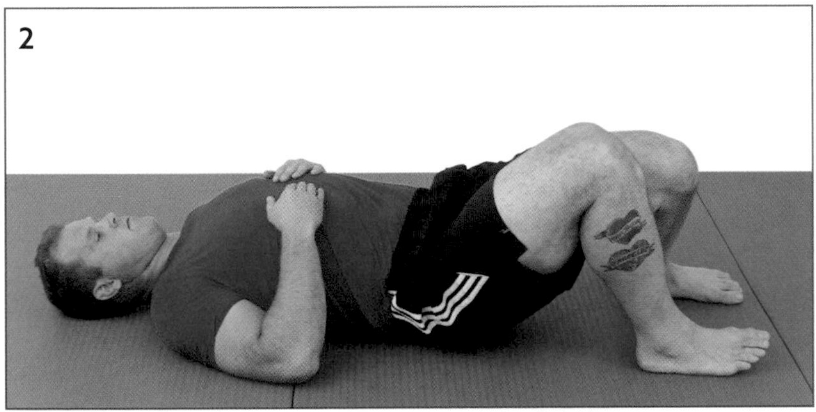

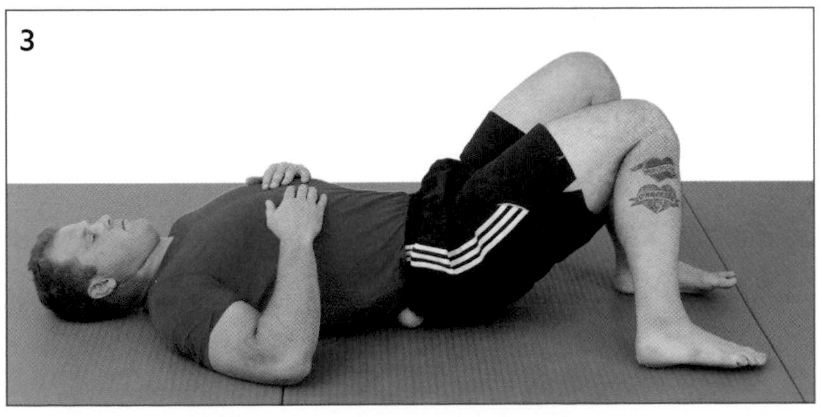

TARGET AREA

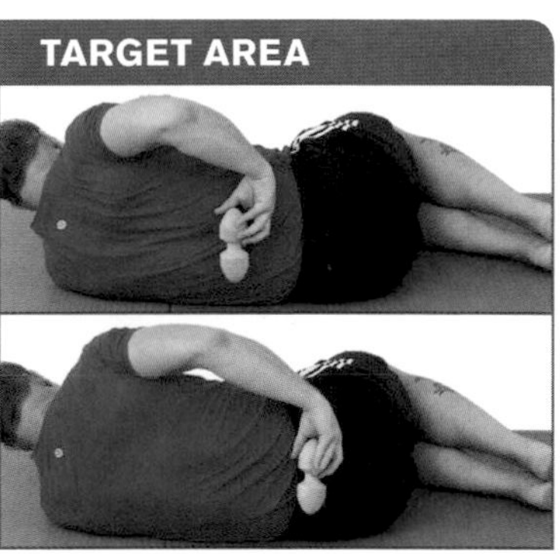

The idea is to hit each motion segment of your spine stretching from the base of your ribcage to your pelvis.

1. Position a double lacrosse ball on your lower back between the motion segments of your vertebrae. To avoid breaking into overextension, keep your midline engaged and your hips off the ground. A helpful cue is to think about creating a long spine as you drop your knees toward the ground. If you want to increase the pressure, you can post your feet up on a box or chair or lift your legs into the air.

2. Drop your left knee toward your right side and rotate your hips slightly.

3. With your motion segments still blocked, rotate your hips and drop your right knee toward your left side. It's important not to over-rotate and lose shoulder contact with the ground. Rotate from side to side until you feel some change, and then move up or down to the next motion segment.

Low Back Smash: Option 3

TARGET AREA

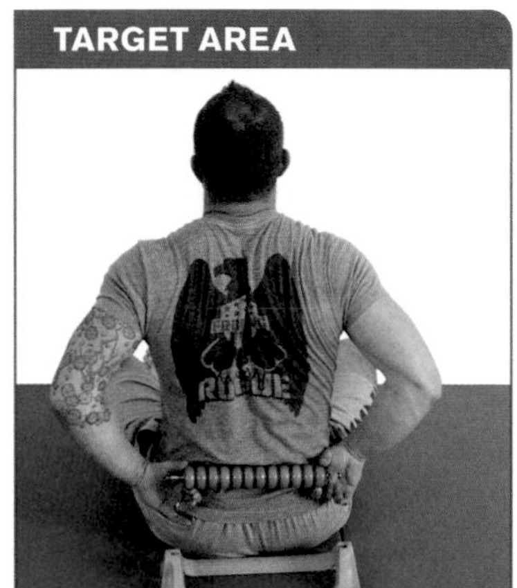

The Little Battlestar is another great tool for smashing your low back because it captures the musculature and fascia including your erectors, quadratus lumborum (QL), oblique, and thoracolumbar fascia, as well as targets the motion segment vertebra of your lumbar spine. However, unlike option 2, which has a mobilization target area stretching from the base of your ribcage to your pelvis, you want to stay just above your iliac crest (hip bone). Mobilize any higher than that and you run the risk of overextending, which—as you know—is never ideal.

What's more, the Little Battlestar is not designed to target each individual motion segment of your spine. In this situation, you're primarily targeting your lumbosacral joint (junction)—the disk between the lower lumbar vertebral body and the uppermost sacral vertebral body. This motion segment is supported by several interconnected components, providing a strong and stable base for your spine. Put simply, as long as you stay near the base of your spine, you're not going to cause damage by overextending. In fact, getting movement through this area is important because a stiff lumbosacral joint is a common source of low back pain and sciatica.

As with the previous techniques, the key is to keep your shoulders pinned to the mat as you roll your hips and legs from side to side.

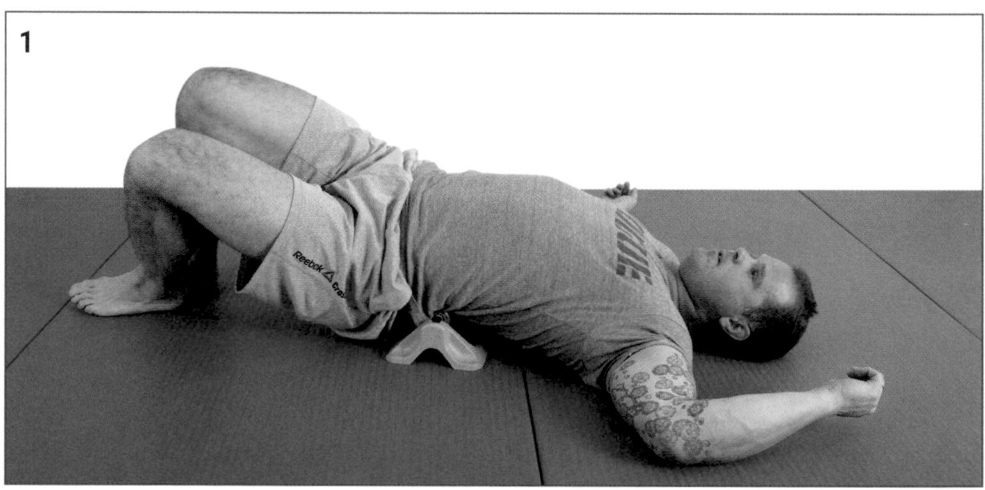

1

2

1. Position a Little Battlestar on your low back just above your iliac crest (hip bone).

2. Keeping your shoulders rooted to the ground, turn your hips and let your legs fall to the side. The idea is to rotate your hips back and forth, working the tissue across the upper glute and low back region.

Erector Side Smash

This mobilization targets your erector spinae—the muscles responsible for straightening your back and for side-to-side rotation—through your lumbar region. This area gets especially ropy when you sit, stand, or lift in flexed or overextended positions. Here's what happens: When you adopt an overextended or flexed position, your abdominals typically go offline—meaning you're not engaging your abdominal muscles to brace your trunk—and your erectors, quadratus lumborum (QL), and psoas (to mention a few) are forced to pick up the slack. This is why you target the muscles surrounding the hip and low back complex when your back hurts: These muscles get put on tension (pulled and stretched in different directions), which can manifest as generalized low back pain.

It's important to note that tight and ropy erectors not only open the door to low back pain, but also compromise your ability to rotate from side to side. So if you play golf, tennis, or any sport that requires a lot of rotation, this is a great mobilization to implement.

As you can see in the photos below, the idea is to position the Gemini, double lacrosse ball, or Yoga Tune Up balls next to your lumbar spine at the base of your ribcage and slowly slide your hips from side to side. You may capture some of your QL and maybe even some of your oblique, but the idea is to scrub back and forth across your erector. You can also rotate your hips, allowing your legs to fall to the side to emphasize rotation. This will not only improve sliding surfaces for your erectors, but also get some motion through your thoracic spine.

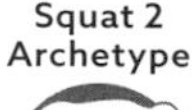

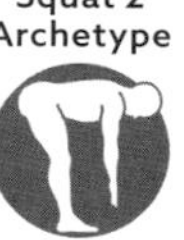
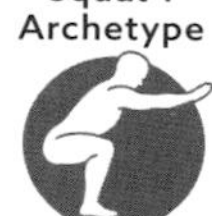

This mobilization will help improve the above archetypes.

IMPROVES:

Low back pain and stiffness
Lumbar joint mechanics
Global rotation

METHODS:

Pressure wave
Contract and relax

TARGET AREA

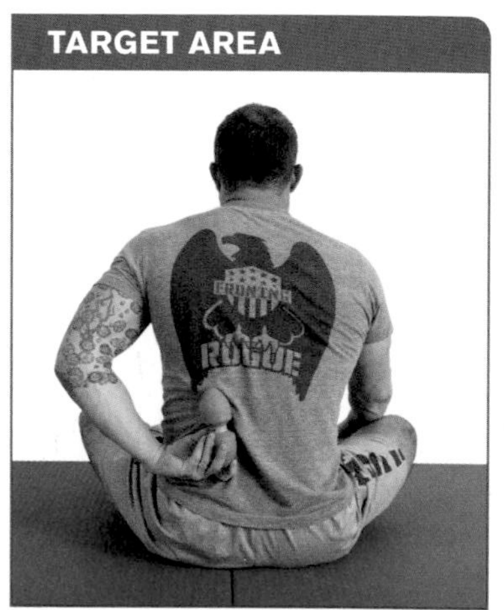

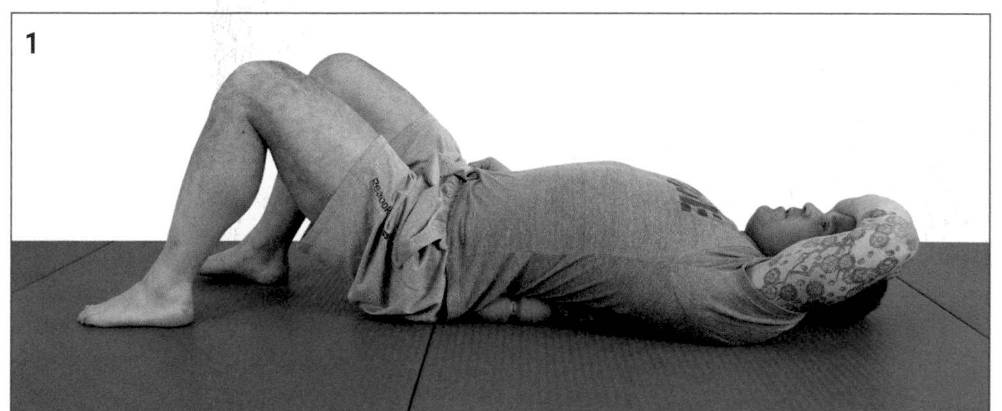

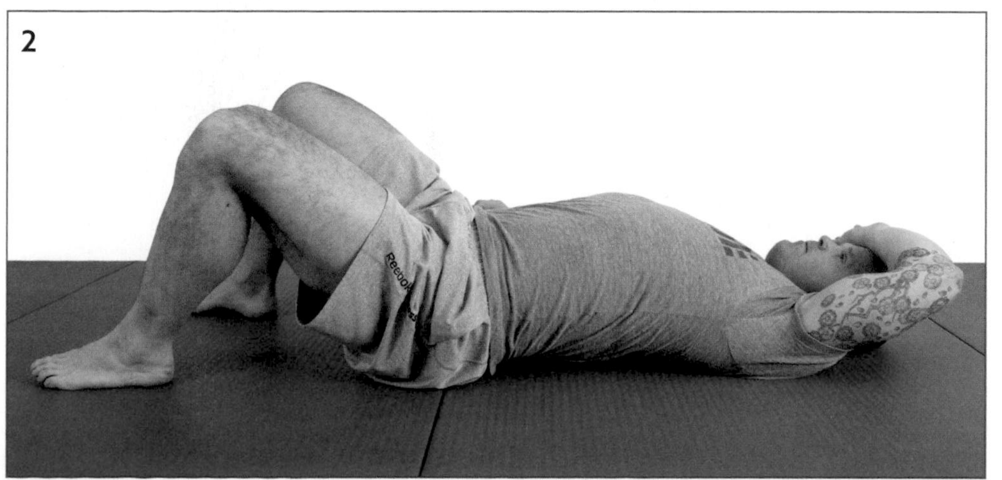

1. Position the Gemini, double lacrosse ball, or Yoga Tune Up balls next to your spine, between your hip bone and ribcage.

2. Keeping your back as flat as possible, slide your hips laterally, scrubbing across your erector. To emphasize rotation, you can rotate your hips and allow your legs to drop to the side.

QL Side Smash

Squat 2 Archetype

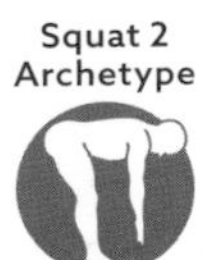

Squat 1 Archetype

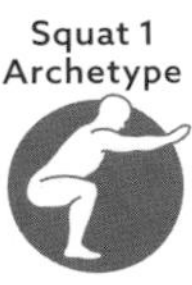

This mobilization will help improve the above archetypes.

IMPROVES:

Low back pain and stiffness
Lumbar joint mechanics
Global rotation

METHODS:

Pressure wave
Contract and relax

TARGET AREA

The quadratus lumborum, or QL—like the erector spinae—is a source of low back pain when prolonged sitting and poor spinal mechanics are the norm. Again, when you're not in a neutral spinal position with your abs engaged (braced), the muscles that connect your spine to your pelvis, like the QL, psoas, and erector spinae (to mention the few), pick up the slack. Stated differently, when you're not neutrally braced, these muscles have to work extra hard to keep you upright. What happens? Those muscles get stiff and become hypertonic (overly tensioned).

The goal with this mobilization is to sink into that QL, which runs from the bottom of your ribcage to the top of your pelvis, using a large ball such as a Supernova or softball. If you are having pelvic positioning issues or low back pain, you sit a lot, or you're an athlete who lifts a ton of heavy weight, this mob is for you.

Note: If you want a more aggressive, elbowlike pressure, you can use a lacrosse ball. However, you'll need to elevate your hips off the ground to get enough pressure. You can do so in one of three ways:

1. Prop your feet up on a box or against a wall.
2. Position the lacrosse ball over a yoga block and extend over the ball and block.
3. Perform the mob against a wall instead of on the ground.

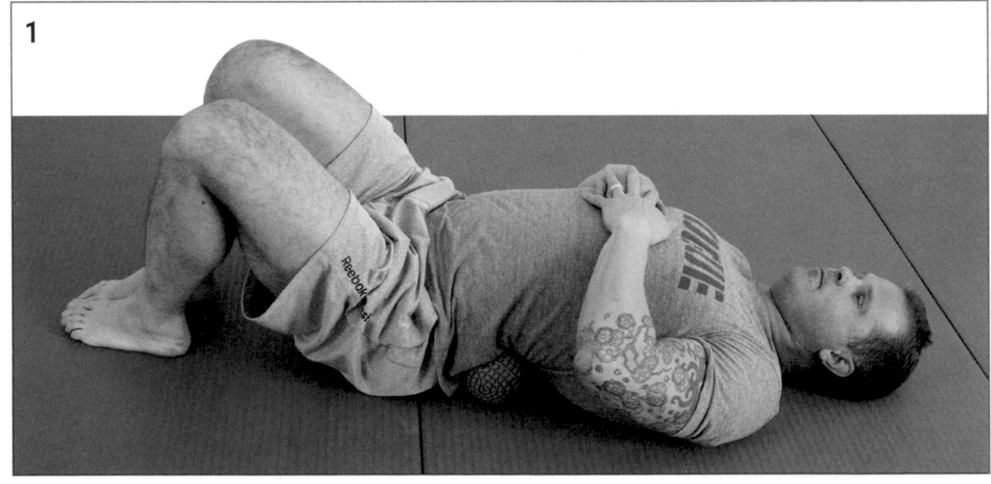

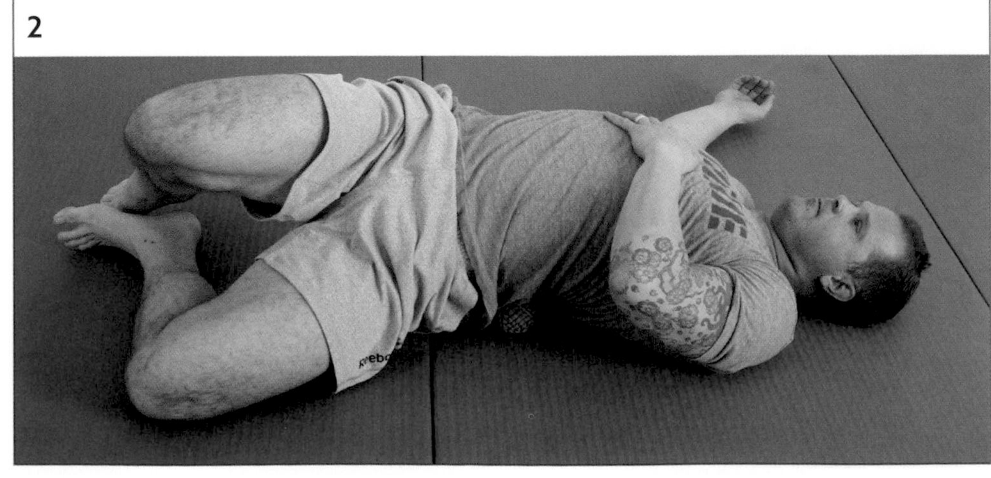

1. Position a ball on the side of your low back between your ribcage and hip bone.

2. There are several ways to mobilize the QL from this position. You can contract and relax, breathing into the area by focusing your inhalations into the ball and relaxing as you exhale. You can also pressure wave by making small oscillations over the QL area and rotating your hips and dropping your legs to the side. *Note:* Rotating your hips back and forth is a great way to emphasize rotation and get movement through the QL and low back regions.

Oblique Side Smash

IMPROVES:
Low back pain
Global rotation
Lateral extension

METHODS:
Pressure wave
Contract and relax

If you're walking around with a tight low back, you need to address all the tissues that tie into that lumbar region. One of the biggest mistakes you can make is to mobilize only the area of localized pain and stiffness. While you obviously want to address any ugliness in the areas where you feel most restricted, you also have to work on the surrounding structures so that you can feed some slack to those tight tissues. In this sequence I demonstrate two simple side smash techniques that target the obliques and other lateral units that tie into the low back structure, like the high glutes and tensor fasciae latae. In most cases, these tissues are very restricted and need to be unglued with some smashing. The best way to do so is to pressure wave back and forth over a roller or ball, positioning the tool between your ribcage and hip bone.

Option 1: Oblique Side Smash (Roller)

Although the Little Battlestar is the preferred tool here, a foam roller or Rumble Roller (a foam roller with protruding studs) will get the job done. The idea is to use something that has ridges or points so that you can penetrate the muscle and dig into the ropy tissue.

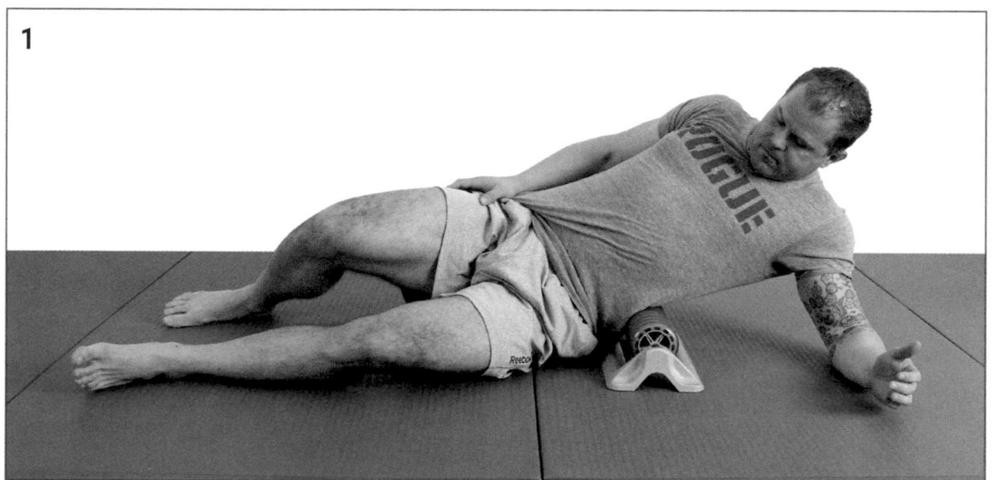

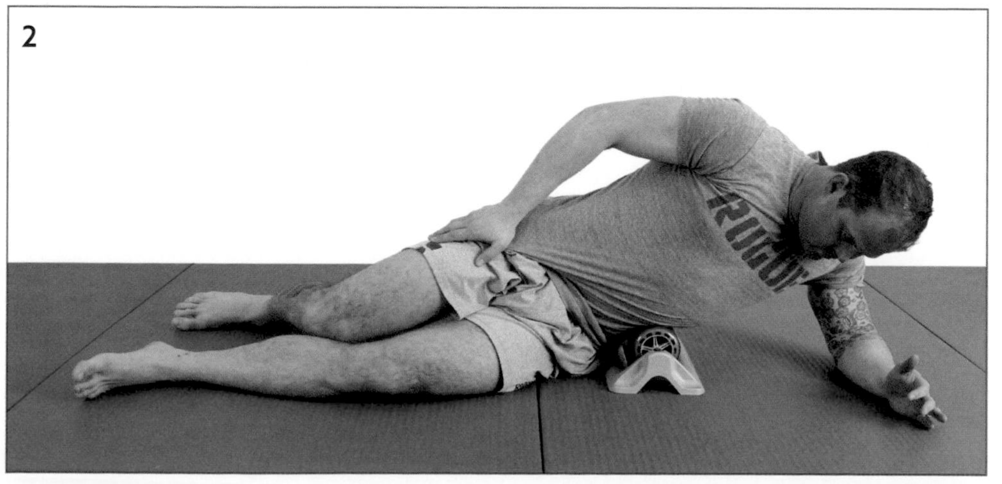

1. Start on your side with a roller positioned between your ribcage and hip bone.

2. Roll toward your belly and twist your torso over the roller. The idea is to seesaw back and forth over your side, smashing your oblique, QL, and high glute. To make this mobilization more aggressive, you can lengthen the tissues by stretching your arm overhead.

Option 2: Oblique Side Smash (Ball)

You can also use a softball, Alpha ball, or Supernova to mobilize your oblique muscles. As with option 1, using a tool that has grooves or ridges is ideal because it grips the skin, which helps delaminate tacked-down muscle tissue and fascia.

You can also perform this mobilization against a wall. While you can't get as much pressure against a wall, it gives you the option of using a smaller ball such as a lacrosse ball, which is a more precise tool.

When implementing this variation, try scouring the border of your hip bone. I'm not going to lie; this is a painful area to mobilize. But it does wonders for alleviating back pain and improving rotational and lateral mobility. If you don't believe me, use the Lateral Hip and Side Openers demonstrated on the following page to test and retest. You'll be amazed.

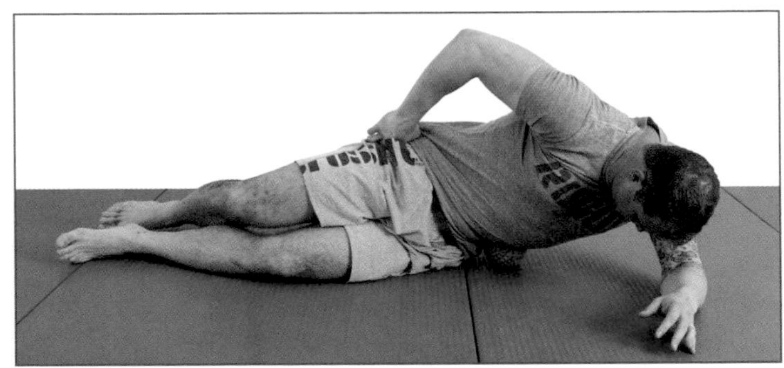

Position the ball between your ribcage and hip bone. Then twist your torso over the ball, keeping as much weight over the ball as you can handle.

Classic Spinal Twist

IMPROVES:
Low back pain and stiffness
Global rotation
Lateral extension

The Classic Spinal Twist is a global mobilization that catches anything that's tight in your low back region. It's not the first stop you want to make when addressing low back and lumbar spine issues, but it's an easy way to relieve stiffness to anything that's tight in that area. It's also a great test and retest model that you can use to assess the effectiveness of the previous mobs.

1. Lie on your back with your feet flat on the mat.

2. Keeping your left shoulder flush with the mat, drop your knees to your right side.

3. Cup your right hand over your left knee, pulling it toward the mat, straighten your left arm, and turn your head toward your left side.

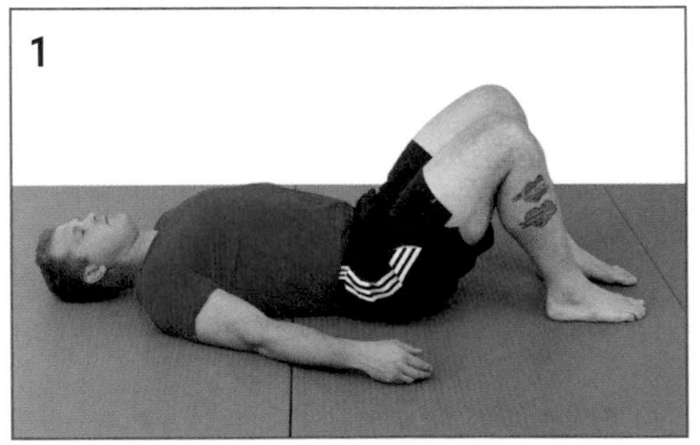

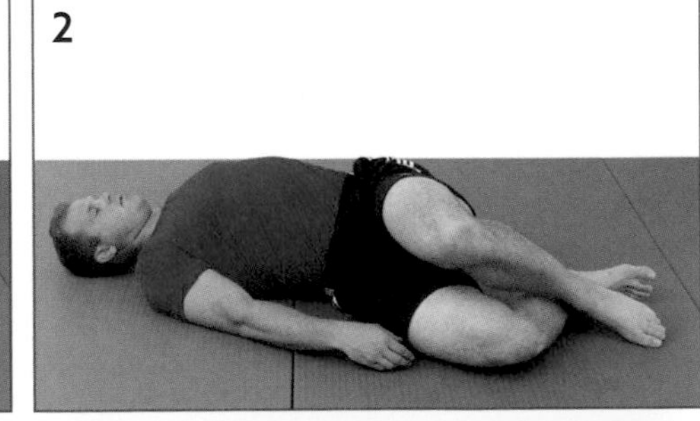

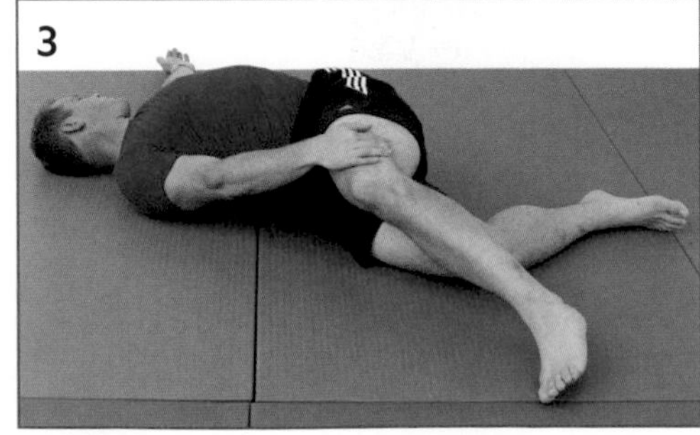

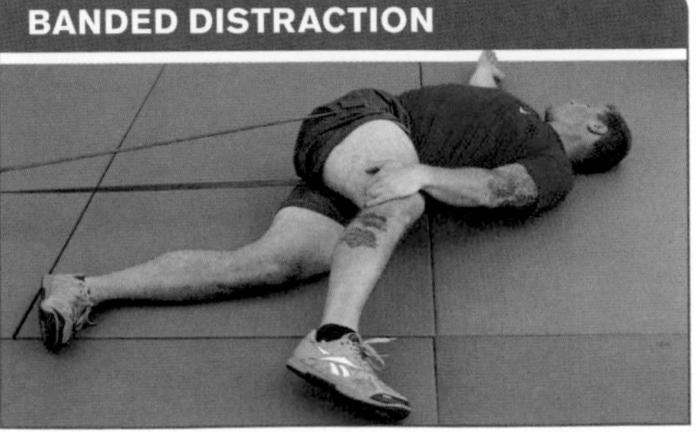

Banded Distraction: Attaching a band to your hip and distracting toward your feet makes this mob 100 times more effective.

Lateral Hip Opener

IMPROVES:
Low back pain and stiffness
Global rotation
Lateral extension

Athletes with low back pain often attack things from the front and back but neglect to work from the side. You must approach the issue from all angles. Performing this basic lateral side bend is just you being responsible for your global stiffness. You'll find that your obliques, ribs, and QL are tacked down and really tight, which contributes to your pain and restriction. This is a simple mobilization that you can drop in after a workout or as you're watching TV. The key is to keep your hips planted on the ground and your torso and arm on the same vertical plane as you fall to the side. Imagine that there are two parallel panes of glass in front of and behind your body, preventing you from folding forward or falling backward. As with all the lateral openers, I recommend using this technique to test and retest the efficacy of the Oblique Side Smash and Low Back Smash mobs.

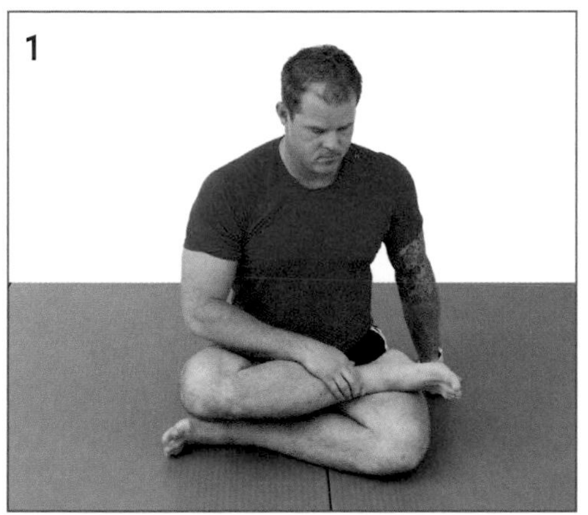

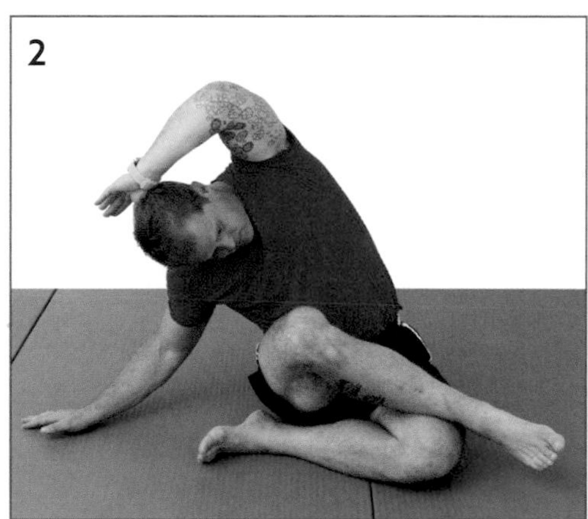

1. From a crossed-legged position, pull your right foot over your left knee.
2. With your right leg holding down your left hip, bring your left arm over your head and fall to your right side. Keep your torso and arm on the same vertical plane as you lean over your right hip.

Lateral Side Opener

IMPROVES:
Low back pain and stiffness
Global rotation
Lateral extension

This is a variation of the previous technique, which mobilizes the lateral compartment encompassing the oblique, QL, ribs, and hip. This mobilization can be performed on a keg, physioball, or medicine ball stacked on some plates. Just like the Lateral Hip Opener, you want to avoid twisting as you bend over your side. Adding rotation will cause you to overextend, which is never okay.

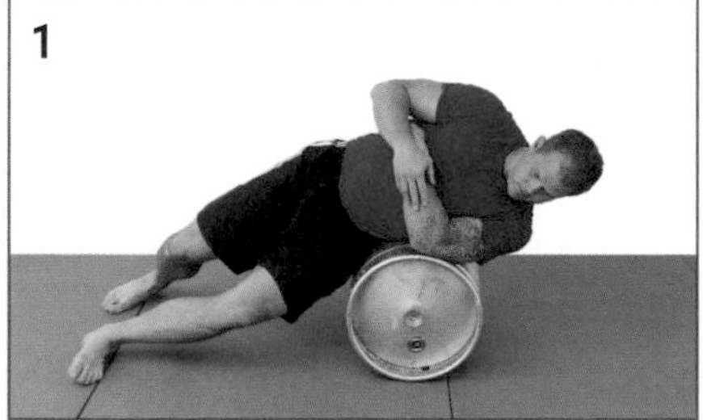

Position your body over a keg.

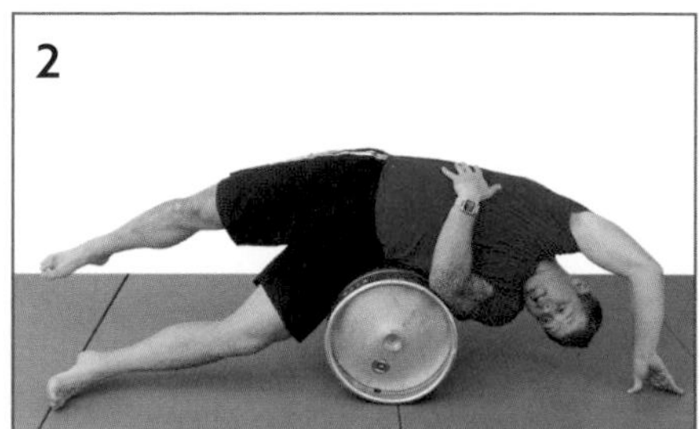

Keeping your midline engaged to avoid rotating, reach your top arm over your head and bend over the keg.

VARIATION

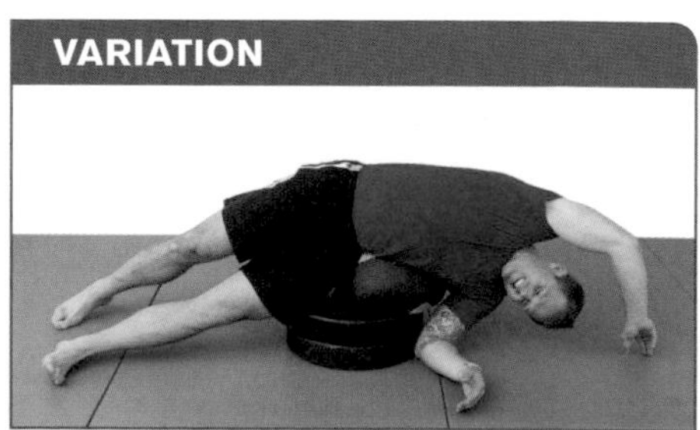

If you don't have a keg or physioball, you can perform this mobilization by stacking a med ball on some bumper plates.

Lunge Archetype

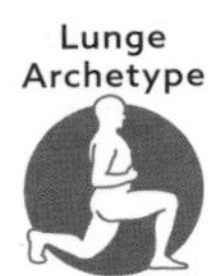

Squat 1 Archetype

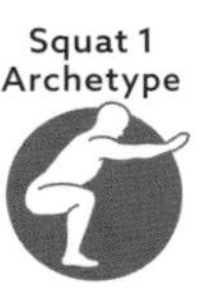

Overhead Archetype

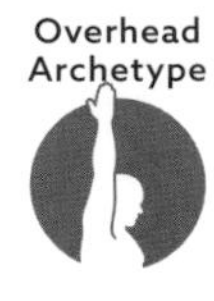

This mobilization will help improve the above archetypes.

IMPROVES:

Hip and low back pain

Sliding surfaces in abdominal musculature

Optimal spinal mechanics

Stabilization of the spine

Flexion and extension of the spine and hip

Rotational capacity

METHODS:

Pressure wave smash (side to side)

Contract and relax

Smash and floss

Targeted Gut Smashing Mobilizations (Psoas and Iliacus)

The trunk is a hardworking system that is bound to get tight, regardless of whether you're organized or disorganized. The simple fact is, you spend a lot of time and energy creating and maintaining stability through your midline, which causes the layers of your abdominal structure, particularly your psoas, to get tacked down and stiff. If you're hanging out or moving in dysfunctional positions, the psoas and surrounding musculature have to work extra hard to stabilize your spine.

The psoas is a big bastard of a muscle that crosses from your diaphragm and lumbar region of the vertebral column to your pelvis and leg. It has the supreme responsibility for stabilizing your spine, flexing your hip, and powering rotation. So if it gets tight and tacked down to the surrounding structures, it's going to cause a lot of problems—like an inflamed low back or cruddy movement patterns. This is another reason why you want to avoid sitting for extended periods. With your hips closed and the muscles of your primary engine turned off, your psoas has to work really hard to keep your spine stabilized.

Imagine bending your arm 90 degrees and then having someone pull on your hand, putting a low-grade tug on your biceps, for 6 hours. What do you think is going to happen to your biceps? It will get brutally tight, causing acute pain in your elbow and shoulder. This is exactly what happens to your psoas when you sit for a long time. Your psoas is under constant tension to maintain an upright position, causing your hips and low back to hurt. This is one of the reasons I encourage people to use some kind of lumbar support that forces the spine into a neutral position. In a neutral position, your psoas isn't overburdened trying to maintain normal lumbar curves.

Always prioritize optimal spinal mechanics by enforcing good positions. You also have to feed some love to the large muscle that supports these structures; otherwise you will end up in pain. In the following sequence, I demonstrate a few different options that you can use to restore suppleness to your psoas. Please note that these are acute, targeted approaches aimed at releasing the superficial layers of stiffness. To get the biggest impact on the psoas, as well as to hammer the surrounding abdominal tissues, use the Global Gut Smash on page 365.

Option 1: Lacrosse Ball Smash and Floss

Although this mobilization represents the lowest form of psoas smashing, it's not a bad place to start, especially if you've never smashed your psoas before. Executing this option first will help prepare you for the more tortuous mobs, as well as tap into some of the superficial layers of the muscle.

TARGET AREA

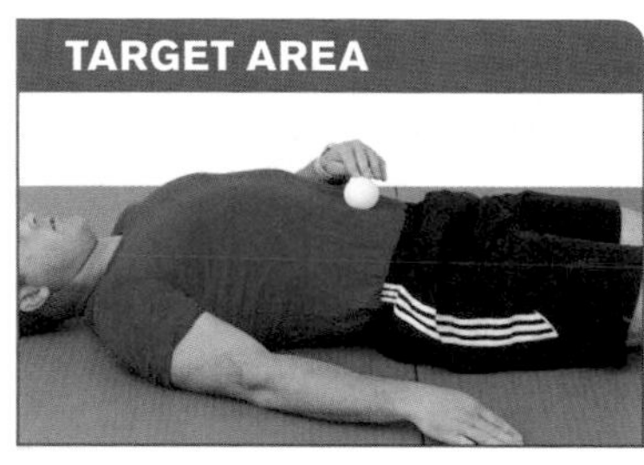

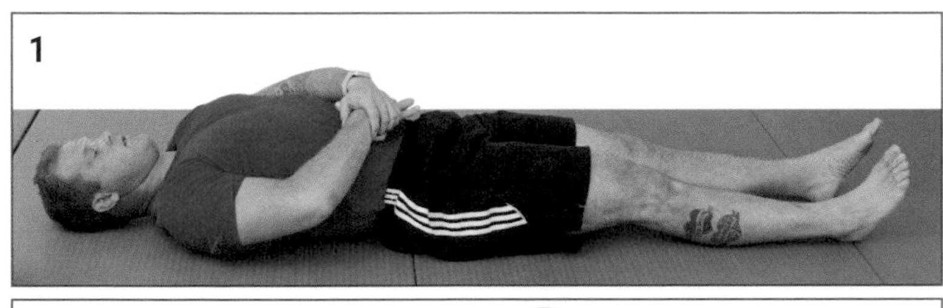

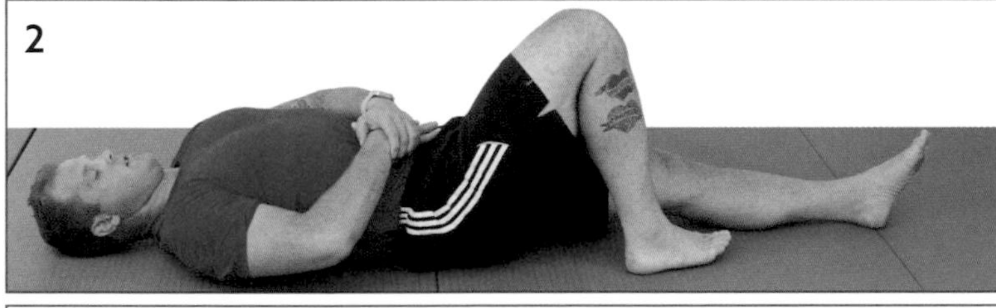

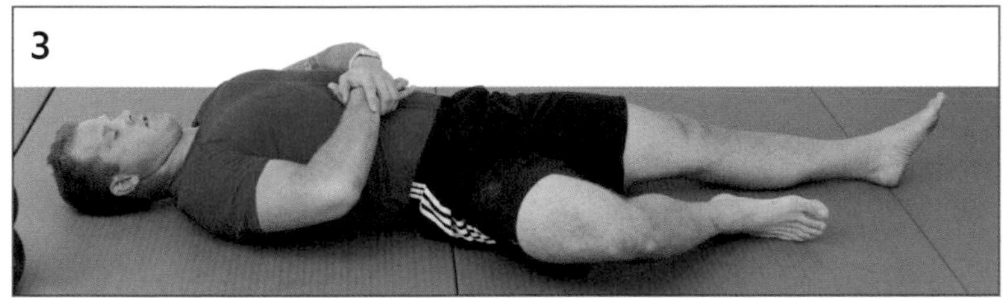

1. Position a lacrosse ball a couple of inches to the outside of your belly button, then use both hands to push the ball into the lateral structures of your abdominals.

2. Having tacked down a piece of your psoas, bring your knee up and try to floss around the belly tissues underneath the ball.

3. Drop your right knee out to the side, keeping downward pressure on the ball. From here, you can move your knee from side to side, straighten your leg, or move on to another area of your psoas. The goal is to find an area that feels painful, tack down the tissue, and then apply a flossing element.

Option 2: Kettlebell + Lacrosse Ball Psoas & Iliacus Smash 1

This is the same idea as option 1, but instead of using your hands, you position a kettlebell over the lacrosse ball to get more acute pressure into the area.

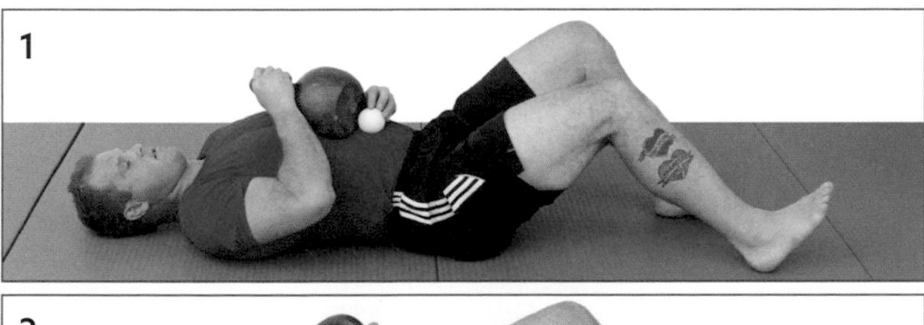

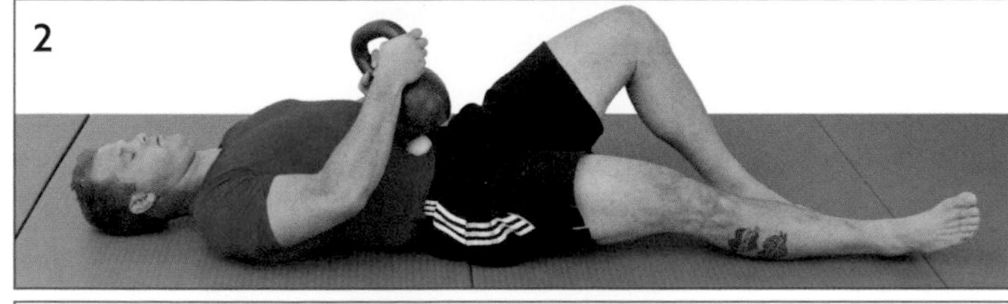

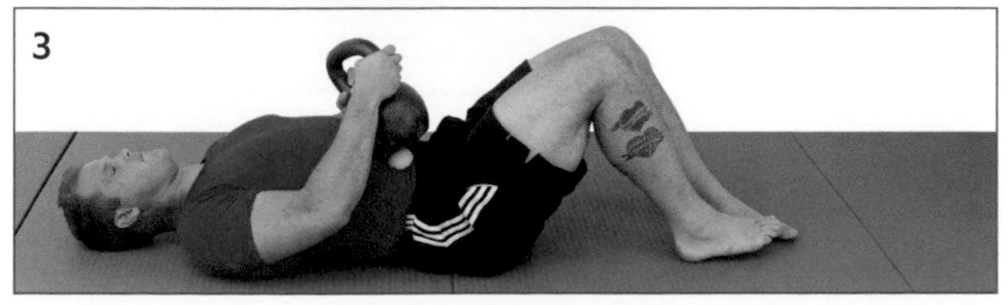

1. Position a lacrosse ball a couple of inches to the outside of your belly button, then position the base of a kettlebell over the ball.

2. With the kettlebell smashing the ball into a stiff spot on your psoas, straighten your leg and begin flossing around the tacked-down tissue.

3. Elevate your knee. From here, you can externally and internally rotate your leg, as well as flex and straighten your knee until you feel some change in the tissue.

Option 3: Kettlebell + Lacrosse Ball Psoas & Iliacus Smash 2

This option gives you a slightly different stimulus by placing your legs up on a box. This takes a bit of tension out of the psoas and iliacus, which allows you to penetrate deep into the pelvic area. The idea here is to extend and flex your leg and pull tension into some of the neural tissues—like the sciatic nerve—to ensure that the nerves are flossing smoothly through the psoas meat tunnel.

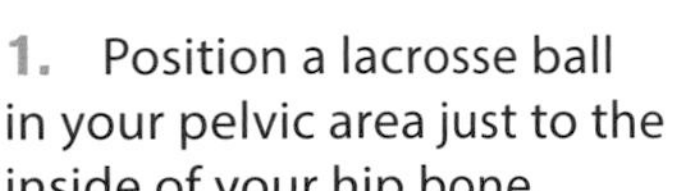

1. Position a lacrosse ball in your pelvic area just to the inside of your hip bone.

2. Add pressure by positioning the base of a kettlebell over the ball.

3. With the weight of the kettlebell driving the ball deep into your pelvic area, straighten your leg and flex your foot. This enables you to floss around the stiff, tacked-down tissues of your psoas.

4. Continue to floss around the tacked-down neural tissues by extending your right foot.

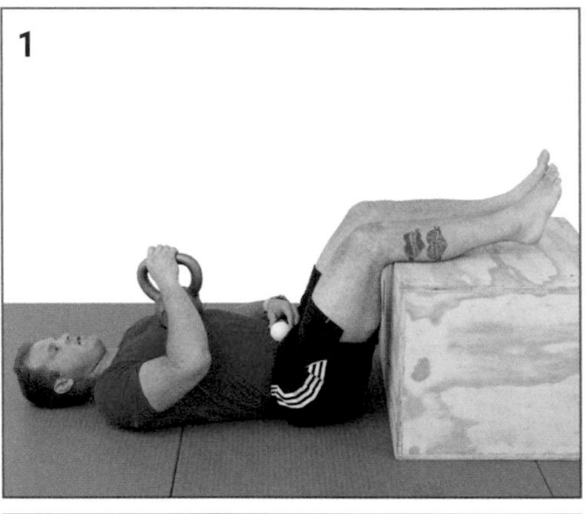

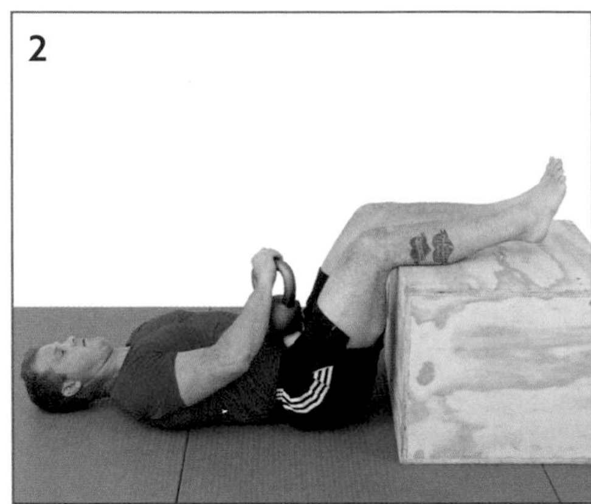

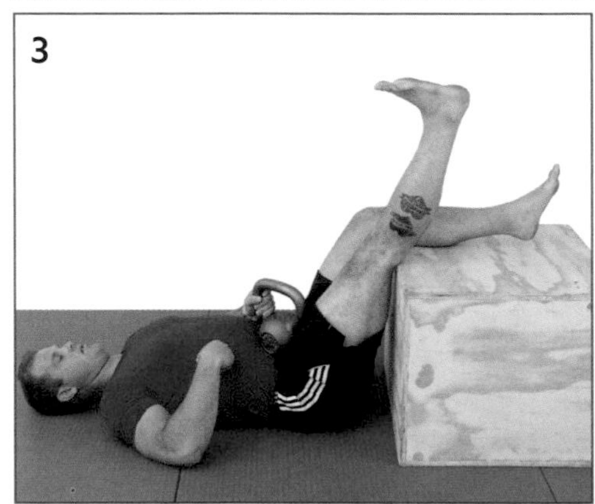

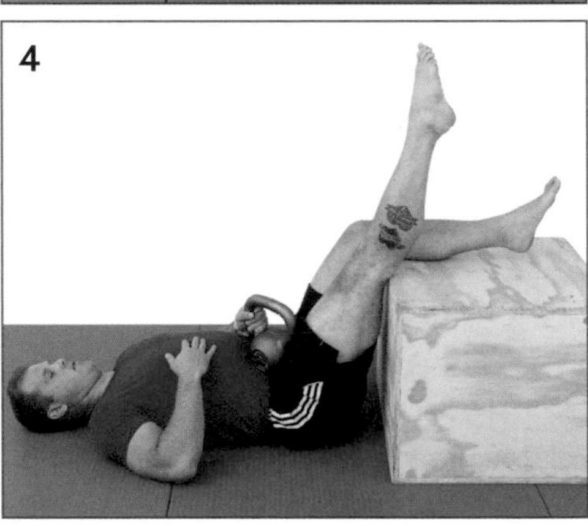

Option 4: Kettlebell + Lacrosse Ball Psoas & Iliacus Smash 3

This variation biases your leg into extension, which stretches or lengths the psoas and iliacus. To get the most out of this mob, take the tension out of your psoas and iliacus by drawing your knee toward your chest. As I mentioned in option 3, this allows the ball to sink deeper into your pelvic region. After a few breaths, drop your leg off the table and put your leg into extension.

1. Raise your leg to take the tension out of your psoas and iliacus, position a lacrosse ball on your pelvic area to the inside of your hip bone, and then add pressure by placing the base of a kettlebell over the ball.

2. Take a few breaths to let the ball sink into your abdomen, then extend your hip, allowing your leg to hang over the edge of the table. From here, you can swing your leg from side to side, extend and flex your knee, contract and relax, and focus your breath into the ball.

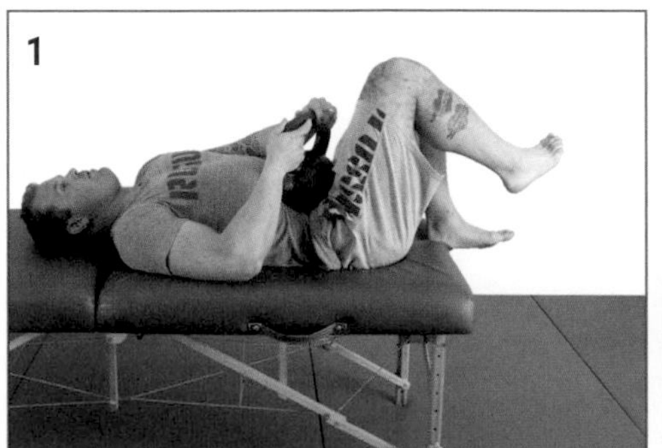

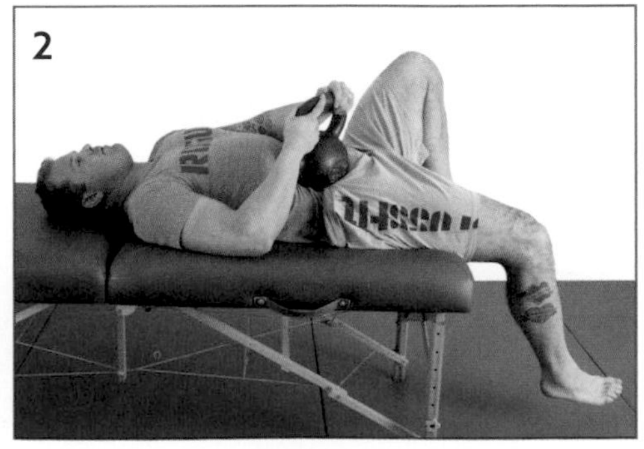

Option 5: Bubo Barbell Psoas & Iliacus Smash

The bubo barbell variation is another great option. As you can see, it's not the most flattering mob, but it definitely gets the job done. The barbell gives you a ton of control because you can twist and shake the bar to delaminate gummed-up tissue.

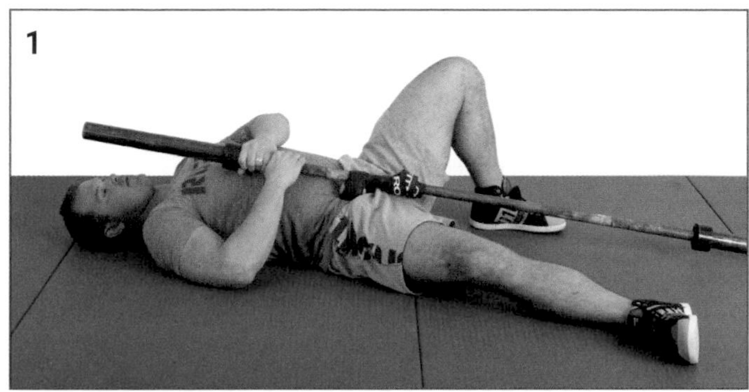

Attach a lacrosse ball to a barbell, then wedge the ball into your pelvic area to the inside of your hip bone.

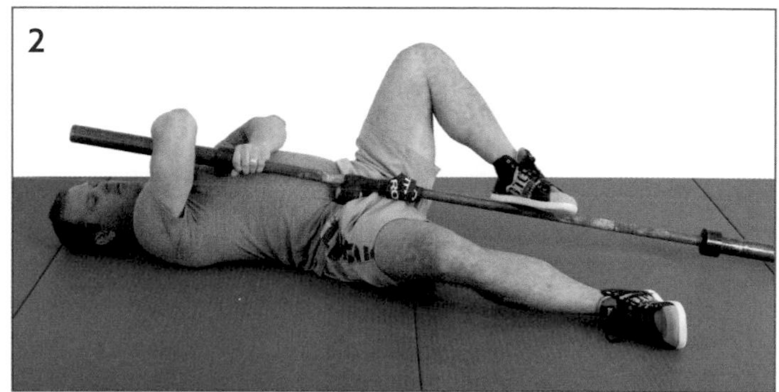

To add pressure, step your foot on the bar and push down with both hands. You can twist the bar and judder it up and down around trigger points.

Option 6: Supernova (Alpha Ball) Smash and Floss

Although it's not as pinpointed, using a larger ball enables you to penetrate deeper into the superficial layers of the psoas and surrounding abdominal tissue. You can use a smash and floss approach by moving your leg around, or you can roll from side to side and explore the outside and inside layers of your abdominal musculature. Basically, anything that makes you feel like vomiting is probably worth your time.

TARGET AREA

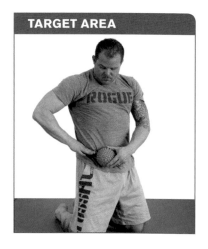

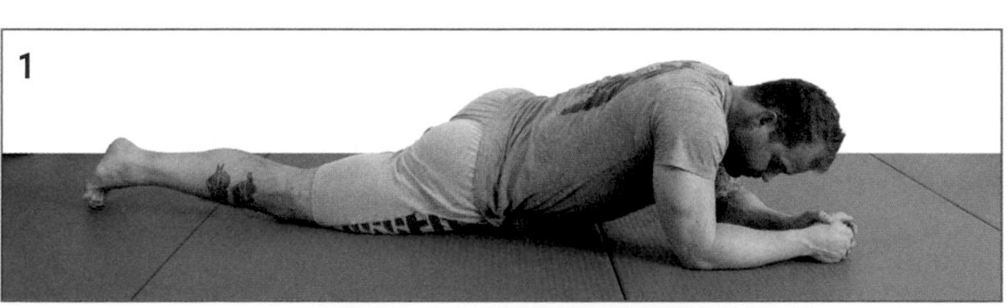

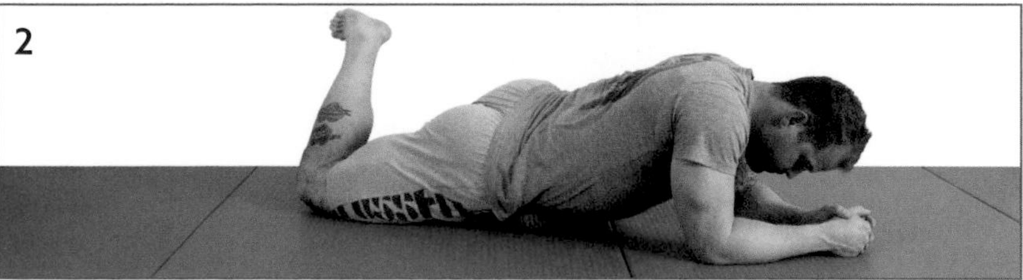

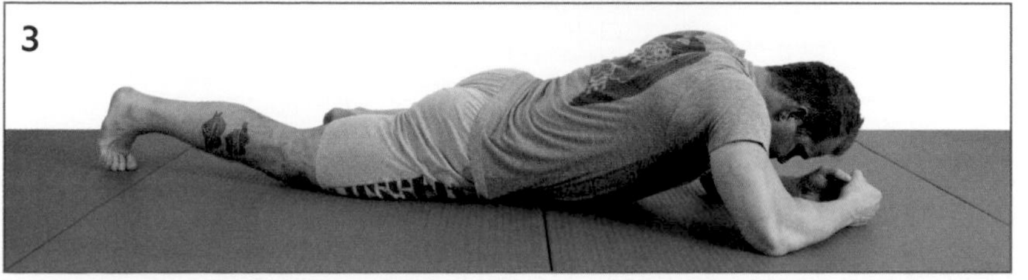

1. Lie down over the ball, positioning it between your belly button and hip bone.

2. After finding a stiff spot, take a big breath, hold it for a few seconds, and then exhale, relaxing into the ball. With your psoas and the surrounding tissue tacked down, floss around it by curling your heel to your butt. You can also move your leg from side to side.

3. Still pressuring your weight into the ball, straighten your leg and then rotate your body slowly to the side to get a pressure wave effect across the tissue.

Option 7: Kettlebell Handle Psoas Smash

This mobilization targets the hard-to-reach iliacus muscle, which is nestled to the inside of your hip bone. Think of the iliacus as the neglected neighbor of the psoas. Often referred to as the iliopsoas because they share a common attachment at the lesser trochanter (upper inner side of the femur), the iliacus—like the psoas—is prone to becoming adaptively short from prolonged sitting or lack of use through a full range of motion (think hip extension). When the psoas and iliacus are not functioning at their normal lengths, trigger points can develop in the muscles and cause mayhem downstream. For example, trigger points in the iliacus can cause referral pains (numbness, tingling, aching, and so on) in the groin, hip, leg, and low back.

Because the iliacus is tucked behind your pelvis, mobilizing the muscle on your own is not easy. To target your iliacus (and groin, for that matter), you have to get creative and use the tools at your disposal. For example, you can get in there with a lacrosse ball (see options 2, 3, and 4), or use the handle of the kettlebell, as demonstrated here.

Note: Be very careful when executing this mob. Don't haphazardly lie on the kettlebell with the full weight of your body. Control the pressure by keeping four points of contact with the ground (all limbs touching the floor), floss cautiously—meaning take it slow—and use breathing in conjunction with the contract and relax method. If you're new to gut smashing, work your way up to this mob using the previous options.

SETUP

Position a kettlebell so the handle is at a 45-degree angle to your body. If you're targeting the right side of your body, turn the handle clockwise. If you're targeting the left side of your body, turn it counterclockwise.

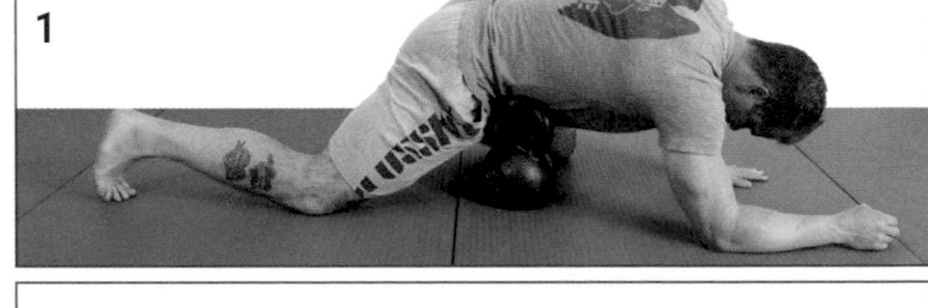

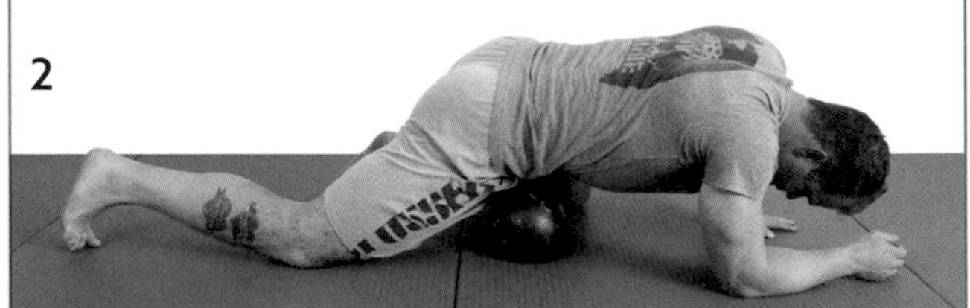

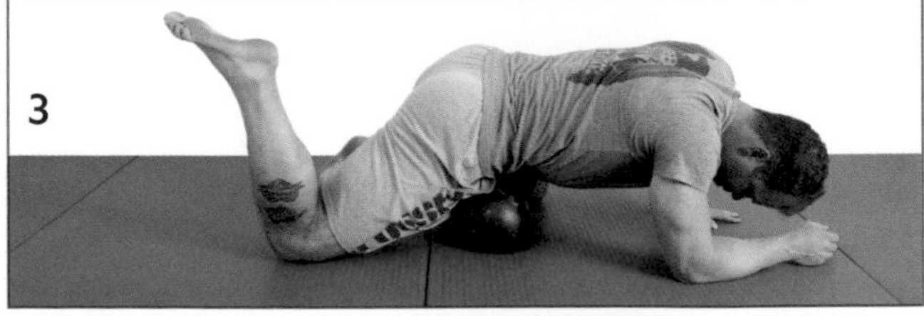

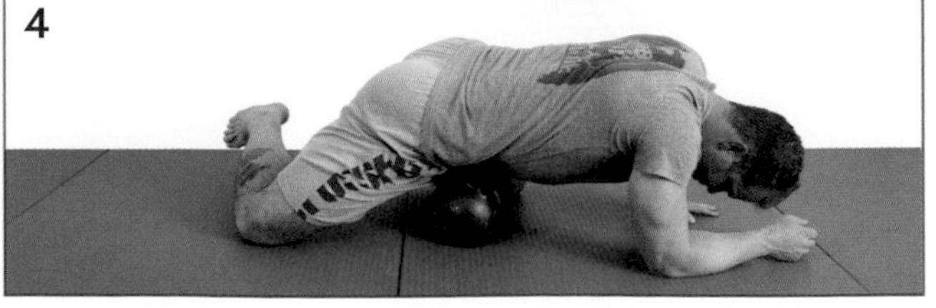

1. Lie down over a kettlebell, positioning it between your belly button and hip bone.

2. After finding a stiff spot, take a big breath in, hold it for a few seconds, and then exhale, relaxing into the kettlebell.

3. With your psoas and the surrounding tissue tacked down, floss around it by curling your heel to your butt. You can also move your leg from side to side.

4. Still pressing your weight into the kettlebell, straighten your leg and then rotate your body slowly to the side to get a pressure wave effect across the tissue.

Diaphragm Gut Smash

The respiratory diaphragm, which is the primary breathing muscle, is the most central muscle in the human body. Yet it is often overlooked when it comes to gut smashing. Understand that your respiratory diaphragm gets stiff just like anything else, especially if you're practicing poor posture. When your ribcage and pelvis are out of alignment, they pull on the respiratory diaphragm, creating trigger points, imbalances, and stiffness throughout the torso. What happens when the muscle that you use to breathe gets stiff and weak? You can't breathe as efficiently, which accelerates fatigue. You can't create as much intra-abdominal pressure (abdominal tension), compromising your ability to brace. What's more, a stiff diaphragm essentially locks you into a sympathetic state. As you might recall from chapter 6, your sympathetic nervous system activates stress functions that prepare your body for action. In other words, a stiff and restricted respiratory diaphragm keeps you in fight-or-flight mode—not exactly ideal when you're trying to relax or get ready for bed.

Addressing the problem requires a twofold approach. First, you have to fix your posture. As discussed in chapter 1, efficient breathing happens naturally when your ribcage and pelvis are in alignment. Stated differently, when you're working from a neutral spinal position, you tend to breathe diaphragmatically. That is, you breathe using your primary breathing muscle—your respiratory diaphragm.

In addition to prioritizing spinal mechanics, you need to spend some time smashing your diaphragm. I recommend that you implement one of these following two options at least once a week, and that you do it right before bed or anytime you're trying to wind down. Doing so will turn on your parasympathetic nervous system, which activates the body functions that prepare your body for rest (the exact opposite of being in a sympathetic state).

Think about it like this: When your respiratory diaphragm is stiff, your breathing is compromised. And when your breathing is compromised, everything is compromised.

IMPROVES:

Diaphragmatic breathing
Spinal mechanics

METHODS:

Smash and floss
Pressure wave
Contract and relax
Tack and spin

TARGET AREA

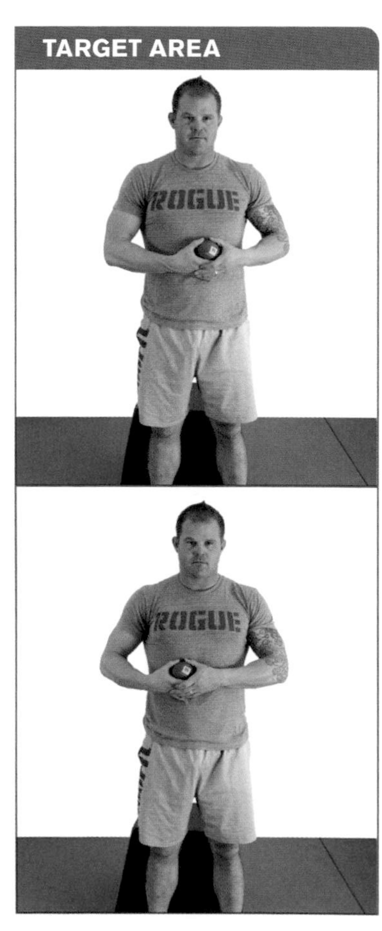

To target your respiratory diaphragm, scour the border of your ribcage, but be careful to avoid your solar plexus (at the center of your ribcage).

Option 1: Elevated Diaphragm Gut Smash

Smashing your diaphragm on an elevated surface such as a box, table, or chair is ideal for two reasons: You can scour the border of your ribcage and control your breath into the ball more effectively than when mobilizing from the ground. Be careful to avoid your solar plexus (at the center of your ribcage).

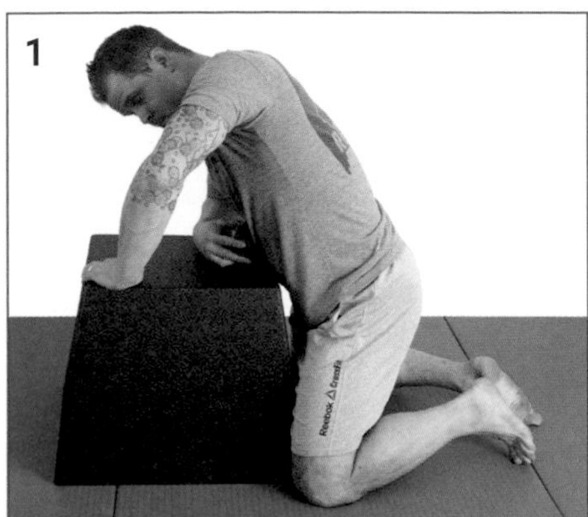

Positioning an Alpha ball, Supernova, or softball at the border of your ribcage, lean over a box, countertop, or chair.

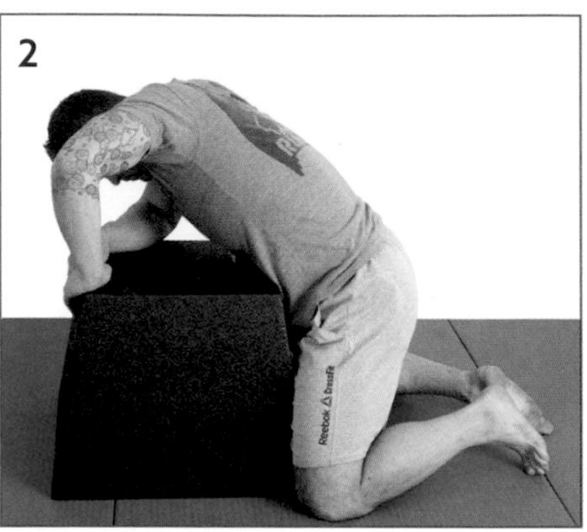

Use your breath in conjunction with your weight to drive the ball deeper into your diaphragm. Do so by taking a big breath, contracting for a few seconds as you hold your breath, and then exhaling, relaxing and allowing your body to sink over the ball.

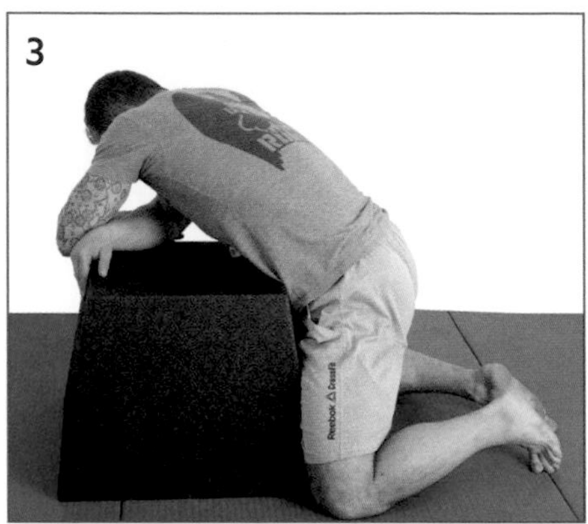

Once you can breathe without pain, try twisting your body from side to side while keeping your weight over the ball. You can also twist the ball to take up the soft tissue slack—see option 2.

Option 2: Grounded Diaphragm Gut Smash

You can also mobilize your diaphragm from the ground. It's not as effective as mobilizing on an elevated surface, but you can still get some quality work done.

TARGET AREA

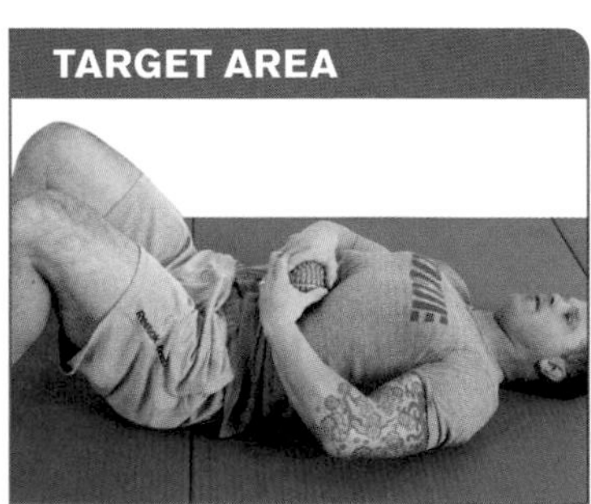

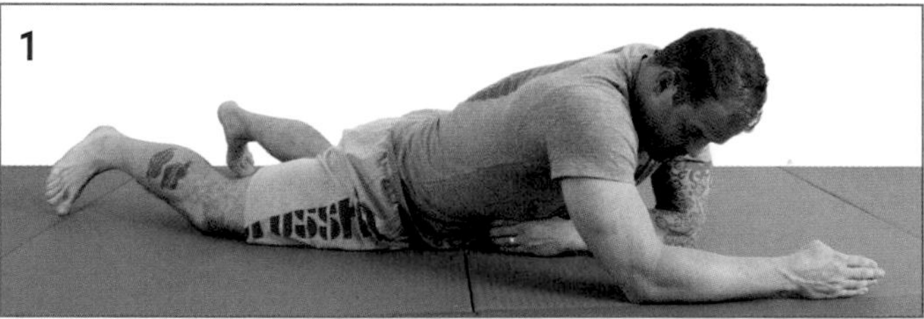

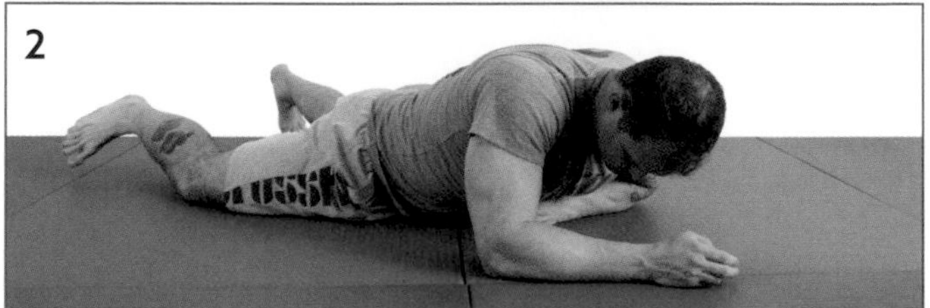

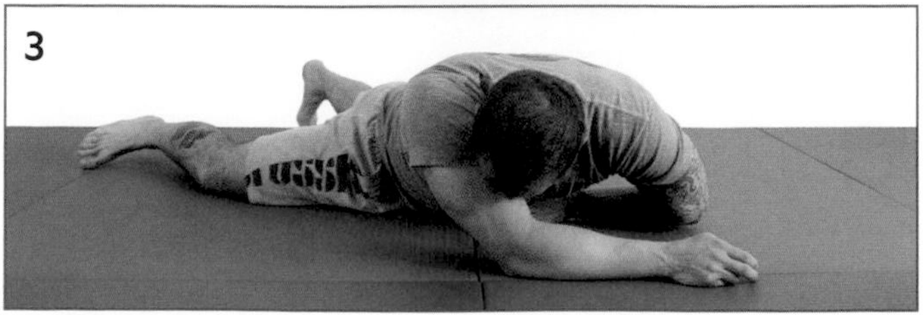

1. Position the ball along the border of your ribcage.
2. To take up the soft tissue slack, twist the ball. From here, you can contract and relax and use your breath to create more pressure.
3. As described above, twist your body from side to side and create movement around the tacked-down tissue.

Global Gut Smash ("The Jilly")

As its name implies, the Global Gut Smash hits all the abdominal musculature surrounding your psoas. Think of it like this: Using a lacrosse ball targets one piece of your psoas like a chisel attacks stone, whereas the Global Gut Smash is like taking a sledgehammer to all the abdominal musculature and tissue surrounding the psoas. Remember, you need these muscles to slide and move over one another unrestricted. If they are matted down and adhered, your entire kinetic system is compromised.

Not only do we rely on these muscles to stabilize, flex, and rotate the spine in our day-to-day lives, but we also spend a ton of our strength and conditioning efforts learning to create and maintain maximum trunk stiffness. Yet we do nothing to "unstiffify" the area. In order for you to be a fully functional elite warrior leopard, that tissue needs to be like filet mignon, not a grisly piece of beef jerky.

This mobilization is especially important if you've had any kind of abdominal surgery. Procedures like C-sections and appendectomies leave behind a lot of scarred layers of tissue that need ungluing. Moreover, if you have a history of low back pain or you sit for long periods, this mob gets a gold star and should be placed near the center of your mobility target.

To execute the Global Gut Smash, use a large ball that has some pliability, like a kid's ball, mini physioball, or soccer ball. Harder balls should be reserved for VooDoo leopard Jedis. As you will soon realize, this mobilization is not pleasant. Don't pass out in the back corner of the pain cave or vomit on your living room floor. That's not cool. Remember, if the layers of your abdominal muscles are sliding as they should, you will feel little pain or visceral symptoms, achiness, pulling, or burning sensations. It will just feel normal. However, if you're a tacked-down mess, expect pain and discomfort. Ten minutes is the minimum commitment to effect change, so pony up.

Note: Don't perform this mobilization before doing any heavy lifting. The last thing you want to do is monkey around with your spinal mechanics before you max deadlift. While I don't think it would cause injury (in fact, you might experience great exercising after this mobilization), it's better to be safe and save it for after your workout.

Lunge Archetype

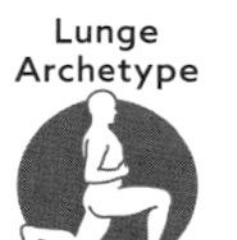

Squat 1 Archetype

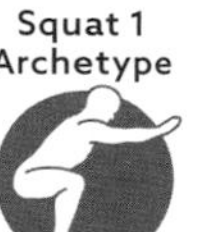

Squat 2 Archetype

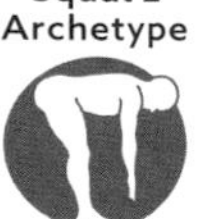

This mobilization will help improve the above archetypes.

IMPROVES:

Hip and low back pain
Sliding surfaces in abdominal musculature
Spinal mechanics
Stabilization of the spine
Flexion and extension of the spine and hip
Rotational capacity

METHODS:

Pressure wave smash (side to side)
Contract and relax
Smash and floss

TOOLS

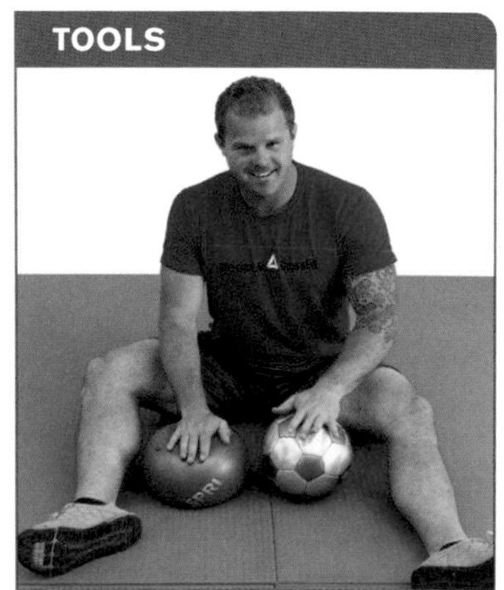

TARGET AREA

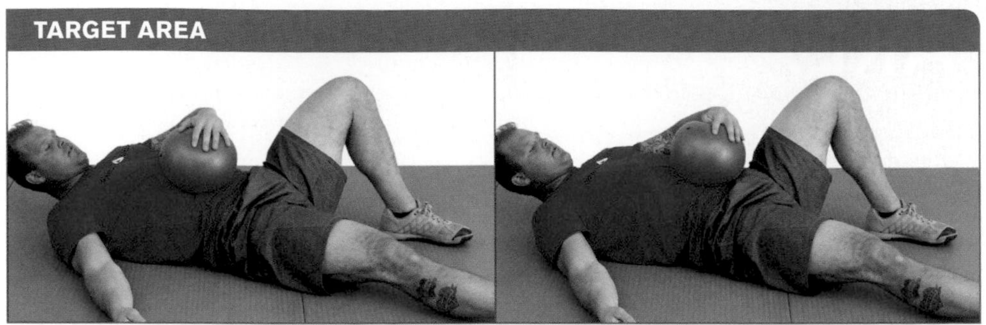

The target area for the Global Gut Smash covers the region from the tops of your hip bones, around your pelvis, up to your diaphragm, and around your ribcage (basically your entire abdominal section).

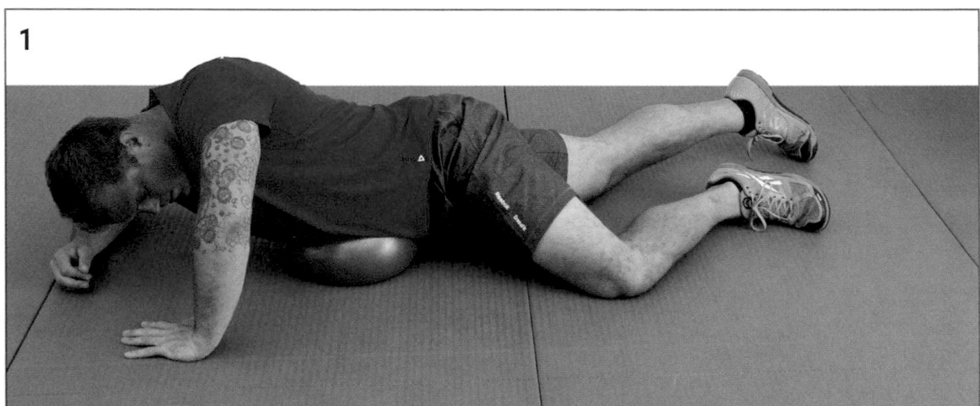

1

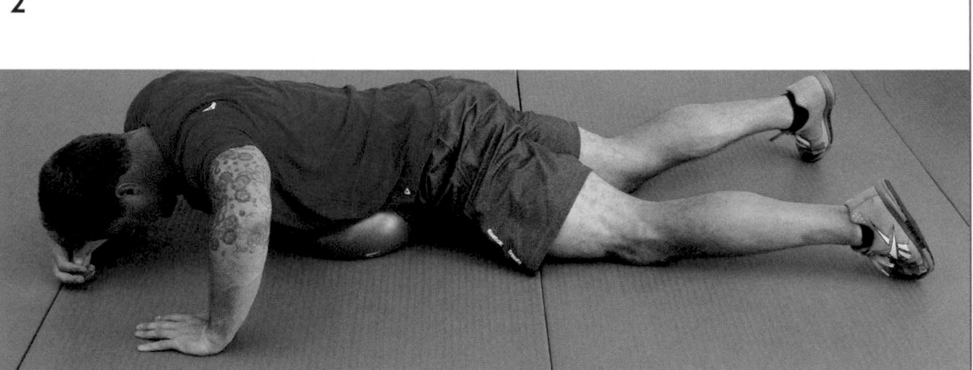

2

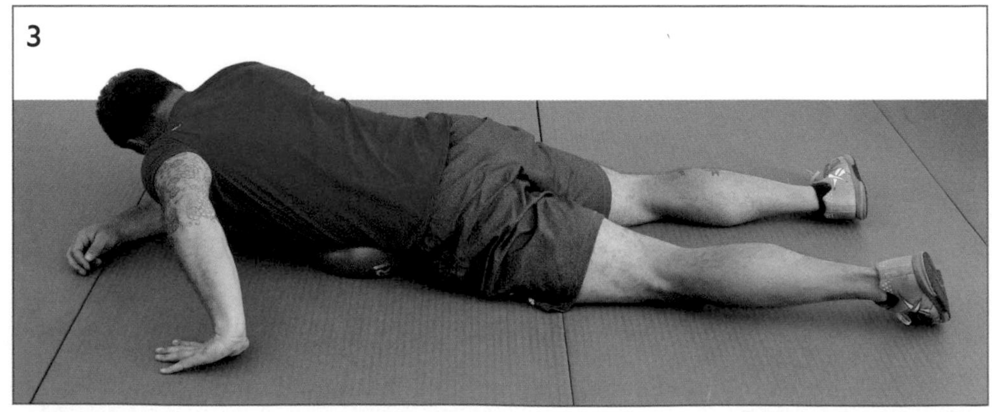

3

1. Lie over the ball, positioning it between your hip bones and ribcage.

2. For the best results, you need to penetrate into the basement level of your tissues by sinking all your weight into the ball. To do so, take a big breath, hold it for a few seconds, and then exhale. As you breathe out, relax your weight over the ball and sink deeper into your gut as if you were a piece of melted cheese.

3. After getting your full weight over the ball, slowly pressure wave. If you find a tight spot, you can contract and relax by holding in air and then exhaling to sink further into the bottom, or implement a smash and floss technique. Spend at least 10 minutes on the area—5 minutes on each side.

AREA 7 GLUTES, HIP CAPSULES

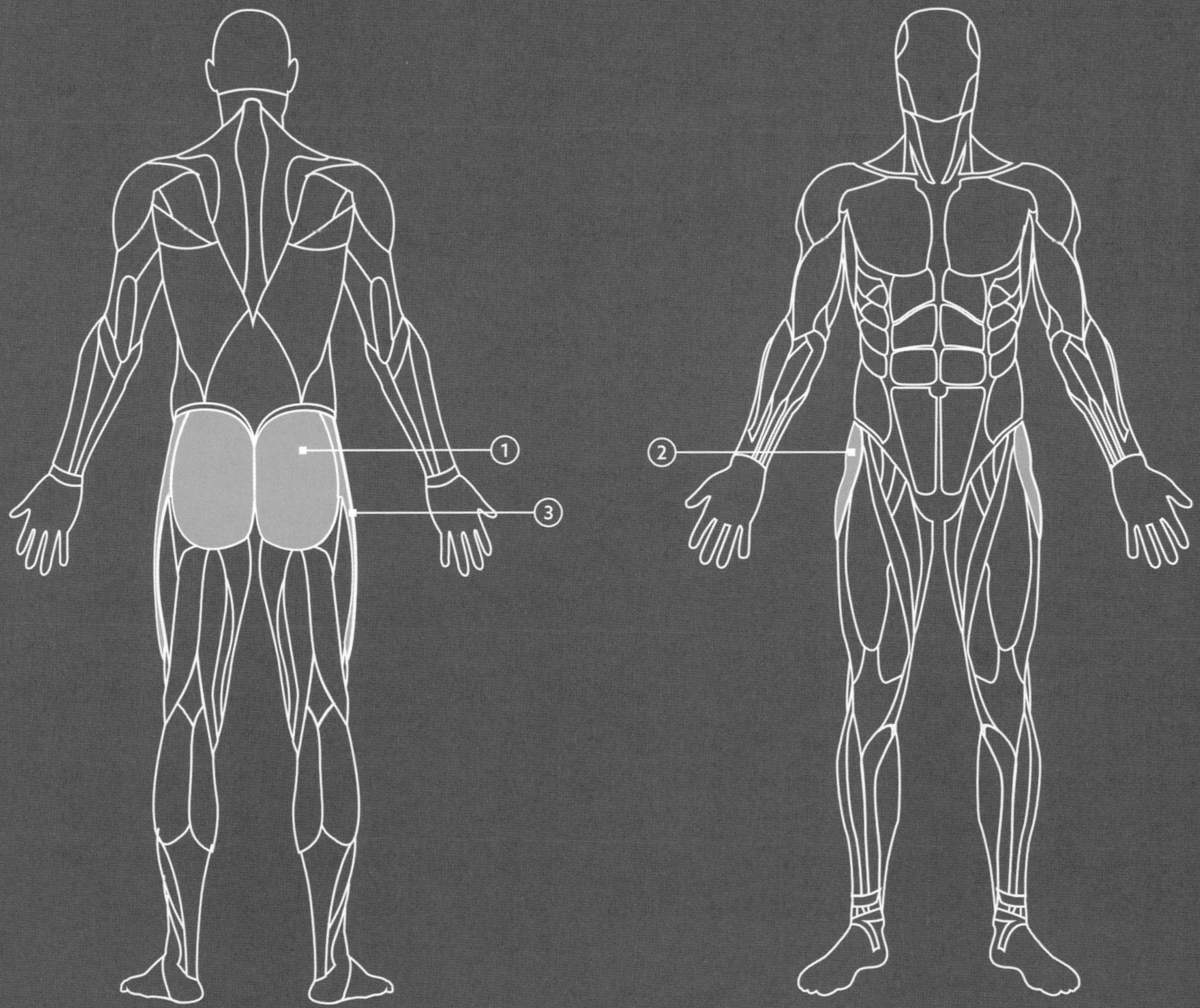

MOBILIZATION TARGET AREAS:

1

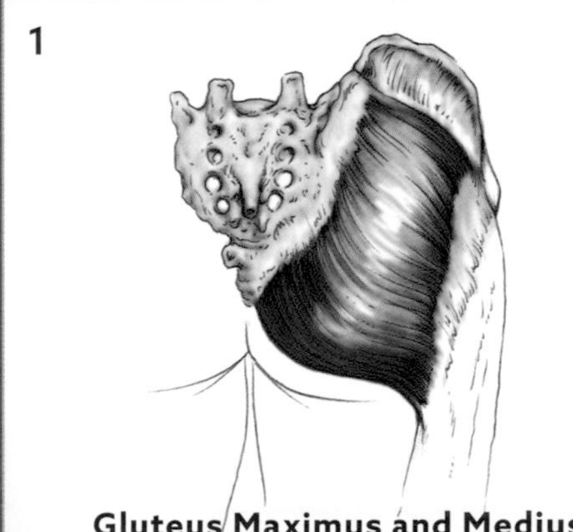

Gluteus Maximus and Medius

2

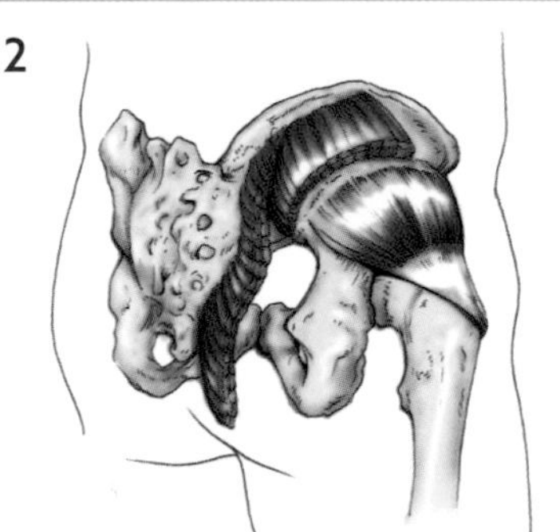

Gluteus Minimus (and cutaways of Maximus and Medius)

3

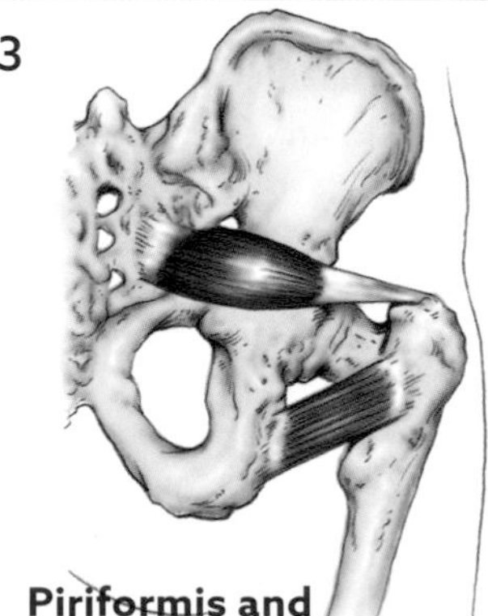

Piriformis and Quadratus Femoris

Squat 1 Archetype | Squat 2 Archetype | Lunge Archetype

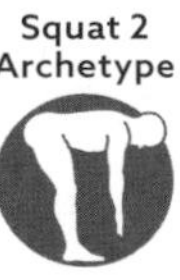
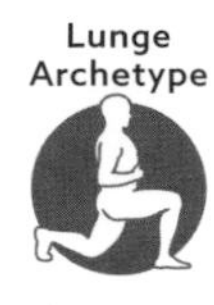

This mobilization will help improve the above archetypes.

IMPROVES:

Hip and low back pain

METHODS:

Pressure wave
Smash and floss
Contract and relax

TARGET AREA

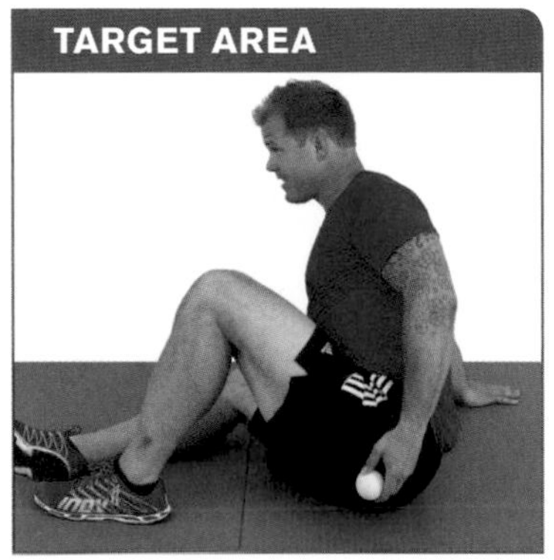

1. Position a lacrosse ball in the side of your hip.
2. With the ball tacking down the underlying muscle, move the surrounding tissue around by externally rotating your leg and dropping your knee to the mat.
3. Continue to floss the tacked-down tissue by pulling your knee in toward your center.
4. In addition to smashing and flossing with internal and external rotation of your leg, slowly roll from side to side across your glute. Focus on pancaking across the grain of the tissue in a pressure wave fashion. If you stumble across a particularly painful area, contract and relax until you get to the bottom of the tissue.

Glute Smash and Floss

Although several habits create stiffness in the high posterior chain, there are two that really mess you up: sitting and assuming an open-foot stance. Sitting creates an inordinate amount of ass lamination, so if you take a long flight, drive for extended periods, or sit at a desk for a living, you have to constantly work on restoring sliding surfaces to the tacked-down quagmire that is your butt. The second issue, which can run parallel to or separate from the sitting paradigm, is standing or walking around with your feet turned out. If you're in a fully externally rotated position with your feet angled outward, the tissues of your posterior high chain are permanently trapped in a shortened state. The result: Your hip external rotators get smoked, and a lot of full-range movements become untenable.

Want to unglue the laminated tissues of your butt? Jam a lacrosse ball in the side of your glute and find an ugly area of trashed tissue. Then use the three sliding surface techniques—pressure wave, smash and floss, and contract and relax. Don't feel like you need to overcomplicate this mobilization by targeting specific muscles. People like to say, "Hit your glute med or short hip rotators." If your last anatomy lesson involved dissecting a frog, this advice might leave you a tad clueless. What's important is that you find your business and put in some quality work, staying on the tight area until you make change. Fundamental stuff.

As with the other large muscle group mobilizations, you don't need to cover the entire glute region in one session. Set a timer for 5 minutes a cheek and put in some work. You'll be surprised at what a difference it makes. To test and retest, employ the butt acuity test. It's easy to do and illuminating. Spend 5 minutes on one cheek, then stand up and squeeze your glutes as hard as you can. You'll find that the side you mobilized contracts with a lot more force than the other. What does that mean? You just got a little bit stronger and more powerful. It's like a free superpower.

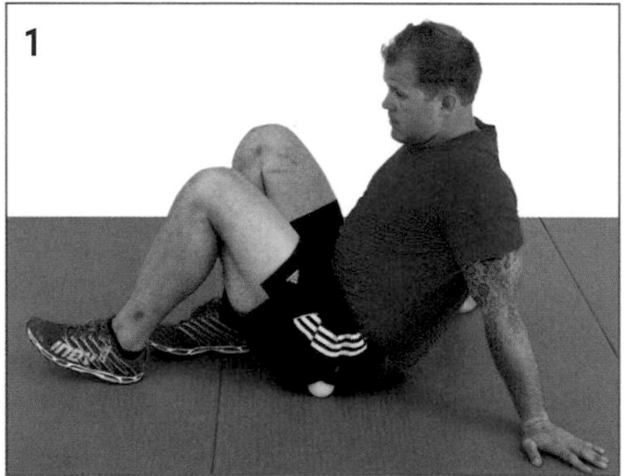

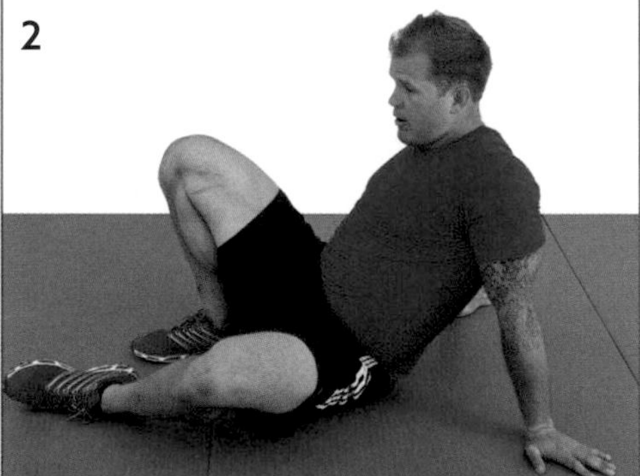

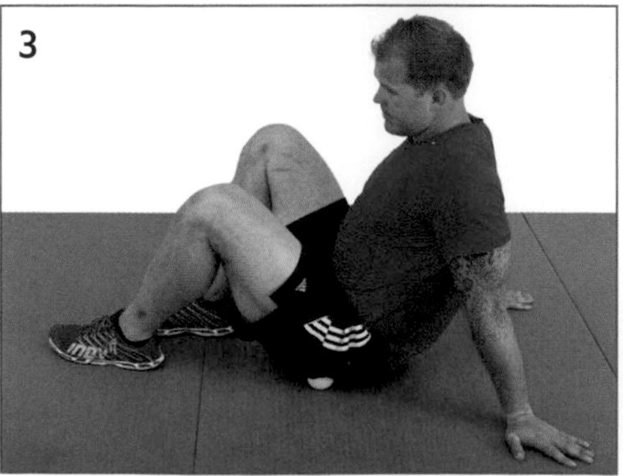

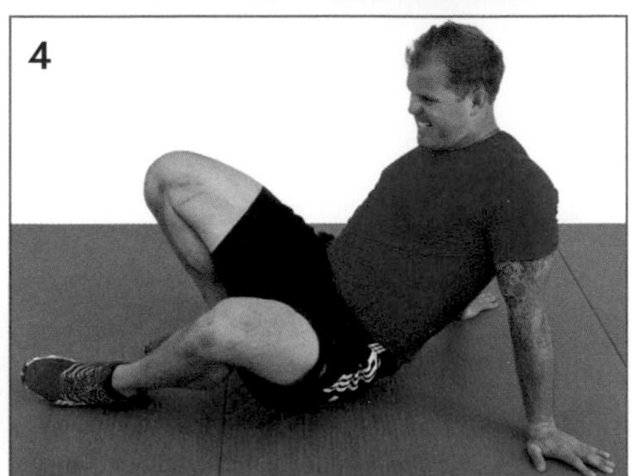

High Glute Smash and Floss

Your glutes are responsible for extending your hips and trunk. When these tissues get tight, generating force through your primary engine becomes difficult. Think about it like this: If you can't open your hips to full extension, the only way to achieve an upright torso is to overextend, forcing the musculature of your trunk and lumbar region to stabilize around your bad position. What happens? You lose your ability to generate force, and you end up with hip and low back pain. By simply ungluing the musculature of your high glute and butt region, you can resolve a lot of your positional mechanics and pain upstream and downstream. In most cases, 10 minutes of good smashing enables you to reclaim a neutral posture, create sufficient external rotation torque, and generate force through your primary engine. Not only that, but you feed slack to the tissue upstream, relieving low back pain.

For the best results, post your feet up on a box or bench. This will allow you to capture the high glute region underneath the back and iliac crest of your hip. Elevating your feet also enables you to get more pressure through the ball and to feather from side to side across the grain of your muscle, which is the best way to break up the tissue and restore suppleness to the region.

Note: This mobilization is often used in conjunction with the single lacrosse ball Low Back Smash (page 349).

Squat 2 Archetype Squat 1 Archetype

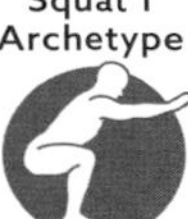

This mobilization will help improve the above archetypes.

IMPROVES:

Hip and low back pain

METHODS:

Pressure wave

Smash and floss

TARGET AREA

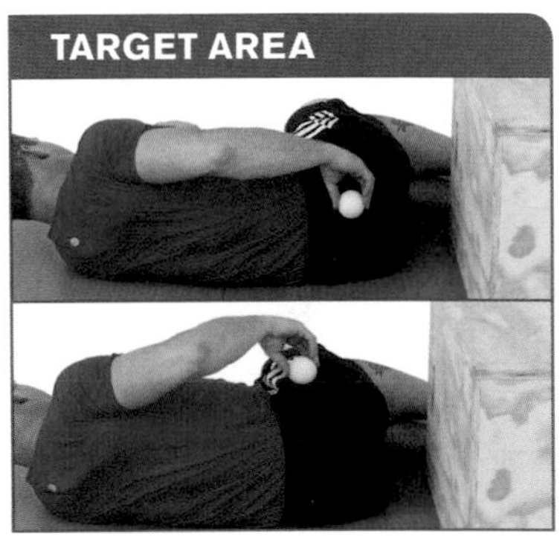

The idea is to hit each motion segment of your spine, stretching from the base of your ribcage to your pelvis.

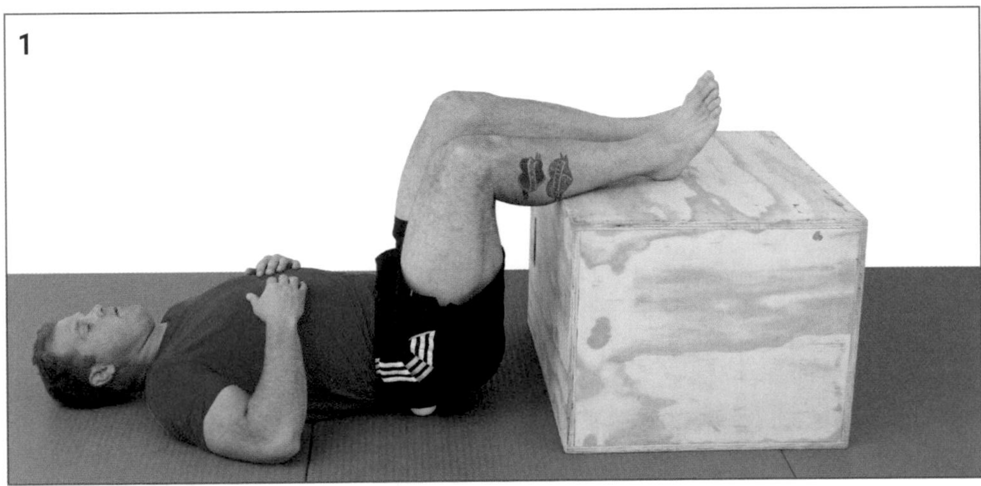

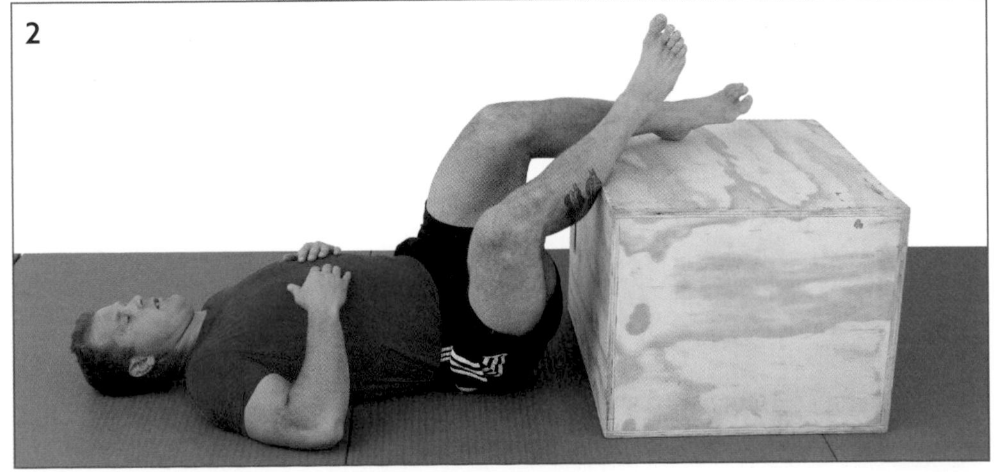

1. Position a lacrosse ball on your upper glute to the outside of your sacrum. To increase the pressure and prevent defaulting into an overextended position, position your feet up on a box.

2. Curling your left heel into the box, slowly roll toward your right side, smashing all the tissues across your upper glute region. The goal is to pressure wave across the grain of the tissue. If you find a really sticky spot, floss around the tacked-down tissue by pulling your knee to your chest and internally and externally rotating your leg.

Squat 2 Archetype · Squat 1 Archetype · Lunge Archetype

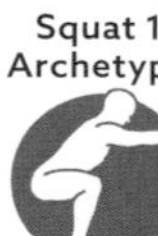
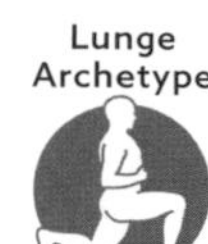

This mobilization will help improve the above archetypes.

IMPROVES:

Hip and low back pain

METHODS:

Pressure wave

Contract and relax

Side Hip Smash

The Side Hip Smash is another easy way to restore hip function as well as feed some slack upstream and downstream of your primary engine (hip). You're trying to capture two areas with this mobilization. As you can see in the photos below, you start on the posterior region of your upper glute, which comes into the top of your hip bone, and rip across that muscle into your hip flexor wad near the front of your hip. This mass, ranging from your posterior glute to the front of your hip, gets chronically stiff and adaptively short. I'm not going to lie: Smashing a lacrosse ball or softball across this stiff tissue is horrible. If you're in public, you might need to cover up that pain face.

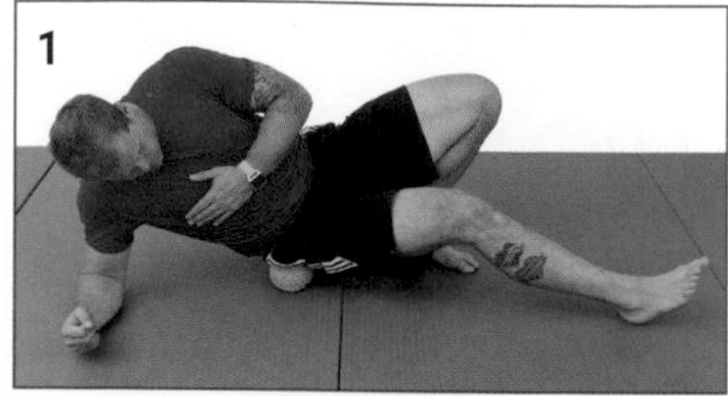
1

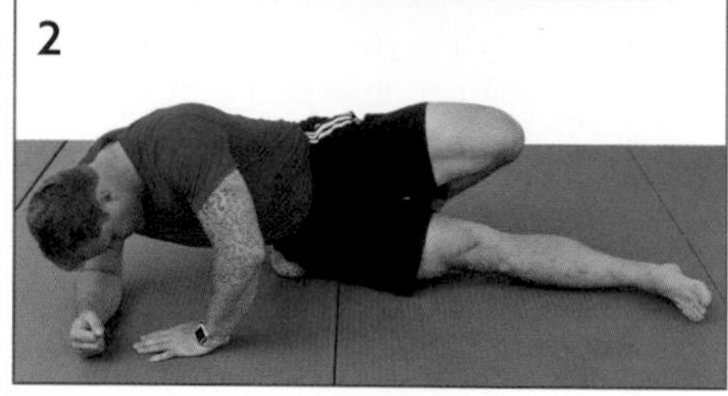
2

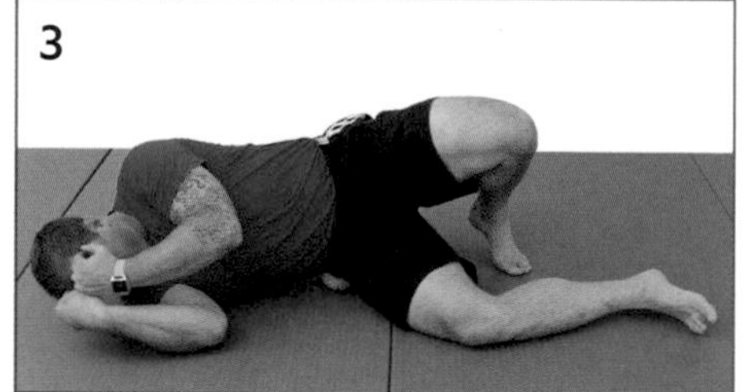
3

1. Position a lacrosse ball or softball on the outside of your high glute, just below your hip bone.

2. Roll onto your belly—distributing as much weight as possible into the ball—and smash the tissue across the muscle fiber.

3. Continue to roll onto your side. For privacy, use both arms to block your pain face from view. Nobody needs to see that.

Squat 2 Archetype · Squat 1 Archetype · Lunge Archetype

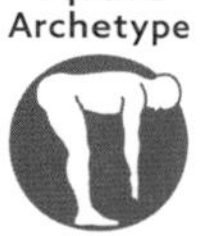
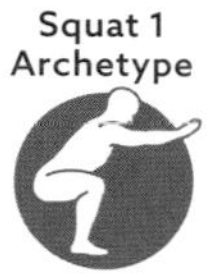
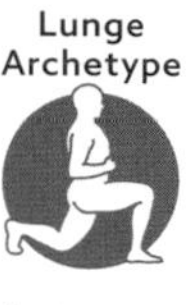

This mobilization will help improve the above archetypes.

METHODS:

Contract and relax

Banded flossing

Single-Leg Flexion with External Rotation

Single-Leg Flexion with External Rotation: Option 1

This mobilization fits perfectly into the model of mobilizing within the context of the movements you're trying to change. Notice in the photos on the following page that I'm essentially mobilizing the bottom of a squat one leg at a time. It doesn't need to be any more complicated than that. If you understand that you're just squatting one leg at a time and trying to mobilize the bottom of the squat position, it becomes simple and easy to understand. There is purpose and intention that goes along with the mob: If you do it, you will squat better.

Here's how to achieve optimal results: First, you have to apply motion to the mobilization by hunting out tight corners and then oscillating in and out of them. Don't just throw your leg up, drop your knee, and hang out. If you're tight in that first position, try capturing the tight pieces of your hip capsule by drawing small circles with your elevated hip. Once you feel like you've made some change, turn away from your elevated leg or rotate your belly button toward your knee while shoving your knee out. You can also shoot your hips back and extend your lead leg, which ties in your hamstring and allows you to hit a different corner of your hip. To put it simply, you want to capture all the different pieces of the tissue by moving your hip into different positions and then "break the paper clip" by moving in and out of end ranges.

The second key is to consider proper squat mechanics as you hunt for tight corners. For example, the most common fault with this mobilization is to let your foot come off the ground as you drive your knee out to the side. Although this is a great way to capture elements of your hip that may be tight (which I demonstrate later), it doesn't necessarily fit into this mobilization. The reason? The moment your foot comes off the ground, you start bleeding torque out of your ankle and biasing a different range, which does not represent proper squatting mechanics. Stapling your foot to the ground allows you to tie in your ankle range and most closely represents what you're trying to change, which is a foot-flat movement in a weight-bearing squat situation. The same rules apply to other faults, like tracking your knee over your foot and breaking at your low back to hit certain corners. If it doesn't make sense mechanically, don't do it.

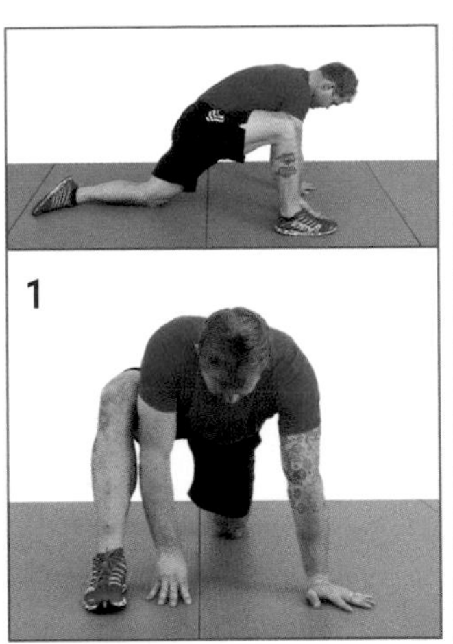
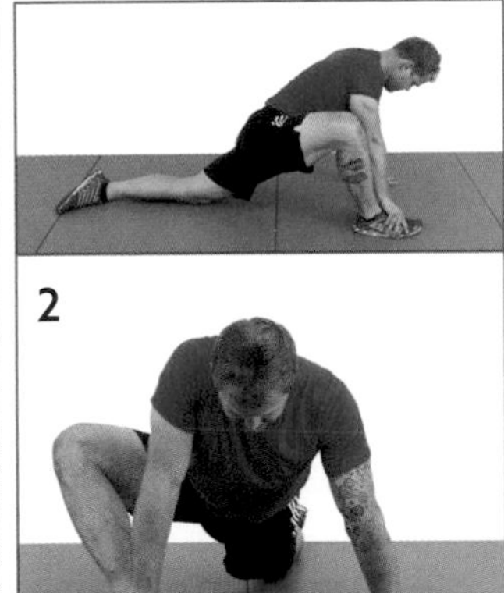
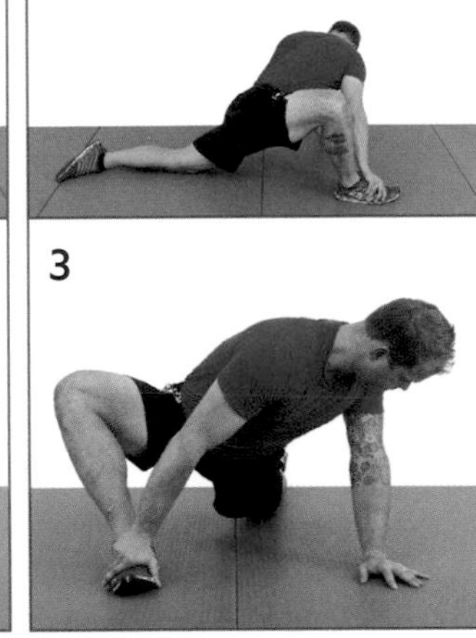
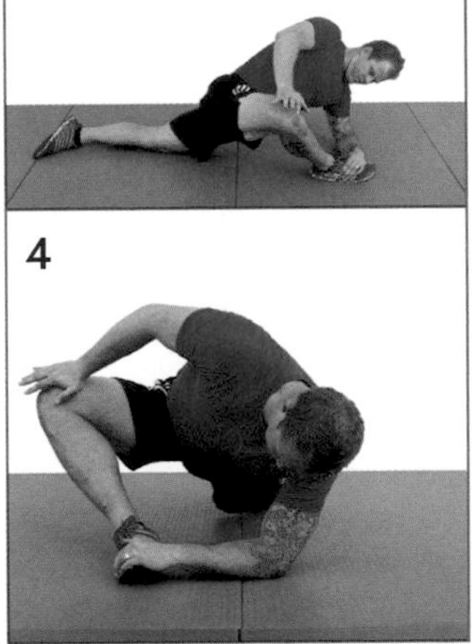
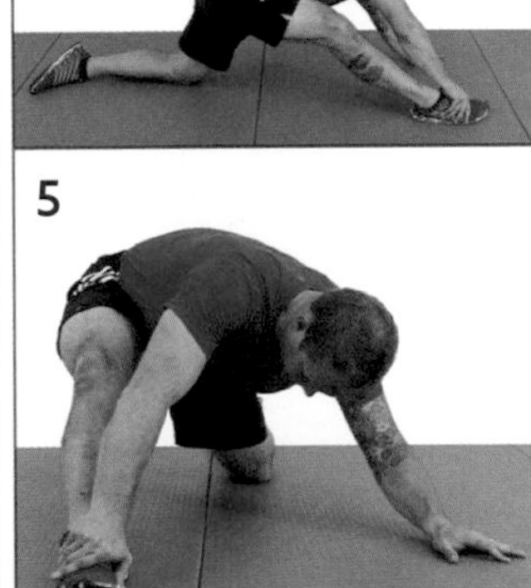
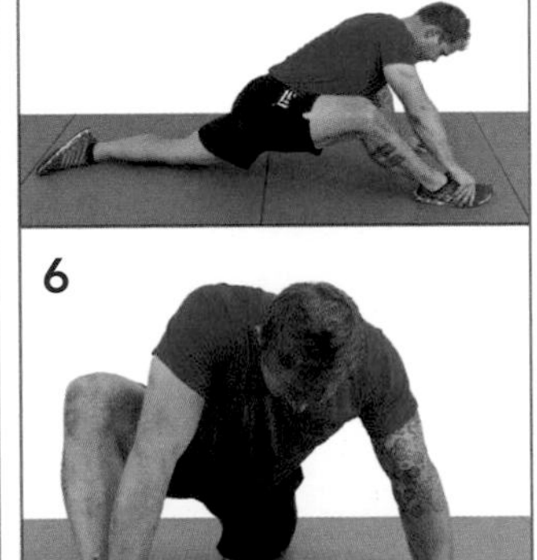

1. Starting on your hands and knees, post your right foot next to your right hand, keeping your right shin vertical.

2. Place your right hand over your right foot, stapling it to the ground. Sprawl your left leg back and drop your left knee to the side. As you do, actively drive your left hip to the ground and flatten your back. From this position, you can oscillate around by driving your weight into the corner of your butt, going in and out of end-range tension.

3. Start hunting for tight corners by rotating your upper body away from your elevated leg.

4. To increase knee-out positioning, drop your left elbow to the mat, cup your left hand over your right foot to pin it to the ground, turn toward your elevated leg, and shove your knee out with your right hand.

5. Drive your hips back. This captures the back of your hip and biases your hamstring into the mobilization.

6. Having loaded your hip into a new position, slide forward and scour for new areas of stiffness.

BANDED DISTRACTION

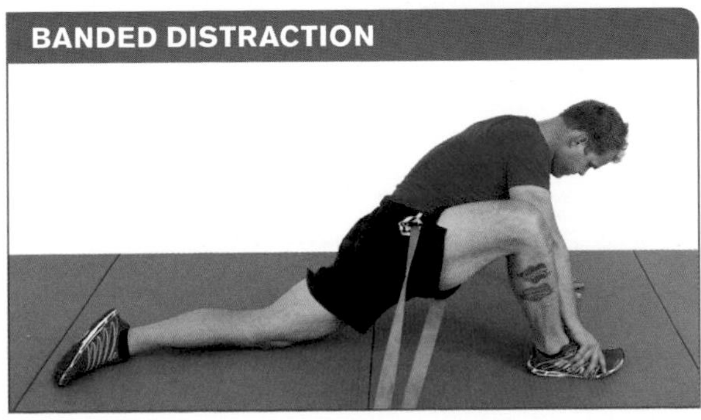

Banded Distraction: Although this mobilization will induce radical change even without a distraction, it's always better to use a band when you can. Creating a distraction multiplies the effectiveness of this mob by a factor of 4 or 5. You can create a distraction in two different directions: You can distract laterally, pulling your hip into the side of your capsule, or you can distract toward your posterior end, pulling your hip to the back of your socket. There's no wrong way. The idea is to change the orientation of the distraction so that you can magnify the stretch and clear any impingements.

Single-Leg Flexion with External Rotation: Option 2

Single-Leg Flexion with External Rotation is a two-for-one mobilization: You're capturing a flexion-with-external-rotation piece with your lead leg and an extension piece with your back leg. A lot of athletes, especially powerlifters the size of highway demolition machines, are restricted in extension when executing this mob on the floor, which prevents them from dropping into deep flexion in the front. In that case, mobilizing with your lead foot up on a box will give you a much better outcome.

Aside from elevating your foot, all the same rules from option 1 apply: Mimic the mechanics of the squat by keeping your lead foot straight and pinned to the box, hunt out stiff corners by forcing your hip into different positions, and apply the paper clip technique as you scour in and out of tight areas.

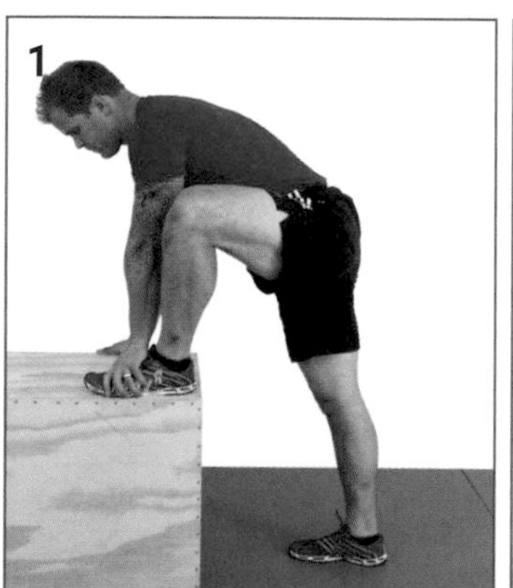

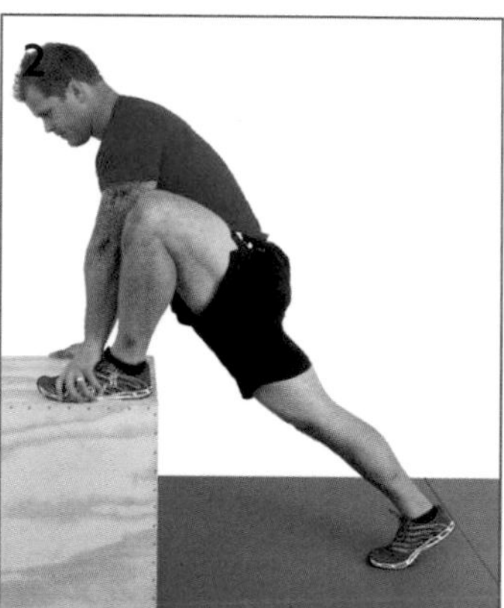

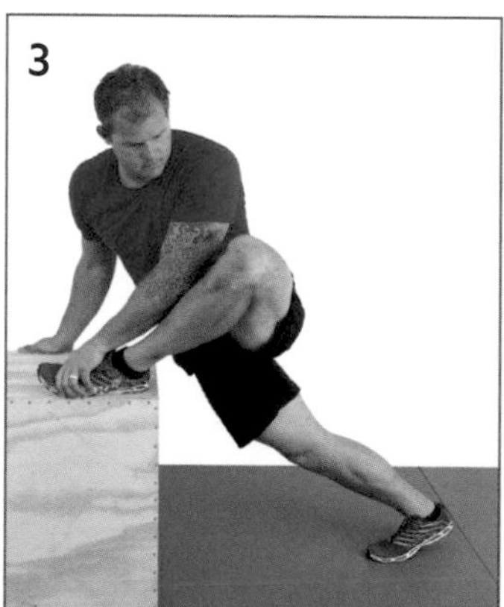

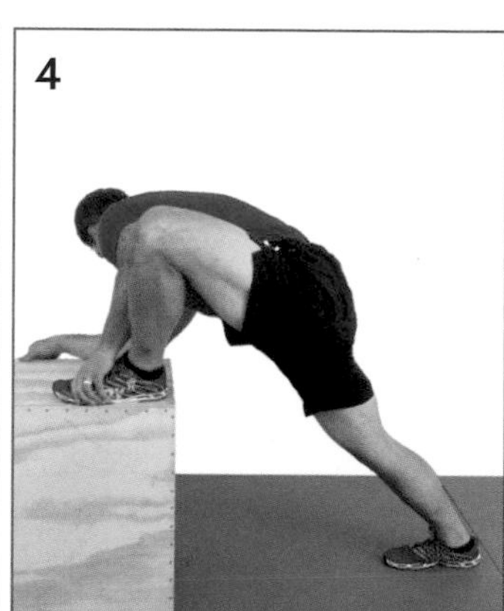

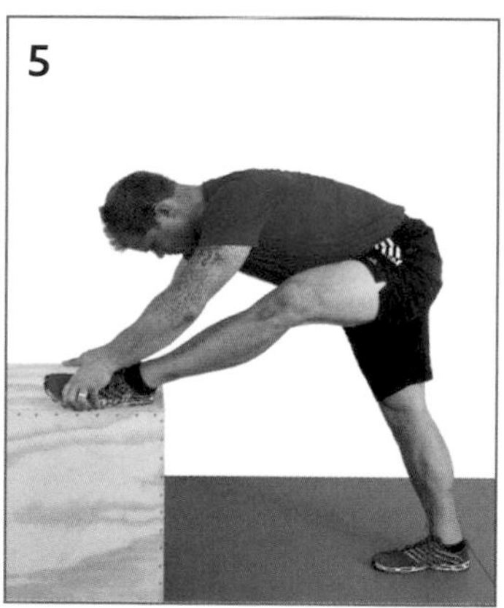

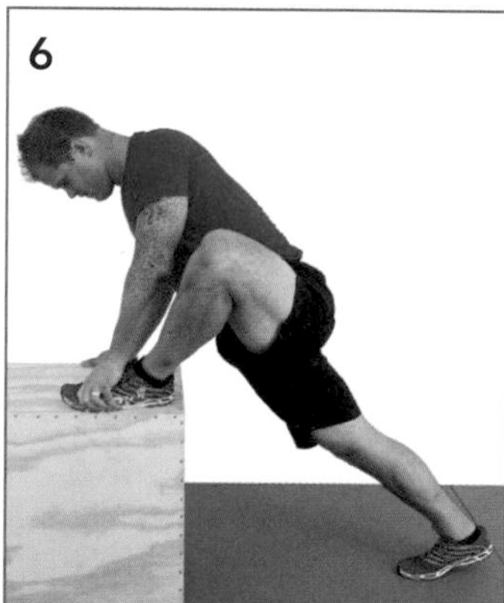

BANDED DISTRACTION

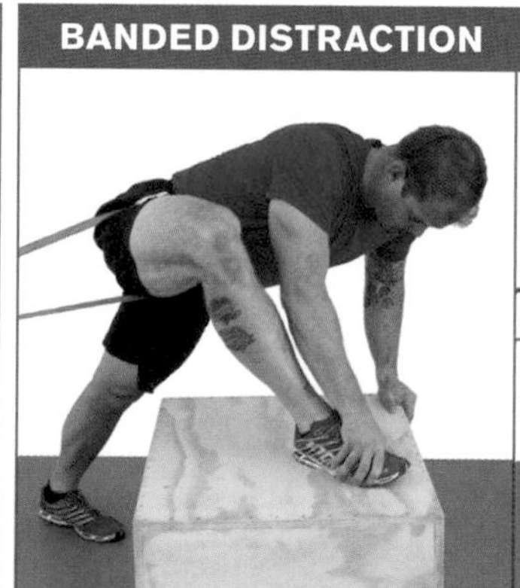

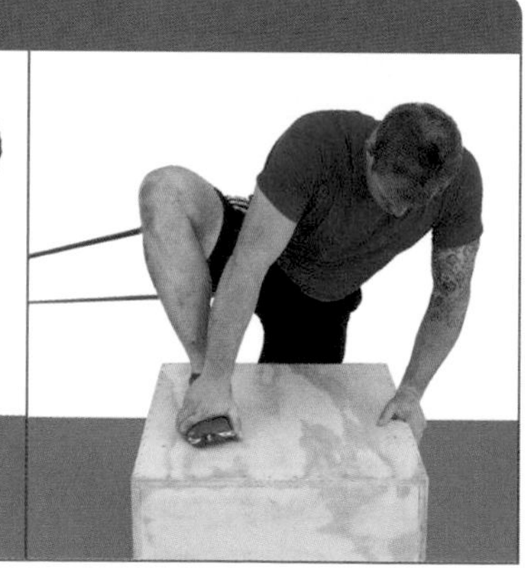

1. Post your left foot up on a box and pin it to the surface with your left hand. To mobilize around a good squat stance, keep your lead shin vertical and your foot straight.

2. Keeping your left foot stapled to the box, slide your right foot straight back and drop your left knee out to the side.

3. Rotate toward your elevated knee. This forces increased knee-out positioning on your left leg and biases an open-hip position on your right hip and leg.

4. To bias more hip flexion, rotate toward your right and drop your chest toward the box.

5. Continue to hunt for stiff corners by driving your hips back. This captures the back of your hip and biases your hamstring into the mobilization.

6. Having loaded your hip into a new position, slide forward and scour for new areas of stiffness.

Banded Distraction: If you have a band, use it! Applying a distraction will dramatically increase the effectiveness of this mobilization. As with option 1, you can distract your hip laterally or toward the back of the capsule.

Hip External Rotation with Flexion

Hip External Rotation with Flexion: Option 1

Squat 2 Archetype

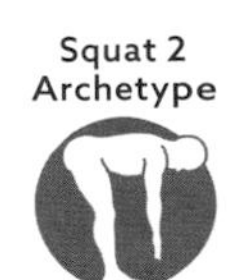

Squat 1 Archetype

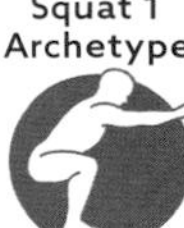

This mobilization will help improve the above archetypes.

METHODS:

Contract and relax

Banded flossing

The previous mobilizations emphasize flexion first and then add external rotation as a tensioner. In this series, you do the opposite. Notice in the photos below that I emphasize external rotation first and then load the position with flexion, which provides a slightly different stimulus. As you can see, this mobilization is very similar to yoga's classic pigeon pose, but with a key difference: You're never going to collapse into a flexed, rounded-forward position. In addition to compromising spinal mechanics, the flexed, rounded-forward position doesn't give you the creative leverage to scour into the deep crevices of your stiffness. By placing one hand on your knee and blocking your foot with your opposite hand, you can load forward with a flat back and hunt for tight corners by rotating from side to side.

Let me caution you here: If you can't position your leg perpendicular to your body because you're restricted, or you experience knee pain at any point, stop what you're doing and implement one of the subsequent variations.

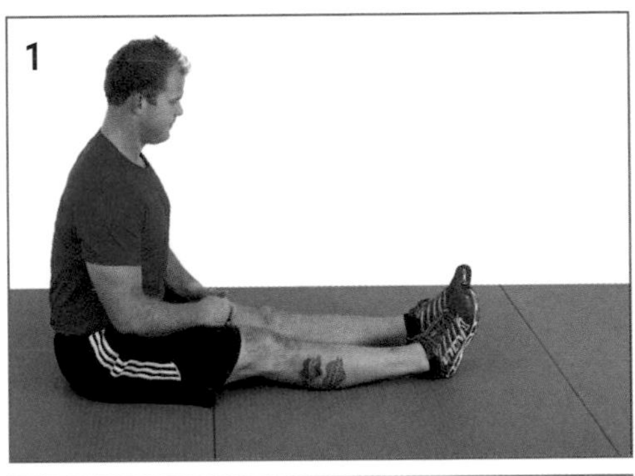

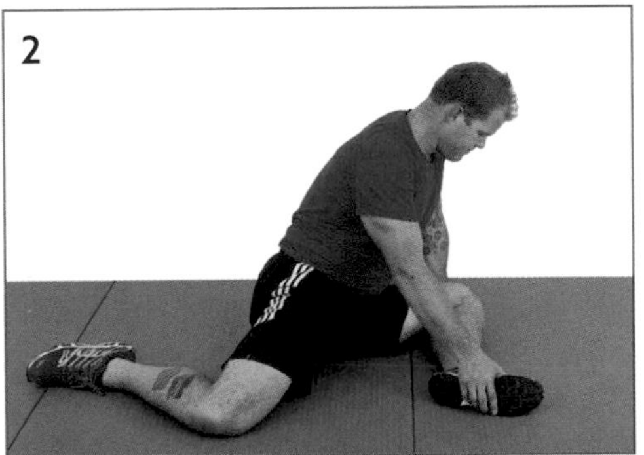

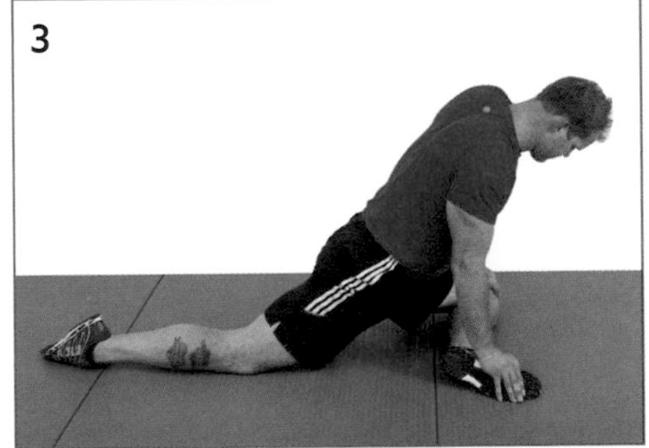

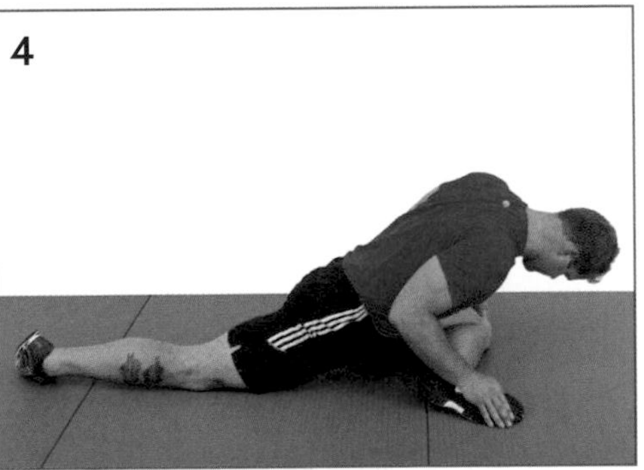

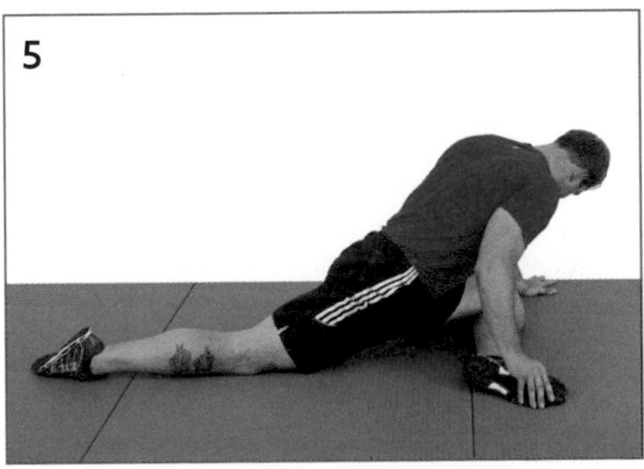

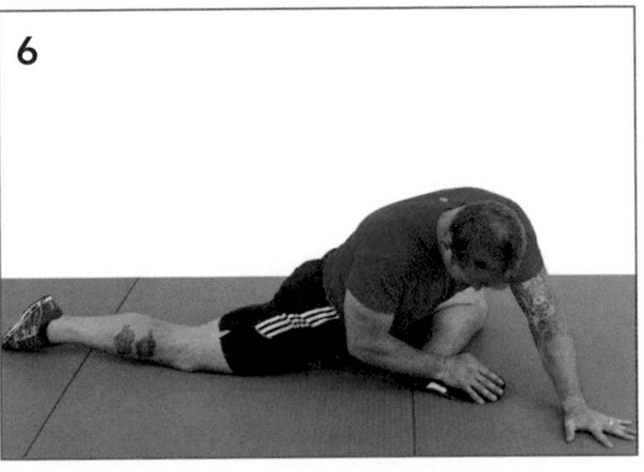

1. Sit upright with your legs straight out in front of you.

2. Lean toward your left and post your left hand on the mat for balance. Swing your right leg behind you, position your lower left leg perpendicular to your body, and post your right hand on your left foot.

3. Place your left hand on your left knee, sprawl your right leg back, and lock out your arms, keeping your shoulders back.

4. Keeping your back flat, lower your chest toward the ground.

5. With your right hand blocking your left foot—which prevents your foot from sliding underneath your body and losing tension in the stretch—rotate toward your left side to hit a different corner.

6. Rotate toward your right side and try to get your belly button over your left foot.

Hip External Rotation with Flexion: Option 2

This is the first mobilization that I recommend to people who experience lateral knee pain in the option 1 position. If you're not flexible enough to get your knee to the ground, you end up pulling your lateral knee joint apart as you load your leg into flexion. Posting up on your foot and then letting your knee drop to the side solves a lot of the knee-gapping issues that cause your knee to flare up. Not only that, but the position is much easier to get into because you're not as restricted by your back leg in extension.

Note: If you continue to experience pain in your knee or ankle, don't try to be tough and grind through it. There are other ways to approach this mobilization without blowing out your knee or putting stress on your ankle joint. Consider options 3, 4, and 5 instead.

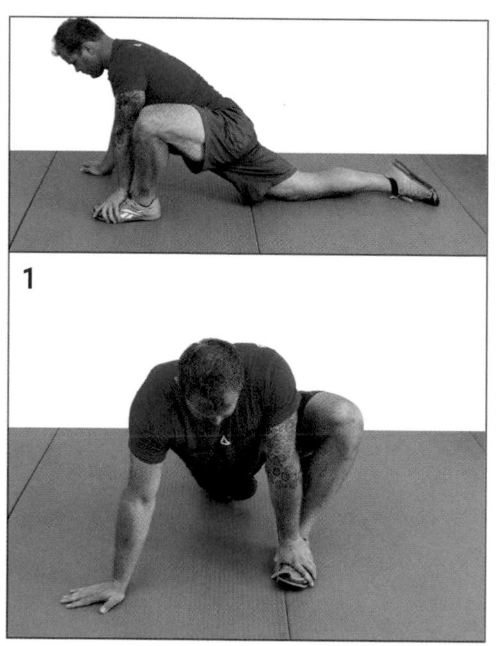

1

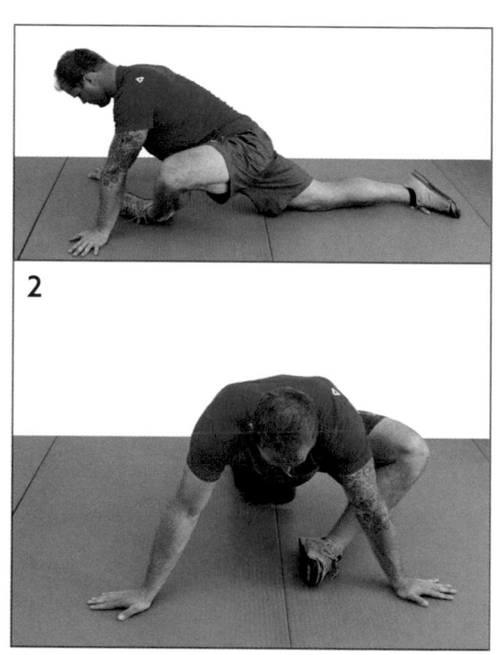

2

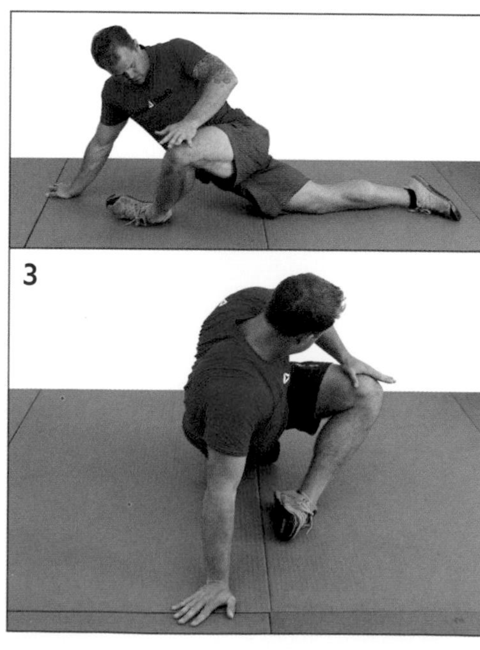

3

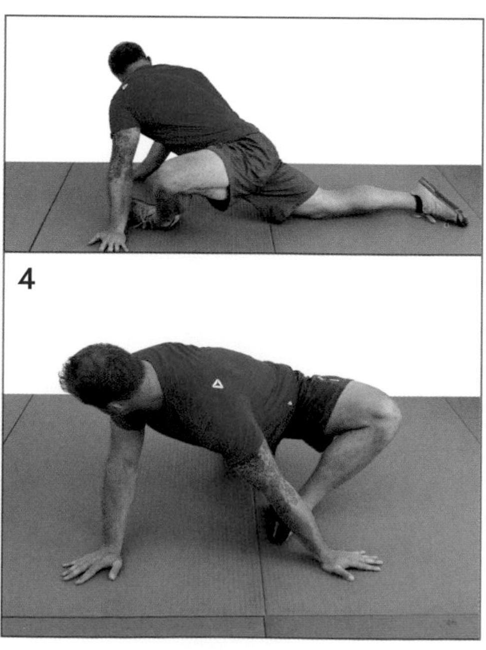

4

1. Set up as you would for the Single-Leg Flexion mobilization (page 370). Post up on your left foot—keeping your shin vertical and your foot straight—and sprawl your right leg back.

2. Post your left hand on the mat for balance and drop your left knee to the side, rolling onto the edge of your left foot.

3. To emphasize external rotation, rotate toward your left side and push your knee farther out using your left hand.

4. Continue hunting out stiff corners by rotating toward your right side.

Hip External Rotation with Flexion: Option 3

This is another option that you can implement if you experience lateral knee pain or struggle to get into an optimal position from the ground. Even if you're not limited by range of motion, positioning your lead leg on an elevated surface is a good option. Although it takes the same shape as the previous variations, it provides a slightly different stimulus. With your lead leg elevated, you can get a little more hip rotation and add a more aggressive flexion load.

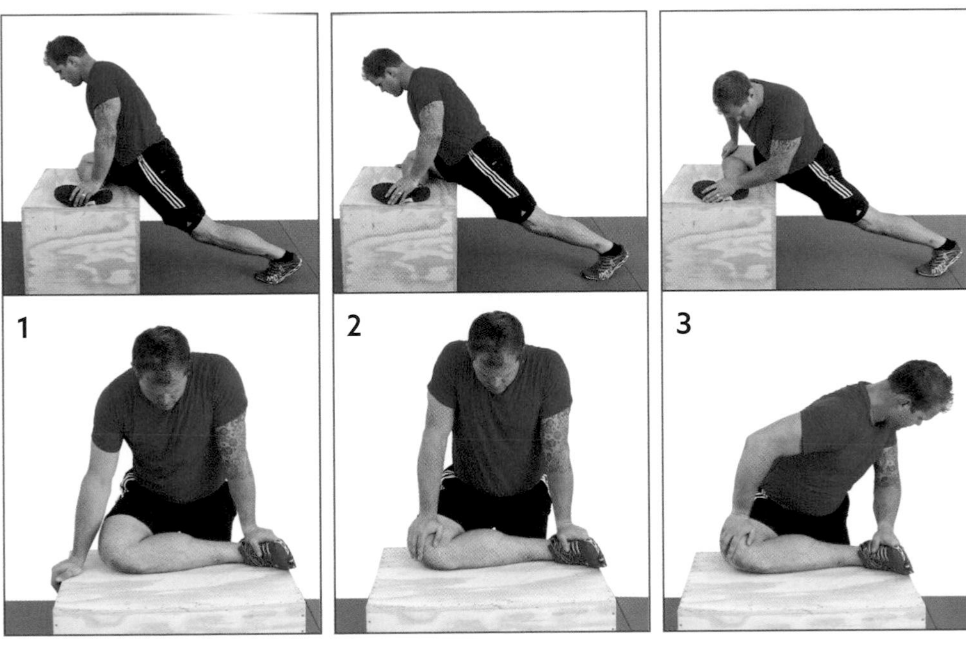

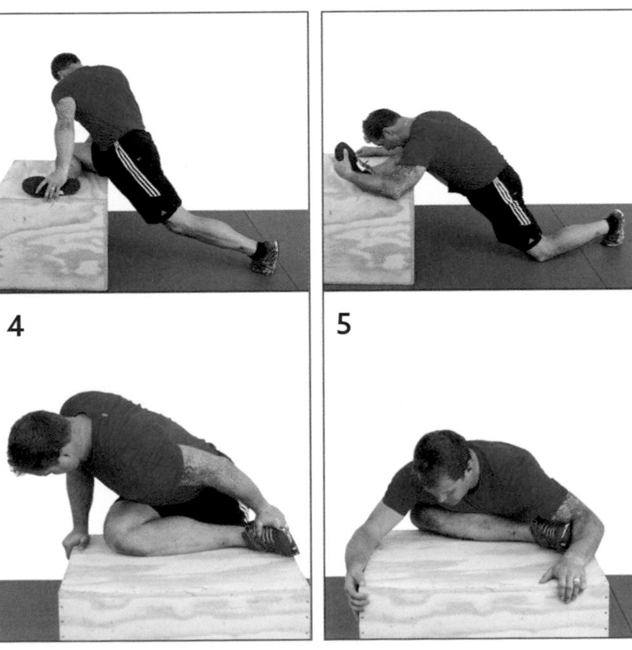

1. Post your right foot on the left side of a box, sprawl your left leg back, and let your right knee drop to the side, positioning your lower right leg across the box. With your lower leg perpendicular to your body, post your left hand on your right foot, pinning it in place.

2. Place your right hand on your right knee. To increase the stretch, flex forward with a level back. From here, apply the paper clip technique by oscillating in and out of end range, folding forward and pushing yourself up.

3. Turn toward your left and try to get your belly button over your foot.

4. Keeping your left foot pinned, rotate toward your right, positioning your chest over your right knee.

5. To hit the deep corners of your hip and capture some of that high hamstring, drop your left knee to the mat and fold forward. This position should be reserved for supple ninjas.

Hip External Rotation with Flexion: Option 4

A lot of athletes are so stiff that they can't get into any of the previous positions without the knee joint ripping apart. If you fall into that category, you need to address the stiffness with some quality quad and hip smashing, and you need to protect your knee joint by dropping your foot off a box. This takes some of the rotational torque off the joint so that you can explore your business without pain.

1. To reduce the load on your knee, sit halfway on a box and drop your right foot off the edge.

2. Fold forward from your hips and lower your chest toward your right knee, creating a stretch in your right posterior hip.

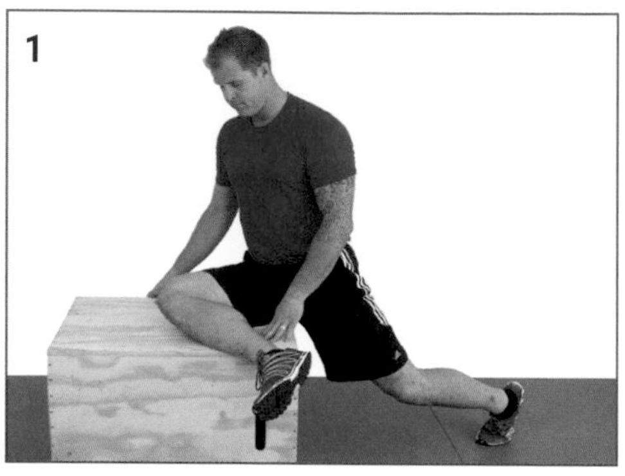

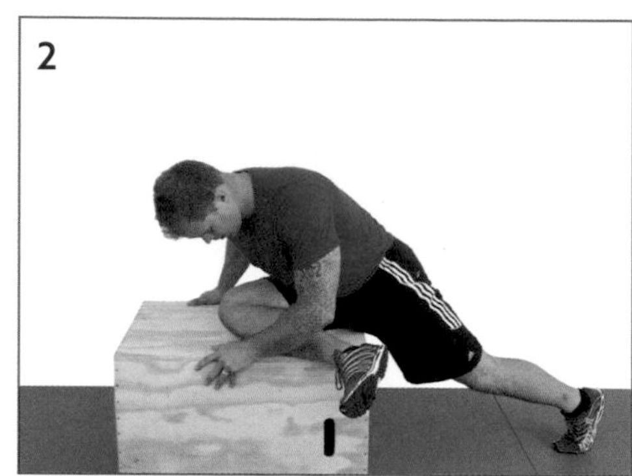

Hip External Rotation with Flexion: Option 5

Here's the last option in the series: Cradle your knee to your chest and add a flexion load by leaning forward. This allows you to bias external rotation of your hip without challenging your knee joint.

1. To protect your knee joint, wrap your arm around the outside of your knee.

2. Cradling your knee to your chest, turn toward your elevated leg and lower your chest toward the box.

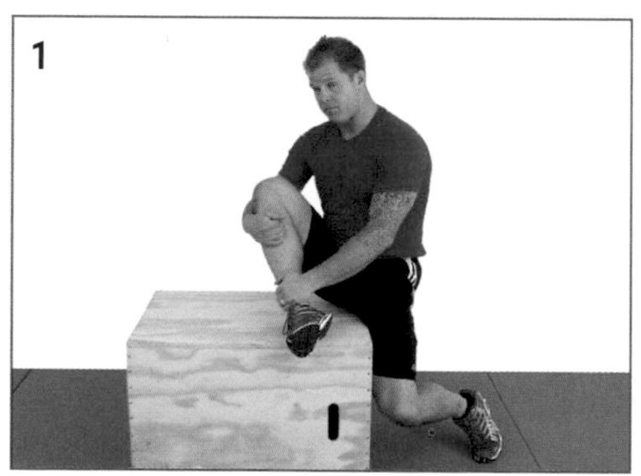

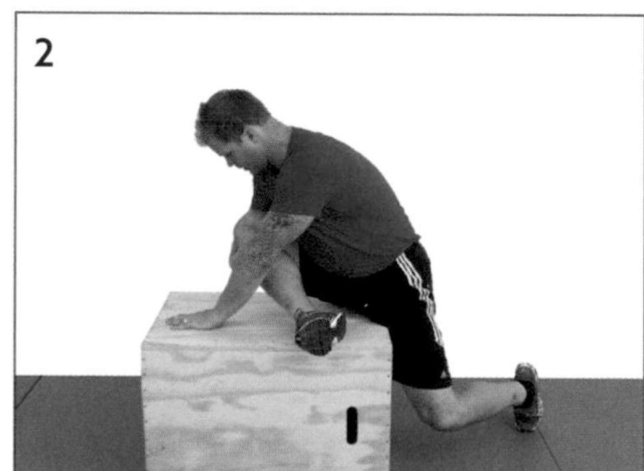

Olympic Wall Squat with External Rotation

This is another oldie-but-goodie hip mobilization that works on flexion and external rotation. Creating a lateral distraction at your hip or wrapping a band around your knees to account for your hip capsule will have a larger impact—which you'll find is true for the other Olympic Wall Squat variations as well.

1. Position your butt as close to a box as possible and assume a squat stance with your feet just outside shoulder width, your shins vertical, and your feet straight.

2. Throw your right leg over your left knee.

3. To increase the aggressiveness of the stretch, pull down on your right instep with your left hand and slide your right foot toward your hip. Use your right hand to push on your right knee.

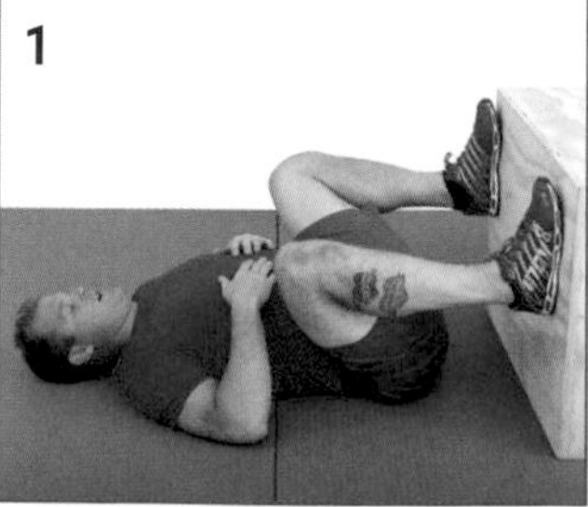

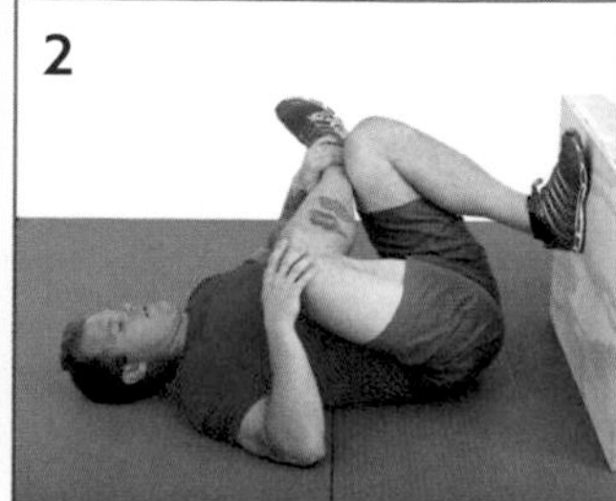

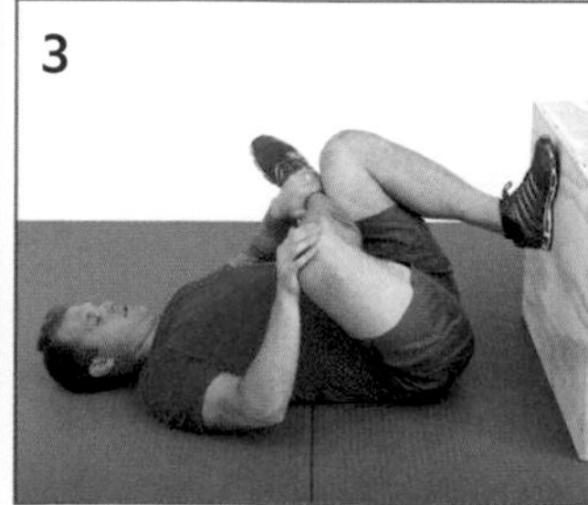

Executive Hip Mobilization

Are you sitting in a chair as you read this book? If the answer is yes, you should:

1. Be ashamed of yourself.
2. At least make the best of a bad situation and get something done—for example, stick a ball into the side of your hip or under your hamstring, or bias some external rotation.

Squat 1 Archetype

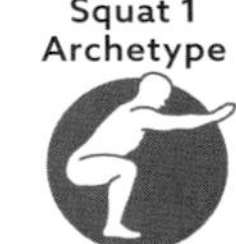

This mobilization will help improve the above archetypes.

METHODS:

Contract and relax

Warriors in the Supple Legion understand the toxic impact that sitting has on performance and do everything in their power to avoid it. However, sometimes you just can't. If you're trapped at a desk or shackled into a Boston-to-LAX window seat, use the following stretches to work on your hip function and try to reverse the slow pending death to your mobility.

Obviously, there are much better ways to work on hip mobility than sitting in a chair and trying to stretch! But something is better than nothing, so putting your hip into these positions and applying the contract and relax method is definitely useful if you're stuck in a chair.

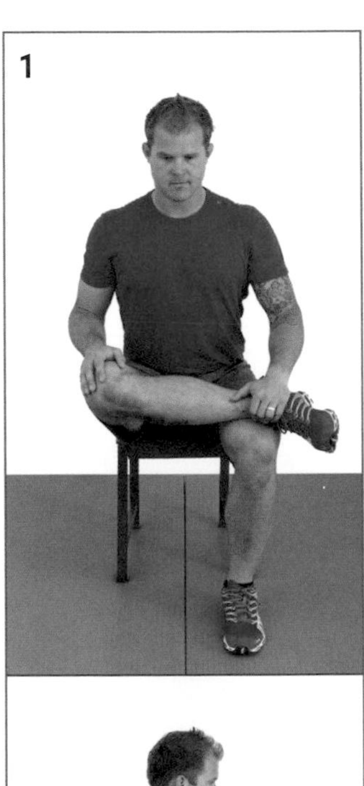

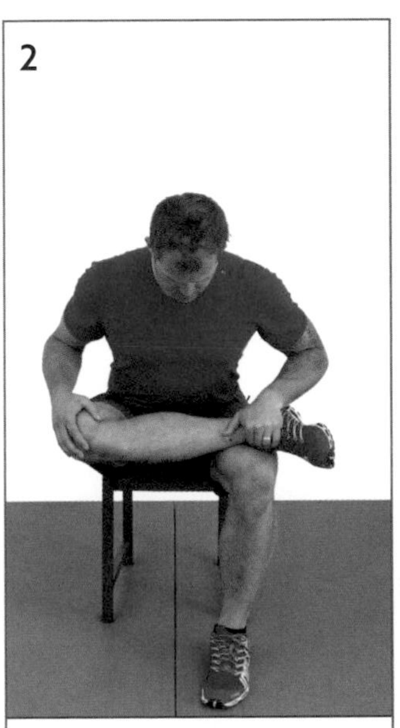

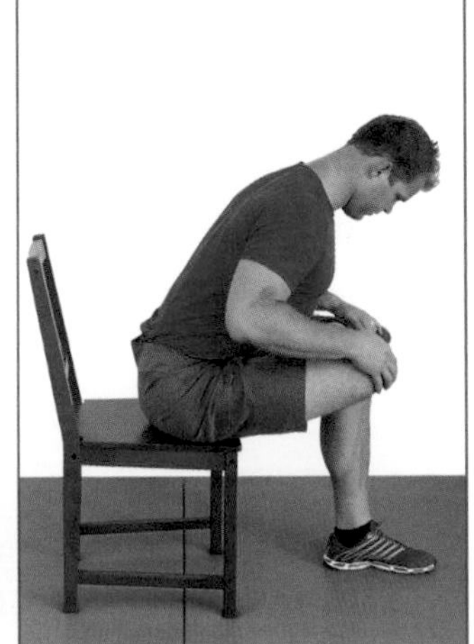

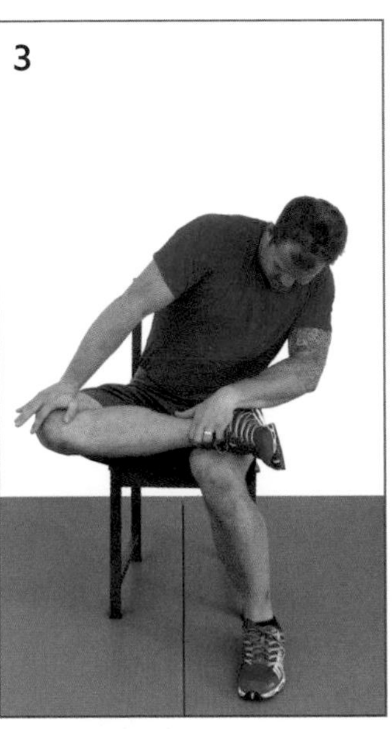

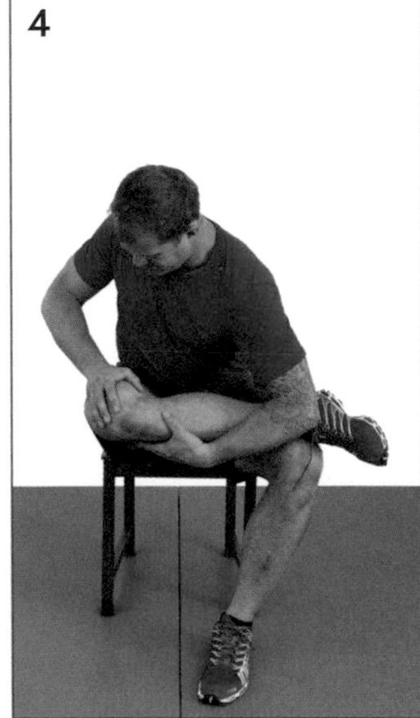

1. Establish a neutral sitting position, then cross your right foot over your left knee.

2. With your right leg biased into external rotation, apply a flexion load by folding forward from your hips with your back flat.

3. Using your left hand to keep your right foot from sliding off your left thigh, push your right knee toward the floor and lock out your arm. This helps tie some of the side abdominal and low back tissues into the stretch.

4. Still pushing your knee toward the floor and keeping your back flat, rotate toward your right hand and lower your chest toward your right knee, capturing another piece of your hip.

Executive Hip Workaround

Sometimes crossing your foot over your knee and adding forward flexion will cause lateral knee pain if you're missing key ranges of motion. If that happens, wrap your arm around your leg and cradle your knee to your chest. This takes the strain off the joint and allows you to rotate from side to side and apply load without pain.

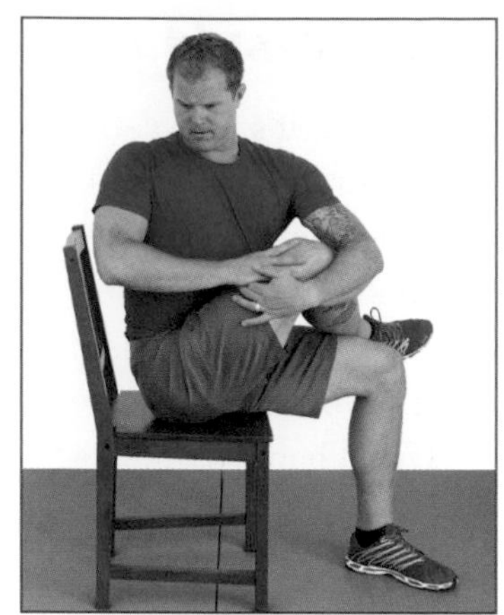

IMPROVES:

Hip and knee pain

Arthritic or inflamed knees and hips

Hip impingement

Gentle Hip Distraction

When I treat people with arthritis or work with athletes who have tweaked a hip or knee, I generally start with a simple banded joint distraction mobilization. These people are dealing with bone-on-bone contact (such as a femur rubbing against a hip joint) and inflamed tissue that cause a lot of pain and discomfort. Wrapping a band around the ankle and adding some tension effectively unimpinges the hip and gives the joints some room to breathe. With any luck, it will alleviate pain and reset the joint to the normal, ideal position.

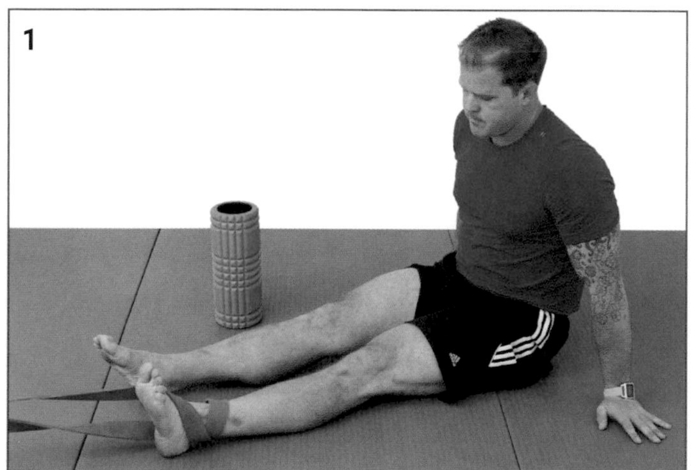

1

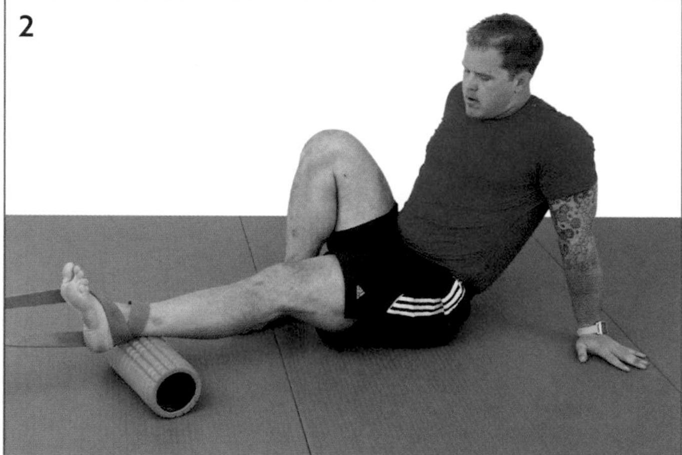

2

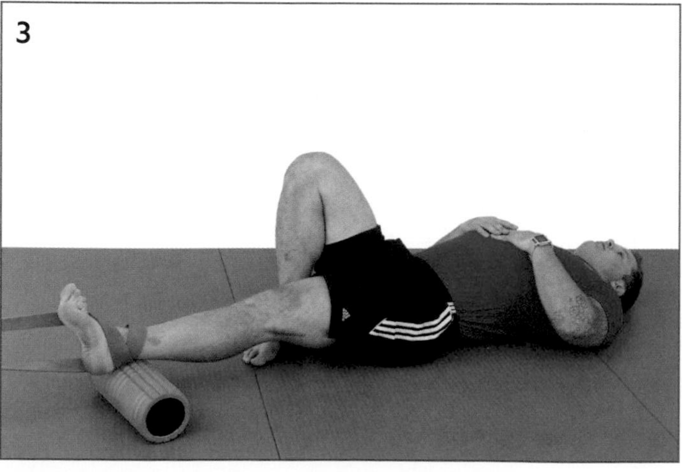

3

1. Hook a band around the top of your foot, then wrap it around the base of your heel.

2. Create tension in the band and then prop your foot up on a foam roller. This helps keep your hip in a neutral position and maximizes the distraction force through your ankle.

3. To encourage a neutral pelvic position and help prevent defaulting into an overextended position, curl your free leg in tight to your body, keeping your foot on the mat, and lie back. The idea is to relax your leg and allow the band to pull and decompress your joints, giving your knee and hip some breathing room.

Hip Capsule Mobilization

Squat 2 Archetype

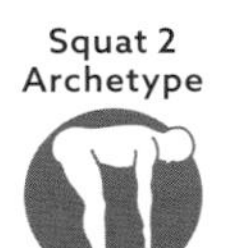

Squat 1 Archetype

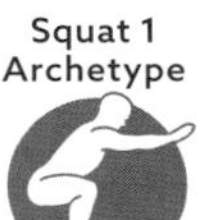

Pistol Archetype

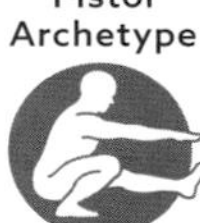

This mobilization will help improve the above archetypes.

METHOD:

Contract and relax

Remember, it's not just your muscles that get tight. Your joint capsule system accounts for a huge chunk of tissue restriction. Here's an example: Say you experience an impingement at the front of your hips when you squat, restricting your range of motion. This is what I refer to as a "flexion wall," which is your femur running into the front of your pelvis. In order to reach end range, you have to compensate by turning your feet out or overextending.

If that happens, one of the first things you should do is reset the position of your hip to the back of the socket by using this mobilization. By aligning your knee directly underneath your hip and loading your weight over your femur, you can drive the head of your femur into the posterior capsule and restore normal hip function. It's a quick and dirty way to improve the efficiency of your hip mechanics without having to see a physical therapist.

The goal here is to spend at least 2 to 3 minutes (or longer if possible), ideally using a band to distract your hip into a good position. To measure your results, you can test and retest by squatting or lifting the knee that you mobilized toward your chest from a standing position. You'll likely find that simply resetting your hip to the back of the socket dramatically improves your hip flexion.

Note: We secretly call this the Donny Thompson World-Record-Breaking Squat Technique because he was able to reclaim a better position and smash the world record squat simply by mobilizing his hip capsule. He did so after failing in three previous attempts. Implementing this mobilization is the only thing that he changed as he prepared for his fourth attempt. Amazing.

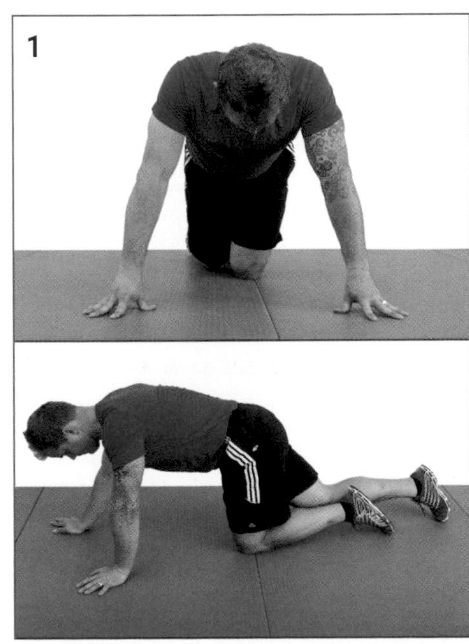

1 Kneel on the ground and shift the majority of your weight onto your left knee, aligning your knee directly under your hip.

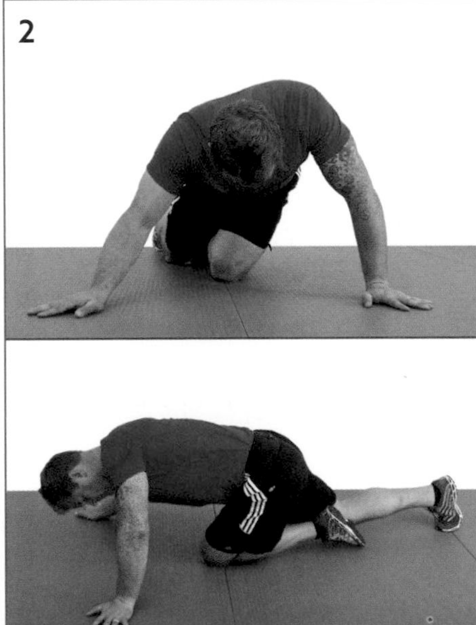

2 Drop your hips toward your left side, keeping your weight loaded over your left knee. Imagine trying to pop the head of your femur out the side of your butt.

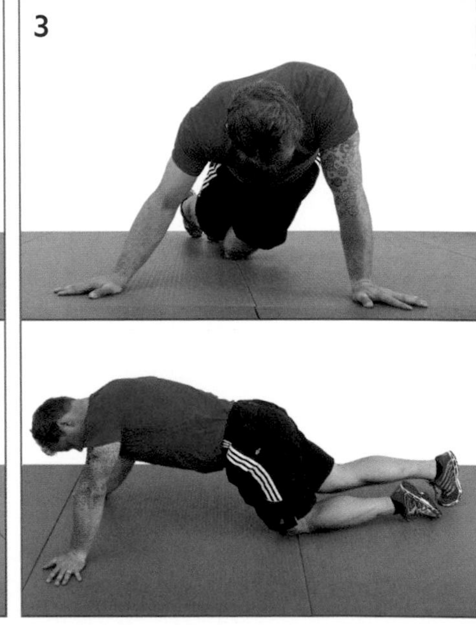

3 Still keeping your weight distributed over your left leg and driving your hips toward your left side, crawl forward and bias the tissues at the front of your hip capsule.

Hip Capsule External Rotation

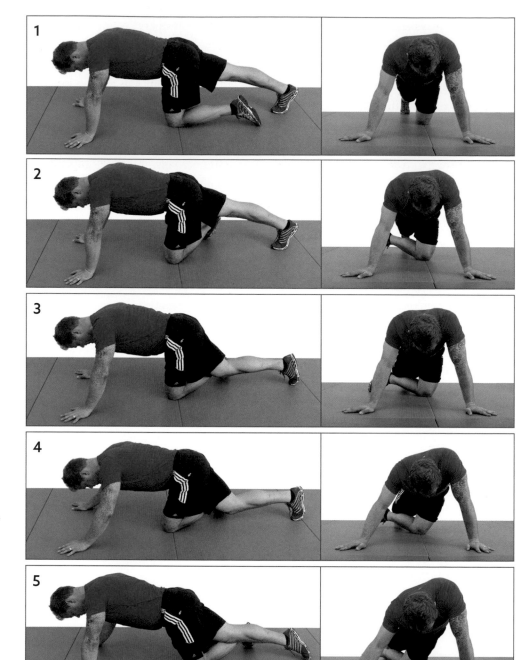

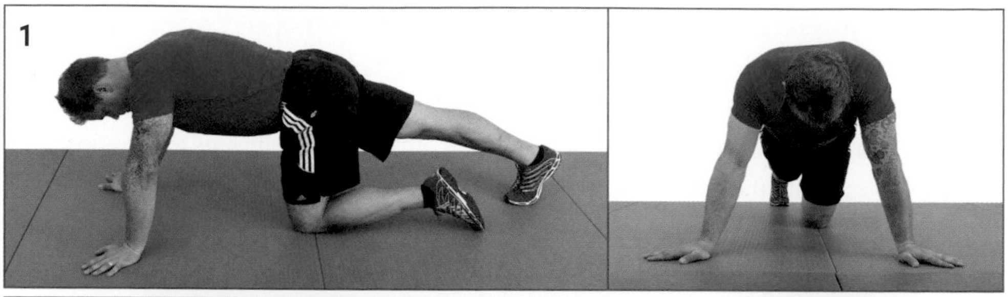

1. Load your weight over your left knee, keeping your femur vertical.

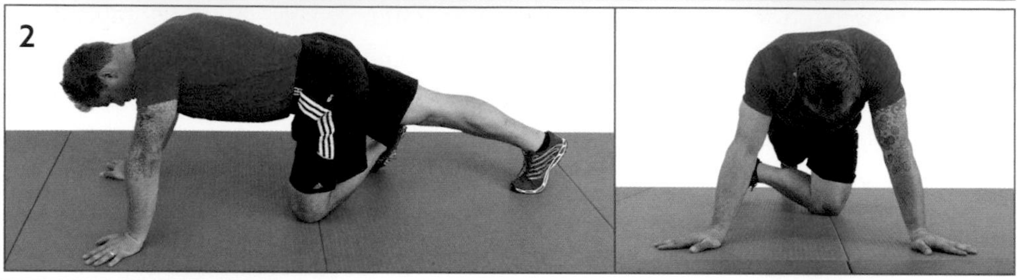

2. With the head of your femur reset to the back of the capsule, swing your left leg across your body.

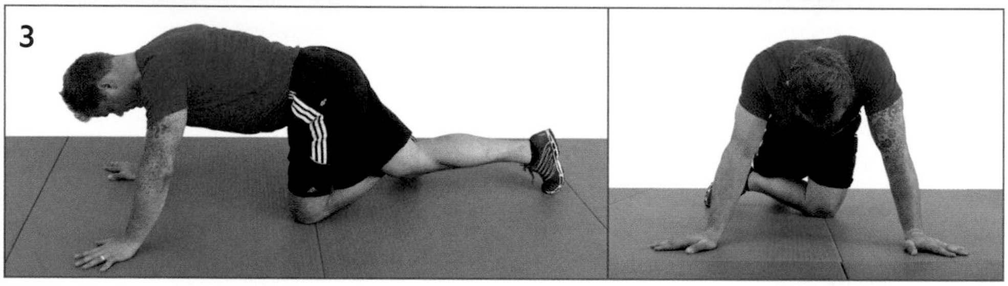

3. Pin your left leg in place using your right knee.

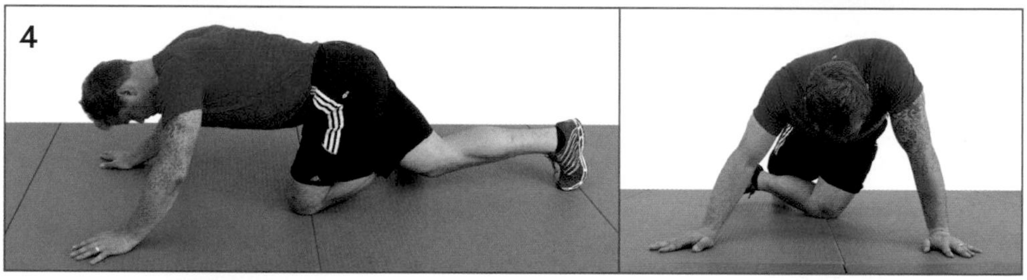

4. Keeping the majority of your weight over your left knee, drop your left hip toward the ground. Again, think about driving the head of your femur through the side of your butt.

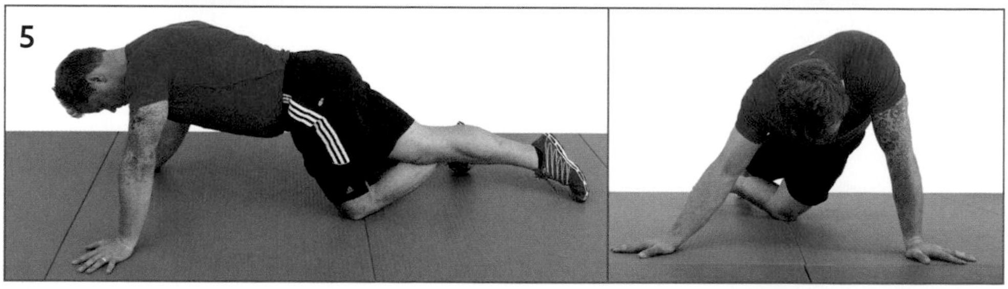

5. After spending a couple minutes in the previous position, crawl forward to capture some of the tissues at the front of your hip capsule.

Banded Distraction: A lot of people feel an impingement in the front of the hip when executing this mobilization. Here's what's happening: The head of the femur is positioned to the anterior edge of the socket, pinching some tissue between the femur and acetabulum (the housing of the hip joint). If this happens, mobilizing without a band is a waste of time. To make an impact on the hip capsule, wrap a band around your hip crease and create a lateral or posterior distraction. This will clear any impingement you may have in the front of the capsule, allowing you to drop your hip to the back of the socket.

BANDED DISTRACTION

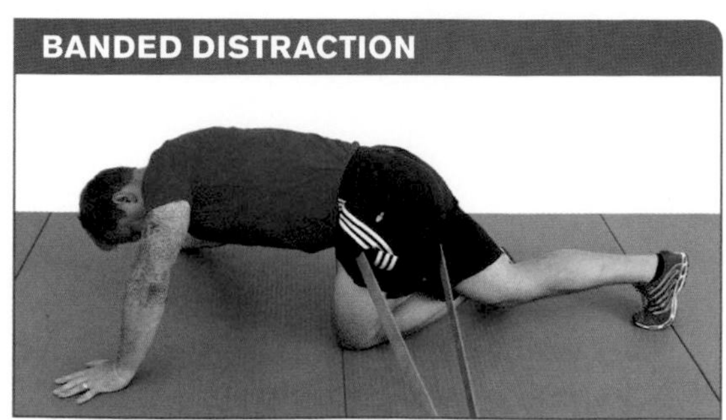

Hip Capsule Internal Rotation

Internal rotational capacity is critical for creating stability when your leg is behind you. It also plays a role in generating torque when your legs are in flexion, such as when you are in the knees-out position in the bottom of a squat. Think of internal rotation as an expression of capsular slack. In other words, if you're missing internal rotation range, you won't be able to externally rotate when your legs are flexion, like when you're squatting, or internally rotate when one leg is behind you in extension, like when you're running or doing a split-jerk. Essentially, you won't be able to create mechanically stable positions or generate power through your primary engine.

This mobilization is an effective way to restore internal rotational capacity. It uses the exact same setup as the Hip Capsule Mobilization, but instead of biasing external rotation by kicking your leg across your body, you swing your leg to the outside of your body and hook your foot on a weight, such as a kettlebell.

Note: To test hip internal rotation, lie on the ground or sit in a chair with your legs bent at a 90-degree angle, and then rotate your leg away from your body, as shown in the photos at right. If you can't get your foot to the outside of your body, chances are you're missing hip internal rotation range of motion.

Squat 2 Archetype

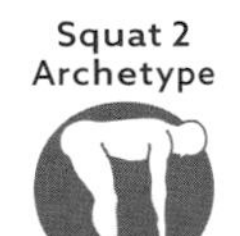

Squat 1 Archetype

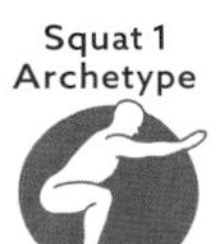

Lunge Archetype

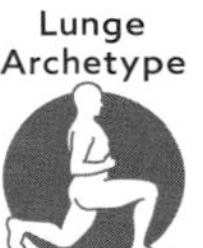

This mobilization will help improve the above archetypes.

METHOD:

Contract and relax

INTERNAL ROTATION TEST 1

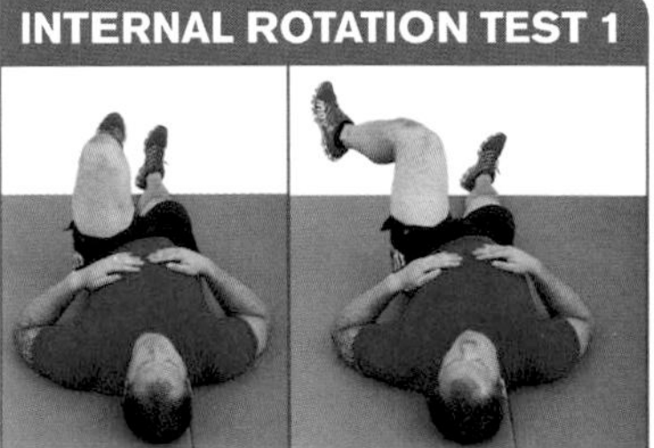

INTERNAL ROTATION TEST 2

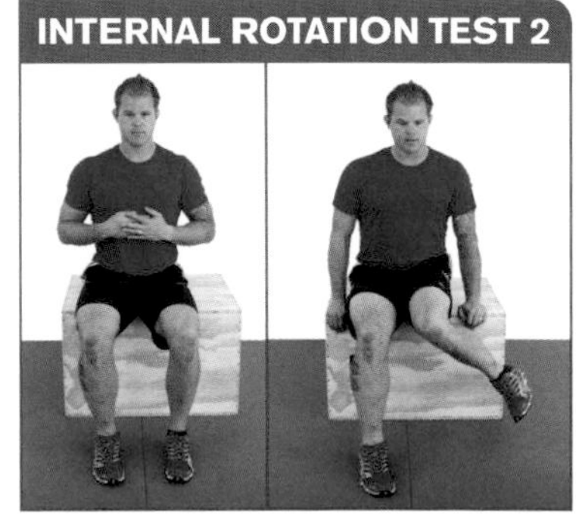

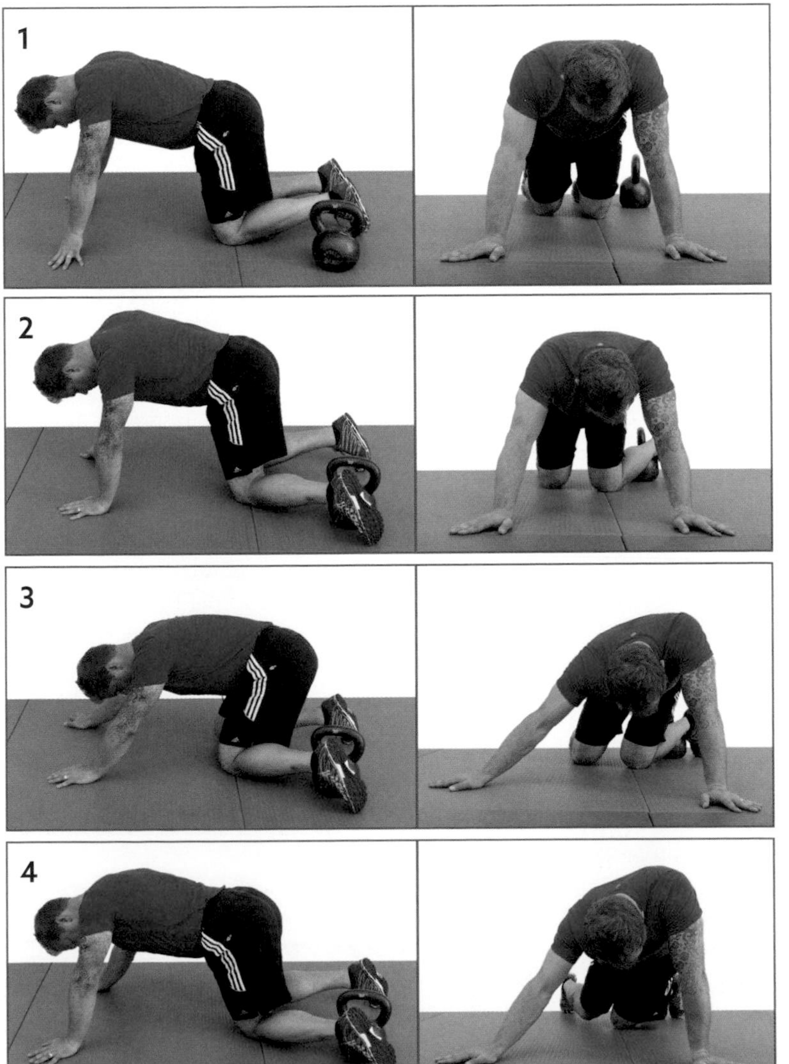

1. Kneel on the ground and shift your weight onto your left knee, making sure your knee is aligned directly under your hip. Position a kettlebell next to your left foot.

2. Hook your left foot around the kettlebell, keeping the majority of your weight over your left knee.

3. Sink your hips back and toward your left side.

4. Still keeping the majority of your weight over your left knee and dropping your left hip toward the ground, crawl forward to capture the front of the hip capsule. If you can use a band to distract the joint, do it!

Cueing Internal Rotation with Distraction

IMPROVES:
Hip pain and impingement

If the head of your femur is jammed into your hip capsule, it's difficult to work on restoring or improving rotational hip range of motion by using the Hip Capsule Internal Rotation mobilization. For some people, wrapping a band around the hip and applying a lateral or posterior distraction is not enough to unimpinge the femur from the hip socket. They still feel a radical pinch at the front of the hip that prevents them from correctly performing the Hip Capsule Mobilization. If that happens, you need to create space within the hip capsule by pulling the joint apart.

In the photos below, notice that I add a distraction from my ankle, roll onto my stomach, and then actively internally rotate my foot. This is the equivalent of distracting your arm overhead and then actively working on external rotation. But in this case, you're working on improving internal rotation capacities with your leg in extension, which is the stable position for your hip when your leg is behind your body.

1. Hook a band around the top of your foot and then wrap it around the base of your heel. Then roll toward your stomach. This biases your leg into extension.

2. Keeping your leg relaxed, internally rotate your leg.

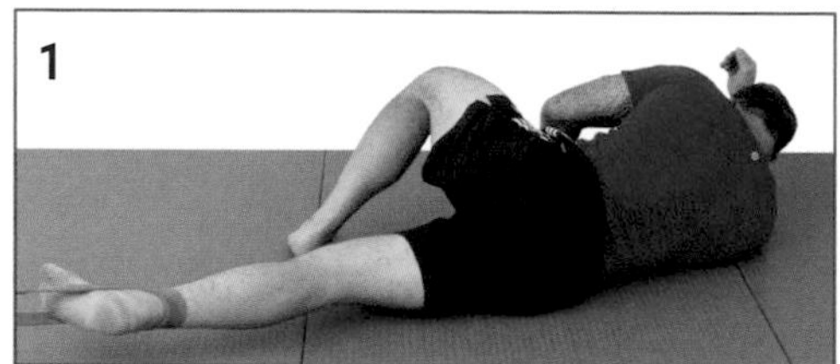

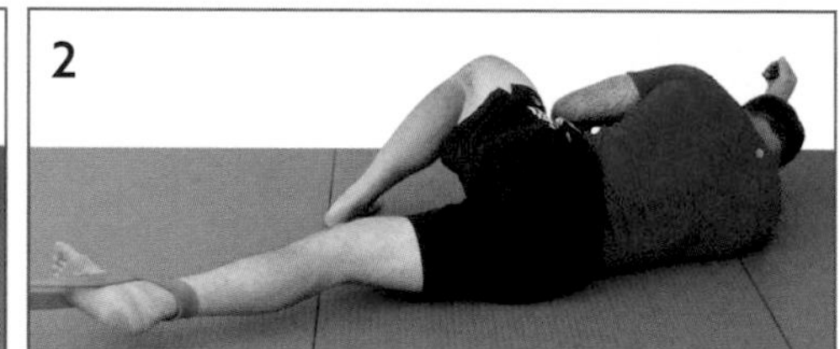

Olympic Wall Squat with Internal Rotation

Lunge Archetype

This mobilization will help improve the above archetype.

METHOD:
Contract and relax

This is another mobilization that improves hip internal rotation. From your back, it's harder to approximate your hip into the back of the socket as you internally rotate, so this mob is less effective than the previous technique. However, it's still useful and can be used in conjunction with the other Olympic Wall Squat variations.

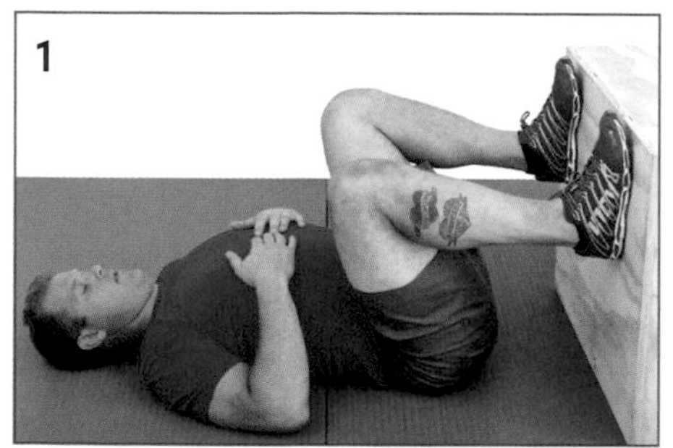

1 Position your butt as close to a box as possible and assume a squat stance, with your feet just outside shoulder width, your shins vertical, and your feet straight.

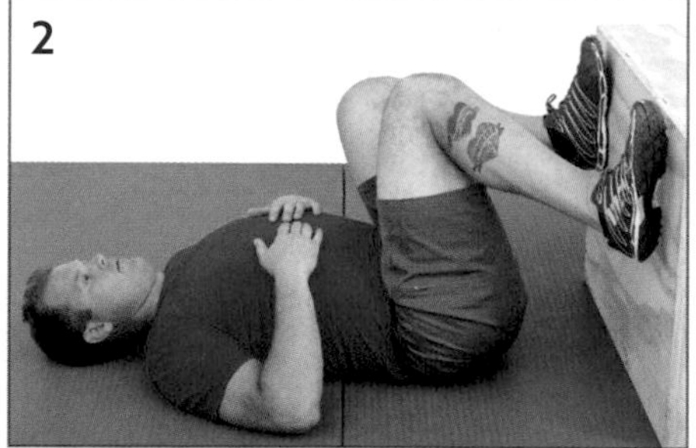

2 Internally rotate your right leg by dropping your right knee toward the left side of your body.

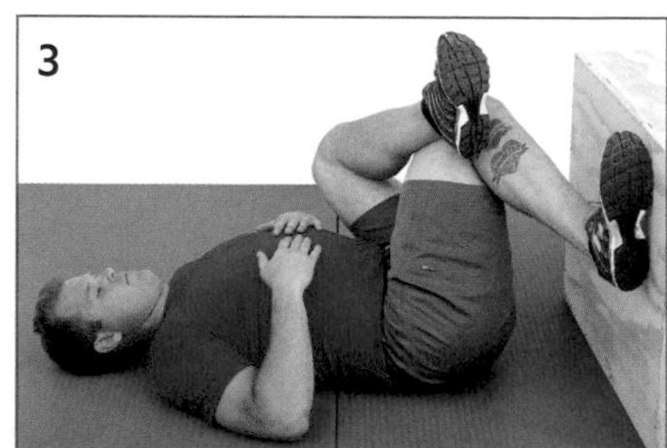

3 Hook your left foot over your right knee to bias internal rotation.

BANDED DISTRACTION

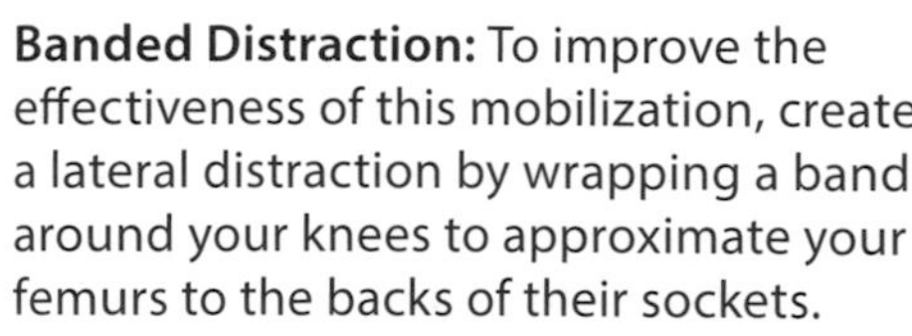

Banded Distraction: To improve the effectiveness of this mobilization, create a lateral distraction by wrapping a band around your knees to approximate your femurs to the backs of their sockets.

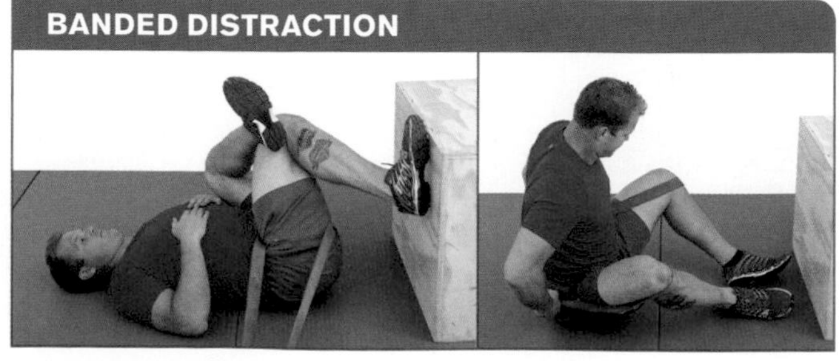

Global Internal Rotation

METHOD:
Contract and relax

Although this technique doesn't have the same impact as the Hip Capsule Mobilization or the Olympic Wall Squat variations, you can do it when you're relaxing on your back watching TV or just hanging out. Adding a lateral distraction on the hip you're mobilizing is ideal.

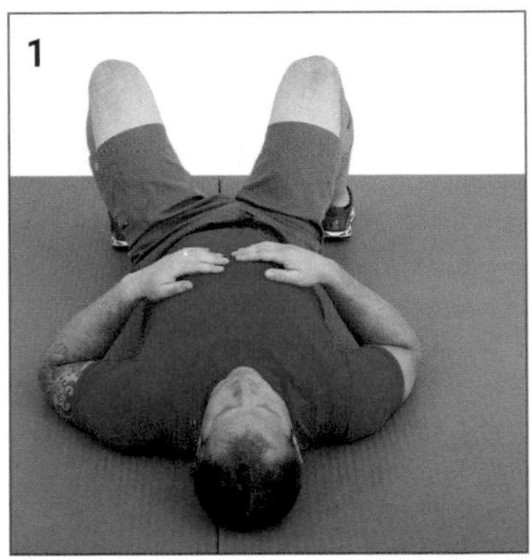

1 Lie on your back with your knees up.

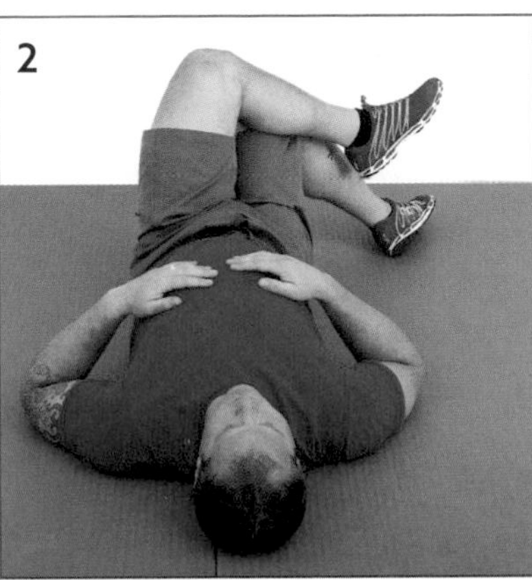

2 Internally rotate your right leg, then cross your left leg over your right knee, anchoring it to the mat.

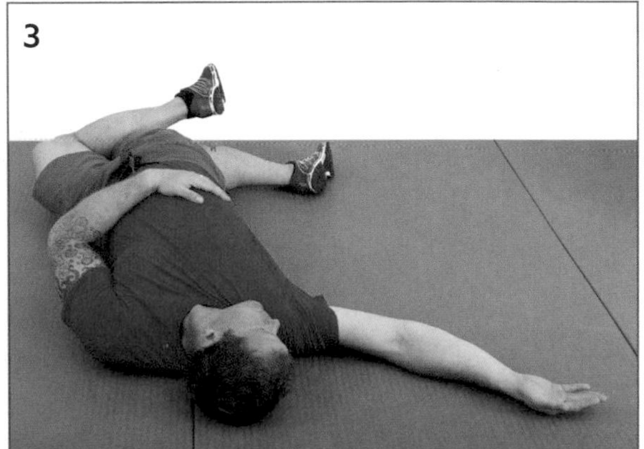

3 As you drop your right knee to the mat, reach your right arm out to the side. This counterbalances your rotation and ties in the musculature of your lower back. It's easy to compensate into an overextended position, so prevent that fault by keeping your butt in contact with the ground.

Internal Rotation Workaround

As with the Executive Hip Workaround, the Internal Rotation Workaround should not be your first stop when mobilizing your hips. In addition to putting the musculature of your trunk on tension, you can't approximate your hips into a good position, making it easier to compensate into a bad position. However, if you're trapped in a chair and you know you're going to be there for a prolonged period, you may as well take a crack at improving internal rotation.

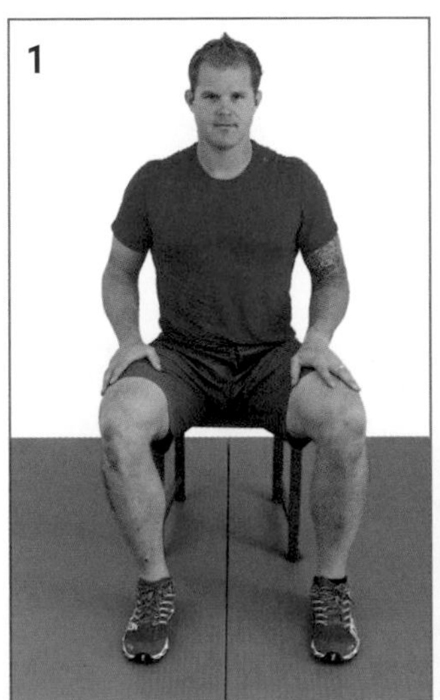

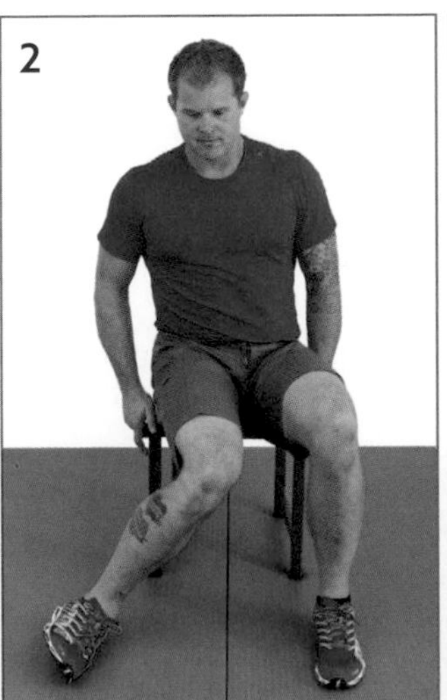

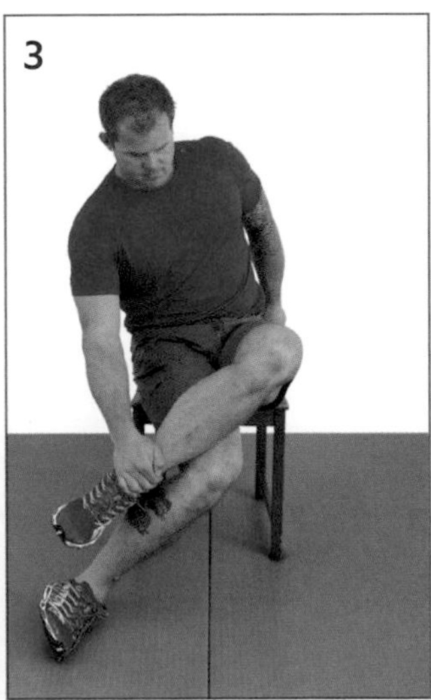

1. Sit upright with neutral posture.

2. Keeping your right foot in contact with the ground, internally rotate your leg by dropping your right knee toward the inside of your body.

3. Cross your left leg over your right knee, grab your left instep with your right hand to hold your foot in place, and then use your left leg to pull your right knee across your body. To involve some of your high hip and low back musculature in the stretch, tilt your upper body toward your right side.

AREA 8 HIP FLEXORS, QUADRICEPS

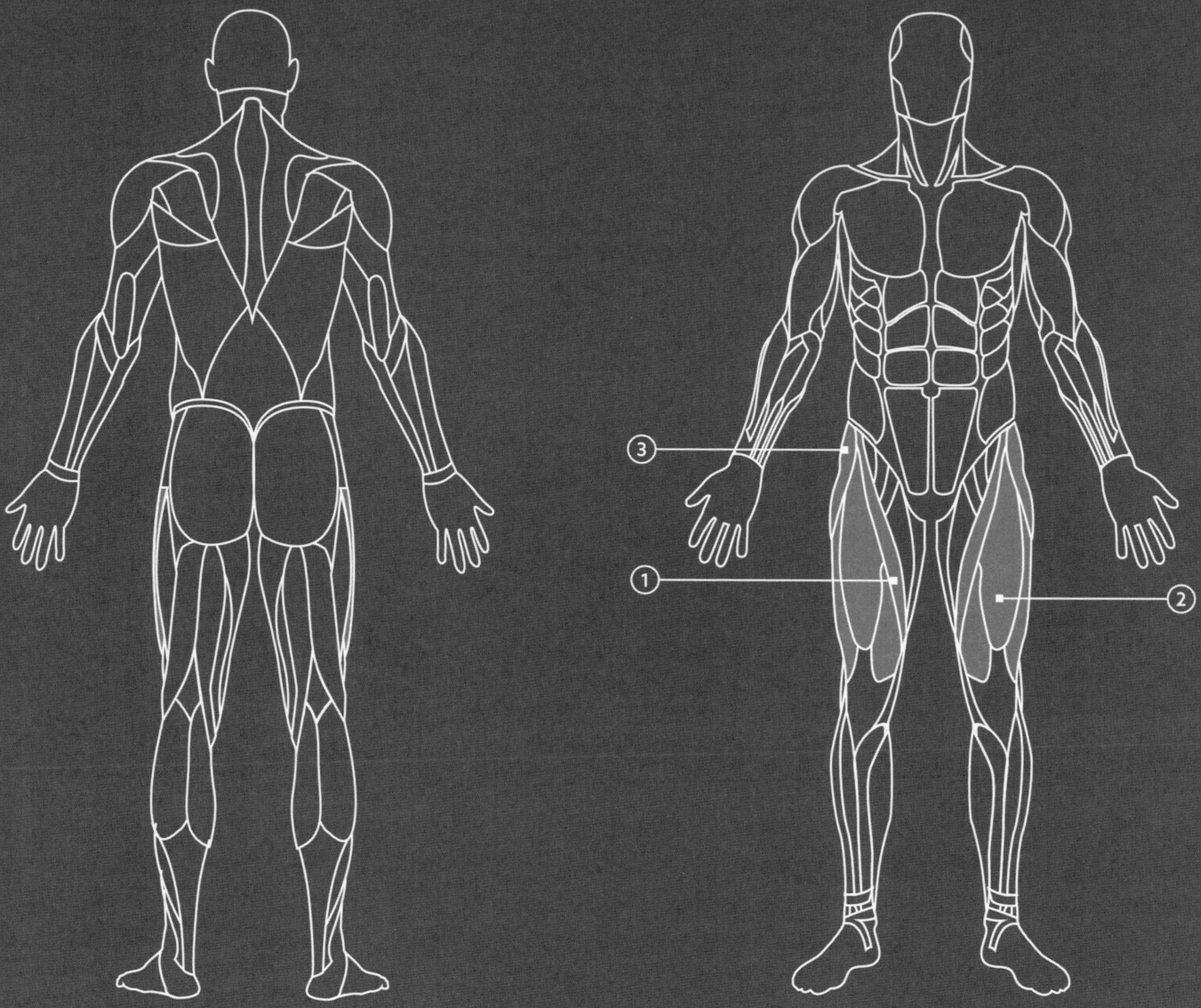

MOBILIZATION TARGET AREAS:

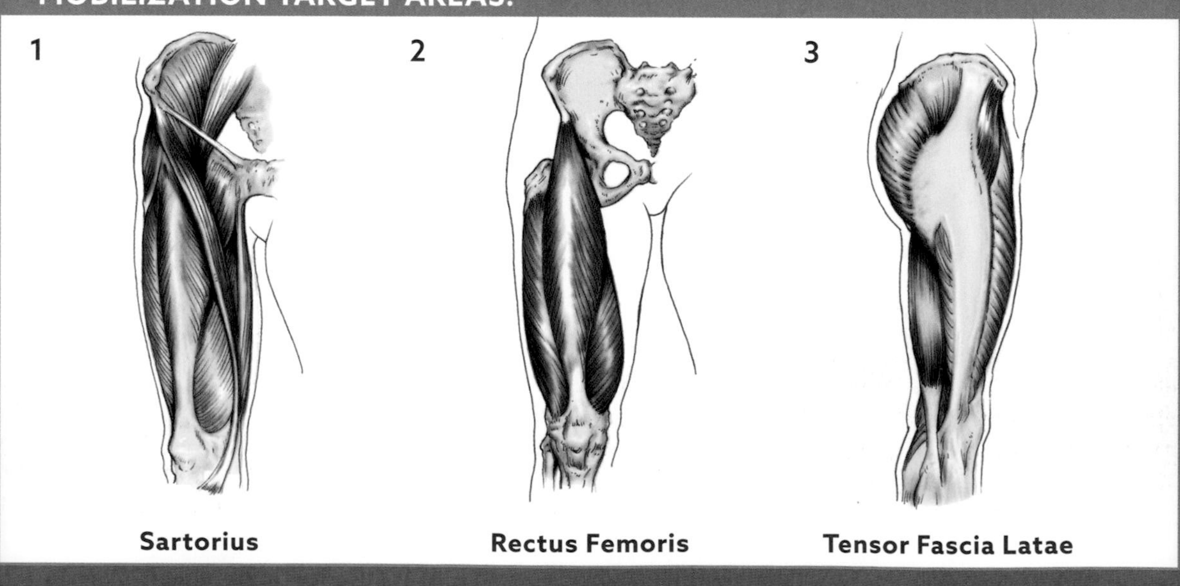

Sartorius

Rectus Femoris

Tensor Fascia Latae

Quad Smash Mobilizations

Lunge Archetype

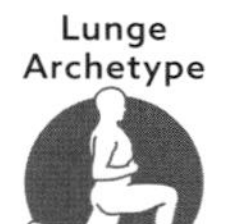

Pistol Archetype

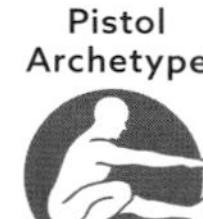

Squat 1 Archetype

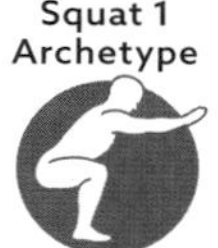

This mobilization will help improve the above archetypes.

IMPROVES:

Knee, hip, and low back pain

METHODS:

Pressure wave (side to side)
Smash and floss
Contract and relax

This is one of my favorite global mobilizations because it has broad range of applications and applies to everyone. CrossFitters, elite-level Olympic weightlifters, tactical athletes, and deskbound workaholics all need tools to address global stiffness in large muscle groups like the quads, hamstrings, and glutes. These muscles are under constant tension, are put under tremendously large loads, and get adaptively short from sitting. Yet many people do little to restore suppleness to the stiff tissue. In this sequence, I demonstrate a potent way to smash your quads and restore normal function to this large bundle of hardworking muscles. However, before you dive in, it's important to revisit some general rules:

Rule #1: Go against the grain of the tissue. Whenever you're dealing with global smashing elements, focus on slow, quality, back-and-forth smashing. As with the T-Spine Smash, rolling up and down the length of the muscle fiber with zero intention is a waste of time. You might as well just do some 1970s-style static stretching and calisthenics, because you're not going to change anything. To produce significant change, create large pressures across the tissue, applying the big three mobilization techniques: pressure wave, smash and floss, and contract and relax.

Rule #2: Stay on the tissue until you make change. The key is to clear a section until it normalizes (meaning it's not painful) before you move up or down the length of the muscle. When I treat athletes in my PT practice, I smash one leg for no less than 10 minutes before switching to the other leg. The point is that you need to commit at least 20 minutes (10 minutes per leg) to ungluing the tissue. If you can't clear the entire leg in 10 minutes, remember where you left off and switch to equal out the other side, and then go back and attack the rest of the first leg.

Rule #3: Use a mobility tool that will make change. To penetrate into deeper layers of tissue, you have to apply large, blunt pressures. If you've never smashed your quads before, starting out with a foam roller is not a bad idea. However, if you're a monster athlete, a foam roller will impact you about as deeply as a bag of marshmallows. If you fall into this category, try using a Battlestar, large pipe, or barbell, or have a Superfriend stand on your quads.

Be warned: Smashing your quads is very painful. You will catch a lot of people hiding in the deep crevices of the pain cave. It may take 20 rolls back and forth before you can take the full pressure of your weight (or a friend's weight) and it stops hurting. So pony up and get some work done.

Option 1: Roller Quad Smash

Smashing your quads over a roller is probably the easiest and most common quad-smashing option. As I mentioned, you can use a foam roller, a PVC pipe, the Big Battlestar, or the Little Battlestar. The Big Battlestar provides broader pressures and is much less aggressive, while the Little Battlestar gives you a more potent, acute stimulus. In general, I recommend using the Big Battlestar for a global smashing effect and the Little Battlestar to target specific knots or trigger points.

TARGET AREA

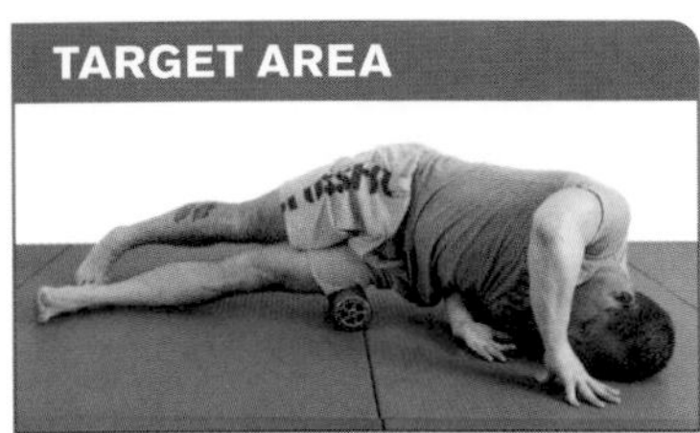

If you're using a Battlestar, you can take the roller out of the cradle and roll from the ground. Positioning the roller on the ground gives you more control over your weight, which allows you to control the pressure, which might reduce the aggressiveness of the mob. It's a matter of personal preference. Try both options and use the one that you feel is more effective.

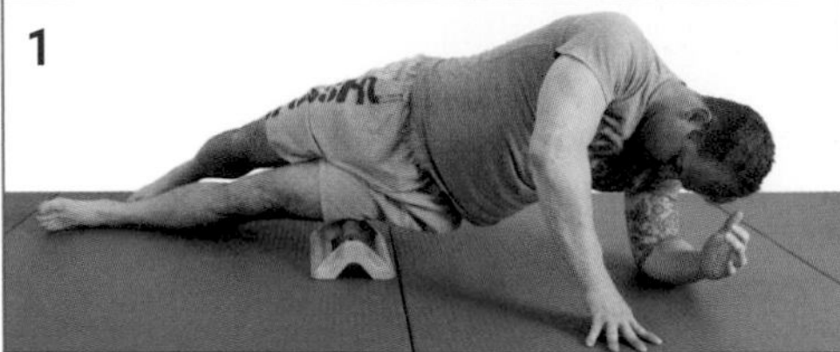

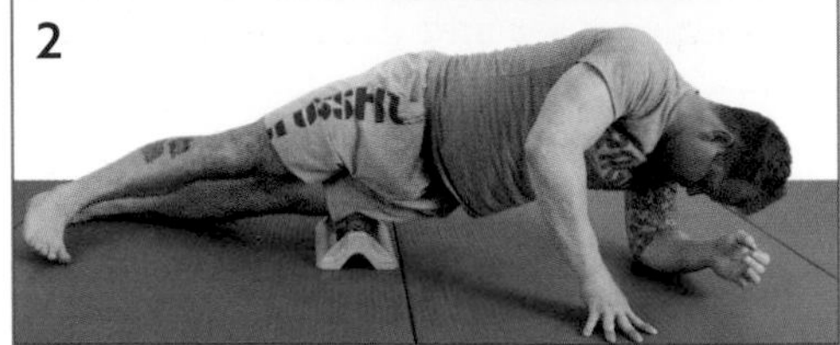

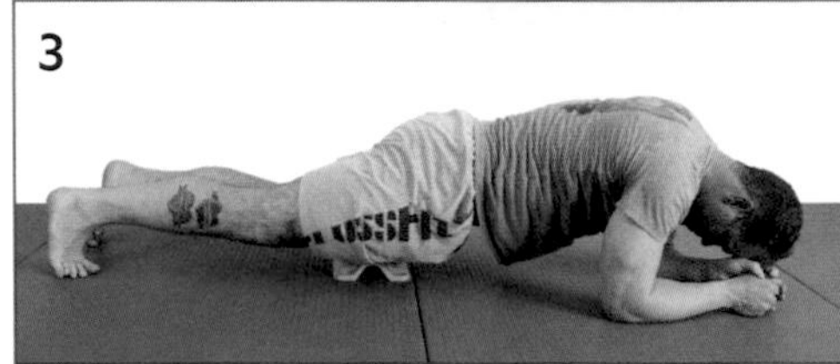

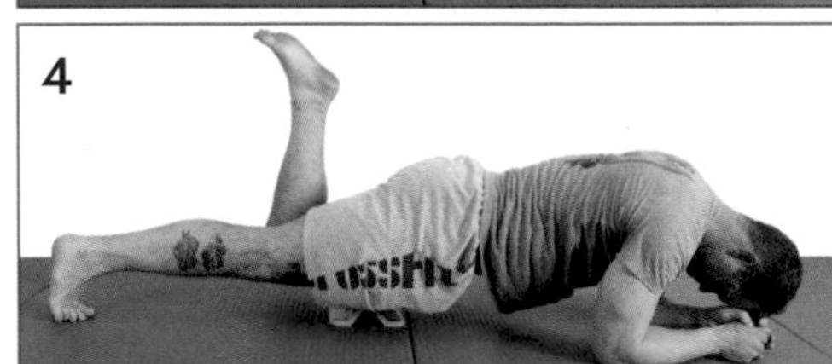

1. Lie on your side over a foam roller, positioning the roller directly under your left leg. To keep your weight distributed over your leg, plant your right foot while supporting the weight of your upper body with your arms.

2. With your weight distributed over your left leg, create a pressure wave across the grain of the tissue by slowly rolling toward your belly.

3. As you roll onto your stomach, plant your right foot on the opposite side of your left leg. From here, you can contract and relax and oscillate on and off of tight spots.

4. Floss around tacked-down tissue by pulling your heel toward your butt. The idea is to stay on the tight area, using the smash and floss and the contract and relax techniques until you no longer feel pain. Once you clear the area, progress up or down your quad to clear another chunk of muscle.

Option 2: Barbell Quad Smash

Using a barbell, rolling pin, or Little Battlestar with X-wing handles is another effective way to tap into the deep tissue stiffness of your quads. As I said, you need large, blunt force to effect change; this is easily done by using a barbell. However, going against the grain of the muscle fiber is difficult using this technique. To restore sliding surfaces to the underlying tissue, be sure to go very slowly, clearing one small area at a time. Think about pressure waving back and forth over stiff muscle bundles until something changes or you stop making change. You can also try rolling your leg from side to side to get the full smashing effect or to tap into different corners.

Note: This mobilization is particularly effective for clearing upper quad stiffness near the hip.

1. Position the sleeve of a barbell over your upper quad. To create pressure, lean forward with a flat back and push the barbell into the meat of your thigh.

2. Slowly roll the barbell down the length of your muscle, maintaining as much downward pressure as possible. Focus on small chunks and go as slowly as you can. The goal is to create a large pressure wave through the tissue. If you encounter a really stiff spot, you can roll your leg from side to side as well as use the contract and relax technique.

3. Pull the barbell back up your thigh, internally rotate your leg, and prepare to attack a new line. For optimal results, create pressure through the barbell only when going down the length of your leg.

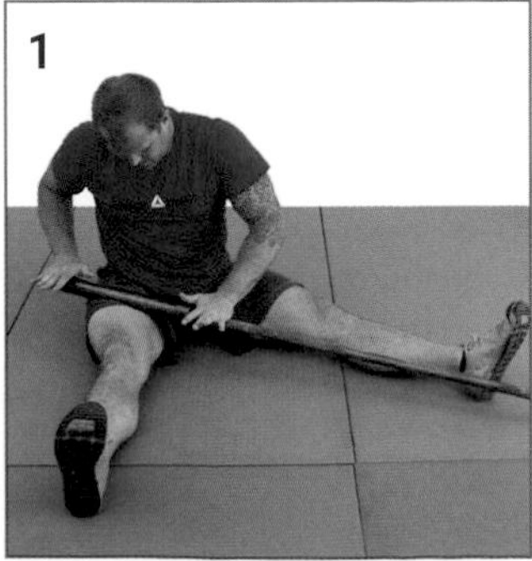

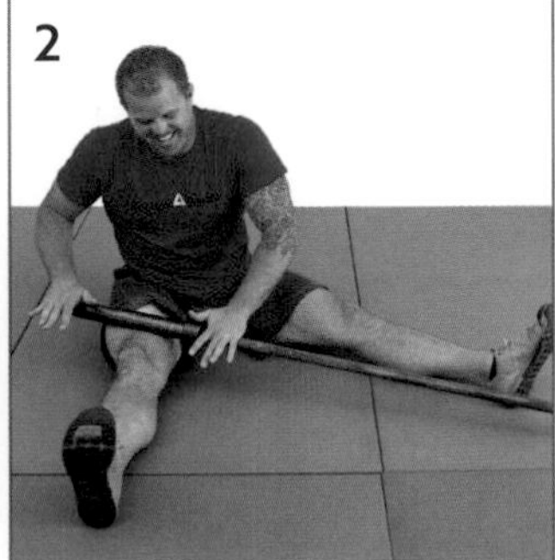

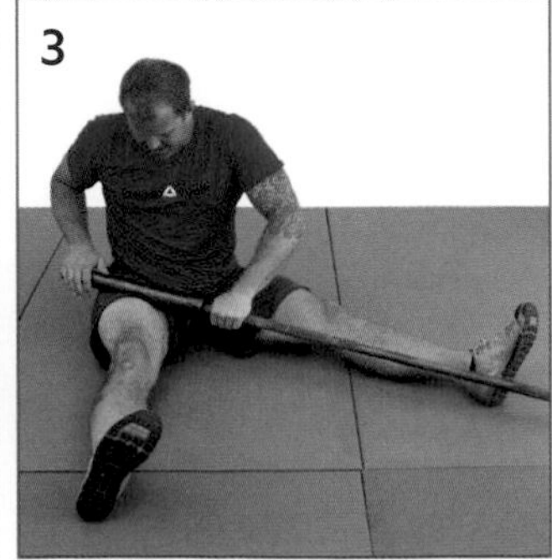

Option 3: Superfriend Quad Smash

The Superfriend Quad Smash is the most efficient way to effect global stiffness change in your quads. While using a barbell, Battlestar, or PVC pipe on yourself is certainly a good idea, the simple fact is that you will never create the same amount of torturous pressure that someone else will. No one is that sick.

To perform this mobilization, have a training partner step on your quad with the arch of his foot and create large downward smashing pressures back and forth across your muscle. If you are the one doing the smashing, avoid using pinpoint, lacrosse ball–like pressures by driving the heel or ball of your foot into the meat. Uncool. The goal is to create a shear force across the muscle in order to restore sliding surfaces to the underlying tissue, as well as make it a little more tolerable for the person getting smashed.

If you're on the receiving end of the smash, fight the urge to overextend. Raising your hips is not going to reduce the pain. Also, don't tap out in submission. It's not a grappling match. However, you probably need to agree on a safe word that will get your training partner to ease up when the pain gets to be too much. Lastly, try to relax your leg as much as possible and go with the pressure. Your leg should roll from side to side as your partner smashes across your quad, as seen in the photos below.

Note: This is a great mobilization to drop into a large group of athletes. In fact, the Chinese weightlifting team has been reported to put on large smashing parties before and after training.

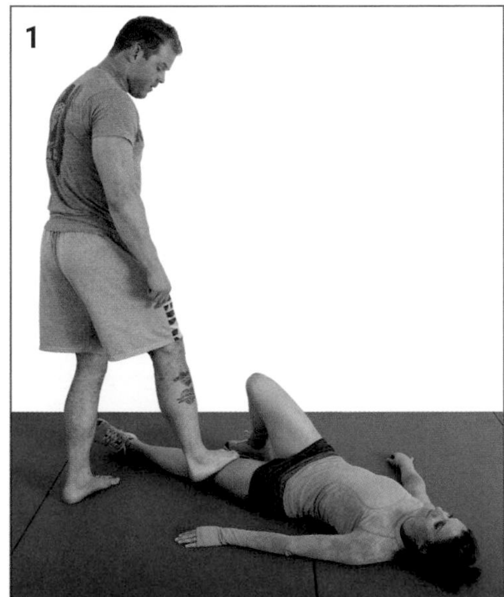

1

As the Superfriend, I position the arch of my foot on Katie's quad. Notice that Katie is posting up on her opposite leg. This helps her maintain a flat back and reduces some of the extension forces (overextending her back) as I smash into her other leg.

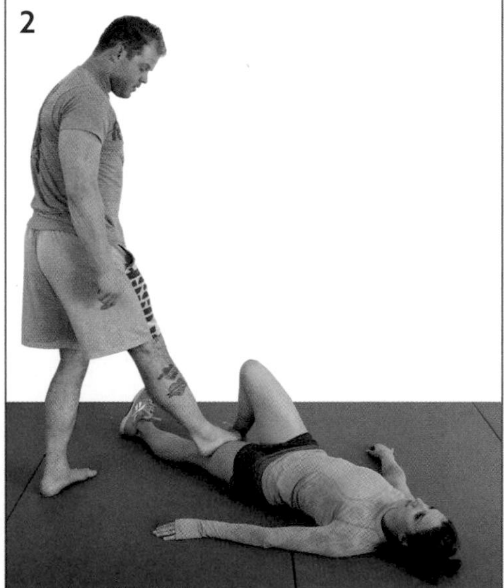

2

I shift my weight forward and create a large shear force across the top of Katie's quad. Notice that her leg rotates as I apply pressure. This is because she's relaxed and not resisting the pressure.

Squat 1 Archetype

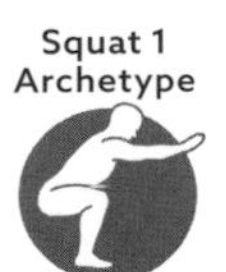

Pistol Archetype

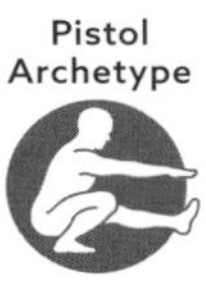

This mobilization will help improve the above archetypes.

IMPROVES:

Knee pain

Knee function

METHODS:

Smash and floss

Pressure wave

Contract and relax

Suprapatellar Smash and Floss

If you're doing a lot of jumping with shins that aren't vertical—that is, your knees are tracking forward when your hips are in flexion—or you're performing sketchy squats where your knees cave in, you will not only experience knee pain, but also burn through duty cycles at an insanely accelerated rate. Don't wait until your knee explodes to do something about it. Feed some slack to the kneecap system so that you can reclaim good knee positions and reduce pain.

To address this issue, snuggle a lacrosse ball into the area just above your kneecap (the suprapatellar pouch), then apply some pressure and smash and floss until something changes. By opening up the area right above your kneecap, you can effectively alleviate joint pain as well as resolve a lot of the knee dysfunction that can occur in deeper ranges of flexion.

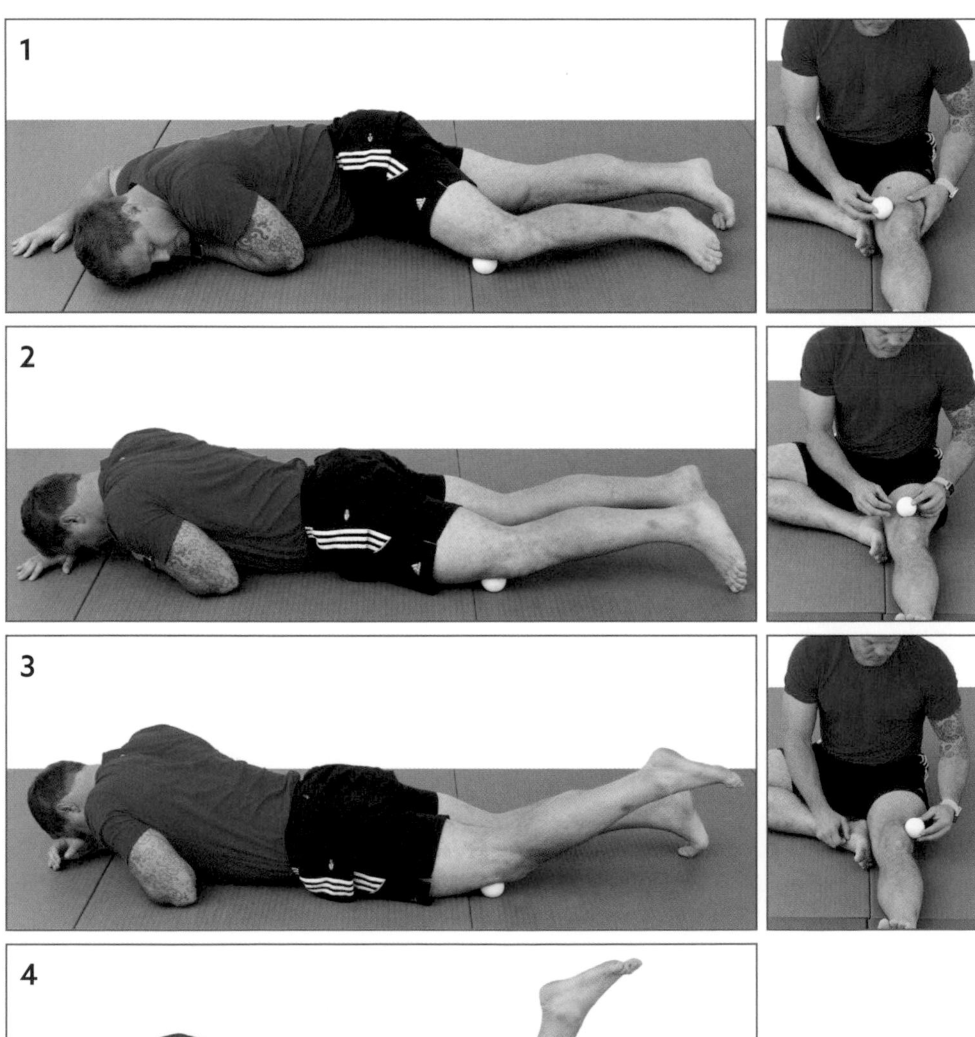

1. Position a lacrosse ball on the inside of your leg, just above your kneecap.
2. Create a pressure wave across your suprapatellar pouch by internally rotating your knee.
3. Continue to smash across your suprapatellar pouch and quad tendon until you reach the lateral part of your knee.
4. If you encounter a hotspot, floss around the stiff tissue by curling your heel toward your butt.

Knee VooDoo

Squat 1 Archetype

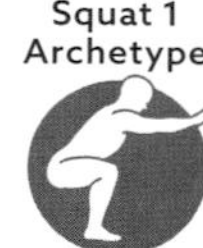

Pistol Archetype

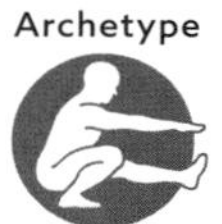

This mobilization will help improve the above archetypes.

IMPROVES:

Knee pain and swelling

Knee sprains or tweaks

METHOD:

VooDoo Floss Band compression

Guess what? Your kneecap does not stretch. The lengths of the ligaments and tendons that make up the knee structure are fixed. The best way to improve knee mechanics (knee out-ness) and reach deeper ranges of flexion is to feed slack to the knee structure by opening up your suprapatellar pouch. In that area, you have the common quad insertion, which shares a large tendon sheath entering into your knee. When this area gets matted down and stiff, it pulls on your knee structure, causing pain and faulty mechanics.

Although the Suprapatellar Smash and Floss works, you're limited to a tiny spot, and you can't get the entire target area. That is why I prefer this VooDoo Floss Band variation as the first step in dealing with upstream and downstream stiffness. It tears open that big, common tendon sheath and clears up the entire area in a very short time.

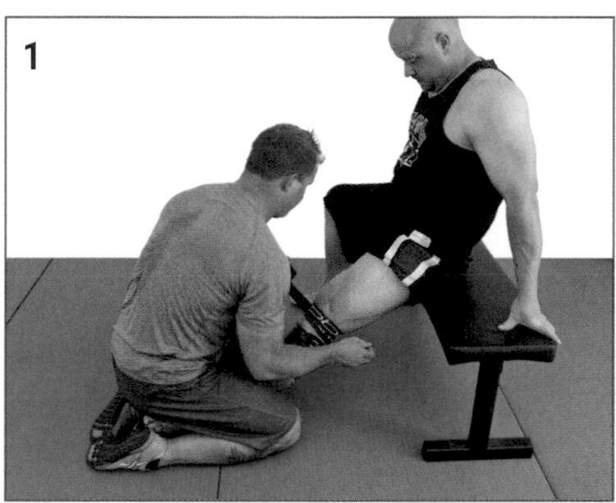

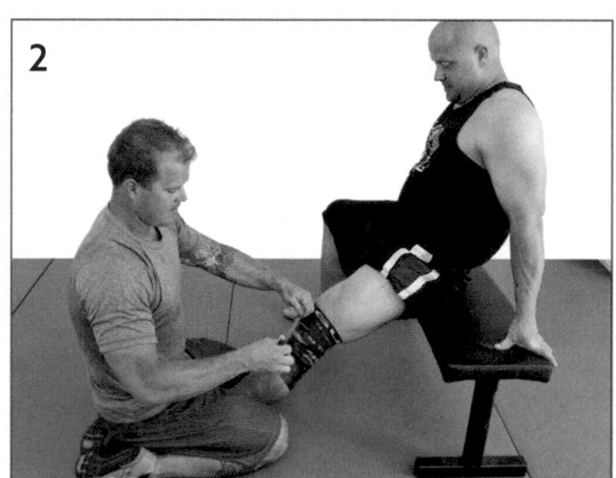

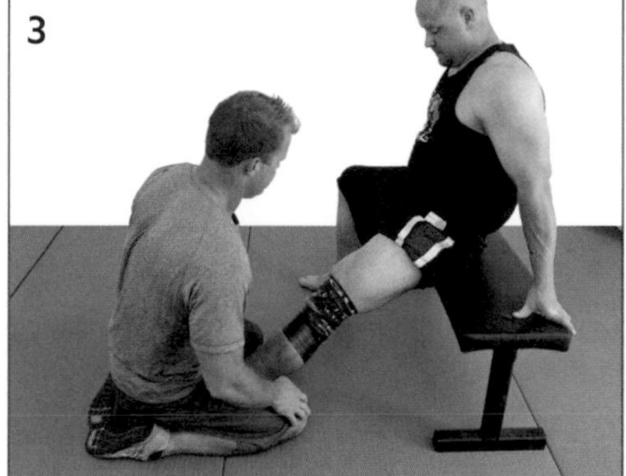

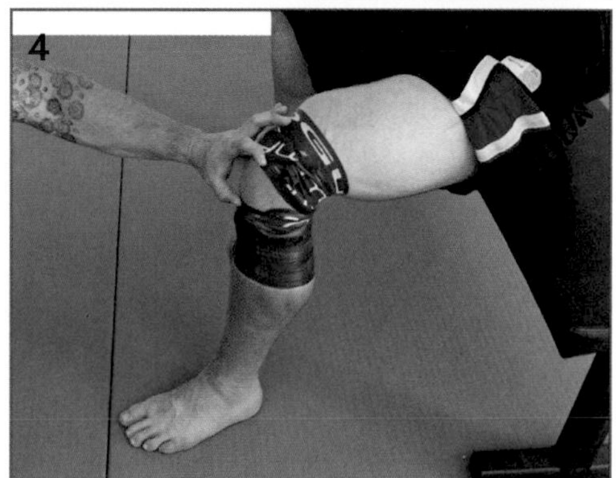

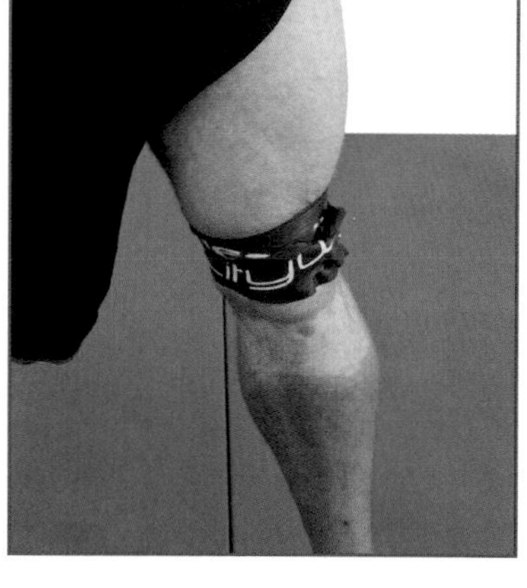

I've wrapped below and above Jesse's knee using two separate VooDoo Floss Bands. You can also wrap the entire knee using one band. To learn the proper wrapping technique, see page 149.

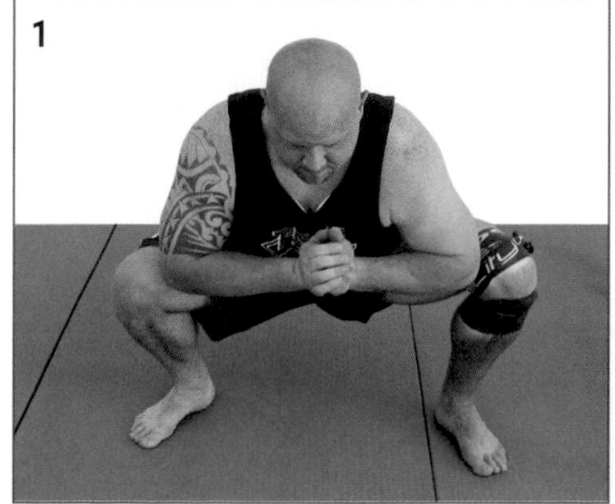

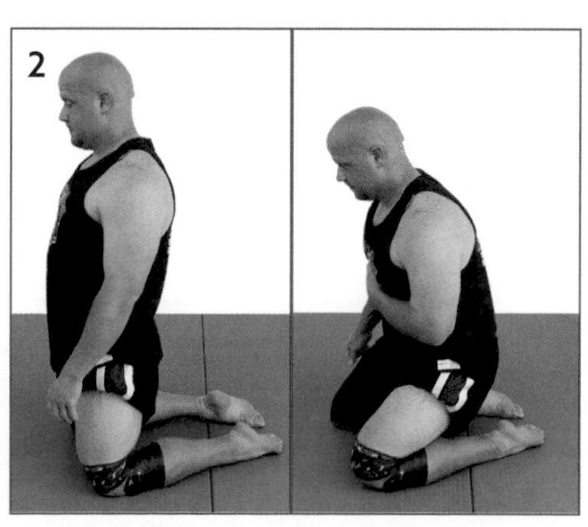

1. With his knee wrapped, Jesse works to floss some of the stiffness away by squatting and biasing knees-out positions. It's important to perform a number of squats, hang out in the bottom position, and force your knee into end-range flexion positions.

2. Jesse continues to force his knee into flexion by kneeling on the ground and sitting his butt to his heels.

Lunge Archetype

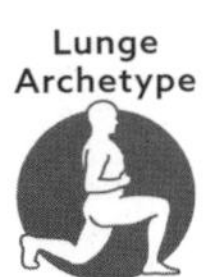

This mobilization will help improve the above archetype.

IMPROVES:

Hip and low back pain

METHOD:

Contract and relax

COMMON FAULT

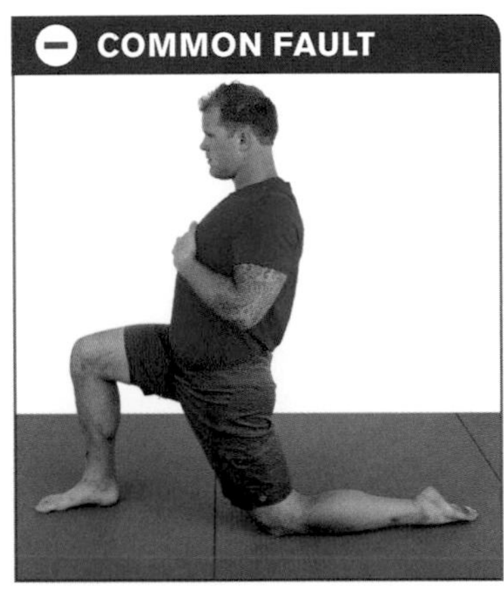

Banded Hip Extension

Opening up the front of your hip while kneeling on the ground is not a new idea. People have been doing this for thousands of years. But there's just one problem: The classic kneeling hip opener (see the Common Fault photo) does not account for the joint capsule, leaving a huge piece of tissue restriction on the table. What's the solution? Simple: Hook your leg through a band, pull the band up to your butt crease, and create a forward distraction. With a large tension force pulling your femur to the front of your hip socket, your joint position is idealized, which not only ties in your anterior hip capsule (y-ligament or iliofemoral ligament), but also makes it easier to mobilize all the musculature at the front of your hip structure.

There are three ways to bias your anterior hip into extension: the Banded Hip Extension, the Banded Hip Extension Lunge, and the infamous Couch Stretch. I'm starting with the most basic, the Banded Hip Extension. To perform this mobilization, you create tension in the band and then slowly shift your body forward while keeping your back flat. A lot of athletes mistakenly arch and hyperextend their back as they open the hip. To avoid this fault, shift your weight over your grounded knee while keeping your posture straight and your butt squeezed.

Note: To capture some of the stiffness in your high anterior hip, put your left arm over your head (if your left knee is on the ground), lean back, and then come back to center. The key is to oscillate back and forth, in and out of end range. As with the classic hip extension, you must keep your butt squeezed to support your lumbar spine. This is just another option that you can infuse into this mobilization. It's a nice way to tear open that high front hip region, which tends to get very nasty.

1

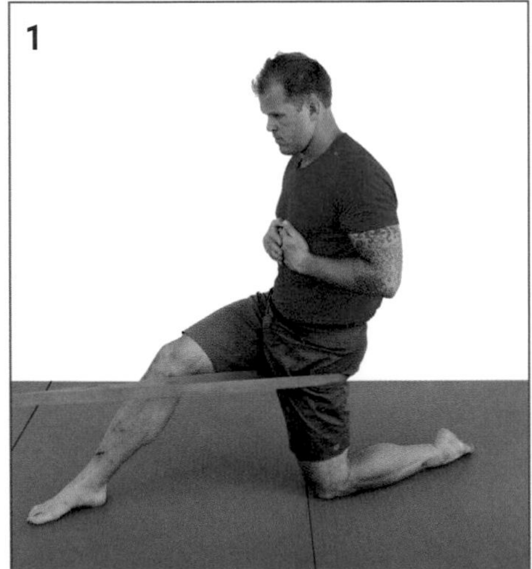

Hook your left leg through a band and step back to create tension, keeping your left foot internally rotated. To avoid breaking into an overextended position, squeeze your left glute and keep your belly tight.

2

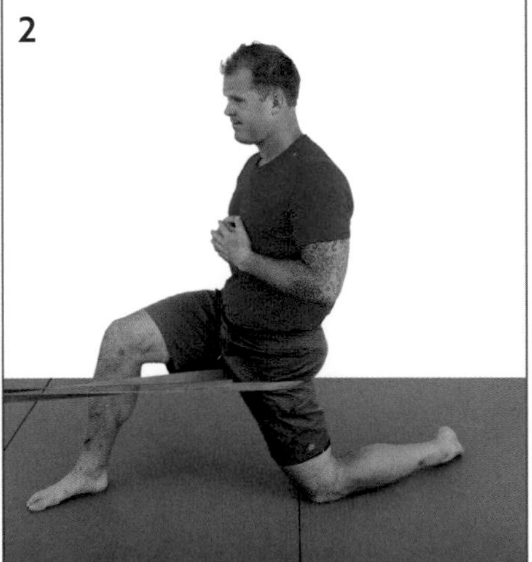

With the band distracting your femur into the front of your hip socket, slowly shift your weight forward over your grounded knee. Notice that I move my entire body rather than thrust my hips forward.

3

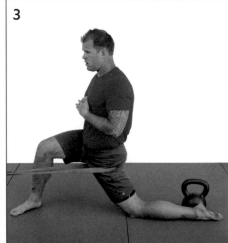

For optimal results, hook your rear foot around a weight so you can bias internal rotation of your hip, which is the stable position for your hip.

Banded Hip Extension Lunge

Mobilizing is a way to deal with muscle stiffness. It restores normal range of motion to tacked-down tissues. It is not a warm-up to exercise. However, some mobilization techniques are appropriate prior to training and competition. The Banded Hip Extension Lunge is a perfect example. As you can see in the photos below, the setup looks a lot like the split-jerk, making it a perfect piece to tie into Olympic lifting or anything else that requires you to open up your hips into full extension.

Lunge Archetype

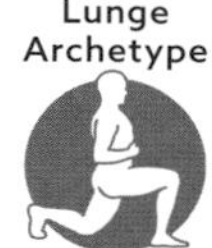

This mobilization will help improve the above archetype.

IMPROVES:

Hip and low back pain

METHOD:

Contract and relax

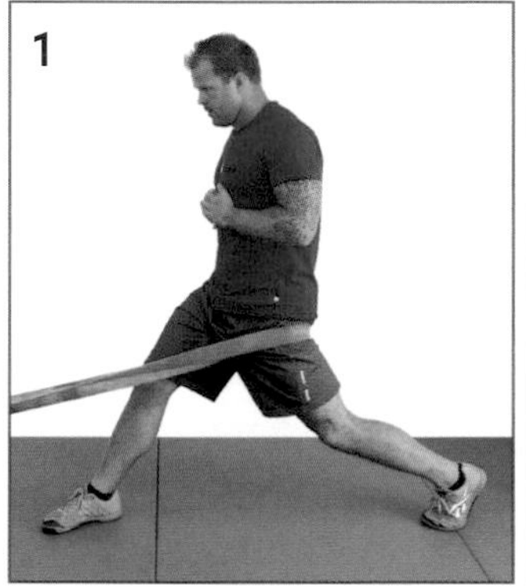

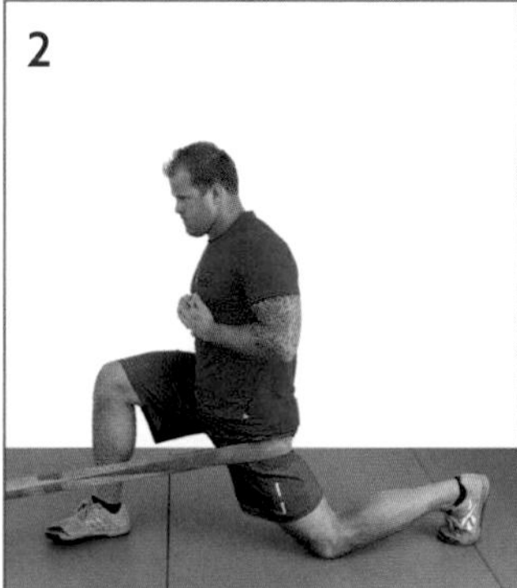

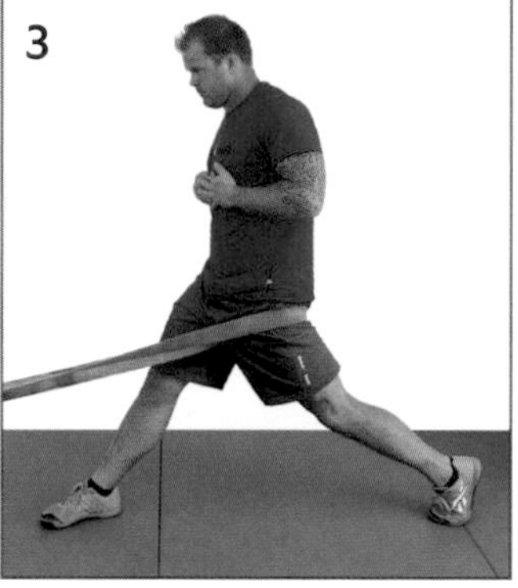

1. Hook a band around your left leg, pull it up to your butt crease, and step back to create a forward distraction on your left hip. To avoid breaking into an overextended position, squeeze your left glute to protect your low back, and brace your trunk.

2. Keeping your left glute squeezed and your belly tight, drop your left knee to the ground. Notice that my right shin does not go past vertical and my torso is upright.

3. Driving off your lead leg, extend both knees and stand up.

Couch Stretch

This mobilization is one of my favorite hip openers, and it's probably the most famous technique in the Movement & Mobility arsenal. Athletes have a real love-hate relationship with the Couch Stretch because it is both effective and horribly painful. When I developed this mob, I had to do it on the couch in front of the TV because:

1. It's an easy way to get your leg into full flexion and open your hips.
2. The TV takes your mind off the pain and keeps you from blacking out.

Although the Couch Stretch is unique to the Movement & Mobility System, it's not a new idea. People have been doing variations of it for a long time. You'd recognize this as the classic standing quad stretch that you did in elementary school (photo 1) or the traditional yogi pose (photo 2), which requires you to grab your foot and pull it to your butt while kneeling on the ground. The problem with these iterations, aside from being difficult to maintain a stable position, is that they do not take you to end range. To effect change, you need to be able to mobilize in a good position and hit end-range knee flexion and hip extension, which the Couch Stretch allows you to accomplish.

Squat 1 Archetype

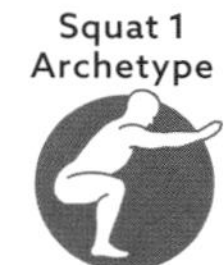

Pistol Archetype

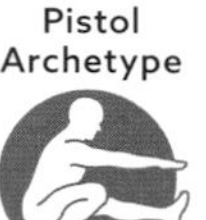

Lunge Archetype

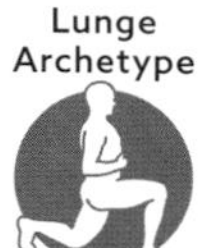

This mobilization will help improve the above archetypes.

IMPROVES:

Hip and low back pain

METHOD:

Contract and relax

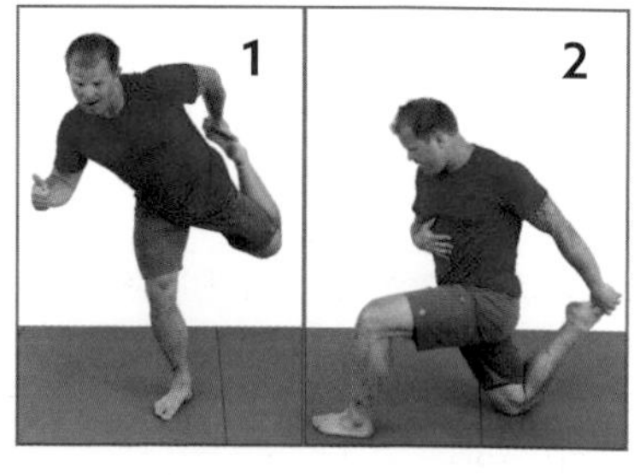

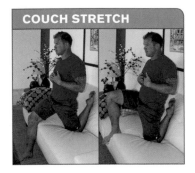

Whether you're trapped at the airport, watching a movie at home, working at your desk, or getting ready to work out, the Couch Stretch is a highly effective way to reclaim range of motion and reduce muscular stiffness in the fronts of your hips and quads.

Note: The positions shown in the photos below are basic physiologic ranges of motion, meaning that everyone should be able to get into these positions without pain or restriction. However, it's just not possible for the majority of people, so this turns into a really quick diagnostic for athletes and coaches alike. If you can't get your leg into the setup position or pull your back to the wall, you know that something is seriously wrong: Your quads and the fronts of your hips are freakishly tight.

COUCH STRETCH

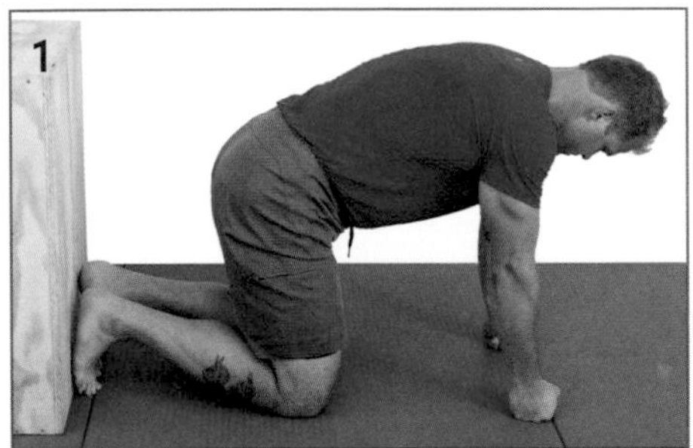
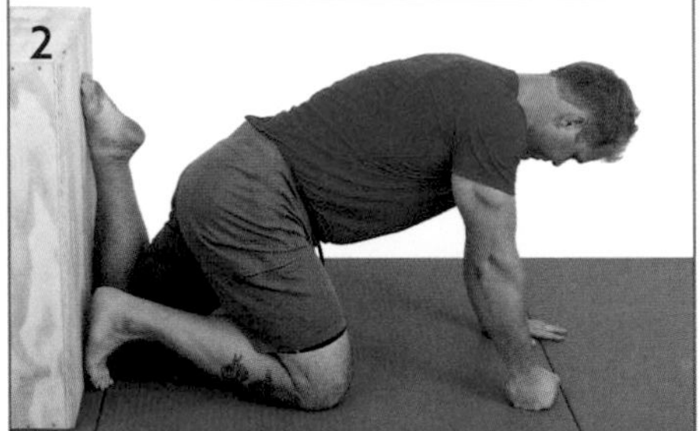
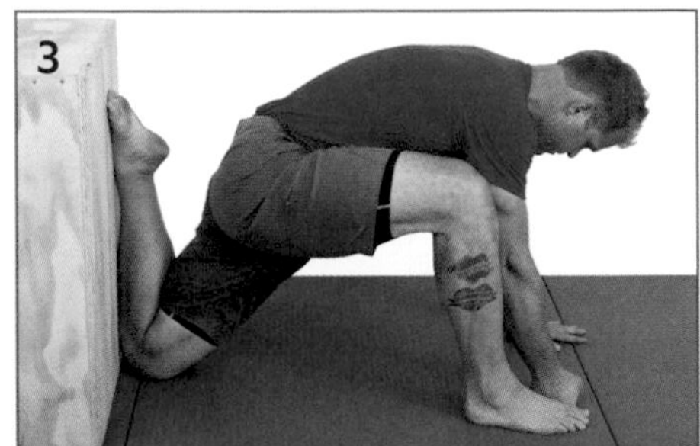
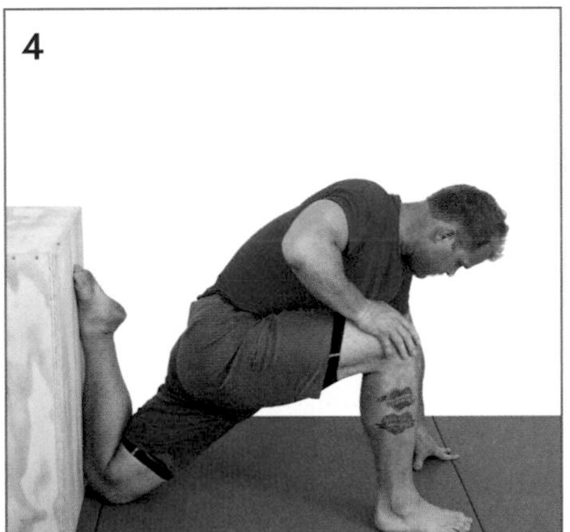
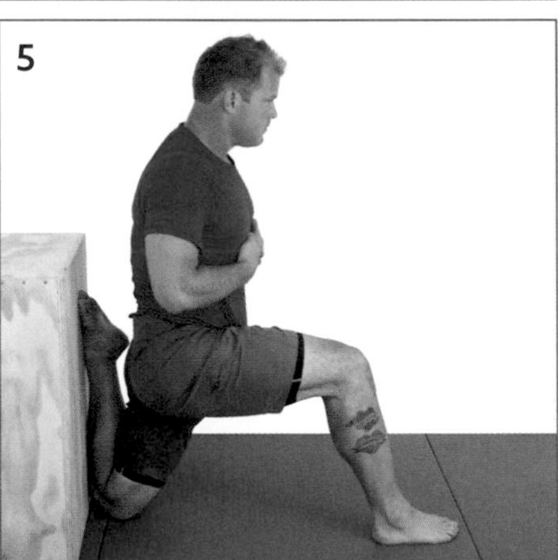

1. On hands and knees, back your feet up to the side of a box.

2. Slide your left leg back, driving your knee into the corner and positioning your left shin and foot flush with the side of the box.

3. Squeezing your left glute to stabilize your lower back, post up on your right foot, keeping your right shin vertical. *Note:* If you're unable to post up on your right leg because you're too stiff, position a small box in front of you for extra stability.

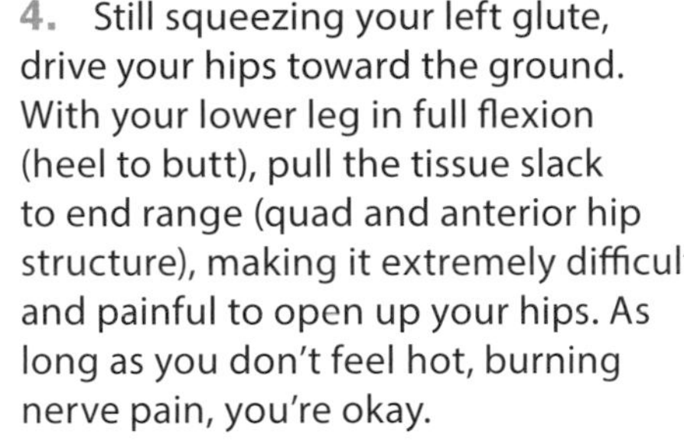

4. Still squeezing your left glute, drive your hips toward the ground. With your lower leg in full flexion (heel to butt), pull the tissue slack to end range (quad and anterior hip structure), making it extremely difficult and painful to open up your hips. As long as you don't feel hot, burning nerve pain, you're okay.

5. After hanging out in the previous position for a minute or two, lift your torso into the upright position. If you find it difficult to support the weight of your upper body from the upright position, position a chair, box, or bench in front of you for extra stability.

COMMON FAULTS

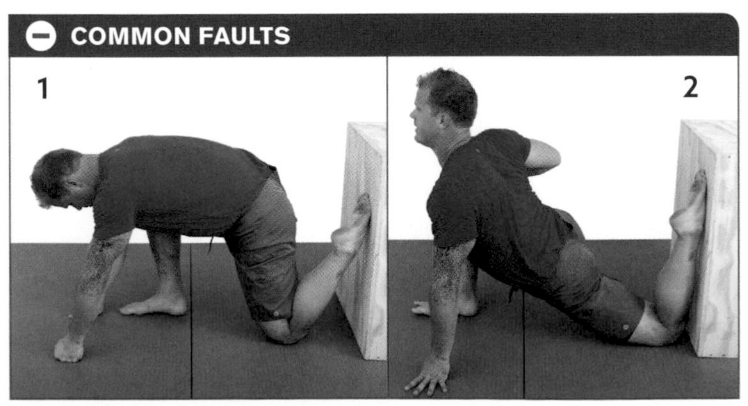

One of the biggest issues people have with the Couch Stretch is that they can't get into the correct positions because they are too tight. It's not uncommon to see an athlete slide his knee out to the side, pull it away from the corner (photo 1), or overextend (photo 2) as a way to circumvent his mobility restriction. If you find it difficult to get into these positions, keep your opposite knee on the ground and stabilize your weight on a box. For the best results, put your knee in full flexion so you can tie in your quads and open up the fronts of your hips. And remember: Don't let your butt go off tension.

Super Couch

The Super Couch is the DEFCON 5 version of the Couch Stretch. Adding a band and creating a forward distraction increases the brutality and effectiveness of this mob by a factor of 10. Remember, anytime you can make a mobilization feel worse, it's probably better. Despite increasing your chances of blacking out, the band opens up your hip capsule and tears into the anterior structures of your quad and hip like nothing else. The results are truly amazing.

Disclaimer: If you don't have full range of motion in your quads and hips, you should probably stick with the Couch Stretch, because adding a band is like dropping a nuclear bomb on your quads and hips. This is the favorite mobilization technique of powerlifter Laura Phelps Sweatt—world champion, world record holder, and one of the greatest strength athletes of our generation—so we commonly refer to the Super Couch as the Laura Phelps.

Note: Wrapping a band around your hip and then positioning your leg against a wall is tricky. Unless you have a $10,000 mobility setup or a large enough box that you can position it next to a pole, you have to get a Superfriend to pull on the other end of the band, which is not ideal. Enter the Coach Roop variation.

Coach Roop Sihota—San Francisco CrossFit super-coach—identified this problem and came up with a solution. In Coach Roop's iteration, you wrap your leg up in a band, pinning your foot to your butt, so that you can implement the Super Couch anywhere. All you need are two bands and a pole. It's genius.

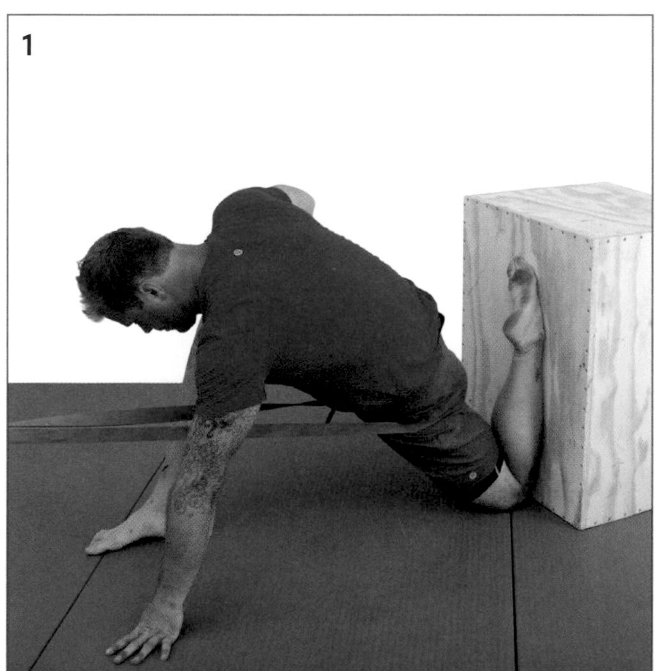

1

Hook your left leg through a band and create a distraction by pulling your left leg back. To prevent the band from pulling you forward, post up on your right foot and then force your left knee into the corner of the box. With your left shin and foot flush with the box, squeeze your left glute with all your might and drive your left hip toward the ground.

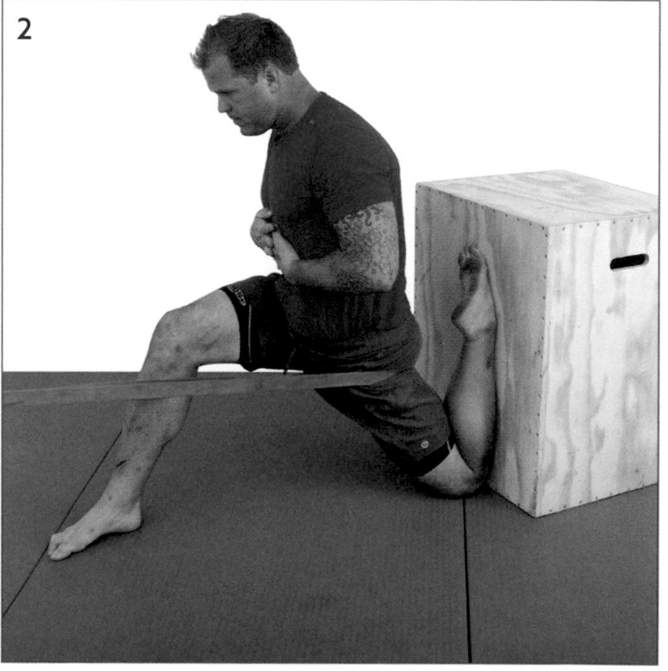

2

Keeping your butt squeezed and your trunk braced, carefully lift your torso into the upright position.

Lunge Archetype

This mobilization will help improve the above archetype.

Trailing Leg Hip Extension

Although the Banded Hip and Couch series is without question the most effective way to mobilize the anterior structures of your hip, you're never really biasing pure hip extension. In other words, if you're always mobilizing with your back leg bent, you never get to open up your hip into full extension. The Trailing Leg Hip Extension is a simple way to remove the flexion component so that you can get your hip into pure extension. This is another mobilization that is only worth doing with a band.

Note: This mob can be used in conjunction with the Banded Hip Extension. For example, you can start in the Banded Hip Extension and then, after a few minutes, slide your trailing leg back and open up your banded hip into full extension.

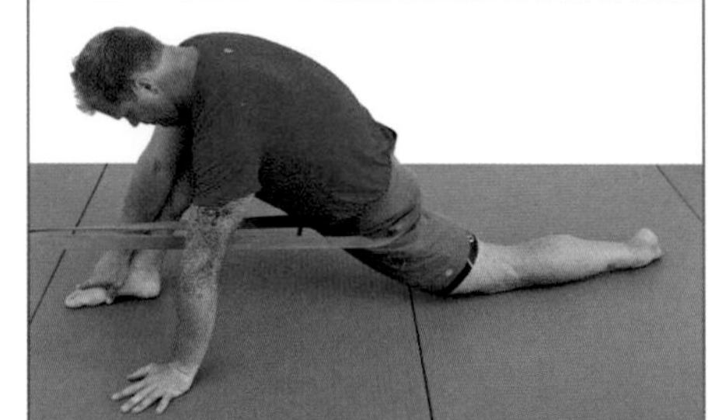

Hook your left leg through a band, positioning the strap around your butt crease, and sprawl your left leg back. To initiate the stretch, squeeze your left glute and drive your left hip toward the ground. From here, you can hunt for stiff areas by dropping your hip to the side and exploring side-to-side ranges. To hit deeper ranges of hip flexion, slide your right leg out or forward (as if you were trying to do the splits) and lower your left hip toward the ground.

METHOD:
Contract and relax

Trailing Leg Hip Extension with Internal Rotation Bias

For this option, you add an internal rotation bias by putting your lead foot up on a box. With your front foot off the ground, you can come up onto the ball of your back foot and rotate your knee toward the inside of your body. This internal rotation bias not only accounts for the stable position of your hip (extension and internal rotation), but also takes on the shape of athletic positions and movements such as the split-jerk, the combat and fighting stance, and sprinting.

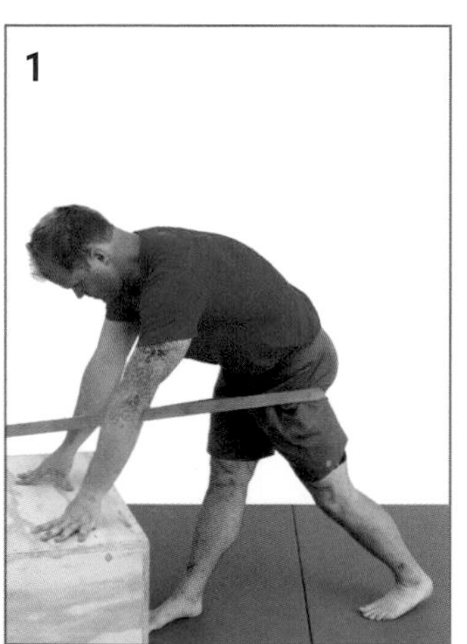

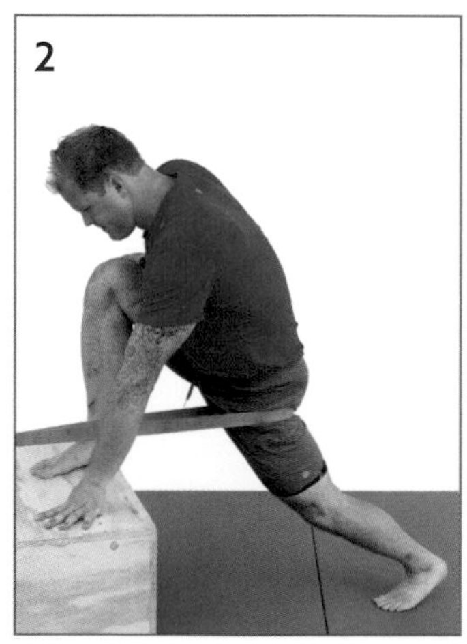

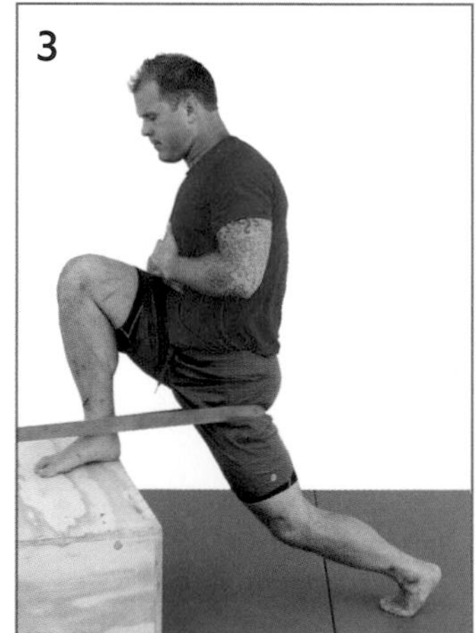

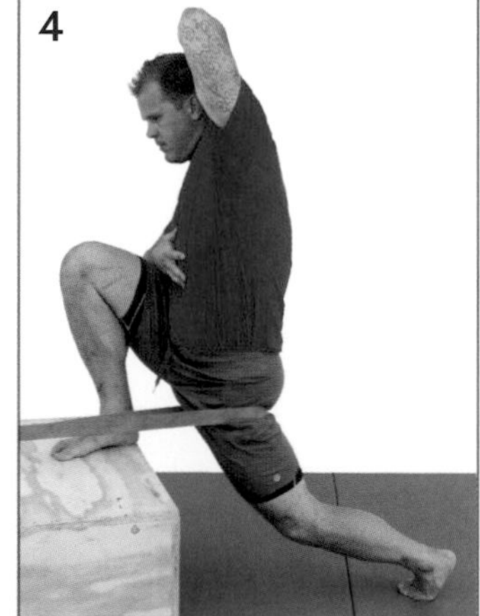

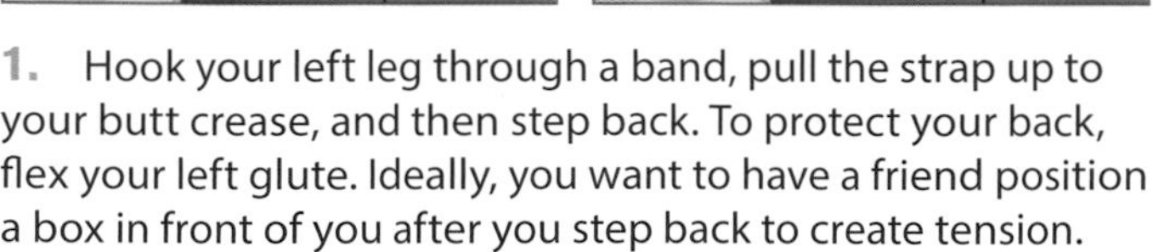
1. Hook your left leg through a band, pull the strap up to your butt crease, and then step back. To protect your back, flex your left glute. Ideally, you want to have a friend position a box in front of you after you step back to create tension.

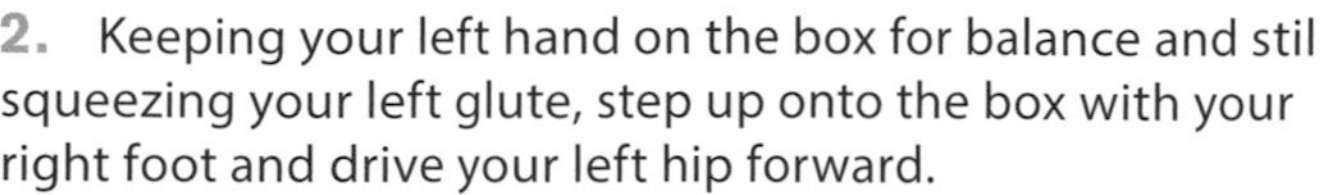
2. Keeping your left hand on the box for balance and still squeezing your left glute, step up onto the box with your right foot and drive your left hip forward.

3. Lift your torso upright, come up onto the ball of your left foot, and bias internal rotation of your trailing leg by rotating your left knee toward the inside of your body.

4. To capture your psoas and encourage more hip extension, throw your left arm over your head.

Reverse Ballerina

The Reverse Ballerina is an easy way to tap into hidden stiffness upstream and downstream of your hips. As you can see in the photos below, this technique takes on the same shape as a lot of kicking movements, making it a great mobilization for sports that involve any kind of leg swing rotational elements—think dance, martial arts, and gymnastics.

In addition, the Reverse Ballerina ties in the adductors (the muscles on the insides of your thighs). When these muscles get tight, they pull your pelvis into a bad position in the bottom of a squat (see the butt wink fault on page 173) and limit your capacity to drive your knees out. By throwing your leg up onto a box, bringing your leg out to the side, and rotating away from your leg, you still get to bias extension and internal rotation, but you add an abduction component, which adds another level of gnarly-ness.

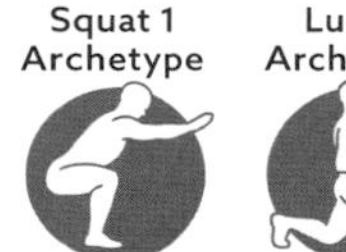

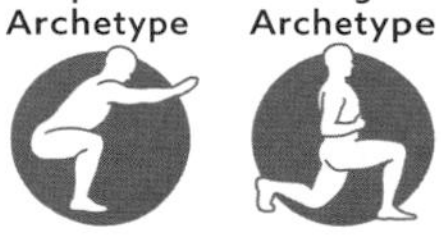

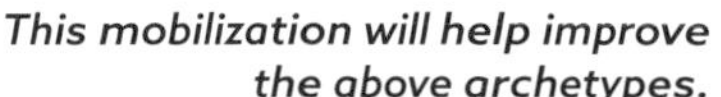

This mobilization will help improve the above archetypes.

METHOD:
Contract and relax

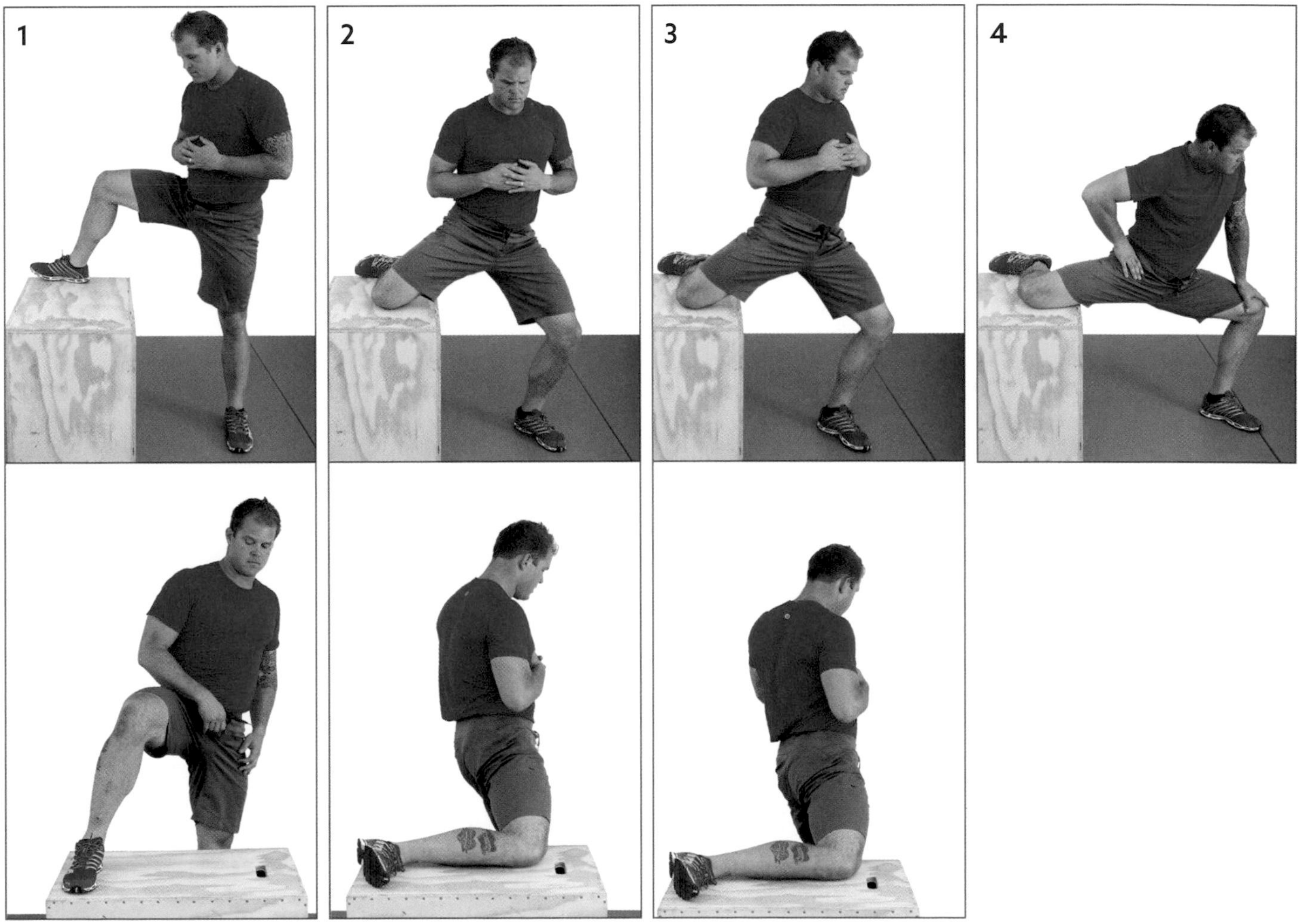

1. Post your right foot up on the far edge of a box.

2. Keeping your right foot open, drop your right knee and ankle to the box and rotate away from your right leg.

3. Driving your knee down into the box, continue to rotate away from that leg. This helps capture some areas in the front of your hip, as well as the musculature running down the inside of your leg.

4. You can hunt for untapped stiffness by lowering your body while twisting away from your right leg. You can also throw your arm over your head, twist around, and scour for hard-to-reach corners.

Squat 1 Archetype

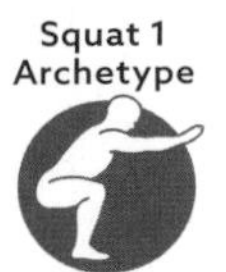

Lunge Archetype

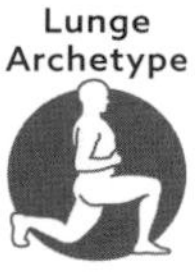

This mobilization will help improve the above archetypes.

METHOD:
Contract and relax

Banded Hurdler

The Banded Hurdler is a spin-off of a classic quad, hip, and hamstring stretch that sports teams and physical education teachers have been implementing for many years. Traditionally, this stretch—commonly referred to as the "hurdler stretch" because the position mimics a runner's shape as she clears a hurdle—was used primarily as a quad and hamstring stretch: Lean back to stretch the quadriceps and anterior hip of the rear leg, and lean forward to stretch the hamstring of the front leg. In this sequence, you do neither. With one leg back and one leg straight out in front of you, you're not in an ideal position to mobilize your quads, hips, or hamstrings. However, attaching a band to your hip with a forward distraction—pulling your leg anteriorly—mobilizes your femur to the front of your hip capsule, turning a not-so-effective classic stretch into a highly effective hip capsule mobilization.

1

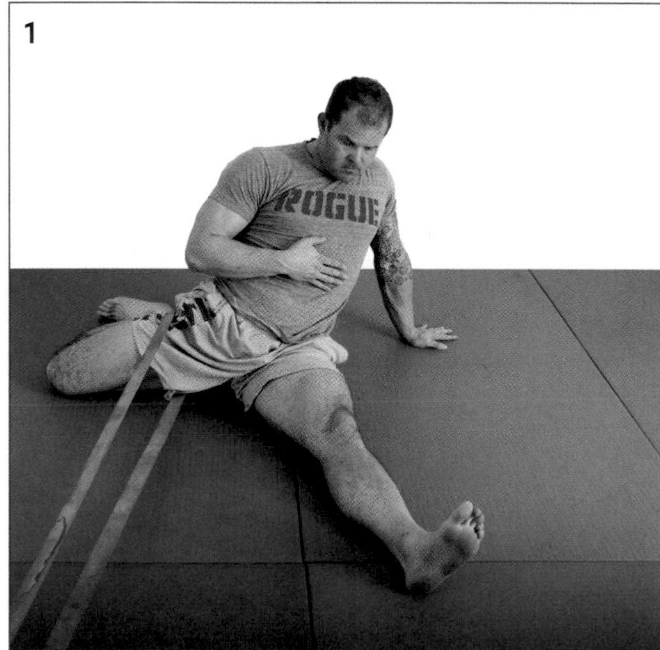

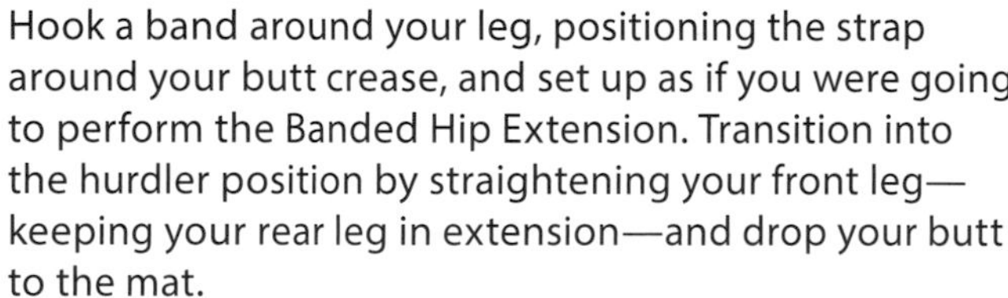

Hook a band around your leg, positioning the strap around your butt crease, and set up as if you were going to perform the Banded Hip Extension. Transition into the hurdler position by straightening your front leg—keeping your rear leg in extension—and drop your butt to the mat.

2

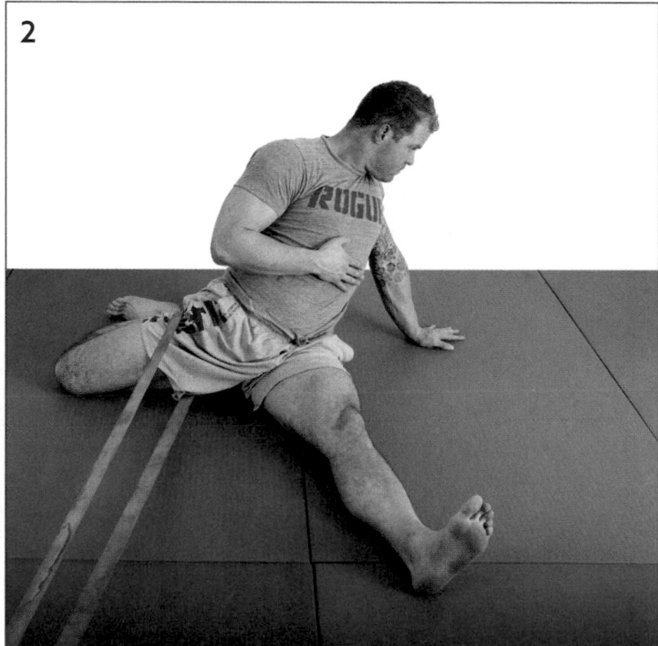

Rotate your upper body away from the leg and hip you're mobilizing. As with the previous techniques, the key is to keep the glute of your banded leg squeezed and your abs engaged to prevent overextension.

AREA 9 ADDUCTORS

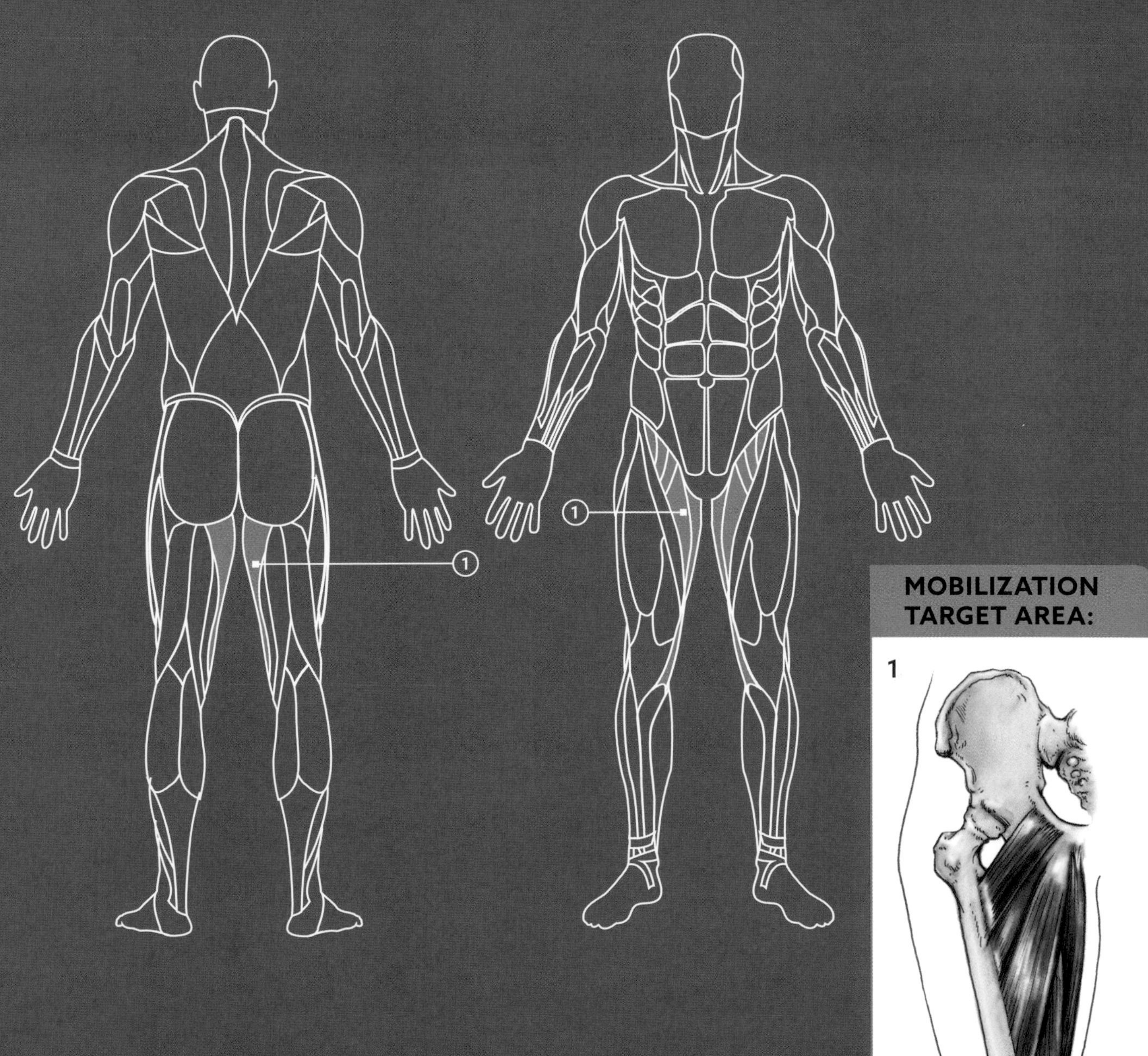

MOBILIZATION TARGET AREA:

1

Adductors (group)

Squat 1 Archetype

This mobilization will help improve the above archetype.

IMPROVES:

Hip and low back pain

METHODS:

Pressure wave
Contract and relax
Smash and floss

Adductor Smash

The adductors—big masses of tissue on the insides of your thighs—are like the undervalued stepchildren of your legs. They play a critical role in the family unit but get ignored and passed over in favor of more important muscle groups like the quads and hamstrings. The fact is, your adductors are responsible for stabilizing your back and pulling your knees back to center as you rise out of a squat. They also give you external rotation slack and stabilize your body laterally when you're standing on one leg, such as when kicking, spinning, or planting.

As I've said, you have to look at your body as a whole and work on solving your mobility issues from all angles. The next time you're having trouble getting your knees out when you squat, don't go straight to your favorite kids—your quads and hamstrings—because there's a good chance that it's your adductors that are limiting your position.

Option 1: Adductor Roller Smash

The roller is the most ubiquitous tool for smashing the adductors. The approach to smashing is the same: Go against the grain of the muscle tissue using a pressure wave, and if you find a trigger point, stop, contract and relax, and floss. Again, you can use a foam roller, which is the least aggressive and consequently least effective, a pipe, the Battlestar, or any hard, round object (such as a wine bottle or metal water bottle).

1

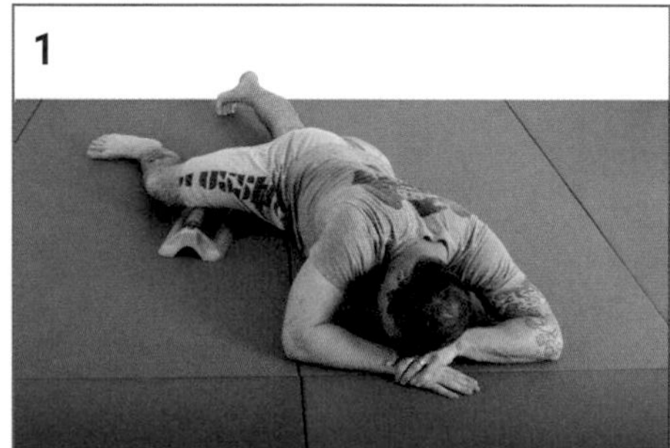

Position the inside of your leg on a roller.

2

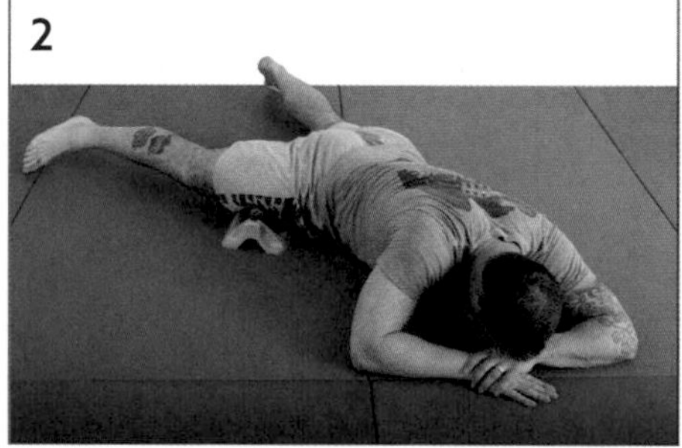

Keeping your leg relaxed, create pressure into the roller by driving your hip toward the ground. Straighten your leg and then turn your knee toward the mat to create a lateral shear force across the muscle fiber.

3

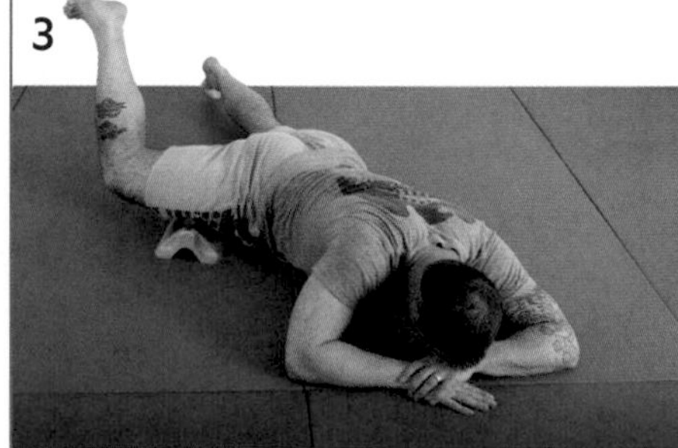

When you roll onto a tight spot, stop, get as much pressure into your leg as possible, and then floss around the tacked-down tissue by pulling your heel toward your butt. Staying on the stiff tissue, move your leg around in all directions to clear the stiffness.

Option 2: Adductor Barbell Smash

As with quad smashing, you can employ several different methods to smash your adductors. You can use a roller or barbell or have a Superfriend step on the inside of your leg. Each has distinct advantages. For example, a roller gives you the freedom to smash and floss around tacked-down tissue; a barbell enables you to isolate pockets of knotted-up muscle by using the pressure wave and contract and relax techniques; and the Superfriend variation unglues more global stiffness than you can ever hope to unglue on your own.

Position the sleeve of a barbell or a Little Battlestar over your adductor. To create pressure, lean forward with a flat back and push the barbell into the meat of your thigh. Slowly roll the barbell down the length of the muscle, maintaining as much downward pressure as possible. Focus on small chunks and go as slowly as you can. The goal is to create a large pressure wave through the tissue. If you encounter a really stiff spot, you can roll your leg from side to side as well as use the contract and relax technique. If you're using a Little Battlestar, you can seesaw back and forth across the muscle.

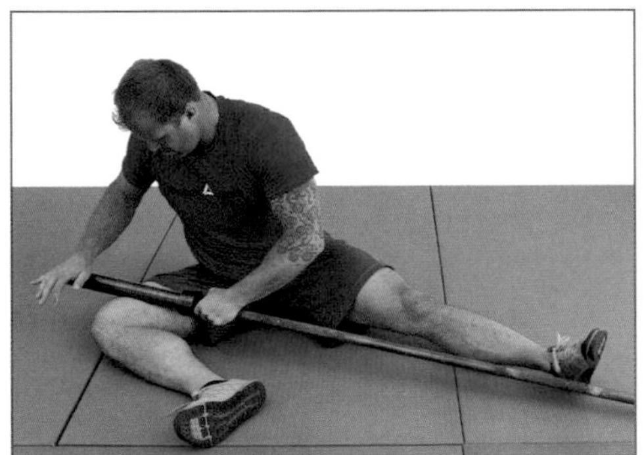

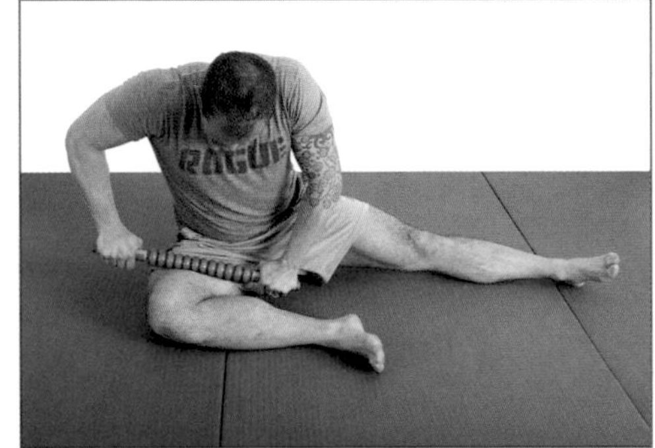

Option 3: Superfriend Adductor Smash

Like the previous technique, the Superfriend Adductor Smash is a great option because it helps delaminate tacked-down tissues with large pressures that you are unlikely to inflict on yourself.

There are two ways to approach this mobilization: You can lie on your back with one leg bent (photo 1) or roll onto your side, crossing one leg over the other (photo 2). The former is great for creating large pressures across the muscle, with your training partner using the arch of his foot, while the latter is ideal for targeting trigger points, with your training partner using his heel.

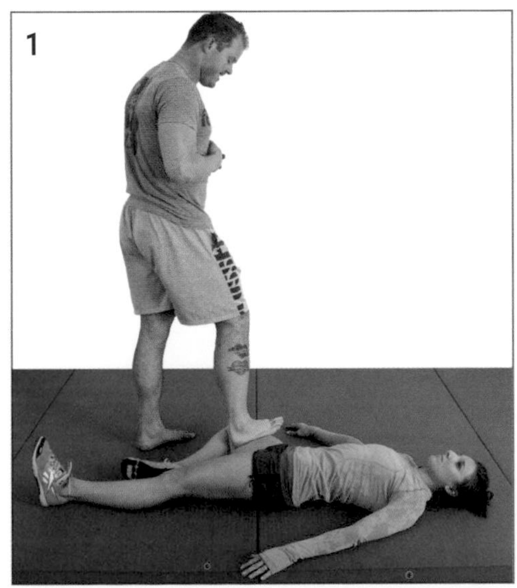
1

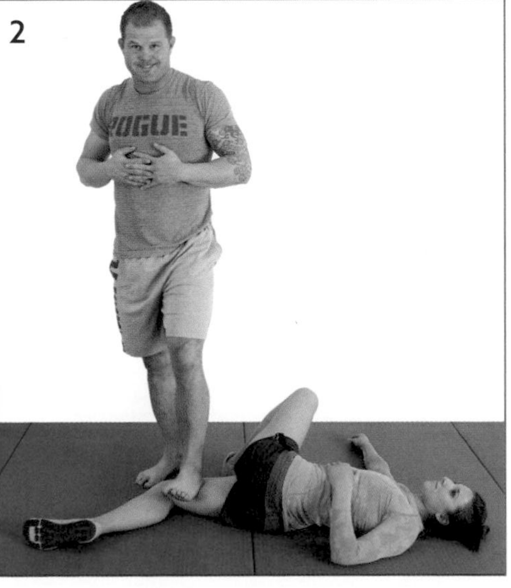
2

Lie on your back and curl your heel toward your hamstring (photo 1). Or roll onto your side by rotating your hips and stepping your opposite leg over your bent leg, which exposes not only your adductors but also your hamstring and groin (photo 2). Have your training partner slowly pressure wave by stepping his foot toward the ground as if he were trying to peel your adductor and hamstring off your leg. If he hits a knotted-up bundle of muscle tissue, contract and relax. He can even rotate his foot from side to side for a smearing effect.

Squat 1
Archetype

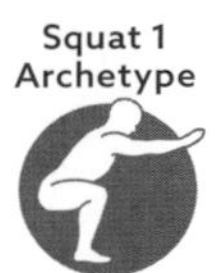

This mobilization will help improve the above archetype.

METHOD:

Contract and relax

Banded Super Frog

The Banded Super Frog is the most effective and consequently the most brutal medial chain (inside of your leg and hip) mobilization in the Movement & Mobility arsenal. For the longest time, I had only the Adductor Smash, the Super Frog, and a few other mobilizations that hit the medial chain of the high hip, adductor, inner hamstring, and groin area. While these techniques yielded good results, I struggled to come up with a way to bias the hip into a good position so that I could account for the joint capsule.

Enter the Banded Super Frog. By hooking your leg through a band hanging from a pull-up bar, sliding it up to your groin, and then placing a bumper plate, barbell, or weight over your banded leg, you can tap into the deep regions of your hip and hit corners of your high hamstring that you didn't even know were there. As with so many of the great mobilizations, this one is not very comfortable. But anything that causes that level of ugliness must be good, right? The fact is, this one mobilization captures multiple systems, which is always the goal. To keep your hip in a good position and protect your back from large extension forces (bridging your hips and hyperextending your back), keep your butt fully engaged.

You can also have a Superfriend step on the weight for an additional level of gnarly-ness. Save this for after your workout, or maybe after a good warm-up, because it is going to create some serious change. Remember, you don't want to monkey around with your pelvic position too much before strenuous activity or heavy lifting.

This mob has also been called the Super Sumo Groin because a lot of our big, strong powerlifters have a hard time locking out while maintaining a good hip position due to this area of the groin and pelvis being short and stiff.

1. Hook your right leg through a skinny band and pull it up to your groin. This sets your femur in a good position within the hip socket, allowing you to tap into tightness in your hip capsule.
2. Set a 45-pound bumper plate over your bent right leg, pinning it to the ground.
3. Squeezing your right glute to support your hip joint and low back, slowly lie back and bring your left foot next to your right foot.
4. Cover your face with your hand so that nobody can see your grisly expression, then lower your left knee toward the ground to add tension. You can contract and relax by driving your right knee into the weight and raise and lower your left knee to control the tension.

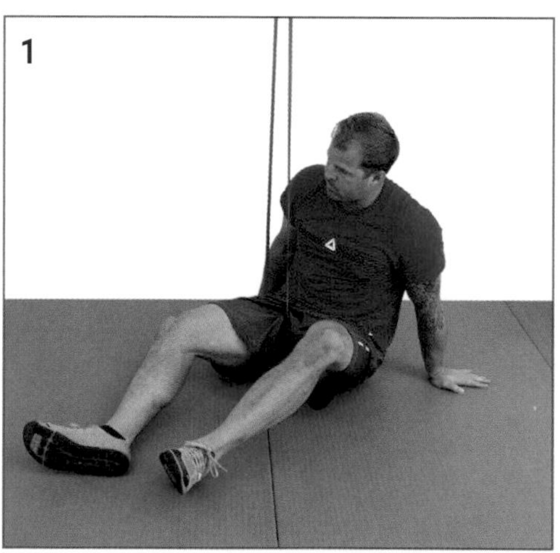

1

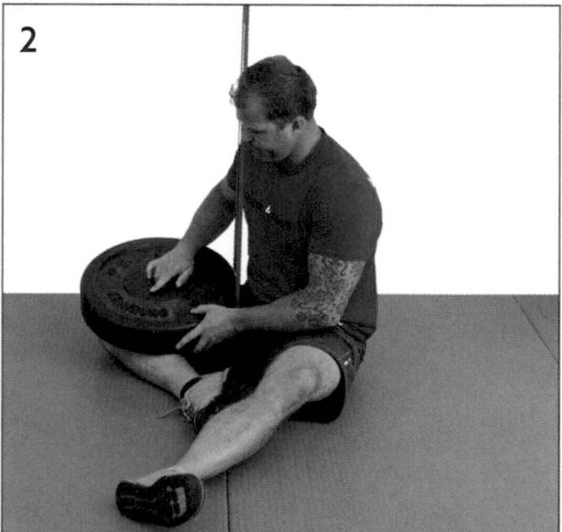

2

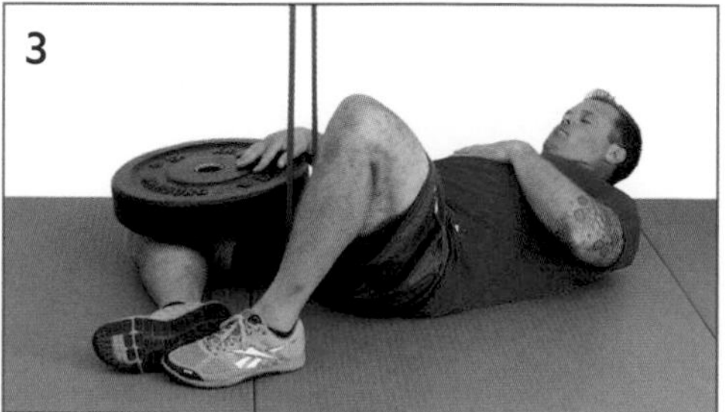

3

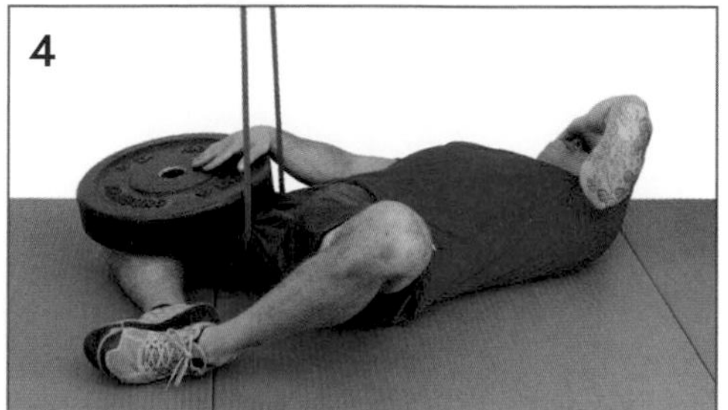

4

Super Frog

If you don't have a band hanging from a pull-up bar, you can still execute the Super Frog. Realize, however, that it won't have the same impact. The band enables you to tap into another system of restriction (your hip capsule). Still, something is better than nothing.

Remember, you have to take a systematic approach when you are trying to improve your position. Failing to account for any of these pieces—motor control, sliding surfaces, muscle dynamics, or the joint capsule—will always leave you a little short when it comes to optimizing movement or restoring function to the tissues you're trying to change. So if you can use a band, do it. But please do not rip down your ceiling fan; it's probably not worth it.

Squat 1 Archetype

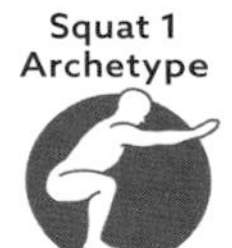

This mobilization will help improve the above archetype.

METHOD:

Contract and relax

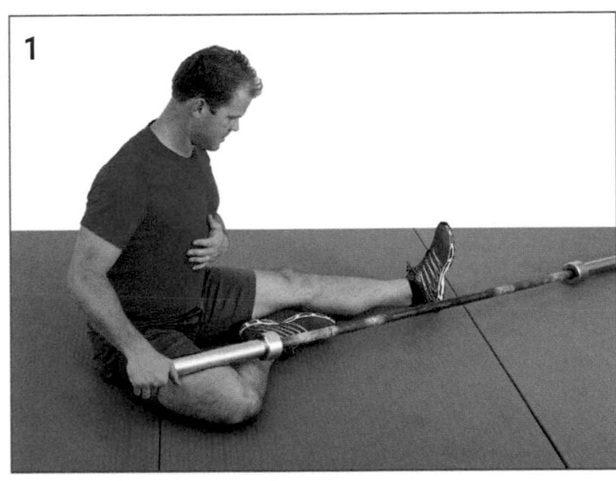

Sitting upright, place the sleeve of a barbell over your right thigh, pinning your knee in place.

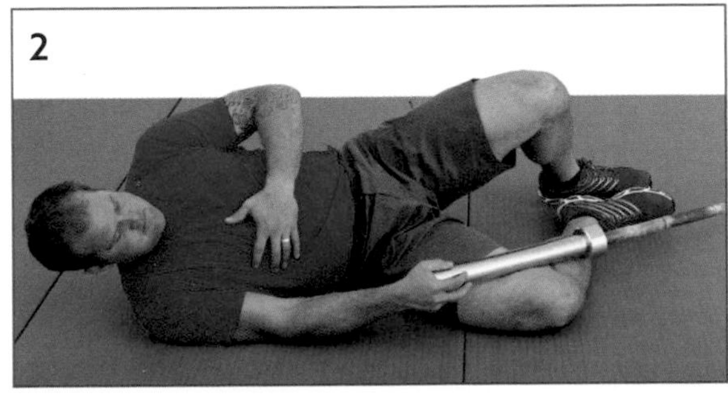

Squeezing your right glute to stabilize your hip and back, lie on your right side and position your left foot next to your right foot.

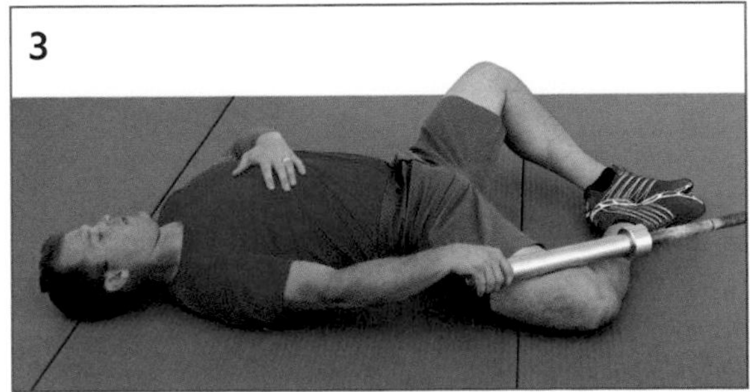

Keeping your right hand on the barbell to keep it positioned over your right leg, lie back and drop your left knee toward the ground to create a greater stretch through your pelvis and medial line (groin).

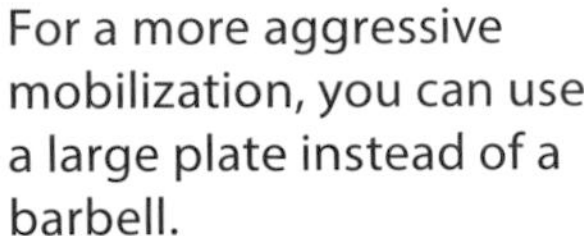

For a more aggressive mobilization, you can use a large plate instead of a barbell.

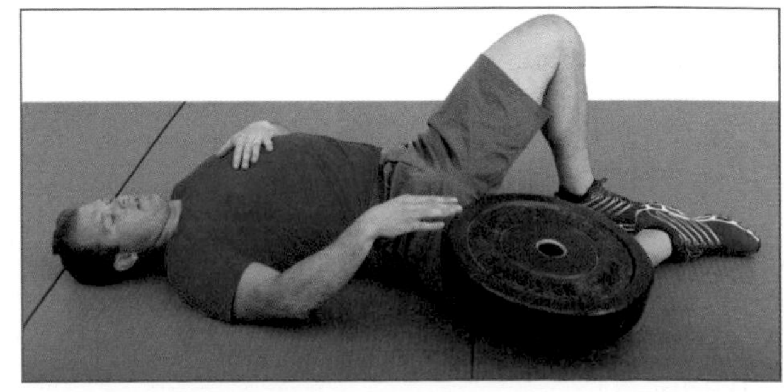

Olympic Wall Squat

Squat 1 Archetype

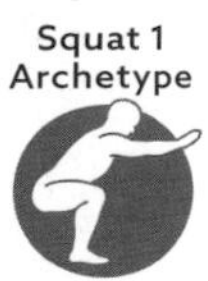

This mobilization will help improve the above archetype.

METHOD:
Contract and relax

I call this mobilization the Olympic Wall Squat because if you turn the position upright, it's like being in the sickest, deepest, most upright squat possible (check out the side-view photo below left).

To execute this mob, you get your butt as close to a wall as possible and position your feet in your squat stance. With your back supported by the ground and the load taken off your legs, you can really feel the areas that are restricting good mechanics. Most people find that their adductors are very tight, limiting their capacity to drive their knees out in the bottom of the squat. You can really feel your feet try to spin out as you drive your knees out.

Although this mobilization can be performed without a distraction, wrapping a band around your back and hooking it around your knees helps set your femurs into the backs of their sockets, allowing you to tap into some of the hip capsule. This compression also helps clear impingements at the front of the hip.

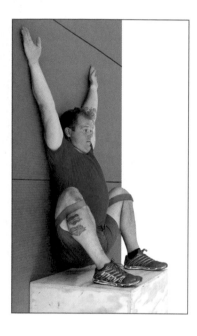

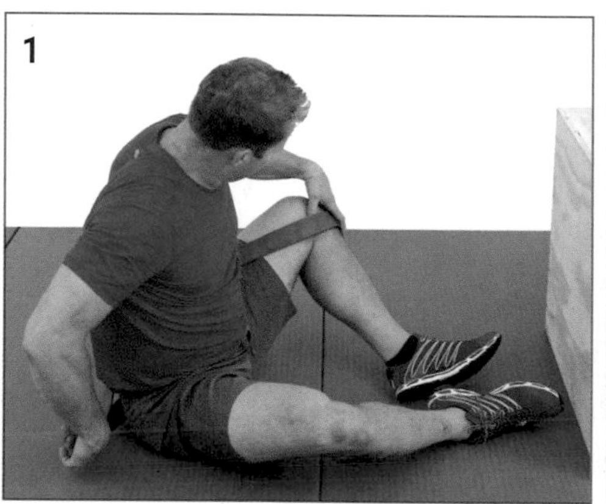

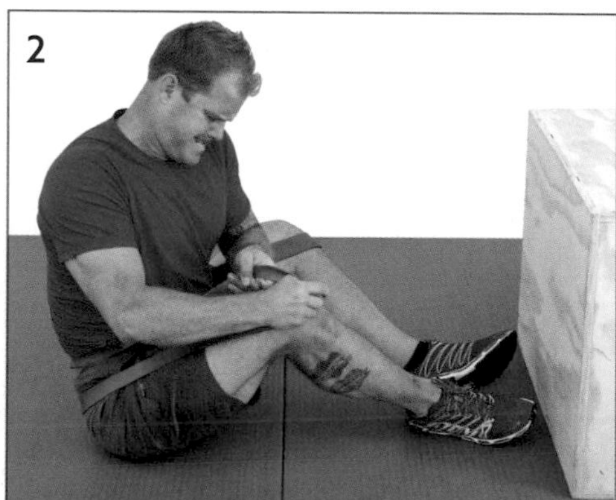

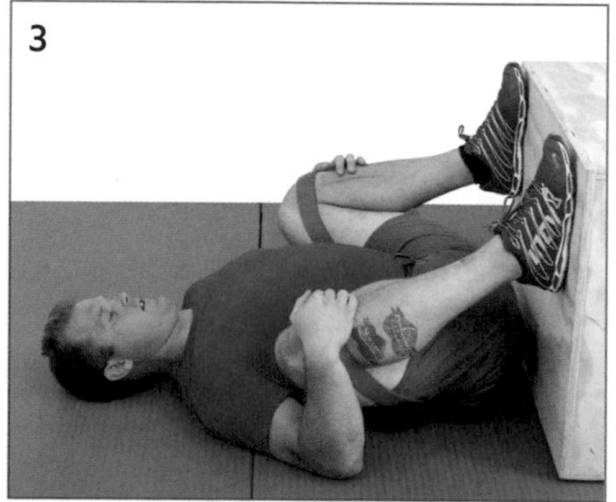

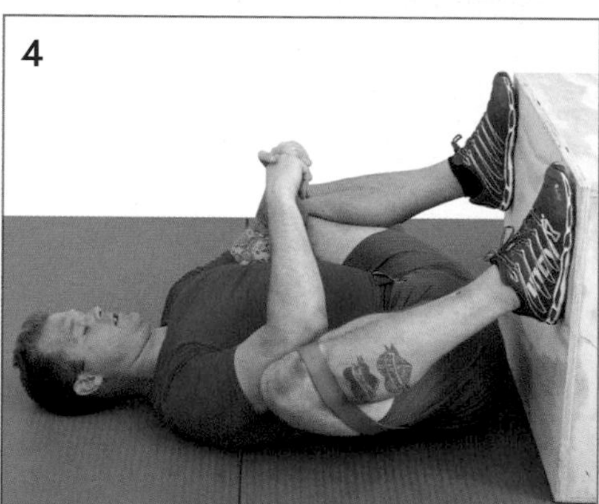

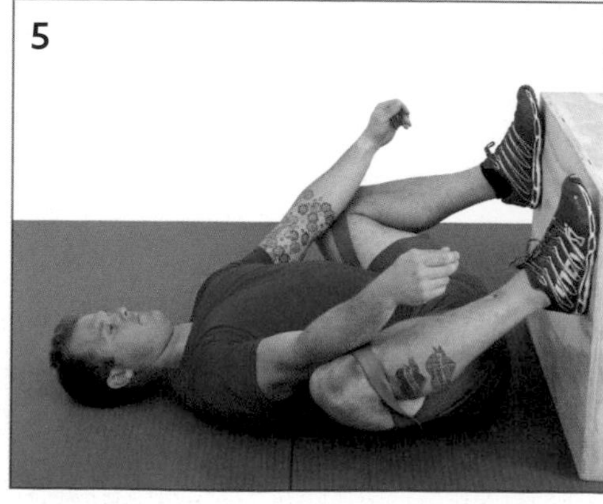

1. Wrap a band around your back—holding it with your right hand—and then hook it around your left knee.

2. Hook the band around your right knee.

3. Position your butt as close to a box as possible and assume your squat stance, keeping your feet as straight as you can. From here, pull down on your knees to increase hip flexion.

4. To tap into your adductors and bias a knees-out position, drive your elbows into the insides of your knees.

5. You can also spread your arms into your knees.

AREA 10 HAMSTRINGS

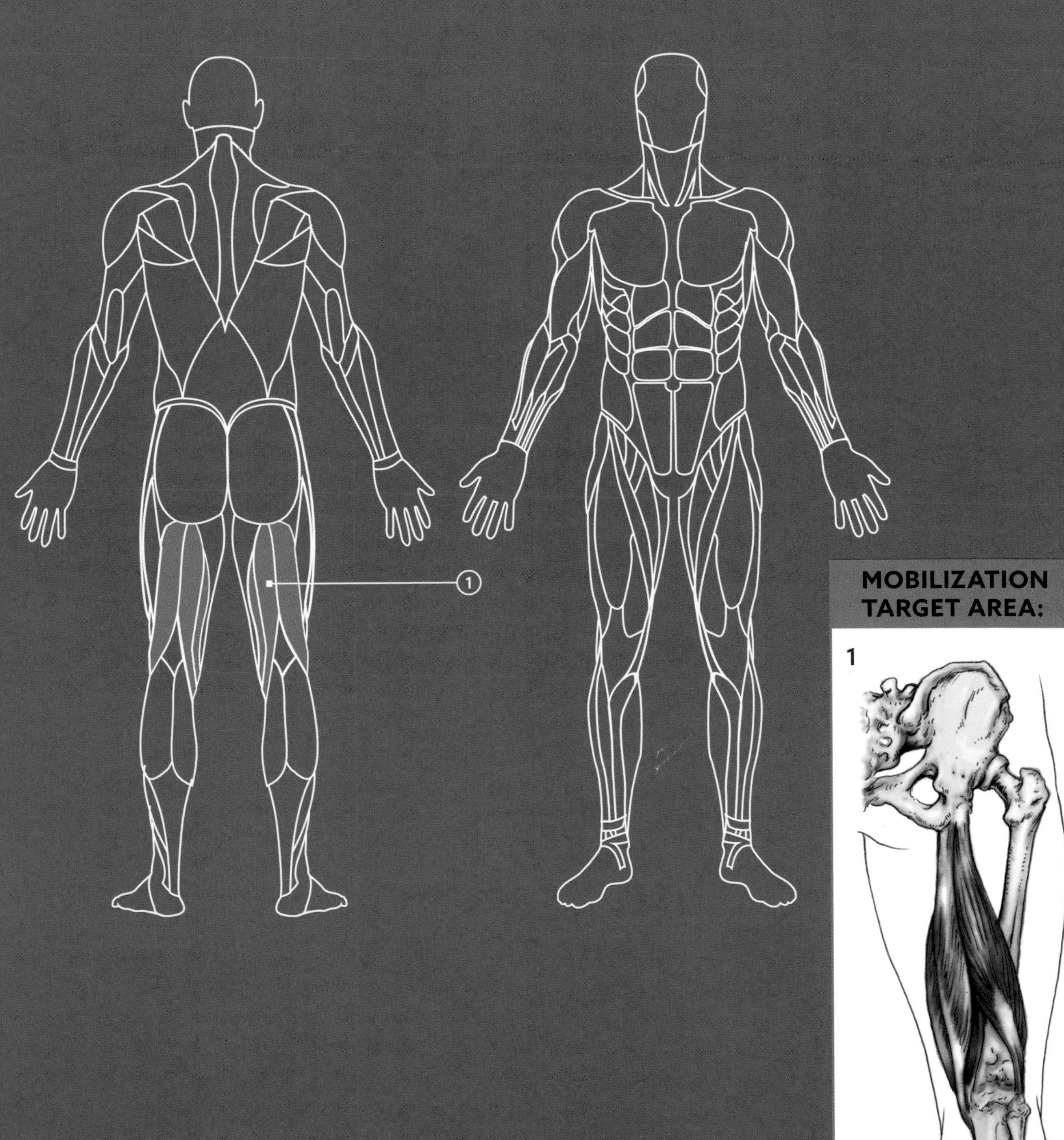

MOBILIZATION TARGET AREA:

1

Hamstring (biceps femoris, semimembranosus. and semitendinosus)

Squat 2 Archetype
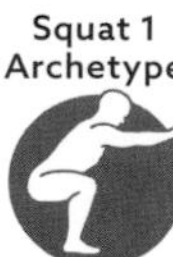

Squat 1 Archetype
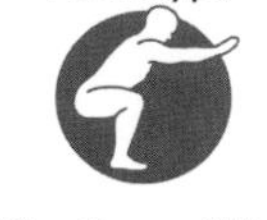

This mobilization will help improve the above archetypes.

IMPROVES:

Hip, low back, and knee pain

METHODS:

Smash and floss

Contract and relax

Pressure wave

Posterior Chain Smash and Floss

Most people train their posterior chain like it's their job. We're talking glutes and hamstrings here, so you know what I mean. The problem is that people put in a ton of work to get the posterior chain strong and then put their muscles to sleep by sitting all day or doing absolutely nothing to restore the sliding surfaces in these tissues.

Three big muscles make up your hamstring—the semimembranosus, semitendinosus, and biceps femoris—all of which arise from different places in your hip and then snake down on different sides of your leg. For your hamstrings to function optimally, you need full range of motion in all these tissues. In other words, you need to schedule a smashing party for your hamstrings every time you put them to work, and especially after long periods of sitting. As you'll see, most of these techniques are done on an elevated surface, for a few reasons.

For starters, mobilizing from an elevated surface—a box, bench, stool, countertop, table, or chair—enables you to get your weight over your leg. It takes a tremendous amount of pressure to make an impact on these stiff posterior chain tissues. If you're mobilizing from the floor, you probably won't be able to get enough weight over your leg to make change.

In addition to adding leverage and weight to the mob, using a box or bench gives you added mobility, giving you access to areas of your hamstrings that are inaccessible when mobilizing from the floor. If you're mobilizing on a box, for example, you can flex and extend your knee for a flossing effect and manipulate your body so that you hit all corners of your hamstrings.

Lastly, mobilizing from an elevated surface is much safer. When you're on the ground, your only option is to sit with your legs straight out in front of you. With your leg locked in extension, you stretch your sciatic nerve, which is embedded within the hamstrings. Smashing your hamstrings in this position can result in numbness and tingly nerve pain. This is why you start with your knee bent on a bench or stool; it gives slack to the sciatic nerve and the surrounding connective tissue.

If you have some down time at work, you're stuck at the airport, or you're cooling off after a workout, find a hard surface (a chair or box) and get some work done.

Option 1: Hamstring Ball Smash

A small ball (such as a lacrosse ball) and a large ball (a softball or Supernova) are the best tools for smashing your hamstrings. As with most ball-smashing techniques, if you hit a hotspot, you should stay on the area while pumping your leg back and forth. It's quick and easy, and it's time well spent. The smaller ball is great for targeting specific trigger points, while the larger ball is great for shearing across muscle interfaces and restoring sliding surfaces to gummed-up connective tissue.

Option 1a: Hamstring Ball Smash

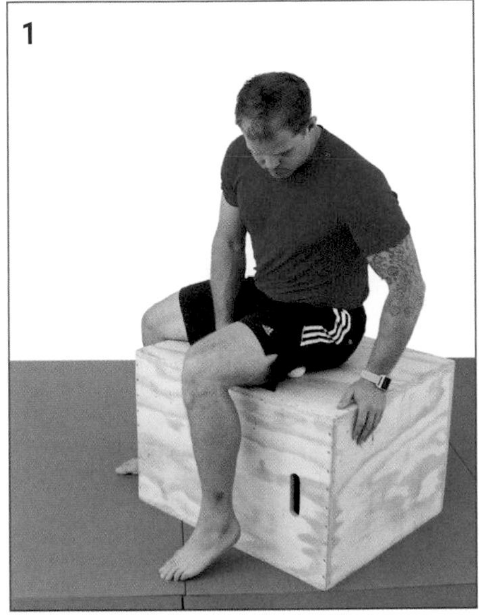

Position a lacrosse ball underneath your leg in the meat of your hamstring and distribute as much weight over the ball as you can handle.

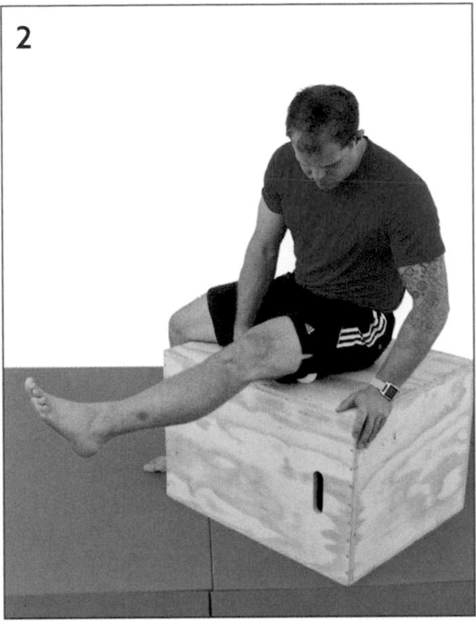

Hunt around for a tight spot, then extend your leg. The idea is to bend and straighten your leg and move it from side to side.

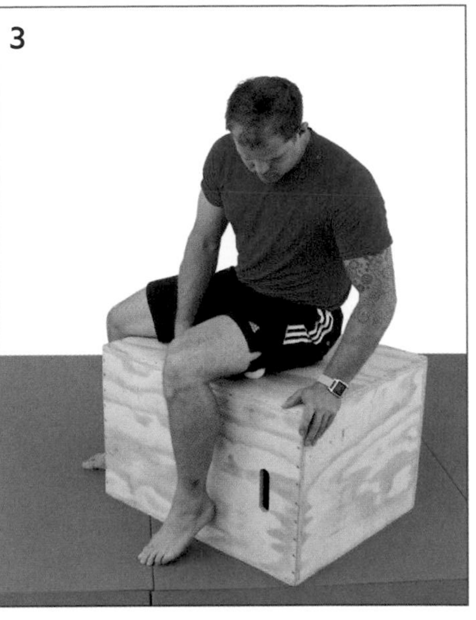

You can also pressure wave across the length of the muscle by shifting your weight over the ball and oscillating on and off pockets of knotted-up tissue.

Option 1b: Hamstring Ball Smash

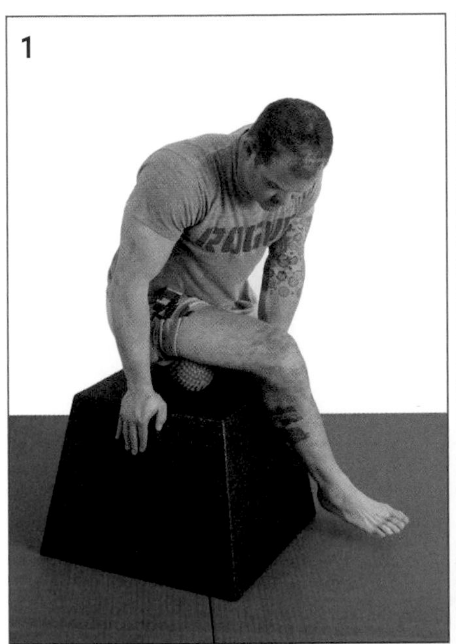

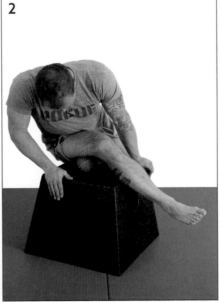

1. Place a softball or Supernova under your hamstring. If you're mobilizing on a box or stool, consider targeting your IT band—the thick band of fascia that runs down the outside of your thigh.

2. Get as much weight over the ball as you can by rotating your body over the leg you're mobilizing. From here, you can contract and relax, floss by extending and flexing your leg, or shear by rolling your hamstring back and forth over the ball. The idea is to create large pressure wave compressions across the muscle fibers, from your IT band to your adductors. If you're using a box or stool, you can circle your leg around while keeping as much weight as you can handle distributed over the ball.

Option 2: Monkey Bar of Death

Remember sitting atop the monkey bars as a kid, with one leg draped over the bar, just swinging back and forth as if it were nothing? I'd be willing to bet that if you did so now, you'd slide into the hellish depths of the pain cave and then scramble away—or worse, black out and plummet off the monkey bars. If you're like the majority of athletes, most of your hamstring stiffness resides near the insertion at your hip, which is a difficult area to target and an extremely painful area to mobilize. Let's face it: Nobody is going to get into your personal regions and work around your business, at least not as effectively as you can do it yourself.

Unless you're looking to get arrested, I wouldn't recommend climbing on the monkey bars where kids play so that you can mobilize around your grundle region. That's just creepy. Instead, set a barbell on a rack at about mid-thigh level. This ends up being a much more aggressive and effective way to break up the tissue and get large pressure into the insertion of your hamstring. Again, the idea is to grind back and forth from side to side against the grain of the muscle tissue.

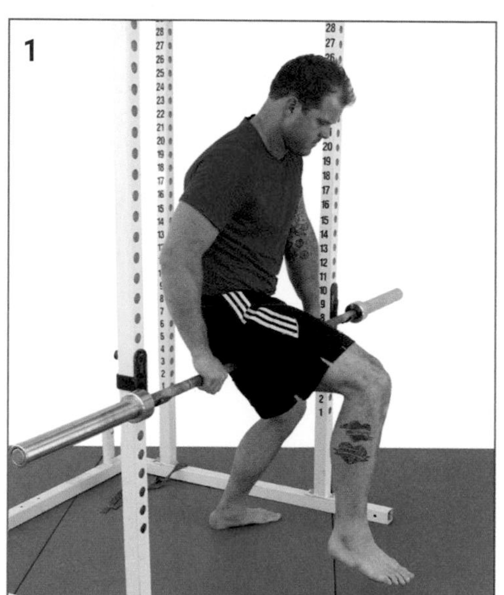

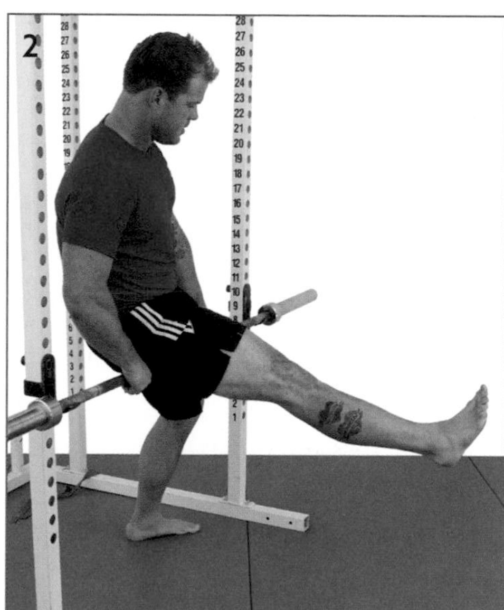

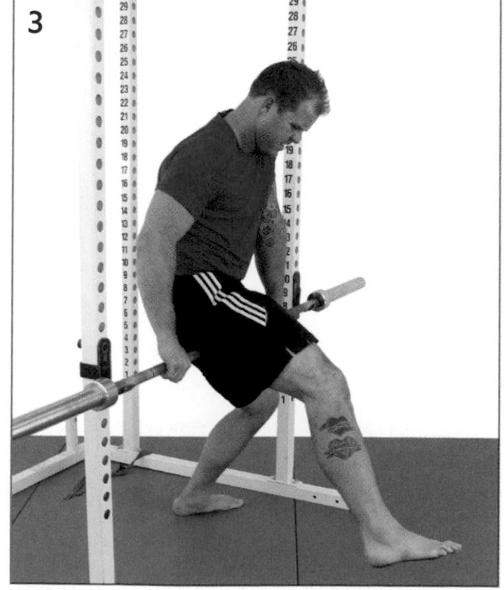

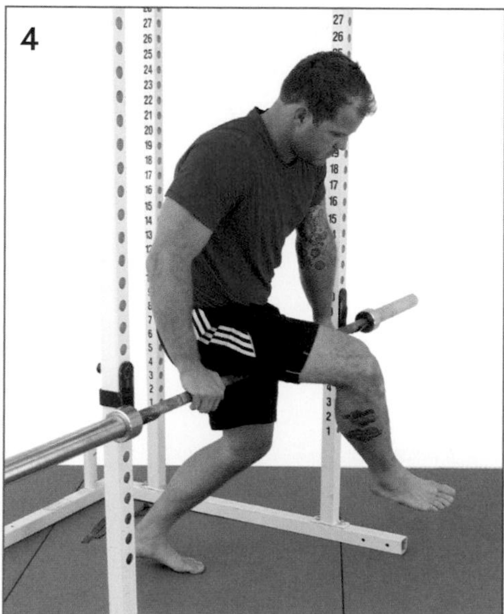

1. Set a barbell on a rack at about mid-thigh level. Throw one leg over the bar, positioning the bar into your high hip, near the insertion of your hamstring.

2. When you find a piece of matted-down tissue (it shouldn't take long), straighten your leg.

3. As you bend your leg, you can shift your weight to the side, rolling across the length of the muscle.

4. You can also rotate your leg from side to side and—using your hands—roll the bar into your sit bones and muscle insertion points.

Option 3: Little Battlestar Smash

This mob is a variation of the Monkey Bar of Death. If you have a Little Battlestar at your disposal, placing it on a box, bench, or chair is a great way to mobilize your hamstrings. Again, the grooves help "break up" tissue more effectively, and the box gives you mobility and control that you don't have when using a barbell.

1

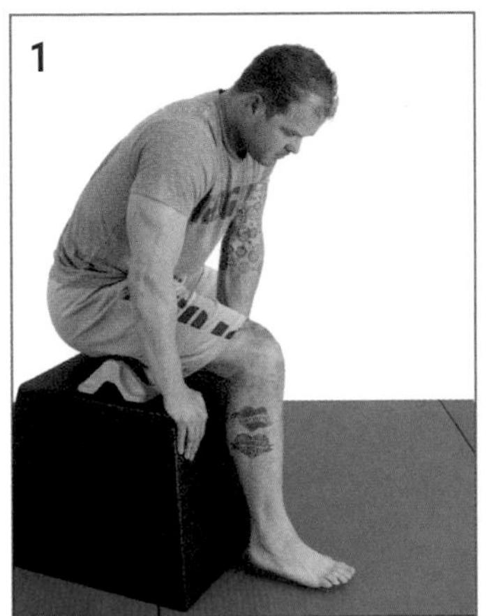

2

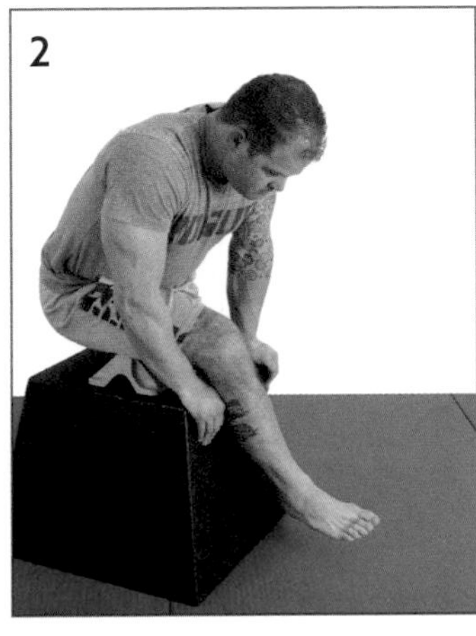

3

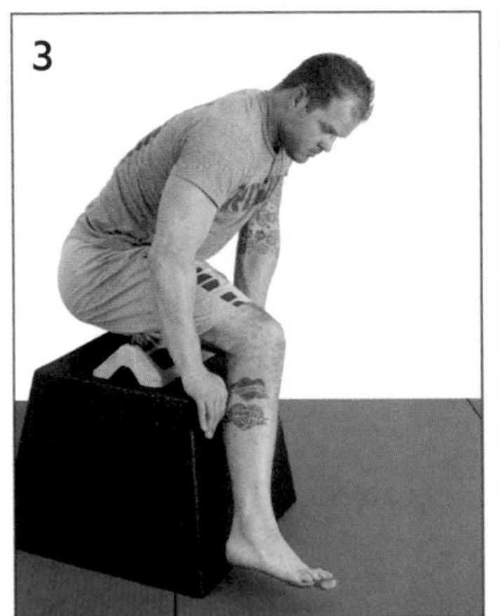

4

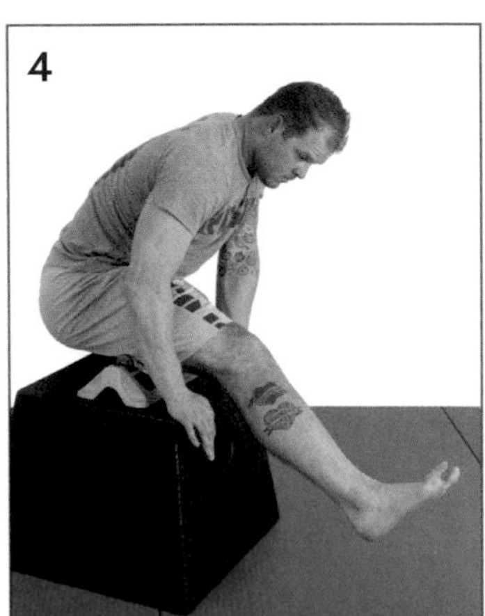

Sit on a Little Battlestar with the roller positioned across your hamstrings. From here, shift your weight back and forth over the leg you're mobilizing while swinging your leg from side to side. For example, if you shift your weight toward your right side, swing your leg toward your left, and vice versa. If you find a tight spot, contract and relax and floss by straightening your leg.

Option 4: Superfriend Hamstring Smash

This is a great mobilization to drop into a big group of people after a hard workout (think football practice or a CrossFit class). The technique is the same as smashing the adductors and quads, in that you use the arch of your foot to create a slow, steady pressure wave across the length of the muscle. The great thing about this mob is that the person being smashed can bury her face in her arms, concealing her pain face from public view.

Note: As the Superfriend, you can stand on either side of your training partner. Standing on the far side of the leg you're smashing, as shown below, is great for targeting the inner hamstring and adductors, while standing on the near side of the leg you're smashing is great for targeting the outer hamstrings and quads.

1

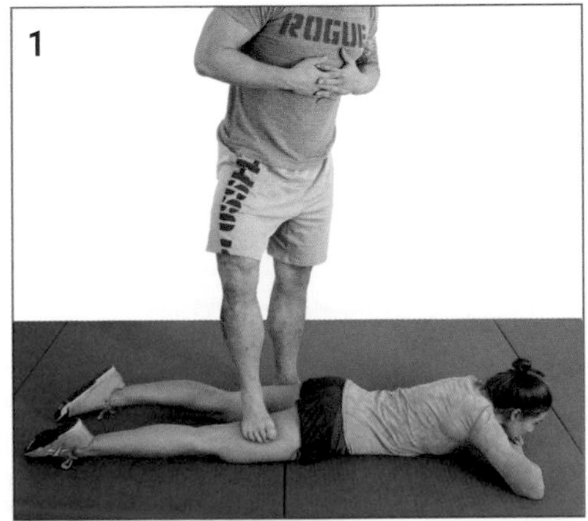

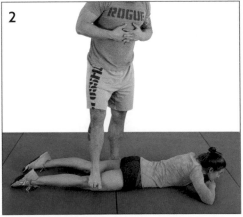

2

As the Superfriend, place the arch of your foot on your partner's hamstring. Then shift your weight forward and drive your foot across the length of the muscle, creating a slow and steady pressure wave. Seesaw your foot back and forth in this manner—working up and down the entire length of the hamstring—until you feel change, you stop making change, or your partner signals you to stop.

VooDoo Groin and Hamstring Wrap

Squat 2 Archetype Squat 1 Archetype

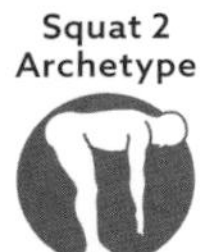
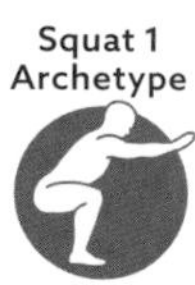

This mobilization will help improve the above archetypes.

IMPROVES:

Scar tissue damage around the groin and hamstring

Hip and low back pain

METHOD:

VooDoo Floss Band compression

Mobilizing with a VooDoo Floss Band offers a few distinct advantages: You can mobilize in the position you're trying to change, you can address multiple systems simultaneously—joint mechanics, sliding surface, and muscle dynamics—and you can capture tissues that are otherwise very difficult to target. For example, smashing or getting enough pressure into the high (proximal) hamstring and adductor area or tapping into your groin and hip flexor region is not easy to do using a conventional mobility tool like a lacrosse ball or roller.

The fact is, people spend a lot of time sitting on their high posterior chain, turning the high hamstring, glute, and groin area into a nexus of junky, matted-down tissue. And when the tissues around the insertion of these muscles get tight, injury follows. As anybody who has strained a groin or hamstring can attest, it's a painful and limiting injury that takes a long time to heal. It affects your ability to generate force and causes a ton of funky movement and tissue adaptations. To make matters worse, it's difficult to get in there and break up the knotted-up scar tissue that starts to form post-injury. This is why VooDoo Flossing is so great: You get a circumferential compression around those hard-to-reach areas. Add some full-range movement to the equation and you have a model for dealing with scar balls (which restrict and compromise movement) and restoring sliding surfaces to matted-down tissues.

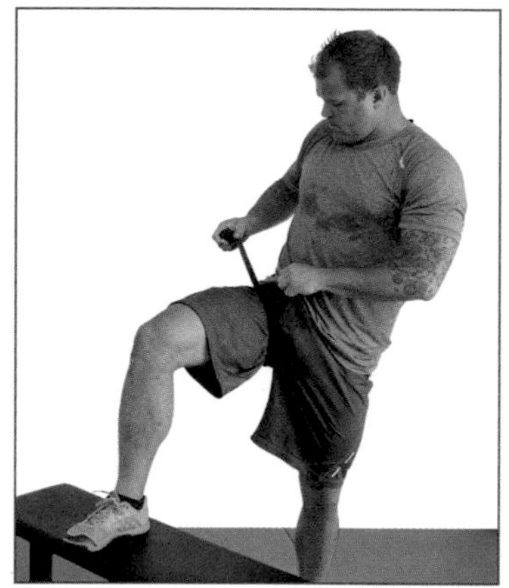

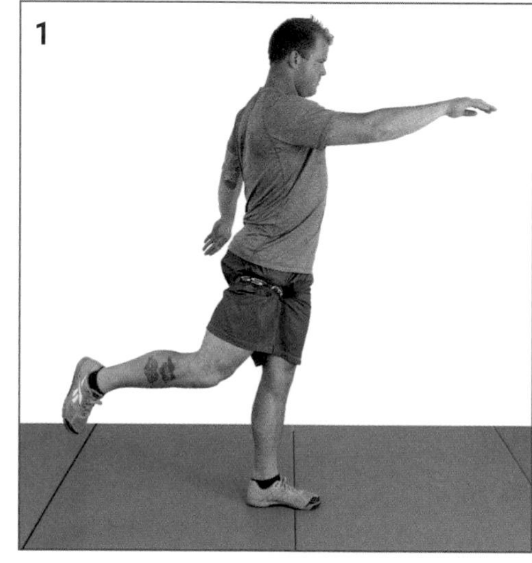
1

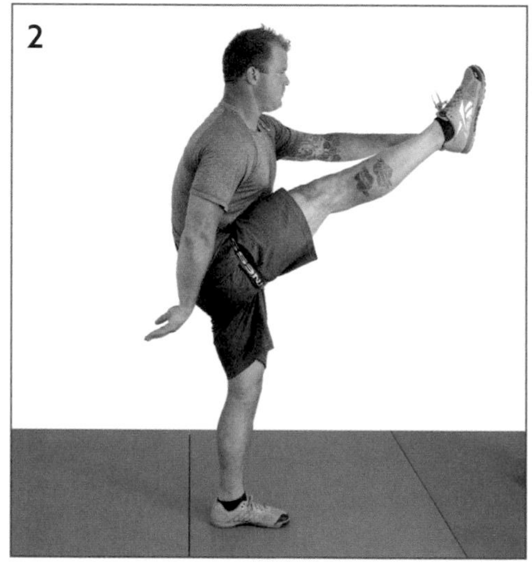
2

Dynamic leg swings are a great way to safely restore sliding surfaces to the high hamstring and groin. Keep your knee straight and foot neutral and swing your leg out in front of you as if you were punting a football.

Posterior Chain Floss

Squat 2 Archetype Squat 1 Archetype

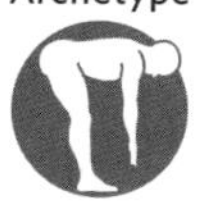
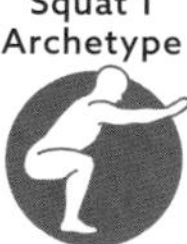

This mobilization will help improve the above archetypes.

IMPROVES:

Hip, low back, and knee pain

METHOD:

Banded flossing

If you're a full-grown adult, you're not going to magically grow new hamstrings. To lengthen these muscles, you need to restore shortened and tight tissues back to their ideal ranges. The bottom line is that stretching is not going to do anything to restore normal range to those steel cables running down the backs of your legs. If you want to make lasting change, you have to take a systematic approach. You have to clear sliding surface dysfunction with aggressive smashing, as well as incorporate end-range mobilization to lengthen the tissue.

One of the key concepts of the Movement & Mobility System is to mobilize tissues into ideal positions and then use them so that the musculature gets appropriately stimulated for normal range development. To be blunt, the best way to lengthen your hamstrings is to use them in a functional setting. The Posterior Chain Floss sequence is a perfect example of a weight-bearing exercise that takes on a shape similar to something you'll actually do (deadlift or pick something up off the ground). As you can see, you have a few different options: You can post your hands on the ground or a box and floss by bending and flexing your knee (options 1 and 2) or hinge forward from your hip (option 3). Whether you use just one option or a combination, the Posterior Chain Floss is a fantastic pregame, preworkout mobilization that will help restore normal range of motion to your hamstrings and hips.

Posterior Chain Floss: Option 1

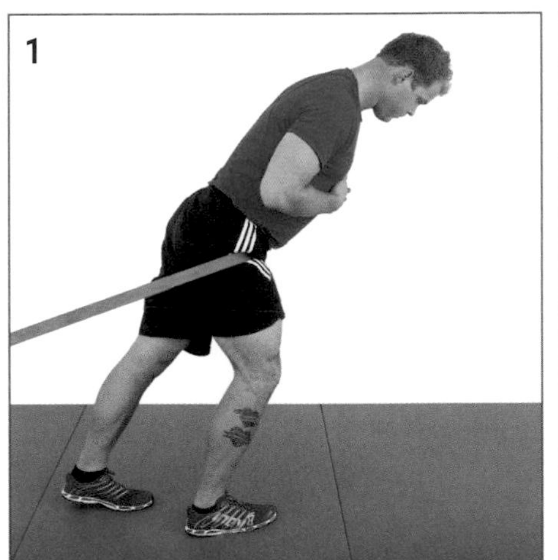

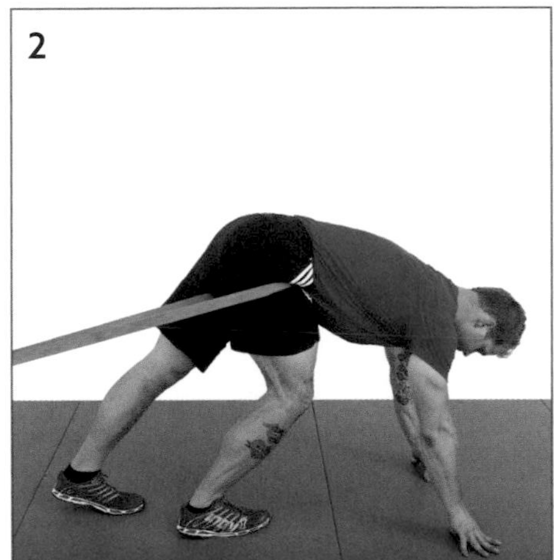

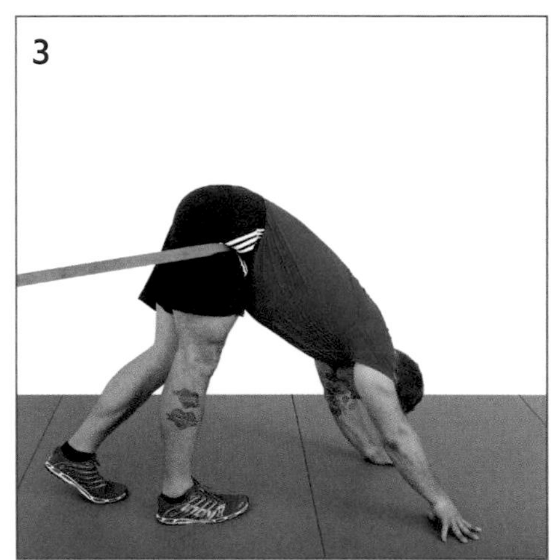

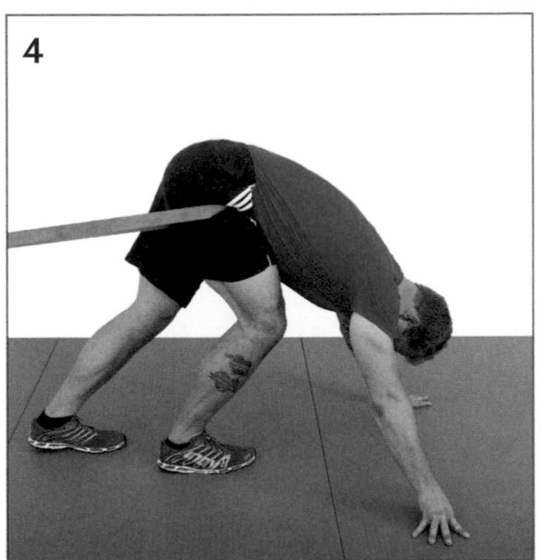

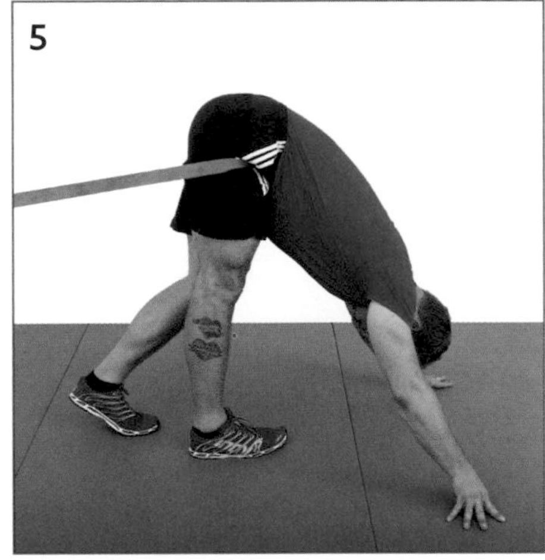

1. Wrap a band around your hip and walk forward to create tension. It helps if your banded leg is positioned slightly in front of your free leg.

2. Fold forward from your hips—keeping your belly tight and back flat—and plant your hands on the ground. If you can't reach the ground without rounding your back, position a box or bench in front of you.

3. Straighten your banded leg and drive your hips back.

4. Keeping your back as flat as possible, bend the knee of your banded leg.

5. Keeping your weight on the heel of your banded leg, continue to floss by extending and flexing your knee. The goal is to put in 20 to 50 knee bends. To capture your high hip (glute region), you can also rotate your hips slightly as you lock out your leg and walk your upper body around your planted foot in either direction.

Posterior Chain Floss: Option 2

1. Wrap a band around your hip and walk forward to create tension.

2. Keeping your belly tight, back flat, and leg straight, hinge forward from your hips until you reach end range.

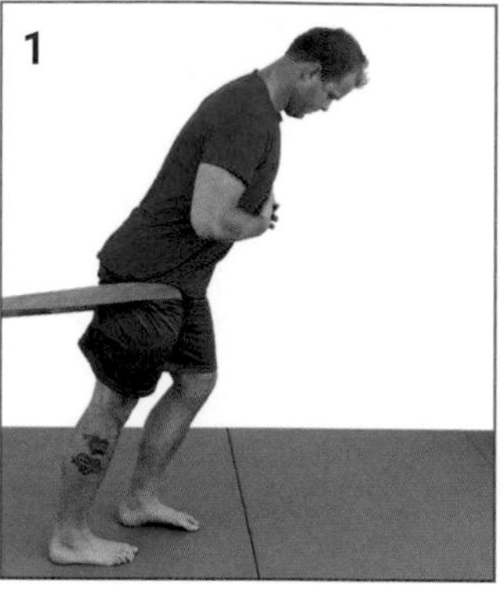

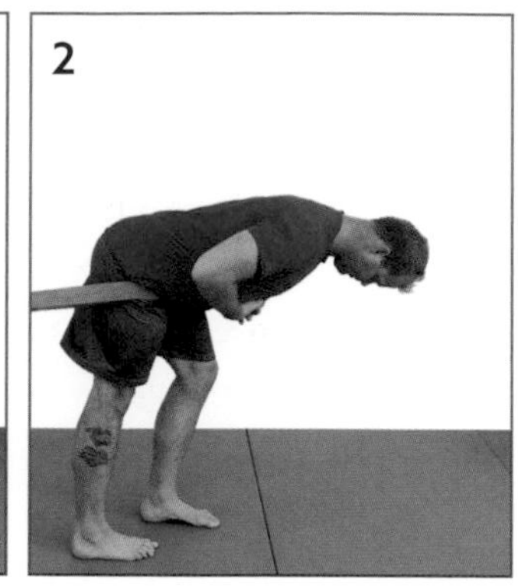

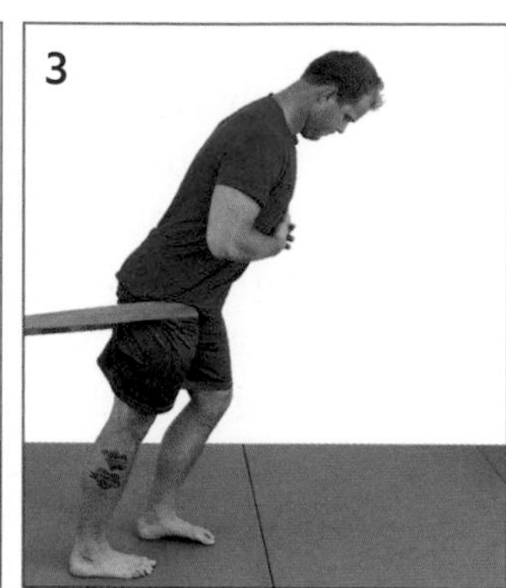

3. Pull yourself back to the upright position. From here, you can continue to bend forward and floss in and out of end-range hip flexion. The idea is to keep your spine rigid, your knee locked out, and your weight centered over your heel.

Posterior Chain Floss: Option 3

Remember, to effect true change, you have to hit your hamstrings from different angles. That means changing your position in order to hunt out hard-to-reach corners of tight muscle. Putting your banded leg on a box gets your leg into a flexed position (think squatting), which allows you to tap into the high hip and hamstring region that is difficult to get.

1. Wrap a band around your hip and plant your foot on a box. You'll probably feel a good stretch in this position, so feel free to scour around for tight corners.

2. Straighten your leg and shoot your hips back. To really capture your high hip region, keep your foot flat on the box until you reach end range, then allow the ball of your foot to come up as you lock out your knee.

3. Slowly bend your knee and shift your weight forward. From here, you can continue to floss by bending and flexing your knee.

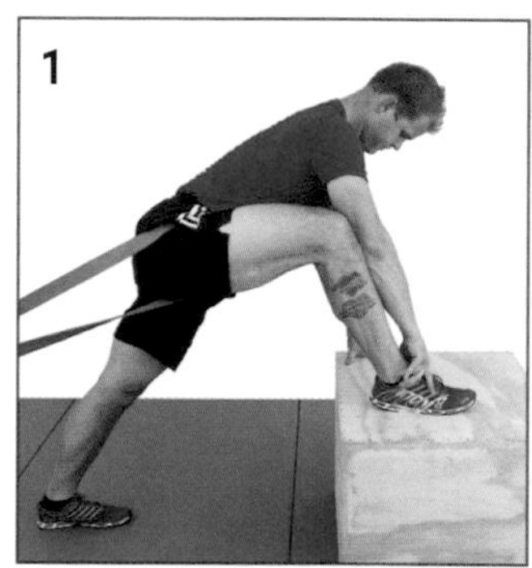

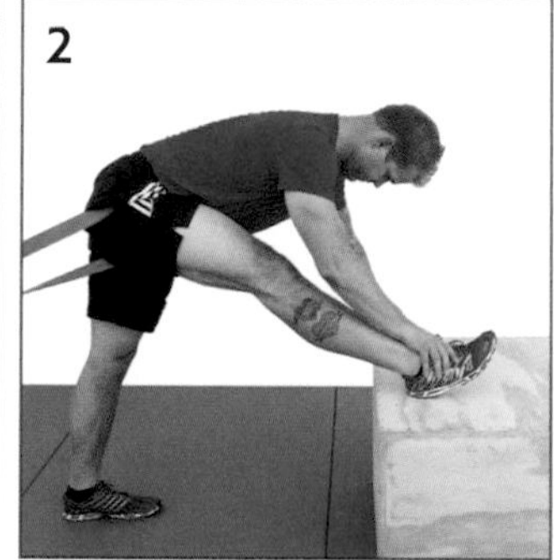

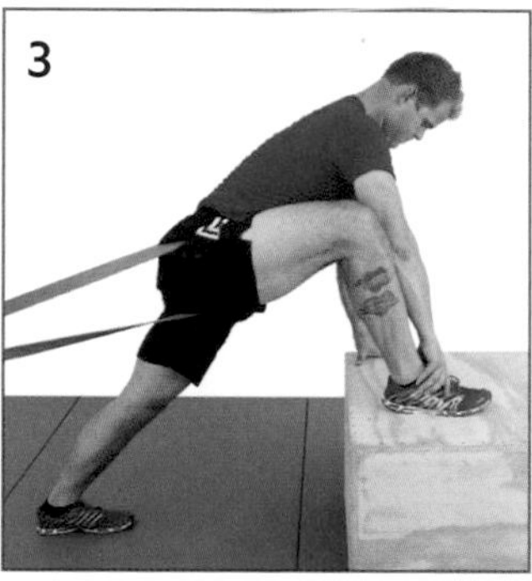

Banded Classic Posterior Chain Mob

Squat 2 Archetype   Squat 1 Archetype

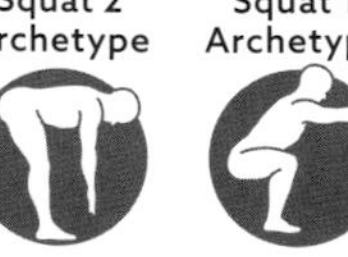

This mobilization will help improve the above archetypes.

IMPROVES:
Hip, low back, and knee pain

METHOD:
Banded flossing

As you know, I'm a big fan of mobilizing in positions that reflect the realities of life and sport. For example, I prefer to mobilize my hamstrings from a standing position because it has a weight-bearing element that reflects the movements that I use in my day-to-day training, like deadlifting. More important, it seems to yield better results. However, that's not to say that you can't apply this method while lying on your back. This classic approach has real value, especially for jiu-jitsu or MMA fighters who utilize this range while lying on their back, fighting from their guard.

What's great about this option is that your spine doesn't bear any weight, so you don't have to work as hard to keep your back in a good position. The key is to approach the stretch as you would when setting up for a deadlift: Load your hip into flexion and then apply tension at your knee by straightening your leg. As I've mentioned, this allows you to capture the corners of your hip and high hamstring, which is where most people are tight. If you straighten your leg first and use your whole leg as a tensioner, which is common, you tend to lose some of the effectiveness.

Another key aspect of this mobilization is adding a posterior distraction. As with the previous techniques, the distraction clears impingements at the front of your hip and helps tie in the musculature of your high hamstring. You can do it in one of two ways. The first is to distract from a pole, which allows you to put a lot of tension into the band, offering a really aggressive distraction. The problem is that hooking a band around a pole isn't always a viable option.

The second option addresses this issue. To set up, loop a band around your foot a couple times, hook it around your hip, and then use your banded foot to create a posterior distraction—see the photos below. This allows you not only to mobilize with your hip in a good position, but also to control the tension with your banded foot. Plus, you can execute this technique in the comfort of your living room or office.

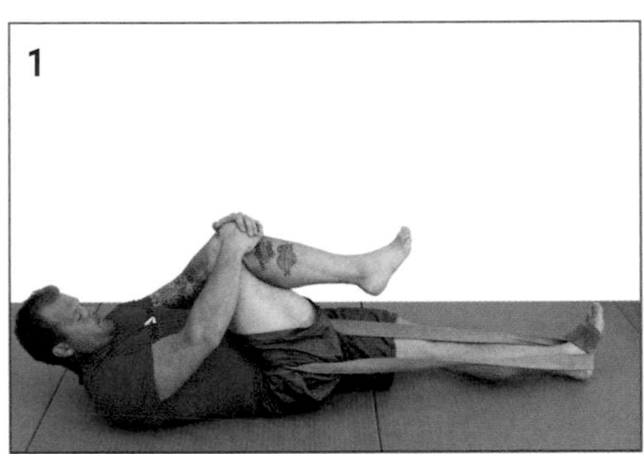

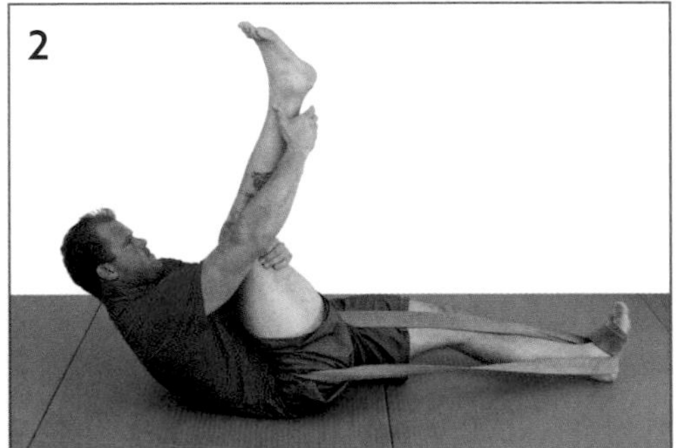

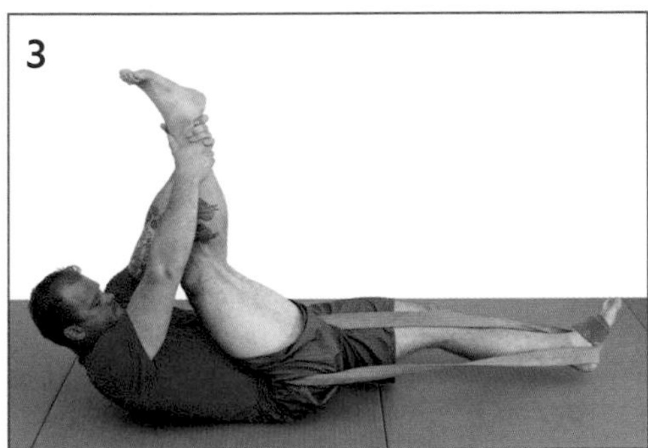

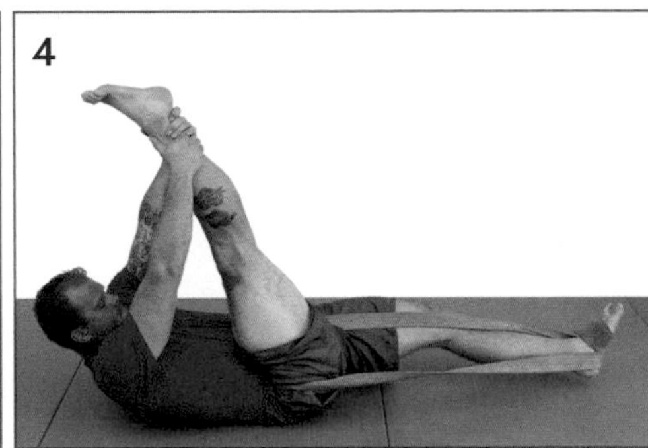

1. Loop a band around the center of your left foot (if it's a thin band, you may need to wrap it a few times), hook it around your right hip, and then pull your knee to your chest. Try to keep your left leg straight. Adding this posterior distraction pulls your femur to the bottom of the capsule, which will clear any impingement you have at the front of your hip. It also allows you to tie in the musculature of your high hamstring.

2. With your hip loaded into a flexed position, wrap your left hand around the back of your right knee, sit up, and grab the back of your right ankle with your right hand.

3. Grab the back of your ankle with both hands.

4. Apply tension by straightening your knee. From here, you can continue to floss by bending and straightening your leg, contract and relax by resisting into your arms, and scour around for tight corners by manipulating your leg to either side of your body.

If you can't reach your foot because you're missing hamstring range of motion, wrapping a band around your foot is a valid idea. Don't flex into a weird position just to grab your foot—that goes against everything I'm trying to teach you. This is also a good alternative if you're sweaty from a workout or your grip is blown, making it difficult to grip your calf.

The key is to keep your foot in a neutral position by hooking the band around the center of your foot. A lot of people mistakenly wrap it around their toes and pull their foot into flexion, creating a big stretch at the back of the knee.

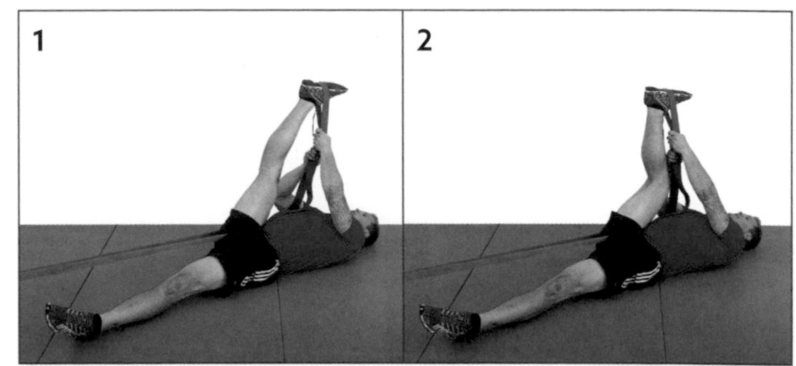

AREA 11 KNEE

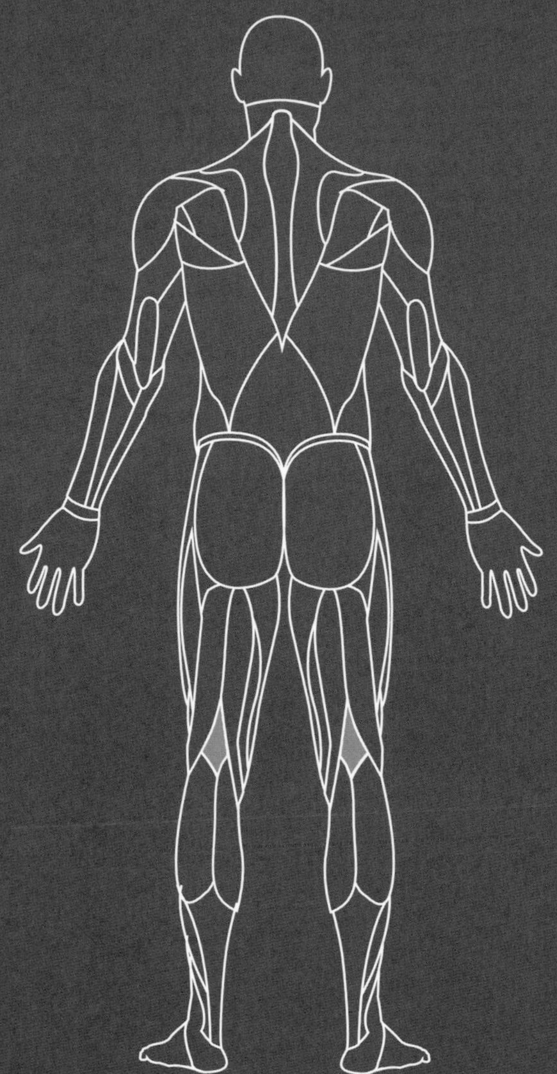

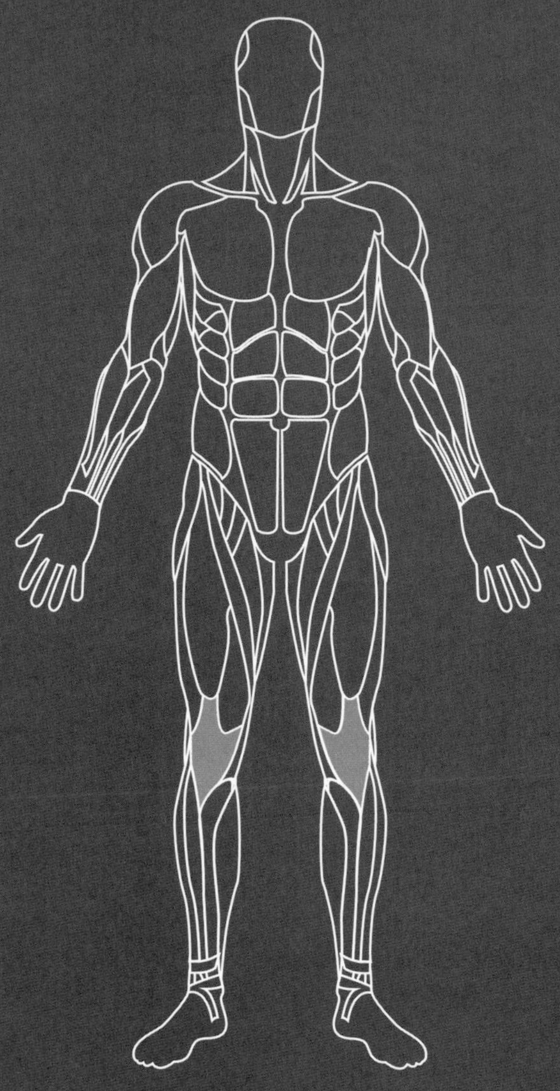

MOBILIZATION TARGET AREA:
Knee and surrounding musculature

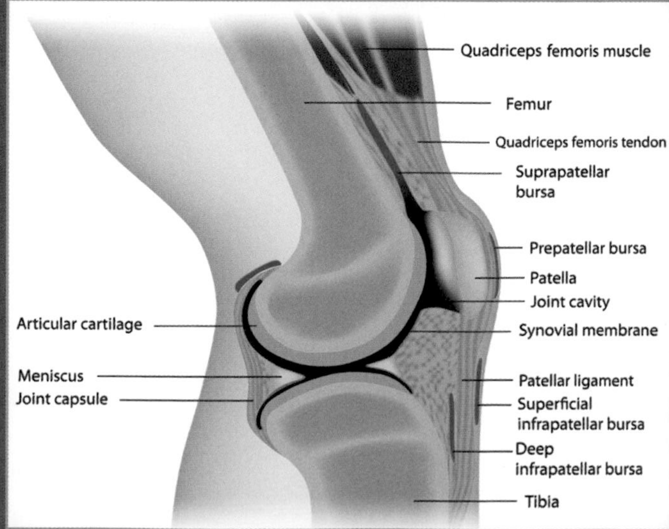

Terminal Knee Extension (Knee Tweak Fix)

IMPROVES:
Knee extension
Knee pain

METHODS:
VooDoo Floss Band compression

When I evaluate athletes for knee pain, one of the first things I check is terminal knee extension. I'm looking to see whether they have full knee range of motion.

An easy way to test this yourself is to sit with your legs out in front of you and then extend one knee by flexing your quad. If you have full knee range of motion, your heel will lift up off the ground and you will see a little bit of hyperextension at the knee joint. If you have a slight bend in your knee or you can't lock out the joint, it's a good indication that you're missing the capacity to achieve terminal knee extension.

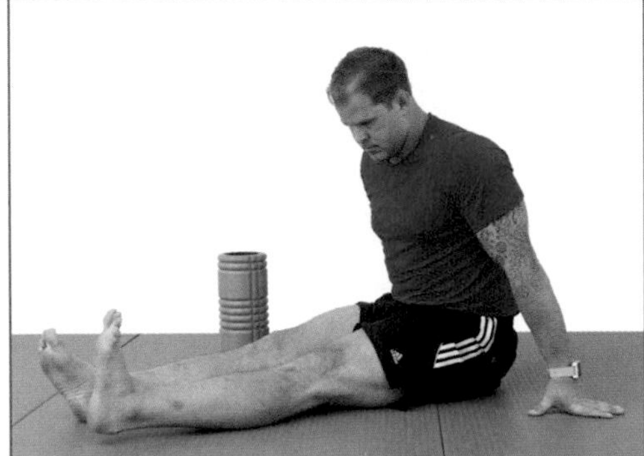

When your knees are stuck in a bent or flexed position, they are under constant tension while you stand. It's the equivalent of being unable to extend your arm and then attempting a handstand. Add 10,000 steps a day and heavily loaded movements to the equation, and you have the smoking gun for knee pain and lost potential. In addition, every movement starts in a preloaded, biomechanically compromised position.

Consider driving your knees forward as you initiate a squat. It's difficult to unload that tension once you've entered the tunnel. It doesn't matter how much tension you have in your hips and hamstrings in this situation; your knees will remain fully loaded. This is why driving your knees forward when you squat or bringing your elbows back when you bench press, dip, or do pushups is a faulty mechanic. These secondary joints are not designed to handle the load. This is a job for the primary engines of your hips and shoulders. You will continuously load your knees and quads instead of your hips and hamstrings every time you hinge from your hips, placing an insane amount of strain on your knees, quads, quad ligaments, patellar tendons, and more.

To restore function and normal range of motion to the joint, you need to pull the joint surfaces apart so that you can reset your knee into a good position. When an athlete is missing knee extension, it's usually because the knee is unlocked and twisted inside its structure. Put simply, there's a kink in the joint that prevents him from opening up the knee. This often stems from a knee fault or tweak of some kind. It's like a door that doesn't swing correctly or open all the way because one of the hinges has a twist in it.

To realign your knee joint, the first thing you need to do is create some space within the joint, which you accomplish by applying a distraction at your ankle. Next, grab your shin and internally rotate your tibia (lower leg bone). This will realign your knee into an ideal position. To restore extension range, apply downward pressure and flex your quad.

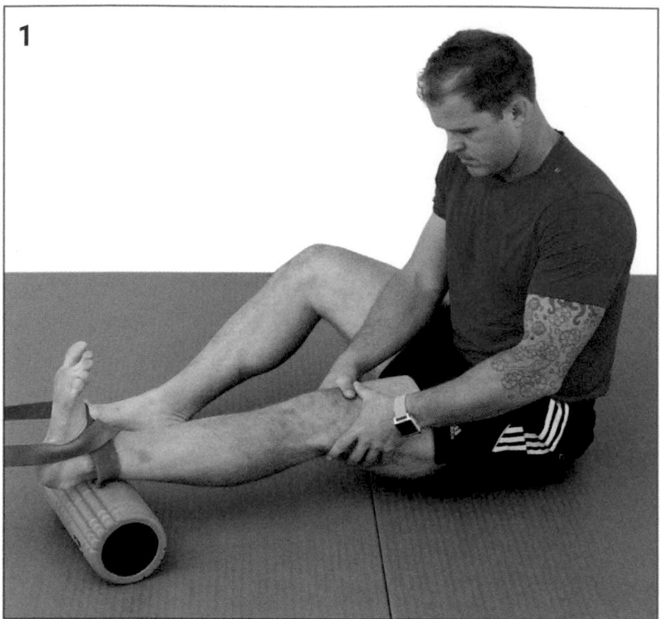

1. Hook a band around the top of your foot and then wrap it around the base of your heel. Then create tension in the band and prop your foot up on a foam roller.

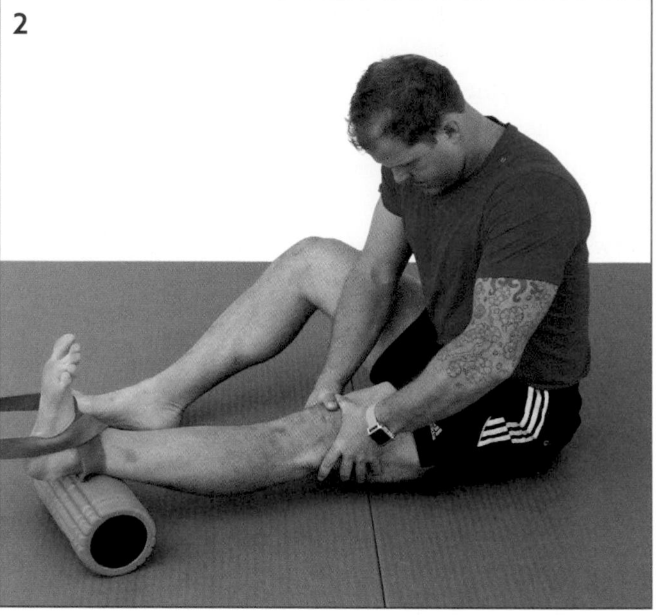

2. Grab above your knee and press down. You're not trying to break your knee in half; apply just enough pressure to achieve full extension and hold it in position for a couple seconds. If you still can't lock out your knee, grab your shin, internally rotate your tibia, and then apply downward pressure in the same manner. Repeat this process until you restore normal function to the joint or experience positive change.

VooDoo Variation

If possible, wrap a VooDoo Floss Band around your entire knee (a couple inches below and a few inches above) before executing this mobilization. Not only will this help reset the joint in a good position, but the compression forces will create a gapping effect. This gives you a little more breathing room within your knee structure, which enables you to press and rotate your knee into newly challenged ranges. Anytime you can use a distraction in conjunction with compression, it's a win.

Grab your shin, internally rotate your tibia, and then apply downward pressure, encouraging your knee into full extension. Having a Superfriend facilitate this motion is ideal.

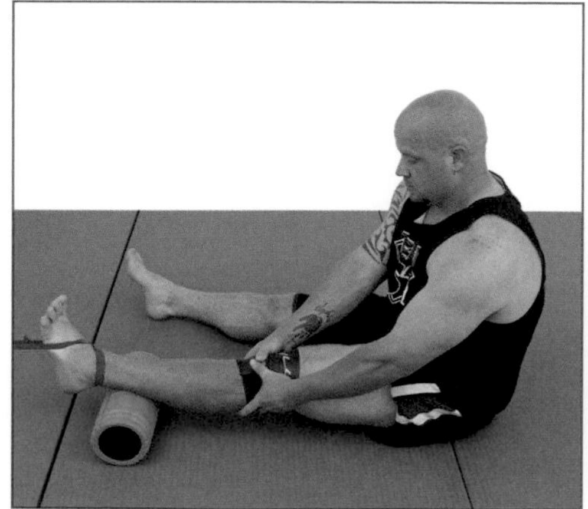

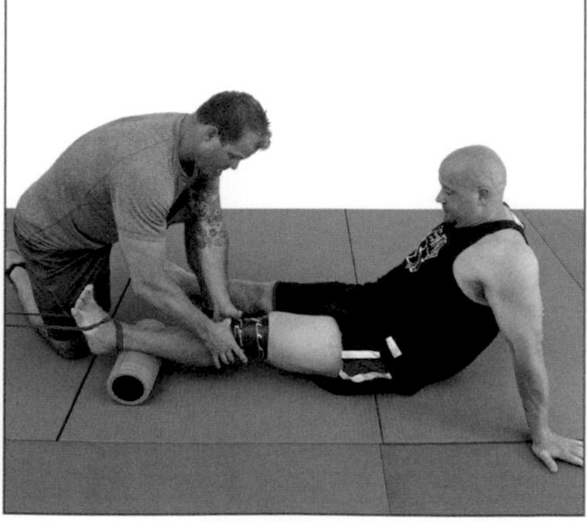

Gap and Smash Mobilizations

If you have knee pain, think this: "I need to mobilize the tissues surrounding my knee joint." Then get to work.

The Gap and Smash is a fast way to hit the areas just behind your knee where your hamstring and calf cross the joint. It's a two-for-one because you hit upstream and downstream of the knee with a single mobilization.

This technique is also great for addressing tight calves. Most people spend tons of time working on their calves at ankle level. What they forget is that the calf crosses two joints: the ankle and the knee. By getting into the high gastrocnemius, you can effectively deal with these tight tissues and feed slack to your knee and ankle.

The idea is to sandwich a ball behind your knee—on either the inside or the outside—creating a large compression force. From there you can implement one of two strategies: You can floss around by moving your foot in all directions, pulling on your shin with both hands; or you can plant your foot on the ground and scoot your butt into your leg. The key is to work the inside and outside of your knee, smashing both sides of your gastroc.

Pistol Archetype

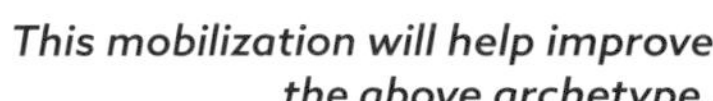

This mobilization will help improve the above archetype.

IMPROVES:

Knee pain

Knee flexion and extension

METHODS:

Smash and floss

Contract and relax

Option 1: Lacrosse Ball Gap and Smash (Inside Line)

This single lacrosse ball option is great because—as with all the single lacrosse ball mobs—you can target specific trigger points and get full compression with your knee in flexion.

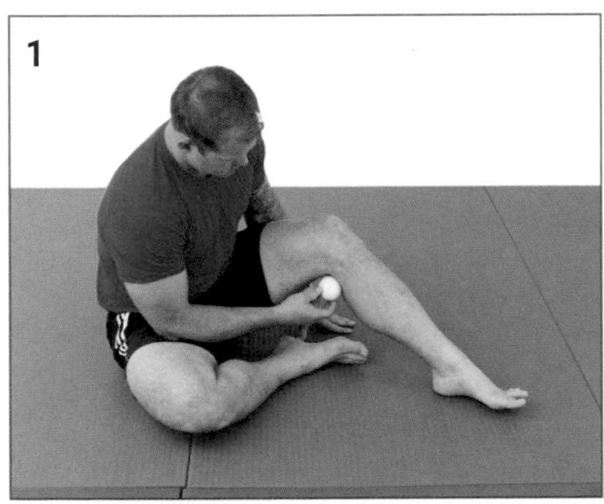
1

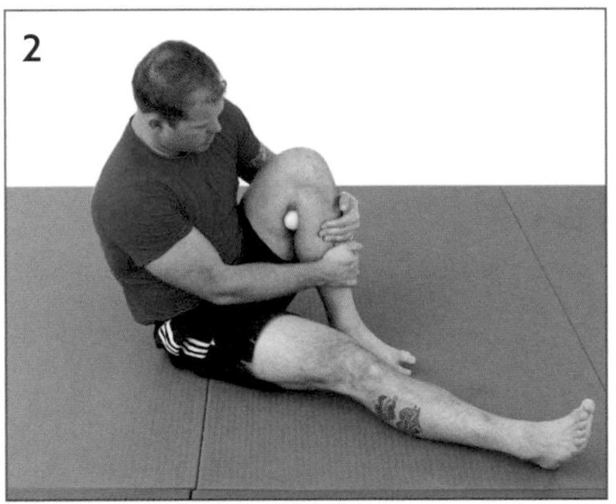
2

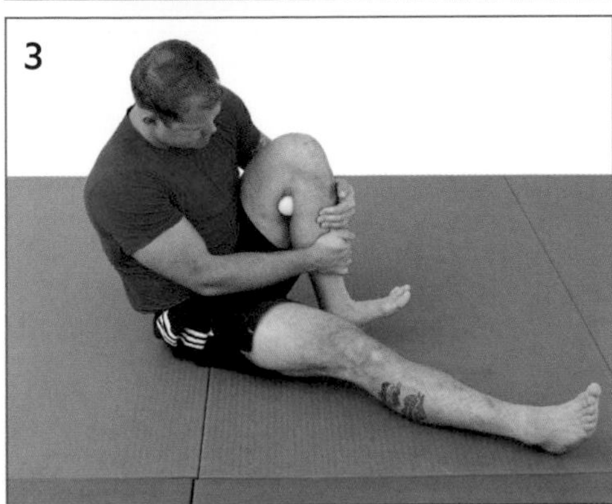
3

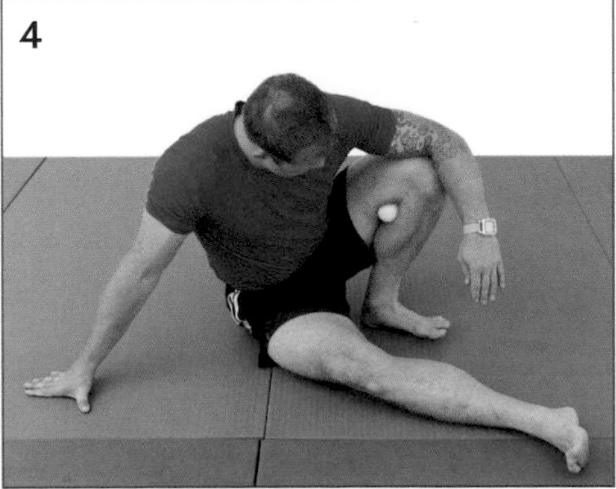
4

1. Position a lacrosse ball behind your knee on the inside of your leg.

2. Curl your heel toward your butt and use both hands to pull your leg in tight. This creates a large compression force that targets your lower hamstring and upper calf.

3. Still pulling on your shin with both hands, start moving your foot around in all directions.

4. To increase the pressure, plant your foot on the ground and scoot your butt toward your heel.

Option 2: Lacrosse Ball Gap and Smash (Outside Line)

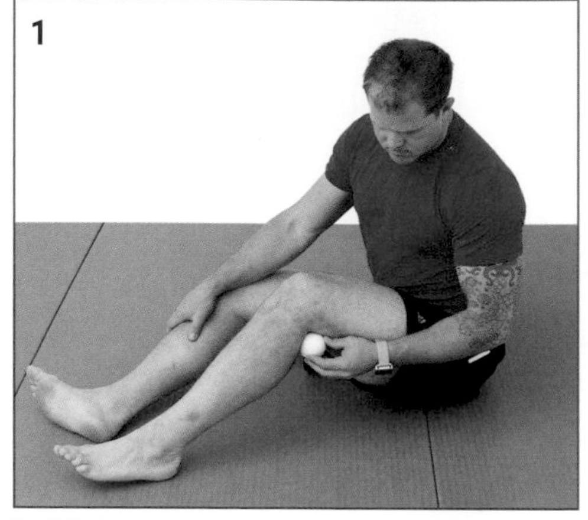

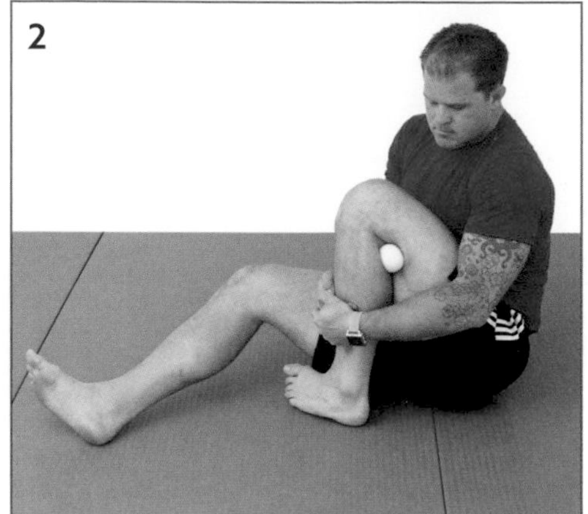

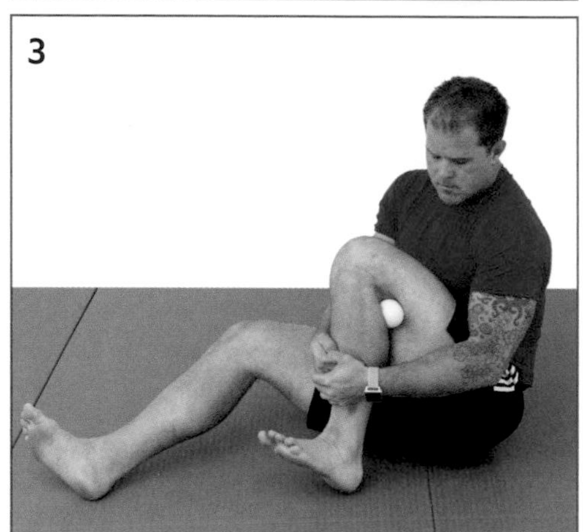

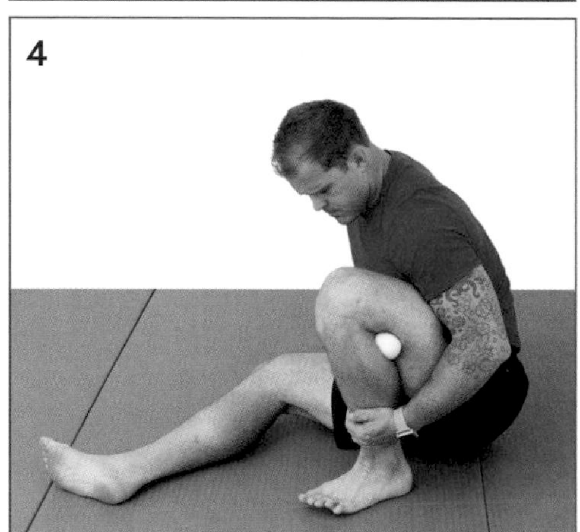

1. Position a lacrosse ball behind your knee on the outside of your leg.

2. Curl your heel toward your butt, cup your hands around your shin, and pull your leg in tight to your body, sandwiching the ball behind your knee.

3. Pulling on your shin to create a large compression force, start moving your foot around in all directions. Tacking down the tissues of your distal hamstring and upper calf will help restore suppleness to the tight tissues that cross your knee.

4. To increase the pressure, plant your foot on the ground and scoot your butt toward your heel.

Option 3: Gemini or Double Lacrosse Ball Gap and Smash

If you have a Gemini or double lacrosse ball, you can hit the inside and outside lines of your calves and hamstrings simultaneously. This option also offers a gapping effect. It doesn't deliver the same precision smashing as options 1 and 2, but it will get the job done.

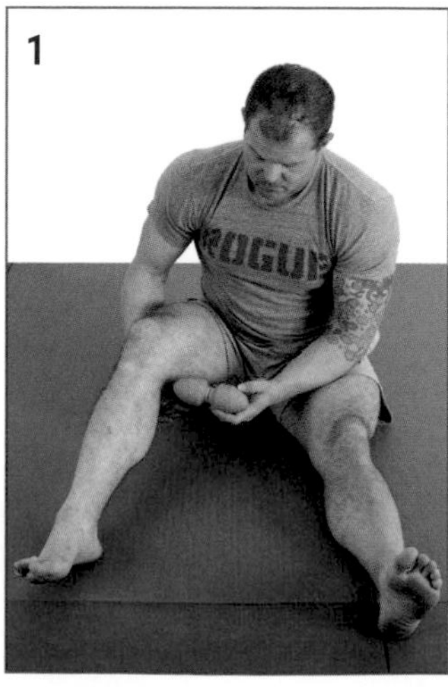

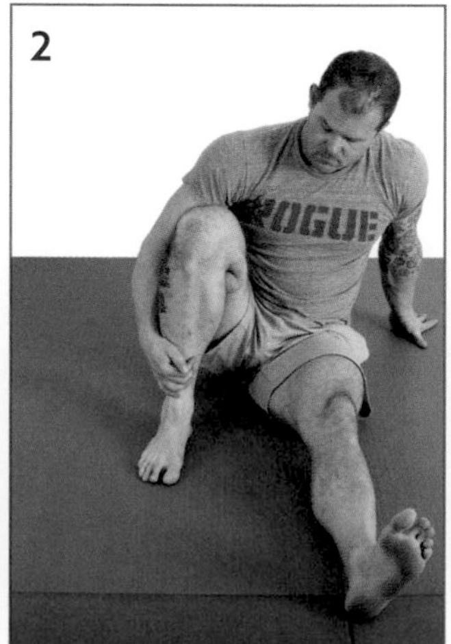

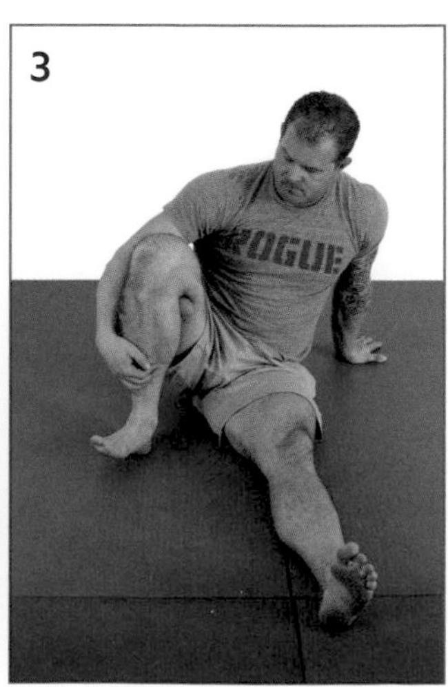

The approach for this mob is simple: Position a Gemini or double lacrosse ball behind your knee, create a compression force by folding your leg around the tool, and then make circles with your foot.

Option 4: Spin and Smash

You can also use a double lacrosse ball or Gemini to mobilize the inside or outside line of your calves and hamstrings, just as you would when using a single lacrosse ball. The idea here is to leave half of the tool exposed so that you can grab the protruding end. This gives you a couple options: You can twist it back and forth as if you were revving a motorcycle engine, or spin it to take up the soft tissue and skin slack and then contract and relax or floss to penetrate the deep muscle layers. It's another creative way to restoring sliding surfaces and release trigger points in the posterior muscles that connect to the knee.

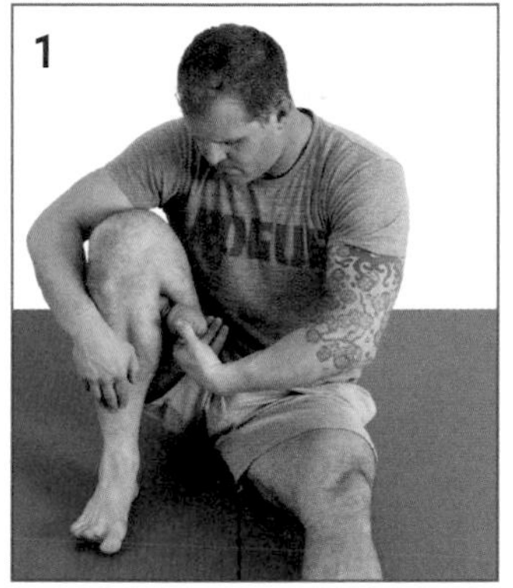

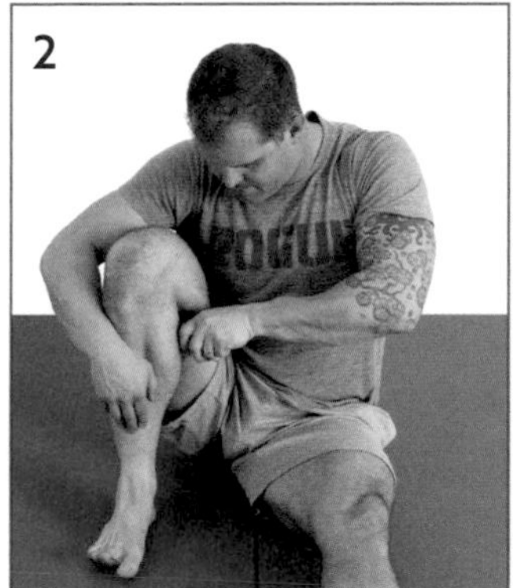

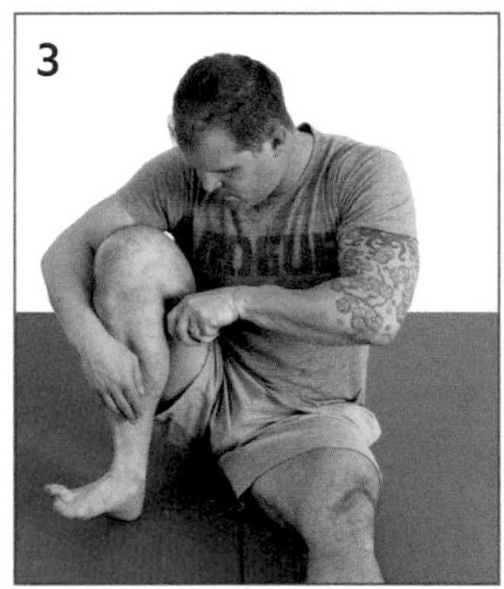

1. Position half of a Gemini or double lacrosse ball on the inside or outside of your knee crease, then create a compression force by folding your leg around the tool.

2. Twist the tool to take up the soft tissue and skin slack. You can turn the tool back and forth to restore sliding surfaces to the superficial layers of skin and muscle tissue.

3. Once you've taken up the slack by rotating the tool, you can contract and relax and floss by moving your foot around in different directions.

Option 5: Knee Stack and Smash

Let's be honest: Mobilizing is not fun. Anytime you can hit two or more areas with one mobilization and reduce the amount of time you spend in the pain cave, it's a win. Like the Forearm Stack and Smash, this is a great way to mobilize multiple areas with a single technique. With a large ball such as a Supernova or softball positioned between your legs and a Gemini or double lacrosse ball positioned underneath your grounded leg, you can hit the inside line of both legs and the outside line of your grounded leg. Although you're targeting three areas, this option is particularly effective for mobilizing the outside of your knee. With the ball positioned between your legs, you can balance your opposite leg over your grounded leg, which adds significant pressure. The fact that you can floss by bending and straightening your legs makes this one of the best lateral knee smashing techniques available.

TARGET AREA

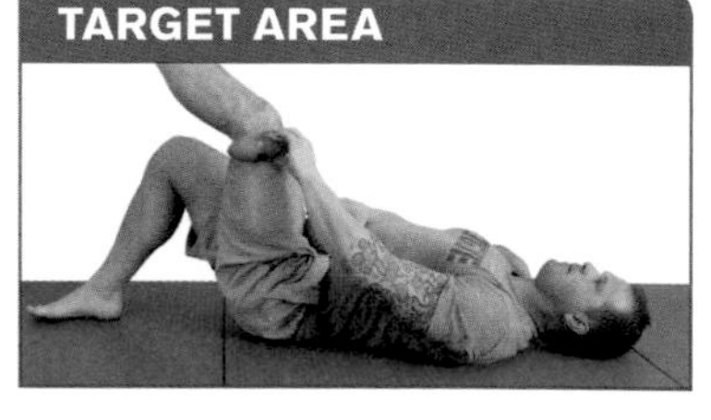

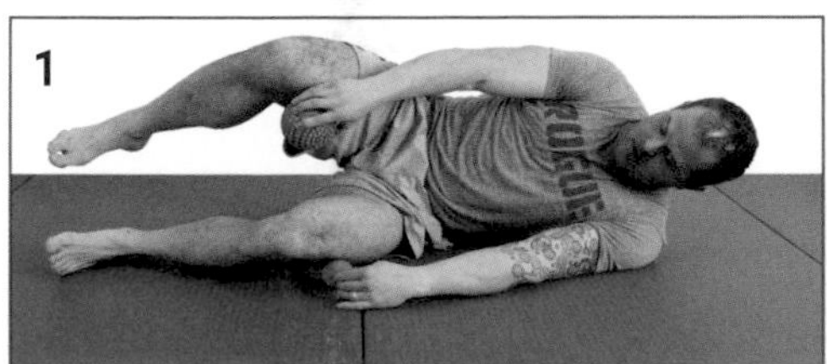

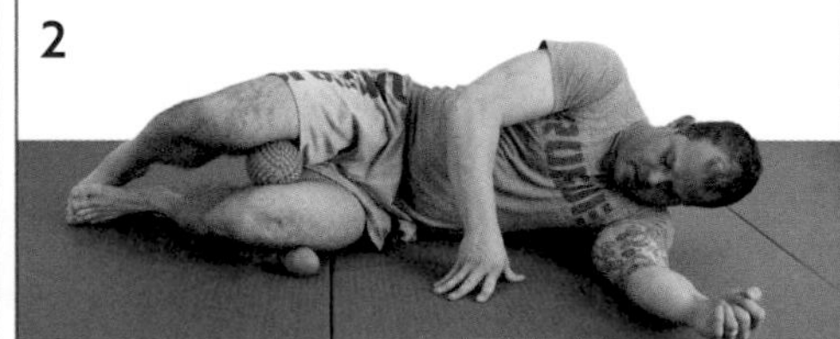

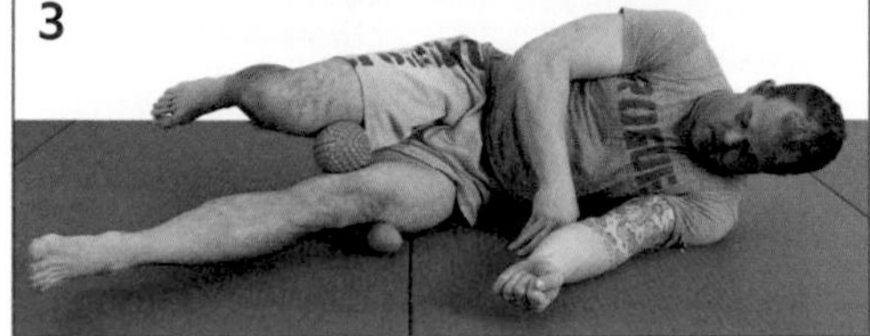

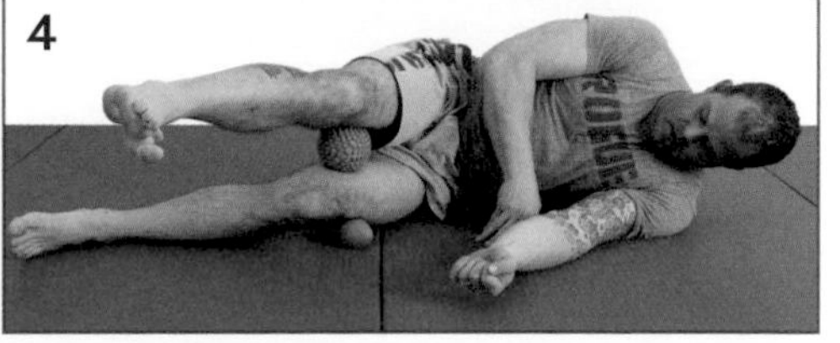

Lying on your side, position a Gemini or double lacrosse ball just above your knee underneath your grounded leg. Then position a large ball between your legs just above your knee. With the balls in position, pinch your knees together and then straighten your bottom leg while simultaneously bending your top leg. The idea is to scissor back and forth—flexing one leg and extending the other—until you experience change. You can also employ the contract and relax technique.

IMPROVES:

Knee flexion and extension

Knee pain

Flexion Gapping

When I work with athletes, I encourage them to think about treating the issues in and around the areas that are giving them trouble. You don't need a background in anatomy to address your business. For example, if you're having knee problems, it's conceivable that one of the structures around your knee is tight or not working correctly. When people have arthritic knees or really stiff knee joints, hinge dust starts to accumulate below the knee. Flexion gapping is a simple way to blow away that dust and restore normal function to the knee joint.

A simple way to screen for knee flexion problems is to sit butt to ankles. You should be able to smash your calves into your hamstrings without pain or restriction. If you're unable to do so, the problem could be quad stiffness, poor ankle range of motion, or a stiff knee capsule. This technique is an easy way to deal with the latter issue. If the joint capsule is restricted, achieving full hip or knee flexion is difficult because there isn't enough space in the front of the knee to accommodate for the rotation of the femur on the tibia. Like the banded distraction iterations, this is an easy way to restore that passive accessory motion and restore normal range of motion to the knee.

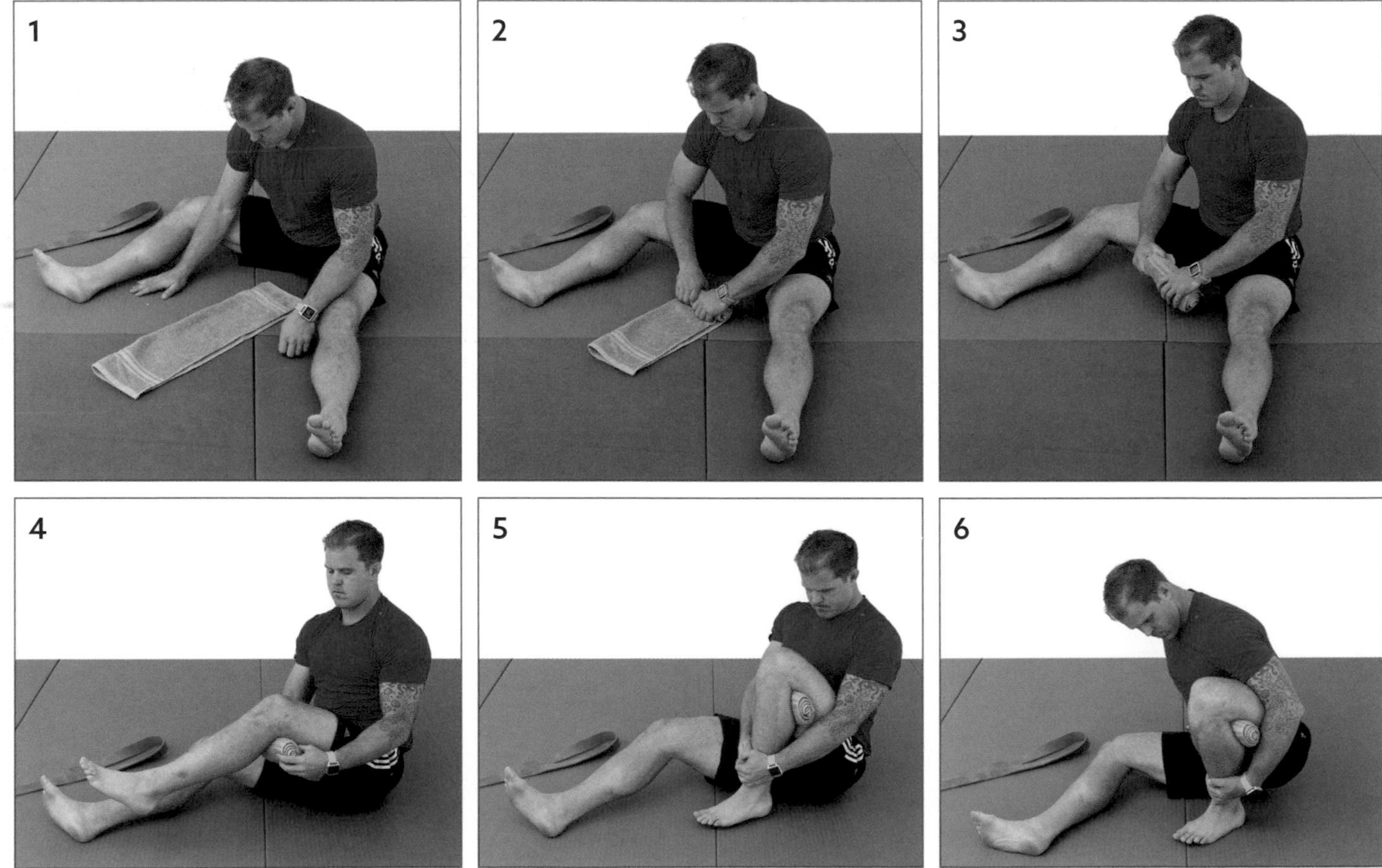

Roll up a small towel and place it behind your knee. Grab your shin, pull your heel toward your butt, and then scoot your butt toward your foot, creating as much pressure as possible. Try to keep your foot straight while oscillating in and out of peak compression.

AREA 12 SHIN

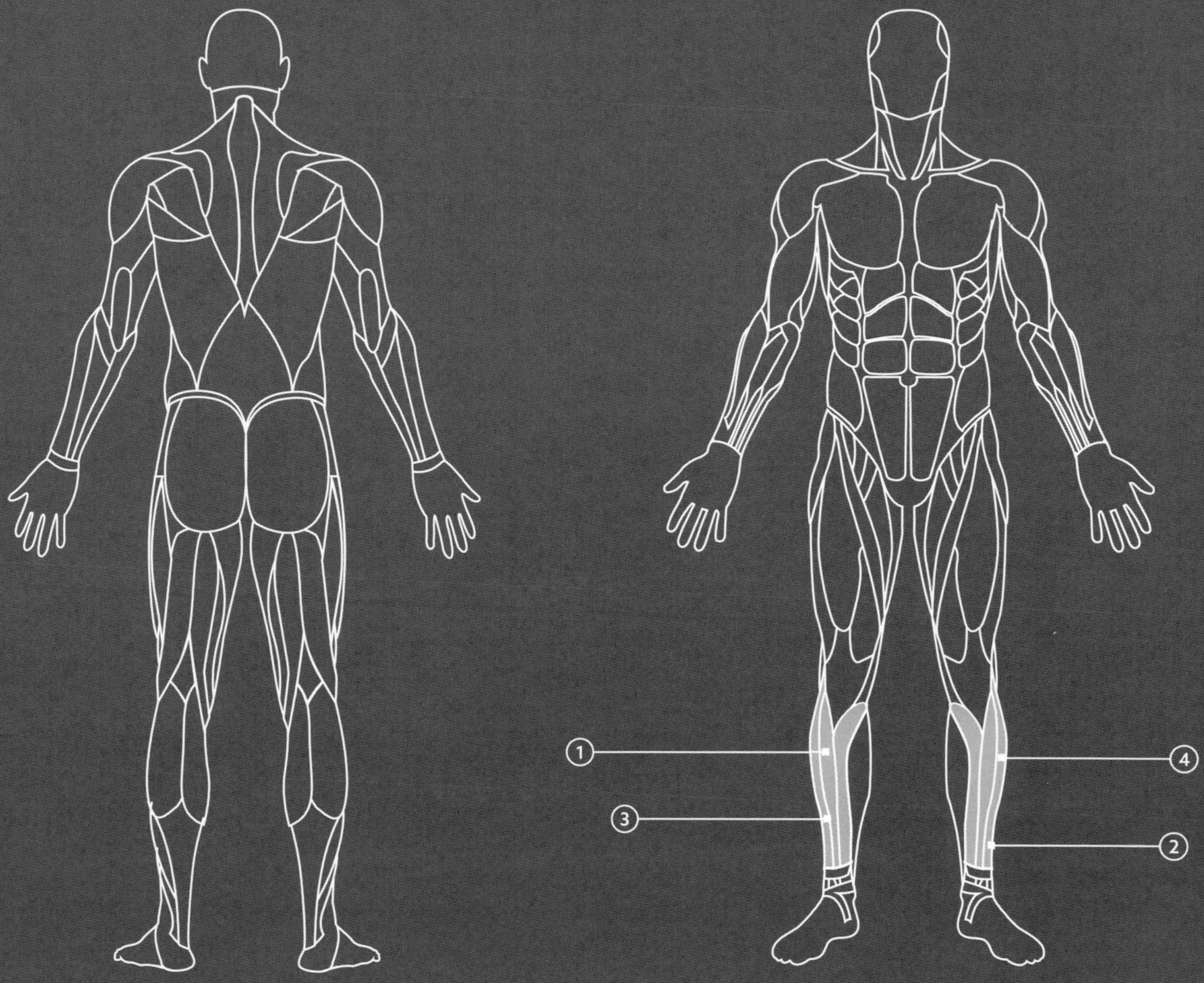

1
3
4
2

MOBILIZATION TARGET AREAS:

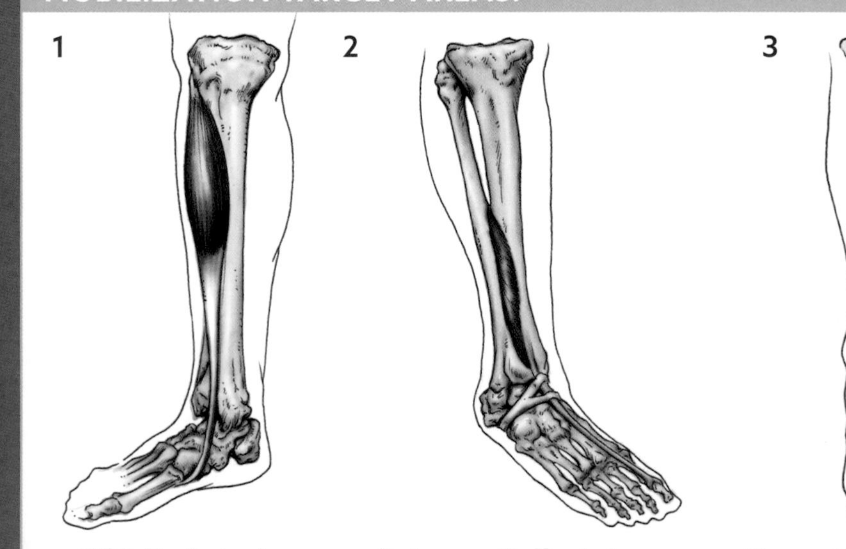

Tibialis Anterior

Extensor Hallucis Longus

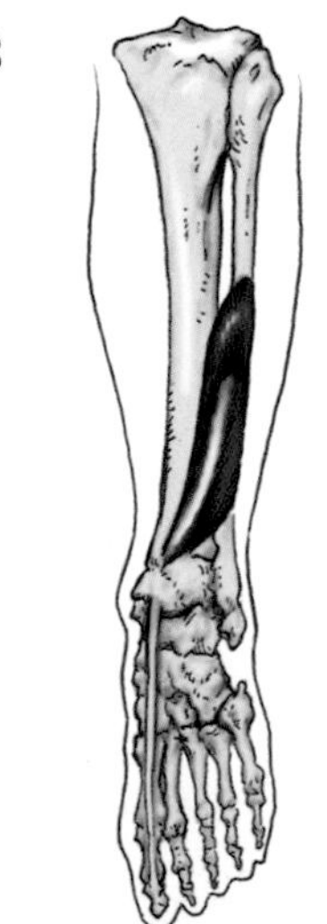

Flexor Hallucis Longus

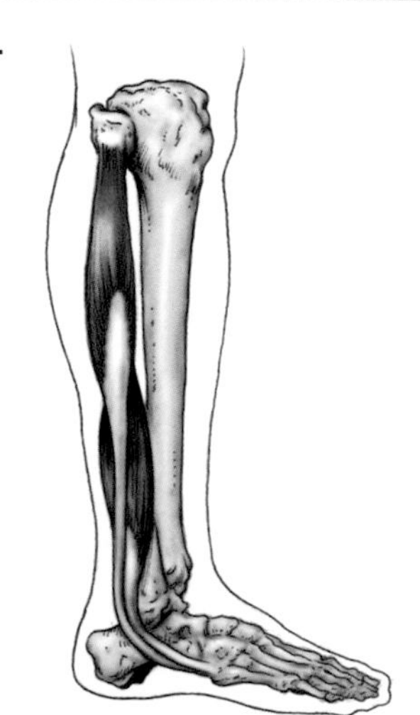

Peroneus Longus

Medial Shin Smash and Floss Mobilizations

Pistol Archetype

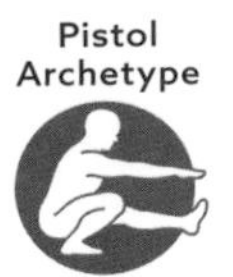

Squat 1 Archetype

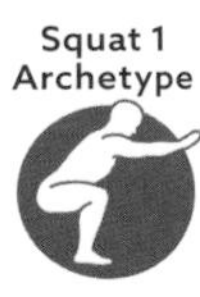

This mobilization will help improve the above archetypes.

IMPROVES:

Ankle function (creating a stable arch)

Knee, ankle, and foot pain

METHODS:

Pressure wave

Contract and relax

Smash and floss

Tack and spin

TARGET AREA

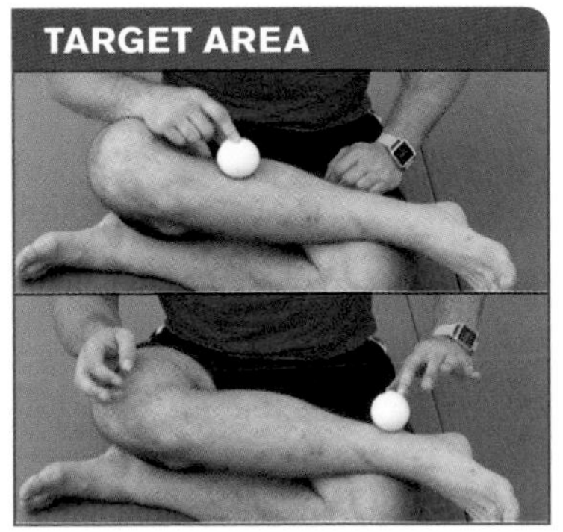

The target area stretches from the base of your knee down to just above the ankle bone along the inside of your shin.

If you run a lot or are on your feet all day, there's a good chance that the tissues of your lower leg are brutally tight and in need of some serious love. The musculature extending from your knee to your ankle along the inside of your shin—specifically the soleus, posterior tibialis, and gastrocnemius muscles—is responsible for giving your foot arch support. Anytime you stand, walk, or run, you are placing a demand on these tissues. As the calf musculature becomes tight and locked up, people start defaulting to an open-foot position, which causes the ankle to collapse and places stress on the upstream tissues.

To restore good positions and normalize these tissues, take a ball and smash it into the inside of your shinbone, working from the base of your knee down to your ankle bone. The idea is to create large pressures and work all the elements. You can pressure wave, contract and relax, and smash and floss by moving your foot through various ranges. People find areas of high pain and areas of low pain. The key is to skip over the low pain and stay on the hot, grody areas behind your shin.

This mobilization should be one of your first stops if you have plantar fascia problems, have posterior tibialis tendonitis, can't get your foot into a good arch, or do a lot of running—especially barefoot-centric running.

Option 1: Lacrosse Ball Shin Smash

There are a few different ways to approach this mobilization. I like to sit on the ground with my legs crossed because it allows for unrestricted flossing—I can move my foot around in all directions—and gives me leverage to pressure the ball into my shin. However, not everyone can comfortably get into this position. If you are physically restricted, you can sit on the ground with your leg extended out to the side (option 2), cross your leg over your knee from a sitting position (option 3), or prop your leg up on an elevated surface such as a bench or tabletop.

1. Pin a lacrosse ball on the inside of your shin and apply downward pressure with both hands.

2. Still applying downward pressure, spin the lacrosse ball into your leg to take up the skin and soft tissue slack, and move your foot around in all directions. You can also pressure wave or implement the contract and relax technique.

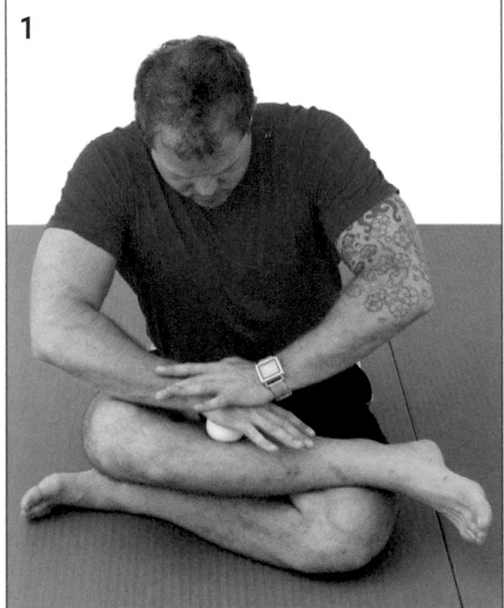

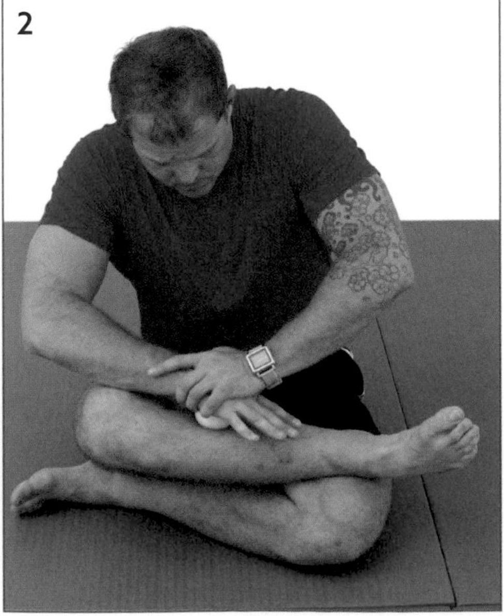

Option 2: Gemini Shin Smash and Spin

You can also use the point of a Gemini (or any tool that has a dull point) to smash the inside line of your shin. This variation is the same as option 1, but with two key differences. Here I'm showing a slightly different leg configuration for people who are unable to cross their foot over the opposite knee, and I'm using the Gemini to illustrate the Smash and Spin technique, for which this tool is well suited.

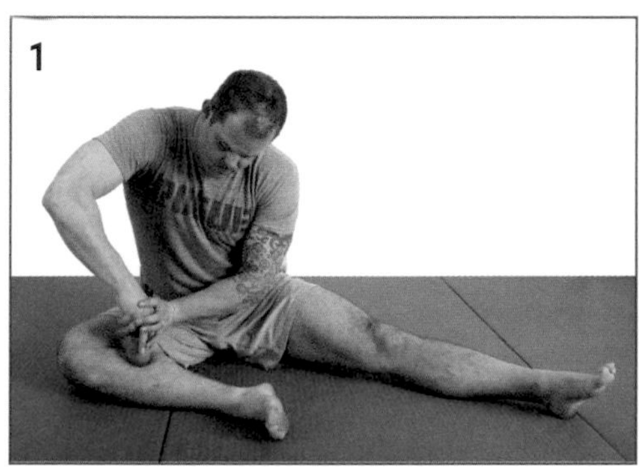

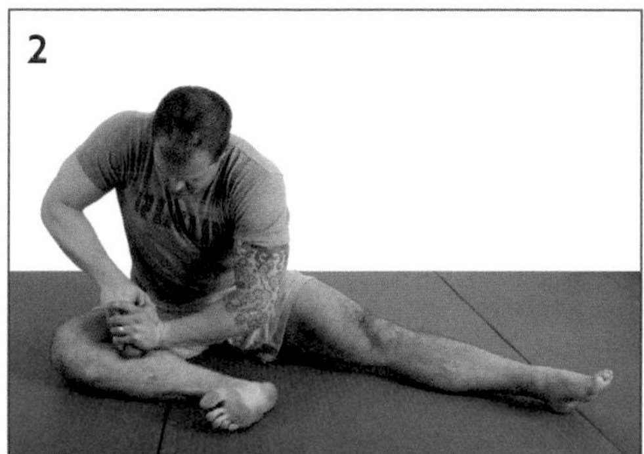

1. For the best results, drive the point of the Gemini into your shin.

2. While maintaining downward pressure, twist the Gemini until you've taken up all the soft tissue and skin slack. Then floss by moving your foot around in all directions or contract and relax to get deeper compression.

Option 3: Executive Medial Shin Smash and Floss

This is a fantastic option for the less mobile. It also serves as a perfect lower body maintenance strategy for deskbound athletes. Anytime you can work on improving your position and mobilizing stiff tissues while trapped in a chair, it's a win.

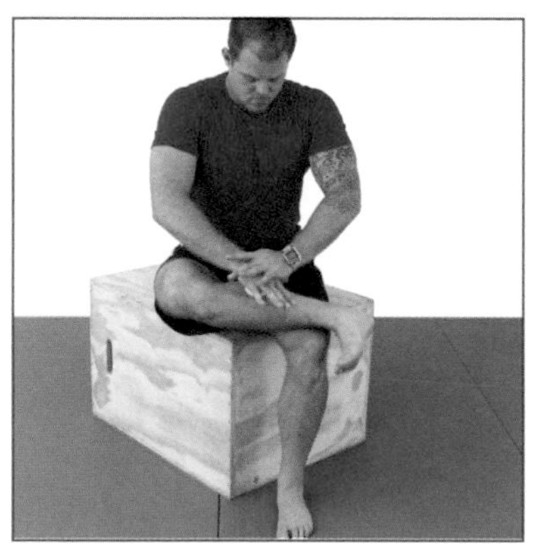

Cross your leg over your knee, wedge a lacrosse ball between your shinbone and calf, and apply downward pressure with both hands. From here, you can contract and relax, roll your foot around in all directions, or apply the pressure wave and tack and spin techniques.

Option 4: Shin Stack and Smash

This option is attractive because it's easy to get into the position, and you can target both sides of your leg. If you're prone to calf stiffness (most people are) or you have foot or ankle pain, consider this a gold star technique.

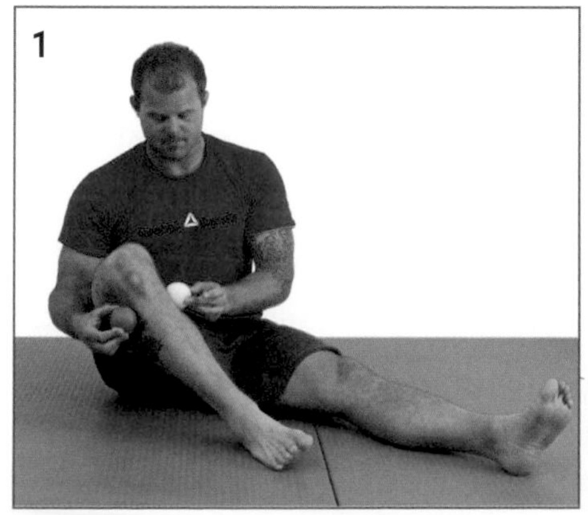

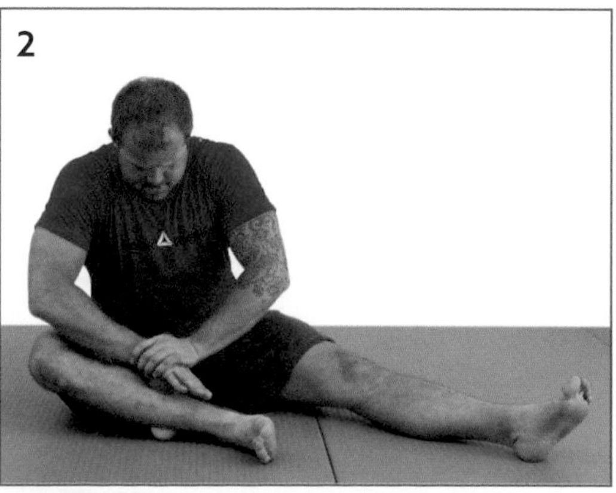

1. Position a lacrosse ball on either side of your leg.

2. Find a tight area, align the top ball over the bottom ball, and apply downward pressure with both hands.

Option 5: Superfriend Medial Shin Smash

Consider this an extension of the Superfriend Adductor Smash, which is done from the same position. If you're on your side, you might as well have a Superfriend hit the entire inseam of your leg. As with the Adductor Smash, the Superfriend uses the outside edge and heel of his foot. It doesn't take a lot of pressure to get the desired results, so be careful and go easy. If you're jerking and squirming like a fish out of water, he's probably smashing too hard.

As the Superfriend, have your partner lie on her side with the inseam of her leg facing the ceiling. Using your heel and the outside edge of your foot, apply light, slow, and steady pressure across the inside of her shin. To "break up" tacked-down tissue, think about smearing your foot around as if you were putting out a cigarette. You can also create a pressure wave across your partner's calf. If you find a trigger point, stay on the area and employ the contract and relax method.

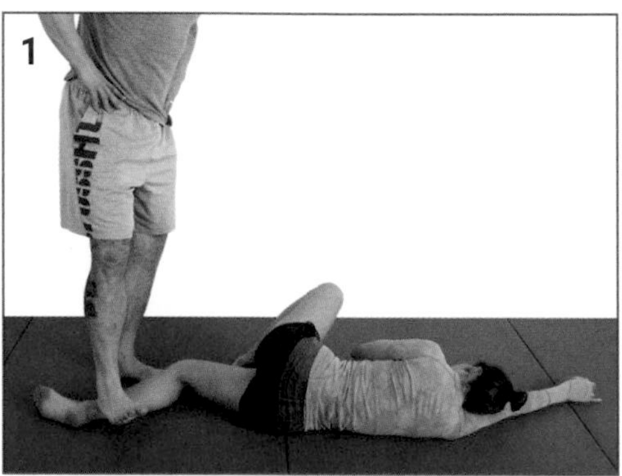

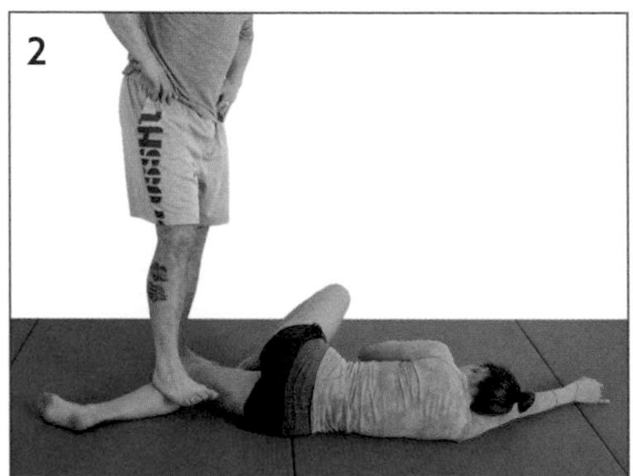

Lateral and Anterior Compartment Shin Mobilization

IMPROVES:

Neutral (straight) foot position

Anterior compartment pain (shin splints)

Knee and ankle pain

METHODS:

Smash and floss

Pressure wave

Contract and relax

If you have foot problems or strange downstream pain, you have to look at your shin and calf. All the tissues that control your feet are housed in your lower leg. The calf and shin are the puppeteers pulling the strings to your feet.

The problem is that people tend to forget about the front of the shin because all the meat is on the back of the leg, which is where most people focus their attention. However, if you do a lot of running, walking, and standing—especially if you heel strike and stand with your feet turned out—those peroneal muscles that run down the outside of your lower leg are on constant tension and will get extremely tight. This is precisely how shin splints develop.

When I treat athletes with shin splints, I ask them, "What are you doing for those tissues?" They usually pause, think for a second, and then say, "Nothing." It's odd, because those tissues are stiff and being pulled off the bone, but more often than not the athlete isn't addressing the area of localized pain. Obviously, working upstream and downstream of the problem is part of the conversation, but to restore those tissues to normal function, you have to get in there and give those stiff tissues some love.

When this anterior compartment of the shin gets tight, the muscles don't contract very well, limiting dorsiflexion range of motion. It also inhibits your ability to point your toes. For this reason, the test and retest is simply to flex and point your foot. If your shin is working efficiently and the sliding surfaces are actually sliding, you will be able to flex and point your toes farther with less discomfort.

TARGET AREA

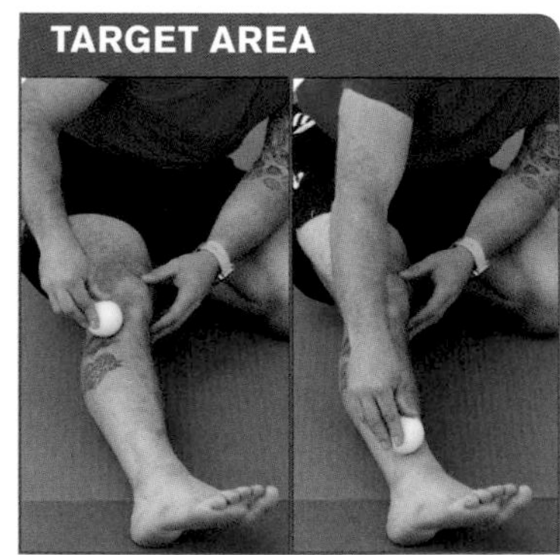

The goal is to work the anterior compartment and lateral compartment (peroneals) along the front of your shin and outside of your leg from knee to ankle.

If you have knee or ankle pain, you're struggling to get your feet into a good position, or the fronts of your shins hurt—meaning that you have shin splints—this mobilization should be at the top of your list. You can attack these tissues in a couple different ways: You can use a rolling pin or stick massager, or pressure your weight over a lacrosse ball or roller, as demonstrated here. The tools that you use are not important, as long as you get the job done.

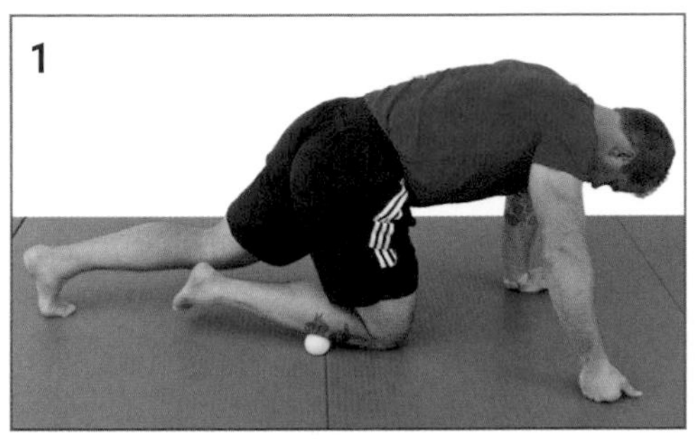

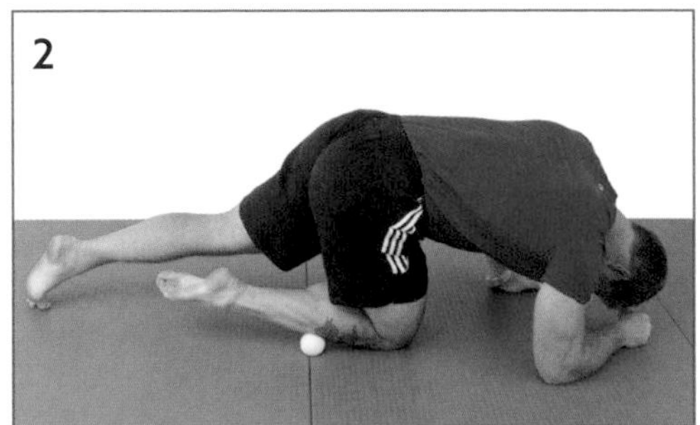

1. Kneel on the ground and position a lacrosse ball on the outside of your shin. To add pressure, you can sit your butt back or reposition your center of mass over the ball.

2. Work across the tissue, pressure waving from the outside to the inside of your leg. If you stumble across a painful spot, stop and move your foot around in all directions. You can also contract and relax to penetrate deeper into the tight tissues.

Roller Variation

You can also use a roller—ideally a Little Battlestar. Work up and down the length of the tissue, hunting out tight areas. When you find a hotspot, rock from side to side across the tissue while moving your foot around in all directions.

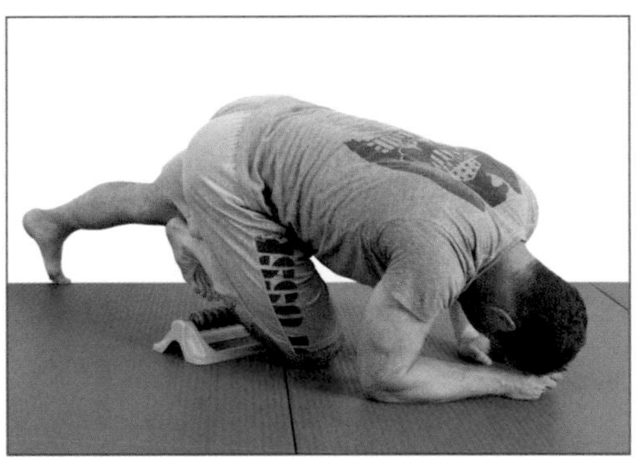

Double-Leg Plantarflexion

IMPROVES:
Anterior compartment pain (shin splints)

This sweet and simple global dorsiflexion technique is a low-budget way to mobilize the fronts of your shins. It's a powerful counter-mobilization to the previous technique that puts the anterior compartment in an end-range position. You can target both legs simultaneously, as shown below, or hit one leg at a time.

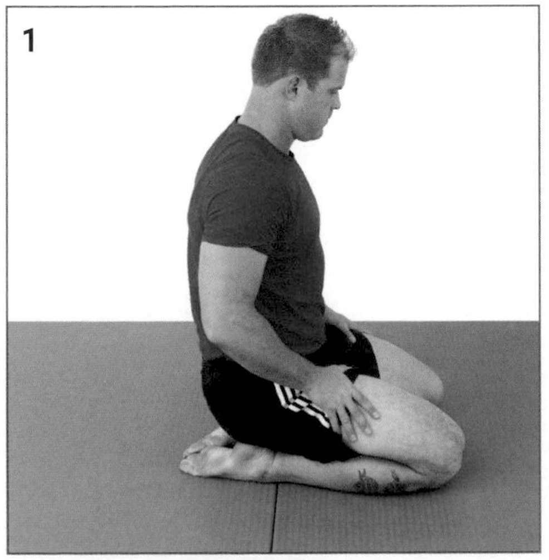

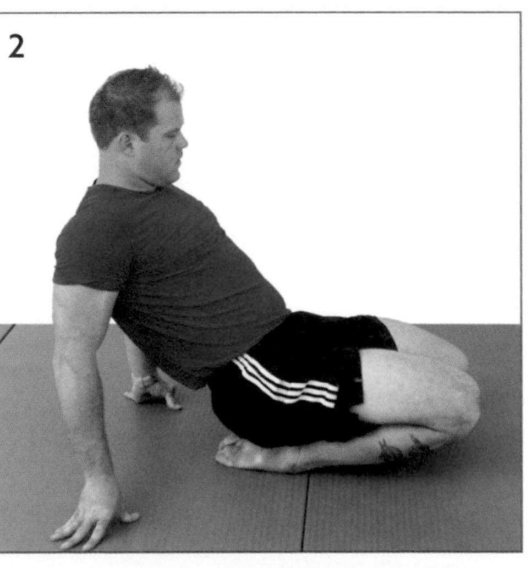

1. Sit on your heels with the tops of your feet flush with the ground and your big toes right next to each other. *Note:* If you want to isolate one leg, plant one foot on the ground. For example, if you want to mobilize your right shin, post up on your left foot and plant your right hand on the mat to counterbalance your weight.

2. Keeping your back flat and your knees straight, lean back and allow your knees to come up off the ground.

AREA 13 CALF

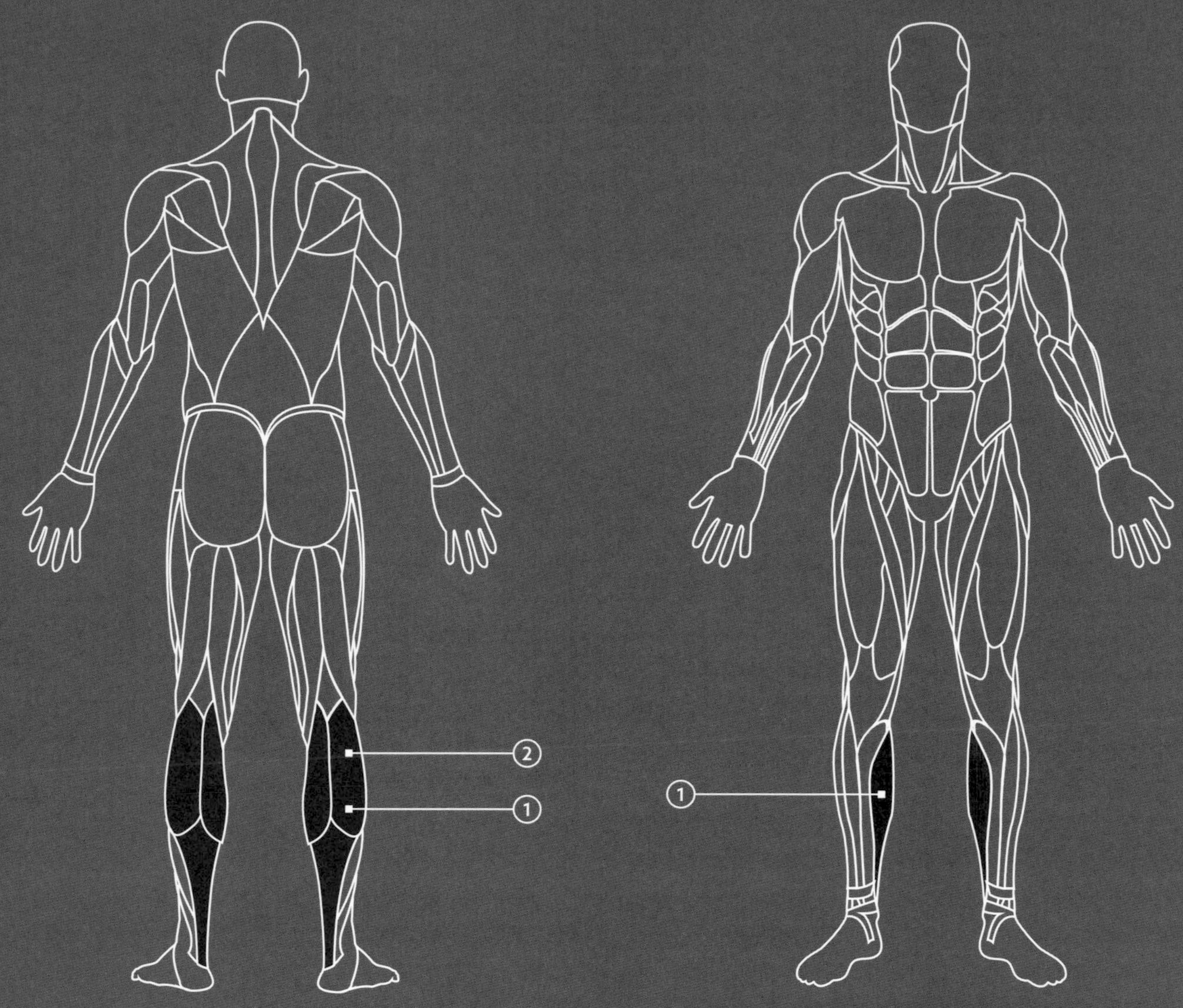

MOBILIZATION TARGET AREAS:

1 Gastrocnemius

2 Soleus

Calf Smash Mobilizations

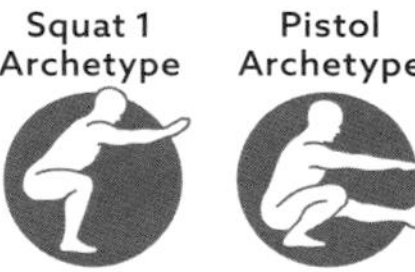

This mobilization will help improve the above archetypes.

IMPROVES:

Knee and ankle pain

METHODS:

Contract and relax
Pressure wave
Smash and floss

Calf muscles have a serious job. An active person takes an average of 10,000 steps per day. That represents 5,000 loads per calf over the course of a single day, and 35,000 loads per calf over the course of a week. This doesn't even include going up and down stairs, running, working out, or playing sports. If you have bad foot positioning, whether you're walking with your feet turned out or wearing shoes that compromise your position, the insidious calf tightness that accumulates is insane. It's no accident that people's calves are in a state of constant stiffness and their heel cords are like steel cables.

If you're missing ankle range of motion, you have no choice but to compensate into an open-foot position, meaning that you stand, walk, run, and move with open knees and collapsed ankles. When this happens, you can't expect everything to be okay. It's the same issue when people are missing wrist extension: They turn their hands out and wonder why their shoulders hurt. If you're missing foot extension or dorsiflexion, you're going to turn your feet out to solve that range of motion problem and buffer the issue. Do this and ultimately say hello to bone spurs, Achilles tendonitis, Achilles ruptures, and a slate of other ankle problems. You can avoid all this if you maintain full ankle range of motion and understand good positioning. You have to make sure that the large drivers of your ankles are full range and supple.

Although the chief problem usually lies in the heel cords, the tightness transmits upstream. The gastroc, which is the powerful lower leg muscle that makes up your calf, is responsible for controlling your ankle. If those tissues get stiff, ankle and knee pain generally follow.

Remember that you have a lot of musculature controlling your feet, and all that tissue runs through a very small space. This is why you need to prioritize some of the smashing techniques when you're trying to deal with knee pain or improve ankle range of motion. You can't just roll around aimlessly on a foam roller. You must smash.

You can incorporate several smashing techniques, ranging from the horribly painful to the mildly uncomfortable. Depending on your level of stiffness and pain tolerance, you may have to start with the most basic, which is the Roller Calf Smash, and work your way up. Just remember, the more uncomfortable the mobilization, the more change you will see, feel, and realize.

Option 1: Roller Calf Smash

This is the most basic calf smashing technique that we use. It's usually reserved for people who are extremely sore. Tight calves are very sensitive, making it tough to mobilize without passing out or vomiting. This is why it's good to have low-level mobilizations that you can throw in as a warm-up to the more aggressive techniques. Remember, in order to make observable and measurable change, you need large, acute pressures, which are difficult to get by using a foam roller.

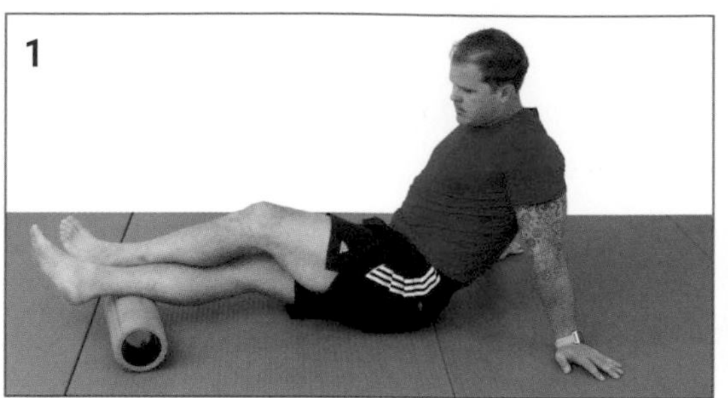

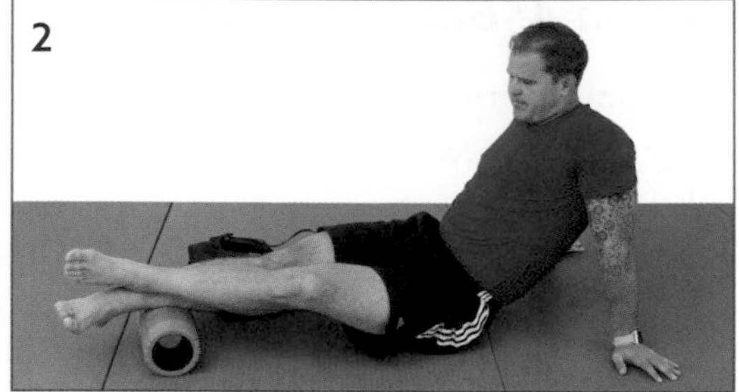

Position your calf and heel cord on a roller or pipe, cross your opposite leg over your shin to add pressure, and then roll your leg from side to side. You can also contract and relax and point and flex your toes.

Option 2: Superfriend Roller Calf Smash

This option is great for two reasons: You can get a ton of pressure into your calf, and you are more likely to tolerate higher compression forces than you would on your own. The bottom line is that there are not too many people out there who will apply the same kind of tortuous pressure to themselves as a Superfriend would. As with the Superfriend Quad Smash, you'll probably want to agree on a safe word that will cue your partner to ease up.

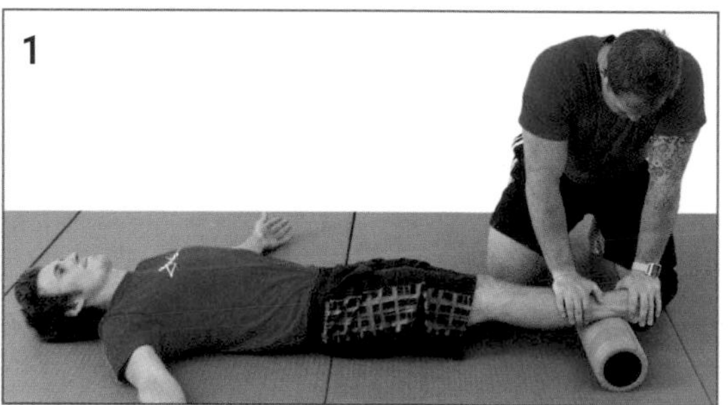

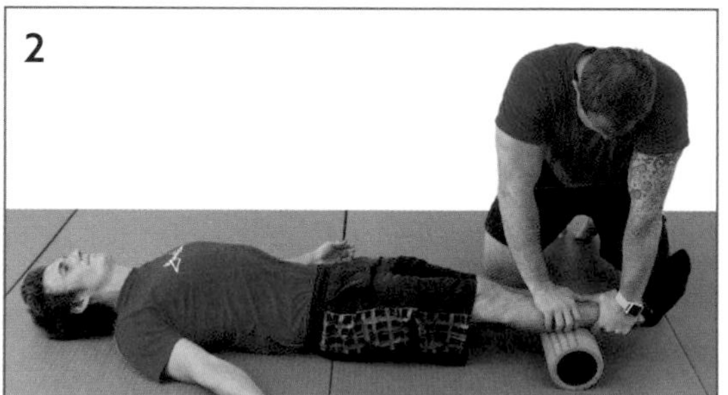

As the Superfriend, grip the top of your partner's shin and ankle, apply downward pressure, and then roll the leg back and forth over the roller.

Option 3: Barbell Calf Smash

This option offers more acute pressure, which is what you want when you're dealing with tight heel cords, because it enables you to restore superficial sliding surfaces to the tissues near the base of your heel and ankle. You can also use a Little Battlestar for this technique.

LITTLE BATTLESTAR VARIATION

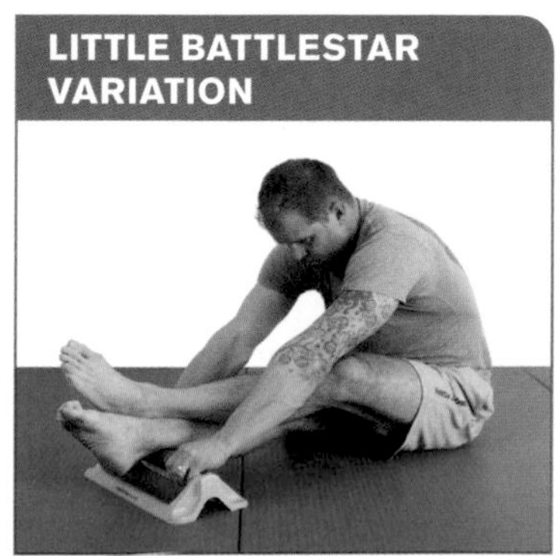

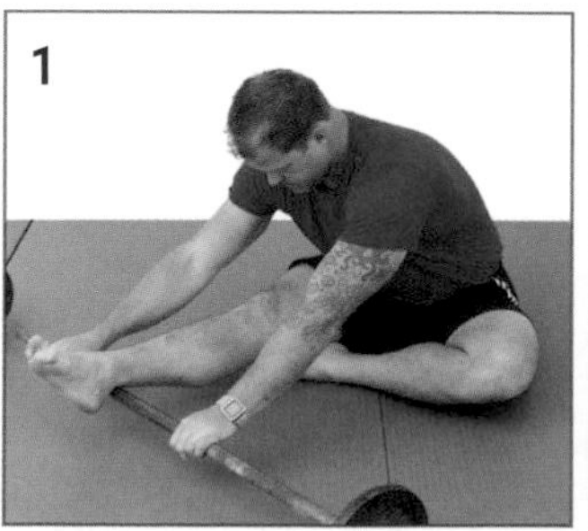

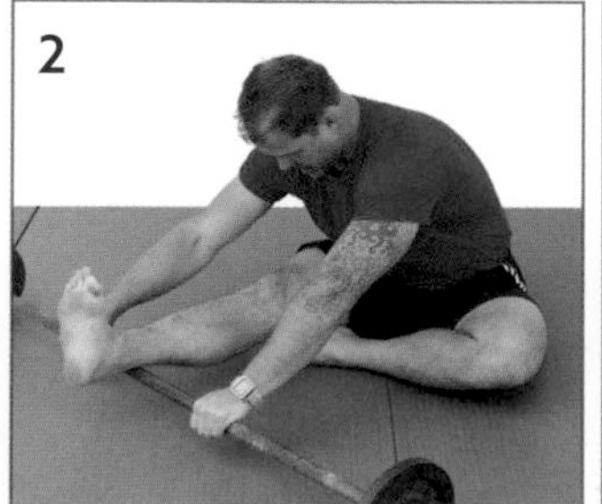

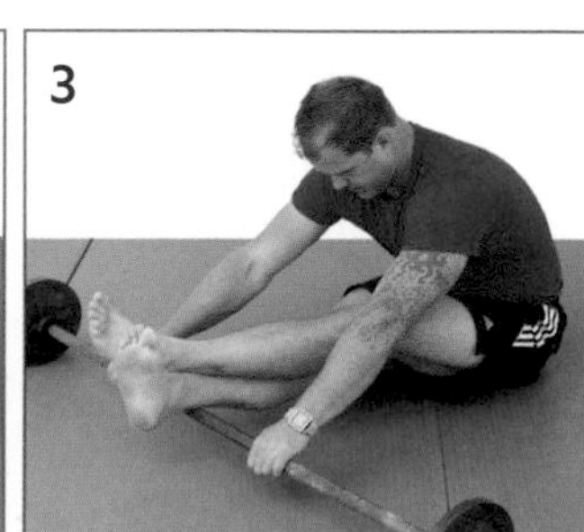

With your heel cord resting on the bar, you can roll your foot from side to side, flex and extend your foot, or twist the barbell up your lower leg to get a pressure wave effect. Crossing your opposite leg over your foot and leaning forward is a great way to add more compression force.

Option 4: Bone Saw Calf Smash

This is my favorite of the Calf Smash Mobilizations, and it's the first one I use when I have calf and heel cord tightness or ankle- or knee-related issues. But I'm not going to lie: It's pretty nasty.

By placing your instep over a foam roller or pillow and positioning your shin over your leg, you can get large pressures working through the back of your calf. The idea is to slice the blade of your shin into the areas that are tight, oscillating from side to side as if you were playing a fiddle. A roller is the ideal tool here because it elevates your foot. This allows you not only to mobilize with a relaxed leg, but also to "floss" by moving your bottom foot around in different directions. The contract and relax technique also works here.

You can control the pressure by adjusting your weight. Sitting your weight back will increase the compression, while shifting forward will take pressure off your leg.

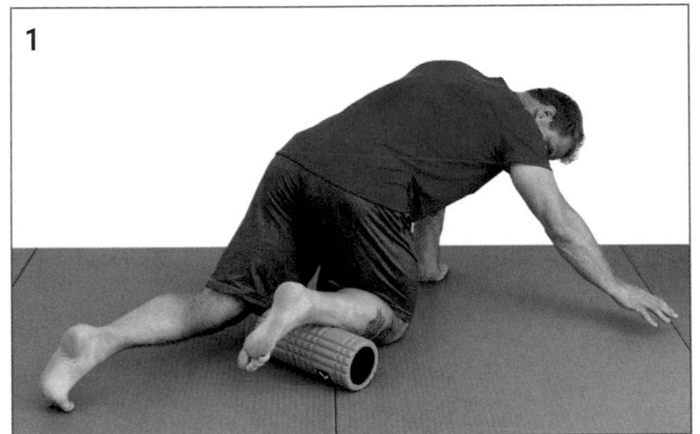
1

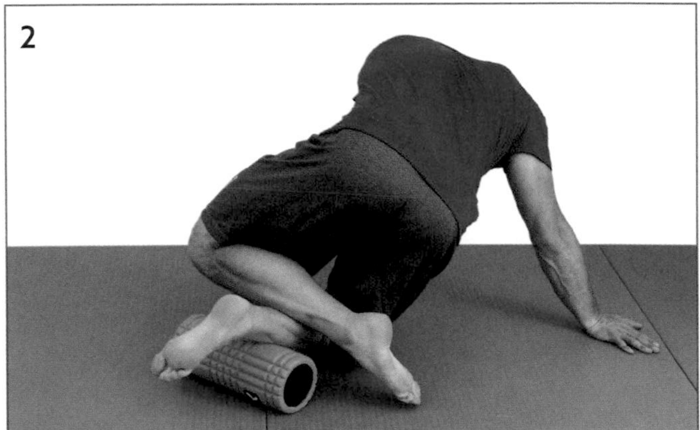
2

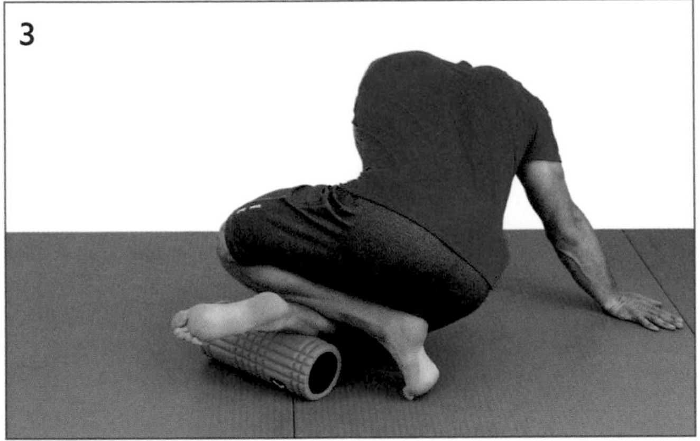
3

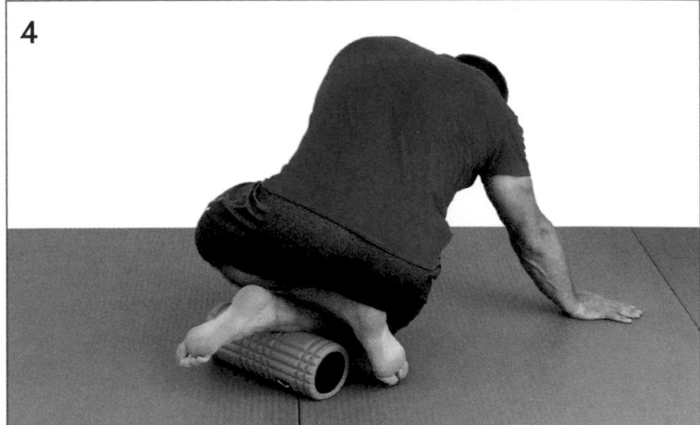
4

1. Kneel and place your instep over a roller or large pillow, keeping your foot neutral.

2. Using your arms to support the weight of your upper body, bring your opposite leg up and place your shin or instep across the tissue you're trying to change.

3. To add a compression force, sit your butt back and shift your weight over your top leg. *Note:* You can control the amount of pressure by shifting your weight forward and backward. The more you sit back, the more aggressive the pressure.

4. Keeping your weight centered over your leg, slowly smash your shin across the back of your calf. The idea is to shear back and forth across the back of your calf. You can also hang out on a tight spot and apply the contract and relax and smash and floss techniques.

Option 5: Superfriend Calf Smash

The Superfriend Calf Smash is another easy way to restore suppleness to the heel cords and calves. As with most of the Superfriend smashes, you want to create a cross-fiber shear using the arch of your foot. To protect your partner's ankle, place an ab mat or pillow underneath her shin.

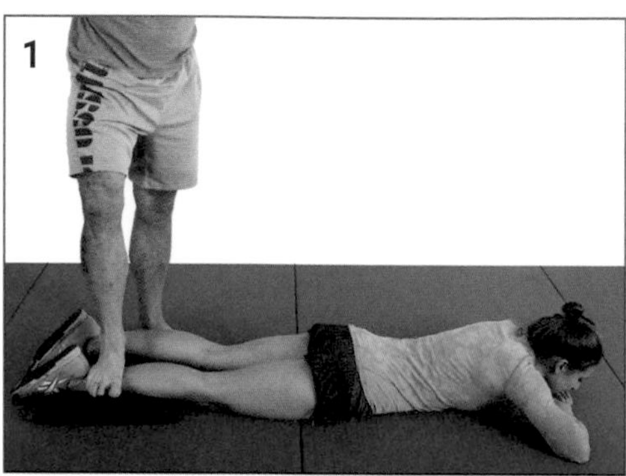

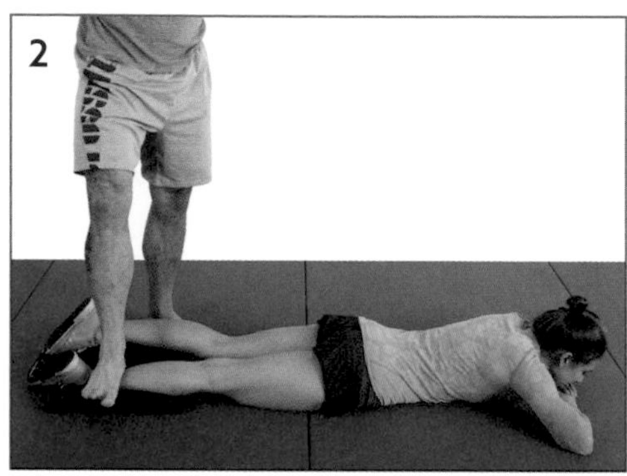

As the Superfriend, place a pillow underneath your partner's ankle. Using the arch of your foot, create slow and steady pressure across her heel cord and calf.

Squat 1 Archetype

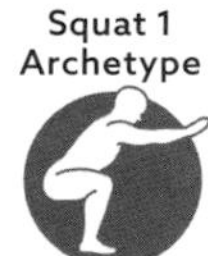

Pistol Archetype

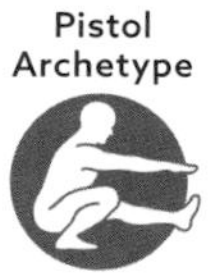

This mobilization will help improve the above archetypes.

IMPROVES:

Knee and ankle pain

Calf stiffness (releasing trigger points)

METHOD:

VooDoo Floss Band compression

VooDoo Calf Mobilization

If you had to consume a human being (not that you ever would), the calf muscle would be one of the worst pieces to eat. It is so thick and fibrous that you would have to boil it for eight hours to break down the grisly muscle tissue. As I said, the calf undergoes an intense number of loading cycles: Walking, playing sports, lifting, wearing high heels, and running all add up. Not to mention that most people spend very little time undoing all that insidious, accumulated stiffness.

The bottom line is this: Your calves are prone to sliding surface restrictions. Left untreated, that stiffness aggregates into intramuscular adhesions and knotted-up scar balls that compromise mechanics and increase the potential for injury.

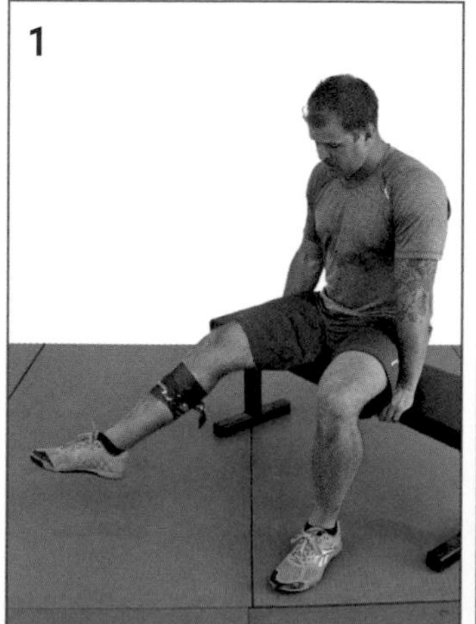

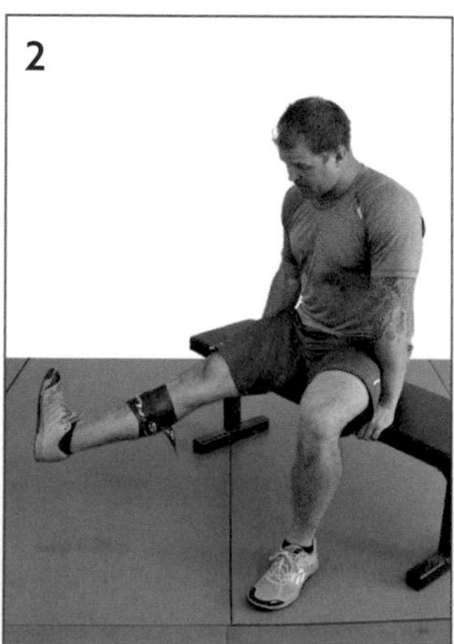

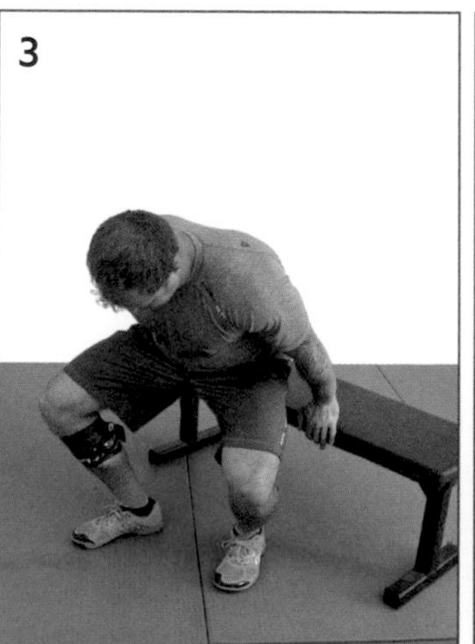

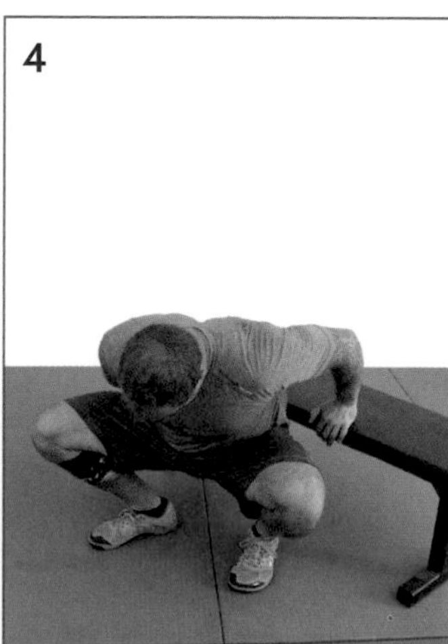

Wrap a band around the area you're trying to change, then move your foot through as much flexion and extension range as possible.

Classic Calf Mobilization

When people have tight calves, their first thought is generally to throw their foot on a wall or curb. It's a classic approach that can be done anywhere, anytime, and with zero equipment aside from shoes. (The shoe helps support your foot and provides traction on the wall so that you can keep the ball of your foot in place.) However, there are a couple of notable problems with this classic calf stretch.

The first problem is that it's difficult to change tissues by hanging out in a static position. These muscles are very, very strong and can handle large loads for extended periods. It's like hanging on a piece of steel cable hoping that it will stretch.

The second issue is that it doesn't take a systematic approach. That is, you're addressing only muscle dynamics and not your ankle capsules or sliding surfaces. You are putting yourself into a physiologic range and then hoping that you can create enough pressure to make change. For these reasons, it's imperative to prioritize the previous mobilizations and, if possible, attach a band around your ankle to tie in the joint capsule.

What's great about this mobilization is that it challenges your heel cord and calf at full range and serves as an excellent supplement or counter-mobilization to the previous techniques. You can also focus on the tissues at the base of your heel by bending your knee and loading the soleus complex. Just be sure to keep your foot in a good position and maintain a good arch as you hunt around for tight areas.

Squat 1 Archetype

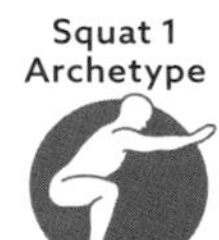

Pistol Archetype

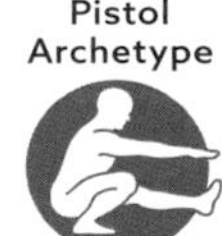

This mobilization will help improve the above archetypes.

IMPROVES:

Knee and ankle pain

METHOD:

Contract and relax

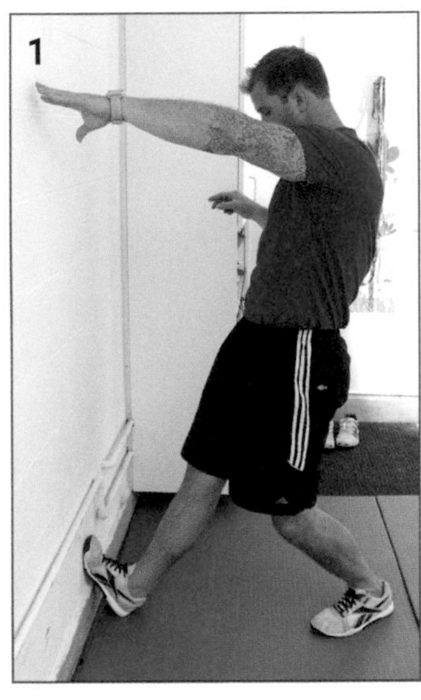

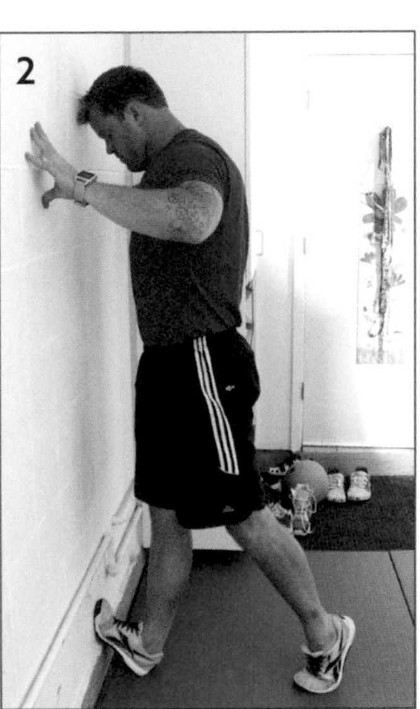

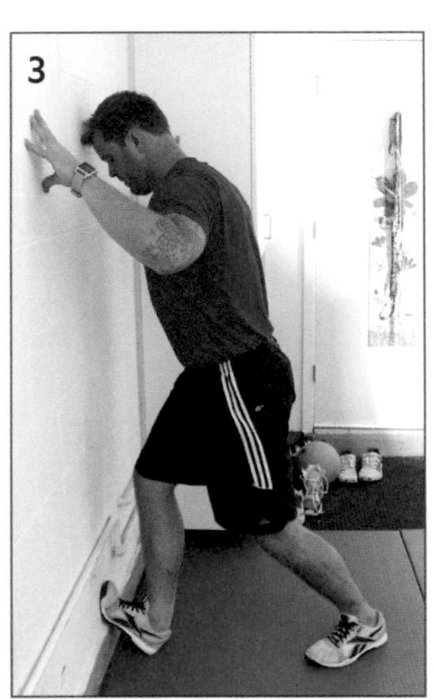

BANDED DISTRACTION

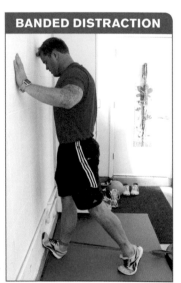

1. Standing a couple feet away from a wall, lower into a quarter or half squat and place the ball of your foot as high up on the wall as possible—keeping your heel in contact with the ground, your foot neutral, and your glute squeezed. Sometimes it's easier to start high up on the wall and slide your foot down until your heel touches. Once your foot is in position, straighten your knee. Don't try to bend your foot.

2. Keeping your foot pinned in place, stand tall and drive your weight toward the wall. With your leg straight, mobilize both your heel cord and calf (gastroc). Remember to keep your glute engaged and your belly tight as you move your hip toward the wall.

3. To explore different ranges of stiffness, lower your elevation by bending your leg and scour around for tight areas by externally and internally rotating your knee.

Banded Distraction: It's a bit tricky to set up, but rigging a band and applying a posterior distraction will increase the effectiveness of this mobilization twofold. Anytime you can apply a distraction to tie in the joint capsule, you turn a good stretch into a great stretch.

Squat 1 Archetype

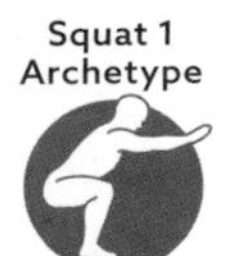

Pistol Archetype

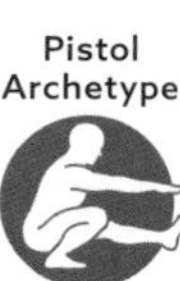

This mobilization will help improve the above archetypes.

IMPROVES:

Ankle pain

Ankle impingement

METHOD:

Banded flossing

1. Hook a band around the front of your ankle and create as much tension in the band as possible. You want your entire foot in contact with the ground and your foot straight. This allows you to generate a little bit of external rotation force to stabilize your ankle in a good position.

2. Drive your knee forward. The idea is to oscillate in and out of end range until you experience positive change.

3. You can also prop the ball of your foot on a weight to challenge more end-range dorsiflexion.

Banded Heel Cord: Anterior Bias

A lot of people report an impingement at the front of their ankle when they perform a classic calf stretch or pull their toes toward their knee. This is the equivalent of an anterior hip impingement. When your femur is resting at the front of your hip socket (usually from too much sitting), it runs into your acetabulum during deep flexion-based movements like squatting. The idea here is the same, but in this situation the bones of your ankle are resting at the front of the joint capsule, causing that familiar pinch at the front of the socket. As with the banded hip distraction, this is a simple way to clear that impingement and restore normal function and range of motion to the joint.

For the best results, create as much posterior tension as you can handle, drive your knee forward and out to the side—keeping your entire foot in contact with the ground—and oscillate in and out of end range until you experience change.

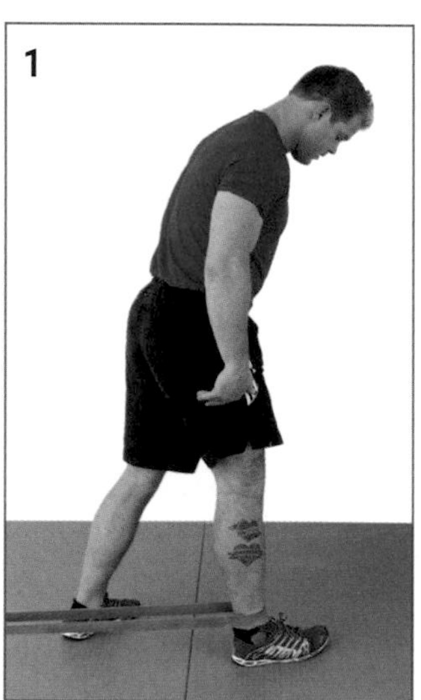

1

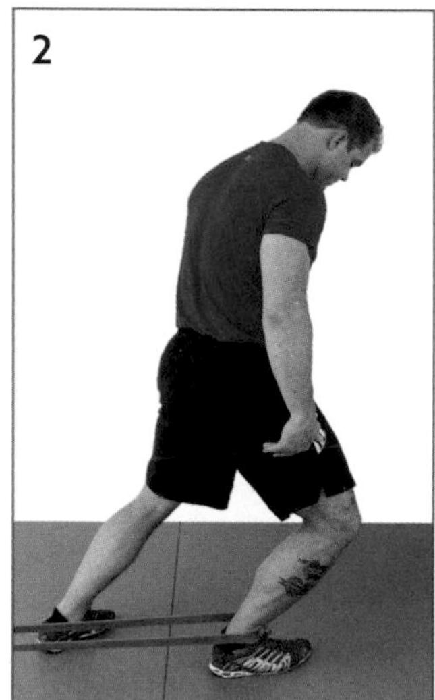

2

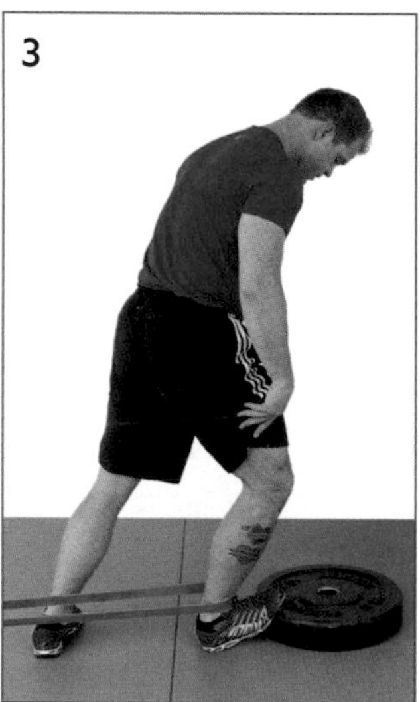

3

IMPROVES:

Sliding surfaces around the heel cord

Achilles pain

METHOD:

Banded flossing

Banded Heel Cord: Posterior Bias

The Banded Heel Cord will tack down the tight tissues at the base of your heel and restore sliding surfaces to the area. If this region gets tight, the skin will literally adhere to the underlying tendon, which restricts range of motion and causes an onslaught of other problems. This is a simple yet cogent way to unglue that matted-down tissue and help restore normal range of motion to your ankle.

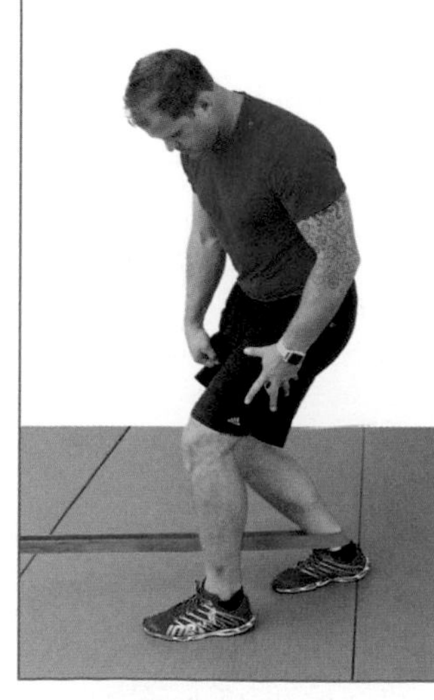

Hook a band around the base of your heel and create as much tension in the band as possible. Keeping your entire foot in contact with the ground, drive your knee forward and toward the outside of your body, oscillating in and out of end range. The idea is to maintain a slight external rotation force to prevent your ankle from collapsing inward.

AREA 14 ANKLE, FOOT, AND TOES

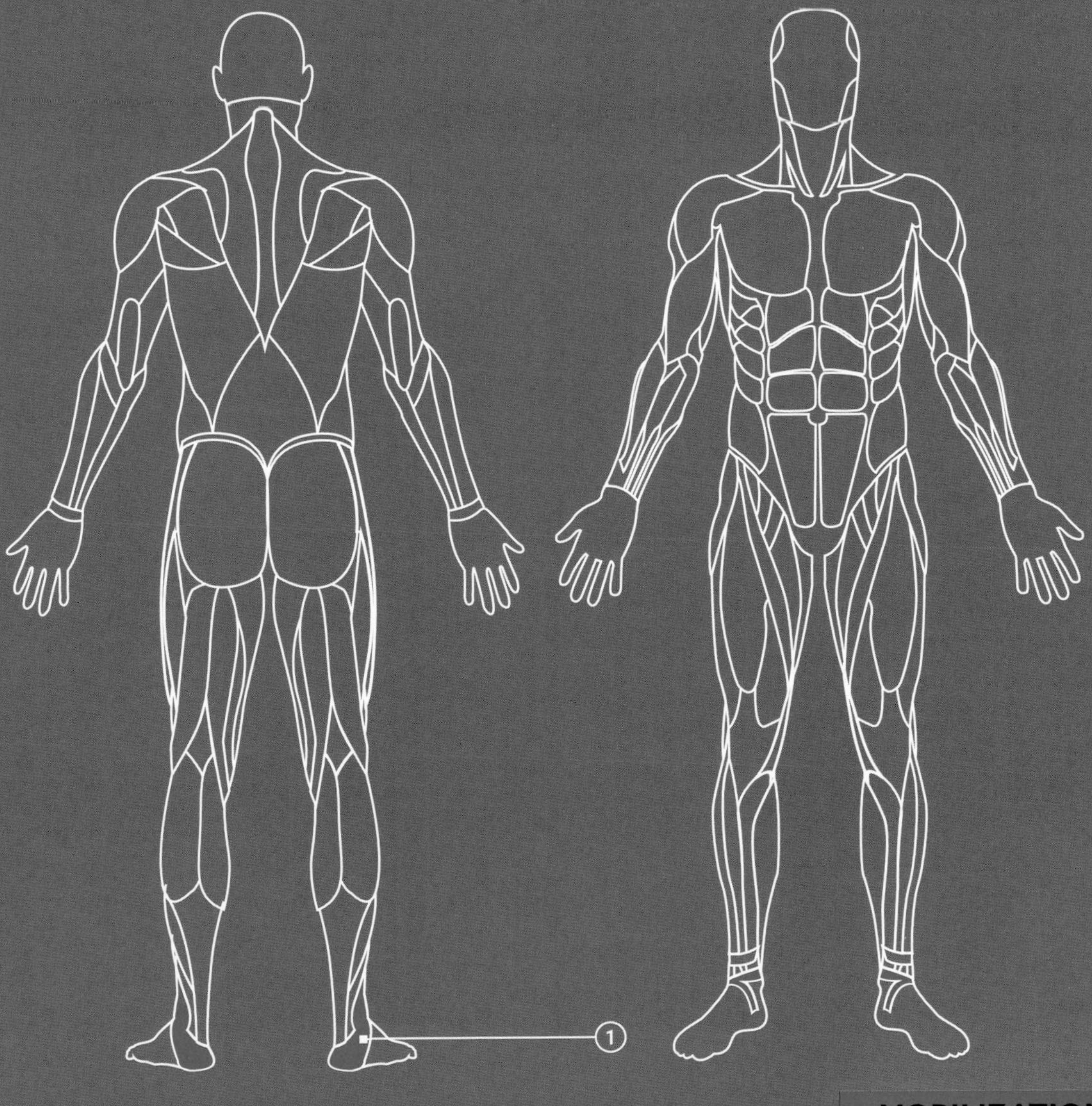

1

MOBILIZATION TARGET AREA:

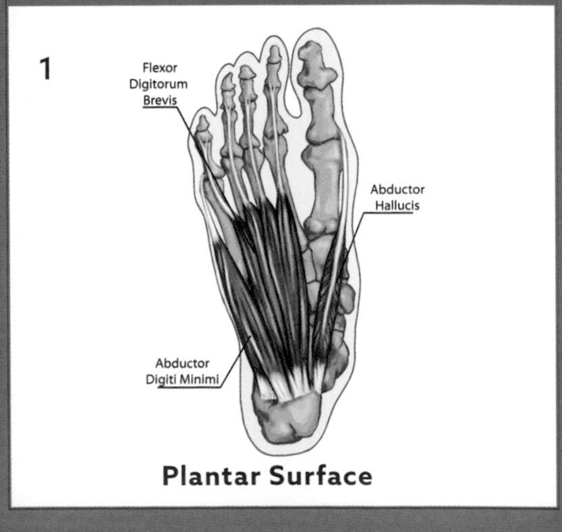

Plantar Surface

Squat 1 Archetype

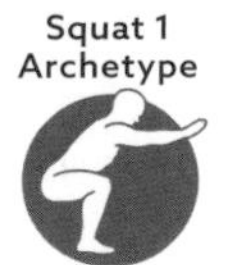

Pistol Archetype

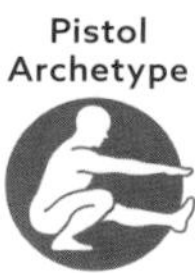

This mobilization will help improve the above archetypes.

IMPROVES:

Sliding surfaces around the ankle
Achilles and ankle pain

Ball Whack

When I see someone in my physical therapy practice who is missing ankle range of motion, this is one of the first techniques I use. It's cheap, easy, and fast, and it yields freakishly good results. The best part is that you don't need a PhD in anatomy to figure out where your skin slides over your bones. Bend your knee. Does your skin slide smoothly over the iliotibial (IT) band? Flex your elbow. Does your skin slide over your elbow without restriction? Flex your foot. Does your skin slide over your ankle bones and tendons? If it doesn't, you should immediately recognize that as a problem and work on restoring sliding surfaces to that tacked-down skin.

To use the Ball Whack to restore sliding surfaces to the skin over the bony prominence and tendons of your foot, pin a ball on the inside and outside of your ankle bone and around your heel cord and give it a firm whack. This momentarily stretches the skin, peeling it off the underlying surfaces.

Although you can do this mobilization on your own, it's difficult to generate sufficient force. For this reason, I recommend enlisting the help of a Superfriend.

Note: You can apply this technique anywhere your skin stretches over a body structure—specifically your elbow or the IT band at your knee.

Inside Ankle

1

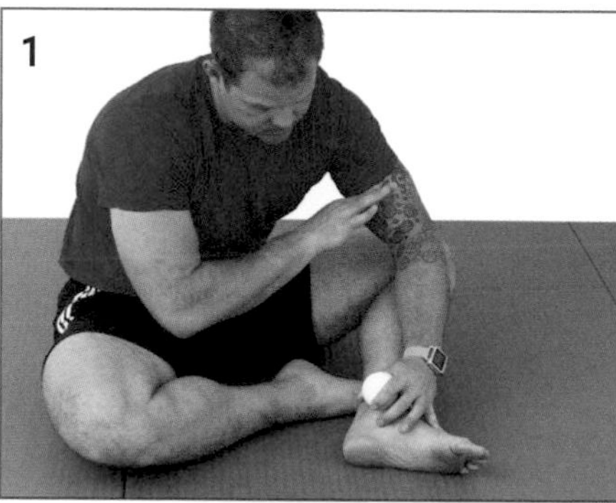

2

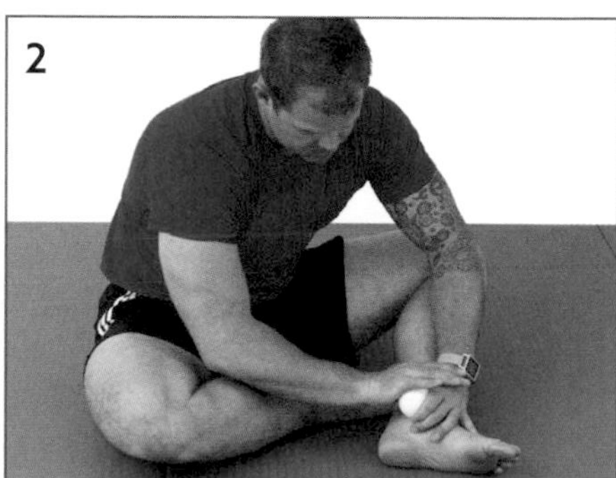

Heel Cord

1

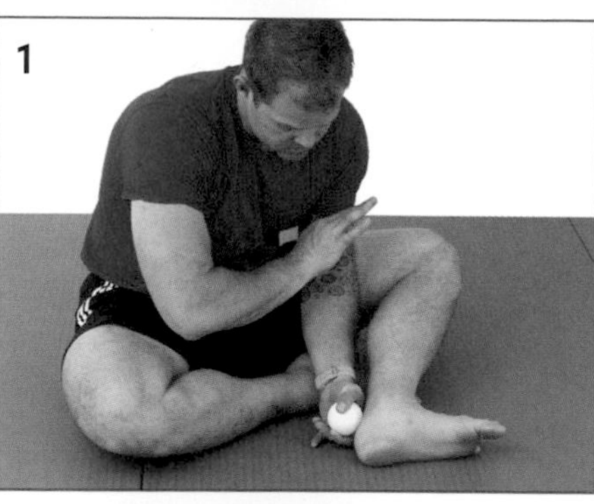

2

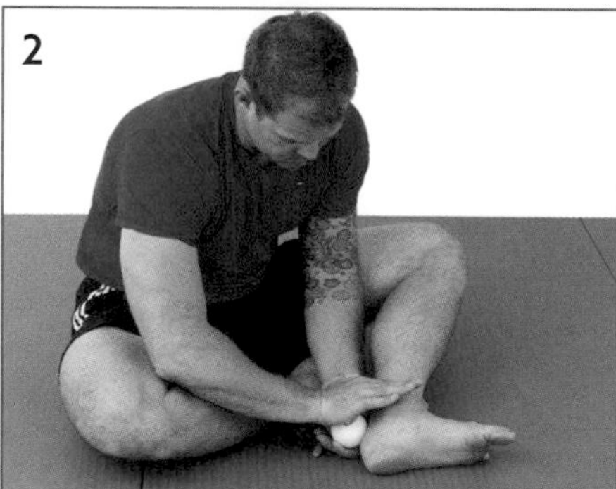

Outside Ankle

1

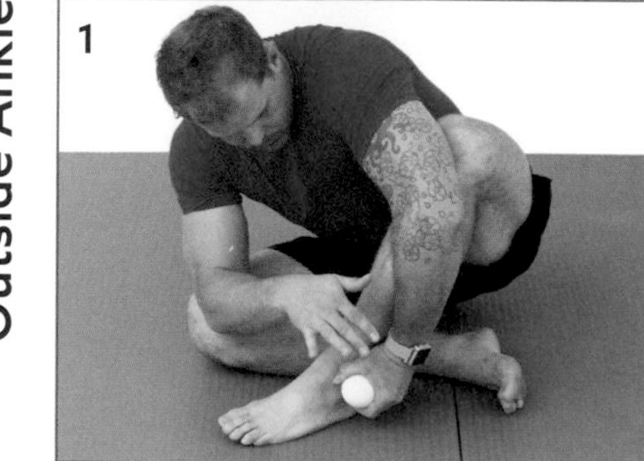

2

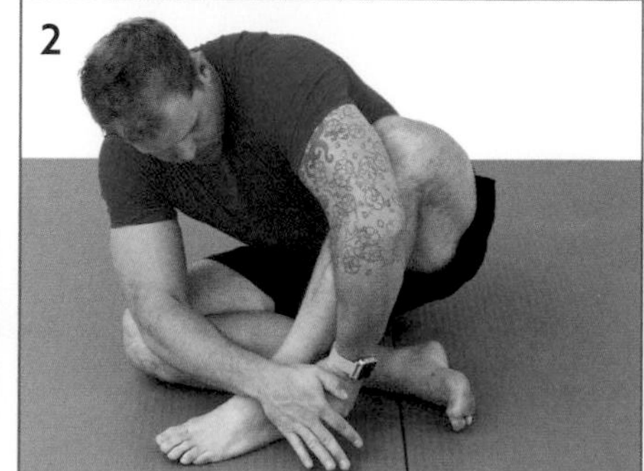

Pin the ball on an area of tacked-down tissue—focusing your attention on your ankle bone, heel cord, and the surrounding areas—and then give the ball a firm smack. You can also try applying pressure with the ball and then rapidly pushing it. Don't limit yourself to one direction, either. To restore sliding surfaces, you need to hit or push the ball in every direction. Do so until the skin starts to slide smoothly over the underlying surfaces. It doesn't take too many whacks get there.

Lateral Malleolus/Heel Smash Mobilizations

The lateral malleolus—the bony knuckle on the outside of your ankle, formed by the lower end of the fibula (calf bone)—needs to slide backward to allow for full dorsiflexion. If it's sticky or stiff—say, due to an old ankle injury—it acts like a doorjamb, limiting ankle range of motion. To restore full ankle mechanics, you have to free up this joint.

A healthy ankle will allow for eversion (tilting your heel toward the outside of your body) and inversion (tilting your heel toward the inside of your body), or twisting of the ankle. When your range of motion is restricted, it can radically affect your ability to get into a stable ankle position. The fact is, some of the accessory movements of your joints are a little tricky to restore, but you should by all means take a crack at it.

Remember, if you have what appears to be a mechanical limitation (not motor control), you should always follow these two simple rules: If something is not in the right place, put it in the right place. And if something isn't moving, get it moving. These ankle mobs follow that line of thinking.

Note: Do not try this mob with a lacrosse ball; it's not pliable enough. Use a Yoga Tune Up ball or a ball that is soft enough to cushion your ankle bone, like a tennis ball or racquetball.

Squat 1 Archetype   Pistol Archetype

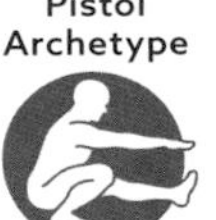

This mobilization will help improve the above archetypes.

IMPROVES:

Ankle function (creating a stable arch)

Ankle pain

METHOD:

Smash and floss

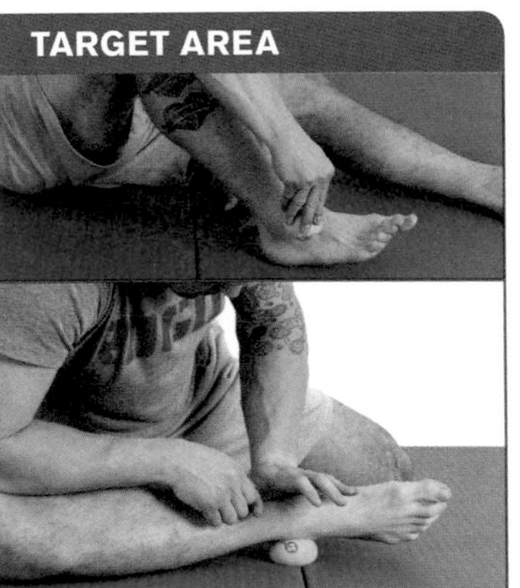

Position the ball in front of your malleolus (ankle bone)—the knuckle on the outside of your ankle.

Option 1: Single Ball

The single ball option is great for getting movement through the malleolus (anklebone). This looks a lot like the manual therapy technique that I use in my PT practice, but you can do it yourself. Do this mob while killing time in front of the TV or anytime your ankle feels restricted.

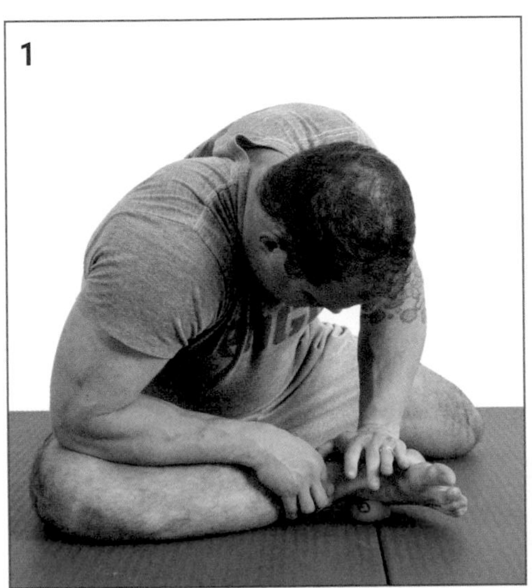

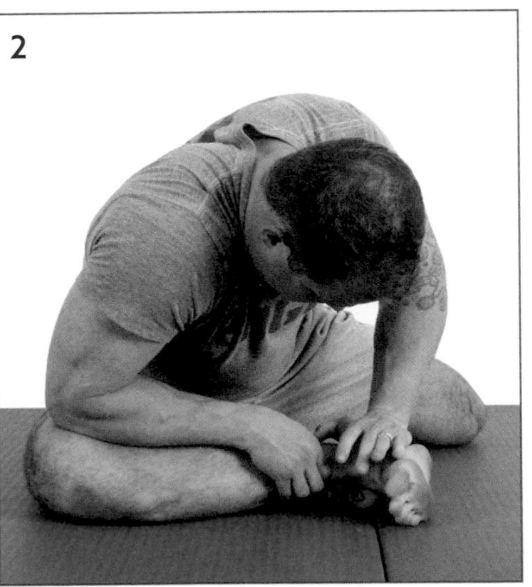

1. Here, you want the ball to push your ankle bone backward. Apply downward pressure to your lower leg using your hands and the weight of your upper body. With the ball blocking your ankle bone, try to push your ankle bone over the ball. Repeat this process—applying downward pressure and pushing your ankle bone over the ball—until you get some movement through the joint.

2. You can also floss by bending and straightening your foot.

Option 2: Double Ball

Using two balls—either two Yoga Tune Up balls in their tote or two tennis balls or racquetballs taped together—is another great option. With your ankle supported on both sides of the ankle bone, it's easier to get up-and-down movement through your ankle joint.

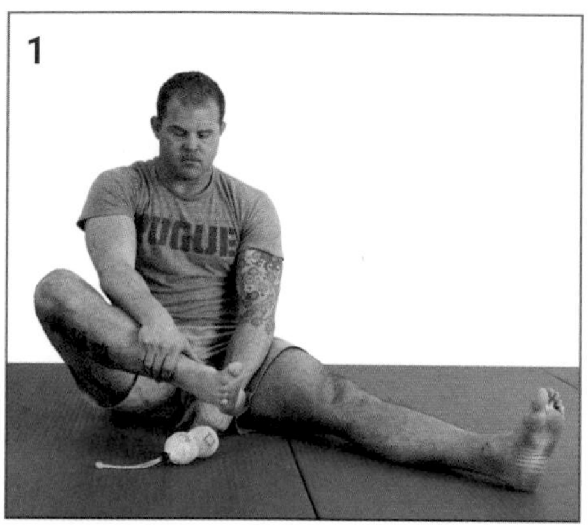

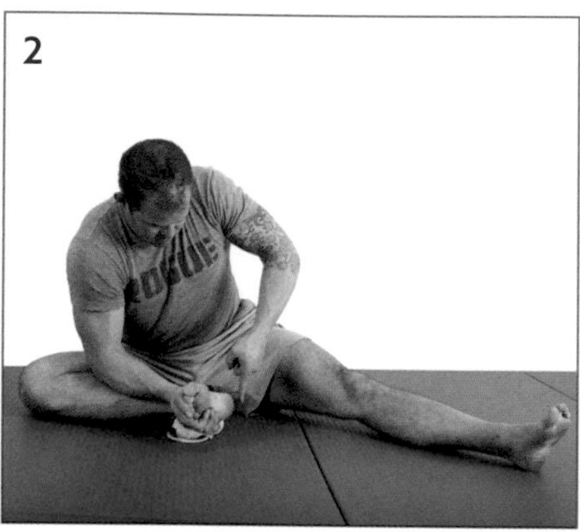

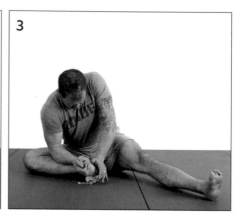

Position the balls so that your ankle bone is supported on both sides. One ball should be positioned in front of your ankle bone, and the other should be positioned behind your ankle bone, on your heel. Then pull up on your forefoot with one hand while simultaneously pushing down on your heel with the other. The idea is to get as much motion through your ankle joint as possible.

Medial Heel Bone Smash

Squat 1 Archetype

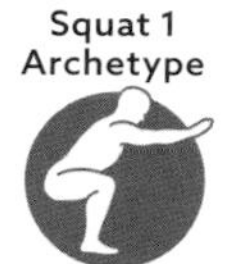

Pistol Archetype

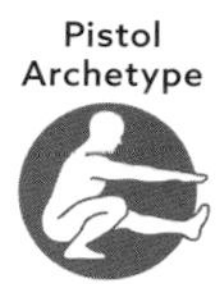

This mobilization will help improve the above archetypes.

IMPROVES:

Ankle function (creating a stable arch)

Ankle pain

METHOD:

Smash and floss

This is a great mobilization for people who have flat feet or who struggle to create an arch through the mid-foot when they screw their feet into the ground.

As a quick recap, screwing your feet into the ground is a cue for creating stability in your ankles and upstream joints. To be clear, you're not spinning your feet outward; you're just exerting force in an outward direction. (This force stems from hip external rotation.)

When I assess an athlete's foot position—say, during a squat—I look for an arch through the mid-foot, which represents the stable position for the ankle. If the athlete can't bring his foot into a stable arch position, it's a good indication that the skin, fascia, muscles, and tendons running along the inside of his foot are tacked down. For example, if the flexor retinaculum—the band of tissue that holds the ankle together—is tight and short, creating an arch by screwing your feet into the ground is difficult, if not impossible.

Remember, if your ankles are collapsed, it's harder to keep your knees, hips, trunk, and shoulders in a stable position. In other words, if your base of support is compromised, everything upstream is compromised. Don't wait for your Achilles tendon to rupture or your ankle to start hurting to do something about it. Get a kettlebell or ball and smash the inside of your heel—or, better yet, employ a Superfriend to do it for you. Test and retest by screwing your feet into the ground.

Option 1: Kettlebell Smash

A kettlebell is one of the best tools for smashing the inside of your heel. What's great is that you can use the handle to spin the base of the kettlebell, providing a smash and spin effect. As you can see in the photos below, the idea is to tack down the tissue, spin the kettlebell to take up the skin slack, and then move your foot around in all directions. By "all directions," I mean not only side to side (internal and external rotation) and up and down (dorsiflexion and plantarflexion), but also tilting the sole of your foot outward (eversion) and inward (inversion).

TARGET AREA

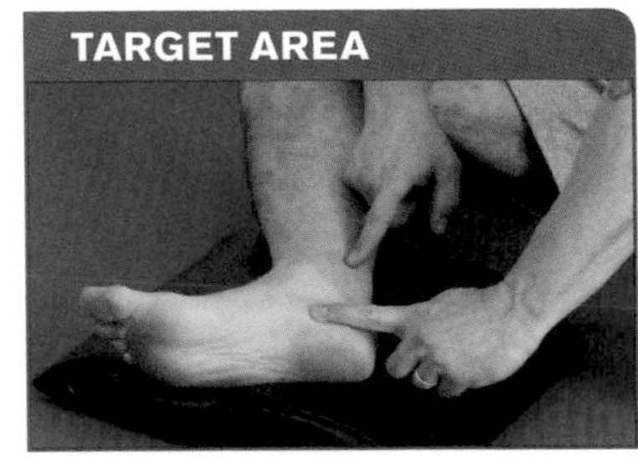

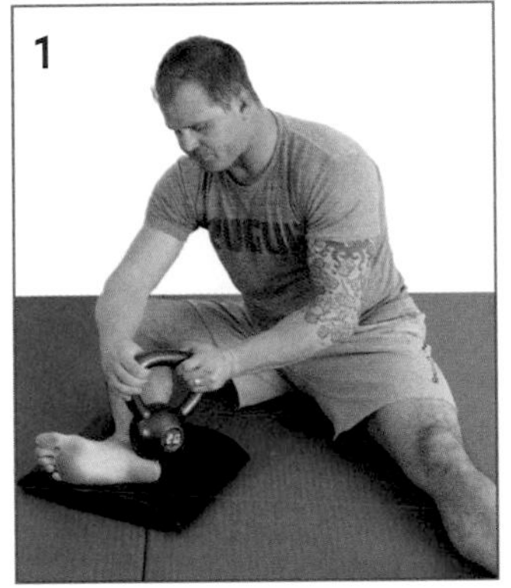

1

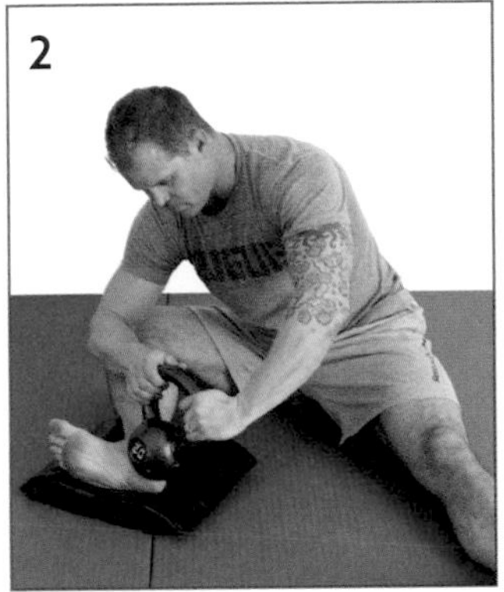

2

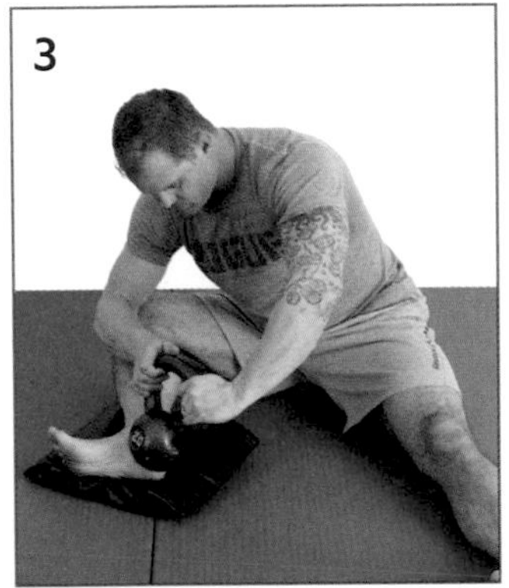

3

To protect your ankle bone, place an ab mat or pillow under your foot. Position the base of a kettlebell on your heel or below your ankle bone and then twist the kettlebell. You can twist it back and forth to restore sliding surfaces, or take up the skin slack with a half-twist and then floss by moving your foot around in all directions.

Ball Variation

You can also use a ball, such as a lacrosse ball, Yoga Tune Up ball, or Supernova. The approach is exactly the same: create pressure to tack down the tissue, rotate the ball into your foot, and then move your foot around in all directions.

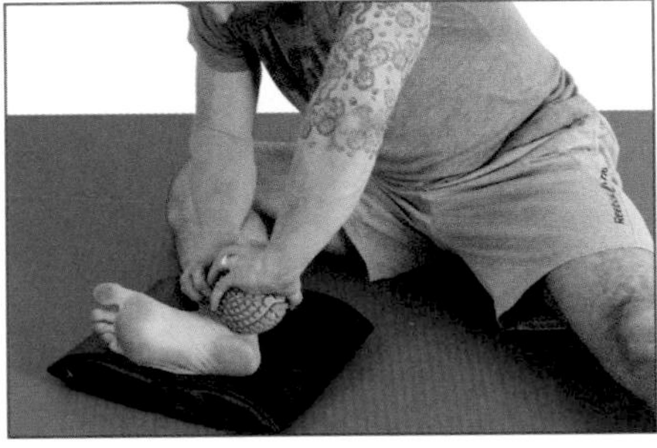

Option 2: Superfriend Foot Smash

The Superfriend Foot Smash is the best way to free up your heel and restore sliding surfaces to the inside of your ankle. Don't get me wrong: You can certainly take a crack at it on your own using a kettlebell or ball, but nothing compares to the Superfriend variation. Notice in the photos that I'm sliding the inside of my foot over Katie's heel. This peeling action not only captures the tissue systems (skin, muscle, fascia, and so on), but also gets movement through the calcaneus (heel bone) and ankle, which is difficult to do when you're mobilizing on your own.

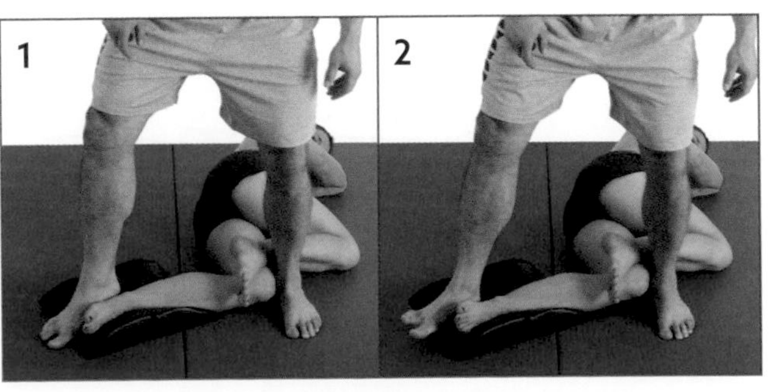

1 2

With your partner's foot resting on an ab mat and the inside of her ankle facing the ceiling, step the inside of your heel/instep over the inside of your partner's heel/instep, then slide your heel over her foot as if you were trying to peel her heel off her foot. Repeat this process—sliding your heel/instep over her heel/instep—until you get motion through the heel and ankle. You can also try smearing your heel over the inside of your partner's ankle (as if you were putting out a cigarette with your heel) by flexing your foot and rotating it from side to side while maintaining downward pressure.

Ankle VooDoo

Pistol
Archetype

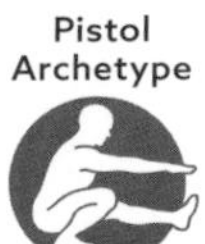

This mobilization will help improve the above archetype.

IMPROVES:

Ankle and foot pain
Swelling
Sliding surfaces around the ankle

METHOD:

VooDoo Floss Band compression

VooDoo Flossing your ankle is one of the most effective ways to restore sliding surfaces to your heel cord, ankle, and forefoot. As I mentioned before, you can approach this mobilization from a couple different angles. If you're treating a swollen (sprained) ankle, start near your toes and cover your entire foot, keeping about 50 percent tension in the band. If you're dealing with sliding surface dysfunction and trying to improve ankle range of motion, you don't have to wrap your entire foot. Instead, focus your attention on the restricted areas, which for most people are around the ankle and heel cord. The key is to keep around 75 percent tension in the band and force your foot through the full range of motion. You can prop your foot up on a bumper plate, implementing one of the calf stretching techniques, or simply hang out in the bottom of a squat.

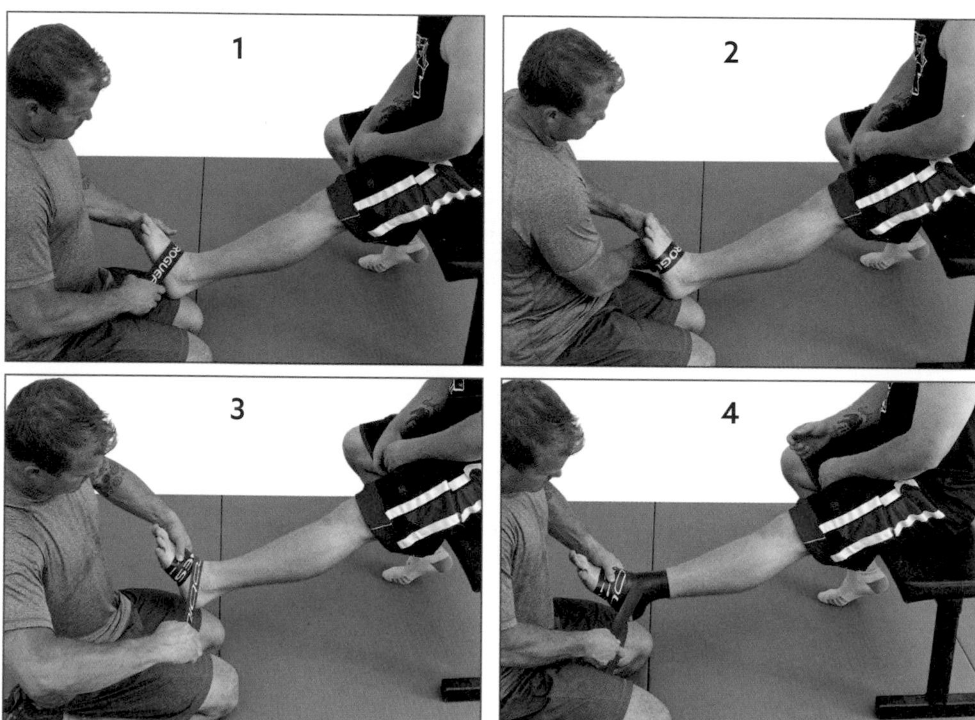

Whether you're trying to clear inflammation or restore sliding surfaces, start on the forefoot and wrap up the leg. Keep about a half-inch (or half of the band) overlap and cover all the restricted areas of the foot.

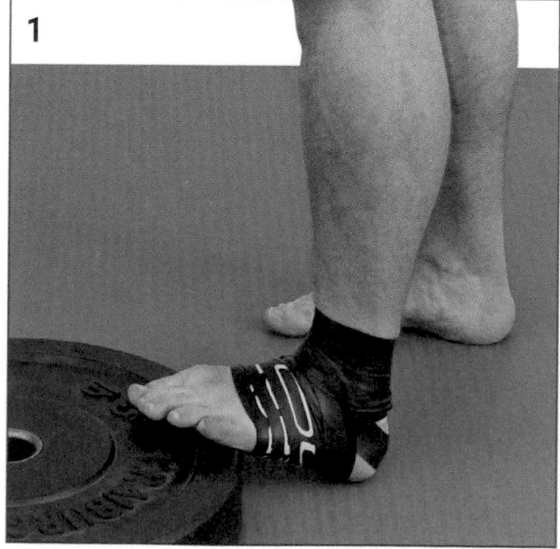

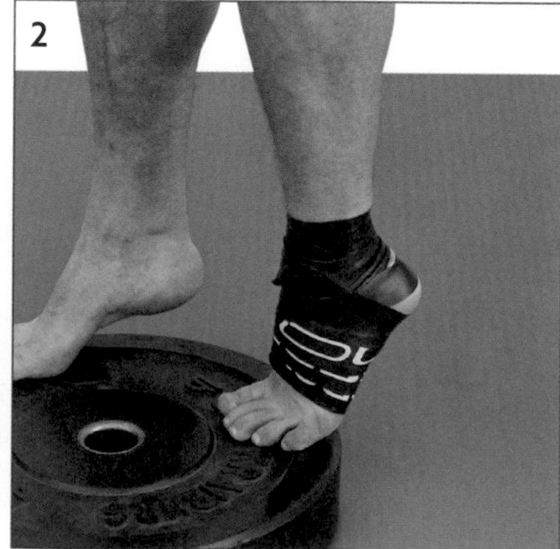

Move your ankle through as much range of motion as possible. You can implement the previous calf mobilization techniques (the Banded Heel Cord is a great option), or prop your foot up on an elevated surface like a bumper plate. An even better option is to perform the movement you're trying to change (run, squat, etc.).

Plantar Surface Smash

This is a great mobilization for the common, dreaded foot disease plantar fasciitis. Although other mechanisms can trigger plantar surface problems—posterior tibialis, caught nerve endings, and so on—plantar fasciitis is the catchall term used to describe any kind of pain on the bottom of the foot. The people who are most susceptible to plantar fascia issues are athletes, especially those who gravitate toward barefoot and Pose-centric running practices, and people who move with their feet turned out and stand with their arches collapsed.

The plantar fascia is a big sheet of connective tissue that runs along the bottom of the foot, from the ball to the heel. As anyone who has had plantar fascia problems can attest, inflammation or stiffness in this area causes a ton of pain and discomfort.

One of the best ways to resolve pain and restore suppleness to the plantar surfaces is to roll your foot over a lacrosse ball. The idea is to put in some quality smashing by slowly pressure waving up and down your plantar fascia. You can also think about strumming the musculature of your foot by moving from side to side. If you hit a hotspot, stay on it, contract and relax, and pressure wave into the ropy tissue. You can do this while you're sitting at your desk at work, or you can stand up and get some pressure into your foot. Either way, don't wait until your foot hurts to address the issue. Fix your foot position, and make sure that your skin slides and glides over your plantar fascia and that the bottoms of your feet are supple.

Lunge Archetype

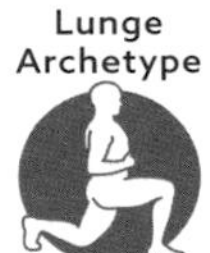

This mobilization will help improve the above archetype.

IMPROVES:

Foot pain (plantar fasciitis)

METHODS:

Pressure wave

Contract and relax

TARGET AREA

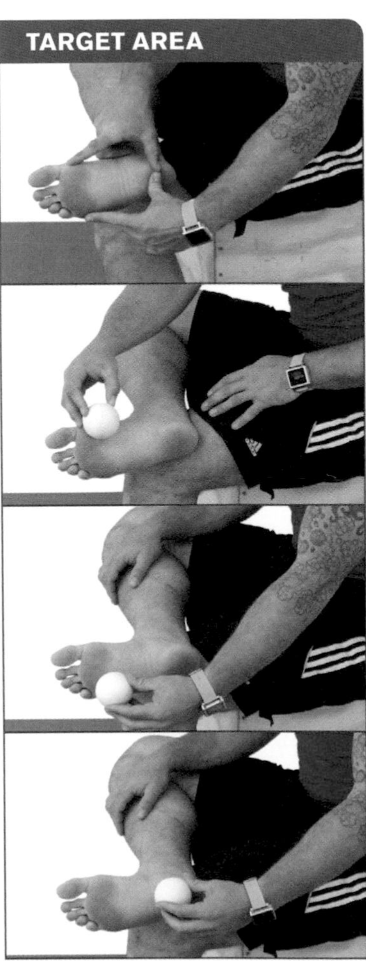

The target area encompasses the plantar surfaces of the bottom of your foot, from the ball of your foot to your heel.

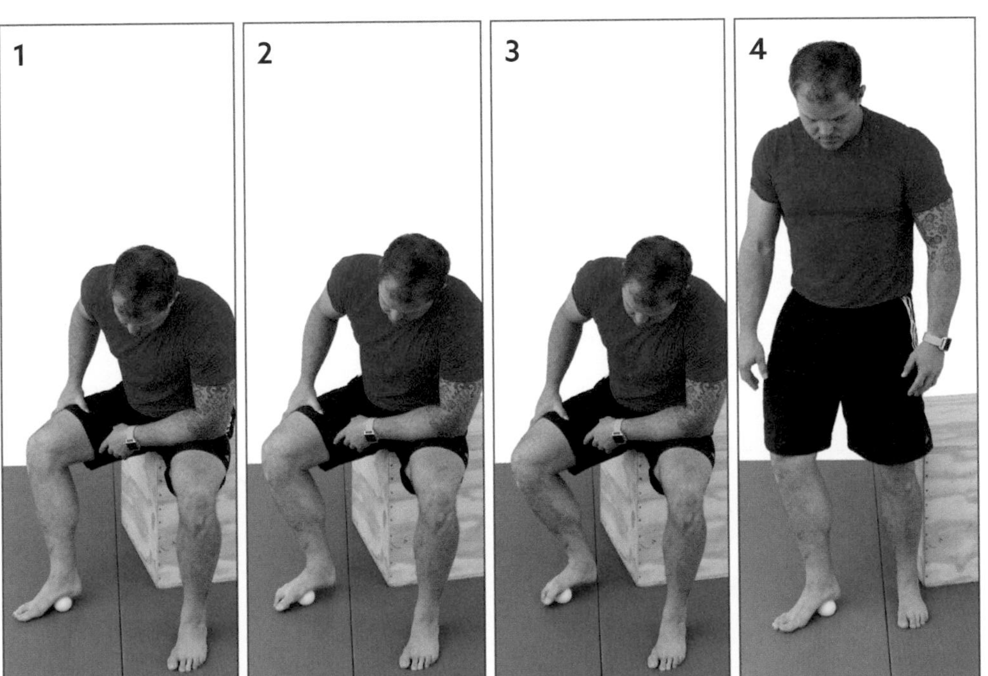

Step on a lacrosse ball, positioning it anywhere on your plantar surface, and apply as much pressure as you can handle. You can contract and relax on stiff areas and pressure wave up and down or across the tissue. The key is to take your time and focus on quality smashing. One of the biggest mistakes that people make is to roll their foot over a ball with zero intention. It should take you at least a minute to traverse the length of your foot. To get more weight over the ball and increase pressure, do this mobilization while standing.

Plantar Surface Smash Variation

Another great technique is to twist your foot into a ball or roller (ideally a Little Battlestar). This creates a cross-directional shear across the plantar surface tissue, which is great for restoring sliding surfaces to the bottom of your foot.

Position your foot over a roller or soft ball such a Yoga Tune Up ball, then smear your foot around as if you were trying to put out a cigarette with the arch of your foot. The goal is to rotate your foot in both directions while maintaining downward pressure. Also work on curling your toes over the roller or ball, which will help "break up" matted-down tissue and restore suppleness to your toes and forefoot.

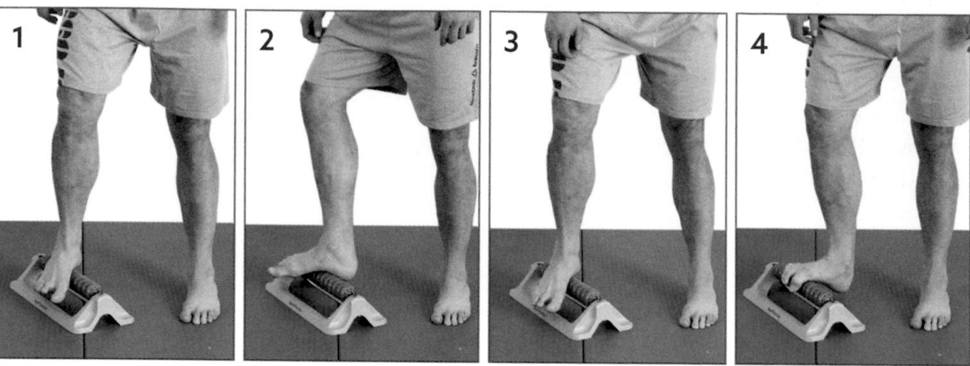

Forefoot Mobilization

IMPROVES:

Ankle and foot function (creating a stable arch)

Foot pain (plantar fasciitis)

This is another effective foot mobilization that can be used in conjunction with the Plantar Surface Smash.

There is a big joint in the middle of your foot that is responsible for providing arch support. When this mid-joint gets ropy and stiff—from either poor foot mechanics or barefoot running—it limits your ability to externally rotate and create a good arch. This is one of the reasons people's feet pop up when they squat: They lack rotational capacity in the mid-joint, so when they try to create external rotation by screwing their feet into the ground, the whole foot rolls up on the outside.

If you grab your forefoot around the base of your toes, you should have slight independent rotation from your heel. Think about it like this: Your hand is pretty flexible, right? Well, if the palm of your hand is really stiff, you won't be able to mold and shape it to gripping and grabbing. All you're doing here is making sure that your foot is a little bit moldable so that you can create a good arch.

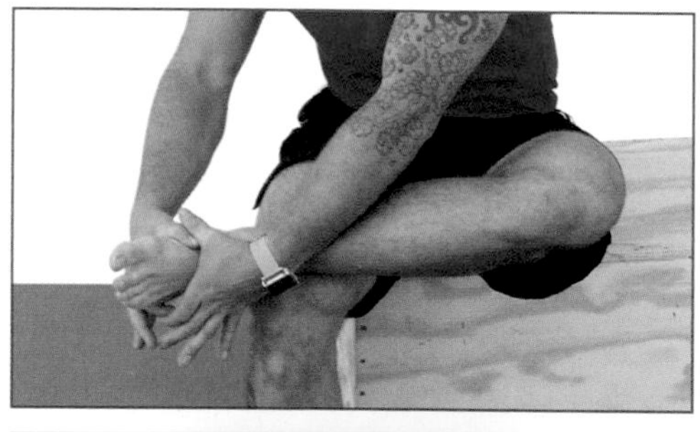

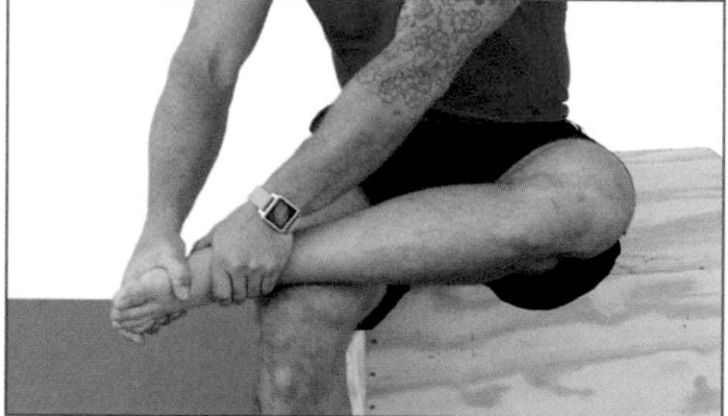

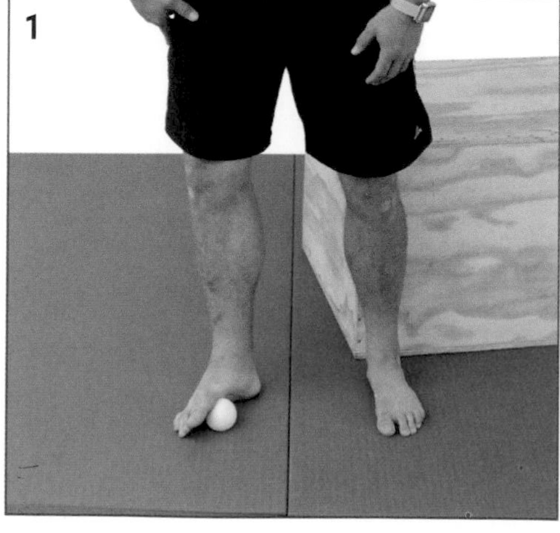

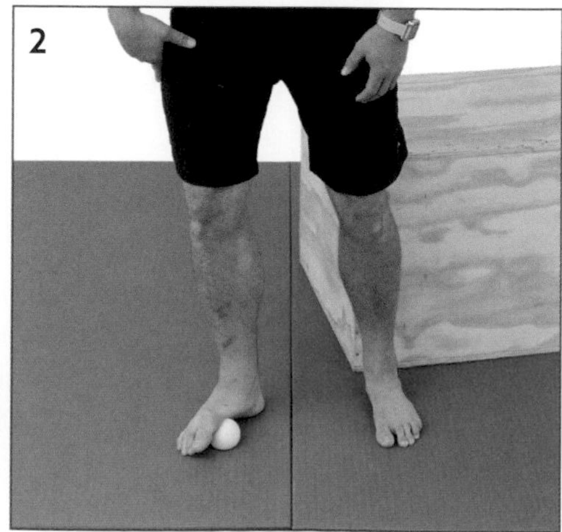

1. Step on a lacrosse ball with the inside of your forefoot. Notice that the outer edge of my foot is flush with the ground. The idea is to block the front of your foot toward the ball and try to collapse down on it. Block the joint and shear past it.

2. Applying downward pressure, create a shear force across the inside of your foot. Think about collapsing your foot over the ball.

Roller Forefoot Strumming

IMPROVES:

Ankle and foot function (creating a stable arch)

Foot pain (plantar fasciitis)

Unlike the Forefoot Mobilization, which is a more pinpointed smash, Roller Forefoot Strumming captures the entire arch. Put simply, it's an inaccurate global smashing technique that captures all the structural layers of your foot. For the best results, slowly collapse your foot over a roller as if you were trying to peel off the edge of the roller with your foot.

1. Place the inside of your foot over the edge of a roller, targeting the inside line of your forefoot.

2. Apply slow and steady downward pressure. Think about trying to peel off the edge of the roller with your foot.

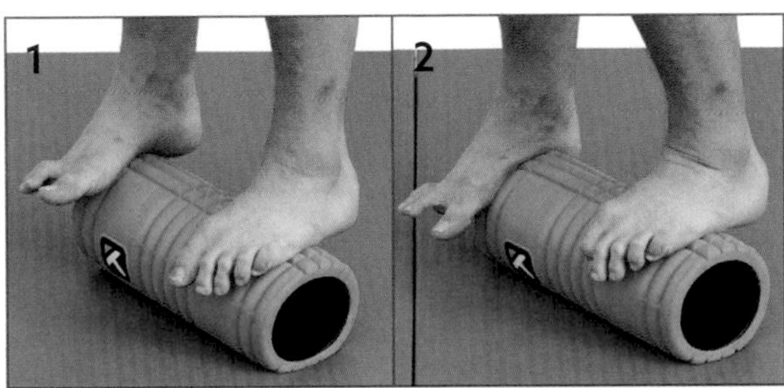

Toe Re-animator Mobilizations

Lunge Archetype

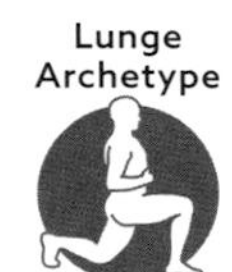

This mobilization will help improve the above archetype.

IMPROVES:

Proprioception

Foot and toe pain

Turf toe

Bunions

Collapsed arches

Foot mobility

These mobs focus on an often-neglected area of the foot. Your toes help you balance while walking and are especially susceptible to abuse and deformation. Consider the average dress shoe, boot, or high-heeled shoe. It's like a Chinese foot-binding torture device that constricts and terrorizes your foot. As if that isn't bad enough, I'd be willing to bet that you do very little to repair or minimize the damage.

Stiff feet (including toes) compromise athletic performance by throwing off your proprioception and can affect your quality of life. (You can't stand or walk comfortably if you have bunions or turf toe, for example.) The good news is that you can rebuild your feet in a relatively short period. Unless your navicular bone has collapsed or your foot is structurally deformed, you can rebuild a strong arch and restore suppleness within a year's time. But it takes consistency and patience.

First, make an effort to go barefoot as much as possible. Resolve to ditch those tight, constrictive shoes and flip-flops (that's right, flip-flops destroy toe and foot function, too) and replace them with barefoot shoes that give your toes plenty of breathing room. You also need to perform daily (or at least weekly) maintenance on your feet and toes by employing one or more of the techniques in this section. As with the other foot mobilizations, this kind of bodywork is great when you're just hanging out killing time, like watching TV. These mobs are easy to do and require zero equipment, so there are no excuses.

Make these mobs part of your prescription if you are on your feet all day; you suffer from turf toe, bunions, or collapsed arches; or your feet are simply stiff and junky. Perform all the options together as a single sequence.

Option 1: Finger Splice

This great foot sequence was lifted from the brilliant physio-mind of Kit Laughlin, the creator of Stretch Therapy. Unless you have a structural deformation (such as webbed toes), you should be able fit your fingers between your toes with zero pain or discomfort. If it's painful, it's a good indication that your fascia is locked up and your toes have weakened. The idea is to splice your fingers between your toes and then twist your foot in both directions. This is a great way to rebuild proprioception and get a big stretch in the fascia at the top and bottom of your foot.

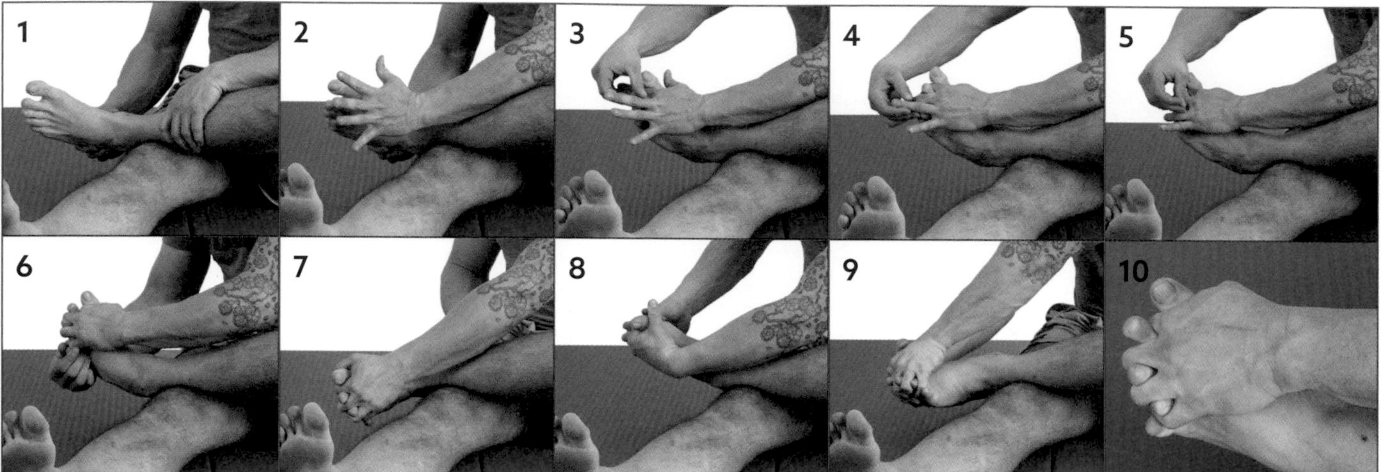

To begin, intertwine your fingers and toes by inserting your index finger between your big toe and index toe, your middle finger between your index toe and middle toe, your ring finger between your middle toe and fourth toe, and your pinky between your fourth toe and pinky toe. You can do this by intertwining your left hand over the top of your left foot, as shown, or by intertwining your right hand around the bottom of your foot. With your fingers and toes interlocked, twist your mid-foot joint back and forth several times. Notice that I use my opposite hand to assist with the twisting. You can also contract against the twist, then relax to go a bit farther.

Option 2: Spread and Pull

As an extension of the Finger Splice, you can spread your toes out by pulling them in different directions. For example, you should not only pull each toe laterally or outward, but also spread them up and down and from side to side. This is a great way to mobilize the fascia between your toes and wake up the proprioceptors (sensory receptors on nerve endings that provide information about the movement and positioning of your body in space) in your feet.

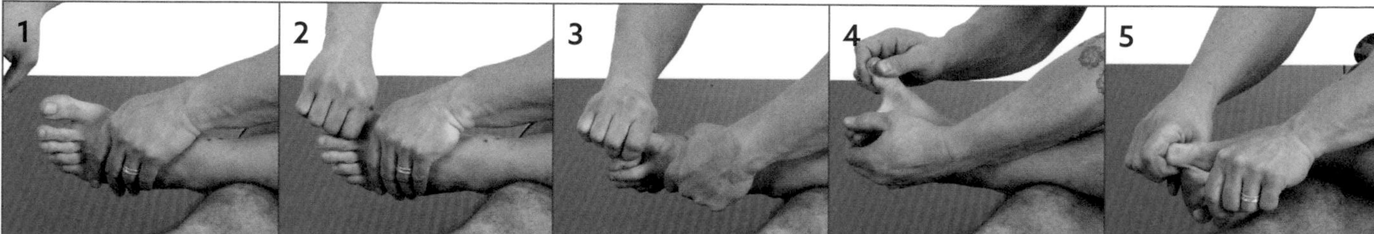

If you're mobilizing your left foot, grip the top of your forefoot with your left hand, latch onto your big toe with your right hand, and then gently pull your toe away from your other toes. Slowly and gently twist your foot and toe in opposite directions as if you were wringing out a towel. The process is the same if you're mobilizing your right foot; the only difference is that you switch your grip. After you've spent some time mobilizing your big toe and mid-foot joint, spread each toe apart in opposite directions. Switch back and forth, spreading your toes up and down and from side to side. Be sure to target every pair of toes, starting with your big toe and index toe, then your index toe and middle toe, and so on.

Option 3: Toe Dorsiflexion

As you will recall from chapter 4, having full range of motion in your foot includes 90 degrees of toe dorsiflexion—see page 114. This is a simple way to mobilize the Lunge Archetype as it relates to your foot.

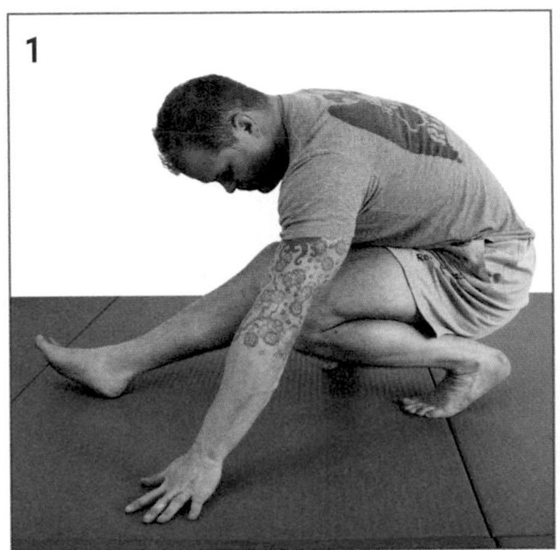

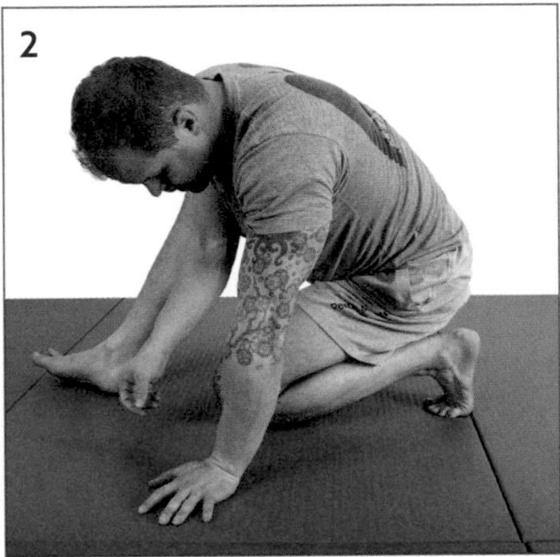

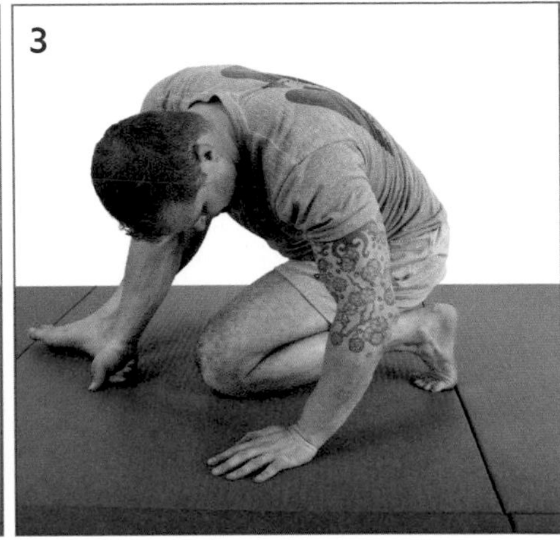

Kneel on the ground as if you were getting into the pistol archetype and come up onto the ball of your foot. Keeping the ball of your foot in contact with the ground, lower your knee toward the floor. The goal is to get to 90 degrees of toe dorsiflexion. The key here is to keep your foot straight or neutral and your weight distributed over the center of your foot. You can certainly roll onto the outside of your toes and explore different ranges, but focus most of your attention on keeping your foot straight so you get a big stretch through the arch of your foot.

Option 4: Toe Plantarflexion

If you're down on the ground working on Toe Dorsiflexion, you might as well hit a counter-mobilization by targeting the top of your foot. You might notice that this same mob is used to target the anterior compartment of the shin (see page 422). I'm including it here as well because it's one of the few positions in which you can mobilize the top of your foot and toes.

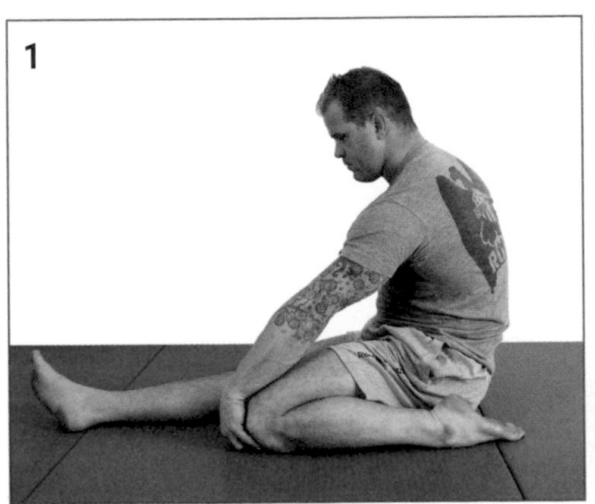

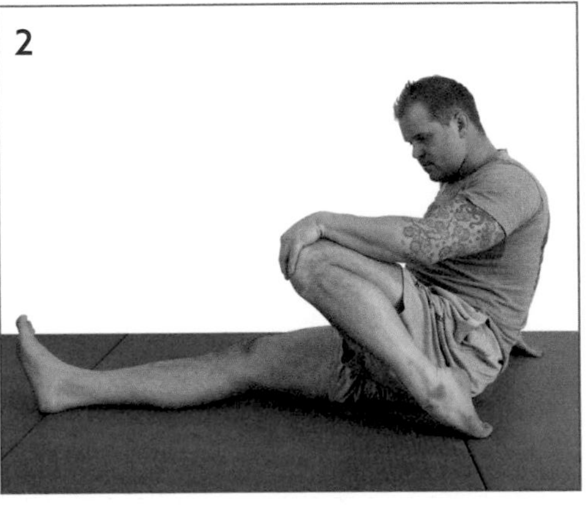

Sit on the ground with one leg straight out in front of you and the other leg folded behind you. Then lean back and lift your bent leg off the ground. Notice how I'm using my left hand to help elevate my left knee. The key is to get enough elevation that you come up onto the top of your toes. With your foot in end-range plantarflexion, you can tilt your leg to the side, roll your foot away from your body, or roll your foot toward the inside of your body.

PART 4 MOBILITY PRESCRIPTIONS

This section of the book can be used in two different ways. If you've read the first three parts of the book and have specific issues that you would like to address, the prescriptions lie on the coming pages. For example, if you took the body archetype quick tests in part 1 (see pages 100–115) and found an archetype that you need to work on, you can use the general body archetype mobility prescription to improve that archetype as a whole. If you discover that you have a fault with one of the movements described in part 2 of the book, you can attack that fault using the appropriate troubleshooting body archetype mobility prescription(s).

If you've come to this part of the book first, there are a number of ways to get started. If you'd like to treat a certain pain, for example, you can use the pain-based prescriptions on pages 467–469. If you simply want to get started mobilizing without reading the whole book, you can use the 14-Day Whole-Body Mobility Overhaul on pages 470–471 to create your own customized mobility program, or follow one of the sample 14-day programs on pages 472–473.

On the opposite page I offer a more detailed breakdown of how this part of the book is organized. But before I delve into that, I want to emphasize one thing: The sample prescriptions are just that—samples. My goal is to equip you with the knowledge and skill to construct your own daily mobility prescription. And if you study this book from front to back, you will acquire that knowledge and skill. Remember that everyone moves differently and has different restrictions. To get the most performance out of your body, you must tailor your mobility workouts to your personal goals and your individual brand of stiffness.

General Body Archetype Mobility Prescriptions

As explained in chapter 4, the functional positions for the hips and shoulders can be categorized into seven body archetypes. To move the way your body is designed to move, you need to have full range of motion in each of these archetypes. On pages 100–115, I included some quick tests to help you determine whether you are lacking in any of these positions. If you took these tests and came up short, or if you simply want to improve upon a particular position, I suggest you start with the general body archetype mobility prescriptions. Included in these prescriptions are a number of mobilization techniques from part 3 that will improve that archetype as a whole. Following these prescriptions will make you more efficient and safe not only when performing the associated movements in the gym, but also in everyday activities that include those archetypes. For example, following the General Squat Archetype Mobility Prescription will make you more efficient at squatting in the gym, but also at getting up and down off of the ground.

Troubleshooting Body Archetype Mobility Prescriptions

Following the general body archetype mobility prescription will do wonders to improve every aspect of that position, but you may have specific limitations. In part 2, I described a host of common faults associated with each movement, and many of those faults arise due to specific restrictions in a particular archetype. For example, say you can raise your arms overhead, but you can't fully extend your elbows. While following the General Overhead Archetype Mobility Prescription might help with this limitation, it may be more beneficial to hone in on the trouble spot. After each of the general body archetype prescriptions, I offer a number of troubleshooting mobility prescriptions to resolve the most common restrictions. If you can perform a particular archetype with ease, but one aspect keeps troubling you or causing you pain, these troubleshooting prescriptions are for you.

Pain-Based Prescriptions

Following the general body archetype mobility prescriptions and attacking your weak areas with the troubleshooting body archetype prescriptions will help get you moving as you were intended to move, reducing the amount of pain and injury you will acquire over time. However, it is nearly impossible in the modern world to move correctly at all times. Simply sitting at a desk for long hours, even if you move correctly while standing, can cause a host of nagging problems. In this section, I offer general mobility prescriptions to treat and resolve minor tweaks, painful joints, and pain-related symptoms such as tension headaches, low back pain, and carpal tunnel. As with all the mobilizations, they will help you master movement, but they are not grouped together to benefit one particular archetype or a specific issue within that archetype. They are grouped simply to help you solve specific pain-related issues.

14-Day Whole-Body Mobility Overhaul

There is no one-size-fits-all prescription when it comes to programming for mobility. Everyone has unique issues that contribute to mobility limitations, poor movement mechanics, and pain. You are a system of systems. Your tight quads might prevent you from getting your knees out when you squat, but the cause could also be your tacked-down heel cords, tight hamstrings, or brutally stiff adductors (to mention a few possibilities). To ensure that all body parts are maintained, it's important to cycle through all the archetypes and body areas over the course of a couple weeks. To help with this, I've included a 14-Day Whole-Body Mobility Overhaul as a general guide (see pages 470–471). You can use this template to construct a well-balanced, all-encompassing mobility program. If you're eager to get started and you just want a mobility program that you can follow, the sample programs on pages 472–473 are for you.

General Overhead Archetype Mobility Prescription

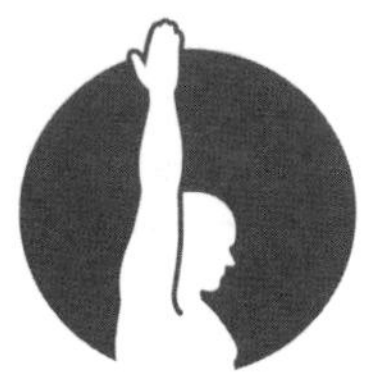

RELATED EXERCISE MOVEMENTS:

Overhead squat (page 192)
Strict press (page 220)
Handstand pushup (page 226)
Pull-up (page 229)
Push-press (page 236)
Kettlebell swing (American variation) (page 240)
Burpee (page 259)
Turkish getup (page 262)
Clean (page 264)
Snatch (page 278)

EVERYDAY EXAMPLES:

Lifting something overhead
Grabbing something off a high shelf
Hanging from a bar

The overhead archetype is an expression of flexion and external rotation of the shoulders and extension of the elbows, and it encompasses any position or movement that requires you to stabilize your arms over your head. In this section, I offer a number of mobilizations that will help you improve the overhead archetype. Here's how it works:

1. Create your own mobility sequence by selecting 3 or 4 mobilizations from the list of techniques on the opposite page. For the best results, perform each mobilization for at least 2 minutes per side, for a total of 10 to 15 minutes of mobility work.

2. Test the position before performing the mobility sequence. After completing the sequence, retest the position to see if you have made change. This test and retest model will illuminate the success of your prescription and help you isolate the most effective mobilizations.

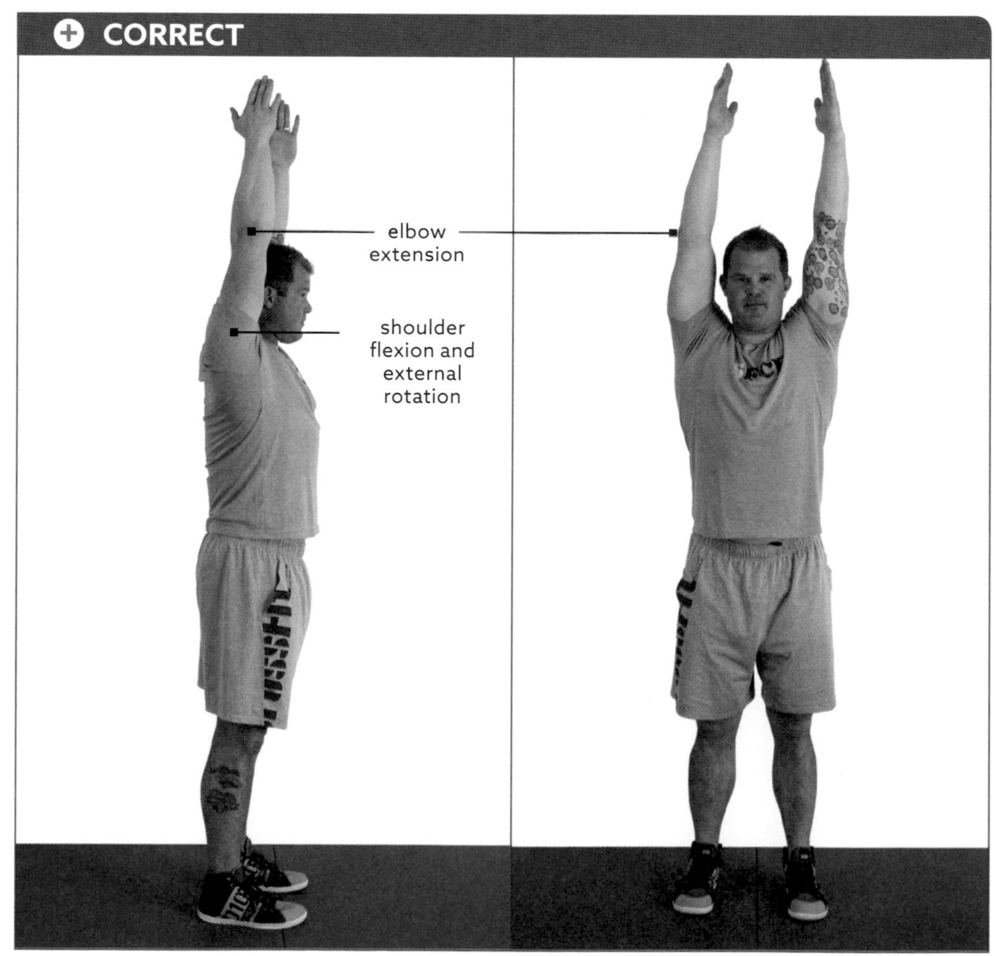

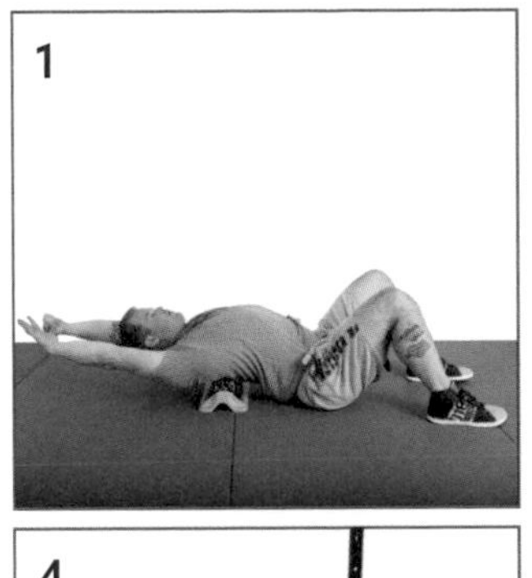

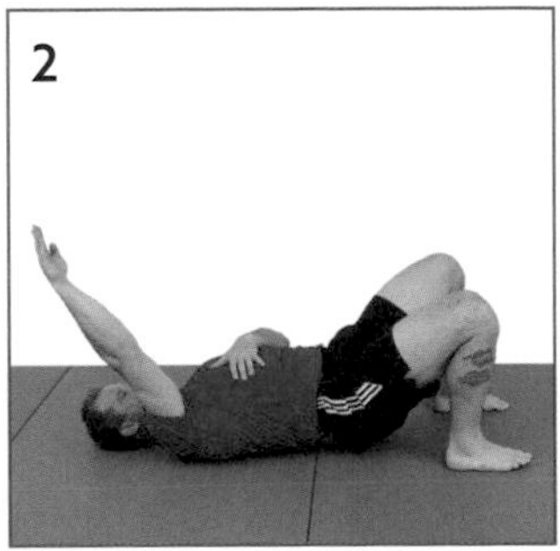

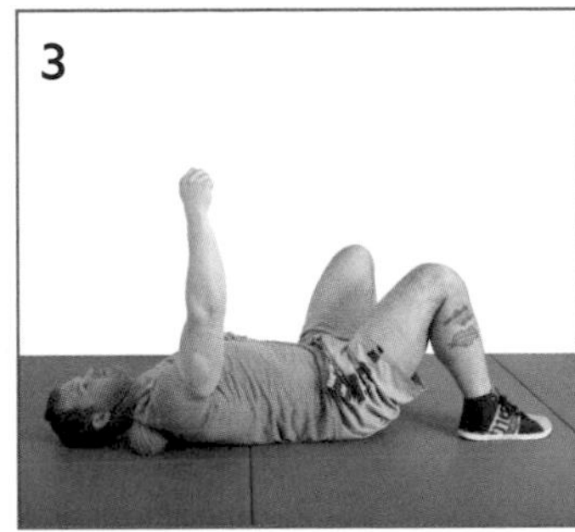

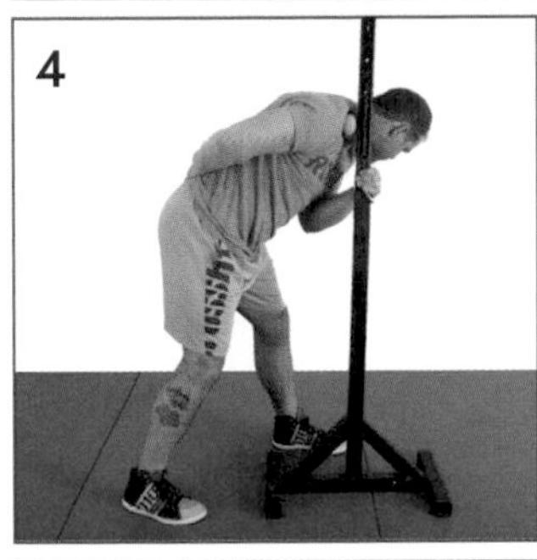

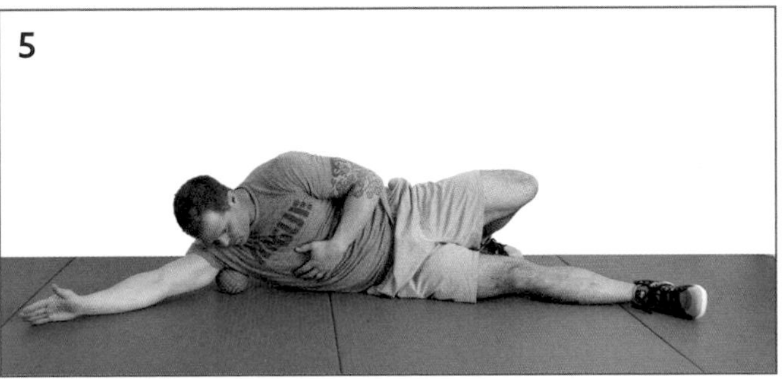

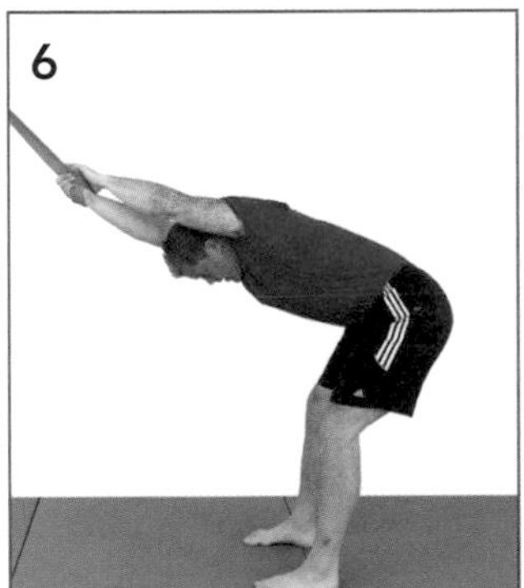

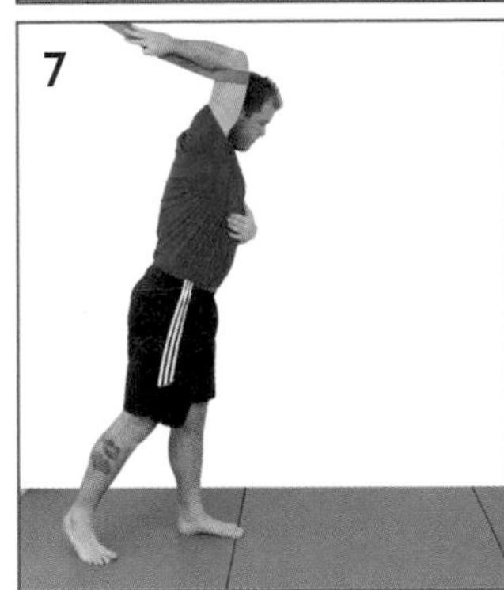

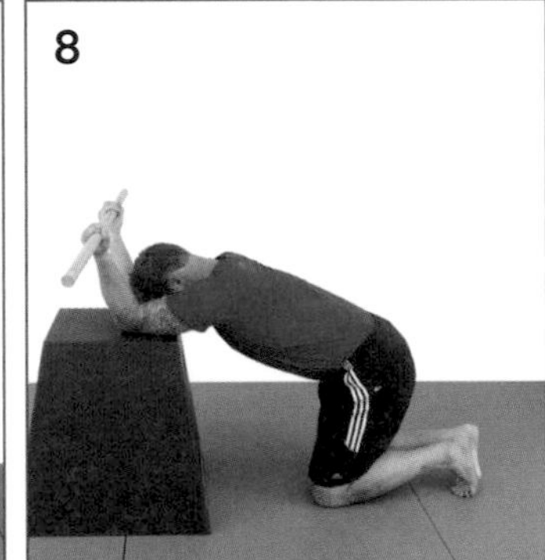

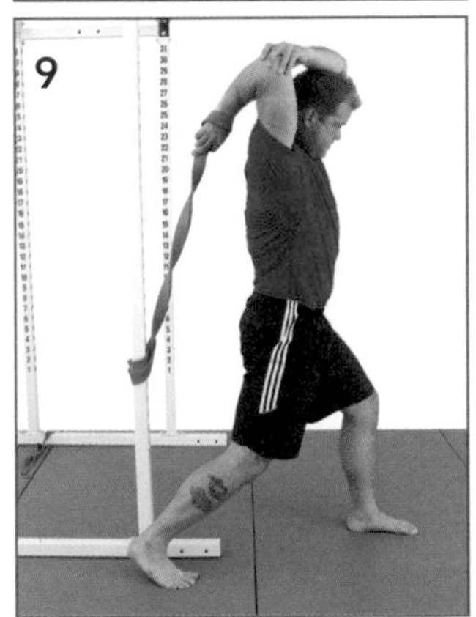

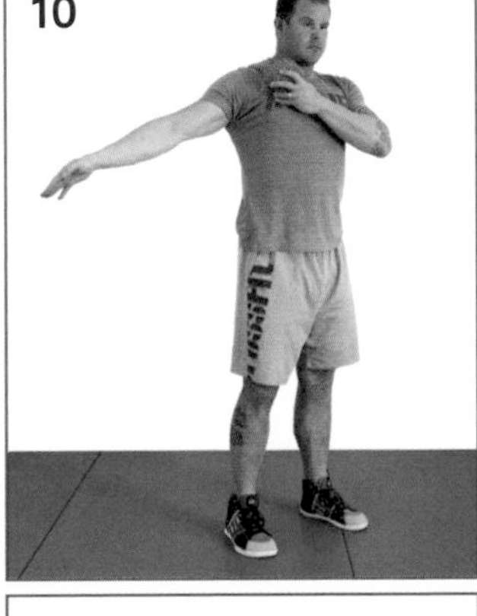

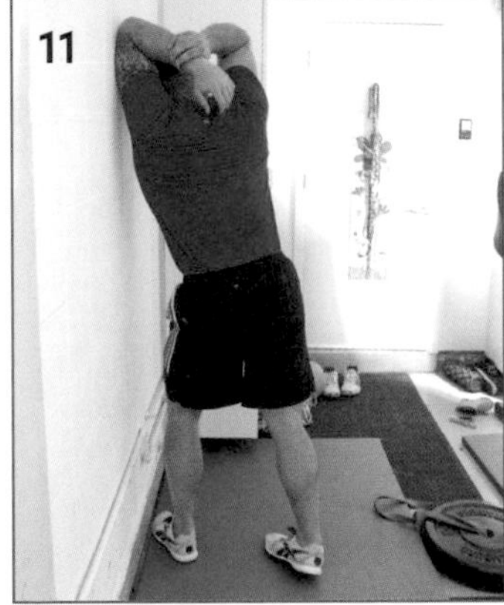

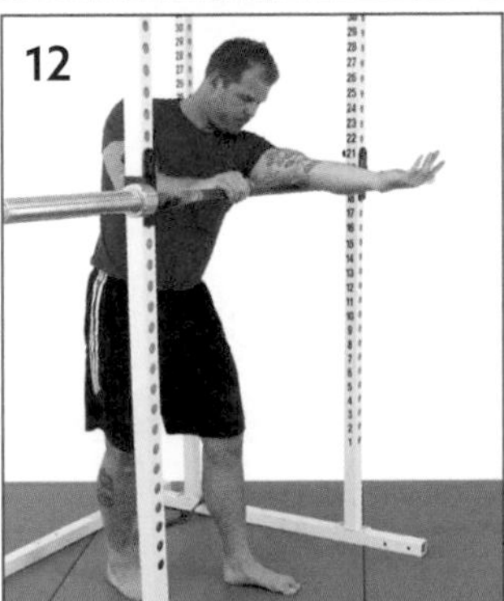

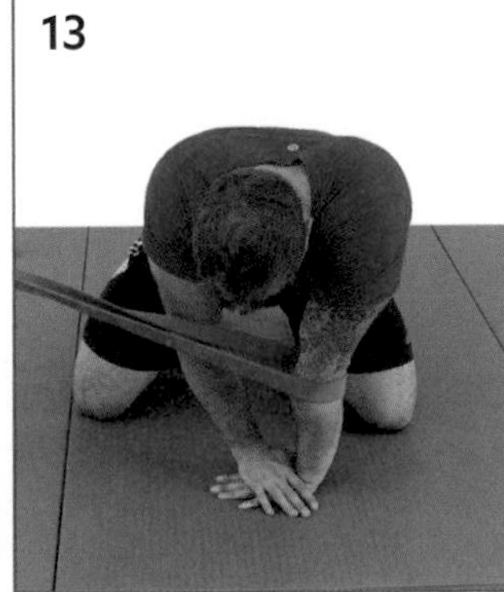

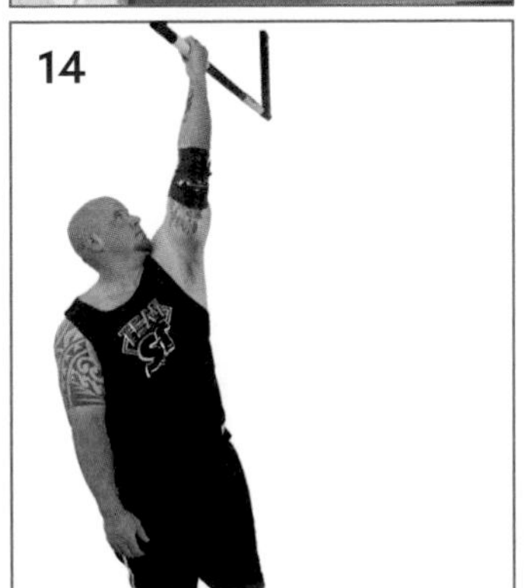

MOBILIZATION LIST:

1. *T-Spine Overhead Extension Smash Mobilizations (page 297)*
2. *Overhead Rib Mobilization (page 301)*
3. *Trap Scrub (page 304)*
4. *First Rib Mobilizations (page 305)*
5. *Overhead Tissue Smash Mobilizations (page 313)*
6. *Banded Overhead Distraction (page 317)*
7. *Overhead Distraction with External Rotation Bias (page 318)*
8. *Bilateral Shoulder Flexion (page 319)*
9. *Super Front Rack (page 320)*
10. *Anterior Compartment Mobilizations (page 323)*
11. *Classic Triceps and Lat Stretch (page 321)*
12. *Triceps Extension Smash (page 336)*
13. *Banded Elbow Extension (page 341)*
14. *Elbow VooDoo (page 339)*

Troubleshooting Overhead Archetype Mobility Prescriptions

People encounter three primary limitations with the overhead archetype: shoulder flexion, shoulder external rotation, and elbow extension. Any of the movement faults in part 2 that are tagged with the overhead archetype icon are likely due to one of these three restrictions. Below I break down these restrictions and offer two sample prescriptions for each.

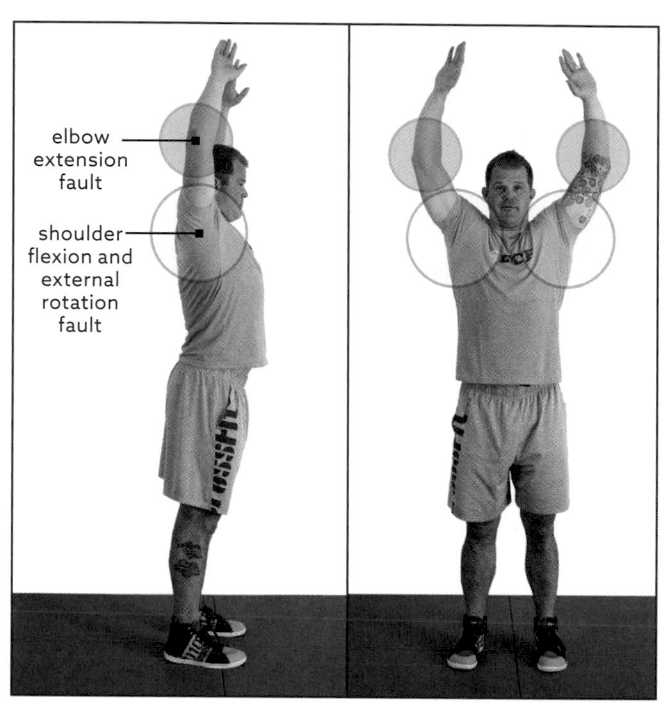

□ Shoulder Flexion and External Rotation Prescriptions

If your shoulders roll forward and your elbows flare outward when you attempt to raise your arms overhead, you are likely missing shoulder flexion range of motion. If you are able to raise your arms overhead but can't rotate your arms forward into a stable position (position your armpits forward), you are likely missing shoulder external rotation. The mobility prescriptions below will help with both issues, so I've lumped them together. Neither prescription is better or more advanced than the other. I offer two prescriptions to give you options and because some people respond better to certain mobilizations than others.

PRESCRIPTION A	TIME
T-Spine Overhead Extension Smash: Option 1 (page 297)	2 minutes
Overhead Tissue Smash Mobilizations (page 313; choose one option)	2 minutes on each side
Banded Overhead Distraction (page 317)	2 minutes on each arm
	10 MINUTES

PRESCRIPTION B	TIME
Overhead Rib Mobilization (page 301)	2 minutes on each side
First Rib Mobilizations (page 305; choose one option)	2 minutes on each side
Overhead Distraction with External Rotation Bias (page 318)	2 minutes on each side
	12 MINUTES

■ Elbow Extension Prescription

If you can't lock out your elbows overhead or your elbows flare outward when you attempt to raise your arms overhead, you are likely missing elbow extension range of motion. The mobility prescriptions below will help with this issue.

PRESCRIPTION A	TIME
Triceps Extension Smash (page 336)	2 minutes on each arm
Banded Elbow Extension (page 341)	2 minutes on each arm
	8 MINUTES

PRESCRIPTION B	TIME
Elbow VooDoo (page 339) (see page 146 for VooDoo Flossing wrapping technique)	1–2 minutes of compression, perform 2 to 3 cycles on each arm
	4–12 MINUTES

General Press Archetype Mobility Prescription

The press archetype is an expression of shoulder extension and elbow flexion. It looks like the bottom position of the pushup, dip, and bench press. In this section, I offer a number of mobilizations that will help you improve the press archetype. Here's how it works:

1. Create your own mobility sequence by selecting 3 or 4 mobilizations from the list of techniques on the following page. For the best results, perform each mobilization for at least 2 minutes per side, for a total of 10 to 15 minutes of mobility work.

2. Test the position before performing the mobility sequence. After completing the sequence, retest the position to see if you have made change. This test and retest model will illuminate the success of your prescription and help you isolate the most effective mobilizations.

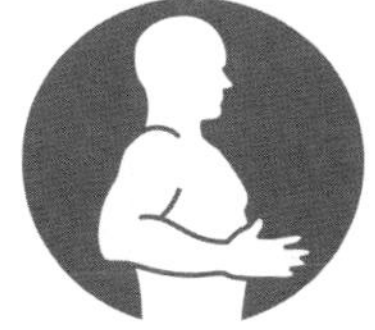

RELATED EXERCISE MOVEMENTS:

Pushup (page 204)
Bench press (page 209)
Dip (page 216)
Burpee (page 259)

EVERYDAY EXAMPLES:

Getting up off the ground from your belly
Pushing against something
Carrying something at your side with a bent arm

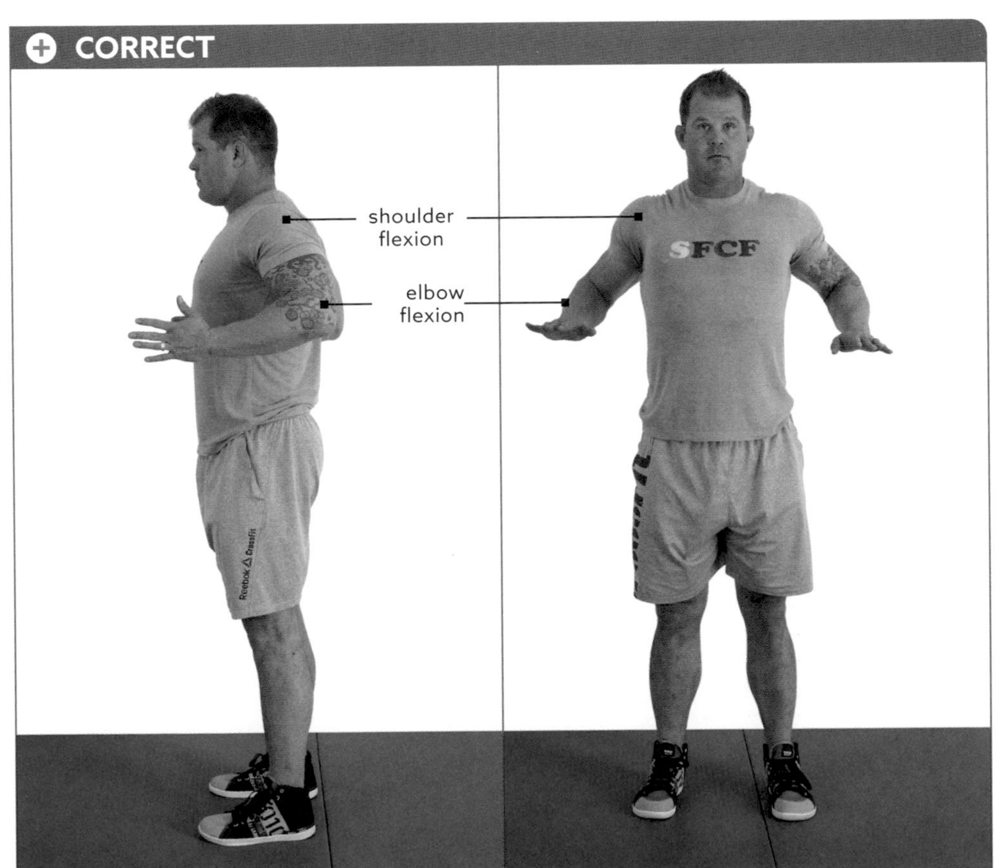

MOBILIZATION LIST:

1. *T-Spine Roller Smash Mobilizations (page 293)*
2. *Shoulder Capsule Mobilization (page 310)*
3. *Trap Scrub (page 304)*
4. *Shoulder Rotator Smash and Floss (page 312)*
5. *Serratus Smash (page 316)*
6. *Anterior Compartment Mobilizations (page 323)*
7. *Forearm Smash Mobilizations (page 344)*
8. *Barbell Shoulder Shear (page 327)*
9. *Bully Extension Bias (page 332)*
10. *Sink Mobilization (page 333)*
11. *Banded Lateral Opener (page 334)*
12. *Banded Elbow Distraction (page 343)*

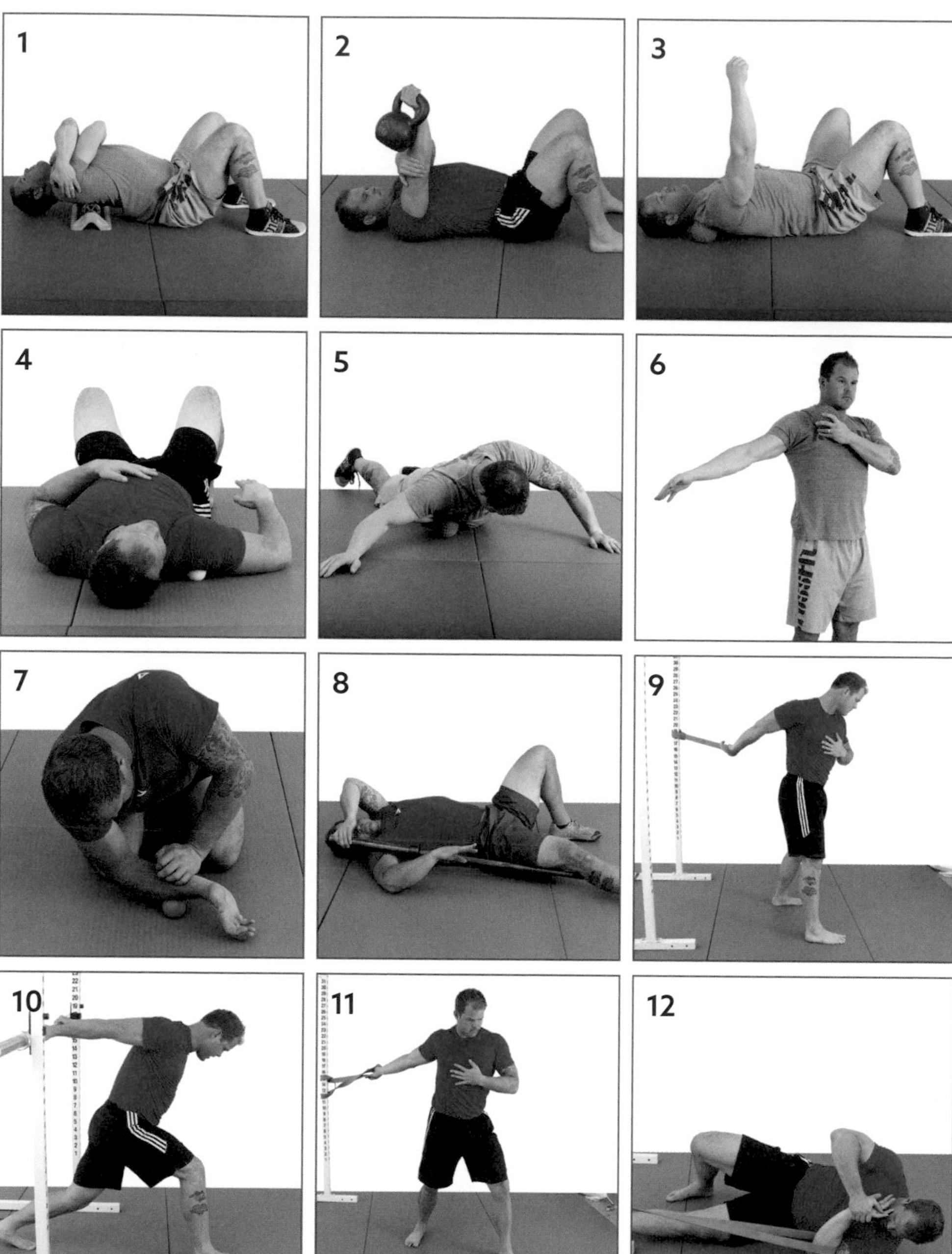

Troubleshooting Press Archetype Mobility Prescriptions

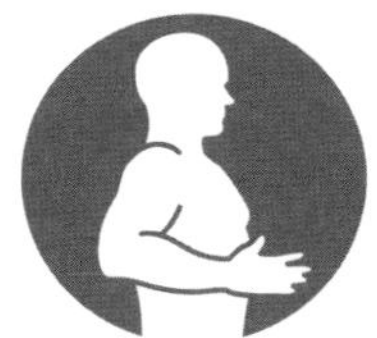

Missing shoulder extension range of motion is the primary limitation that people encounter with the press archetype. Any of the movement faults in part 2 that are tagged with the press archetype icon are likely due to this restriction.

☐ Shoulder Extension Prescriptions

If your shoulders roll forward and your elbows flare outward when you get into the press archetype, you are likely missing shoulder extension range of motion. The mobility prescriptions below will help with this issue. Neither prescription is better or more advanced than the other. I offer two prescriptions to give you options and because some people respond better to certain mobilizations than others.

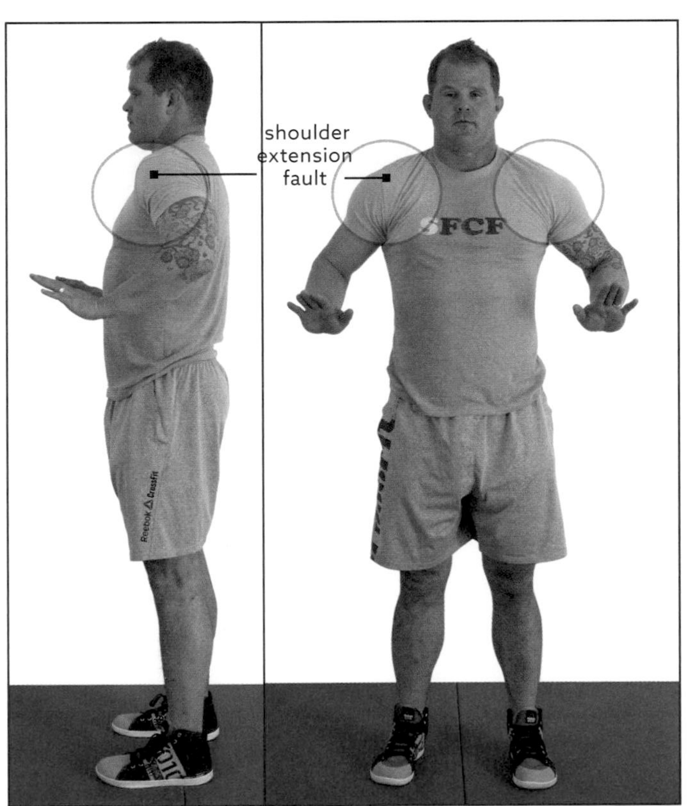

PRESCRIPTION A	TIME
Shoulder Capsule Mobilization (page 310)	2 minutes on each side
T-Spine Roller Smash Mobilizations (page 293; choose one option)	2 minutes
Barbell Shoulder Shear (page 327)	2 minutes on each side
Bully Extension Bias (page 332)	2 minutes on each side
	14 MINUTES

PRESCRIPTION B	TIME
Anterior Compartment Mobilizations (page 323; choose one option)	2 minutes on each side
Serratus Smash (page 316)	2 minutes on each side
Sink Mobilization (page 333)	2 minutes
Banded Lateral Opener (page 334)	2 minutes on each side
	14 MINUTES

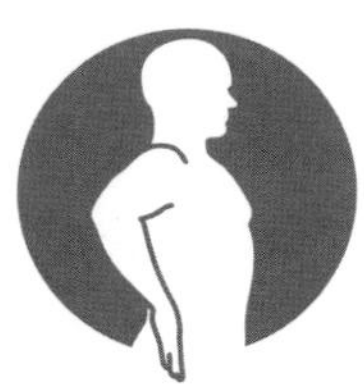

RELATED EXERCISE MOVEMENTS:

Deadlift (page 196)
Dip (page 216)
Clean (page 264)
Snatch (page 278)

EVERYDAY EXAMPLES:

Standing with your arms by your sides

Standing with your hands in your pockets

Carrying something at your side with your arm extended

General Hang Archetype Mobility Prescription

The hang archetype encompasses all movements and positions for your shoulders when your arms are down by your sides. This includes the resting position for your shoulders when your arms are hanging at your sides; the setup position for pulling movements like the deadlift, clean, and snatch; and the finish position for most throwing movements (think pitching). In this section, I offer a number of mobilizations that will help you improve the hang archetype. Here's how it works:

1. Create your own mobility sequence by selecting 3 or 4 mobilizations from the list of techniques on the opposite page. For the best results, perform each mobilization for at least 2 minutes per side, for a total of 10 to 15 minutes of mobility work.

2. Test the position before performing the mobility sequence. After completing the sequence, retest the position to see if you have made change. This test and retest model will illuminate the success of your prescription and help you isolate the most effective mobilizations.

CORRECT

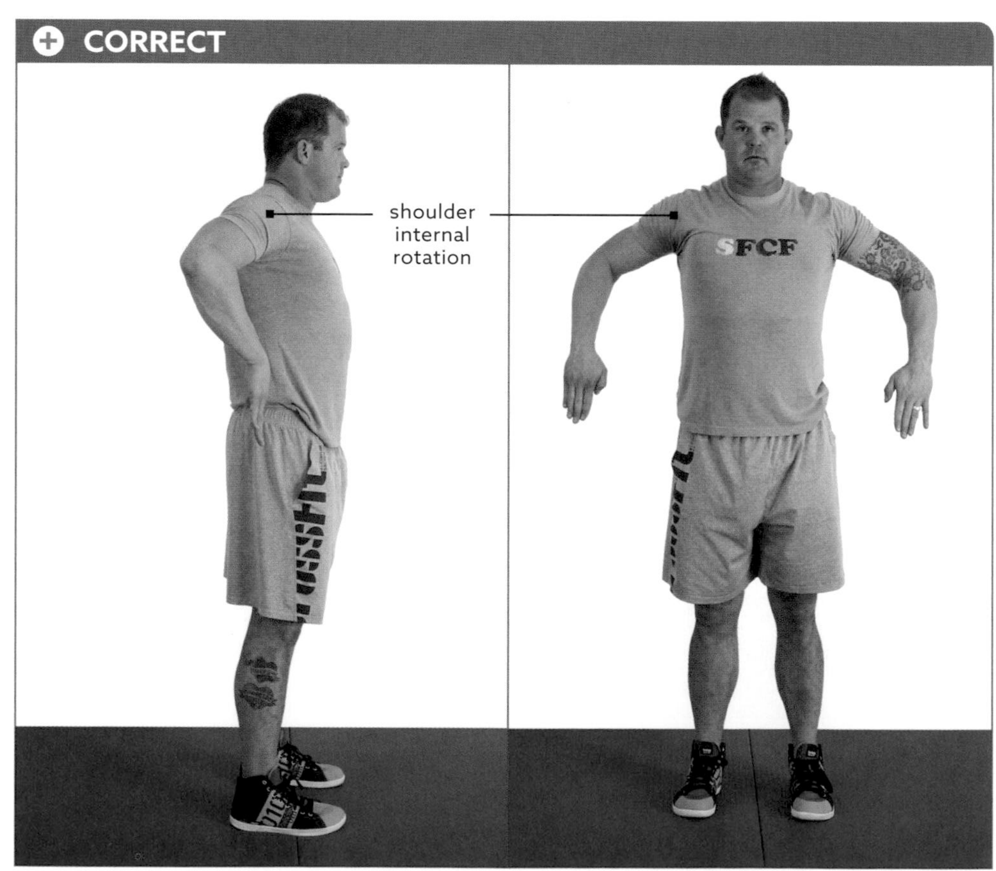

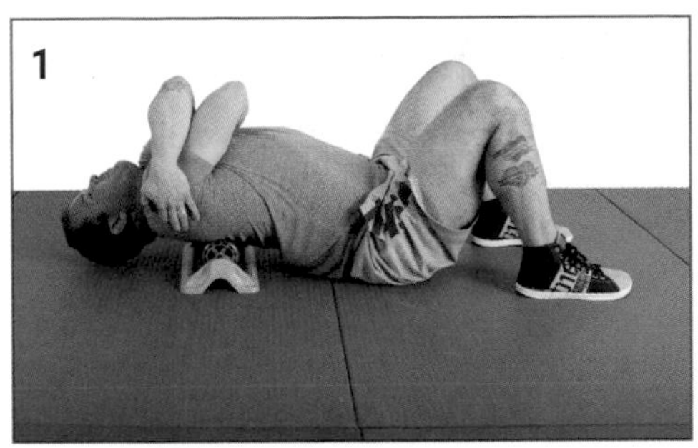

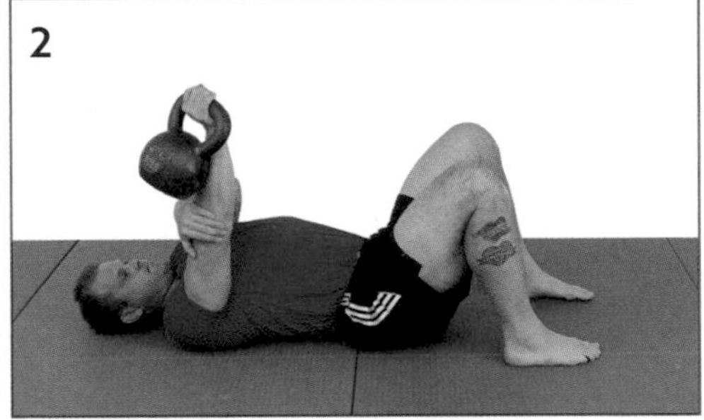

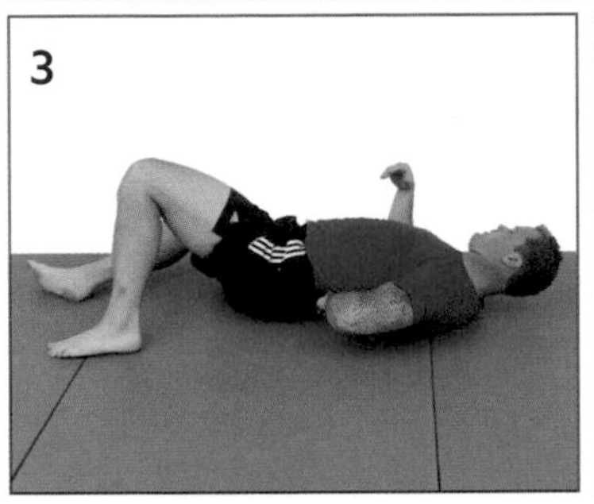

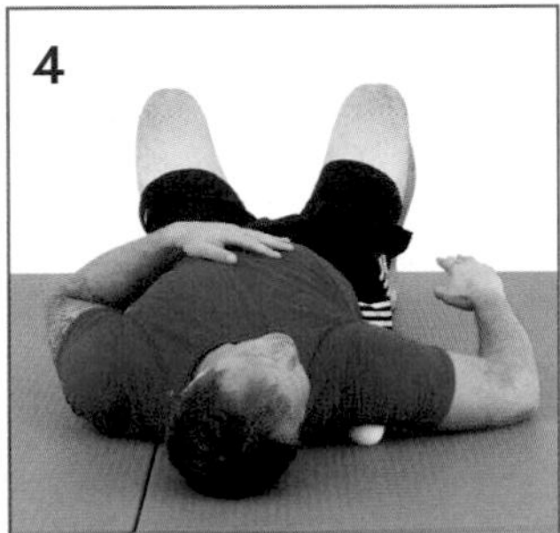

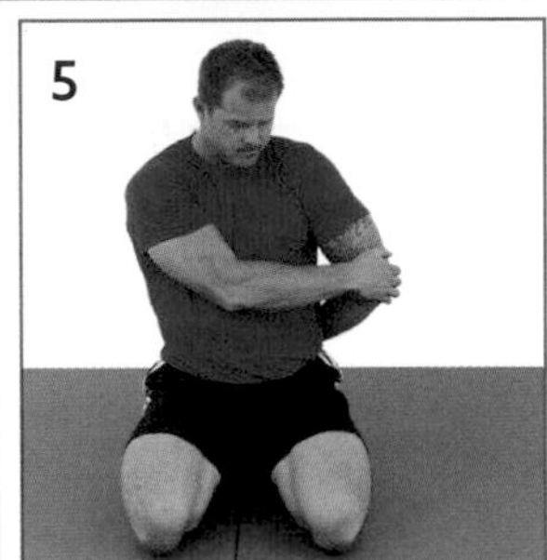

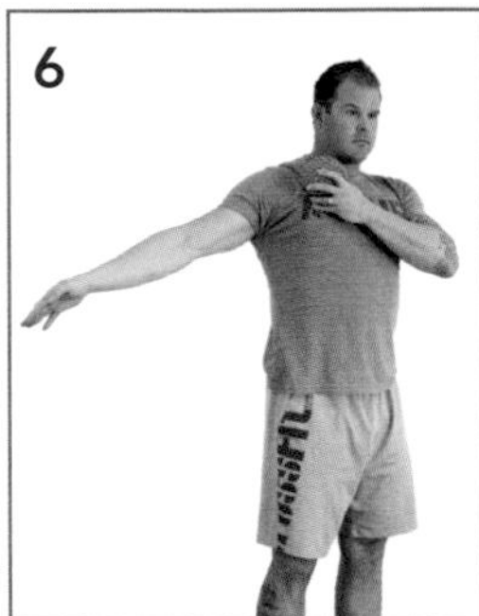

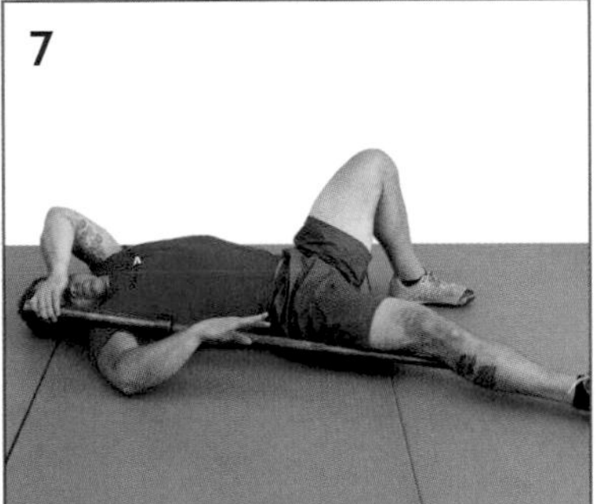

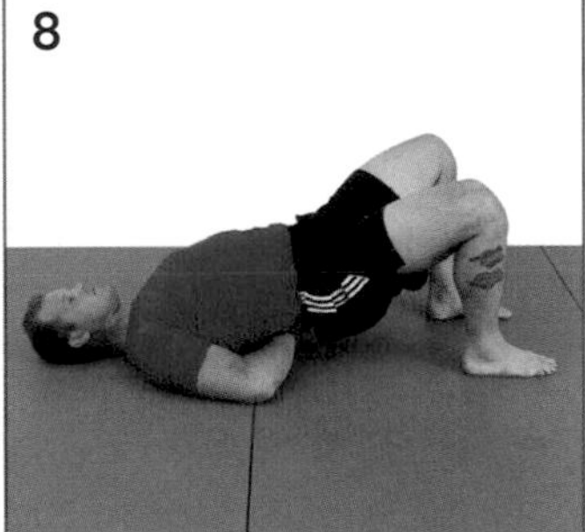

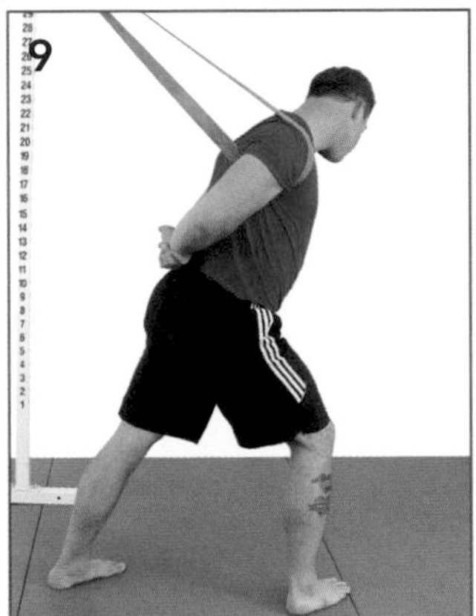

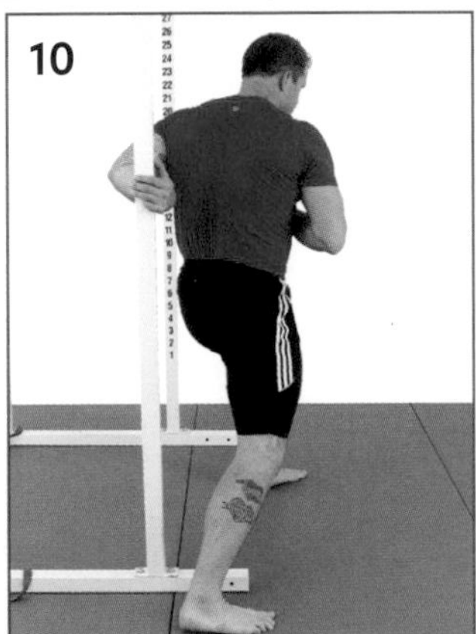

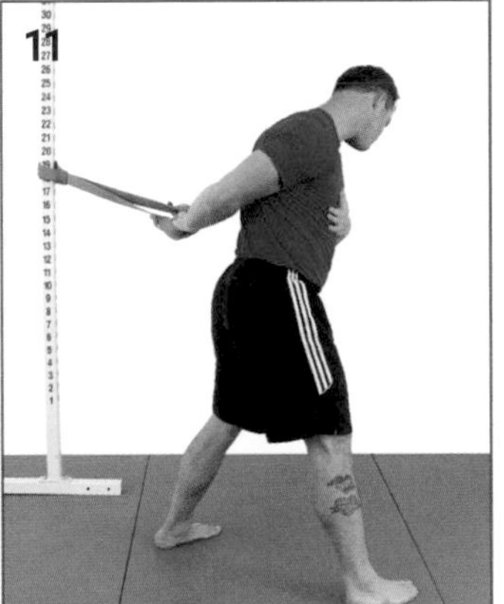

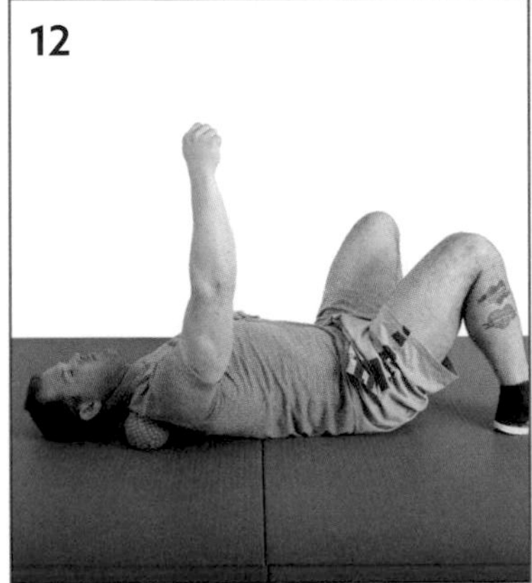

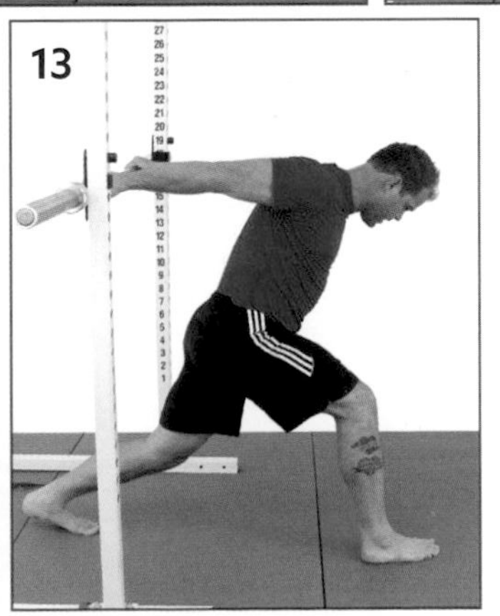

MOBILIZATION LIST:

1. *T-Spine Roller Extension Smash (page 293)*
2. *Shoulder Capsule Mobilization (page 310)*
3. *Lower Rib Smash: Internal Rotation (page 303)*
4. *Shoulder Rotator Smash and Floss (page 312)*
5. *Reverse Sleeper Stretch (page 321)*
6. *Anterior Compartment Mobilizations (page 323)*
7. *Barbell Shoulder Shear (page 327)*
8. *Bilateral Internal Rotation Mobilization (page 329)*
9. *Banded Bully (page 330)*
10. *Triple Bully (page 331)*
11. *Bully Extension Bias (page 332)*
12. *Trap Scrub (page 304)*
13. *Sink Mobilization (page 333)*

Troubleshooting Hang Archetype Mobility Prescriptions

Missing shoulder internal rotation is the primary limitation that people encounter with the hang archetype. Any of the movement faults in part 2 that are tagged with the hang archetype icon are likely due to this restriction.

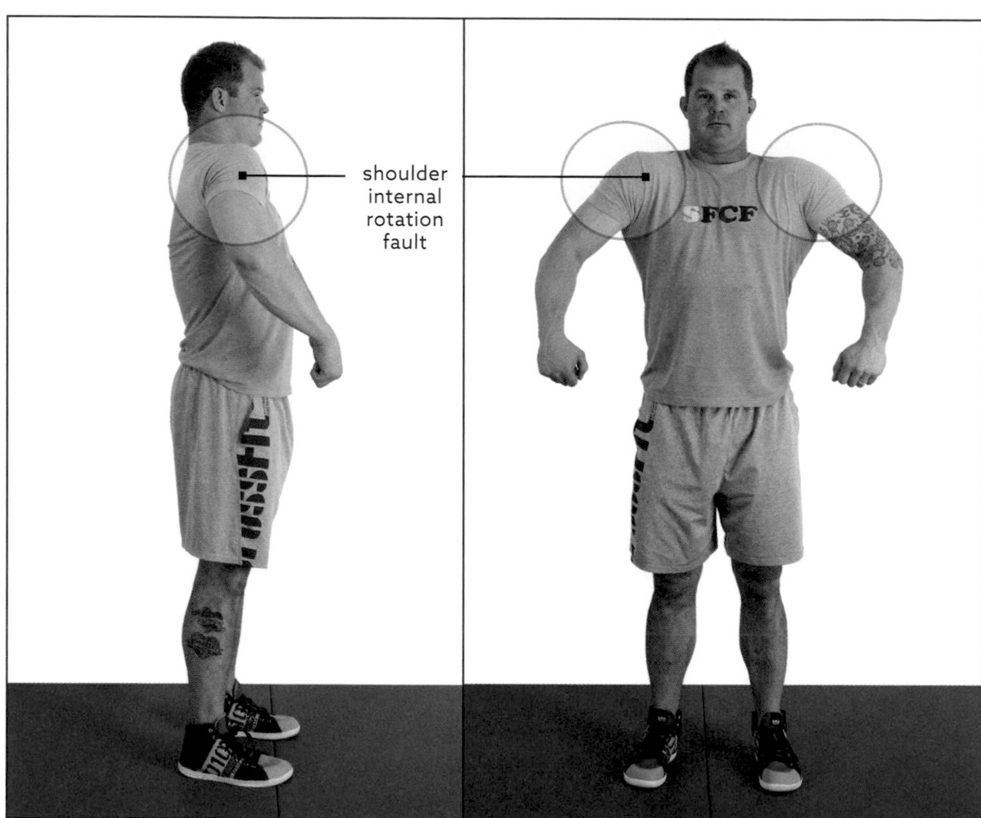

☐ Shoulder Internal Rotation Prescriptions

If your shoulders roll forward and your elbows flare outward when you get into the hang archetype, you are likely missing shoulder internal rotation range of motion. The mobility prescriptions below will help with this issue. Neither prescription is better or more advanced than the other. I offer two prescriptions to give you options and because some people respond better to certain mobilizations than others.

PRESCRIPTION A	TIME
T-Spine Roller Smash Mobilizations (page 293; perform all options)	4 minutes
Shoulder Rotator Smash and Floss (page 312)	2 minutes on each side
Bilateral Internal Rotation Mobilization (page 329)	2 minutes on each side
	12 MINUTES

PRESCRIPTION B	TIME
Anterior Compartment Mobilizations (page 323; choose one option)	2 minutes on each side
Barbell Shoulder Shear (page 327)	2 minutes on each side
Triple Bully (page 331)	2 minutes on each side
	12 MINUTES

General Front Rack Archetype Mobility Prescription

There are two shapes associated with this archetype: arms extended straight out in front of you (Front Rack 1) and arms bent (Front Rack 2). Front Rack 1 captures the stable position for your shoulders when you're pushing or pulling with your arms extended in front of you. Front Rack 2 captures the stable position for your shoulders when you're carrying a load on your shoulder, holding something at chest level, or talking on the phone. This archetype is also buried in a lot of gym-based movements: You start in Front Rack 1 when you set up for the pushup and bench press. You come into Front Rack 2 as the start position for the front squat and overhead press and the finish position for the pull-up and clean. Remember, your elbow moves independently of your shoulder. So when your arm is extended (straight) out in front of you—say, in the start position for the pushup—you're expressing the same stable front rack shoulder position. In this section, I offer a number of mobilizations that will help you improve the front rack archetypes. Here's how it works:

1. Create your own mobility sequence by selecting 3 or 4 mobilizations from the list of techniques on the following page. For the best results, perform each mobilization for at least 2 minutes per side, for a total of 10 to 15 minutes of mobility work.
2. Test the position before performing the mobility sequence. After completing the sequence, retest the position to see if you have made change. This test and retest model will illuminate the success of your prescription and help you isolate the most effective mobilizations.

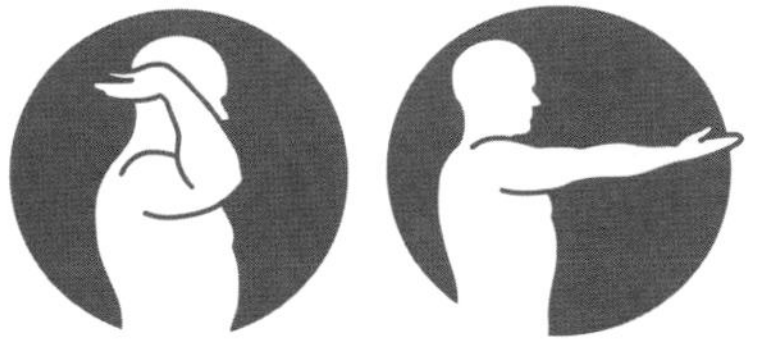

RELATED EXERCISE MOVEMENTS:

Front squat (page 187)
Strict press (page 220)
Pull-up (page 229)
Push-press (page 236)
Turkish getup (page 262)
Clean (page 264)

EVERYDAY EXAMPLES:

Pushing or pulling with your arms extended out in front of your body
Holding or carrying something at chest level or on your shoulder
Talking on the phone

CORRECT (FRONT RACK 1)

elbow extension
shoulder flexion and external rotation

CORRECT (FRONT RACK 2)

wrist extension
shoulder flexion and external rotation
elbow flexion

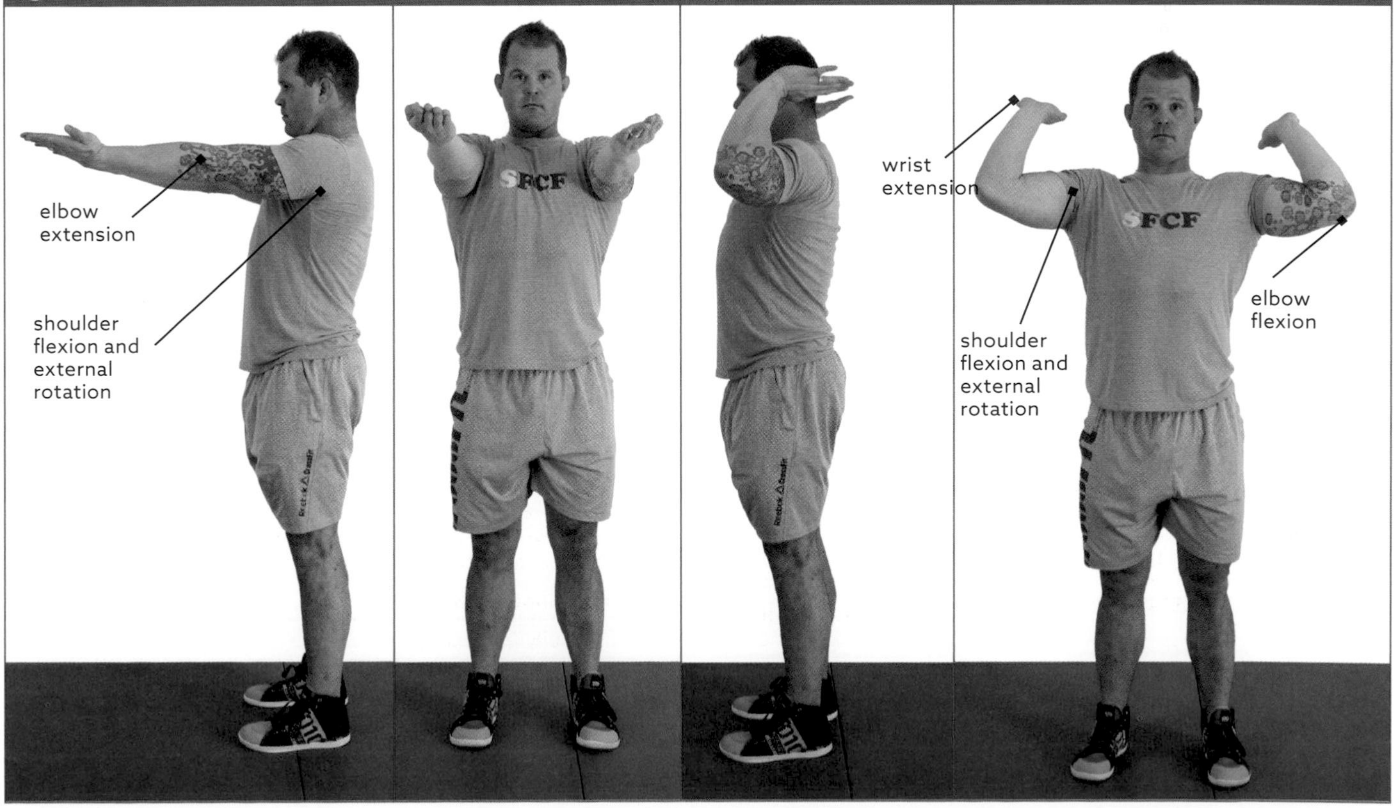

MOBILIZATION LIST:

1. *T-Spine Roller Smash Mobilizations (page 293)*
2. *Shoulder Capsule Mobilization (page 310)*
3. *Shoulder Rotator Smash and Floss (page 312)*
4. *Barbell Bubo Armpit Smash (page 315)*
5. *Overhead Distraction with External Rotation Bias (page 318)*
6. *Super Front Rack (page 320)*
7. *Classic Triceps and Lat Stretch (page 321)*
8. *Banded Lateral Opener (page 334)*
9. *Anterior Compartment Mobilizations (page 323)*
10. *Triceps Extension Smash (page 336)*
11. *Banded Elbow Extension (page 341)*
12. *Banded Elbow Distraction (page 343)*
13. *Forearm Smash Mobilizations (page 344)*
14. *Wrist Tack and Spin (page 346)*
15. *Banded Wrist Distraction (page 347)*

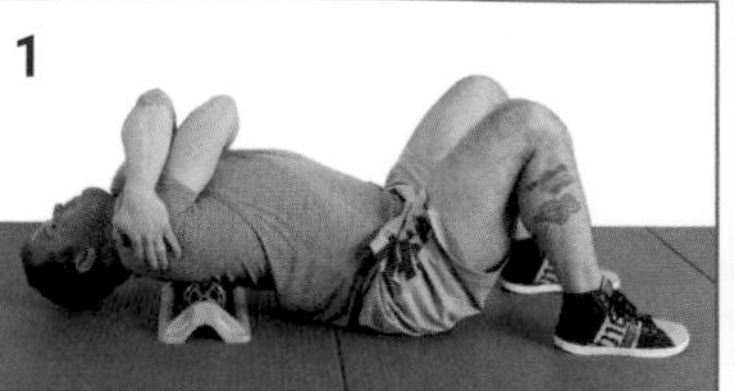
1

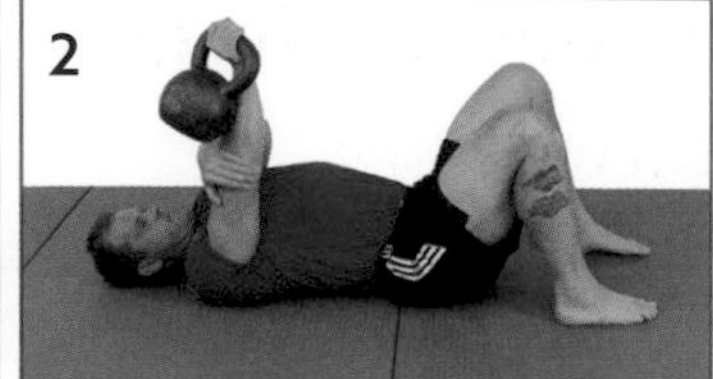
2

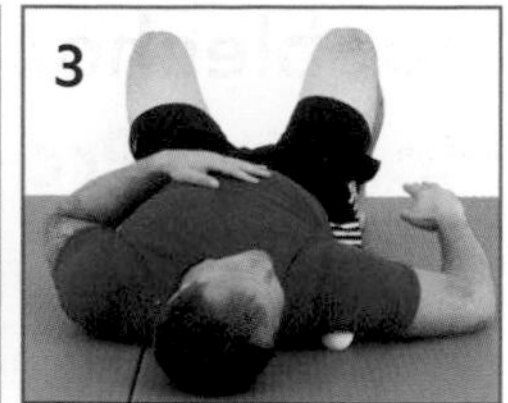
3

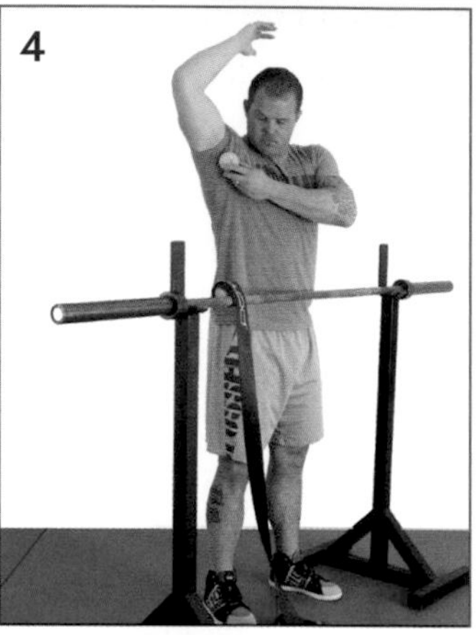
4

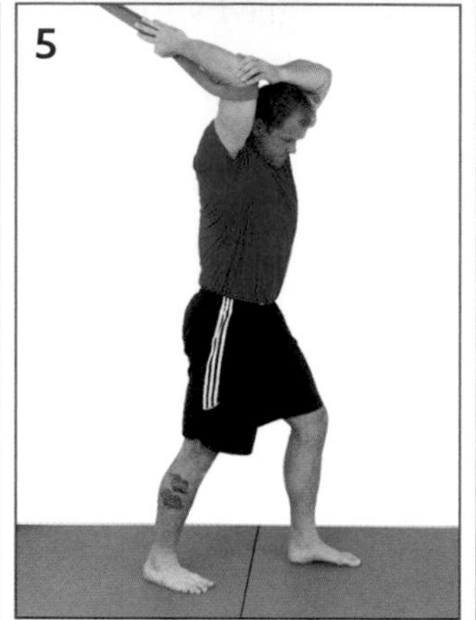
5

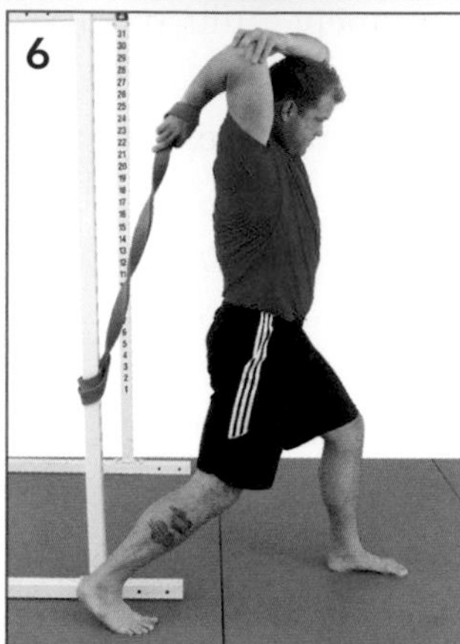
6

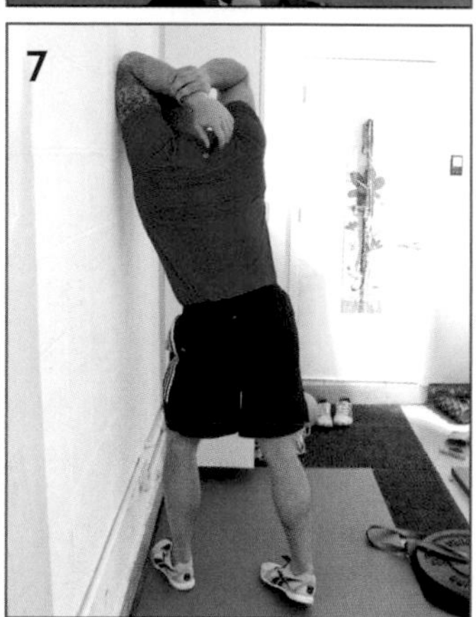
7

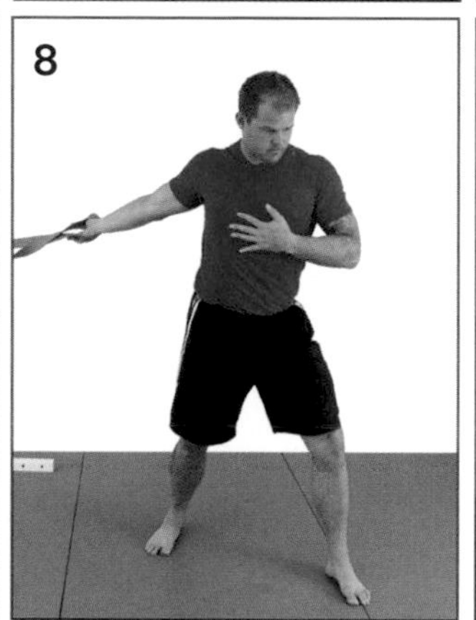
8

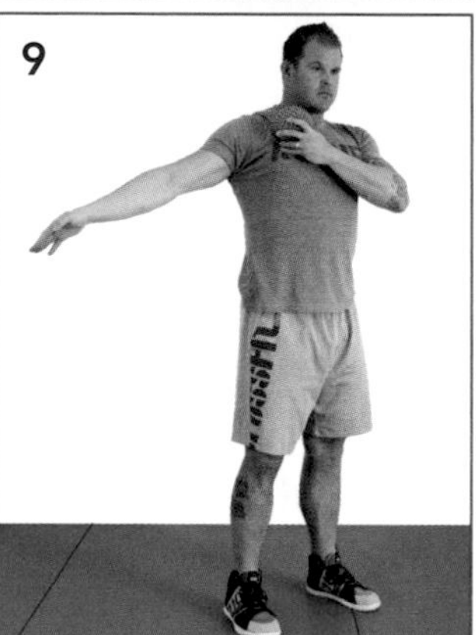
9

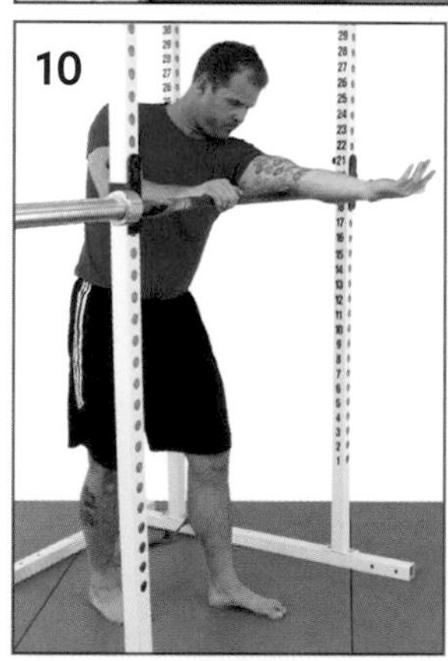
10

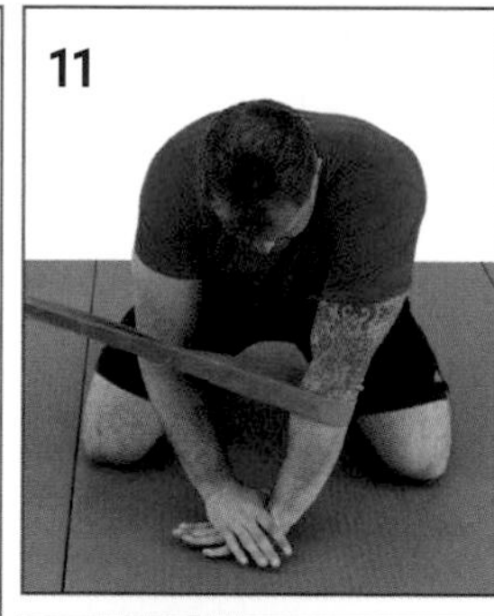
11

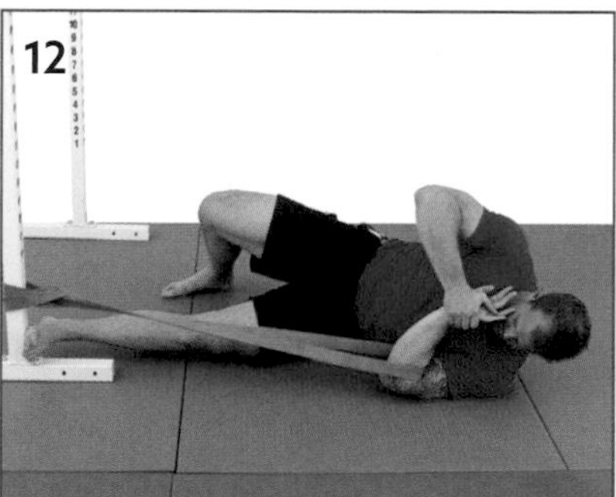
12

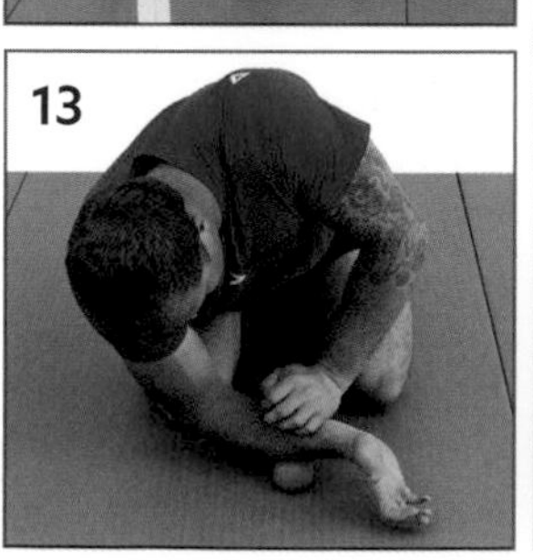
13

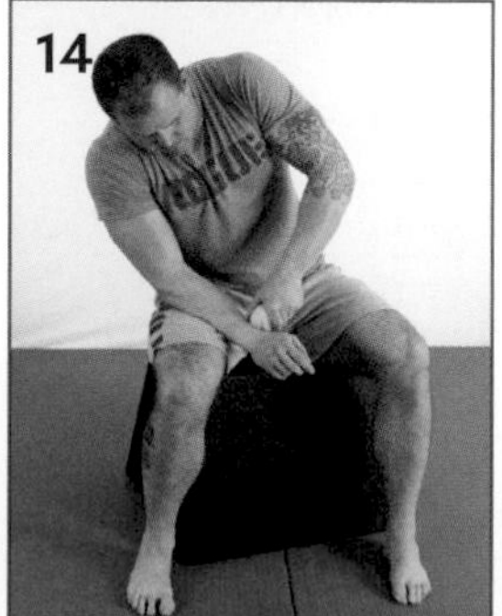
14

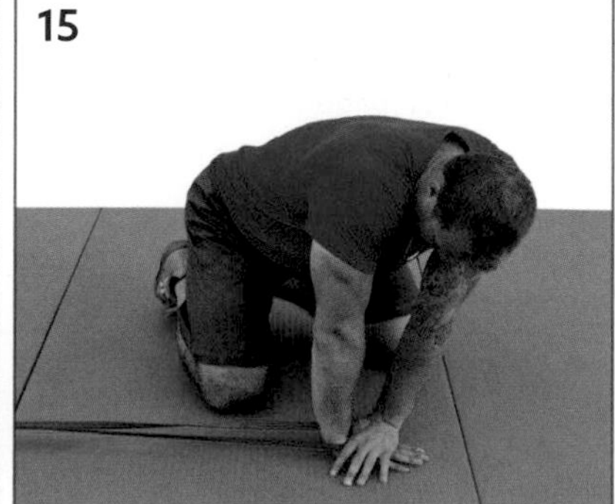
15

Troubleshooting Front Rack Archetype Mobility Prescriptions

People encounter four mobility restrictions with the front rack archetype: shoulder external rotation, elbow flexion, elbow extension, and wrist extension. Any of the movement faults in part 2 that are tagged with the front rack archetype icons are likely due to one of these restrictions. Below I break down these restrictions and offer a sample prescription for each.

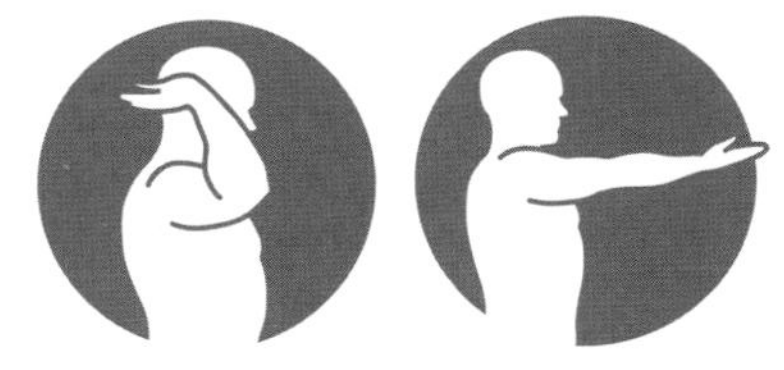

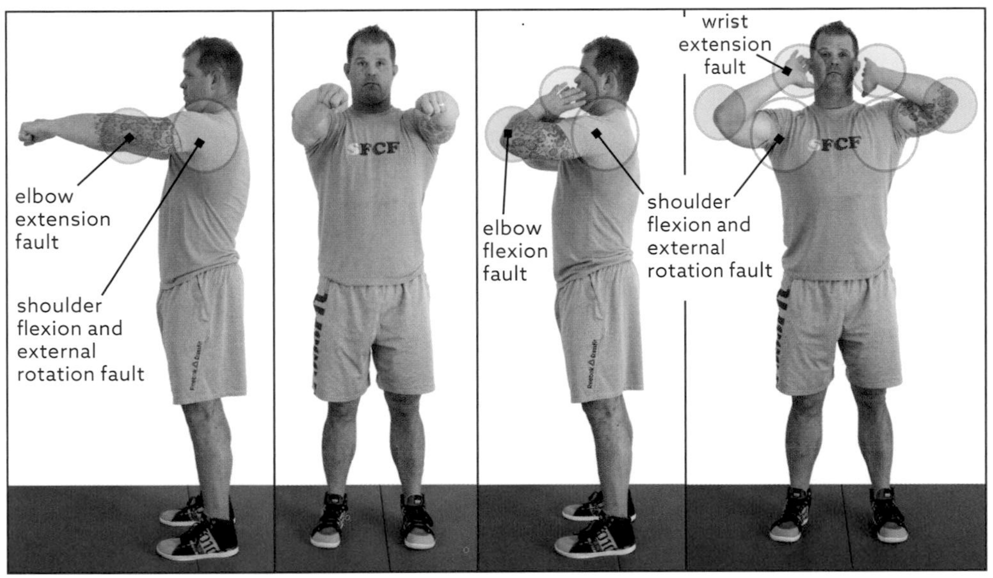

Shoulder External Rotation Prescriptions

If your shoulders roll forward and your elbows flare outward when you get into the front rack position, there's a strong possibility that you're missing shoulder external rotation range of motion. The mobility prescriptions below will help with this issue. Neither prescription is better or more advanced than the other. I offer two prescriptions to give you options and because some people respond better to certain mobilizations than others.

PRESCRIPTION A	TIME
T-Spine Roller Smash Mobilizations (page 293; perform all options)	4 minutes
Overhead Distraction with External Rotation Bias (page 318)	2 minutes on each side
Super Front Rack (page 320)	2 minutes on each side
	12 MINUTES

PRESCRIPTION B	TIME
Shoulder Capsule Mobilization (page 310)	2 minutes on each side
Anterior Compartment Mobilizations (page 323; choose one option)	2 minutes on each side
Banded Lateral Opener (page 334)	2 minutes on each side
	12 MINUTES

Elbow Flexion and Elbow Extension Prescriptions

If your elbows flare outward or your elbows hurt when you get into the front rack position, chances are you are missing either elbow flexion or elbow extension range of motion. If you're missing elbow flexion range of motion, perform prescription A. If you're missing elbow extension range of motion, perform prescription B.

PRESCRIPTION A: ELBOW FLEXION	TIME
Triceps Extension Smash (page 336; choose one option)	2 minutes on each arm
Banded Elbow Distraction (page 343)	2 minutes on each arm
	8 MINUTES

PRESCRIPTION B: ELBOW EXTENSION	TIME
Banded Elbow Extension (page 341)	2 minutes on each arm
Elbow VooDoo (page 339) (see page 146 for VooDoo Flossing wrapping technique)	1–2 minutes of compression, perform 2 to 3 cycles on each arm
	8–15 MINUTES

Wrist Extension Prescription

If your wrists collapse inward when you get into the front rack, chances are you are missing wrist extension range of motion. The prescription below will help with this issue.

PRESCRIPTION	TIME
Wrist Tack and Spin (page 346)	2 minutes on each side
Banded Wrist Distraction with VooDoo Wrist Sequence (page 347)	1–2 minutes on each wrist
	6–8 MINUTES

General Squat Archetype Mobility Prescription

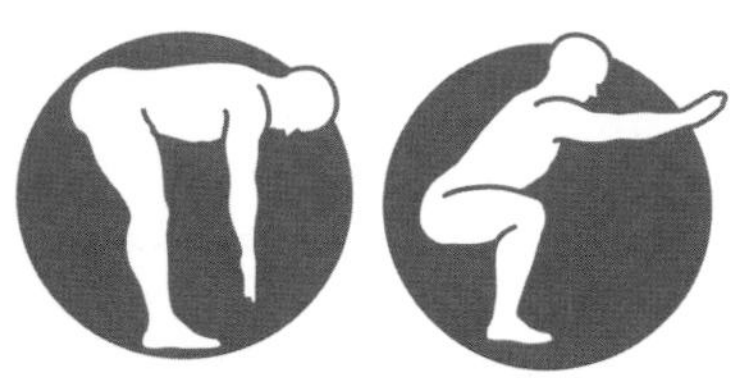

RELATED EXERCISE MOVEMENTS:

Air squat (page 162)
Box squat (page 176)
Back squat (page 178)
Front squat (page 187)
Overhead squat (page 192)
Deadlift (page 196)
Wall ball (page 234)
Jumping and landing (page 238)
Kettlebell swing (page 240)
Snatch balance progression (page 254)
Burpee (page 259)
Clean (page 264)
Snatch (page 278)

EVERYDAY EXAMPLES:

Sitting down into and getting up out of a chair
Getting down to and up from the ground
Bending over

The squat archetype is one of the most fundamental human shapes. Most of the movements that we perform in the gym and in life involve some iteration of the squat. It doesn't matter how your feet are oriented—wide or narrow stance—or whether your torso is upright or tilted forward; the function and position of your hips are relatively the same. This archetype captures flexion and external rotation of the hips.

When it comes to gym movements, the squat archetype is a part of the deadlift, the squat (front squat, back squat, etc.), and the setup for Olympic lifts. There are two basic tests for this archetype: the hips-just-below-knee-crease squat (Squat 1) and the deadlift (Squat 2). The differences are the orientation of your torso and the degree of knee or leg flexion. These distinctions are important because both movements, though similar in shape, test range of motion in different areas: The deadlift tests posterior chain straight-legged movements—specifically your hips and hamstrings—range of motion, while the squat tests hip external rotation and hip, knee, and ankle flexion.

In this section, I offer a number of mobilizations that will help you improve the squat archetype. Here's how it works:

1. Create your own mobility sequence by selecting 3 or 4 mobilizations from the list of techniques on the opposite page. For the best results, perform each mobilization for at least 2 minutes per side, for a total of 10 to 15 minutes of mobility work.

2. Test the position before performing the mobility sequence. After completing the sequence, retest the position to see if you have made change. This test and retest model will illuminate the success of your prescription and help you isolate the most effective mobilizations.

CORRECT (SQUAT 1)

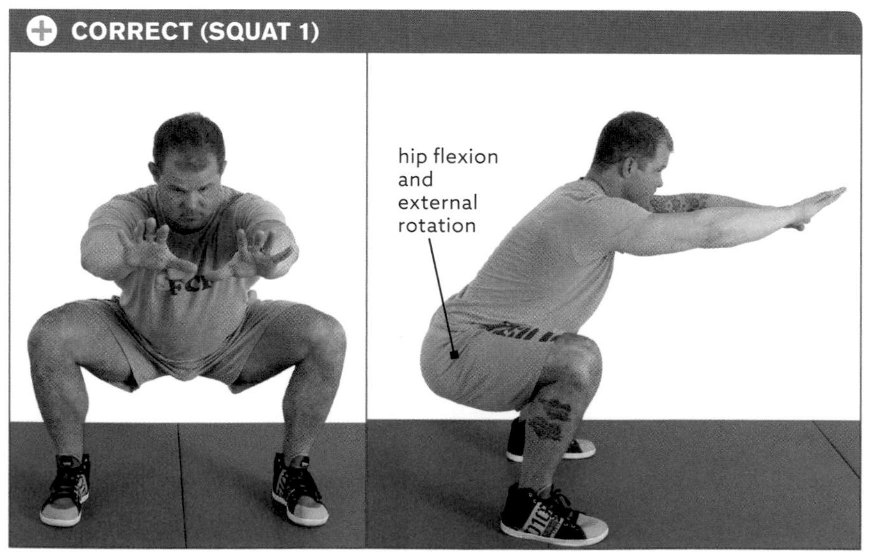

CORRECT (SQUAT 2)

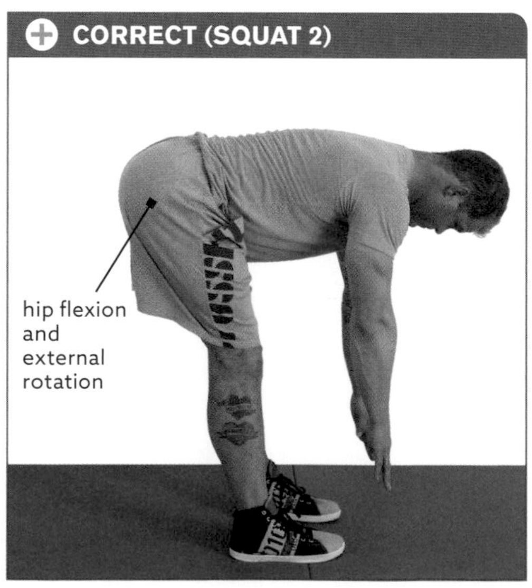

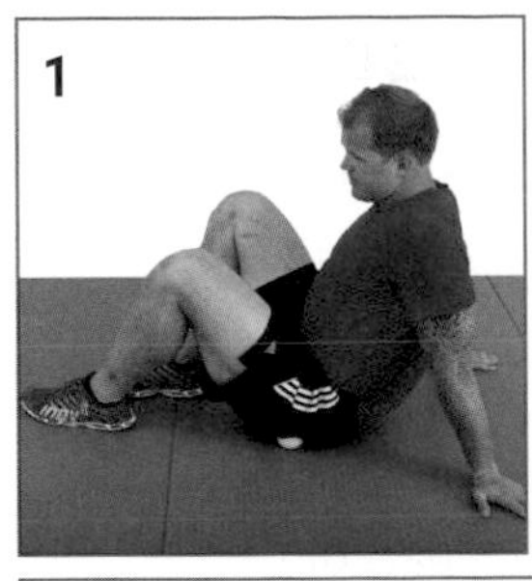
1

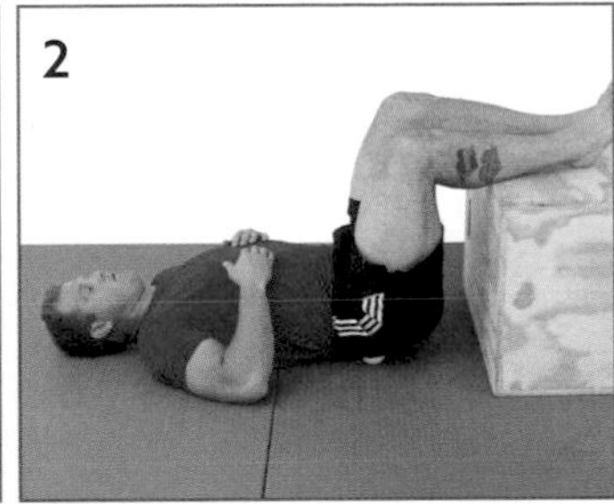
2

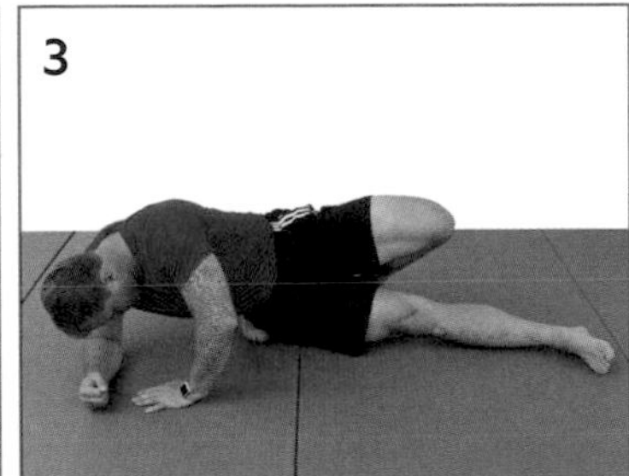
3

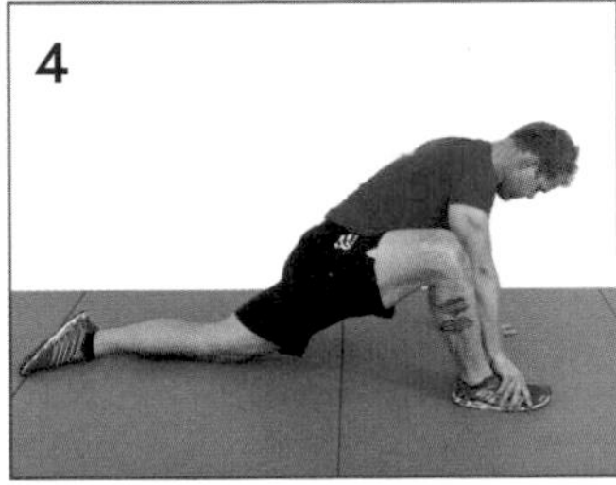
4

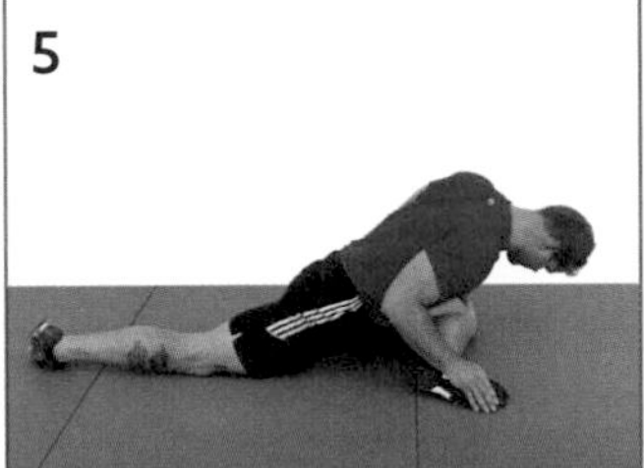
5

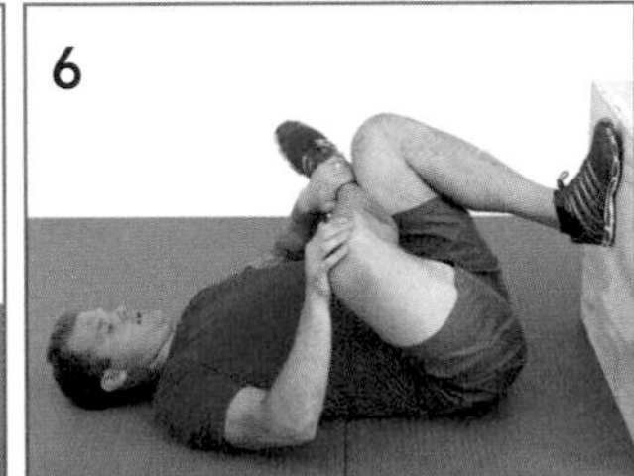
6

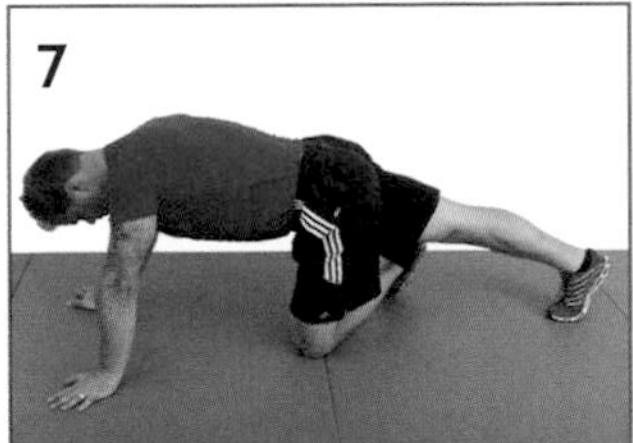
7

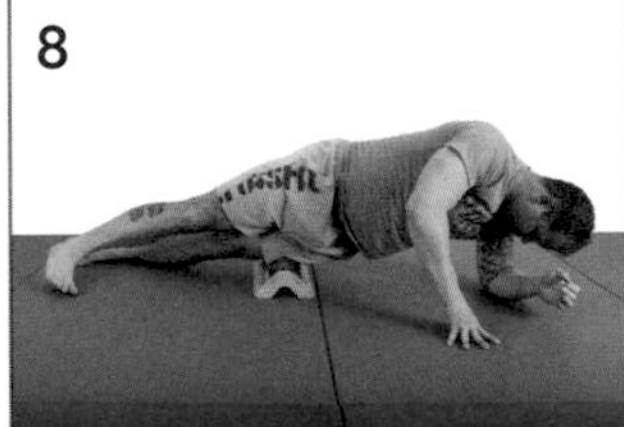
8

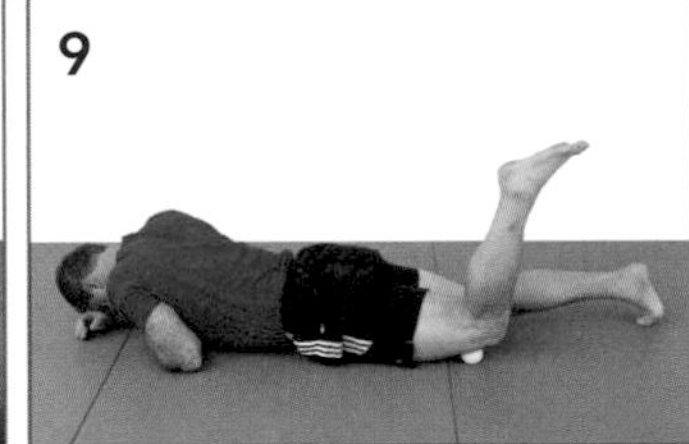
9

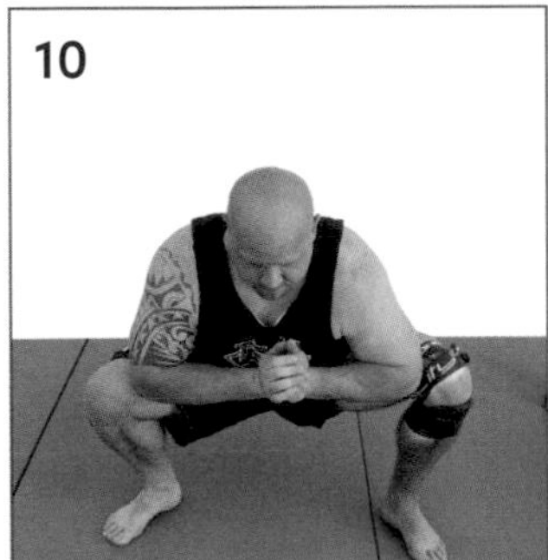
10

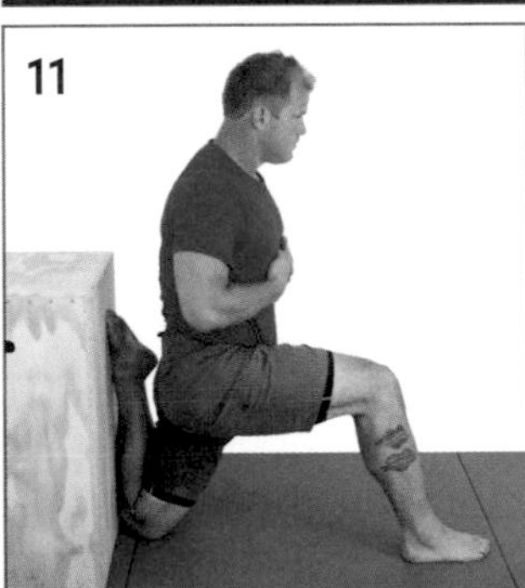
11

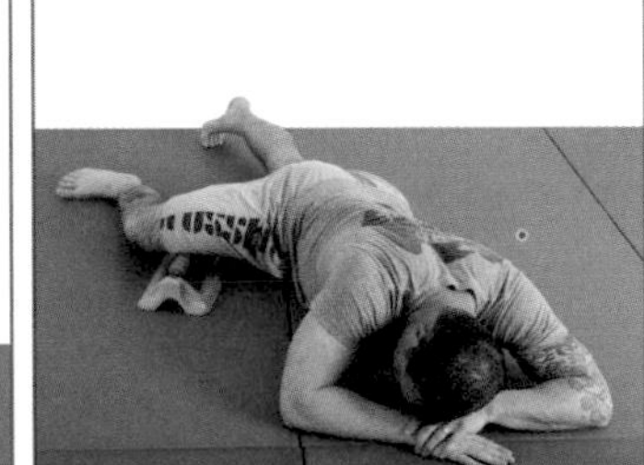
12

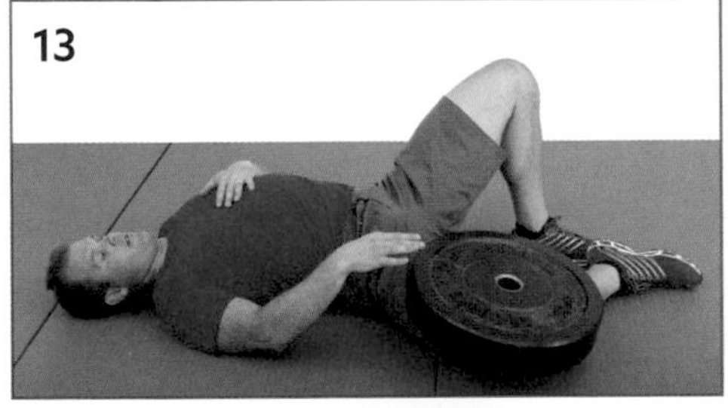
13

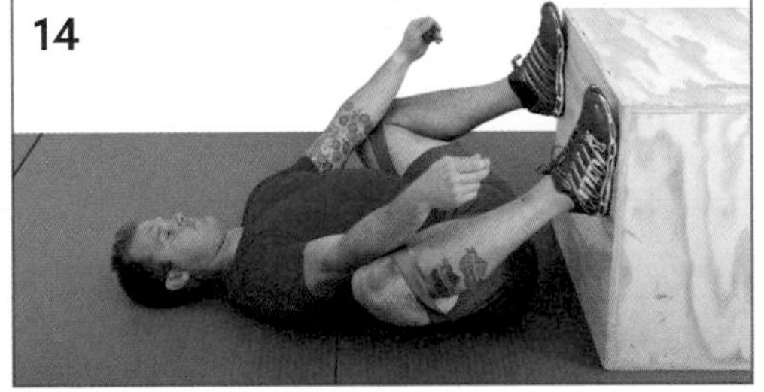
14

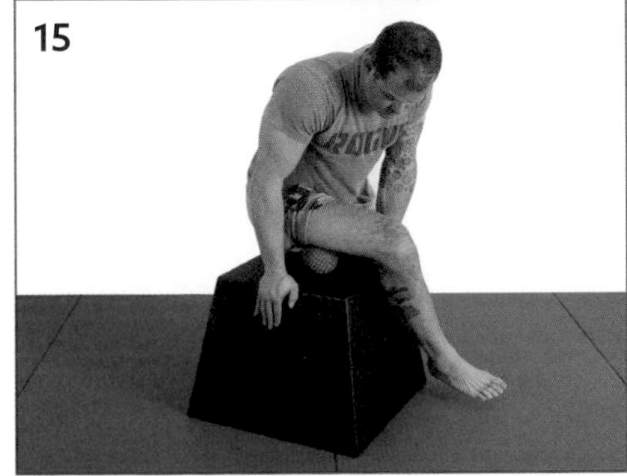
15

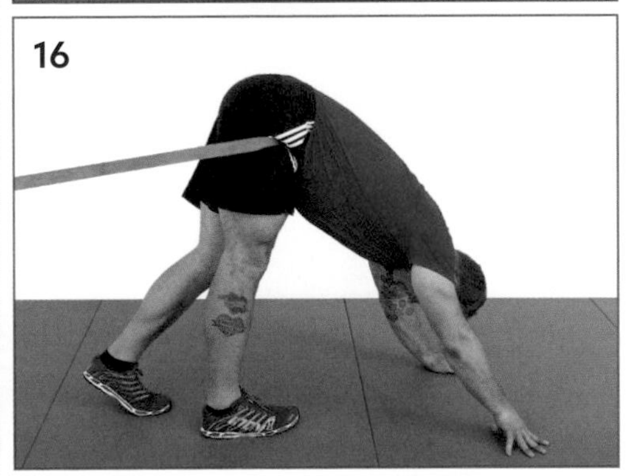
16

MOBILIZATION LIST:

1. *Glute Smash and Floss (page 368)*
2. *High Glute Smash and Floss (page 369)*
3. *Side Hip Smash (page 370)*
4. *Single-Leg Flexion with External Rotation (page 370)*
5. *Hip External Rotation with Flexion (page 373)*
6. *Olympic Wall Squat with External Rotation (page 376)*
7. *Hip Capsule Mobilization (page 379)*
8. *Quad Smash Mobilizations (page 385)*
9. *Suprapatellar Smash and Floss (page 388)*
10. *Knee VooDoo (page 389)*
11. *Couch Stretch (page 391)*
12. *Adductor Smash (page 398)*
13. *Super Frog (page 401)*
14. *Olympic Wall Squat (page 402)*
15. *Posterior Chain Smash and Floss (page 404)*
16. *Posterior Chain Floss (page 408)*

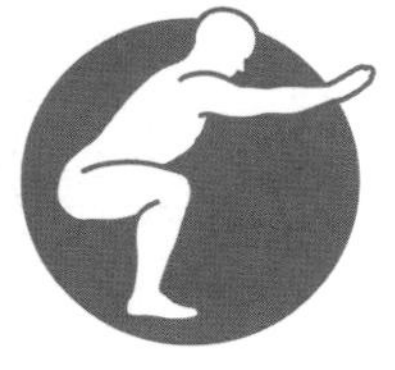

Troubleshooting Squat 1 (Squat Position) Mobility Prescriptions

People encounter two primary limitations with the Squat 1 position: hip flexion and hip external rotation. Any of the movement faults in part 2 that are tagged with the squat 1 archetype icon are likely due to one of these two restrictions.

It's important to note that ankle dorsiflexion range of motion plays a critical role in your ability to squat to full depth (hips below knee crease). If your ankles are the limiting factor, flip to the General Pistol Archetype Mobility Prescription on page 460.

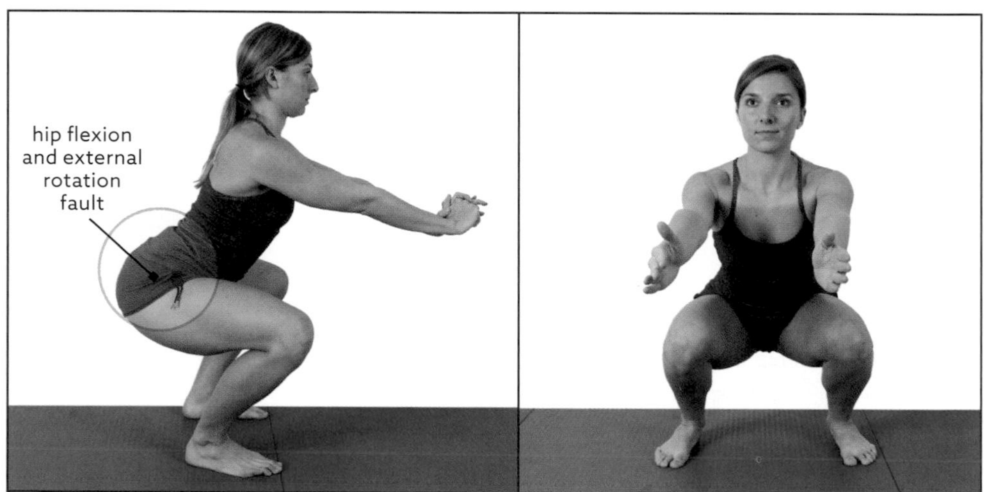

☐ Hip Flexion and External Rotation Prescriptions

If you're having trouble keeping your pelvis from tilting forward and backward (see the butt wink fault on page 173) or your knees are positioned to the inside of your ankles as you descend to or rise from the bottom of the squat, there's a strong chance that you are missing hip flexion and hip external rotation range of motion. The mobility prescriptions below will help with these issues. Neither prescription is better or more advanced than the other. I offer two prescriptions to give you options and because some people respond better to certain mobilizations than others.

PRESCRIPTION A	TIME
Glute Smash and Floss (page 368)	2 minutes on each side
Quad Smash Mobilizations (page 385; choose one option)	2 minutes on each side
Single-Leg Flexion with External Rotation (page 370; choose one option)	2 minutes on each side
	12 MINUTES

PRESCRIPTION B	TIME
Adductor Smash (page 398; choose one option)	2 minutes on each side
Suprapatellar Smash and Floss (page 388)	2 minutes on each side
Olympic Wall Squat (page 402)	2 minutes on each side
	12 MINUTES

Troubleshooting Squat 2 (Deadlift/Pulling Position) Mobility Prescription

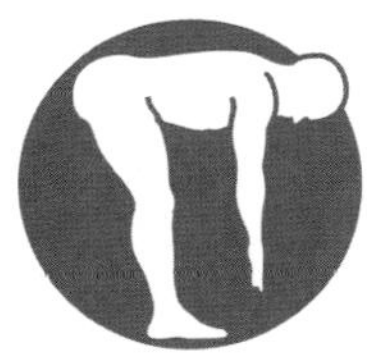

Missing hamstring range of motion is the primary limitation that people encounter with the deadlift/pulling position. Any of the movement faults in part 2 that are tagged with the squat 2 archetype icon are likely due to this restriction.

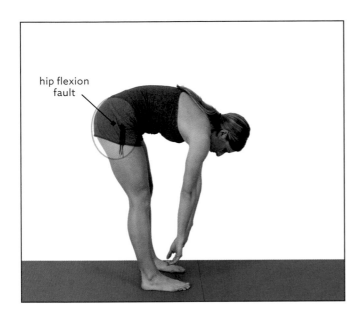

☐ Hip Flexion Prescription: Hamstring Restriction

If you can't bend over and touch a barbell or the ground while keeping your spine neutral, the muscles of your posterior chain, specifically your hamstrings, are the limiting factor. The mobility prescription below will help with this issue.

PRESCRIPTION	TIME
High Glute Smash and Floss (page 369)	2 minutes on each side
Posterior Chain Smash and Floss (page 404; choose one option)	2 minutes on each side
Posterior Chain Floss (page 408; choose one option)	2 minutes on each side
	12 MINUTES

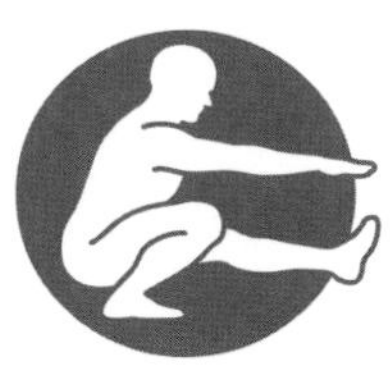

RELATED EXERCISE MOVEMENTS:

Turkish getup (page 262)

EVERYDAY EXAMPLES:

Getting up off the ground from a seated position

Sitting in a deep squat (such as while gardening)

Moving on the ground

Stepping up onto a high platform

Lowering yourself down from a high step

General Pistol Archetype Mobility Prescription

The pistol (single-leg squat) shape captures all the ankle mobility you need to be a fully functional human being. It requires full hip flexion plus full ankle dorsiflexion. So, if you can get into the pistol shape, chances are you have full ankle dorsiflexion and full hip flexion range of motion.

Stated differently, the pistol is the fullest expression of a deep squat. When you squat with your feet apart, for example, you never take your hip or ankle into full flexion. The pistol archetype, on the other hand, expresses full range of motion around the primary engines and the associated joints (knee and ankle).

Anytime you're low to the ground—say, when getting up from a seated position or while gardening or break-dancing—you're expressing a close iteration of this archetype. In this section, I offer a number of mobilizations that will help you improve the pistol archetype. Here's how it works:

1. Create your own mobility sequence by selecting 3 or 4 mobilizations from the list of techniques on the opposite page. For the best results, perform each mobilization for at least 2 minutes per side, for a total of 10 to 15 minutes of mobility work.

2. Test the position before performing the mobilization sequence. After completing the sequence, retest the position to see if you have made change. This test and retest model will illuminate the success of your prescription and help you isolate the most effective mobilizations.

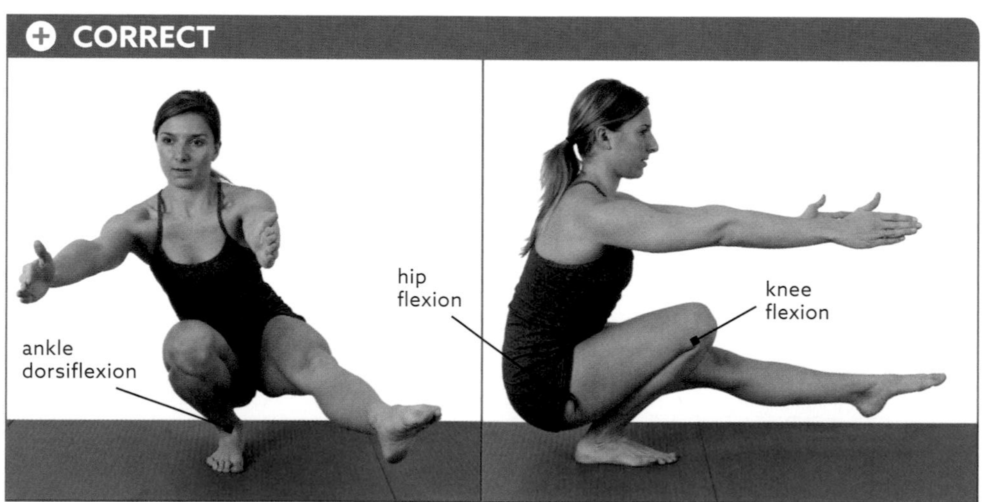

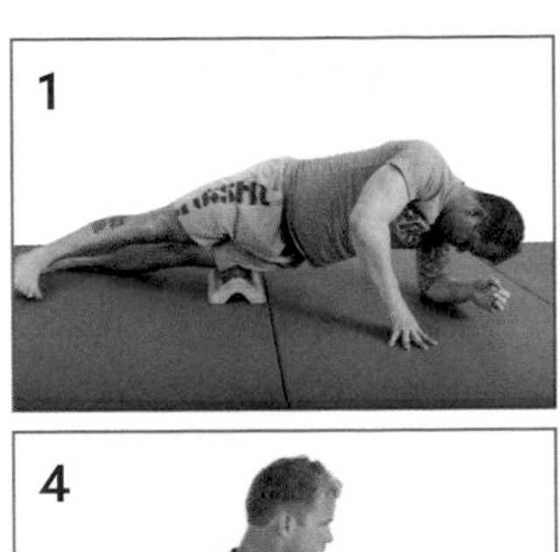

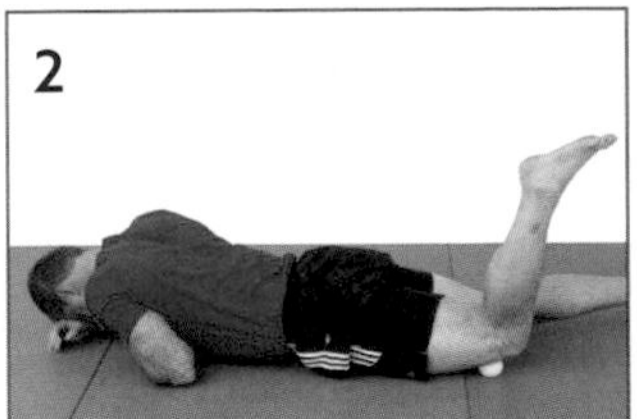

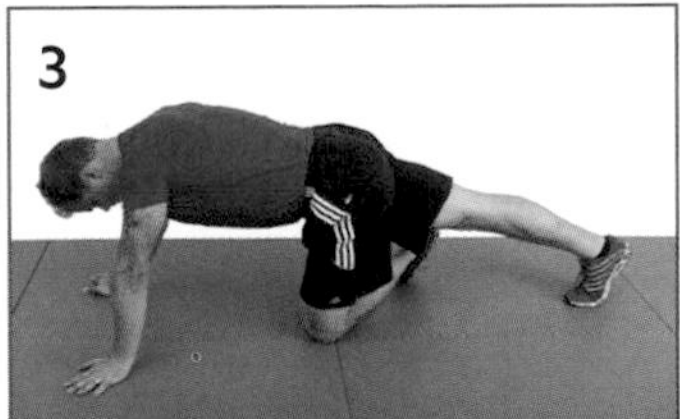

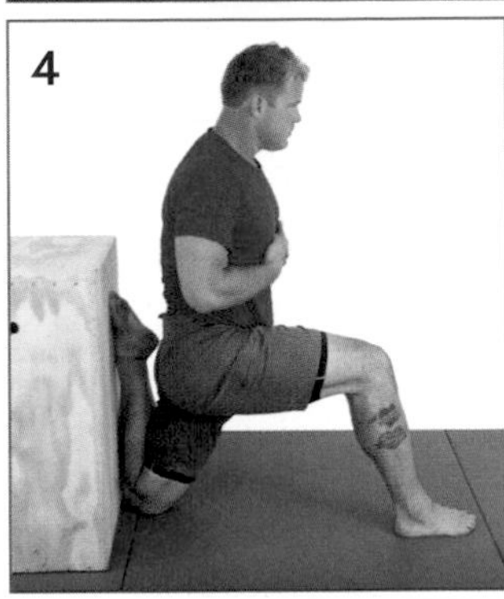

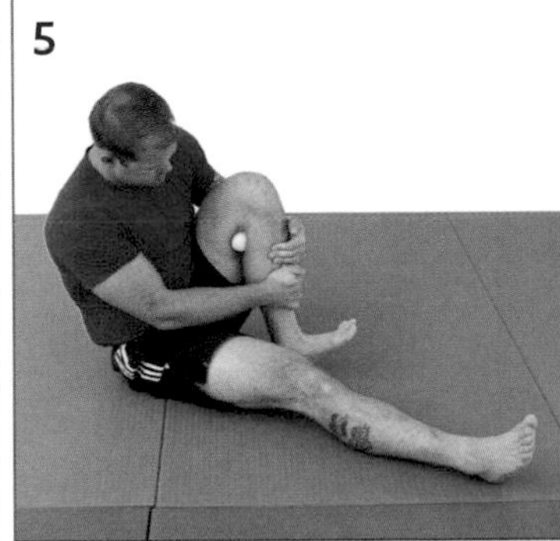

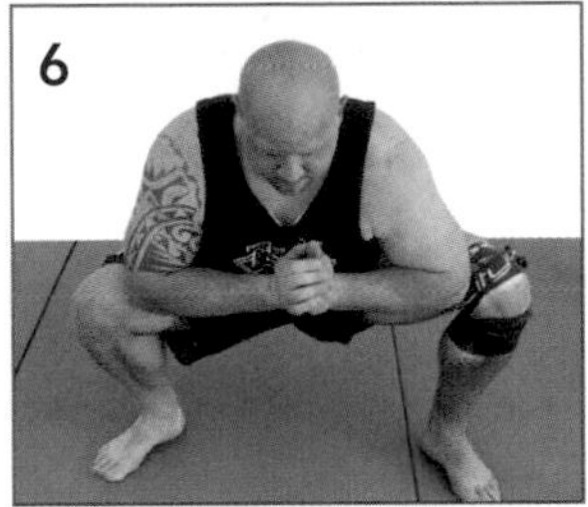

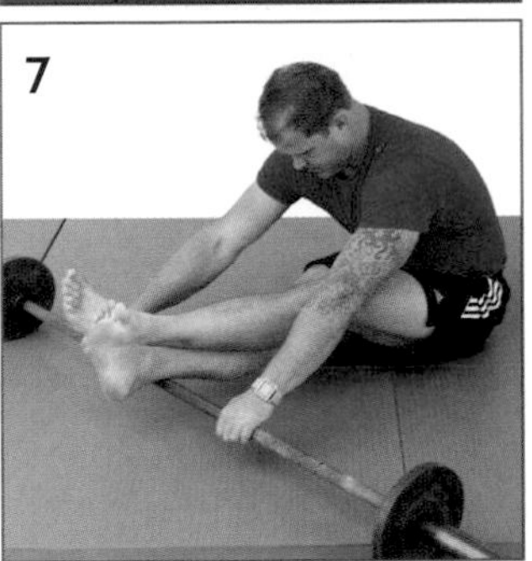

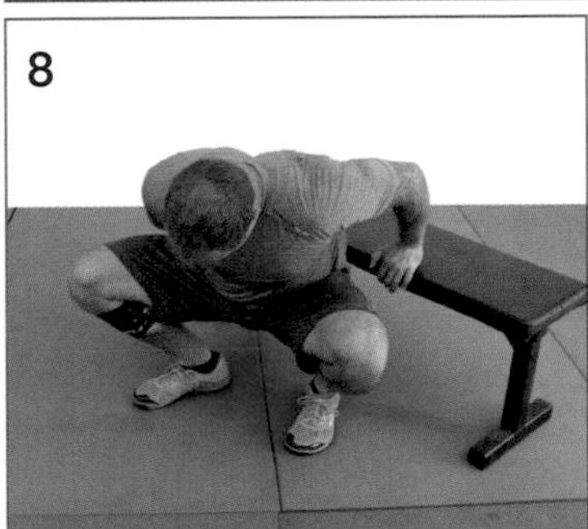

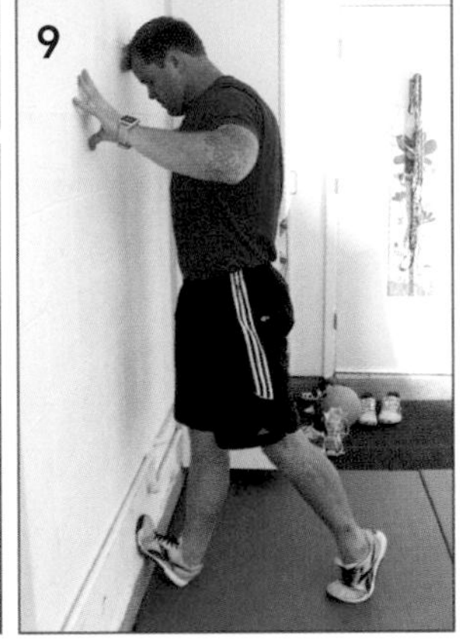

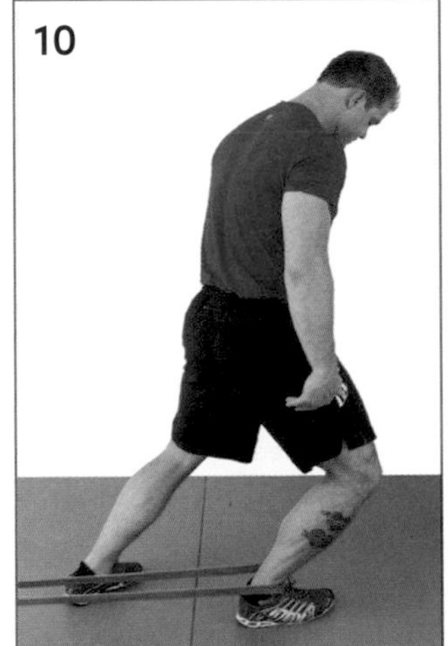

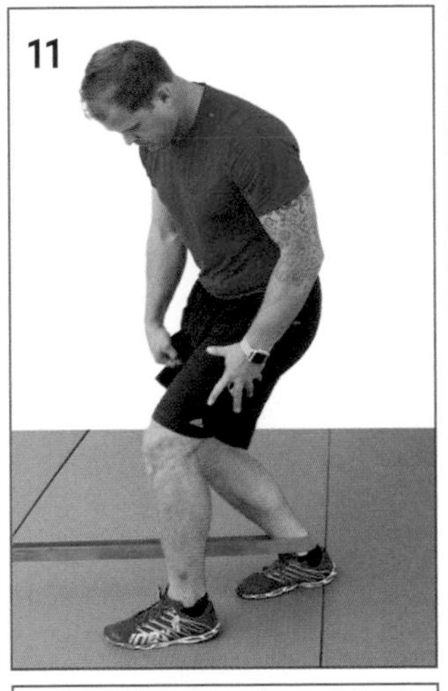

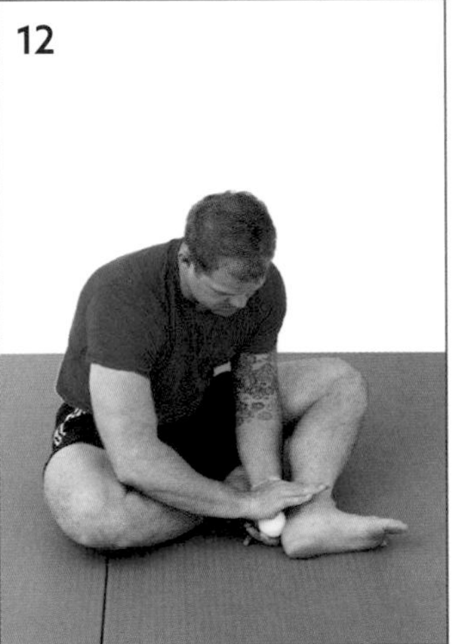

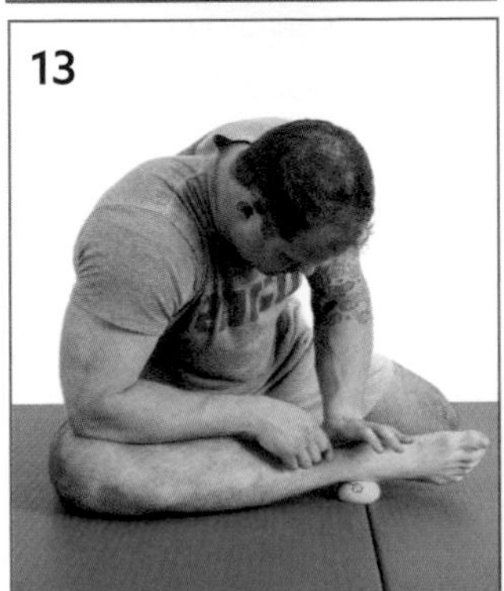

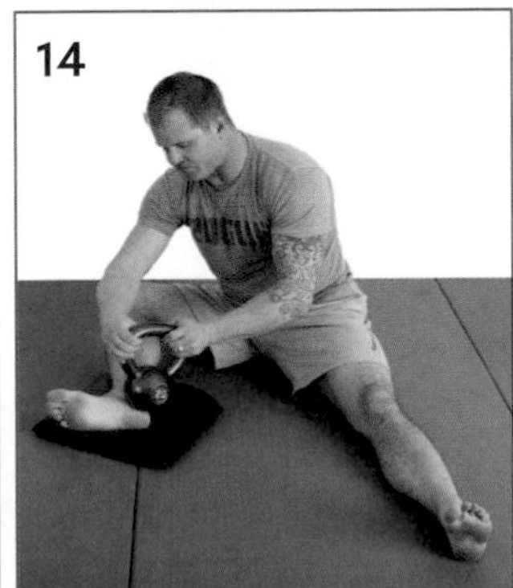

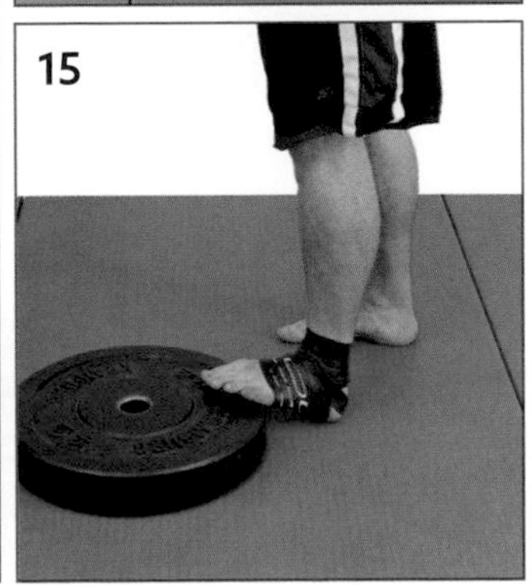

MOBILIZATION LIST:

1. *Quad Smash Mobilizations (page 385)*
2. *Suprapatellar Smash and Floss (page 388)*
3. *Hip Capsule Mobilization (page 379)*
4. *Couch Stretch (page 391)*
5. *Gap and Smash Mobilizations (page 415)*
6. *Knee VooDoo (page 389)*
7. *Calf Smash Mobilizations (page 425)*
8. *VooDoo Calf Mobilization (page 428)*
9. *Classic Calf Mobilization (page 429)*
10. *Banded Heel Cord: Anterior Bias (page 430)*
11. *Banded Heel Cord: Posterior Bias (page 430)*
12. *Ball Whack (page 432)*
13. *Lateral Malleolus/Heel Smash Mobilizations (page 433)*
14. *Medial Heel Bone Smash (page 434)*
15. *Ankle VooDoo (page 436)*

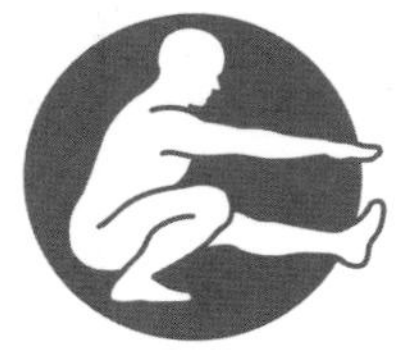

Troubleshooting Pistol Archetype Mobility Prescriptions

People encounter three primary limitations with the pistol archetype: hip flexion, knee flexion, and ankle dorsiflexion. Any of the movement faults in part 2 that are tagged with the pistol archetype icon are likely due to one of these three restrictions. Below I break down these restrictions and offer a sample prescription for each.

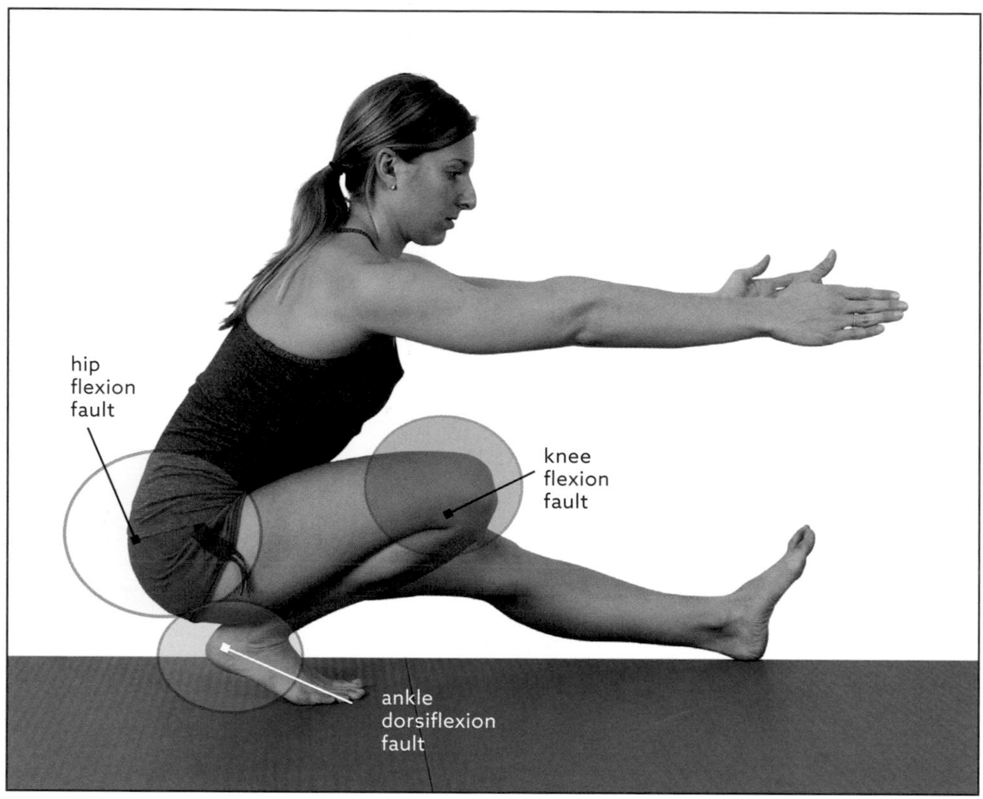

■ Knee Flexion Prescription

If you are unable to comfortably compress your knee into a fully flexed position or you experience knee pain in the pistol position, you might be missing critical corners of knee flexion. The mobility prescription below will help with this issue.

PRESCRIPTION	TIME
Suprapatellar Smash and Floss (page 388)	2 minutes on each side
Gap and Smash Mobilizations (page 415; choose one option)	2 minutes on each side
Lateral and Anterior Compartment Shin Mobilization (page 422; choose one option)	2 minutes on each side
	12 MINUTES

Hip Flexion Prescription

Sitting for prolonged periods locks your hips in a shortened position. As your muscles and tissues adapt to this position, they create a cast around your hips that limits hip flexion and extension range of motion. If you're missing hip flexion and extension range of motion, you are more susceptible to overextending as you lower into the pistol position. You are also more likely to feel a hip impingement (this is your femur running into your hip socket). The mobility prescription below will help with this issue.

PRESCRIPTION	TIME
Hip Capsule Mobilization (page 379)	2 minutes on each side
Single-Leg Flexion with External Rotation (page 370; choose one option)	2 minutes on each side
Couch Stretch (page 391)	2 minutes on each side
	12 MINUTES

Ankle Dorsiflexion Prescription

If you fall backward onto your butt or you can't comfortably get your heel flush to the ground, restricted ankles are probably to blame. The mobility prescriptions below will improve ankle dorsiflexion range of motion. Neither prescription is better or more advanced than the other. I offer two prescriptions to give you options and because some people respond better to certain mobilizations than others.

PRESCRIPTION A	TIME
Calf Smash Mobilizations (page 425; choose one option)	2 minutes on each side
Banded Heel Cord: Anterior Bias (page 430)	2 minutes on each side
Classic Calf Mobilization (page 429)	2 minutes on each side
	12 MINUTES

PRESCRIPTION B	TIME
Ball Whack (page 432)	2 minutes on each side
Lateral Malleolus/Heel Smash Mobilizations (page 433)	2 minutes on each side
Medial Heel Bone Smash (page 434)	2 minutes on each side
	12 MINUTES

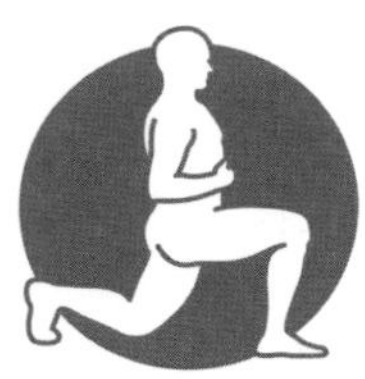

RELATED EXERCISE MOVEMENTS:

Turkish getup (page 262)
Split-jerk (page 274)

EVERYDAY EXAMPLES:

Running and walking
Stepping
Getting up off the ground

General Lunge Archetype Mobility Prescription

The lunge archetype captures extension and internal rotation of the hip. Anytime your leg is behind your body—whether you're running, throwing, fighting, etc.—you're expressing a close iteration of this archetype. The split-jerk and the lunge are the best exercise examples of this shape. In this section, I offer a number of mobilizations that will help you improve the lunge archetype. Here's how it works:

1. Create your own mobility sequence by selecting 3 or 4 mobilizations from the list of techniques on the opposite page. For the best results, perform each mobilization for at least 2 minutes per side, for a total of 10 to 15 minutes of mobility work.

2. Test the position before performing the mobilization sequence. After completing the sequence, retest the position to see if you have made change. This test and retest model will illuminate the success of your prescription and help you isolate the most effective mobilizations.

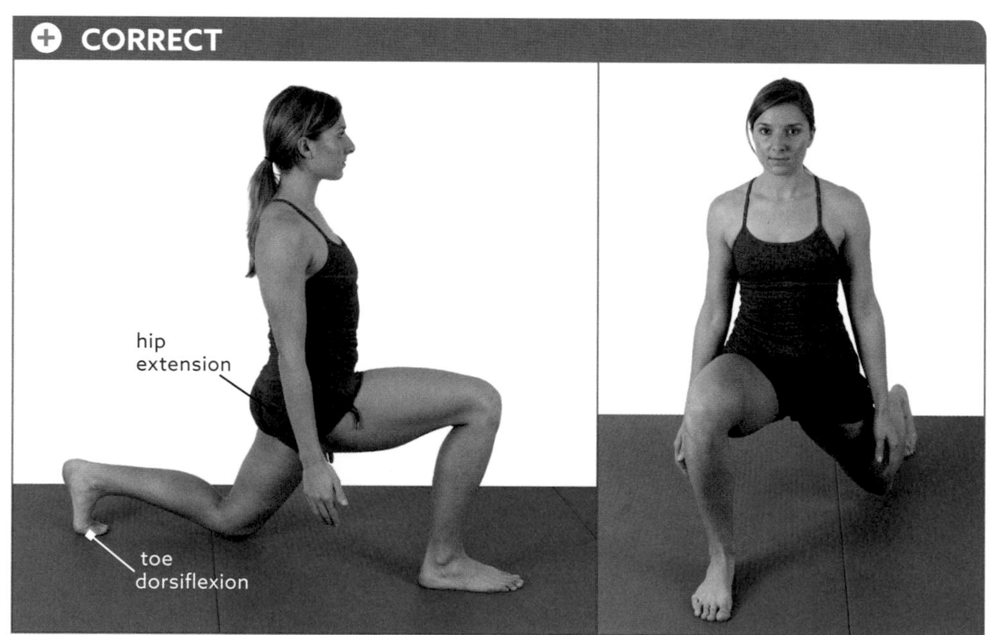

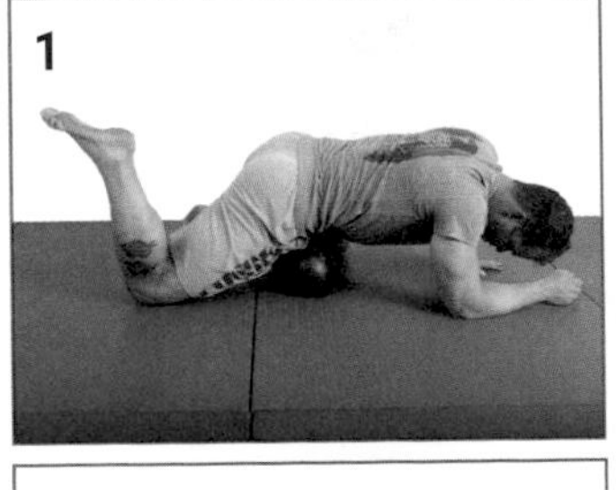
1

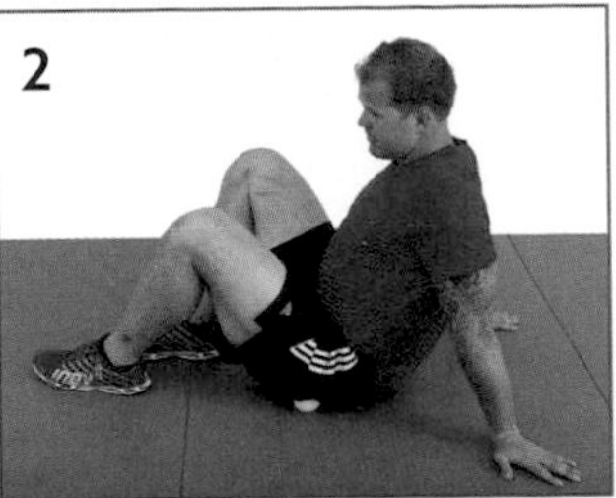
2

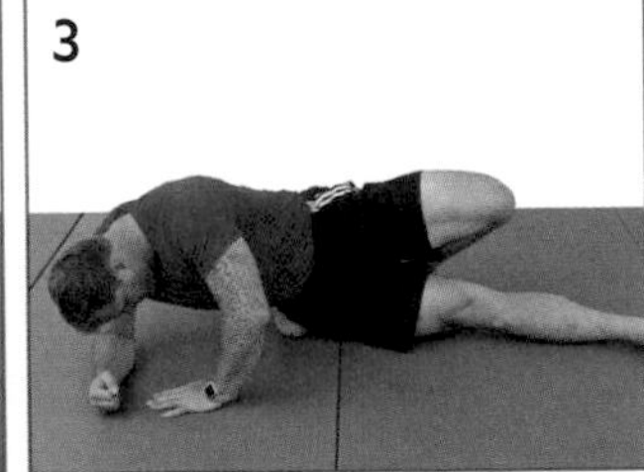
3

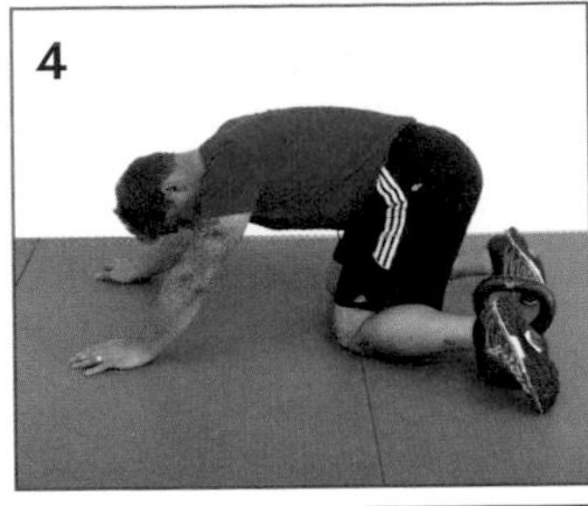
4

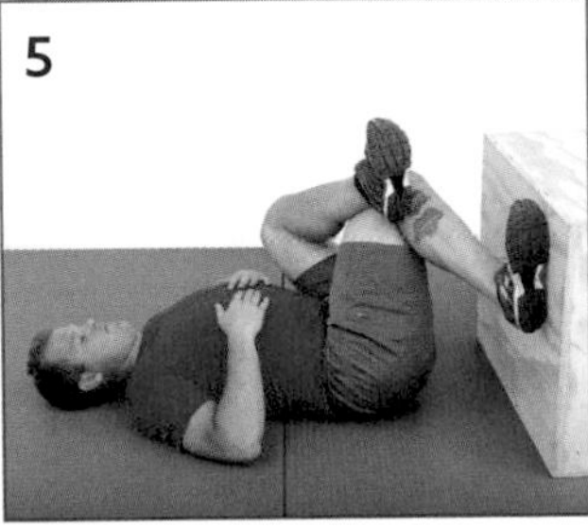
5

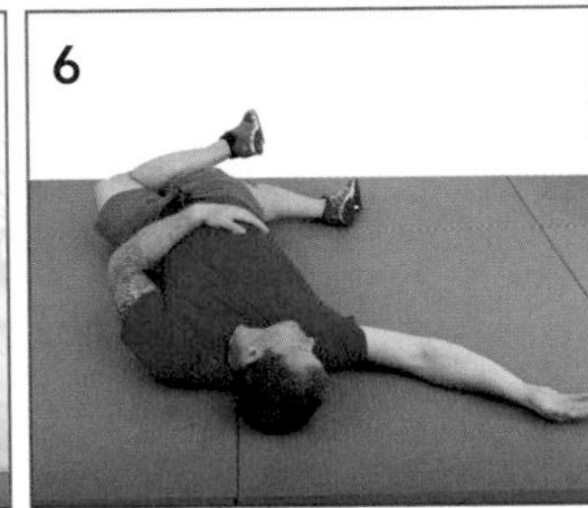
6

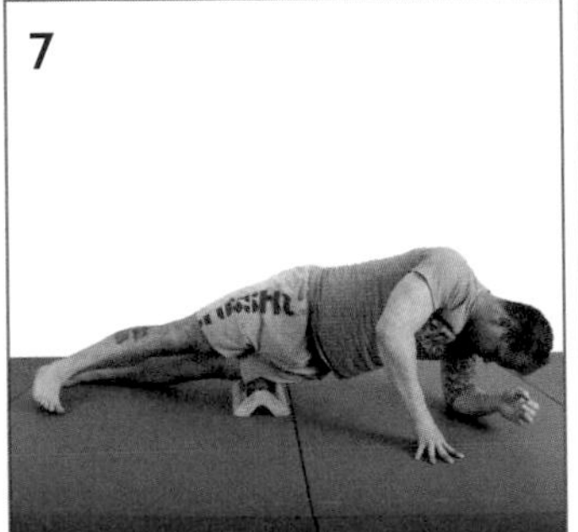
7

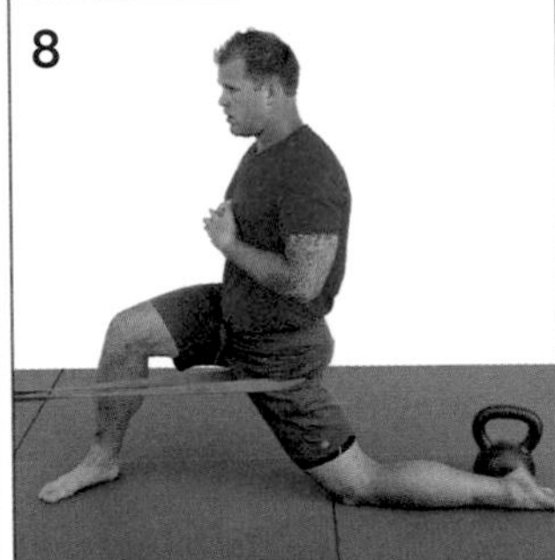
8

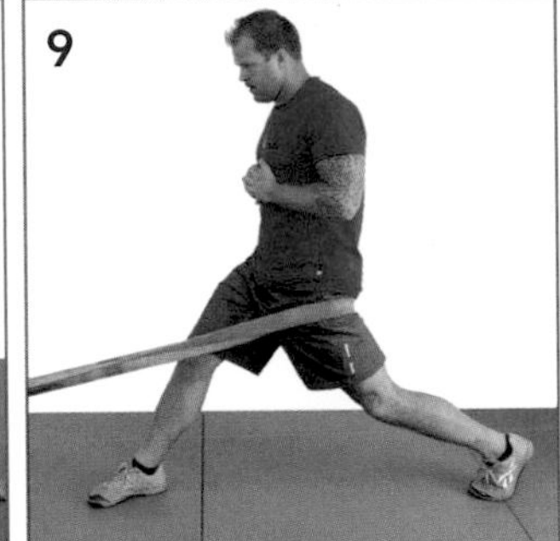
9

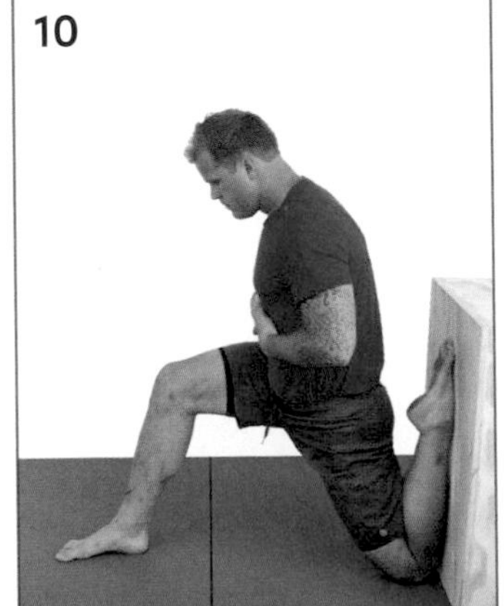
10

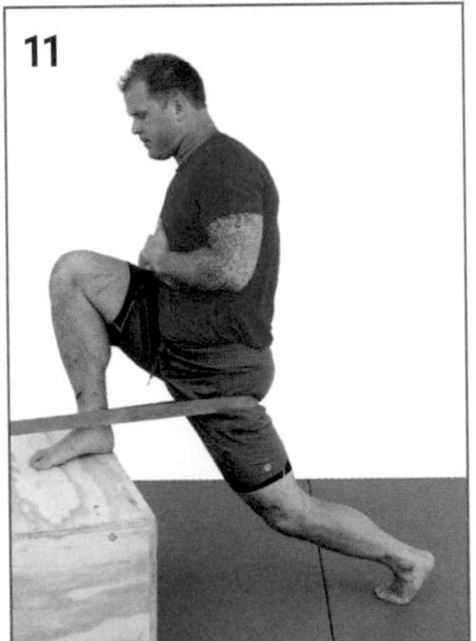
11

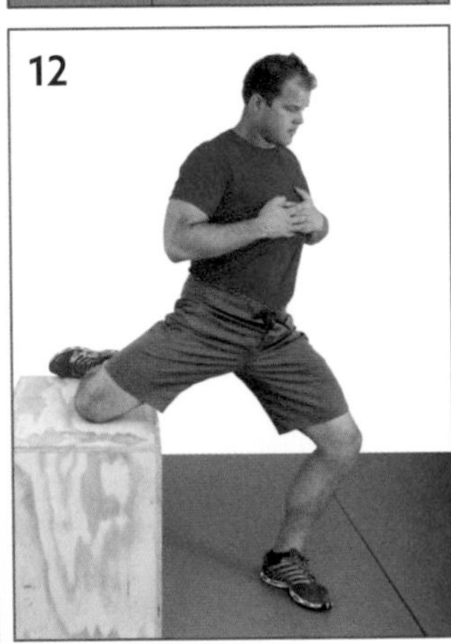
12

MOBILIZATION LIST:

1. *Targeted Gut Smashing Mobilizations (page 358)*
2. *Glute Smash and Floss (page 368)*
3. *Side Hip Smash (page 370)*
4. *Hip Capsule Internal Rotation (page 381)*
5. *Olympic Wall Squat with Internal Rotation (page 382)*
6. *Global Internal Rotation (page 383)*
7. *Quad Smash Mobilizations (page 385)*
8. *Banded Hip Extension (page 390)*
9. *Banded Hip Extension Lunge (page 391)*
10. *Couch Stretch (page 391)*
11. *Trailing Leg Hip Extension (page 394)*
12. *Reverse Ballerina (page 395)*
13. *Plantar Surface Smash (page 437)*
14. *Forefoot Mobilization (page 438)*
15. *Toe Re-animator Mobilizations (page 439)*
16. *Single-Leg Flexion with External Rotation (page 370)*

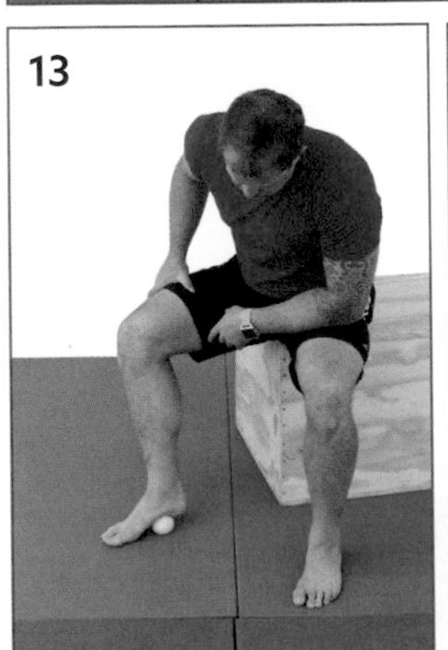
13

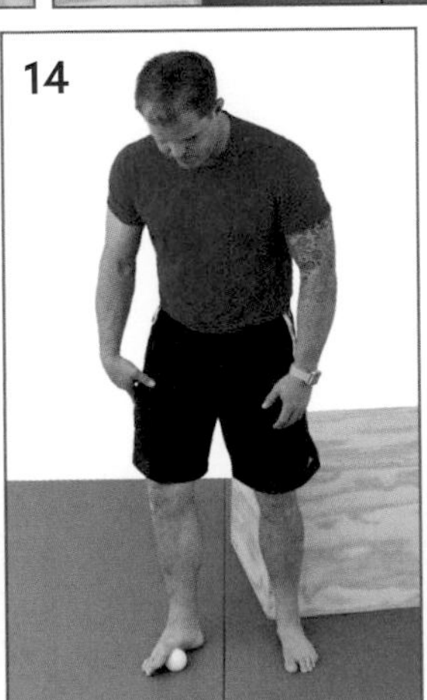
14

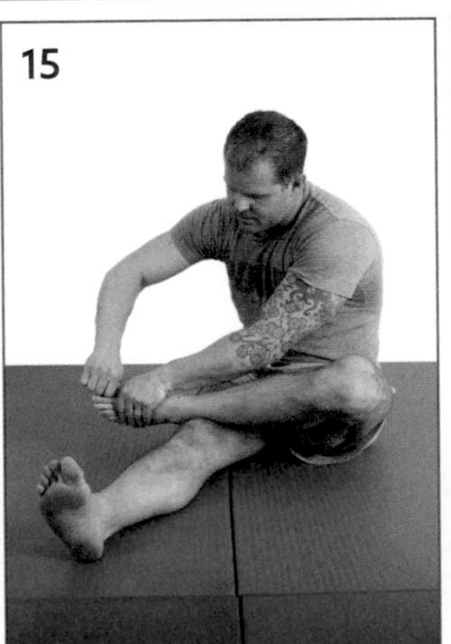
15

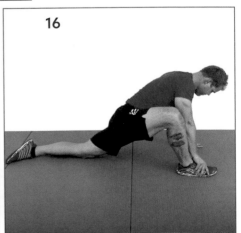
16

Troubleshooting Lunge Archetype Mobility Prescriptions

People encounter two primary limitations with the lunge archetype: hip extension and toe dorsiflexion. Any of the movement faults in part 2 that are tagged with the lunge archetype icon are likely due to one of these two restrictions. Below I break down these restrictions and offer a sample prescription for each.

■ Toe Fault Prescription

If you are unable to get the ball of your foot flush with the ground or you experience toe pain in the lunge position, stiff toes are probably to blame. The mobility prescription below will help with this issue.

PRESCRIPTION	TIME
Plantar Surface Smash (page 437)	2 minutes on each side
Toe Re-animator Mobilizations (page 439; perform all options)	2–4 minutes on each side
	8–12 MINUTES

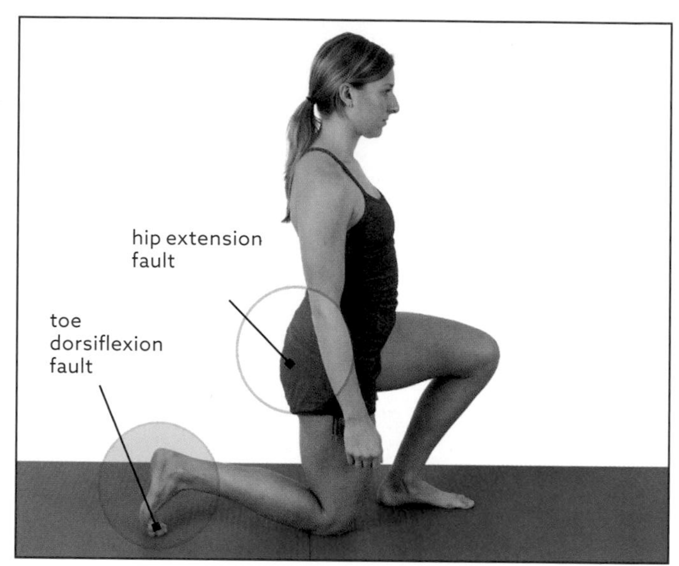

□ Hip Extension and Internal Rotation Prescriptions

If you are unable to position your knee behind your hip, or your leg externally rotates (flares outward) when you move it behind your body, chances are you are missing hip extension or hip internal rotation range of motion. The mobility prescriptions below will help with these issues.

PRESCRIPTION A Missing Hip Extension	TIME
Quad Smash Mobilizations (page 385; choose one option)	2 minutes on each side
Trailing Leg Hip Extension (page 394; choose one option)	2 minutes on each side
Couch Stretch (page 391)	2 minutes on each side
	12 MINUTES

PRESCRIPTION B Missing Hip Internal Rotation	TIME
Side Hip Smash (page 370)	2 minutes on each side
Hip Capsule Internal Rotation (page 381)	2 minutes on each side
Olympic Wall Squat with Internal Rotation (page 382)	2 minutes on each side
	12 MINUTES

Joint and Body Area Prescriptions (Pain)

Have a minor tweak, painful joint, or pain-related symptom such as tension headache, low back pain, or piriformis syndrome? Here I provide sample prescriptions to treat and resolve them. As with the archetype troubleshooting sequences, these prescriptions are just sample programs. Don't limit yourself to what is shown. You have the knowledge and the ability to treat your own symptoms: Correct the position that is causing pain, and then work upstream and downstream of the problem area.

Headache/Neck Pain/TMJD

PRESCRIPTION	TIME
Jaw Mob (page 288)	1-2 minutes on each side
Head Mob (page 288)	1-2 minutes on each side
Anterior Neck Mob (page 289)	2 minutes
Posterior Neck Mob (page 290)	2 minutes
	8-12 MINUTES

Posterior Neck Pain/ Tension and Exertion Headache

PRESCRIPTION	TIME
T-Spine Ball Smash Mobilizations (page 295; choose one option)	2-4 minutes
Basic First Rib Smash and Floss (page 306)	2 minutes on each side
Posterior Neck Mob (page 290)	2 minutes
	8-10 MINUTES

Posterior Shoulder Pain

PRESCRIPTION A	TIME
T-Spine Ball Smash Mobilizations (page 295; choose one option)	2 minutes
Shoulder Capsule Mobilization (page 310)	2 minutes on each arm
Overhead Rib Mobilization (page 301)	2 minutes on each side
	10 MINUTES

PRESCRIPTION B	TIME
Trap Scrub (page 304)	2 minutes on each side
Shoulder Rotator Smash and Floss (page 312)	2 minutes on each side
Overhead Tissue Smash Mobilizations (page 313; choose one option)	2 minutes on each side
	12 MINUTES

Anterior Shoulder Pain

PRESCRIPTION	TIME
Anterior Compartment Mobilizations (page 323; choose one option)	2 minutes on each side
Barbell Shoulder Shear (page 327)	2 minutes on each shoulder
Bilateral Internal Rotation Mobilization (page 329)	2 minutes
	10 MINUTES

Elbow Pain (Tennis Elbow)

PRESCRIPTION A	TIME
Elbow VooDoo (page 339) (see page 146 for VooDoo Flossing wrapping technique)	1-2 minutes of compression; perform 2 to 3 cycles on each arm
	4-12 MINUTES

PRESCRIPTION B	TIME
Triceps Extension Smash (page 336)	2 minutes on each arm
Forearm Smash Mobilizations (page 344; choose one option)	2 minutes on each arm
Banded Elbow Distraction (page 343)	2 minutes on each arm
	12 MINUTES

Wrist Pain (Carpal Tunnel)

PRESCRIPTION A	TIME
Banded Wrist Distraction (page 347) (see page 146 for VooDoo Flossing wrapping technique)	1-2 minutes of compression; perform 2 to 3 cycles on each wrist
	4-12 MINUTES

PRESCRIPTION B	TIME
Forearm Smash Mobilizations (page 344; choose one option)	2 minutes on each arm
Wrist Tack and Spin (page 346)	2 minutes on each wrist
Banded Wrist Distraction (page 347)	2 minutes on each wrist
	12 MINUTES

Upper Back Pain (Trap Tweak Sequence)

PRESCRIPTION	TIME
T-Spine Ball Smash Mobilizations (page 295; choose one option)	2–4 minutes
Overhead Rib Mobilization (page 301)	2 minutes on each arm
Trap Scrub (page 304)	2 minutes on each arm
	10–12 MINUTES

Low Back Pain

PRESCRIPTION A (Low Back Tweak)	TIME
Pelvic Reset (page 350)	1–2 minutes
Global Gut Smash (page 365)	4 minutes
QL Side Smash (page 354)	2 minutes on each side
Quad Smash (page 385; focus on rectus femoris or front of upper leg)	2–4 minutes on each side
	13–15 MINUTES

PRESCRIPTION B	TIME
Targeted Gut Smashing Mobilizations (page 358; choose one option and focus on the iliacus)	2 minutes on each side
Adductor Smash (page 398; choose one option)	2 minutes on each side
Couch Stretch (page 391)	2 minutes on each side
	12 MINUTES

PRESCRIPTION C	TIME
Low Back Smash: Option 1 (page 349)	2 minutes on each side
High Glute Smash and Floss (page 369)	2 minutes on each side
Oblique Side Smash (page 355; choose one option)	2 minutes on each side
	12 MINUTES

PRESCRIPTION D	TIME
Erector Side Smash (page 353)	2 minutes on each side
Posterior Chain Smash and Floss (page 404; choose one option)	2 minutes on each leg
Posterior Chain Floss (page 408)	2 minutes on each side
	12 MINUTES

SI Pain (Sacroiliac Joint Pain)

PRESCRIPTION	TIME
Glute Smash and Floss (page 368)	2 minutes on each side
Targeted Gut Smashing Mobilizations (page 358; choose one option)	2 minutes on each side
Hip Capsule Mobilization (page 379)	2 minutes on each side
	12 MINUTES

Diaphragm Dysfunction (Breathing Sequence)

PRESCRIPTION	TIME
T-Spine Ball Smash Extension (page 295)	4 minutes
Diaphragm Gut Smash (page 363)	4 minutes
	8 MINUTES

Posterior Hip Pain (Piriformis Syndrome/Sciatica Pain)

PRESCRIPTION A	TIME
Glute Smash and Floss (page 368)	2 minutes on each side
High Glute Smash and Floss (page 369)	2 minutes on each side
Adductor Smash (page 398)	2 minutes on each side
	12 MINUTES

PRESCRIPTION B	TIME
VooDoo Groin and Hamstring Wrap (page 408) (see page 146 for VooDoo Flossing wrapping technique)	1–2 minutes of compression; perform 2 to 3 cycles on the problem area
	4–12 MINUTES

Anterior Hip Pain

PRESCRIPTION	TIME
Side Hip Smash (page 370)	2 minutes on each side
Targeted Gut Smashing Mobilizations (page 358; choose one option)	2 minutes on each side
Banded Hip Extension (page 390)	2 minutes on each side
	12 MINUTES

Hip Impingement

PRESCRIPTION	TIME
Gentle Hip Distraction (page 378)	2 minutes on each side
Cueing Internal Rotation with Distraction (page 382)	2 minutes on each side
Hip Capsule Mobilization (page 379)	2 minutes on each side
	12 MINUTES

Knee Pain

PRESCRIPTION A (Knee Tweak)	TIME
Terminal Knee Extension: VooDoo Variation (page 414) (see page 146 for VooDoo Flossing wrapping technique)	1–2 minutes of compression; perform 2 to 3 cycles on each knee
Gap and Smash Mobilizations (page 415; choose one option)	2 minutes on each knee
	8–15 MINUTES

PRESCRIPTION B	TIME
Suprapatellar Smash and Floss (page 388)	2 minutes on each knee
Calf Smash Mobilizations (page 425; choose one option)	2 minutes on each knee
Classic Calf Mobilization (page 429)	2 minutes on each leg
	12 MINUTES

PRESCRIPTION C	TIME
Posterior Chain Smash and Floss (page 404; choose one option)	2 minutes on each leg
Knee Stack and Smash (page 417)	2 minutes on each knee
Medial Shin Smash and Floss Mobilizations (page 420; choose one option)	2 minutes on each knee
	12 MINUTES

PRESCRIPTION D	TIME
Quad Smash Mobilizations (page 385; choose one option)	2 minutes on each leg
Lateral and Anterior Compartment Shin Mobilization (page 422)	2 minutes on each shin
Knee VooDoo (page 389) (see page 146 for VooDoo Flossing application)	1–2 minutes of compression; perform 2 to 3 cycles on the problem area
	12–15 MINUTES

Shin Splints

PRESCRIPTION	TIME
Medial Shin Smash and Floss Mobilizations (page 420; choose one option)	2 minutes on each leg
Lateral and Anterior Compartment Shin Mobilization (page 422)	2 minutes on each leg
Double-Leg Plantarflexion (page 423)	2 minutes
	10 MINUTES

Ankle Pain (Achilles Pain)

PRESCRIPTION A	TIME
Calf Smash Mobilizations (page 425; choose one option)	2 minutes on each calf
Banded Heel Cord: Anterior Bias (page 430)	2 minutes on each ankle
Banded Heel Cord: Posterior Bias (page 430)	2 minutes on each ankle
	12 MINUTES

PRESCRIPTION B	TIME
Ball Whack (page 432; perform all options)	2 minutes on each calf
Lateral Malleolus/Heel Smash Mobilizations (page 433)	2 minutes on each ankle
Medial Heel Bone Smash (page 434)	2 minutes on each ankle
	12 MINUTES

PRESCRIPTION C	TIME
Ankle VooDoo (page 436) (see page 146 for VooDoo Flossing wrapping technique)	1–2 minutes of compression; perform 2 to 3 cycles on each ankle
	4–12 MINUTES

Foot Pain (Plantar Fasciitis)

PRESCRIPTION	TIME
Plantar Surface Smash (page 437)	2 minutes on each foot
Forefoot Mobilization (page 438)	2 minutes on each foot
Toe Re-animator Mobilizations: Option 3: Toe Dorsiflexion (page 441)	2 minutes on each foot
	12 MINUTES

Turf Toe/Bunion Sequence

PRESCRIPTION	TIME
Toe Re-animator Mobilizations (page 439; perform all options)	
	5–10 MINUTES

14-Day Whole-Body Mobility Overhaul

When it comes to mobilizing, you're responsible for maintaining everything under your hairline. The goal is to spend at least 10 to 15 minutes a day, every day, on solving your mobility restrictions. Over the course of two weeks, you should visit each area of your body at least once and cycle through all the body archetypes at least twice.

Most people mobilize only one region of the body, or they have a few go-to mobilizations that they do every day, but that's it. Don't make these mistakes. If you're having trouble hitting all the body areas and archetypes, you can use the template below as a general guide. Think of it as a blueprint for constructing a whole-body mobility program.

Here's how it works: To begin, pick a mobilization, ideally one that will resolve or improve one of your weaknesses. Maybe your low back hurts from driving all day, or you want to spend extra time working on your squat. The key is to dedicate at least one mobilization to the problem of the day, whether it's a position that needs work or a pain-related issue. Next, choose one mobilization from the general archetype list and one mobilization from the listed body area. For example, on Monday you would choose one mobilization that focuses on the problem of the

WEEK 1

	MONDAY	TUESDAY	WEDNESDAY
MOB 1 (PERSONAL PICK)	**Choose** one mobilization from part 3 (pages 282–441) that focuses on the problem of the day, a personal weakness, or a position you want to improve.	**Choose** one mobilization from part 3 (pages 282–441) that focuses on the problem of the day, a personal weakness, or a position you want to improve.	**Choose** one mobilization from part 3 (pages 282–441) that focuses on the problem of the day, a personal weakness, or a position you want to improve.
MOB 2 (ARCHETYPE)	**Overhead Archetype** Choose one mobilization from the overhead archetype list (page 445) or one mobilization from part 3 that is tagged with the overhead archetype icon.	**Squat Archetype** Choose one mobilization from the squat archetype list (page 457) or one mobilization from part 3 that is tagged with the squat archetype icon.	**Hang Archetype** Choose one mobilization from the hang archetype list (page 451) or one mobilization from part 3 that is tagged with the hang archetype icon.
MOB 3 (BODY AREA)	**Area 1: Jaw, Head, and Neck** Choose one mobilization from Area 1 (pages 287–291).	**Area 13: Calf** Choose one mobilization from Area 13 (pages 424–430).	**Area 2: Upper Back** Choose one mobilization from Area 2 (pages 292–308).

WEEK 2

	MONDAY	TUESDAY	WEDNESDAY
MOB 1 (PERSONAL PICK)	**Choose** one mobilization from part 3 (pages 282–441) that focuses on the problem of the day, a personal weakness, or a position you want to improve.	**Choose** one mobilization from part 3 (pages 282–441) that focuses on the problem of the day, a personal weakness, or a position you want to improve.	**Choose** one mobilization from part 3 (pages 282–441) that focuses on the problem of the day, a personal weakness, or a position you want to improve.
MOB 2 (ARCHETYPE)	**Overhead Archetype** Choose one mobilization from the overhead archetype list (page 445) or one mobilization from part 3 that is tagged with the overhead archetype icon.	**Squat Archetype** Choose one mobilization from the squat archetype list (page 457) or one mobilization from part 3 that is tagged with the squat archetype icon.	**Hang Archetype** Choose one mobilization from the hang archetype list (page 451) or one mobilization from part 3 that is tagged with the hang archetype icon.
MOB 3 (BODY AREA)	**Area 5: Arm** Choose one mobilization from Area 5 (pages 335–347).	**Area 9: Adductors** Choose one mobilization from Area 9 (pages 397–402).	**Area 10: Hamstrings** Choose one mobilization from Area 10 (pages 403–411).

day, one mobilization from the overhead archetype list (see page 445), and one mobilization from body area 1 (see pages 287–291).

As you start piecing together your own program, feel free to rearrange the body areas and archetypes. Like the sample prescriptions, this template is not set in stone.

As a final reminder, try to find ways to build mobility work into your day. If you're strapped for time, break your mobility sessions into smaller chunks and bury them in your schedule. For example, you can make them a part of your cool-down after training or do them while watching television. The key is to take a systematic approach. As a quick recap, joint mechanics mobilizations are great to work on before training, muscle dynamics mobilizations are great for post-training, and sliding surface mobilizations are great for post-training and before bed. So on Monday you could perform the Overhead Rib Mobilization and a mobilization of your choosing after your training session, and then perform the Posterior Neck Mob at night as you wind down for bed. In short, it doesn't matter how you choose to break up your mobility sessions. As long as you're putting in the daily maintenance, you will experience long-term change.

THURSDAY	FRIDAY	SATURDAY	SUNDAY
Choose one mobilization from part 3 (pages 282–441) that focuses on the problem of the day, a personal weakness, or a position you want to improve.	**Choose** one mobilization from part 3 (pages 282–441) that focuses on the problem of the day, a personal weakness, or a position you want to improve.	**Choose** one mobilization from part 3 (pages 282–441) that focuses on the problem of the day, a personal weakness, or a position you want to improve.	**Choose** one mobilization from part 3 (pages 282–441) that focuses on the problem of the day, a personal weakness, or a position you want to improve.
Front Rack Archetype Choose one mobilization from the front rack archetype list (page 454) or one mobilization from part 3 that is tagged with the front rack archetype icon.	**Pistol Archetype** Choose one mobilization from the pistol archetype list (page 461) or one mobilization from part 3 that is tagged with the pistol archetype icon.	**Lunge Archetype** Choose one mobilization from the lunge archetype list (page 465) or one mobilization from part 3 that is tagged with the lunge archetype icon.	**Press Archetype** Choose one mobilization from the press archetype list (page 448) or one mobilization from part 3 that is tagged with the press archetype icon.
Area 6: Trunk Choose one mobilization from Area 6 (pages 348–366).	**Area 12: Shin** Choose one mobilization from Area 12 (pages 419–423).	**Area 14: Ankle, Foot, and Toes** Choose one mobilization from Area 14 (pages 431–441).	**Area 3: Posterior Shoulder, Lat, Serratus** Choose one mobilization from Area 3 (pages 309–321).

THURSDAY	FRIDAY	SATURDAY	SUNDAY
Choose one mobilization from part 3 (pages 282–441) that focuses on the problem of the day, a personal weakness, or a position you want to improve.	**Choose** one mobilization from part 3 (pages 282–441) that focuses on the problem of the day, a personal weakness, or a position you want to improve.	**Choose** one mobilization from part 3 (pages 282–441) that focuses on the problem of the day, a personal weakness, or a position you want to improve.	**Choose** one mobilization from part 3 (pages 282–441) that focuses on the problem of the day, a personal weakness, or a position you want to improve.
Front Rack Archetype Choose one mobilization from the front rack archetype list (page 454) or one mobilization in part 3 that is tagged with the front rack archetype icon.	**Pistol Archetype** Choose one mobilization from the pistol archetype list (page 461) or one mobilization in part 3 that is tagged with the pistol archetype icon.	**Lunge Archetype** Choose one mobilization from the lunge archetype list (page 465) or one mobilization in part 3 that is tagged with the lunge archetype icon.	**Press Archetype** Choose one mobilization from the press archetype list (page 448) or one mobilization in part 3 that is tagged with the press archetype icon.
Area 11: Knee Choose one mobilization from Area 11 (pages 412–418).	**Area 7: Glutes, Hip Capsules** Choose one mobilization from Area 7 (pages 367–383).	**Area 8: Hip Flexors, Quadriceps** Choose one mobilization from Area 8 (pages 384–396).	**Area 4: Anterior Shoulder and Chest** Choose one mobilization from Area 4 (pages 322–334).

14-DAY WHOLE-BODY SAMPLE PROGRAM (BEGINNER)

WEEK 1

	MONDAY	TUESDAY	WEDNESDAY
MOB 1 (PERSONAL PICK)	Choose a mobilization that addresses a personal weakness	Choose a mobilization that addresses a personal weakness	Choose a mobilization that addresses a personal weakness
MOB 2 (ARCHETYPE)	**Overhead Archetype** T-Spine Overhead Extension Smash Mobilizations: Option 1 (page 297)—2 minutes	**Squat Archetype** Single-Leg Flexion with External Rotation: Option 2 (page 372)—2 minutes on each leg	**Hang Archetype** Reverse Sleeper Stretch (page 321)—2 minutes on each arm
MOB 3 (BODY AREA)	**Area 1: Jaw, Head, and Neck** Posterior Neck Mob (page 290)—2 minutes	**Area 13: Calf** Calf Smash Mobilizations: Option 1 (page 425)—2 minutes on each calf	**Area 2: Upper Back** T-Spine Roller Smash Mobilization: Option 1 (page 293)—2 minutes

WEEK 2

	MONDAY	TUESDAY	WEDNESDAY
MOB 1 (PERSONAL PICK)	Choose a mobilization that addresses a personal weakness	Choose a mobilization that addresses a personal weakness	Choose a mobilization that addresses a personal weakness
MOB 2 (ARCHETYPE)	**Overhead Archetype** Overhead Tissue Smash Mobilizations: Option 2 (page 314)—2 minutes on each side	**Squat Archetype** Posterior Chain Floss (page 408)—2 minutes on each leg	**Hang Archetype** Bilateral Internal Rotation Mobilization (page 329)—2 minutes on each side
MOB 3 (BODY AREA)	**Area 5: Arm** Triceps Extension Smash (page 336)—2 minutes on each arm	**Area 9: Adductors** Olympic Wall Squat (page 402)—2 minutes	**Area 10: Hamstrings** Posterior Chain Smash and Floss: Option 1 (page 404)—2 minutes on each leg

14-DAY WHOLE-BODY SAMPLE PROGRAM (INTERMEDIATE)

WEEK 1

	MONDAY	TUESDAY	WEDNESDAY
MOB 1 (PERSONAL PICK)	Choose a mobilization that addresses a personal weakness	Choose a mobilization that addresses a personal weakness	Choose a mobilization that addresses a personal weakness
MOB 2 (ARCHETYPE)	**Overhead Archetype** Overhead Rib Mobilization (page 301)—2 minutes on each arm	**Squat Archetype** Single-Leg Flexion with External Rotation: Option 1 (page 370)—2 minutes on each leg	**Hang Archetype** Barbell Shoulder Shear (page 327)—2 minutes on each shoulder
MOB 3 (BODY AREA)	**Area 1: Jaw, Head, and Neck** Posterior Neck Mob (page 290)—2 minutes	**Area 13: Calf** Calf Smash Mobilizations: Option 4 (page 427)—2 minutes on each calf	**Area 2: Upper Back** T-Spine Ball Smash Mobilizations: Option 1 (page 295)—2 minutes

WEEK 2

	MONDAY	TUESDAY	WEDNESDAY
MOB 1 (PERSONAL PICK)	Choose a mobilization that addresses a personal weakness	Choose a mobilization that addresses a personal weakness	Choose a mobilization that addresses a personal weakness
MOB 2 (ARCHETYPE)	**Overhead Archetype** T-Spine Overhead Extension Smash Mobilizations: Option 2 (page 298)—2 minutes	**Squat Archetype** Hip External Rotation with Flexion: Option 1 (page 373)—2 minutes on each leg	**Hang Archetype** Shoulder Rotator Smash and Floss (page 312)—2 minutes on each shoulder
MOB 3 (BODY AREA)	**Area 5: Arm** Triceps Extension Smash (page 336)—2 minutes on each arm	**Area 9: Adductors** Adductor Smash: Option 1 (page 398)—2 minutes on each leg	**Area 10: Hamstrings** Posterior Chain Smash and Floss: Option 2 (page 406)—2 minutes on each leg

THURSDAY	FRIDAY	SATURDAY	SUNDAY
Choose a mobilization that addresses a personal weakness	Choose a mobilization that addresses a personal weakness	Choose a mobilization that addresses a personal weakness	Choose a mobilization that addresses a personal weakness
Front Rack Archetype Classic Triceps and Lat Stretch (page 321)—2 minutes on each arm	**Pistol Archetype** Banded Heel Cord: Anterior Bias (page 430)—2 minutes on each ankle	**Lunge Archetype** Banded Hip Extension (page 390)—2 minutes on each side	**Press Archetype** Sink Mobilization (page 333)—2 minutes
Area 6: Trunk Global Gut Smash (page 365)—5 minutes	**Area 12: Shin** Double-Leg Plantarflexion (page 423)—2 minutes on each leg	**Area 14: Ankle, Foot, and Toes** Plantar Surface Smash (page 437)—2 minutes on each foot	**Area 3: Posterior Shoulder, Lat, Serratus** Shoulder Rotator Smash and Floss (page 312)—2 minutes on each shoulder

THURSDAY	FRIDAY	SATURDAY	SUNDAY
Choose a mobilization that addresses a personal weakness	Choose a mobilization that addresses a personal weakness	Choose a mobilization that addresses a personal weakness	Choose a mobilization that addresses a personal weakness
Front Rack Archetype Banded Lateral Opener (page 334)—2 minutes on each arm	**Pistol Archetype** Classic Calf Mobilization (page 429)—2 minutes on each leg	**Lunge Archetype** Olympic Wall Squat with Internal Rotation (page 382)—2 minutes on each side	**Press Archetype** Banded Bully (page 330)—2 minutes on each side
Area 11: Knee Flexion Gapping (page 418)—2 minutes on each side	**Area 7: Glutes, Hip Capsules** Glute Smash and Floss (page 368)—2 minutes on each side	**Area 8: Hip Flexors, Quadriceps** Couch Stretch (page 391)—2 minutes on each side	**Area 4: Anterior Shoulder and Chest** Anterior Compartment Mobilizations: Option 2 (page 325)—2 minutes on each side

THURSDAY	FRIDAY	SATURDAY	SUNDAY
Choose a mobilization that addresses a personal weakness	Choose a mobilization that addresses a personal weakness	Choose a mobilization that addresses a personal weakness	Choose a mobilization that addresses a personal weakness
Front Rack Archetype Super Front Rack (page 320)—2 minutes on each arm	**Pistol Archetype** Medial Heel Bone Smash (page 434)—2 minutes on each ankle	**Lunge Archetype** Trailing Leg Hip Extension (page 394)—2 minutes on each side	**Press Archetype** Serratus Smash (page 316)—2 minutes on each side
Area 6: Trunk Targeted Gut Smash: Option 7 (page 362)—2 minutes on each side	**Area 12: Shin** Lateral and Anterior Compartment Shin Mobilization (page 422)—2 minutes on each leg	**Area 14: Ankle, Foot, and Toes** Plantar Surface Smash (page 437)—2 minutes on each foot	**Area 3: Posterior Shoulder, Lat, Serratus** Shoulder Capsule Mobilization (page 310)—2 minutes on each shoulder

THURSDAY	FRIDAY	SATURDAY	SUNDAY
Choose a mobilization that addresses a personal weakness	Choose a mobilization that addresses a personal weakness	Choose a mobilization that addresses a personal weakness	Choose a mobilization that addresses a personal weakness
Front Rack Archetype Overhead Distraction with External Rotation Bias (page 318)—2 minutes on each arm	**Pistol Archetype** Ankle VooDoo (page 436)—1–2 minutes on each ankle	**Lunge Archetype** Hip Capsule Internal Rotation (page 381)—2 minutes on each side	**Press Archetype** Triple Bully (page 331)—2 minutes on each side
Area 11: Knee Gap and Smash Mobilizations: Options 1 and 2 (pages 415–416)—2 minutes on each side	**Area 7: Glutes, Hip Capsules** Side Hip Smash (page 370)—2 minutes on each side	**Area 8: Hip Flexors, Quadriceps** Super Couch (page 393)—2 minutes on each side	**Area 4: Anterior Shoulder and Chest** Anterior Compartment Mobilizations: Option 2 (page 325)—2 minutes on each side

INDEX